Peripheral Vascular Diseases

Peripheral Vascular Diseases

Edited by

JESS R. YOUNG, M.D.
Chairman, Department of Vascular Medicine
The Cleveland Clinic Foundation
Cleveland, Ohio

ROBERT A. GRAOR, M.D.
Department of Vascular Medicine
The Cleveland Clinic Foundation
Cleveland, Ohio

JEFFREY W. OLIN, D.O.
Department of Vascular Medicine
The Cleveland Clinic Foundation
Cleveland, Ohio

JOHN R. BARTHOLOMEW, M.D.
Department of Vascular Medicine
The Cleveland Clinic Foundation
Cleveland, Ohio

539 illustrations

Mosby
Year Book

St. Louis Baltimore Boston Chicago London Philadelphia Sydney Toronto

Mosby
Year Book
Dedicated to Publishing Excellence

Editors Anne Patterson and Stephanie Manning
Assistant editor Anne Gunter
Project manager Karen A. Edwards
Production editor Amy Adams Squire
Production assistant Ginny Douglas
Design Dave Zielinski

Printed in the United States of America

Mosby–Year Book, Inc.
11830 Westline Industrial Drive
St. Louis, MO 63146

Library of Congress Cataloging-in-Publication Data

Peripheral vascular diseases / edited by Jess R. Young . . . [et al.].
p. cm.
Includes bibliographical references.
Includes index.
ISBN 0-8016-6115-3
1. Peripheral vascular diseases. I. Young, Jess R., 1928-
[DNLM: 1. Vascular Diseases. WG 500 P445]
RC694.P487 1991
616.1'31—dc20
DNLM/DLC
for Library of Congress 90-13568
CIP

GW/MV/MV 9 8 7 6 5 4 3 2 1

Peripheral Vascular Diseases

Edited by

JESS R. YOUNG, M.D.
Chairman, Department of Vascular Medicine
The Cleveland Clinic Foundation
Cleveland, Ohio

ROBERT A. GRAOR, M.D.
Department of Vascular Medicine
The Cleveland Clinic Foundation
Cleveland, Ohio

JEFFREY W. OLIN, D.O.
Department of Vascular Medicine
The Cleveland Clinic Foundation
Cleveland, Ohio

JOHN R. BARTHOLOMEW, M.D.
Department of Vascular Medicine
The Cleveland Clinic Foundation
Cleveland, Ohio

539 illustrations

Mosby
Year Book

St. Louis Baltimore Boston Chicago London Philadelphia Sydney Toronto

Mosby
Year Book
Dedicated to Publishing Excellence

Editors Anne Patterson and Stephanie Manning
Assistant editor Anne Gunter
Project manager Karen A. Edwards
Production editor Amy Adams Squire
Production assistant Ginny Douglas
Design Dave Zielinski

Printed in the United States of America

Mosby–Year Book, Inc.
11830 Westline Industrial Drive
St. Louis, MO 63146

Library of Congress Cataloging-in-Publication Data

Peripheral vascular diseases / edited by Jess R. Young . . . [et al.].
p. cm.
Includes bibliographical references.
Includes index.
ISBN 0-8016-6115-3
1. Peripheral vascular diseases. I. Young, Jess R., 1928-
[DNLM: 1. Vascular Diseases. WG 500 P445]
RC694.P487 1991
616.1'31—dc20
DNLM/DLC
for Library of Congress 90-13568
CIP

GW/MV/MV 9 8 7 6 5 4 3 2 1

CONTRIBUTORS

WALID ARRABI, M.D.
Department of Vascular Medicine
Cleveland Clinic Foundation
Cleveland, Ohio

WILLIAM R. BELL, M.D.
The Johns Hopkins Hospital
Baltimore, Maryland

EDWIN G. BEVEN, M.D.
Department of Vascular Surgery
Cleveland Clinic Foundation
Cleveland, Ohio

SETH D. BILAZARIAN
The John's Hopkins Hospital
Baltimore, Maryland

EARL Z. BROWNE, Jr., M.D.
Department of Plastic and Reconstructive Surgery
Cleveland Clinic Foundation
Cleveland, Ohio

LEONARD H. CALABRESE, D.O.
Department of Rheumatic and Immunologic Disease
Cleveland Clinic Foundation
Cleveland, Ohio

GUY M. CHISOLM, Ph.D.
Department of Vascular Cell Biology and Atherosclerosis
Cleveland Clinic Foundation
Cleveland, Ohio

JOHN D. CLOUGH
Chairman, Department of Rheumatology and Immunology
Cleveland Clinic Foundation
Cleveland, Ohio

JAY D. COFFMAN, M.D.
Professor of Medicine
Chief, Peripheral Vascular Section
University Hospital, Boston University Medical Center
Boston, Massachusetts

ANTHONY J. COMEROTA, M.D.
Professor of Surgery
Chief of Vascular Surgery, Department of Surgery
Temple University School of Medicine
Philadelphia, Pennsylvania

MICHAEL D. CRESSMAN, D.O.
Lipid Research and Referral Clinic
Cleveland Clinic Foundation
Cleveland, Ohio

RALPH G. DePALMA, M.D.
Professor and Chairman, Department of Surgery
George Washington University Medical Center
Washington, D.C.

PAUL E. DiCORLETO, Ph.D.
Department of Vascular Cell Biology and Atherosclerosis
Cleveland Clinic Foundation
Cleveland, Ohio

L. ALLEN EHRHART, Ph.D.
Department of Vascular Cell Biology and Atherosclerosis
Cleveland Clinic Foundation
Cleveland, Ohio

PAUL L. FOX, Ph.D.
Department of Vascular Cell Biology and Atherosclerosis
Cleveland Clinic Foundation
Cleveland, Ohio

PATRICK J. GINLEY III, R.N.
Department of Vascular Medicine
Cleveland Clinic Foundation
Cleveland, Ohio

PETER GLOVICZKI, M.D.
Consultant, Section of Vascular Surgery
Mayo Clinic and Mayo Foundation
Assistant Professor of Surgery
Mayo Medical School
Rochester, Minnesota

BRUCE H. GRAY, D.O.
Department of Vascular Medicine
Cleveland Clinic Foundation
Cleveland, Ohio

HENRY F. HOFF, Ph.D.
Department of Brain and Vascular Research
Cleveland Clinic Foundation
Cleveland, Ohio

BYRON J. HOOGWERF, M.D.
Lipid Research and Referral Clinic
Cleveland Clinic Foundation
Cleveland, Ohio

JOHN W. JOYCE, M.D.
Associate Professor of Medicine, Department of Cardiovascular Diseases and Internal Medicine
Mayo Medical School
Mayo Clinic
Rochester, Minnesota

KANDICE KOTTKE-MARCHANT, M.D., Ph.D.
Department of Pathology
Cleveland Clinic Foundation
Cleveland, Ohio

LEONARD P. KRAJEWSKI, M.D.
Department of Vascular Surgery
Cleveland Clinic Foundation
Cleveland, Ohio

ERIC LEEFMANS, M.D.
Subspeciality Resident in Vascular Surgery, Department of Surgery
Temple University School of Medicine
Philadelphia, Pennsylvania

MARVIN E. LEVIN, M.D.
Professor of Clinical Medicine, Department of Medicine/ Division of Metabolism
Washington University School of Medicine
St. Louis, Missouri

RICHARD E. MORTON, Ph.D.
Department of Vascular Cell Biology and Atherosclerosis
Cleveland Clinic Foundation
Cleveland, Ohio

ANDREW C. NOVICK, M.D.
Chairman, Department of Urology
Cleveland Clinic Foundation
Cleveland, Ohio

THOMAS F. O'DONNELL, Jr., M.D.
Professor of Surgery, Tufts University School of Medicine
Chief of Vascular Surgery, New England Medical Center
Boston, Massachusetts

PATRICK J. O'HARA, M.D.
Department of Vascular Surgery
Cleveland Clinic Foundation
Cleveland, Ohio

MALCOLM O. PERRY, M.D.
The H. William Scott, Jr. Professor of Surgery
Chief, Division of Vascular Surgery
Department of Surgery; Division of Vascular Surgery
Vanderbilt University School of Medicine
Nashville, Tennessee

NORMAN B. RATLIFF, M.D.
Director of Cardiovascular Pathology, Department of Pathology
Cleveland Clinic Foundation
Cleveland, Ohio

HENRY H. ROENIGK, Jr., M.D.
Professor and Chairman, Department of Dermatology
Northwestern University Medical School
Chicago, Illinois

THOM W. ROOKE, M.D.
Division of Cardiovascular Diseases and Internal Medicine
Mayo Clinic
Rochester, Minnesota

WILLIAM F. RUSCHHAUPT III, M.D.
Department of Vascular Medicine
Cleveland Clinic Foundation
Cleveland, Ohio

ALEXANDER SCHIRGER, M.D.
Consultant, Division of Cardiovascular Diseases and Internal Medicine, Mayo Clinic and Mayo Foundation
Professor of Medicine, Mayo Medical School
Rochester, Minnesota

FREDERICK J. SCHWAB, M.D.
Assistant Professor of Radiology
George Washington University Medical Center
Washington, D.C.

JOHN A. SPITTELL, Jr., M.D.
Consultant, Department of Cardiovascular Disease and Internal Medicine
Mayo Clinic
Rochester, Minnesota

PETER C. SPITTELL, M.D.
Senior Clinical Fellow, Cardiovascular Division
Mayo Clinic
Rochester, Minnesota

ANTHONY W. STANSON, M.D.
Associate Professor of Diagnostic Radiology
Mayo Clinic
Rochester, Minnesota

D. EUGENE STRANDNESS, Jr., M.D.
Professor of Surgery, Department of Surgery
University of Washington School of Medicine
Seattle, Washington

DONALD G. VIDT, M.D.
Chairman, Department of Hypertension and Nephrology
The Cleveland Clinic Foundation
Cleveland, Ohio

J. TRACY WATSON, M.D.
Division of Orthopaedic Traumatology
Henry Ford Hospital
Detroit, Michigan

CHERYL E. WEINSTEIN, M.D.
Lipid Research and Referral Clinic
Cleveland Clinic Foundation
Cleveland, Ohio

PATRICK WHITLOW, M.D.
Departments of Cardiology and Vascular Medicine
The Cleveland Clinic Foundation
Cleveland, Ohio

PREFACE

Peripheral vascular diseases are common and have a major impact on health. With the aging of the U.S. population, we are seeing more and more patients suffering from vascular diseases. Unfortunately, training in the diagnosis and treatment of these conditions generally has not been included or emphasized in medical schools or during postgraduate training. The number of nonsurgical specialists who deal solely with peripheral vascular disorders has not been increasing significantly. With the exception of physicians in a small number of medical centers, there are few medical specialists for the diagnosis and treatment of these disorders. Instead, vascular surgeons, general surgeons, cardiologists, internists, and family physicians have assumed the specialist's role. Vascular surgeons have had to become familiar with many of the nonsurgical vascular diseases by default.

Several factors have produced a renewed interest in peripheral vascular diseases. As mentioned, the aging of the U.S. population has resulted in an increased prevalence of these disorders. The emergence of new methods of treating hyperlipidemia; new techniques and drugs for thrombolytic therapy; new methods of opening occluded, or stenosed, peripheral arteries; and the increased availability of the noninvasive vascular laboratory have all served to increase interest in these conditions. In addition, there has been an explosion of growth in the field of vascular biology. A great body of knowledge is accumulating regarding vasoactive factors and growth factors produced by the blood vessels and regarding blood coagulation and thrombolysis. Because this research is linked to clinical applications in vascular medicine, the growth of this field will accelerate.

Although many texts on vascular surgery are now available, most patients with vascular disease will never need the services of a vascular surgeon. While several books on the noninvasive diagnosis of vascular disease are also available, the practicing physician needs to know when to send patients to a vascular laboratory and when to refer them to a specialist in vascular disease.

The "Bible" for this specialty, *Peripheral Vascular Diseases,* compiled by physicians at the Mayo Clinic and published in five editions since 1946, has had no new edition since 1980. Since there were no immediate plans for further editions, we undertook this text. We have several contributors from the Mayo Clinic and have tried to duplicate the high standards of quality found in their book.

This is a clinically oriented text written mainly by practicing clinicians. We have attempted to cover the various vascular disorders in a practical and topical manner. It is intended for all physicians interested in caring for patients with vascular diseases, including internists, family physicians, general surgeons, vascular surgeons, cardiologists, orthopaedic surgeons, plastic surgeons, dermatologists, interventional radiologists, and podiatrists.

Jess R. Young
Robert A. Graor
Jeffrey W. Olin
John R. Bartholomew

CONTENTS

Part I

BASIC CONSIDERATIONS

Chapter 1

CLINICAL CLUES TO PERIPHERAL VASCULAR DISEASE

Jess R. Young

Physicians are not well acquainted with peripheral vascular diseases. Vascular medicine is a field that is poorly taught in medical schools and in postgraduate programs. The signs and symptoms of vascular disease can therefore be quite confusing to most physicians. However, vascular medicine is a specialty that lends itself to solving problems by using the powers of observation. The clinical clues to vascular disease are usually there for the trained clinician to discover.

ARTERIAL DISEASE

Cold hands and cold feet are not good indicators of arterial insufficiency. Tense patients and patients with an overactive sympathetic nervous system can have impressively cold hands and feet in spite of excellent arterial circulation to the extremities. Some of these tense patients may also have vasomotor instability with cyanosis or mottling of the hands and feet during exposure to cold or with increased tension.

Poor hair growth, poor skin condition, and deformed or slowly growing toenails are frequently mentioned as signs of arterial insufficiency. However these are not reliable signs. *Ischemic fissures* of the feet (Fig. 1-1), *decubitus ulcers* of ankles (Fig. 1-2) and heels (Fig. 1-3), and *ischemic ulcers* (Fig. 1-4) are much more reliable signs of arterial insufficiency.

Tendinous (Fig. 1-5) *and tuberous* (Fig. 1-6) *xanthomas* may be clues that the patient has hypercholesterolemia and therefore may have an increased tendency to develop arteriosclerosis obliterans. *Xanthelasma* of the eyelids (Fig. 1-7) is associated with hypercholesterolemia in approximately 50% of the persons who have xanthelasma. The other

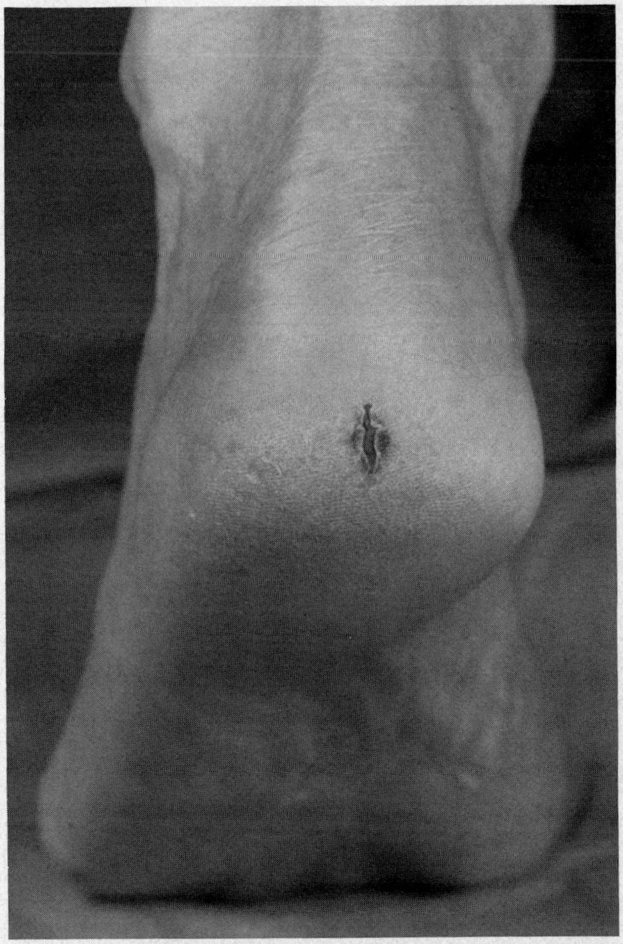

Fig. 1-1. Ischemic heel fissure in a patient with arteriosclerosis obliterans. This is often a precursor of a heel ulcer.

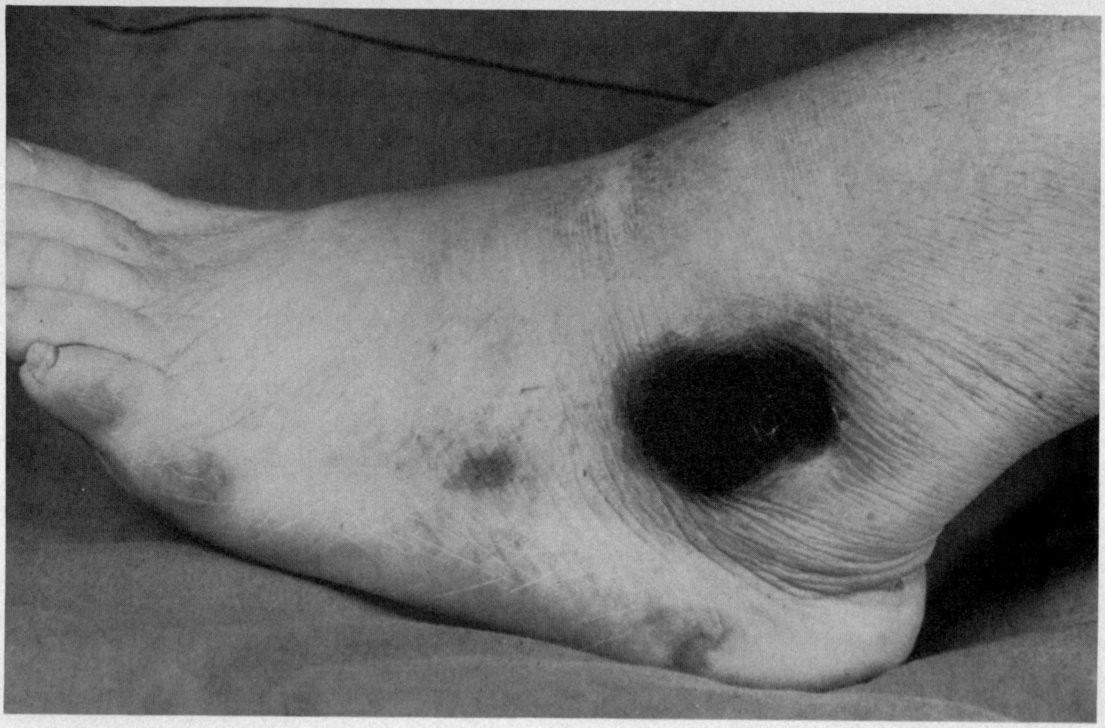

Fig. 1-2. Necrotic area over lateral malleolus in a patient with impaired arterial circulation. The lesion occurred secondary to prolonged pressure while lying in bed.

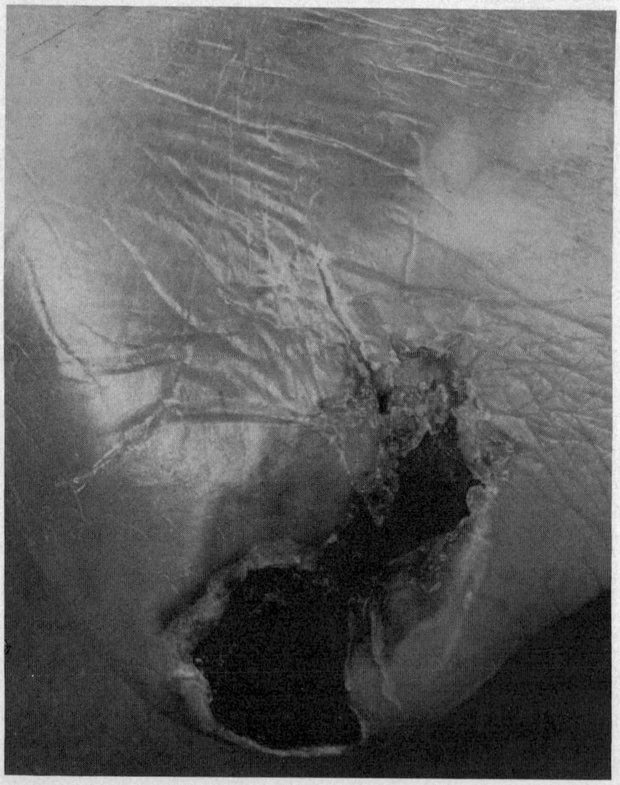

Fig. 1-3. Heel pressure decubitus lesion in a patient with arteriosclerosis obliterans.

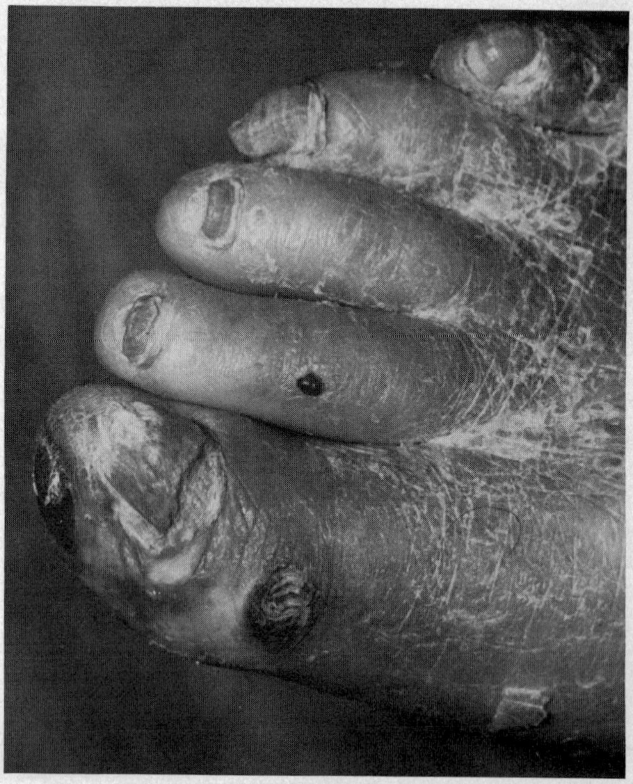

Fig. 1-4. Painful dry ischemic digital ulcers in a patient with severe arterial insufficiency.

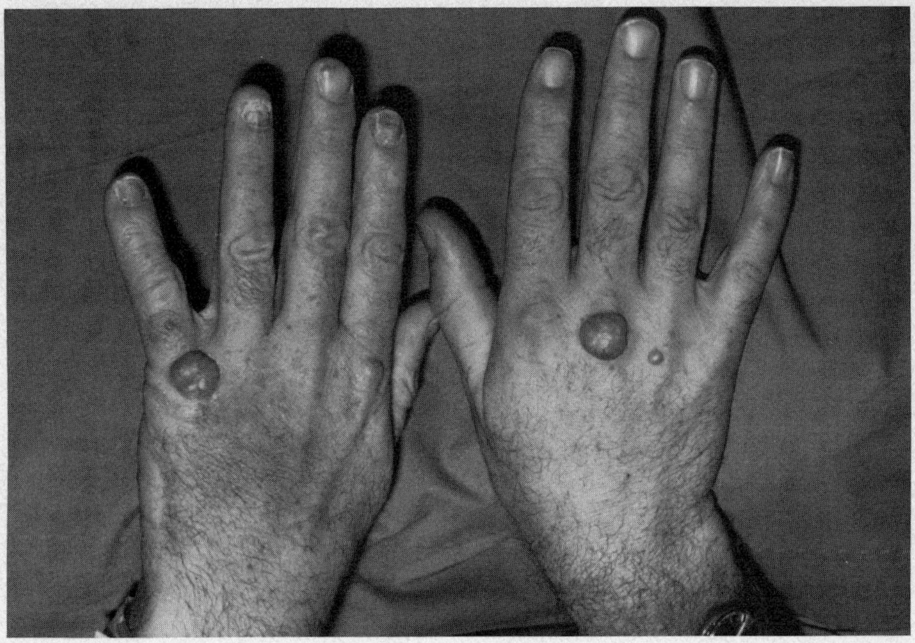

Fig. 1-5. Tendinous xanthomas in a patient with Type IIA hyperlipidemia.

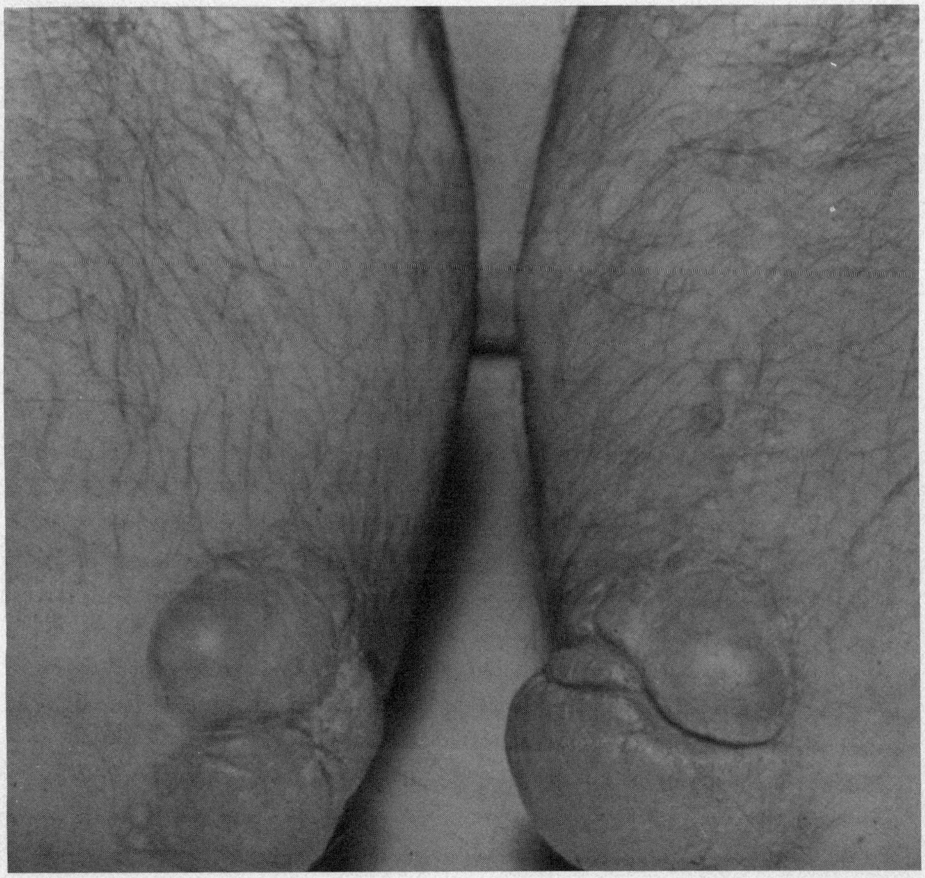

Fig. 1-6. Tuberous xanthomas of the elbows in a patient with Type IIA hyperlipidemia.

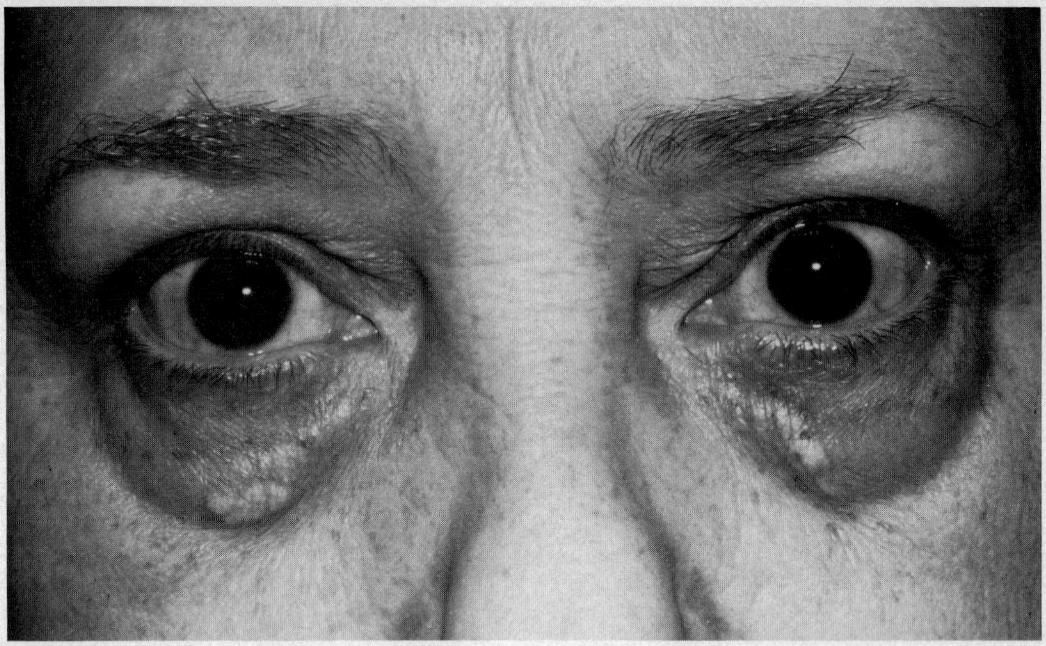

Fig. 1-7. Xanthelasma in a patient with normal total cholesterol and low HDL cholesterol.

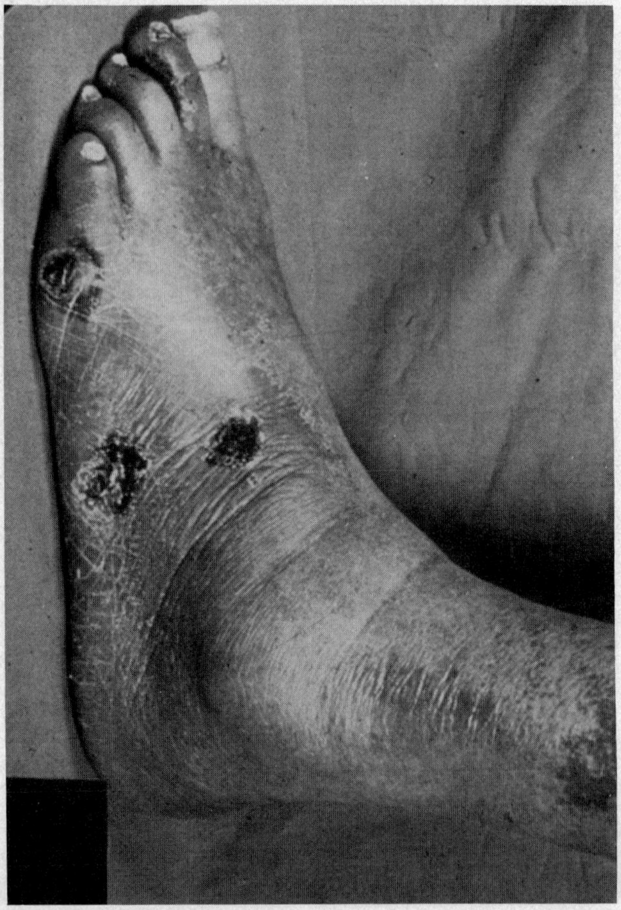

Fig. 1-8. Painful, dry ischemic ulcers on pressure points of the foot of a patient with severe arterial insufficiency.

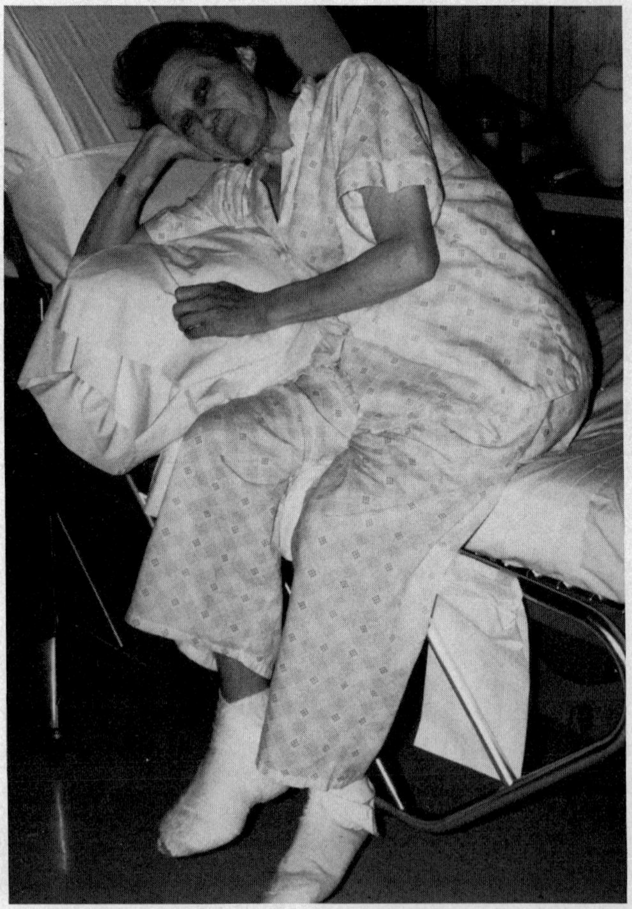

Fig. 1-9. Typical position assumed by a patient with severe arteriosclerosis obliterans and rest pain. The legs are dangled in an attempt to relieve the pain.

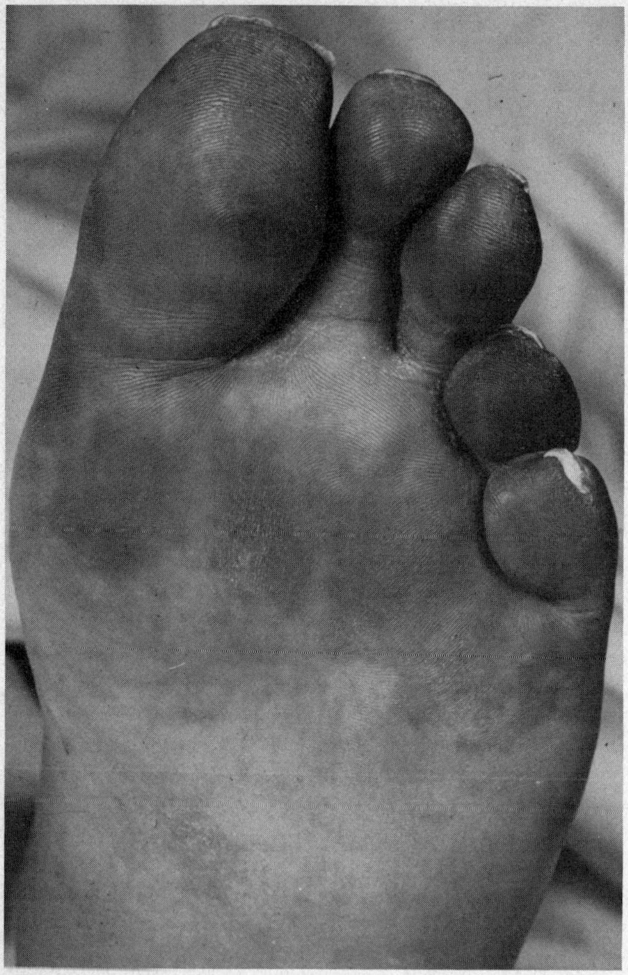

Fig. 1-10. Distal gangrene in a patient with severe arteriosclerosis obliterans.

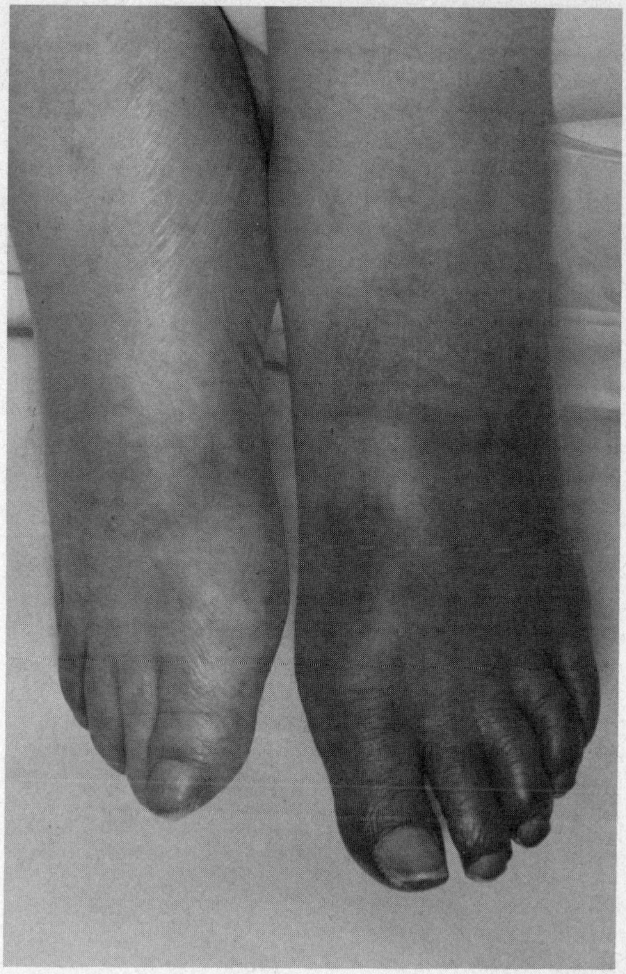

Fig. 1-11. Phlegmasia cerulea dolens (venous gangrene) in a patient with carcinoma of the lung.

50% cannot be considered to have a benign disorder, however, since Bates and Warren[1] found that 94% of their patients with xanthelasma had less than mean levels of high-density lipoprotein (HDL) cholesterol and 69% of the patients had documented cardiovascular disease.

Intermittent claudication is a classic and usually reliable symptom of arteriosclerosis obliterans. Unless the ischemia is severe, the patient is typically distressed only with walking and is relieved within 1 or 2 minutes by stopping and standing in place. The distance that the patient can walk before he must stop varies little from day to day, and he does not need to sit down to get relief from his symptoms.

Increasing numbers of patients are being seen who have *pseudoclaudication* (see Chapter 9) associated with the cauda equina syndrome. This syndrome occurs when there is pressure on the lower spine as a result of lumbar canal stenosis, herniated disk, or hypertrophic ridging. Although the clinical picture can closely mimic true claudication, the distress in a patient with pseudoclaudication may also occur when he straightens his back, either while in bed, standing, or walking. Often the patient will stand or walk slightly bent over in a "gorilla position." The distance that a patient with pseudoclaudication can walk before stopping varies considerably from time to time. The distress is often described with some neurologic component such as a tingling, weakness, incoordination, or clumsiness, as well as the classic symptoms of aching or cramping. A final differentiating point is that the patient usually must sit or lie for at least 5 or 10 minutes to obtain relief, whereas the patient with true claudication is usually relieved within 2 or 3 minutes of standing in place.

Ischemic rest pain is usually worse at night and may be difficult to differentiate from the pain of peripheral neuropathy. In general, patients with peripheral neuropathy have equal pain in both extremities, and the discomfort is not relieved by dependency. They have signs of peripheral neuropathy with absent or decreased deep tendon reflexes and loss of touch and vibratory sensation. The patient with ischemic rest pain usually does not have symmetric discomfort, does get some relief with dependency, and has no signs of

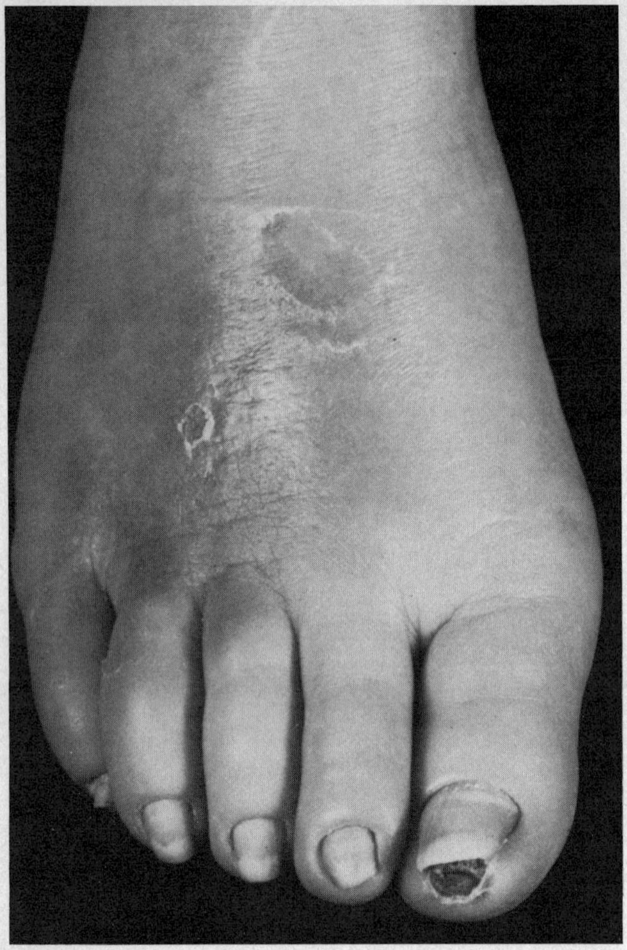

Fig. 1-12. Ischemic lesion of the first toe and superficial thrombophlebitis of the dorsum of the foot in a 38-year-old man with thromboangiitis obliterans (Buerger's disease).

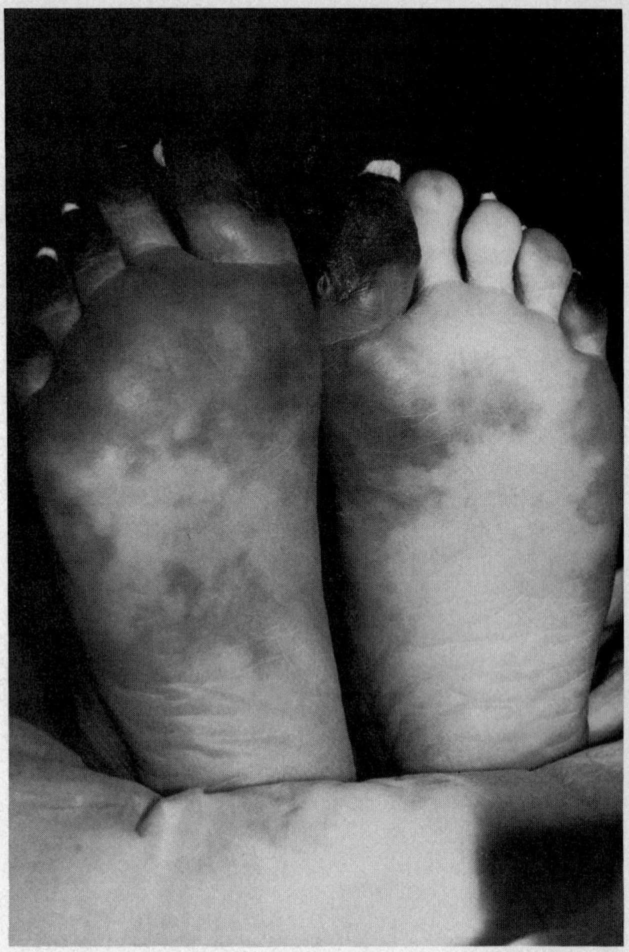

Fig. 1-13. Extensive areas of foot and toe ischemia caused by emboli from an abdominal aortic aneurysm.

peripheral neuropathy. In addition, the patient with ischemic rest pain has other evidence of marked ischemia, including marked pallor on elevation of the legs, marked rubor on dependency, and delayed venous filling time (see Chapter 2).

Ischemic ulcers are painful lesions found distally on the toes or on pressure points of the feet (Fig. 1-8). A patient with ischemic lesions often sits with his legs dangling over the side of the bed (Fig. 1-9) or sits in a chair all night because the dependent position gives him the best possible blood supply to the painful extremities. As a result of prolonged dependency, the extremities can become quite edematous.

The *peripheral gangrene* of severe arterial insufficiency (Fig. 1-10) may be difficult to differentiate from that of venous gangrene (phlegmasia cerulea dolens) (Fig. 1-11). In a patient with venous gangrene marked swelling in the extremity usually occurs early before the onset of frank ischemic changes. In a patient with arterial ischemia the severe ischemic changes usually occur first, followed by edema because the limb is kept in a constant dependent position. If the patient is a poor observer and is seen after ischemia and edema are well established, there may be great difficulty in differentiating these two entities.

Thromboangiitis obliterans (Buerger's disease) (see Chapter 19) usually occurs in young adults less than 40 years of age, but older patients can also be affected. In the past it was thought that only men were afflicted, but recent reports show that 20% to 30% of the patients are women. All patients with thromboangiitis obliterans either smoke tobacco or are exposed to nicotine in some form. The first symptom may be intermittent claudication, but more commonly the more distal arteries are involved so that ulceration and gangrenous changes of the digits may be the initial presentation. The upper extremities are involved in at least 40% of patients with thromboangiitis obliterans. An Allen test should be done to test the patency of the radial and ulnar arteries in anyone suspected of having this condition (see Chapter 2). Thrombophlebitis—usually superficial thrombophlebitis (Fig. 1-12)—occurs at some stage of the

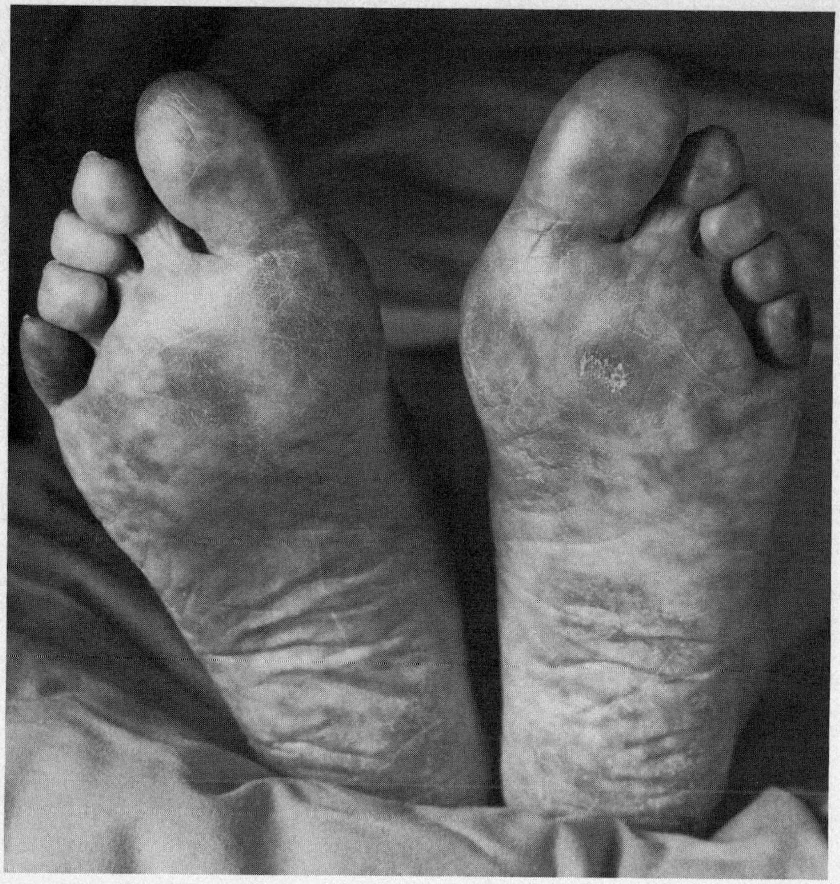

Fig. 1-14. Scattered areas of ischemia in a patient with atheromatous emboli from an atheromatous abdominal aorta.

disease in approximately 40% of the cases.

Arterial embolism (see Chapter 12) is a fairly common cause of occlusion of both large and small arteries of the extremities. The changes produced are often dramatic and at times pathognomonic of embolism, with either acutely ischemic limbs or scattered areas of well-demarcated ischemia (Fig. 1-13). Approximately 90% of large emboli originate in the heart. The cardiac causes include atrial fibrillation, myocardial infarction with mural thrombus, infective or marantic endocarditis, ventricular aneurysm, atrial myxoma, cardiomyopathy, and valve prosthesis. Another 5% of emboli originate in aneurysms of the more proximal arteries. Embolism should be suspected in the patient with an ischemic limb who has a potential source for emboli, who has no previous history of intermittent claudication, and who has good pulses in the uninvolved limb.

Atheromatous embolization (see Chapter 11) is a fairly common problem and produces multiple scattered areas of cyanosis or gangrene in the toes and feet (Fig. 1-14) and occasionally in the calves, thighs, and buttocks. A livedo reticularis pattern, representing emboli to the dermal vessels, can be seen at times in the involved areas. Extensive embolization can result in ischemic ulcers and gangrene. Atheromatous emboli may also cause myocardial infarctions, transient ischemic attacks, strokes, pancreatitis, renal infarctions and failure, gastrointestinal bleeding, and bowel ischemia.

The scattered areas of fixed mottling in the toes associated with atheromatous embolization must be differentiated from the lesions of *chronic pernio* (chilblains) (see Chapter 33). These lesions typically begin as reddish-blue or violet blisters on the toes or dorsum of the feet, then later form superficial painful ulcers (Fig. 1-15). Pernio lesions appear in the fall at the onset of cold weather and usually disappear in the spring in warm weather.

Aneurysms (see Chapter 17) may initially be seen clinically as one of three complications: rupture, thrombosis, or embolization. Uncomplicated aneurysms may be seen as a visible or palpable pulsating mass (Fig. 1-16) or be detected as a result of pressure on surrounding structures, including long bones, vertebrae, nerves, veins, or ureters.

Abdominal aortic aneurysms can rupture into the intraab-

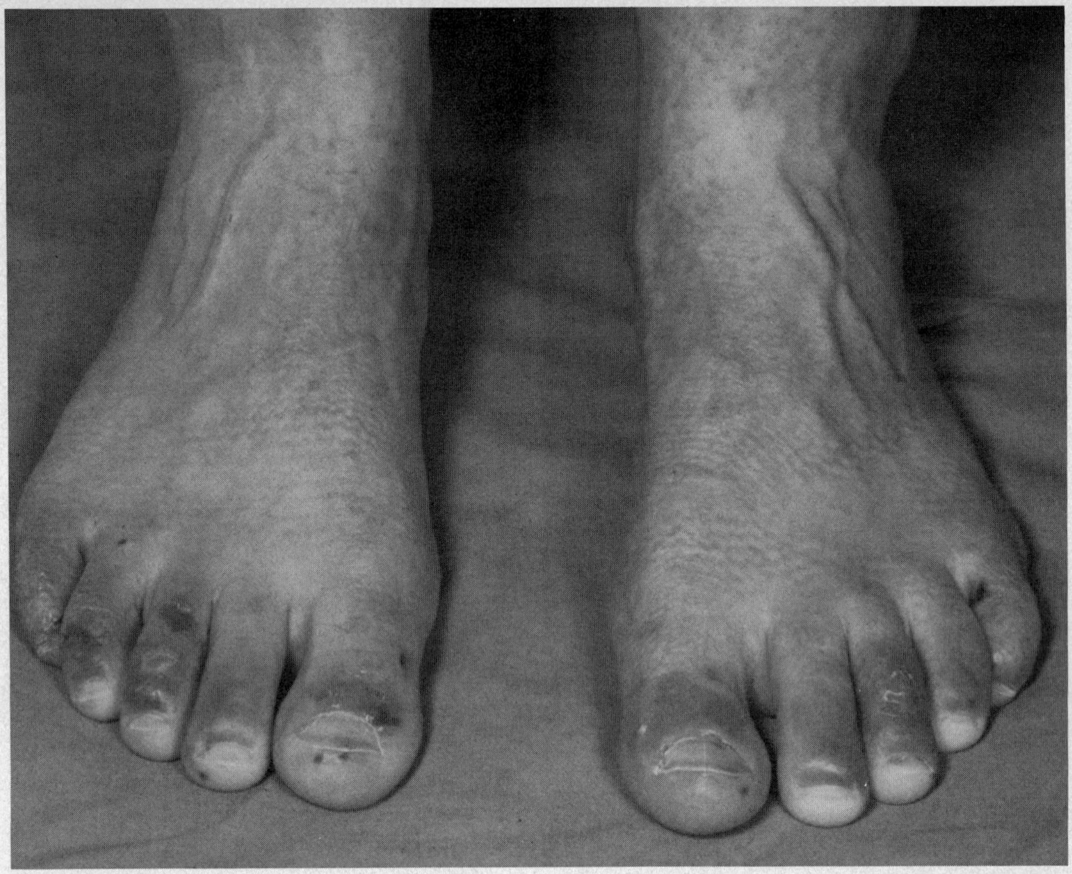

Fig. 1-15. Reddish blue and violet blisters, some with eschars, in a patient with chronic pernio (chilblains).

dominal cavity and become evident as sudden abdominal pain and shock. They can rupture in the retroperitoneal area and result in severe back pain, pain of renal colic, or hypotension. Rupture into the inferior vena cava can produce sudden edema of the extremities and acute congestive failure. Rupture into the gastrointestinal tract can produce an acute gastrointestinal bleed. *Mycotic aneurysms* or a secondarily infected aneurysm can give the clinical picture of a pulsating mass in a patient with a fever of unknown origin.

Aneurysms of the carotid arteries are rare. In some patients, especially middle-aged women with hypertension, the carotid or innominate arteries may be elongated and tortuous. This S-shaped curve of the artery may at first feel like an aneurysm. Careful palpation or duplex ultrasound scanning will confirm that this is a *tortuous carotid, subclavian, or innominate artery* and is not an aneurysm. This "buckling" is far more common than true aneurysms in this area. Another condition that can be mistaken for a carotid aneurysm is a *carotid body tumor*. It usually appears as a mass at the common carotid artery bifurcation and can be diagnosed by arteriography or by duplex ultrasound scan.

The clinical picture seen in a patient with an *aortic dissecting aneurysm* is extremely variable. The event usually starts as severe chest pain, often described as a "tearing" pain. This discomfort may begin in the anterior or posterior chest and may migrate downward. Depending on which arteries and structures are involved, the patient can also have a myocardial infarction if the coronary arteries are involved, congestive failure if the aortic valve is affected, cardiac tamponade, stroke, renal failure, mesenteric ischemia, paraplegia, or ischemia of the extremities. With rupture, death usually results, often as a result of cardiac tamponade. Because of these many clinical manifestations, the diagnosis is often missed because it was never considered.

Vasculitis can produce patterns of change in the extremities varying from palpable purpura to ischemic ulcers in atypical locations or to frank gangrene. Typical locations for ischemic ulcers with arteriosclerosis obliterans or thromboangiitis obliterans would be distally on the toes or on pressure points of the foot, including the ankles, heels, and

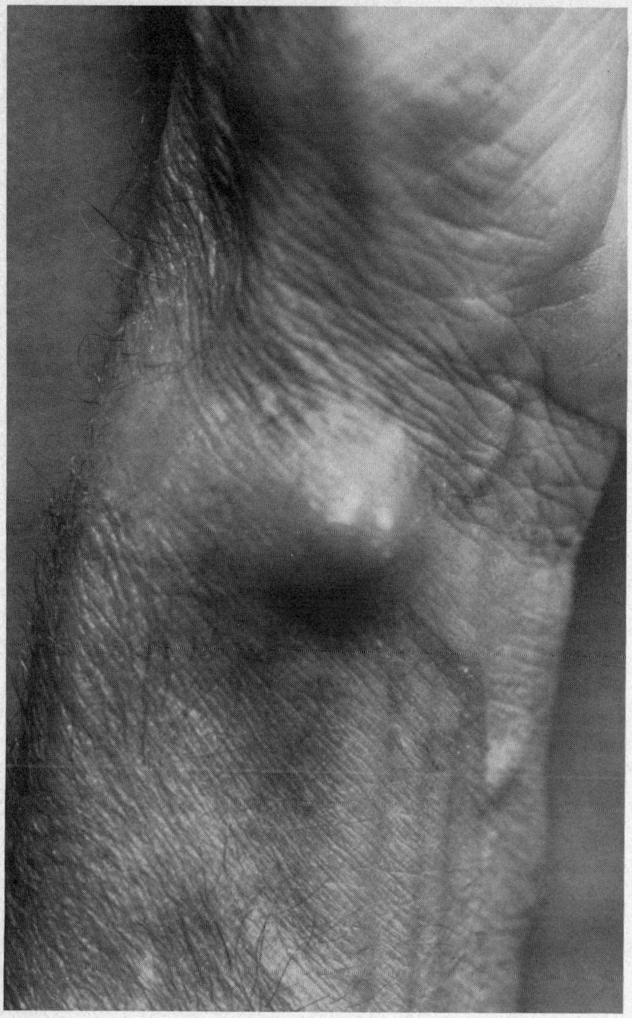

Fig. 1-16. False aneurysm of the radial artery at the site of an arterial puncture for blood gas determinations.

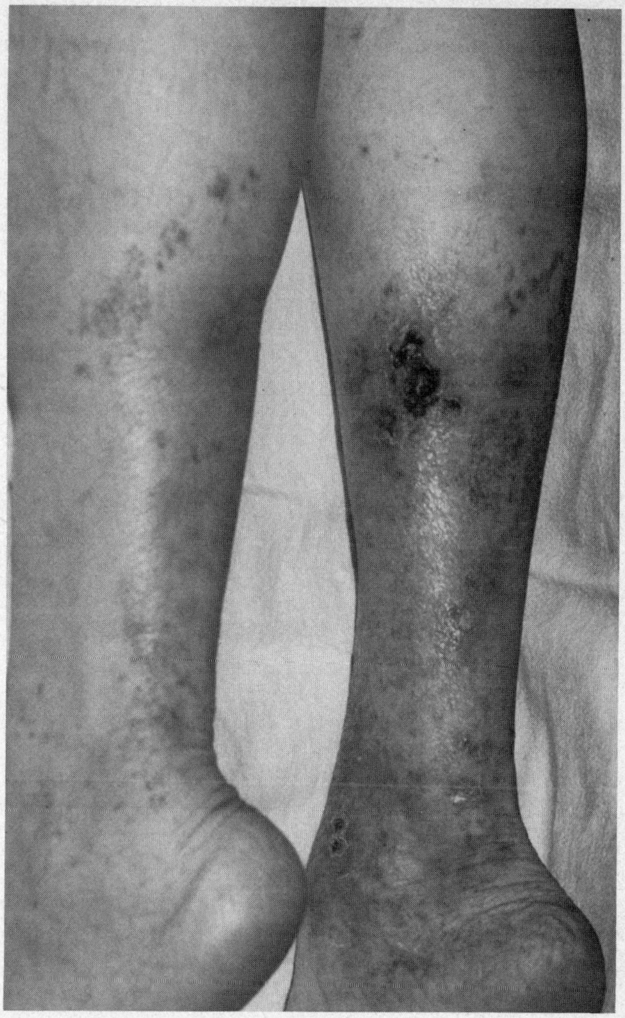

Fig. 1-17. Painful, black ischemic ulcers of the calves in a patient with lupus erythematosus.

tarsal-metatarsal joint areas. Vasculitic ulcers not uncommonly are found higher up on the calf or thigh (Fig. 1-17). In addition to vasculitis, these ischemic ulcers in atypical locations can also be caused by atheromatous emboli or by trauma to an already ischemic limb.

The patient with *Raynaud's phenomenon* (Fig. 1-18) should be examined closely for signs of underlying causes (see Chapter 21). The Allen test (see Chapter 2) may show an occluded radial or ulnar artery that may be a clue to scleroderma, thromboangiitis obliterans, or vasculitis with associated Raynaud's phenomenon. Thickening of the skin of the hands and fingers in patients with scleroderma may be difficult to detect early. An attempt should be made to pinch the skin between the middle and distal knuckles of the fingers (Fig. 1-19). Early in the course of scleroderma the skin at this site is thickened so that it cannot be pinched between the thumb and index finger of the examiner. Superficial, small open or healed ulcerations on the tips of the fingers (Fig. 1-20) or spider angioma (telangiectasia) (Fig. 1-21) can also be early signs of scleroderma.

VENOUS DISEASE

Varicose veins (Fig. 1-22) usually develop because of a hereditary weakness in the structures of the vein walls or valves or both. Contributing factors include pregnancy, obesity, and occupations requiring long periods of standing. When varices appear early in life and without obvious cause, particularly when they are unilateral, arteriovenous fistulas should be suspected. This is especially true if the varices are in an unusual location or are associated with ulceration, a birthmark, elongation of a limb, or distal gangrene.

Superficial thrombophlebitis (see Chapter 24) is usually

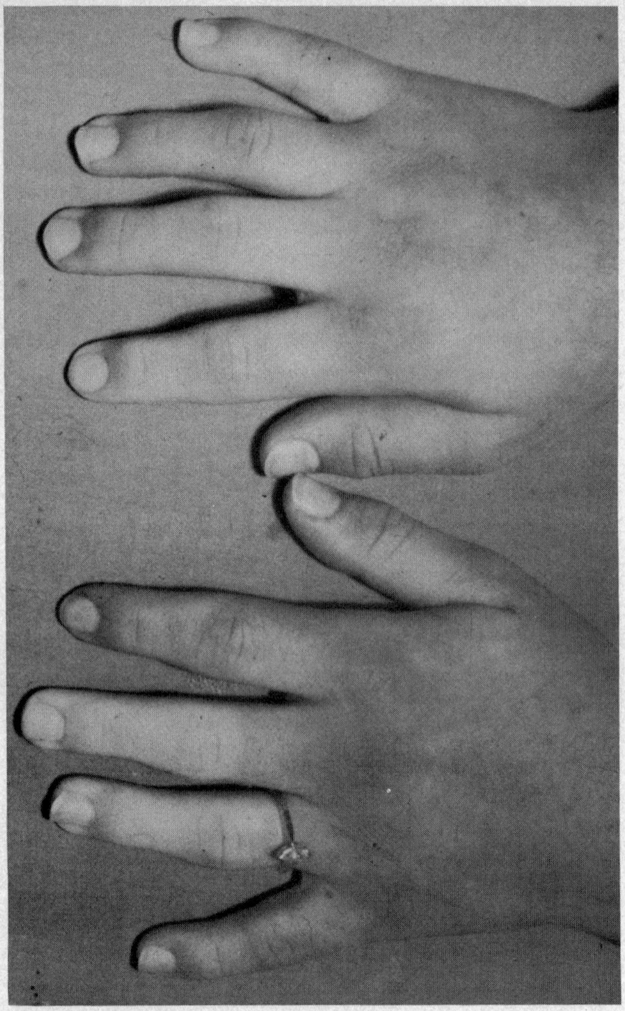

Fig. 1-18. Pallor phase of Raynaud's phenomenon in a young woman with primary Raynaud's disease.

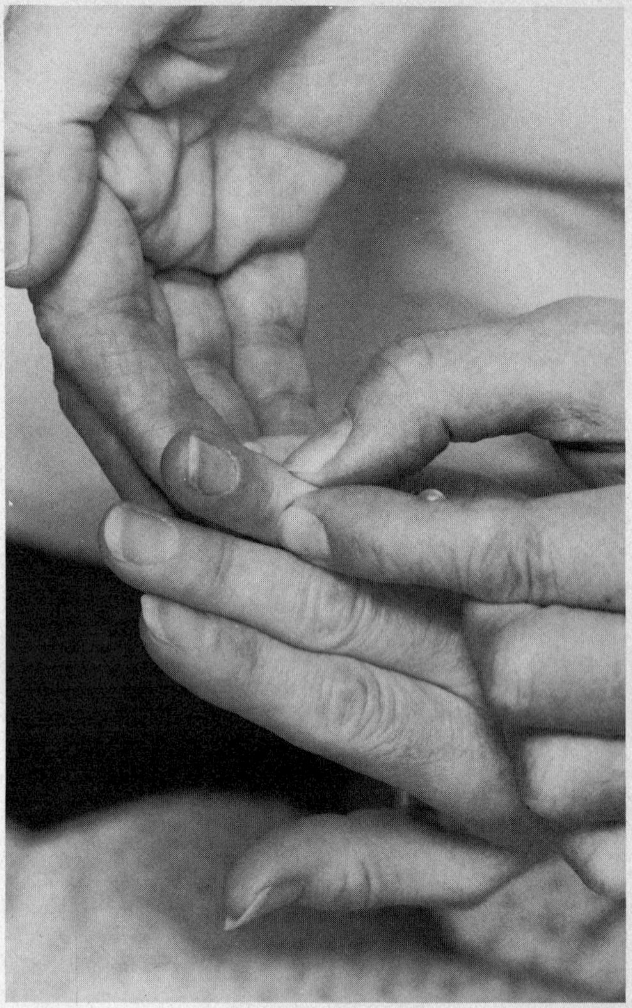

Fig. 1-19. Testing for scleroderma by attempting to pinch the skin between the middle and distal knuckles of a patient with Raynaud's phenomenon.

an easily diagnosed condition. A raised, red, slightly indurated, warm tender cord is usually present along the course of the involved vein (Fig. 1-23). Erythema nodosum or lymphangitis can produce a somewhat similar picture, although lymphangitis is usually associated with cellulitis and sepsis.

Deep venous thrombosis (DVT) (see Chapter 24) may be present with no clinical signs or symptoms in 50% to 80% of patients. Therefore in a proper setting any change at all in an extremity should be considered venous thrombosis until proven otherwise. Swelling is the most common sign, but any new discomfort in a leg or any increased temperature, any change in color, ranging from pink to reddish-blue, or any increased prominence of the superficial veins (Fig. 1-24) should raise the possibility of DVT. A temperature up to 38° C is compatible with DVT, but a higher temperature or the appearance of shaking chills is not associated with venous thrombosis unless the patient has septic thrombosis. The higher temperature and shaking chills usually indicate that the patient has *cellulitis and lymphangitis*. Localized areas of erythema would also suggest cellulitis (Fig. 1-25) rather than deep venous thrombosis. Erythema of the skin in venous thrombosis should be generalized in the extremity and not localized.

Patients with *phlegmasia cerulea dolens* (venous gangrene) (see Chapter 24) usually present a striking clinical picture (Fig. 1-26). The involved extremity may be markedly swollen, at least distally. The skin is taut, shiny, and deeply cyanotic. Superficial gangrene is followed by more extensive gangrene. Distal pulses are decreased or absent.

Chronic venous insufficiency (see Chapter 26) is most

Text continued on p. 18.

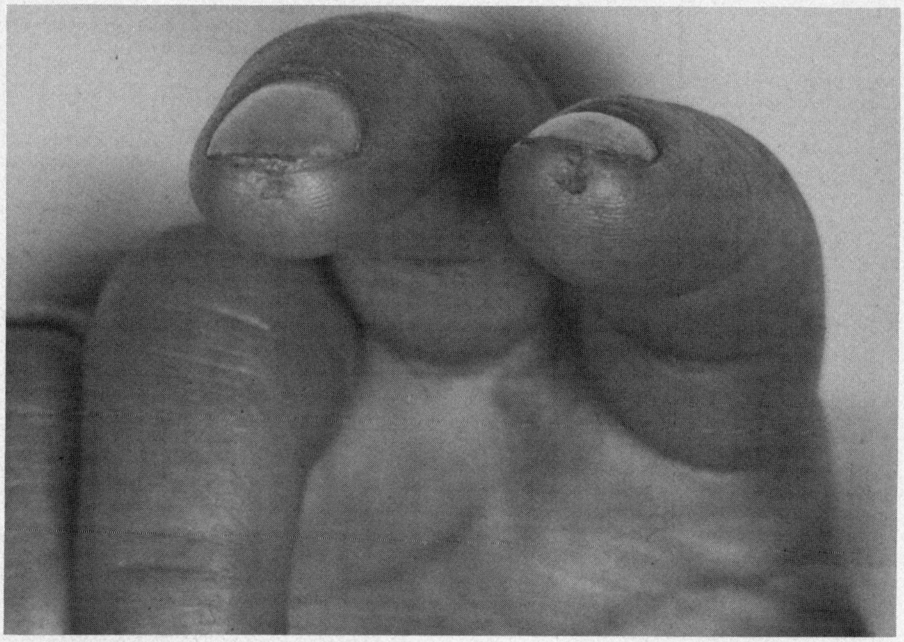

Fig. 1-20. Small healed fingertip ulcers in a patient with scleroderma.

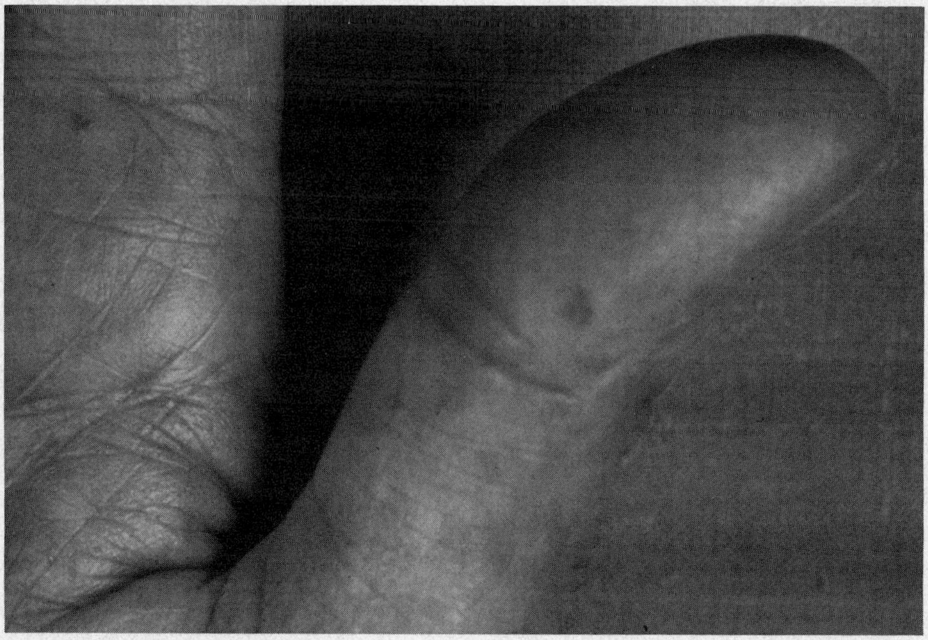

Fig. 1-21. Telangiectasias of the thumb and palm in a patient with scleroderma.

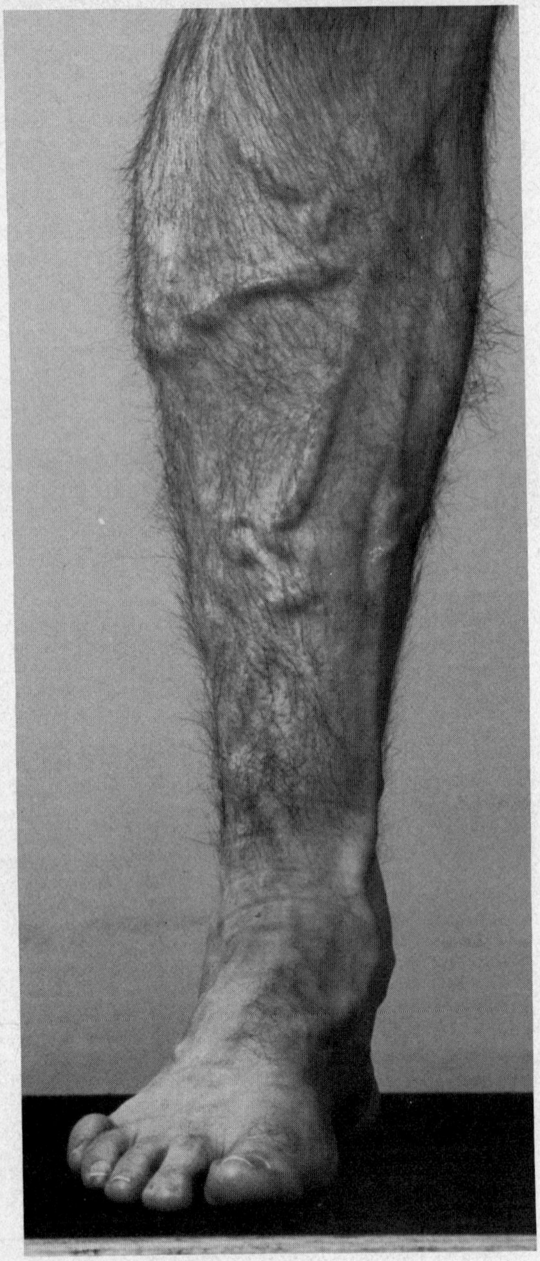

Fig. 1-22. Varicose veins involving branches of the greater saphenous vein.

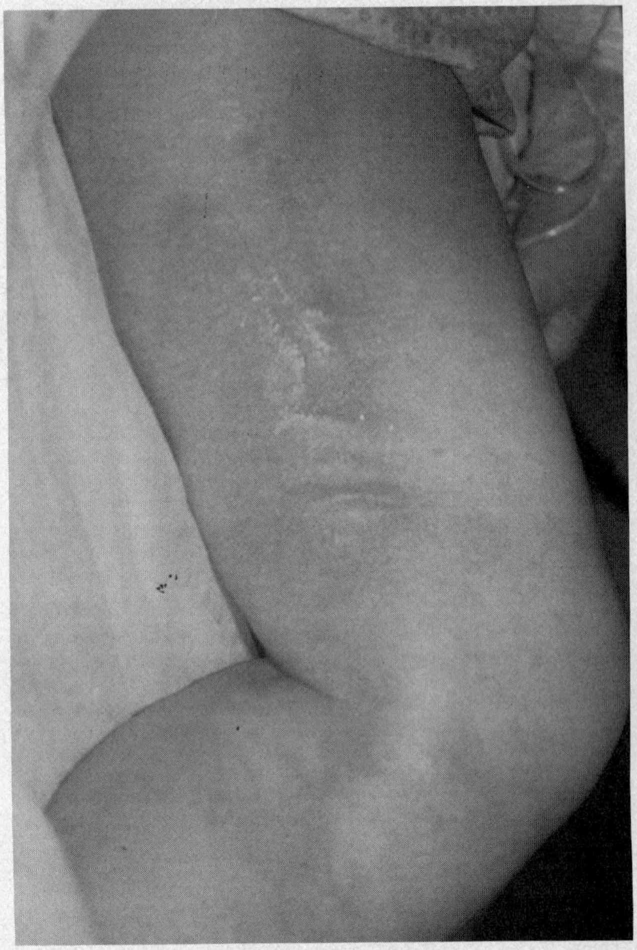

Fig. 1-23. Superficial phlebitis of the greater saphenous vein, presenting as a raised, red, tender, indurated cord.

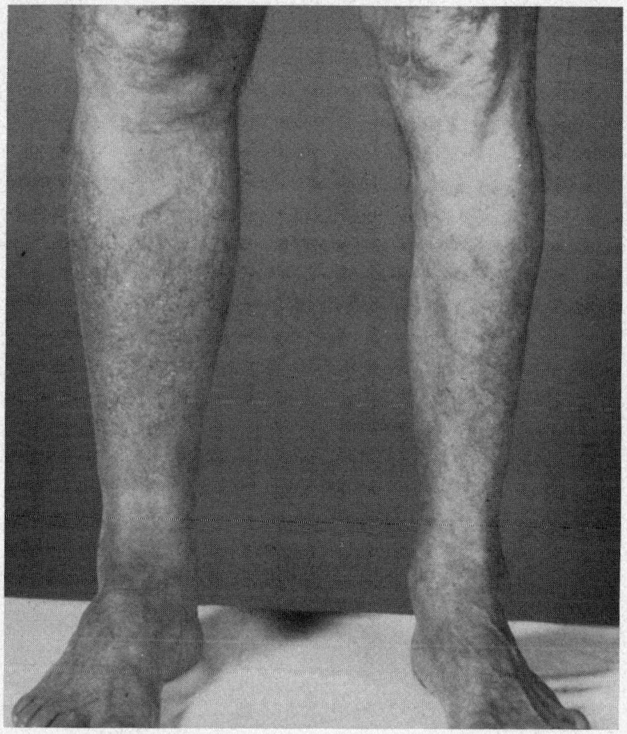

Fig. 1-24. Edema, reddish cyanotic color, and dilated pretibial vein in a patient with acute deep venous thrombosis involving the popliteal vein.

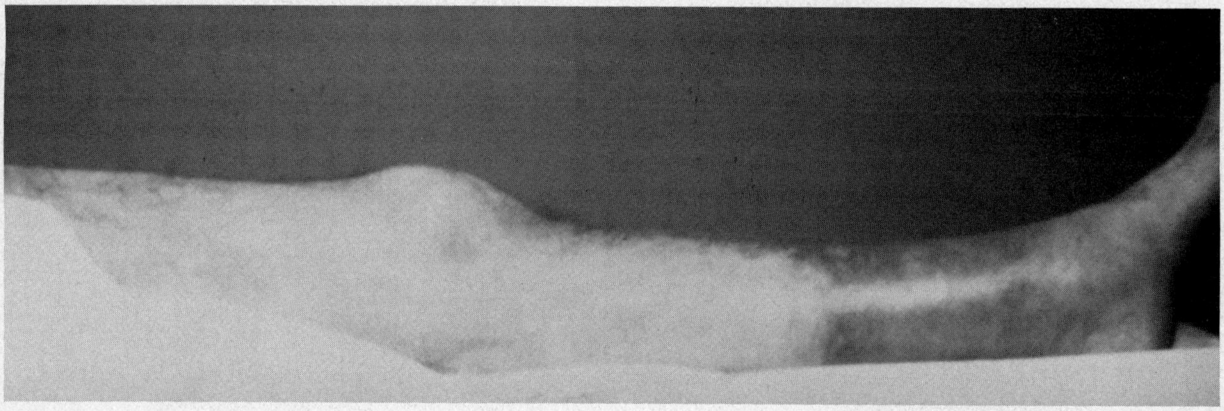

Fig. 1-25. Cellulitis of the leg with a localized area of erythema, heat, and tenderness in distal calf.

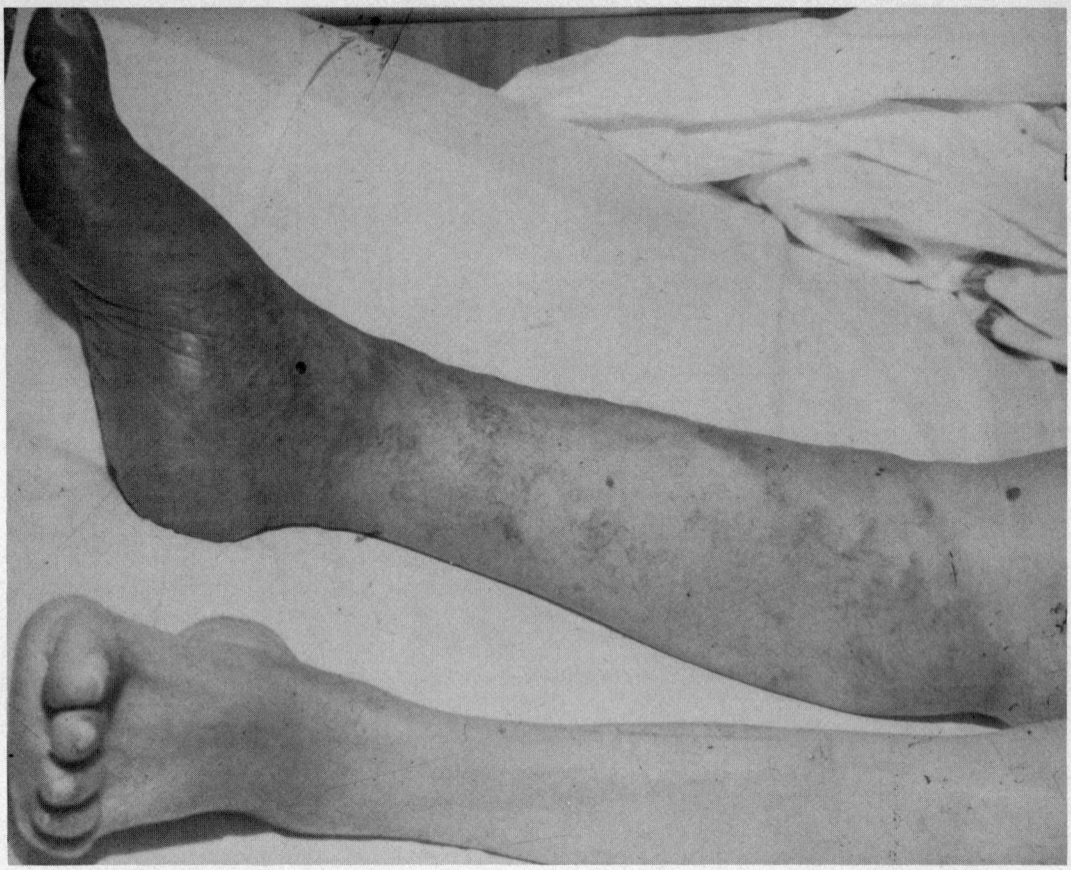

Fig. 1-26. Marked swelling of the leg with severe distal ischemia in a patient with phlegmasia cerulea dolens.

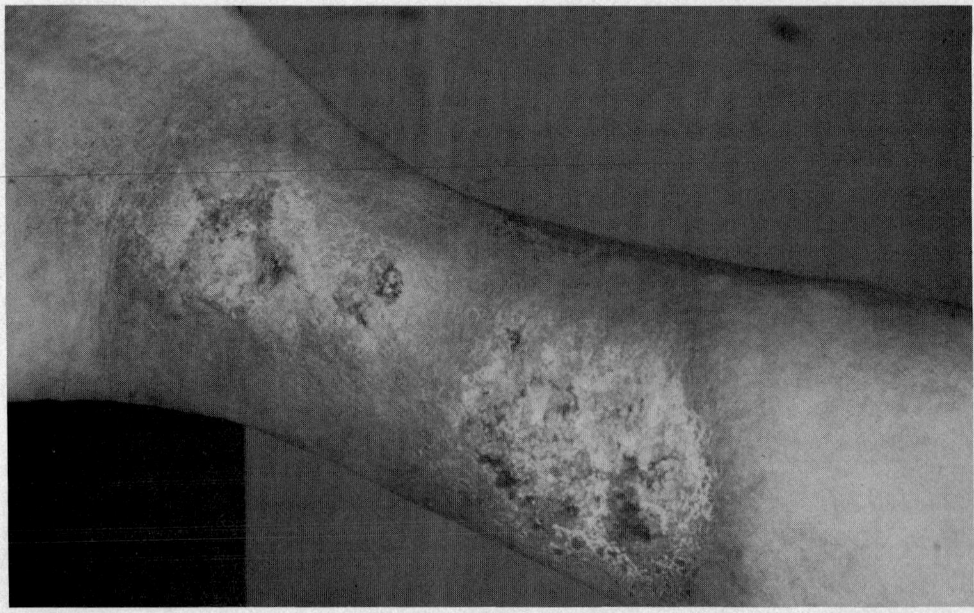

Fig. 1-27. Stasis pigmentation, dermatitis, and ulcerations in a patient with chronic venous insufficiency.

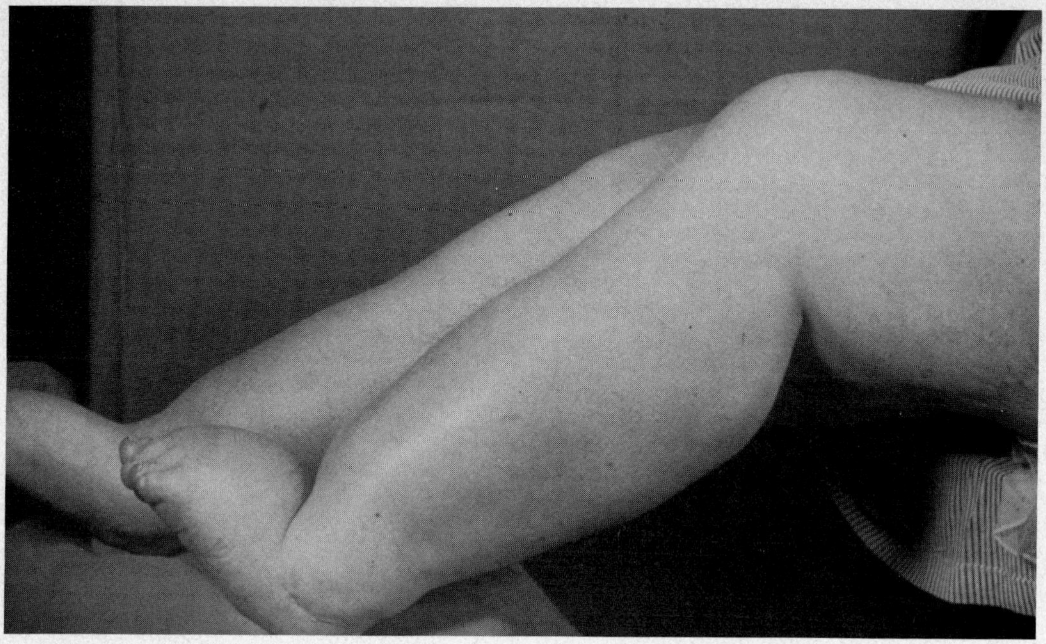

Fig. 1-28. Typical hump of swelling on the dorsum of the feet of a young woman with lymphedema praecox.

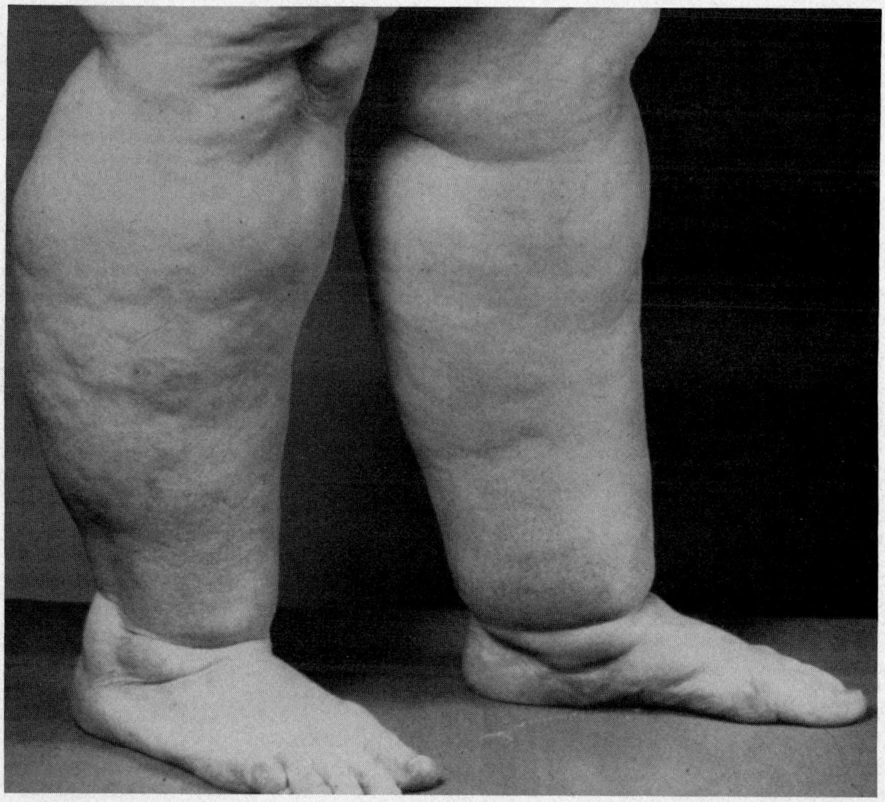

Fig. 1-29. Typical absence of swelling on the dorsum of the feet in this patient with lipedema.

commonly the result of venous valvular damage secondary to remote deep thrombophlebitis. The first sign of venous insufficiency is edema. Prominent superficial veins may also be present. Later, pigmentation, induration, and dermatitis may occur. A painful, tender, red area of chronic indurated cellulitis can develop up and down the lower calf on the medial side. Venous stasis ulcers usually occur in the region of the ankle in the vicinity of the malleoli, especially the medial malleolus (Fig. 1-27). There is usually brown pigmentation in the surrounding skin, and the leg is often edematous. The ulcers may be moderately painful but are never as painful as ischemic ulcers. The differential diagnosis of leg ulcer is covered in Chapter 35.

LYMPHATIC DISEASE

Lymphedema usually occurs gradually over a period of weeks, months, or even years. It starts as a slight hump of swelling on the dorsum of the foot and swelling around the ankle (Fig. 1-28), then later involves the leg itself. Stasis pigmentation is not present, and usually no superficial veins are visible in the lymphedematous leg. If lymphedema is extensive and long-standing and has been neglected as far as elastic supports are concerned, the tissue may be firm and resistant to pitting because of extensive fibrosis. In this stage the skin may be thickened and verrucous.

Lymphedema should be differentiated from *lipedema*, a painless, symmetric, bilateral deposition of fat in the lower extremities that affects women almost exclusively. The buttocks may also be involved. There is often a history of lipedema in other female members of the family. The distinguishing feature in lipedema is that the adipose tissue, which does not pit, always stops at the ankle thus sparing the foot (Fig. 1-29). For a more extensive differential diagnosis of the swollen leg, see Chapter 36.

A yellow discoloration of the fingernails and/or toenails in a patient with lymphedema may indicate the presence of *"yellow nail syndrome"* (see Chapter 27) with associated chylothorax or chylous ascites.

Patients with lymphedema have an increased susceptibility to episodes of cellulitis. The portals of entry include fissured skin from athlete's foot, ingrown toenails, or trauma to the skin or nails. Typically the patient suddenly experiences a severe shaking chill with a fever of 38° C to 41° C. This may be preceded by a short period of distress in the involved extremity or proximal lymph nodes. Soon a localized area of erythematous, inflamed skin appears on the extremity and rapidly increases in size. Reddened streaks may occur along the course of inflamed lymphatic vessels, and the proximal lymph nodes are often enlarged, tender, and painful. The response to antibiotic therapy is usually rapid.

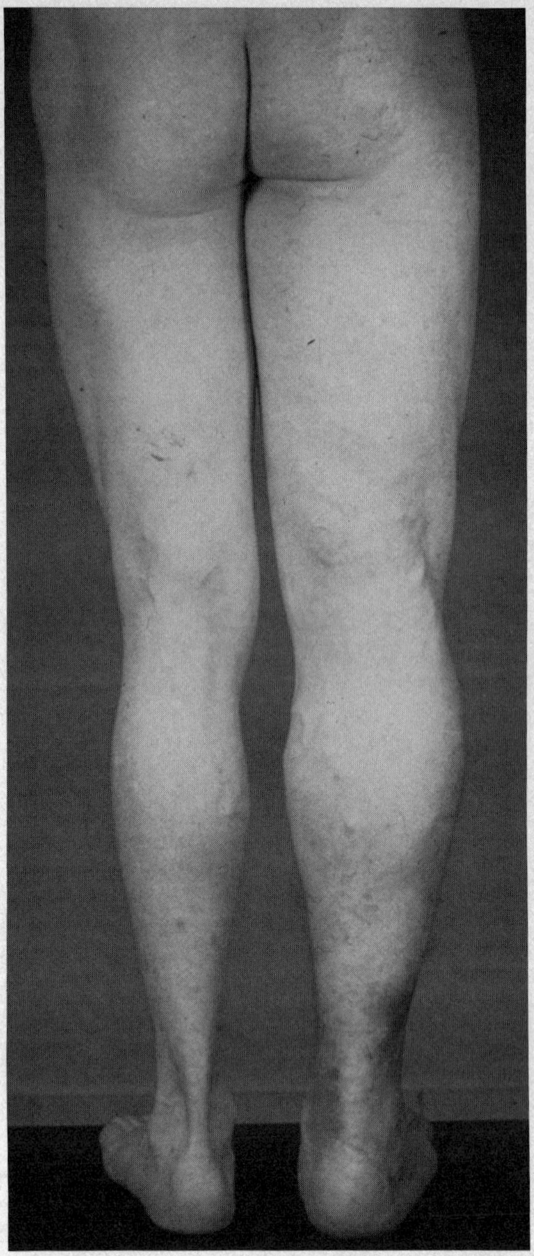

Fig. 1-30. Young man with Klippel-Trenaunay-Weber syndrome, demonstrating the triad of muscular hypertrophy, varicose veins, and port-wine stain.

ARTERIOVENOUS FISTULAS

Arteriovenous fistulas that affect the limbs (see Chapter 30) can be either congenital or traumatic in origin. A traumatic arteriovenous fistula may be associated with edema of the extremity, prominent veins, and congestive heart failure if the fistula is large enough. Thrills and bruits are

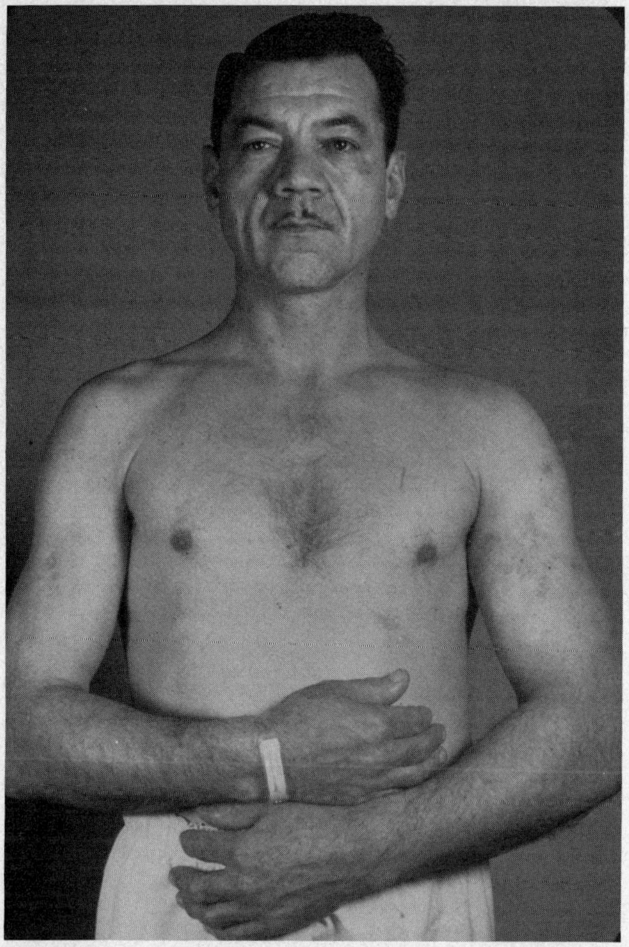

Fig. 1-31. Edema and dilated veins of left arm in a patient with subclavian vein thrombosis secondary to thoracic outlet syndrome.

common. Congenital arteriovenous fistulas are usually associated with the presence of varicose veins. Thrills and bruits are usually not present. The involved limb may have an increased length and increased muscular development. The temperature of the skin is usually higher than that of the normal extremity. Ulcerations and gangrene may affect the distal parts of the limb.

Birthmarks are present in approximately half the patients with congenital arteriovenous fistulas involving the extremities. They are either port-wine stains (nevus flammeus) or more diffuse hemangiomas. The *Klippel-Trenaunay-Weber syndrome* comprises a triad of port-wine stain, muscular hypertrophy, and varicose veins (Fig. 1-30). The patients may also have congenital arteriovenous fistulas or localized areas of agenesis of the deep venous system.

THORACIC OUTLET SYNDROME

The great majority of patients who have evidence of arterial compression during thoracic outlet maneuvers has no symptoms at all. However, symptoms can be produced by compression of the artery, vein, nerves, or combinations of them (see Chapter 28).

Neurologic symptoms are the most common clinical manifestations of thoracic outlet syndrome. Numbness, tingling, or weakness of the fingers, hand, and arm may be intermittent or constant and may or may not be associated with position of the arms above the shoulder level. Arterial symptoms associated with thoracic outlet syndrome include intermittent claudication when working with the arms above shoulder level, Raynaud's phenomenon, and distal ischemia caused by emboli from a mural thrombosis of the subclavian artery. A subclavian artery aneurysm can be caused by trauma at the thoracic outlet and can, in turn, cause ischemia as a result of an embolism or thrombosis. Finally, ischemia can be caused by thrombosis of the subclavian artery itself. Cerebral embolism secondary to retrograde extension of a subclavian artery thrombosis can occur. Venous compression can produce intermittent obstruction of the subclavian vein with intermittent swelling and cyanosis of the arm. Subclavian venous thrombosis, the so-called "effort" thrombosis, can also occur and is the most common cause, other than iatrogenic, of subclavian and axillary venous thrombosis. Clinically, this thrombosis can result in edema of the involved arm and dilated superficial veins and venules (Fig. 1-31).

REFERENCE

1. Bates MC and Warren SG: Xanthelasma: clinical indicator of decreased levels of high-density lipoprotein cholesterol, South Med J 82:570

Chapter 2

PHYSICAL EXAMINATION

Jess R. Young

Despite new developments in the noninvasive vascular laboratory, new imaging techniques with ultrasound duplex studies, and new arteriographic and venographic techniques, the basic foundation for diagnosis in vascular disease remains a good history and a thorough physical examination. Unfortunately, these skills are rarely adequately taught in medical schools and in residency programs. In this chapter the basic examination of the patient with vascular disease is reviewed.

HEAD AND NECK

In checking for arterial disease of the head and neck, the eyes must also be examined carefully. Xanthelasma of the lids may be an indicator that the patient has either hypercholesterolemia or a low level of high-density lipoprotein (HDL) and therefore may be prone to develop atherosclerosis. An arcus senilis in a younger patient may be a sign of premature atherosclerosis. The fundi may reveal evidence of severe hypertension, diabetes mellitus, extensive atherosclerosis, or atheromatous embolization.

Pulse palpation should begin with the temporal artery. The pulsation is always found just anterior to the tragus of the ear (Fig. 2-1). The strength of the pulse should be gauged, and the artery should be examined for the thickening or inflammation found in temporal arteritis. Aneurysms of the temporal artery are also occasionally found.

When palpating for the carotid arteries, the carotid bifurcation area high in the neck should be avoided. Palpation in this area can cause dislodgment of atheromatous emboli that most commonly develop at the bifurcation. Palpation near the carotid sinus at the bifurcation may also produce marked bradycardia or asystole if a hypersensitive carotid sinus reflex is present. The carotid artery can be palpated low in the neck by hooking the fingers or thumb of the examining hand around in front of the sternocleidomastoid

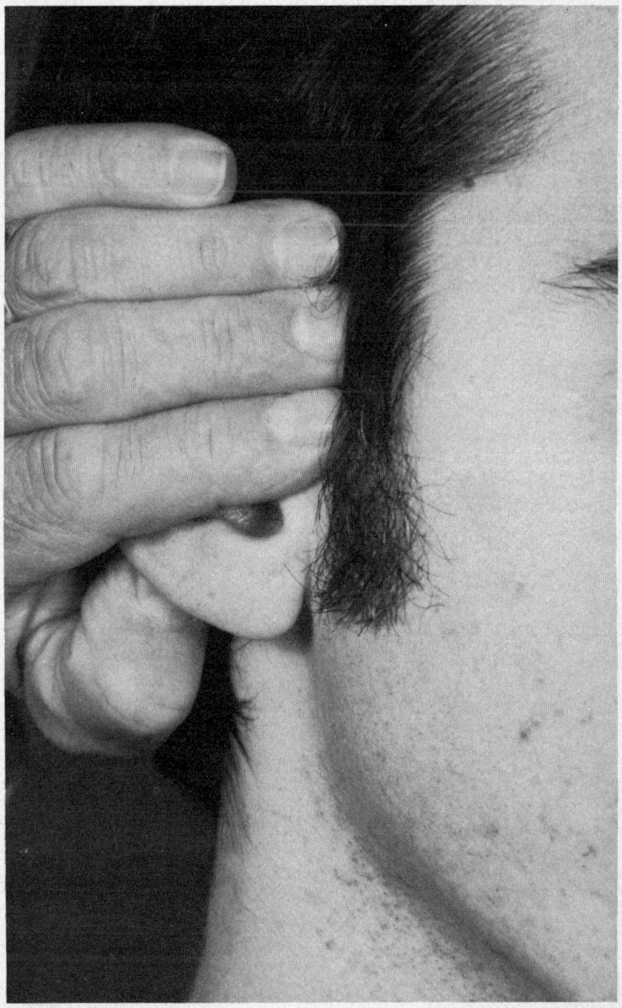

Fig. 2-1. The temporal artery pulse is palpated just anterior to the tragus of the ear.

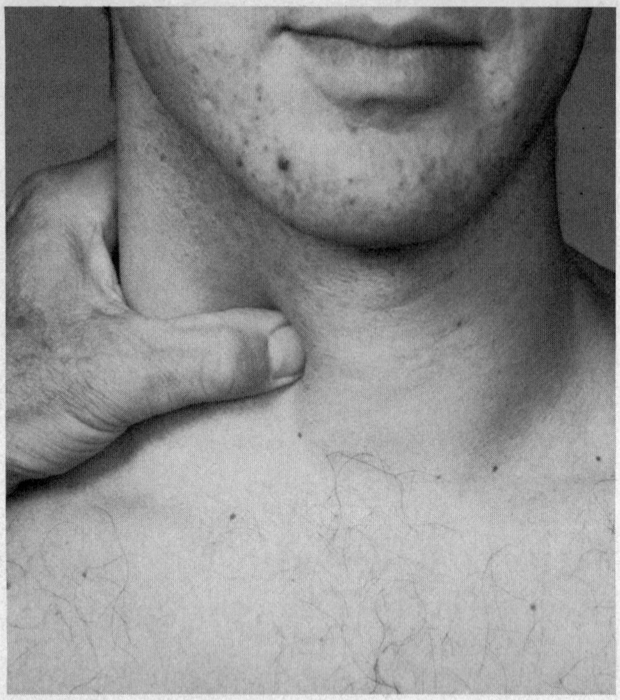

Fig. 2-2. The common carotid pulse should be palpated low in the neck.

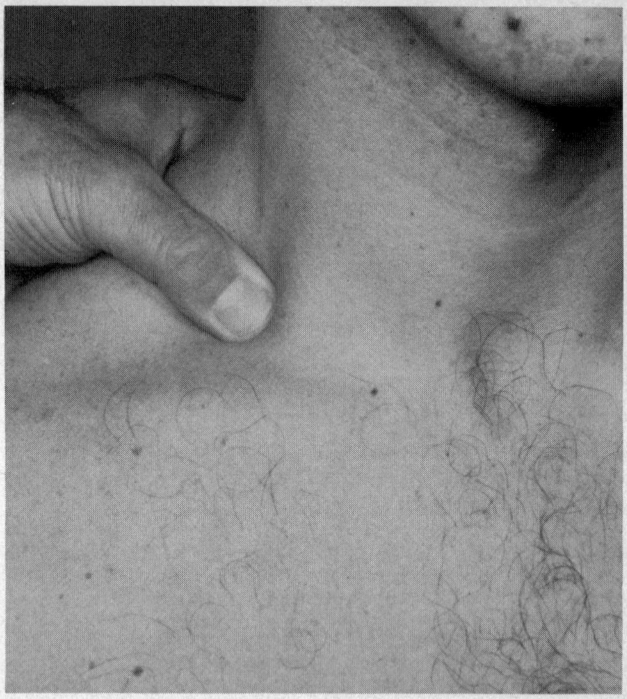

Fig. 2-3. Subclavian artery palpation.

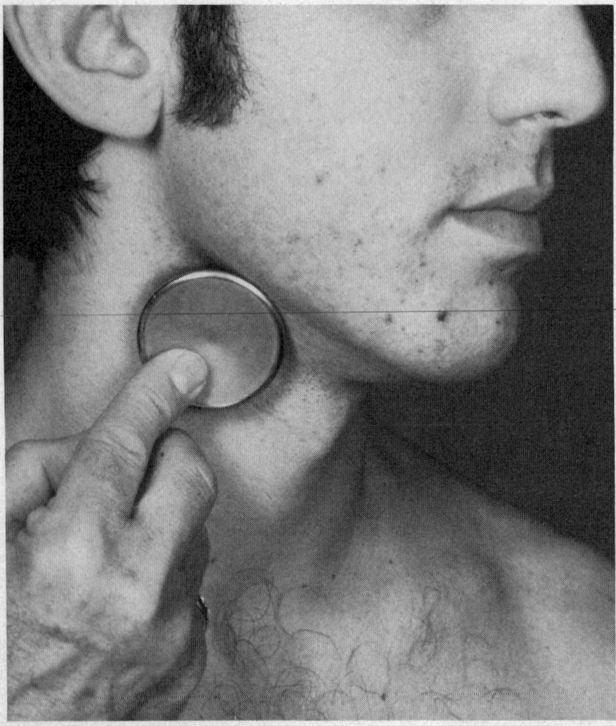

Fig. 2-4. Auscultation for bruits at the carotid bifurcation.

muscles (Fig. 2-2). The subclavian artery pulse is most easily appreciated by palpation with the thumb, with the remaining fingers braced behind the neck (Fig. 2-3). As with pulses elsewhere, the strength of the pulsation on one side of the body should be compared with the pulse on the other side.

Bruits can best be heard with the bell of the stethoscope. The bell fits better in the various areas of the neck and the globe of the eye that will be examined, and low rumbling bruits are heard better with the bell. Bruits heard over the eyeball may indicate intracranial carotid artery stenosis. As much care and detail should be given in describing the bruits as is given in describing heart murmurs. The bruit should be rated as to severity, with either four or six categories. The location of the bruit should be described, whether it is low in the neck, in the midneck, at the angle of the mandible, or over the subclavian artery. The quality of the bruit should be described, whether it is low and rumbling, blowing, or high pitched and musical. Notation should be made as to whether the bruit is purely systolic or whether it extends into diastole.

The examination for carotid artery bruits should begin as high in the neck as possible, getting up under the mandible as far as the bell of the stethoscope can reach (Fig. 2-4). After noting the presence or absence of bruits at this lo-

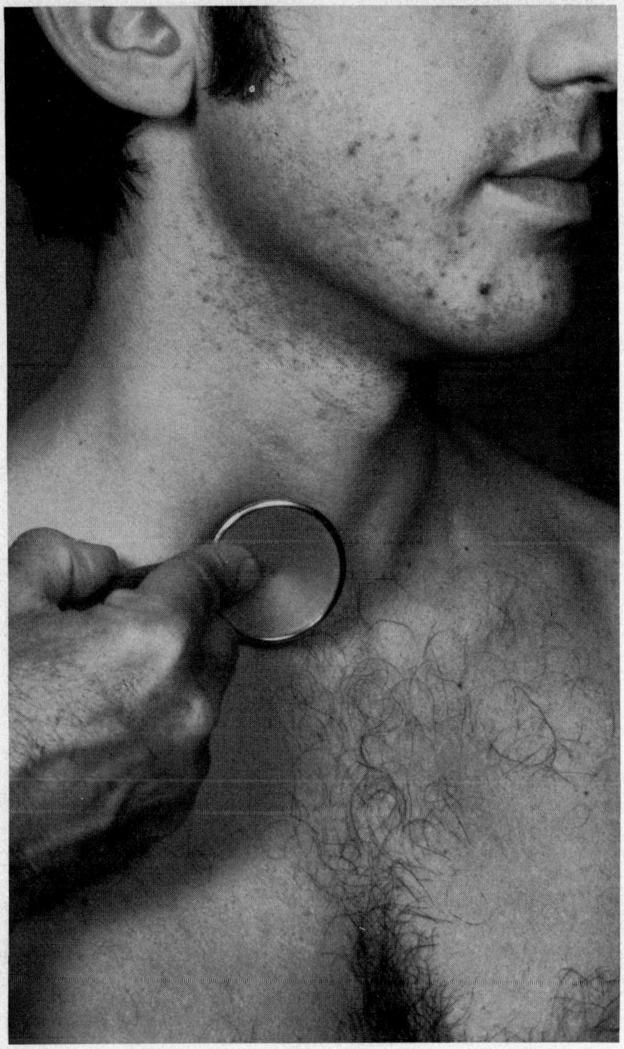

Fig. 2-5. Bruits at the base of the neck can be transmitted from the heart or from carotid, innominate, or subclavian stenosis.

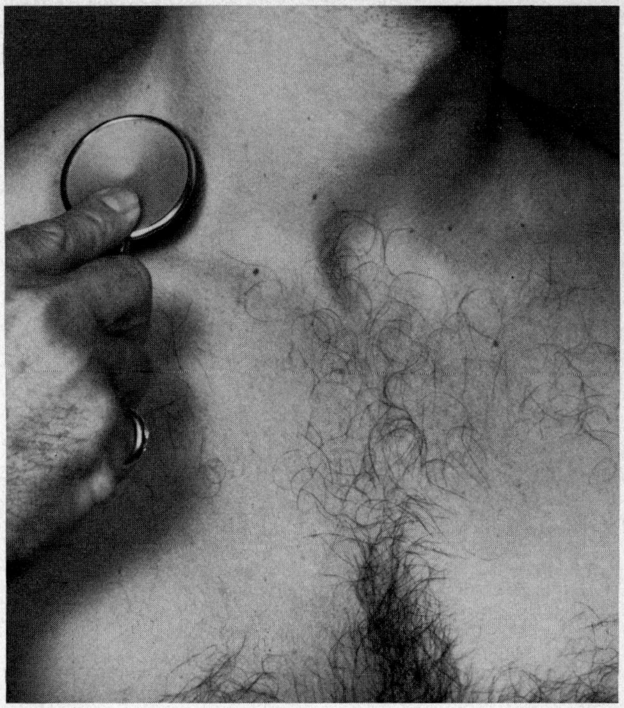

Fig. 2-6. Subclavian artery bruits are usually loudest at the supraclavicular area.

cation, the examiner moves the stethoscope slowly down the course of the common carotid artery to the base of the neck (Fig. 2-5), noting whether the bruit is increasing or decreasing in intensity. After the base of the neck is reached, the stethoscope is moved into the supraclavicular area over the subclavian aartery (Fig. 2-6), and any bruits in this location are noted. Vertebral artery bruits should be looked for in the area posterior to the sternocleidomastoid muscles (Fig. 2-7). Arteriovenous malformations are sometimes heard more posteriorly in the neck and occipital areas (Fig. 2-8). Finally, auscultation at the aortic and pulmonic valve areas over the upper chest (Fig. 2-9) is done to determine whether or not the neck bruits might be transmitted from the heart. Usually a murmur from an aortic stenosis or sclerosis will be transmitted up into all four neck vessels, the subclavian and the common carotid arteries, equally, and the intensity of the bruits will diminish as the stethoscope is moved up the neck.

To determine whether a bruit over the carotid artery is transmitted from a stenosis of the subclavian artery, the examiner compresses the subclavian artery (Fig. 2-10) while listening to the bruit over the carotid. If the bruit disappears, the stenosis is in the subclavian artery and not the carotid artery.

A bruit that is heard during both systole and diastole may indicate a severe arterial stenosis, an arteriovenous malformation, an arteriovenous fistula, or a venous hum. The systolic-diastolic bruit caused by severe carotid stenosis is usually heard at the carotid bifurcation area high in the neck. An important point in this situation is that either a severe stenosis or a complete occlusion of the contralateral internal carotid artery is present in more than 60% of patients.[1] Arteriovenous fistulas are often traumatic in origin. The bruit of an arteriovenous fistula may often be heard in other areas of the head and neck, including the back of the neck and the temple areas. A venous hum is usually heard at the base of the neck. It can be easily detected by lightly compressing the external jugular vein with a finger (Fig. 2-11),

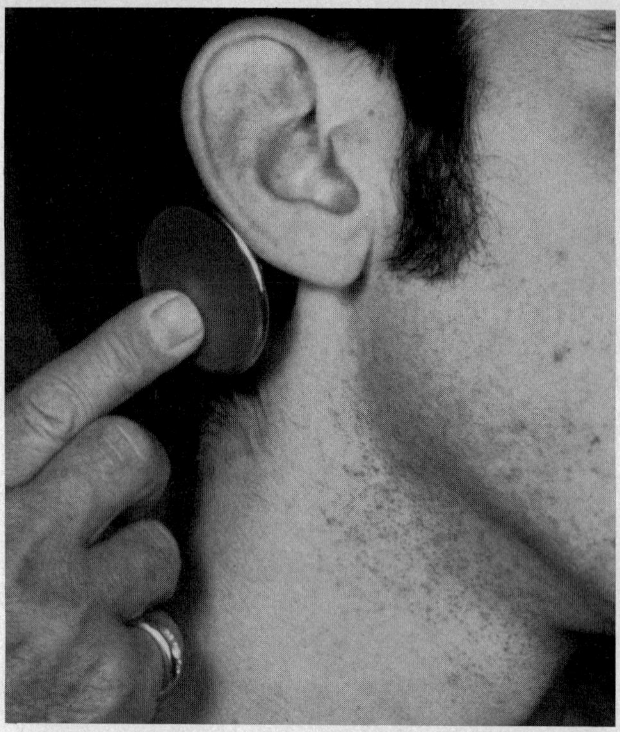

Fig. 2-8. Bruits of arteriovenous malformations may be loudest posteriorly in the neck and occipital areas.

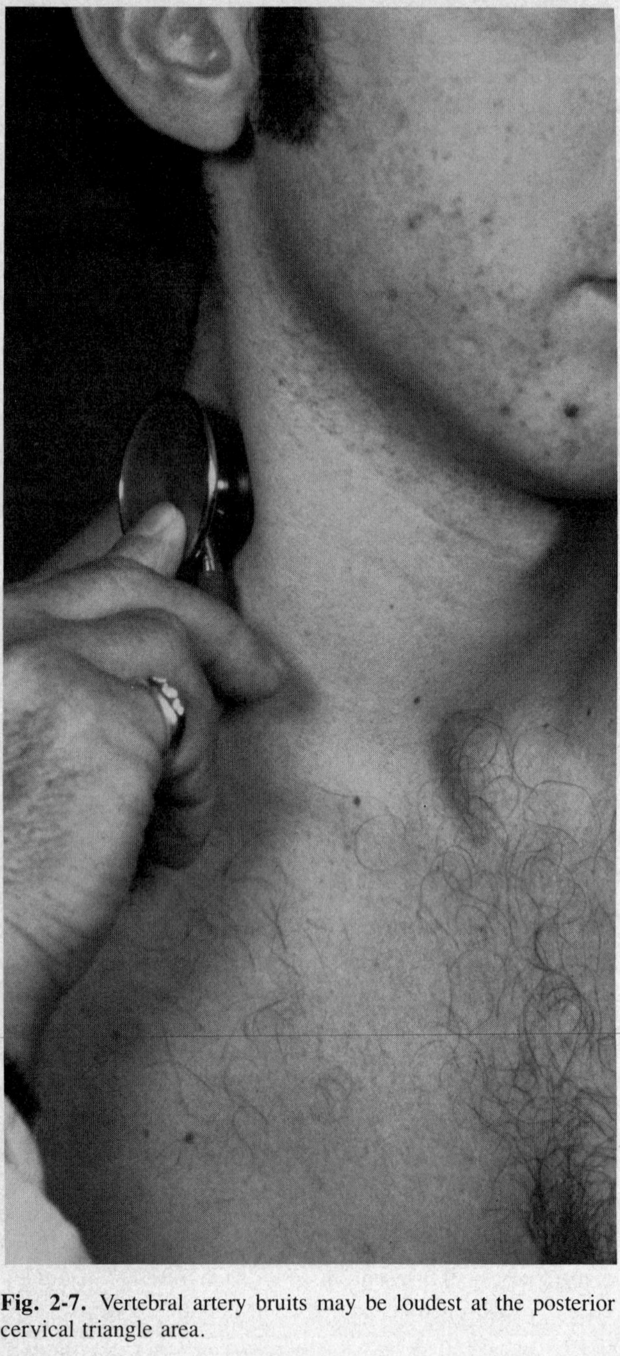

Fig. 2-7. Vertebral artery bruits may be loudest at the posterior cervical triangle area.

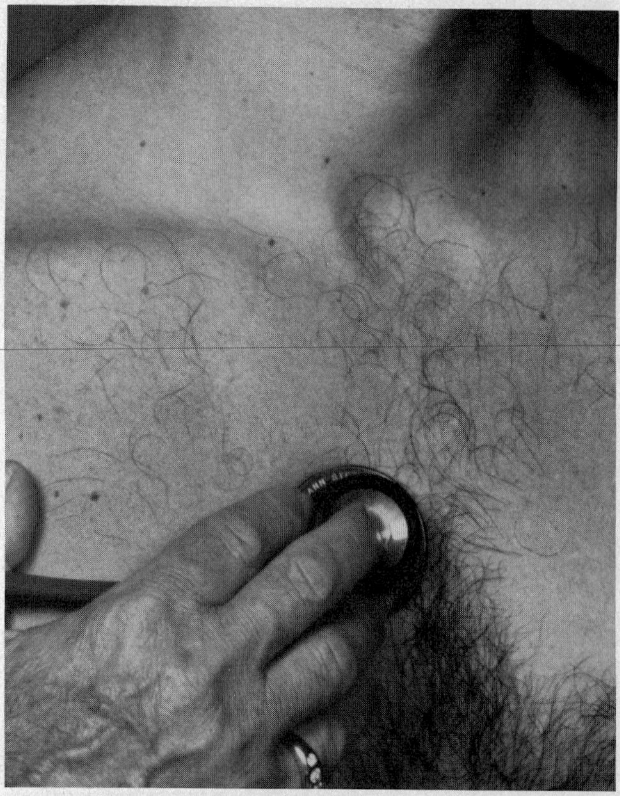

Fig. 2-9. The heart should be checked for murmurs, a possible cause of bruits transmitted to the neck.

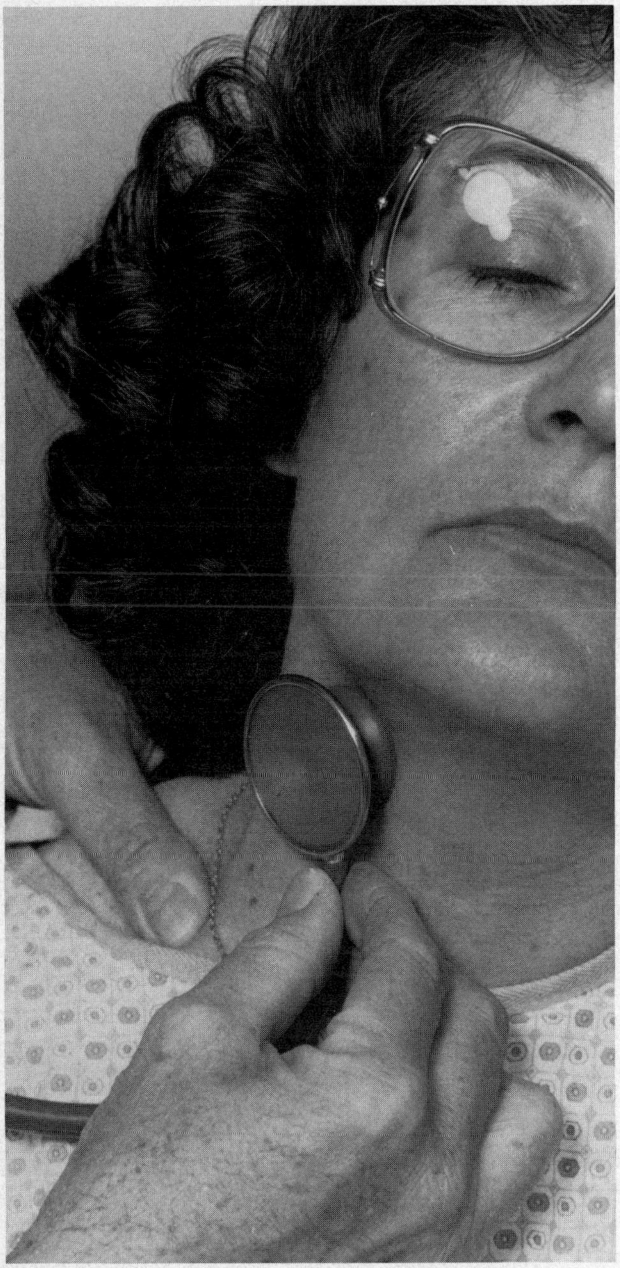

Fig. 2-10. If a subclavian artery bruit is transmitted to the carotid artery area, it will disappear with digital compression of the subclavian artery.

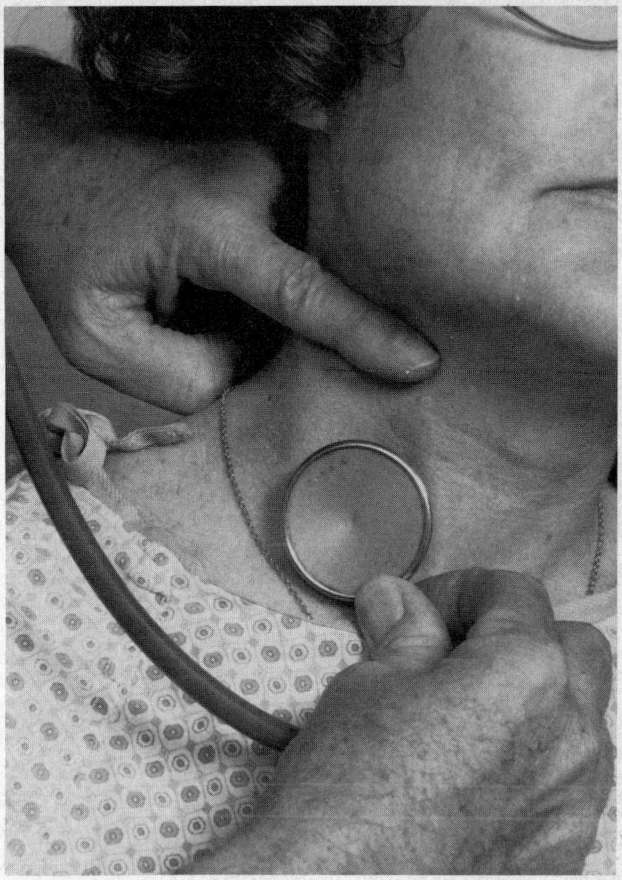

Fig. 2-11. The bruit of a venous hum will disappear with light compression of the external jugular vein.

thus stopping venous flow and immediately eliminating the continuous bruit.

Dilated jugular veins may indicate an arteriovenous fistula (Fig. 2-12), congestive heart failure, or venous occlusion proximal to the dilated vein. If both sides of the neck and both arms have dilated veins, a superior vena caval syndrome can be suspected (Fig. 2-13).

UPPER EXTREMITIES

A blood pressure check should be made in both arms to see if there is a significant difference in pressures. A significant difference (more than 10 mm of mercury) would suggest that one of the subclavian arteries or the innominate artery is narrowed or occluded.

The arms should be examined for symmetry. Asymmetry could indicate congenital hypertrophy or atrophy on one side, previous neurologic disease, an arteriovenous fistula on one side, or edema secondary to lymphedema or venous insufficiency. Edema and dilated superficial veins would suggest a previous deep venous thrombosis on that side.

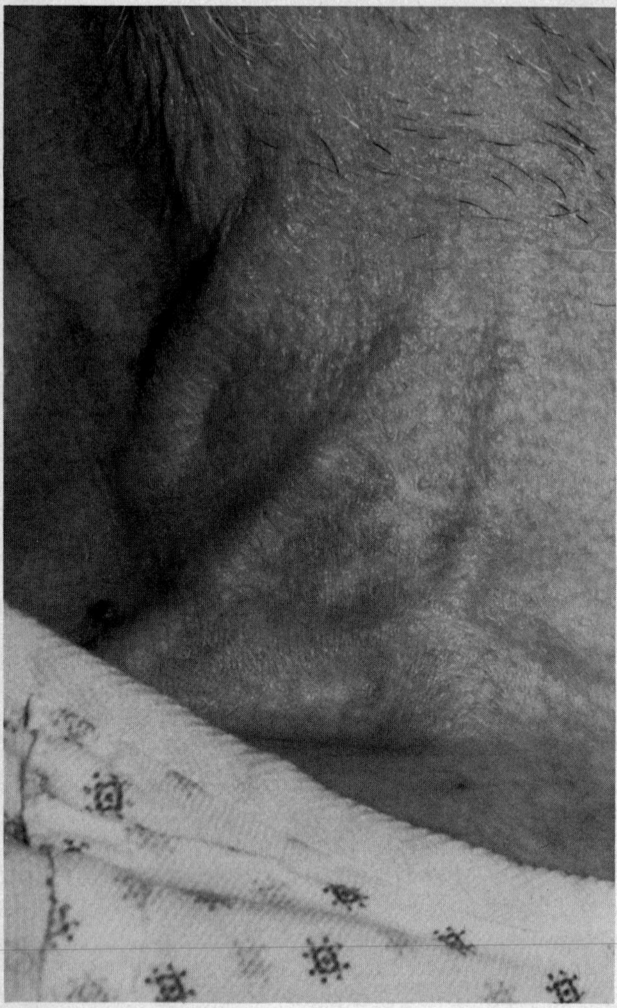

Fig. 2-12. Dilated jugular veins secondary to a traumatic carotid-jugular arteriovenous fistula.

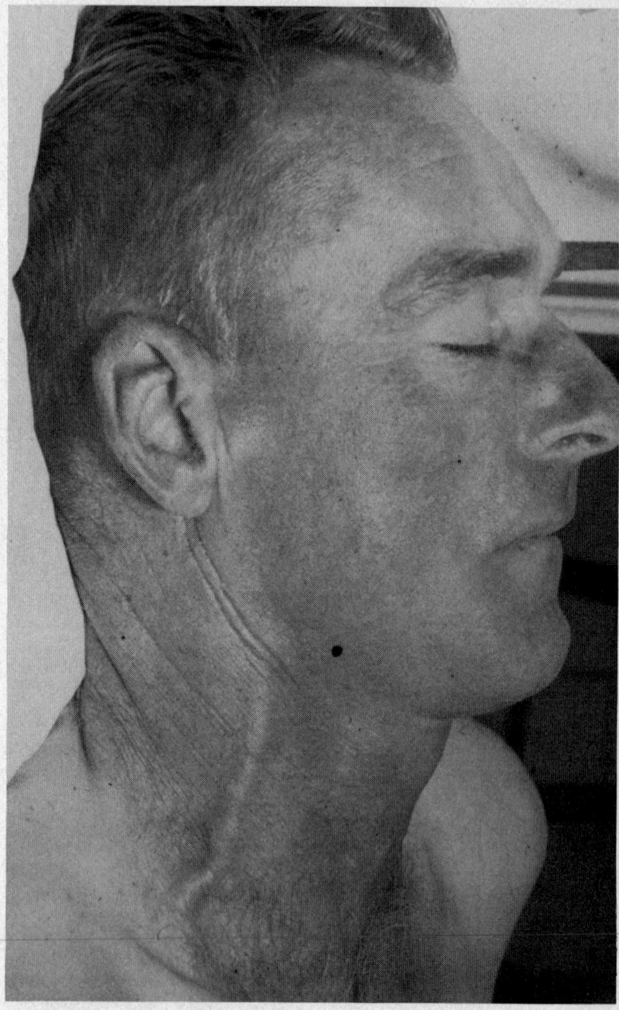

Fig. 2-13. Dilated jugular veins and facial plethora secondary to an acute superior vena cava syndrome caused by an acute dissecting aneurysm.

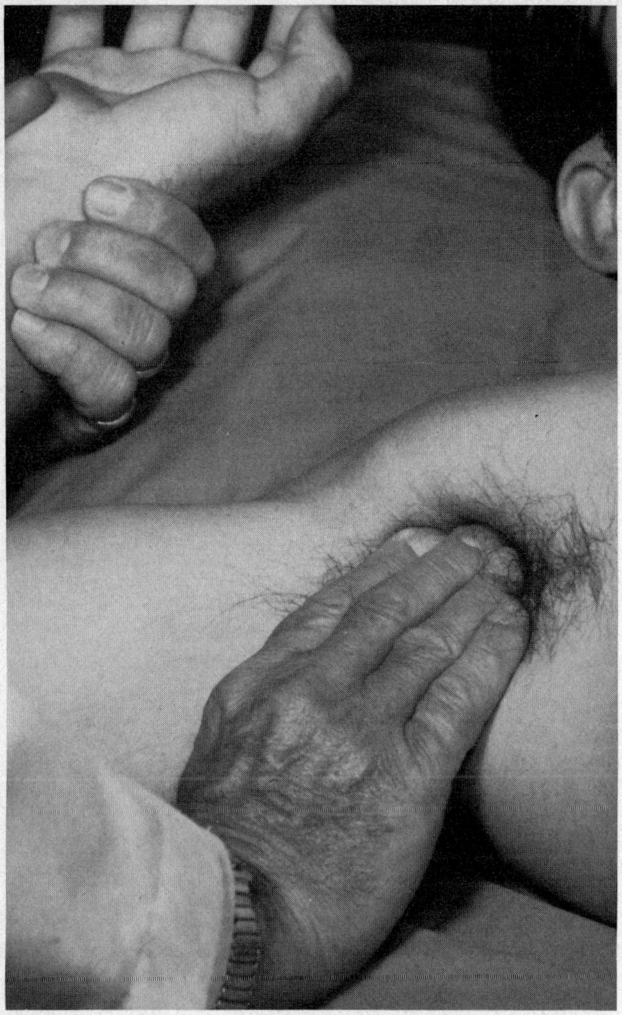

Fig. 2-14. The axillary pulse is felt deep in the axilla.

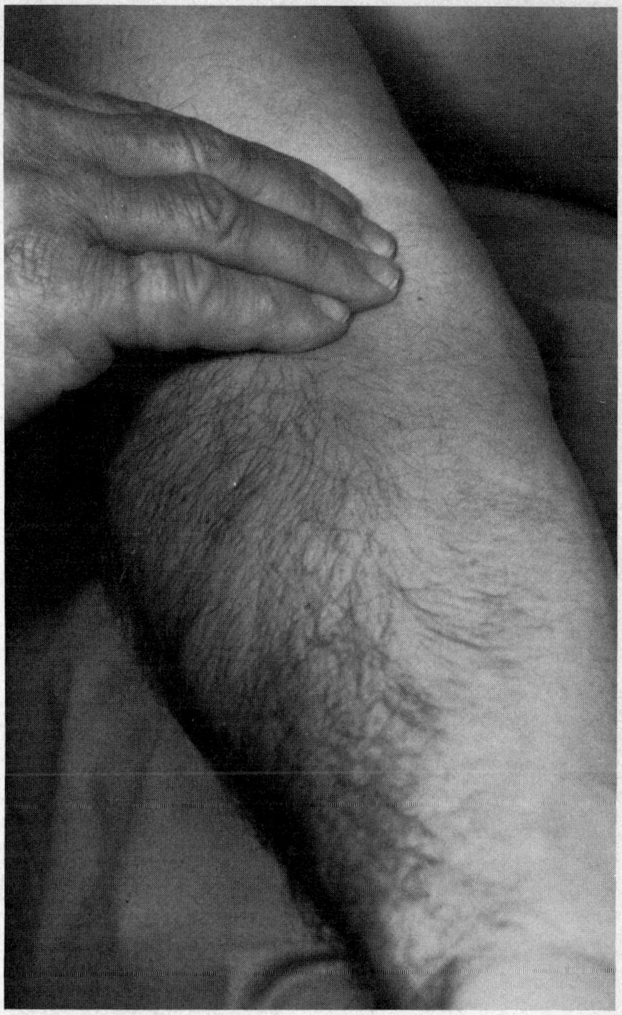

Fig. 2-15. Brachial pulse palpation.

The axillary (Fig. 2-14), brachial (Fig. 2-15), radial (Fig. 2-16), and ulnar pulses (Fig. 2-17) should be palpated. The presence or absence of aneurysms of these arteries should be noted (Fig. 2-18). Auscultation of the arm for bruits that might suggest arterial stenosis or an arteriovenous fistula should be done. The temperature of the skin of the two arms should be compared.

When indicated, thoracic outlet maneuvers should be done. They are best performed by bracing the patient's shoulder with one hand while the other hand abducts and externally rotates the patient's arm (Fig. 2-19). If the pulse does not obliterate or if symptoms are not produced, further checking would include having the patient look first to one side and then to the other with the chin extended (Fig. 2-20). If the test is still negative, the patient should perform a Valsalva maneuver while looking first to the right and then to the left with the chin extended. A thoracic outlet maneuver is positive when the patient's symptoms are reproduced. As a rule, the pulse will also disappear when the patient's symptoms are reproduced, but this is not necessary for a positive test.

If occlusion of the arteries distal to the wrist are suspected, an Allen test should be done. The patient is instructed to make a tight fist, which will empty most of the blood from the hand and fingers except for the thenar and hypothenar eminences. These eminences are drained of blood by the examiner's swiping his thumbs down across the eminences to the wrist and then with the same motion occluding both the radial and ulnar arteries with his thumbs (Fig. 2-21). The patient then opens his hand, making sure that he does not overextend his fingers. Overextension will cause a false-positive Allen's test (Fig. 2-22). After opening

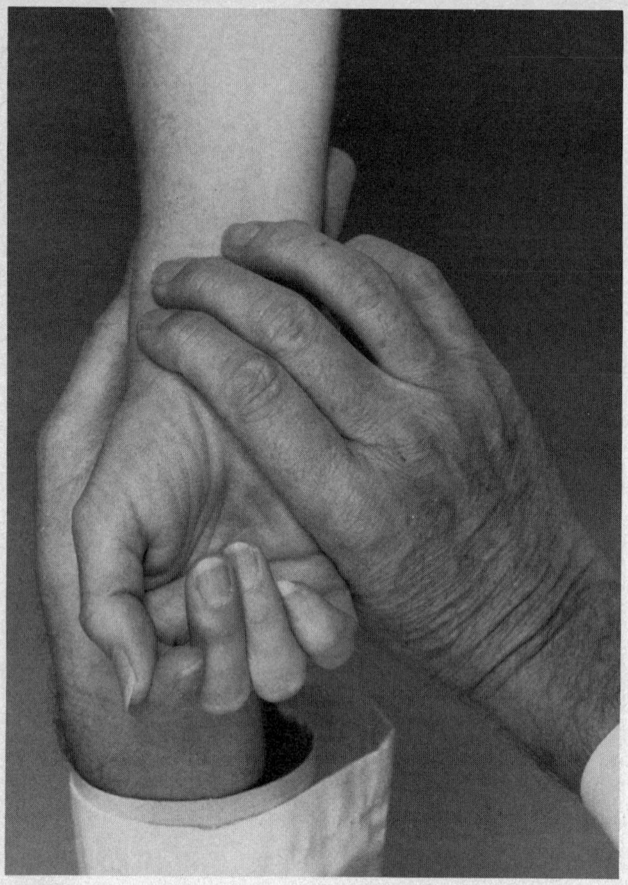

Fig. 2-16. Radial pulse palpation.

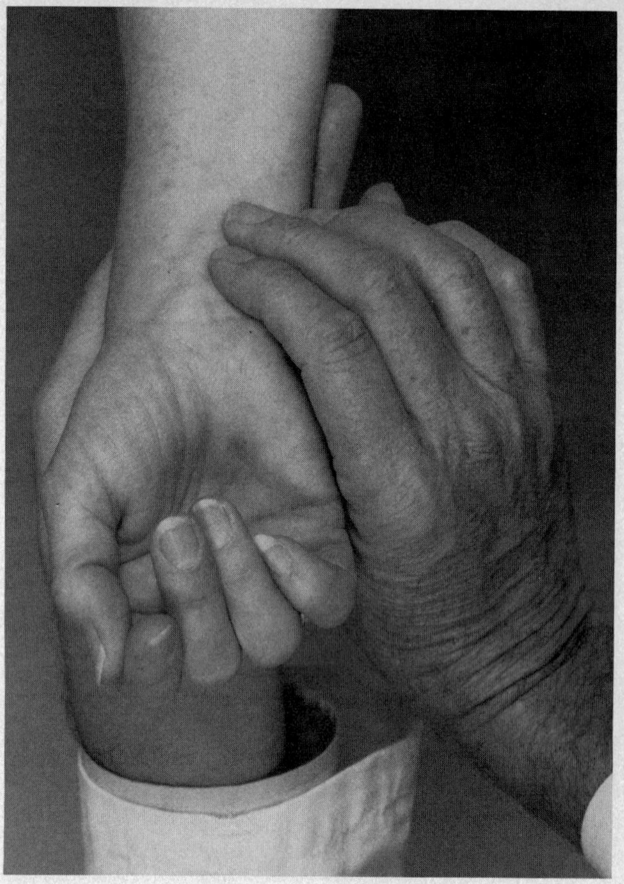

Fig. 2-17. Ulnar pulse palpation.

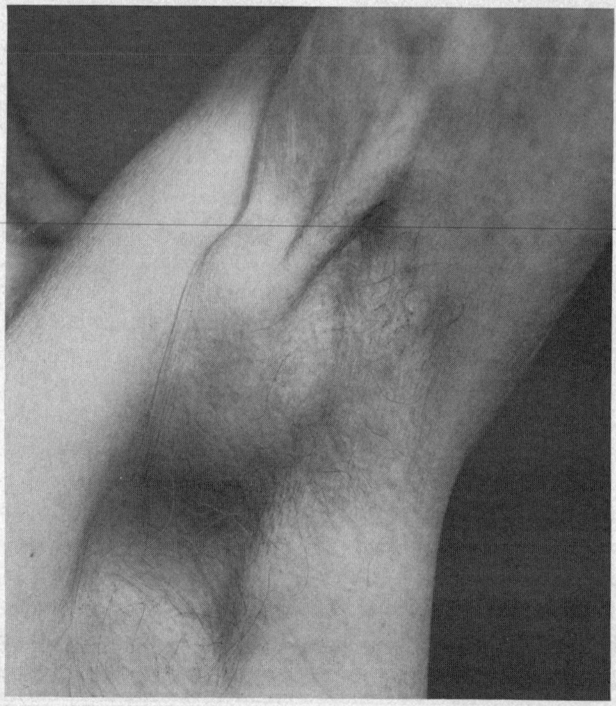

Fig. 2-18. Aneurysm of axillary artery.

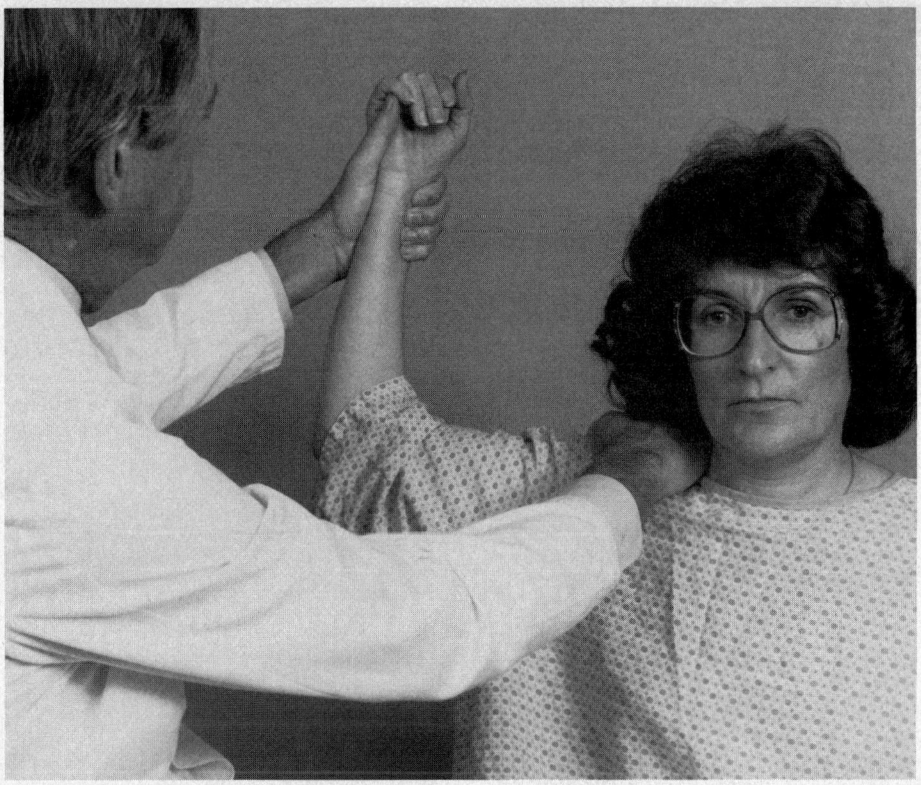

Fig. 2-19. Thoracic outlet maneuver. The patient's shoulder is braced by the examiner's right hand while the left hand abducts and externally rotates the patient's arm. The patient's radial pulse is monitored by the fingers of the examiner's left hand.

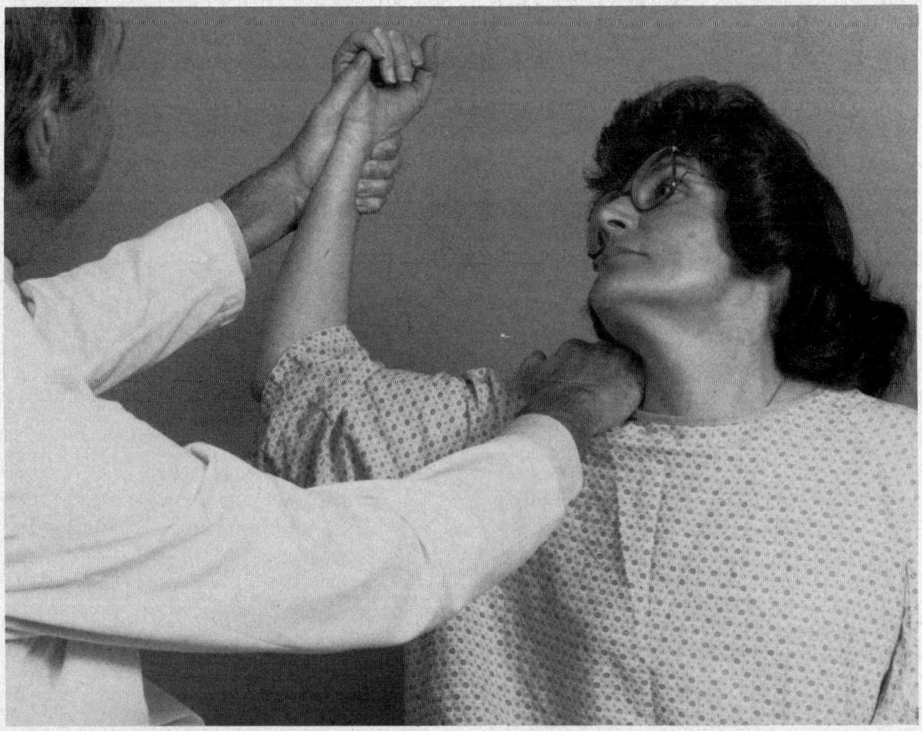

Fig. 2-20. If the routine thoracic outlet maneuver is negative, further testing can be done by having the patient turn the head to one side or the other while extending the chin.

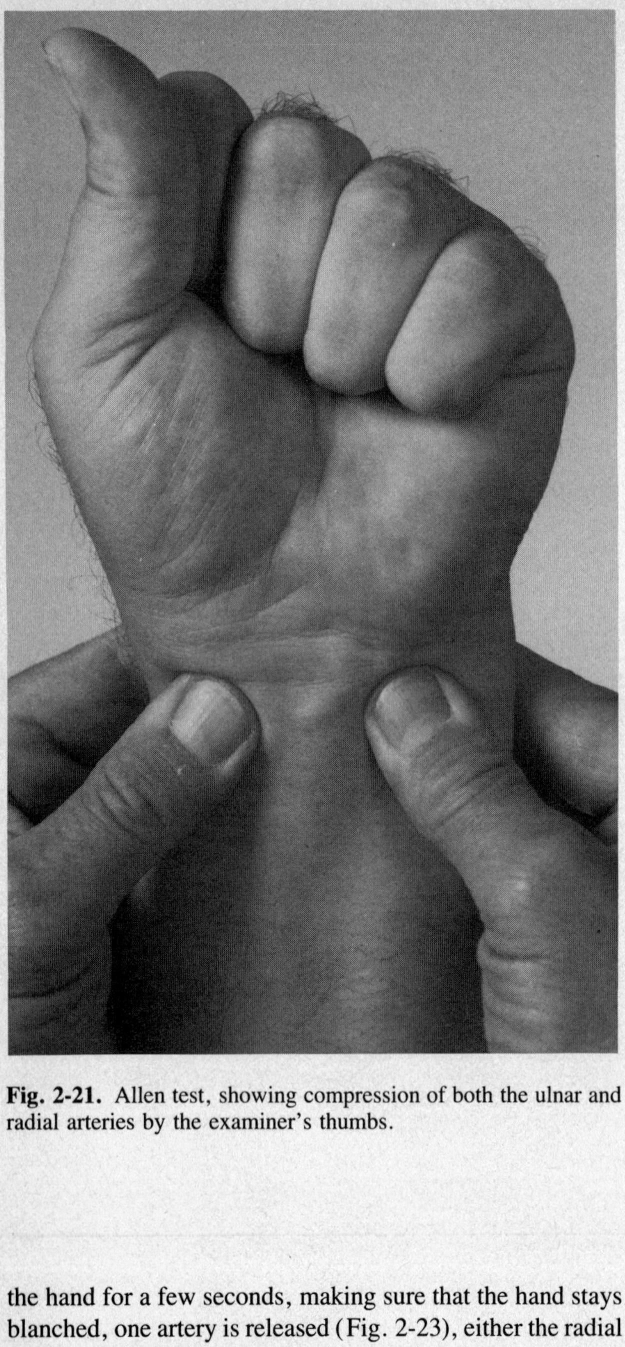

Fig. 2-21. Allen test, showing compression of both the ulnar and radial arteries by the examiner's thumbs.

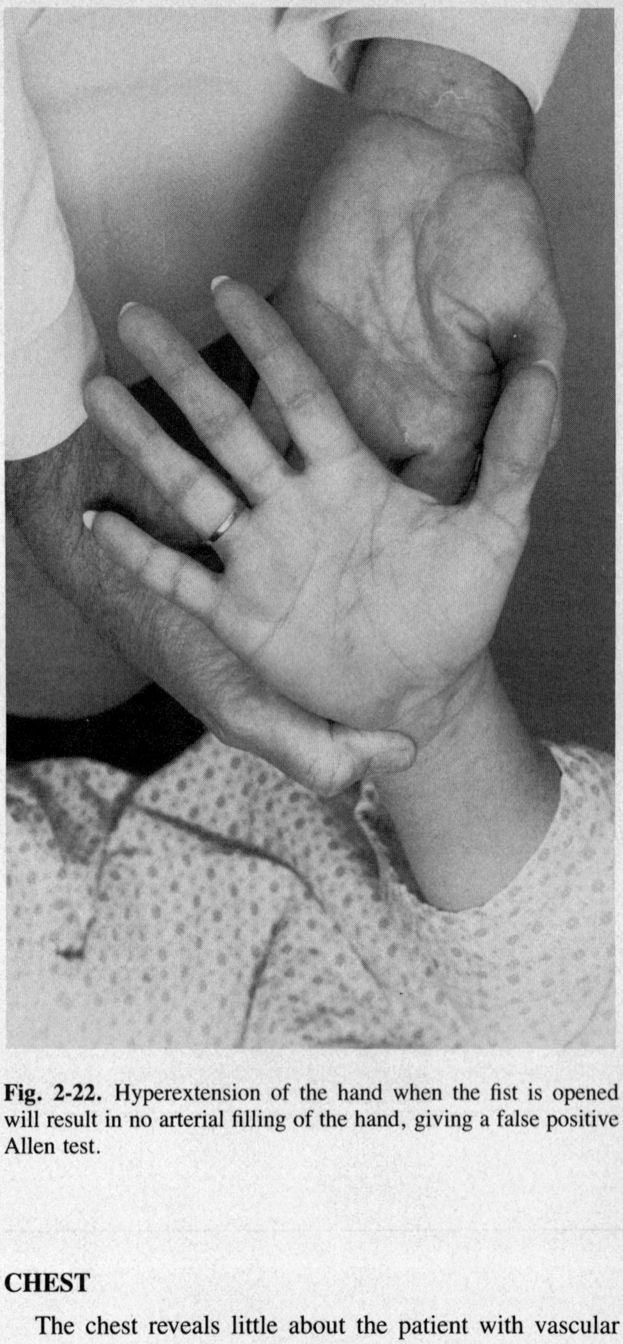

Fig. 2-22. Hyperextension of the hand when the fist is opened will result in no arterial filling of the hand, giving a false positive Allen test.

the hand for a few seconds, making sure that the hand stays blanched, one artery is released (Fig. 2-23), either the radial or the ulnar. If there is prompt filling from that artery with a prompt return of color to the hand, the maneuver is repeated; then the second artery is released (Fig. 2-24). Thus the patency of the radial and ulnar arteries are determined. A positive test results when there is no return of color to the blanched hand when the occluded artery is released (Fig. 2-25).

CHEST

The chest reveals little about the patient with vascular disease. Occasionally a large aneurysm of the ascending aorta may be felt as a pulsation high in the chest near the sternum. The sudden appearance of a murmur of aortic insufficiency may be a clue to the presence of a dissecting aneurysm. The presence of dilated veins on the chest may suggest the presence of an axillary or subclavian venous thrombosis (Fig. 2-26) or a superior or inferior vena caval occlusion.

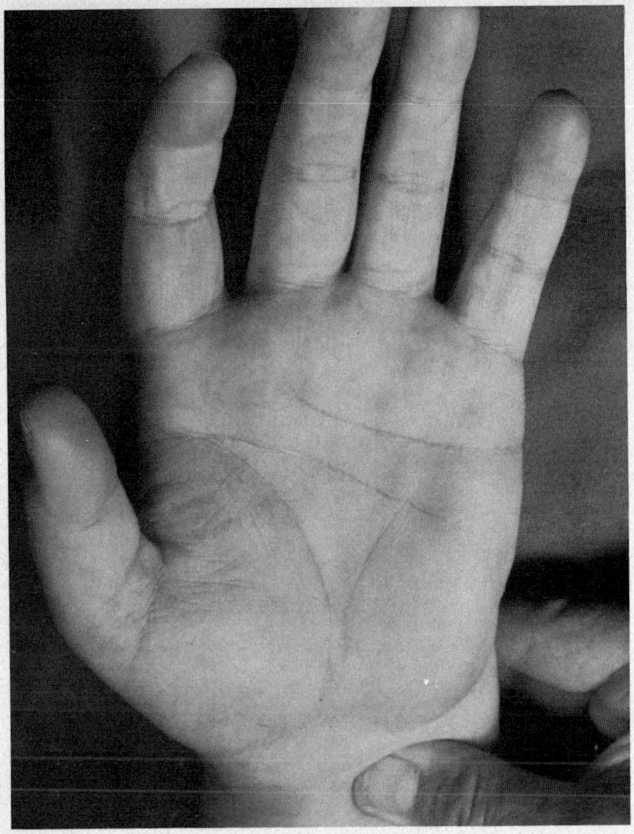

Fig. 2-23. With the hand relaxed, there is rapid arterial filling via the radial artery, with rapid return of color.

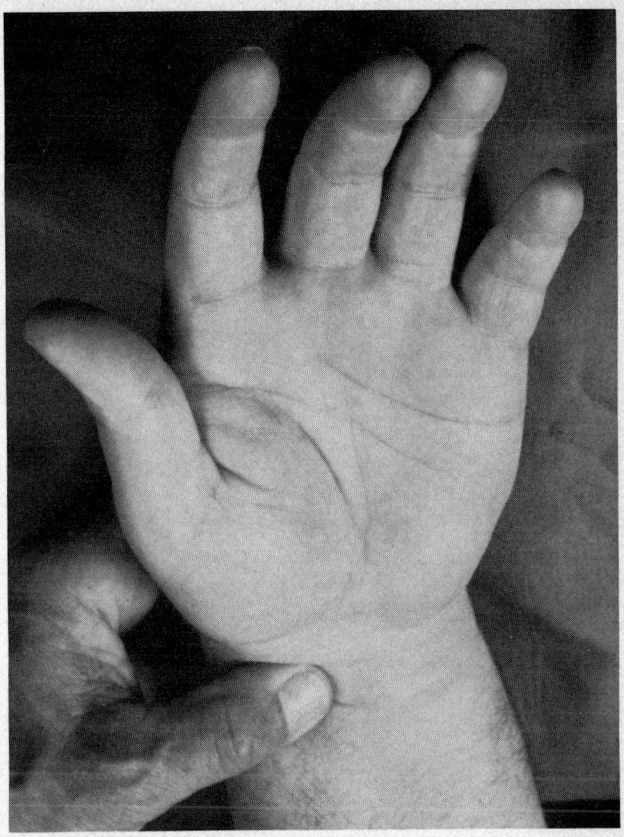

Fig. 2-24. Normal Allen test with rapid return of color when pressure on the ulnar artery is released.

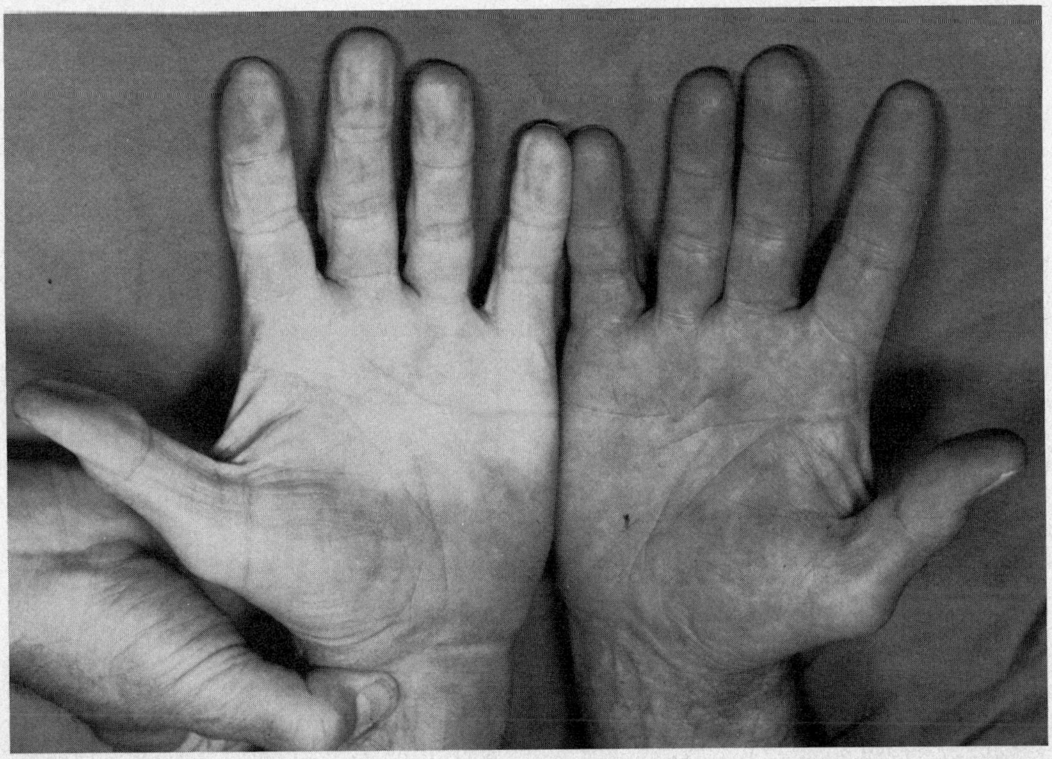

Fig. 2-25. Positive Allen test with no filling via the left ulnar artery.

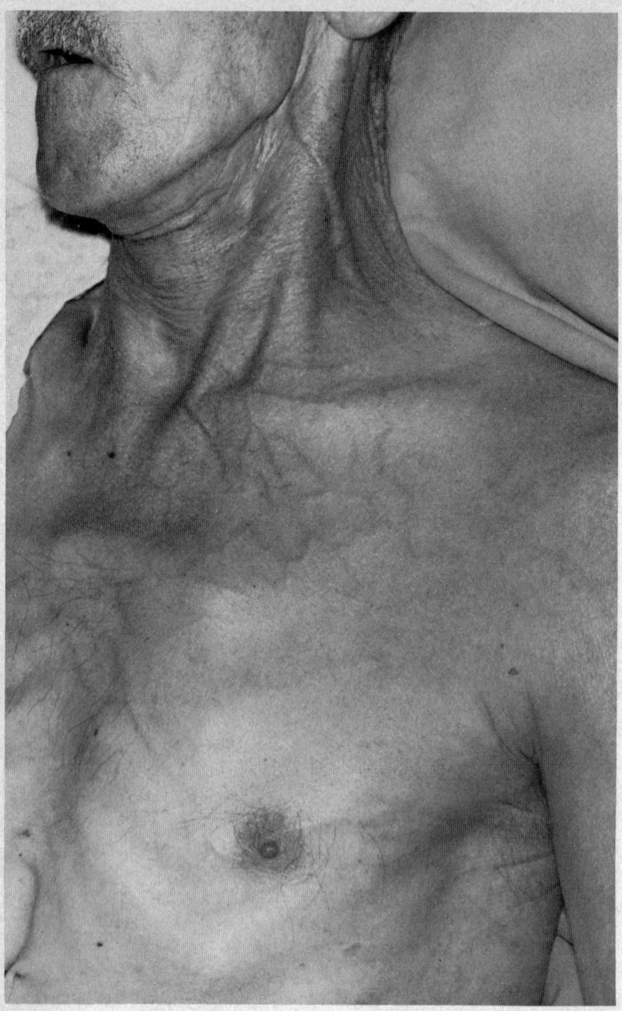

Fig. 2-26. Dilated jugular and left chest veins in a patient with a left subclavian vein occlusion.

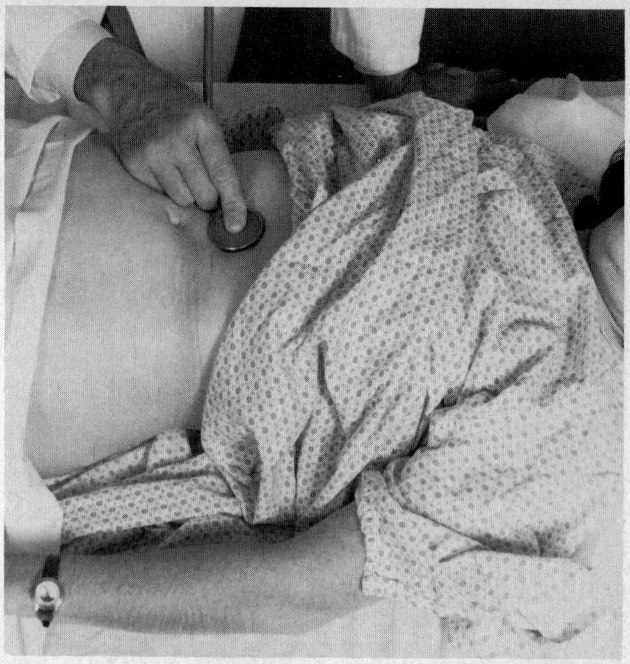

Fig. 2-27. Listening for abdominal bruits, using light pressure on the bell of the stethoscope.

ABDOMEN

In the abdomen a careful check for bruits should be carried out (Fig. 2-27). A systolic-diastolic bruit may indicate a severe stenosis of a renal artery or the presence of an arteriovenous fistula. Bruits are common over atherosclerotic plaques or over aneurysms.

A real attempt should be made to feel the abdominal aorta in all patients. This can be difficult in the obese patient and in the patient with a low pain threshold. The patient must relax his abdominal muscles as much as possible to allow the examiner to feel deep in the abdomen. The aorta should be sought just left of the midline and in the area between the umbilicus and the costal margin. An attempt should be made to measure the width of the abdominal aorta. One hand should try to locate the lateral border of the aorta and the other hand the medial border. Both borders should then be palpated at the same time (Fig. 2-28), using a ruler to get an accurate measurement between the fingertips of the palpating hands. Another maneuver that often is helpful in determining whether the patient has an aneurysm or whether there is merely a tortuous, normal-sized aorta is to roll the aorta back and forth under the fingertips (Fig. 2-29).

A check should be made in the right lower quadrant and left lower quadrant for aneurysms of the iliac arteries.

LOWER EXTREMITIES

The pulse examination of the legs and feet is not difficult, but it takes some practice to develop these skills. While palpating the pulses, the presence or absence of aneurysmal dilation should also be noted.

The femoral pulse is palpated just below the inguinal ligament and approximately midway across this ligament (Fig. 2-30). Firm pressure must be applied to feel the pulse, which is rather deep in the groin in most patients.

Physicians have great difficulty in palpating the popliteal pulse. Generally there are three major errors in technique. One is that the location of the popliteal artery is unknown to the examiner. Normally the pulse should be felt directly below the lateral aspect of the patella. The second error is in bending the knee too much at the time of the examination. The knee should be flexed only approximately 10 degrees (Fig. 2-31). The third error is in not palpating deep enough. Firm pressure must be applied to allow the fingers to go deep in the popliteal space. The pulse should be sought with the pads of the fingers and not the tips of the fingers.

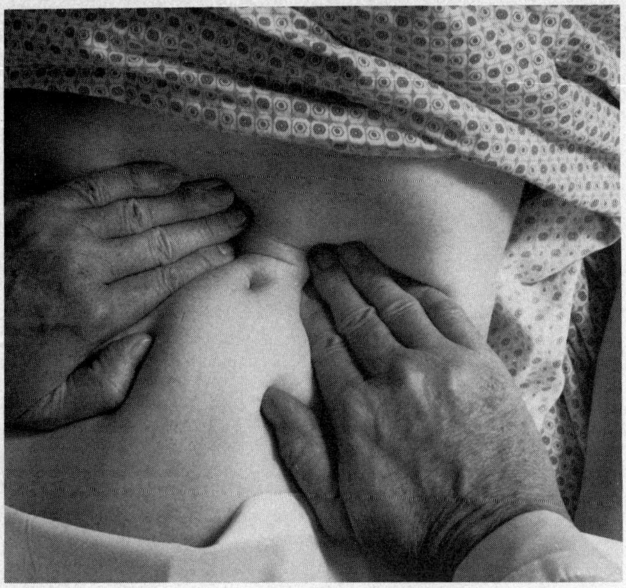

Fig. 2-28. Checking the size of the abdominal aorta.

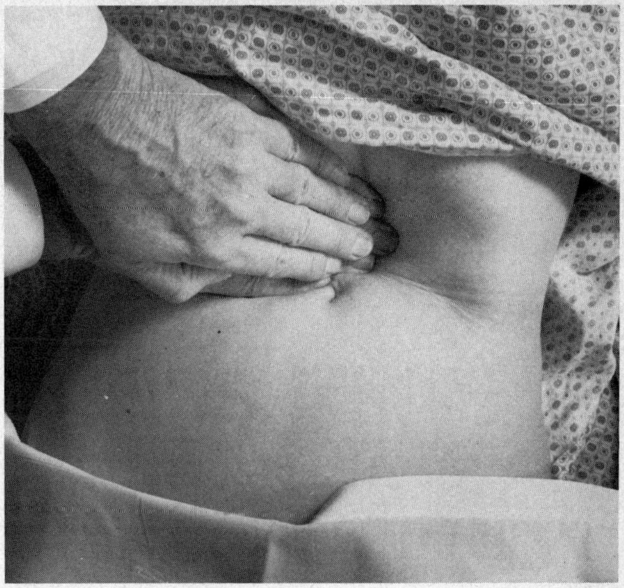

Fig. 2-29. Checking the size of the abdominal aorta by rolling it under the fingertips of the examiner's hand.

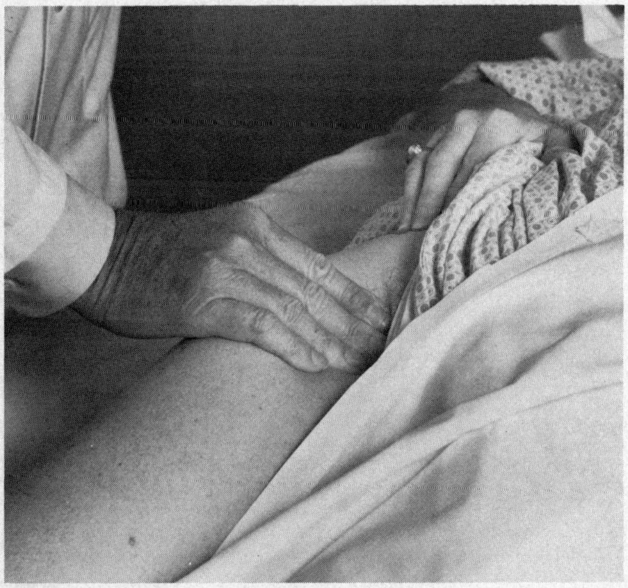

Fig. 2-30. Palpating the femoral pulse just below the inguinal ligament.

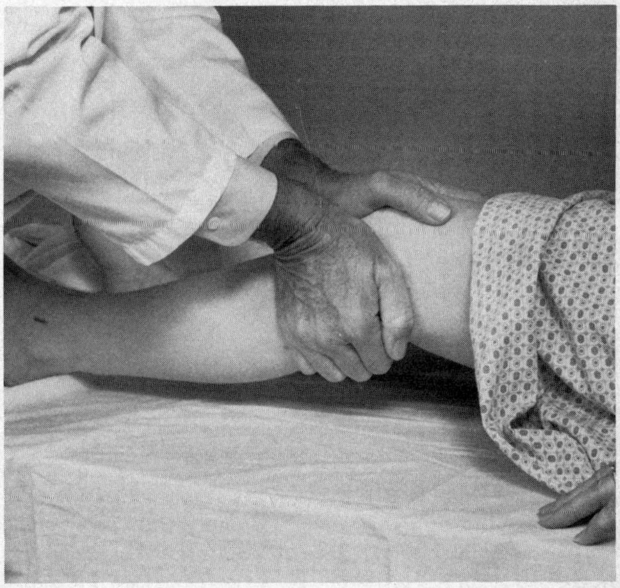

Fig. 2-31. Palpating the popliteal pulse with the patient's knee slightly flexed.

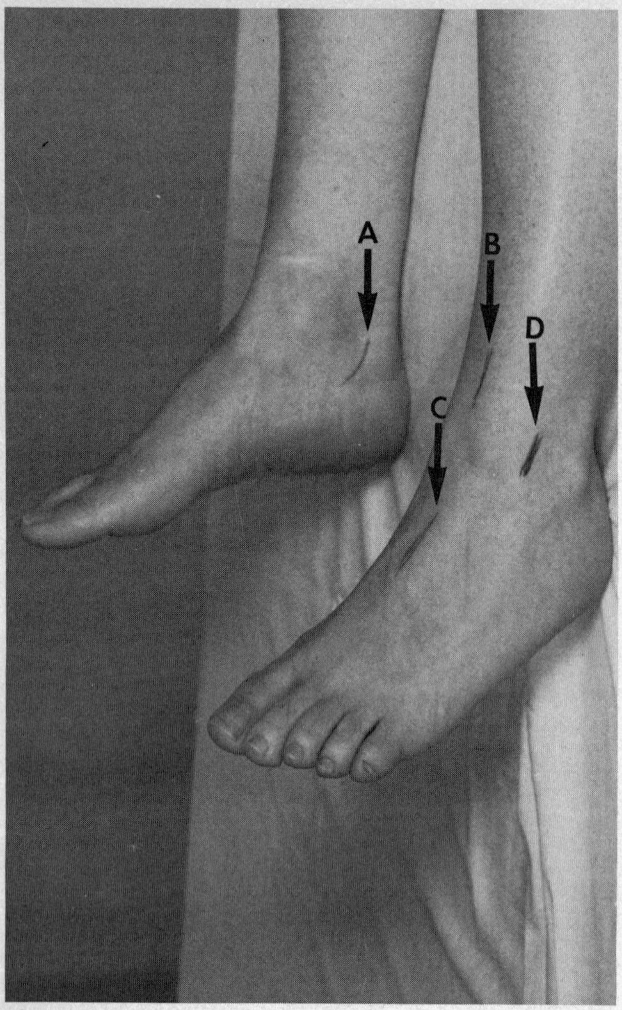

Fig. 2-32. Usual sites for pedal pulses palpation. *A*, Posterior tibial artery. *B*, Anterior tibial artery. *C*, Dorsalis pedis artery. *D*, Perforating branch of peroneal artery.

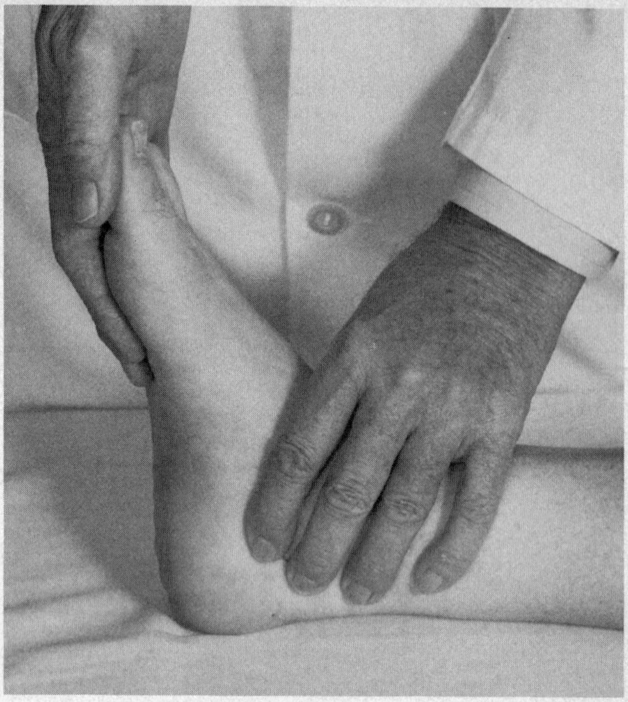

Fig. 2-33. Palpating the posterior tibial artery with the examiner's fingers held slightly apart. The examiner's right hand is used to adjust the angle of the ankle.

The usual sites for palpating foot pulses are demonstrated in Fig. 2-32. The posterior tibial pulse has quite a variable course posterior to the medial malleolus. Once the skills to palpate the femoral and popliteal pulse are honed, the posterior tibial pulse is one of the more difficult ones to find. The patient's right posterior tibial pulse should be sought with the examiner's left hand, for the curvature of the fingers of the left hand fits well into the curve behind the malleolus (Fig. 2-33). The fingers of the examiner's hand should be spread slightly to minimize the possibility of the examiner feeling his own digital pulse and mistaking it for the patient's pulse. The examiner's right hand should be used to adjust the angle of the ankle (see Fig. 2-33), for these adjustments may at times be necessary to feel the pulse more easily. The patient's left posterior tibial pulse should be examined by the examiner's right hand, using the left hand to adjust the angle of the ankle. The dorsalis pedis pulse is usually

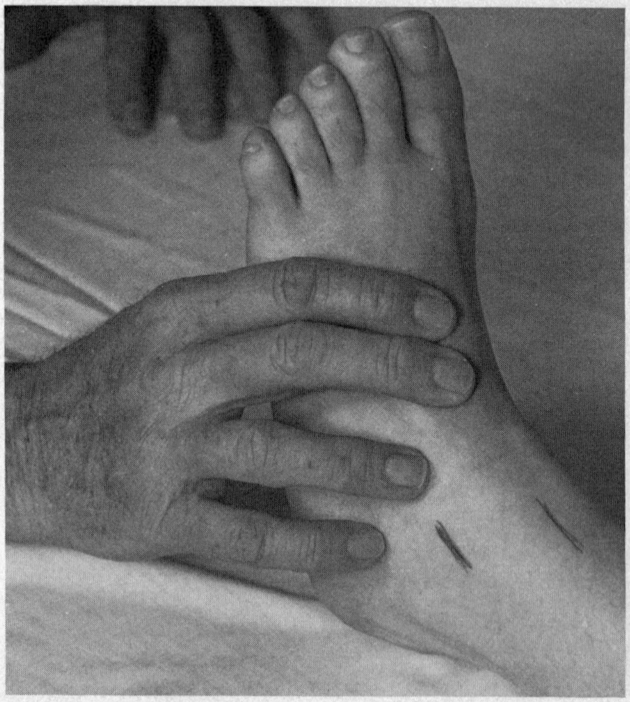

Fig. 2-34. Palpating the dorsalis pedis pulse with a light touch of the pads of the fingers.

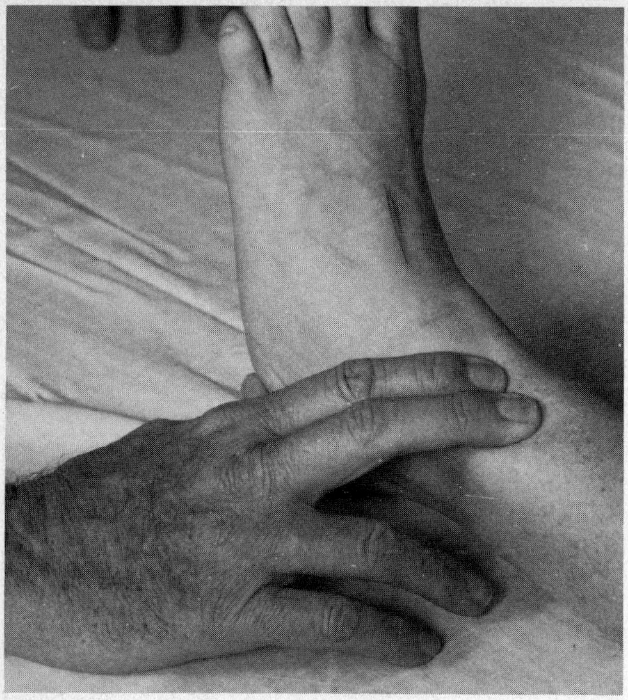

Fig. 2-35. Palpating the anterior tibial pulse with a firm pressure on the pads of the fingers.

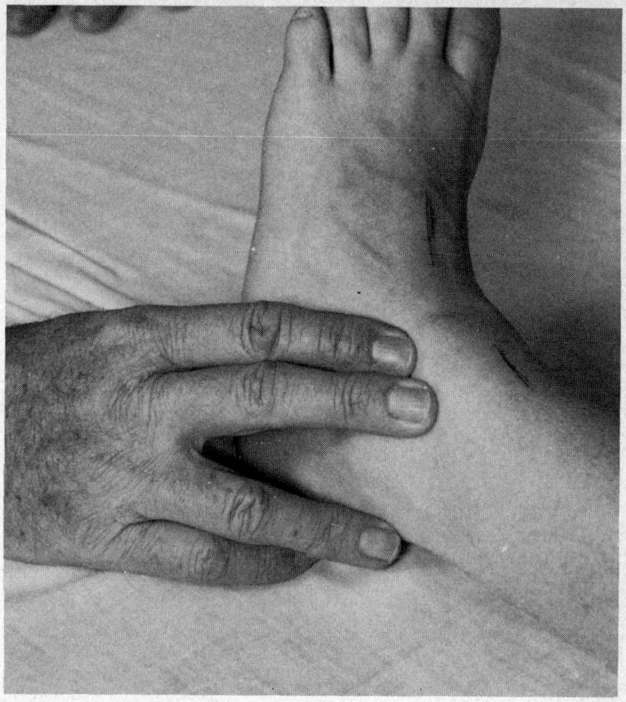

Fig. 2-36. Palpating the perforating branch of the peroneal artery, just anterior to the lateral malleolus.

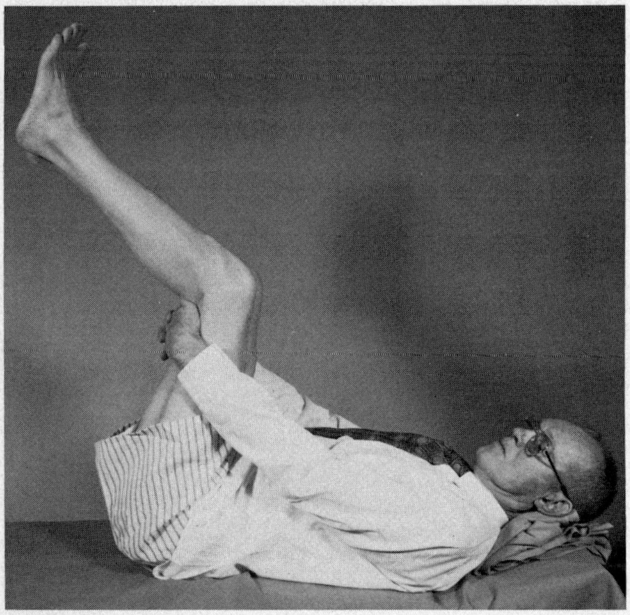

Fig. 2-37. To check for pallor on elevation, the feet must be elevated above the level of the heart.

felt along the line of the second metatarsal bone and is best appreciated by light touch of the pads of the fingers (Fig. 2-34). If the dorsalis pedis pulse cannot be felt, the anterior tibial pulse should be sought (Fig. 2-35). Firm pressure with the pads of the fingers is necessary to detect this pulse. If neither the dorsalis pedis pulse nor the anterior tibial pulse can be felt, the perforating branch of the peroneal artery should be sought. This artery usually runs just anterior to the lateral malleolus (Fig. 2-36).

If arterial insufficiency is suspected, the amount of pallor of the feet on elevation should be determined. Both of the patient's legs and feet should be elevated above the heart level (Fig. 2-37). The color should then be milked from the soles of the feet by gentle pressure; then after approximately 30 seconds the amount of color that reappears is noted. If the patient has significant arterial disease, he will have significant persistent pallor on elevation (Fig. 2-38). This can be graded between 0 and 4+, with 4+ indicating marked pallor.

Following this determination, the patient sits up quickly, and the length of time that it takes the first vein to fill on the dorsum of the foot is recorded (Fig. 2-39). This is the venous filling time, and with normal arterial circulation the first veins should fill within 10 to 15 seconds. In a patient

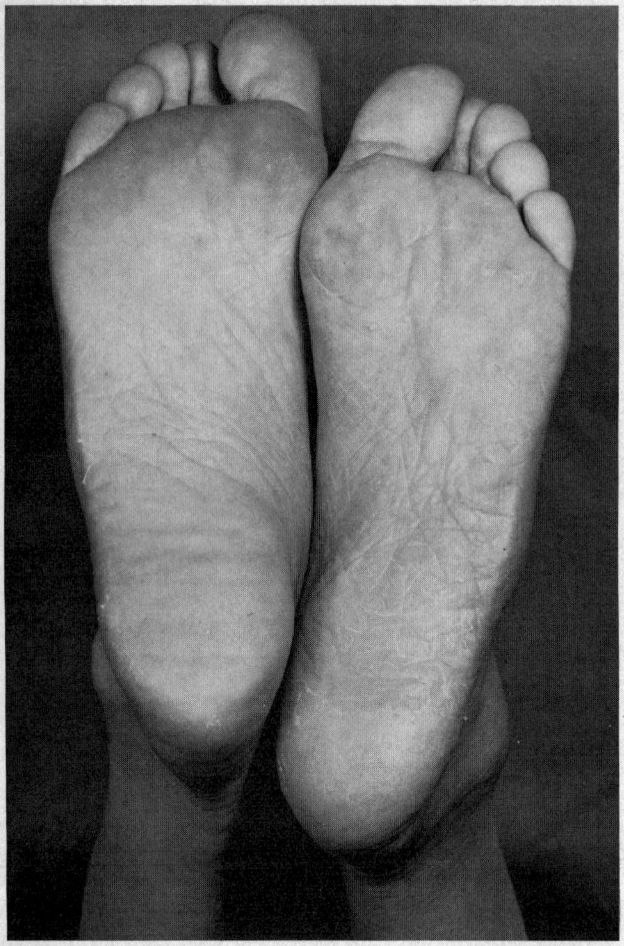

Fig. 2-38. Pallor on elevation is noted in the right foot.

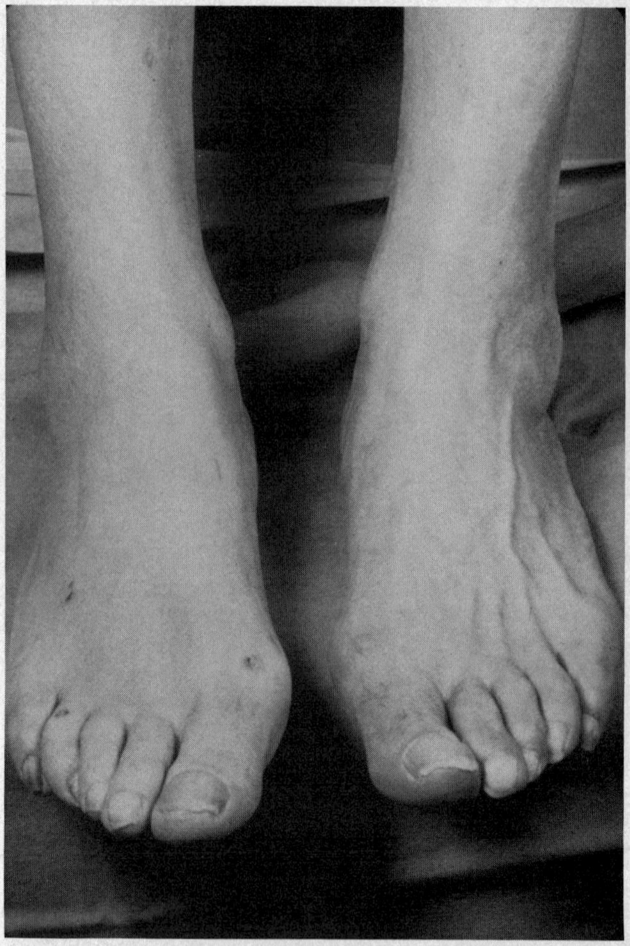

Fig. 2-39. Delay in filling of the veins of the right foot.

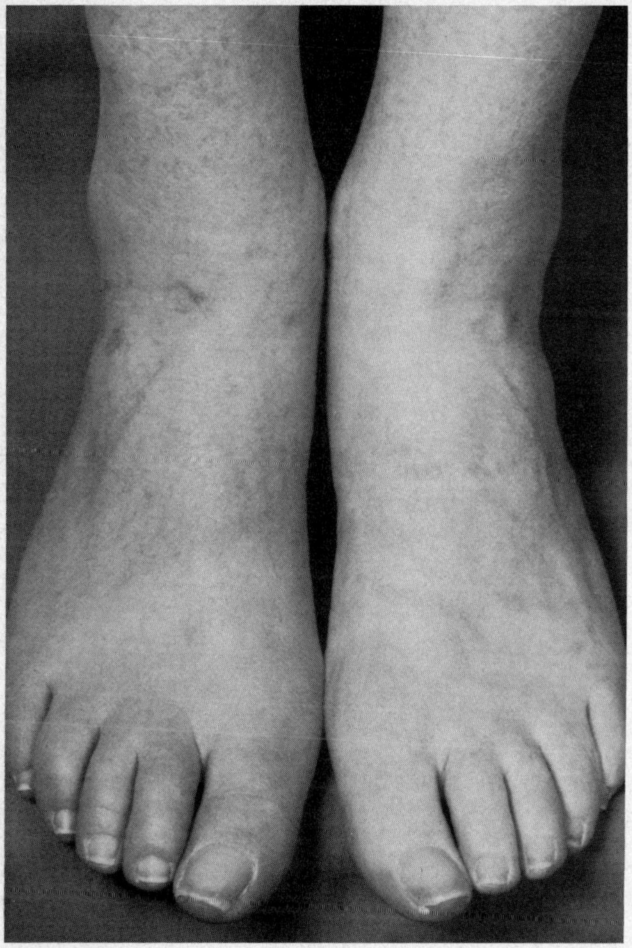

Fig. 2-40. Rubor on dependency is obvious in the right foot.

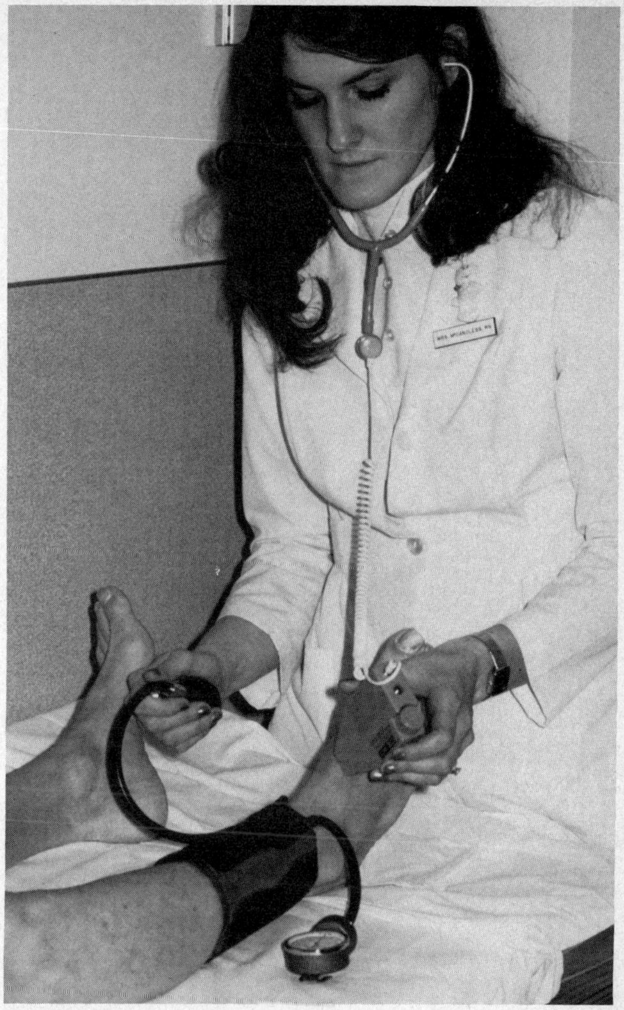

Fig. 2-41. Checking the ankle pressure with a pocket Doppler instrument.

with significant arterial disease there will be a delay in venous filling time up to 30 to 60 seconds or more. After recording the venous filling time, the amount of rubor in the feet after 2 or 3 more minutes should be noted. With significant arterial disease there will be significant rubor on dependency (Fig. 2-40).

For examiners who are not sure of their ability to feel pulses, the investment in a pocket Doppler device (Fig. 2-41) is advisable if patients with vascular disease are being seen in the office. The Doppler systolic pressure at the ankle should be equal to the brachial Doppler systolic pressure. Any decrease in pressure indicates some narrowing of the arteries. A decrease of more than 50% at the ankle as compared to the brachial pressure would indicate quite significant narrowing. If the ankle pressure is less than 20% of the brachial pressure, severe narrowing of the arteries is usually present.

As with the upper extremities, the lower extremities should be examined closely for asymmetry, edema, dilated veins, signs of inflammation, and stasis pigmentation. Although the condition of the skin, the hair, and the nails is not always a good indicator of arterial insufficiency, this observation should be noted. The presence or absence of dermatophytosis should be determined, for the fissures associated with dermatophytosis are often the portals of entry for recurrent cellulitis and lymphangitis.

REFERENCE

1. Graor RA, deWolfe VG, and Elliott I: A clinical vignette: the clinical significance of systolic-diastolic bruits in the carotid arteries, Cleve Clin Q 51:155, 1984.

Chapter 3

NONINVASIVE VASCULAR LABORATORY AND VASCULAR IMAGING

D. Eugene Strandness, Jr.

The objective evaluation of diseases of the circulatory system has been best approached by routine clinical appraisal combined with methods of documenting the site(s) of involvement and the functional significance of the disorder. This is most elegantly done during the evaluation of heart disease in which both noninvasive and invasive methods are used to obtain the maximal amount of information. The same approach has been much slower to develop in the evaluation of diseases of the vascular system for reasons that are easy to understand. Since the 1950s evaluating diseases of the arterial and venous systems has been under the control of the surgeons who, together with the radiologists, possessed all the clinical skills and tools that seemed necessary to approach successfully the majority of problems brought to their attention.

A perception, still present in many circles, was that a well-performed history and a physical examination were all that was required. The diagnosis was easy to make, and its confirmation was a simple matter by making good use of one's eyes, fingers, and ears. If there were any doubt concerning one's impression, it could be complemented by using arteriography, which not only confirmed the clinical suspicions but also provided a road map in case direct arterial surgery was needed.

I became convinced of the need for good noninvasive testing when I tried to assess the outcome of arterial procedures through a review of hospital records. It soon became apparent that it was often difficult to tell from a review of the hospital record whether a patient was indeed improved after surgical therapy and it was difficult to determine the extent of improvement. This led to a search for better methods of evaluation that would provide objective evidence that could be used, not only for evaluating the initial event, but also for follow-up purposes as well.[1] The evolution of the methods of evaluation described in this chapter serves as a suitable outline of the status of the field and what we may anticipate in the future.

To maintain some continuity, the discussion focuses on areas of clinical interest, dealing with the patients as they appear and how the available testing procedures may be of value.

PERIPHERAL ARTERIAL SYSTEM

Those diseases that affect the arterial supply of the upper and lower extremity are discussed in this section. Although the majority of the diseases affects the large- and medium-sized arteries (those with proper names), other disorders that involve the microcirculation also benefit from referral to the vascular laboratory. For the large- and medium-sized arteries the most common disorders include atherosclerosis, aneurysmal disease, and thromboangiitis obliterans. The level and extent of involvement of atherosclerosis and thromboangiitis obliterans are somewhat different, and the questions that need answers are also different. In general, atherosclerosis is a disease of branch points and bifurcations, but for unknown reasons it spares those arteries distal to the origin of the subclavian artery.[2] Thromboangiitis obliterans involves the distal medium-sized arteries of the legs and the palmar and digital arteries of the hand.[3,4] Although a history of instep claudication and cold sensitivity may suggest the diagnosis of thromboangiitis obliterans and serve to distinguish it from atherosclerosis, noninvasive testing may be of some value in making this distinction. Although trauma to the major arteries is common, it is considered under the category of "acute ischemia" since its important clinical manifestations are usually in this area.

For most patients the diagnosis of arterial narrowing and occlusion is made on the basis of a history of intermittent claudication, the presence of arterial bruits, and the detection of pulse deficits. The typical patient with atherosclerosis will have disease that involves major proximal arterial segments (popliteal to aorta), with thromboangiitis involving the arteries of the distal leg, and in approximately one half of cases, the arteries of the distal arm and hand. A very important subset of patients are those with diabetes mellitus (particularly the type II, non-insulin dependent patients) who have a different pattern and distribution of atherosclerosis.[5,6] These patients have less involvement of the aortoiliac segment with equal occurrence in the femoropopliteal segment but more extensive occlusions in the tibial and peroneal arteries. In addition, it is not at all unusual for medial calcification (Mönckeberg's medialsclerosis) to be present in the arteries below the knee. However, medial calcification (while unique to patients with diabetes) bears no relationship to the arteriosclerosis obliterans that frequently involves the same arterial segments.[2]

The information that may be obtained from a referral to the vascular laboratory depends on the patient presentation and the issues to be resolved. The testing procedures used vary in complexity, with each providing information that may or may not be necessary or complementary for the diagnosis and planning of therapy. It is thus important to know what type of information can be obtained and how the data may be of assistance. These tests can be considered in the categories of screening and planning of therapy.

Screening tests

If one assumes that the diagnosis can be made on the basis of the history and physical examination alone, under what circumstances would further testing be needed? The noninvasive tests are done to confirm the diagnosis and provide an estimate of the extent of the involvement. Screening tests include three basic procedures of value: measurement of limb blood pressure, exercise testing, and assessment of velocity patterns.

Limb blood pressure. The measurement of blood pressure is the most commonly applied noninvasive test of cardiovascular function. It is primarily done for detecting high blood pressure but is also of value in evaluating hypotensive states. It may be the best single indicator of how well perfusion is being maintained. Although not often thought of in this manner, acute and chronic arterial occlusion produces regional hypotension, the magnitude of which is determined by the extent of the disease and the status of the collateral circulation. If anything is done to improve the circulation by removing or bypassing the areas of obstruction, this action would be immediately recognized by an increase in the intraarterial pressure distal to the site of involvement.

One of the impediments to the measurement of arterial pressure distal to sites of occlusion is that the usual auscultatory method is not applicable. It is necessary to use sensors distal to a pneumatic cuff that can detect when flow is restored during cuff deflation.[7,8] These methods are able to measure systolic pressure but not diastolic pressure. This is not a major problem since it is the systolic pressure that is the first to fall with arterial narrowing and is the most sensitive to changes in resistance to flow. The most commonly available sensors include the continuous wave Doppler flowmeter, photoplethysmography, and strain-gauge plethysmography. The most common method in use is the Doppler device, which has the advantage of being able to measure pressure in any artery in which flow can be detected.

The measurements of pressure with the Doppler device can be done at the time the patient is first seen. However, the physician, nurse, or technician must know how to do the test properly. For the test to be reliable and useful it must be done in the following manner: (1) the arm systolic pressure should always be measured with the Doppler device as well, for the value obtained by the auscultatory method is not adequate; (2) the pressure must be recorded in both arms and both tibial arteries at the ankle; (3) the systolic pressure is taken at that point at which flow is first detected during cuff deflation and not at the point it disappears during cuff inflation; and (4) both the absolute levels of pressure and the ankle/arm (A/A) index are recorded.[9]

What is normal? The systolic pressure in the arterial system increases from the central aorta to the periphery.[9,10] This is due to the fact that the arteries toward the periphery become stiffer. In addition, reflections from the branch points, bifurcations, and arterioles amplify the systolic pressure. The mean pressure, on the other hand, is decreasing, permitting flow to occur toward the distal limb. Given the fact that the systolic pressure is being amplified, the A/A index is 1.0 or greater in healthy patients. Since there may be some variability in the measurement, we have elected to use a value of greater than 0.95 as normal.

When an area of narrowing exceeds 50% in terms of diameter reduction or occlusion, the systolic pressure will fall beyond the site of involvement (Fig. 3-1). The magnitude of the pressure fall is a reflection of two things—the magnitude of the resistance offered by the stenosis (occlusion) and that offered by the collateral arteries bypassing the area of involvement. If there are multiple levels of stenosis or occlusion, the systolic pressure level measured distal to the last area of involvement will reflect the additive resistances offered by the collateral circuits, which are in series[11] (Fig. 3-2). In general terms, in patients with chronic occlusive arterial disease an A/A index of greater than 0.5 is seen with single segments of occlusion. With levels below this value, it is likely that multiple levels of involvement are present.

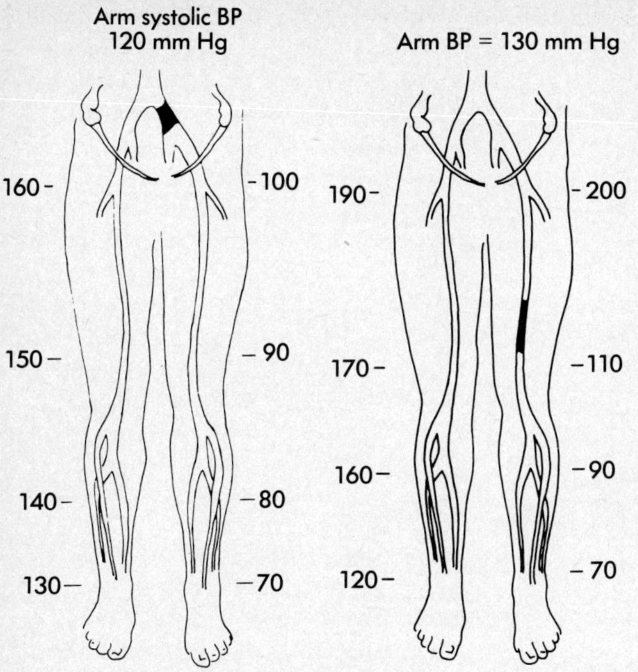

Fig. 3-1. Systolic pressures recorded from two patients with arterial occlusions in the common iliac artery and superficial femoral artery. There is a large drop in systolic pressure across the areas of obstruction. (From Strandness DE Jr: Peripheral arterial disease, Boston, 1969, Little, Brown & Co.)

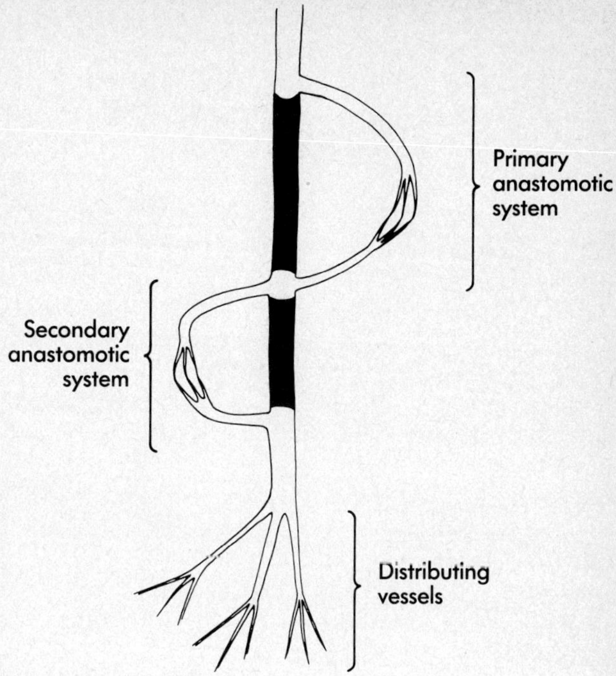

Fig. 3-2. With multiple levels of occlusion the resistance to flow offered by collateral arteries are additive. This explains why the ankle systolic pressures distal to multiple levels of involvement are lower than found with single occlusions.

The absolute levels of pressure at the ankle and the digits may also be useful in providing a rough estimate of the extent of the perfusion. It has been my experience that levels greater than 50 mm Hg are consistent with normal tissue perfusion, whereas levels below this become worrisome, particularly if an open lesion is present and the prospects for healing without intervention become important.

In addition to measuring the blood pressure at the ankle and digits, it is possible to estimate the pressure at the level of the calf and at the low and high thigh.[9,12] This is done by placing the pneumatic cuffs at these levels and inflating them to suprasystolic levels to interrupt flow. The Doppler sensor is placed in the same locations at the ankle that are used to measure ankle pressure. The pressures that are recorded by this method will be artifactually high, and this fact must be taken into account when this procedure is used. This is due to the fact that the cuffs used may not effectively transmit the pressure to the vessels deep in the leg. Those interested in reviewing this problem further are urged to review the work of Carter,[9] who has examined this issue in great detail. The results of measuring systolic limb pressures and their interpretation are summarized in Table 3-1.

Another method used to assess the perfusion at various levels of the limb is the pulse-volume recorder. This device records the pulsatile volume changes that occur in the limb with each heartbeat. The pneumatic cuffs used for this purpose are the same as used for the measurement of limb blood pressures and in the same locations. A measured quantity of air is injected into the cuff until a preset pressure is reached. As the limb expands with each heartbeat, the pressure in the cuff changes, and this can be recorded on a strip chart. In general, a 1 mm Hg pressure change in the cuff will produce a 20 mm chart deflection. The waveform by its phasic characteristics can provide information concerning the nature of the arterial system at that level. Extensive studies have been done establishing PVR categories

Table 3-1. Summary of systolic blood pressures in the limbs and their interpretation

Measurement site	Range of values
Ankle pressure	Normally greater than brachial pressure
Ankle pressure index	Normally 1.0-1.2; hemodynamically significant <0.95
Ankle pressure after exercise	Normally drops <20% of baseline; returns to preexercise levels in 3 minutes or less
Proximal thigh pressure	Normally 30-40 mm Hg higher than brachial pressure
Segmental pressures	Normally <20mm Hg difference between two levels of limb
Toe pressure	Normally 80%-90% of brachial pressure
Toe indexes	Normally 0.8-0.9; hemodynamically significant lesion, <0.64; rest pain, <0.15

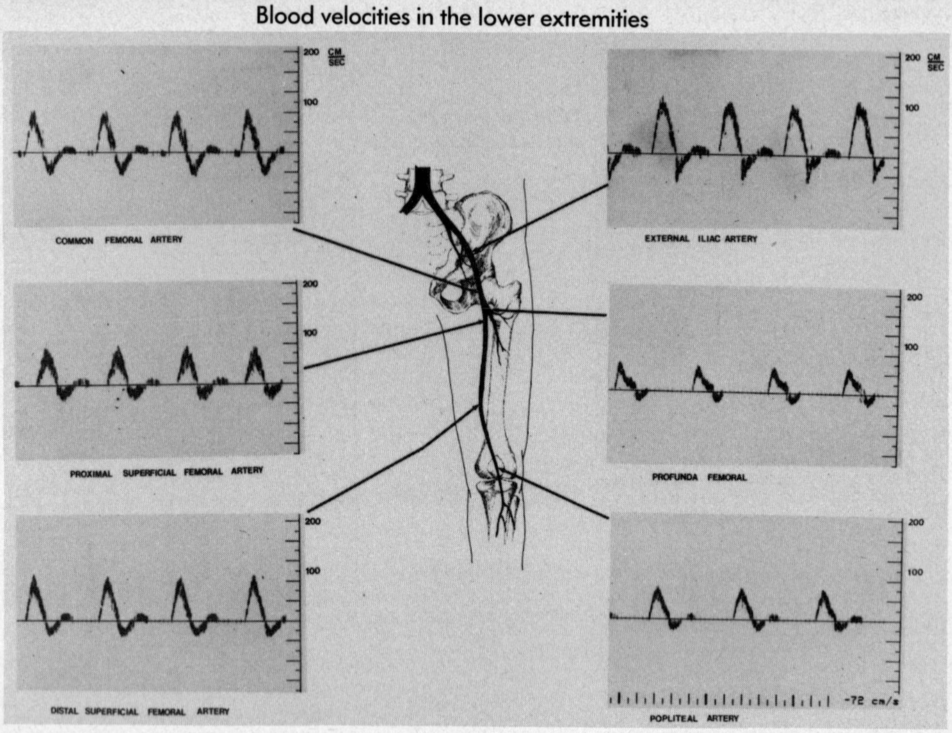

Fig. 3-3. Normal velocity patterns found in peripheral arteries. The triphasic component is seen at all levels.

based on the magnitude of the deflection noted at each level of the limb. They in turn can be related to the location of the occlusive disease, giving rise to the finding. For more complete information the reader is urged to review the work of Raines[13] who was the person who developed this method for clinical use.

Assessment of velocity patterns. Vascular laboratory studies may include a survey with the continuous wave Doppler flowmeter at the following standard sites: (1) external iliac–common femoral artery; (2) proximal, mid, and distal superficial femoral artery; (3) popliteal artery; and (4) tibial arteries at the ankle. By such scanning it is possible roughly to localize the areas of involvement because the method is used without imaging; thus one cannot always be certain the intended vessel is being evaluated. Nonetheless, it does serve a useful purpose for screening. As is discussed shortly, more definitive information can be obtained with duplex scanning of the arterial supply to the lower limbs.

The normal arterial velocity patterns have characteristic features that are altered by the presence of arterial stenoses that exceed 50% (diameter reduction) and total occlusion. The normal patterns from the level of the abdominal aorta to the arteries at the ankle are similar, with three separate and distinct phases easily seen on a hard-copy spectral display of the waveform.[14] They include the forward-flow velocity associated with myocardial contraction, the reverse-flow component that occurs in late systole and early diastole, and a secondary forward-flow component that is seen in late diastole (Fig. 3-3). When there is a high-grade stenosis or total occlusion, blunting of the systolic peak occurs, with loss of the reverse-flow component resulting in a monophasic waveform. If the normal triphasic waveform is noted, it is very unlikely that significant disease is proximal to the recording site. The finding of a monophasic waveform is *certain* evidence of disease proximal to the recording site.

The upper extremity can be assessed in a similar fashion. The waveforms from the subclavian artery commonly show the three components seen in the lower-extremity arteries. However, those recorded from the brachial, radial, and ulnar arteries may not show the reverse-flow component in up to one half of healthy individuals. This may be due to the fact that the resistance to flow is less than that seen uniformly in the lower limbs in which the reverse-flow component is always normally seen. It is also possible to survey the hand's flow patterns in the palmar arch, the digital arteries, and the tip of the fingers. In fact, the most accurate way to determine the status of the palmar arch is to use the continuous wave Doppler sensor. This can be done by listening over the radial and ulnar sides of the palmar arch while the two arteries are sequentially occluded. This is a much better method than using Allen's test, which depends on the appearance of the hand, with clenching and release of the hand when the arteries at the wrist are sequentially occluded. With arterial stenosis and occlusion, the velocity patterns observed are similar to those seen in the lower limbs.

Exercise testing. The typical patient with intermittent claudication has a history of pain in the leg with exercise that is relieved with rest. The major diagnostic features are a walk-pain-rest cycle that is constant from day to day.[15] In addition, the pain is always made worse by an activity that increases the work load such as going up a hill or stairs. When this history is obtained and combined with pertinent physical findings, the diagnosis is nearly certain, with the only remaining questions concerning its severity and how much it interferes with the patient's life-style. Because a frame of reference is needed, it is common to relate the distance walked to city blocks—a very imprecise method because the blocks vary in length and patients walk at different rates of speed. Thus a better more objective standard would be of benefit.

An increasing problem in our society is the aging patient who may develop neurospinal problems that produce pain in the limbs with exercise that may be confused with intermittent claudication.[16,17] The neurospinal problem has several characteristic features that can be recognized on the basis of the history alone. The walk-pain-rest cycle is not constant from day to day; these patients have good days and bad days. In addition, the pain may be brought on by sitting or standing. Some patients also have to lie down for pain relief—something never required for patients who have true claudication.

Stress testing is commonly used for evaluation of cardiac performance because it is recognized that it provides a much better index of myocardial perfusion. The principles are similar for the legs. There are differences in how the test is done and how the performance is estimated. In this regard performance is gauged in two ways: (1) the duration of the walking time and (2) the ankle systolic blood pressure response to the walk.

The work load to which the patient is subjected is modest. The speed and elevation of the treadmill used for this purpose vary in different laboratories. In general, the walking speed is 1½ to 2 miles per hour, with an elevation that ranges from 10% to 12% in terms of the grade. Using this walking speed and elevation, most people can perform the test unless they have cardiac, rheumatologic, or pulmonary problems that are significant. We limit the amount of time the patient walks to 5 minutes. If he can walk this long, he is mildly symptomatic and should rarely be considered for interventional therapy. On the other hand, we have found that walking times less than 1 minute represent severely limiting claudication. For walking times of 3 to 5 minutes, the impact depends on the patient's needs and daily activities. If, for example, the patient is a postman and needs to walk for a living, even mild claudication may be a problem.

To estimate the hemodynamic response to walking, the changes in the ankle systolic blood pressure must be measured, as must the response of the pulse-volume recorder, if used, after the patient resumes the supine position. A healthy person walking at this rate and elevation for 5 minutes will sustain little or no drop in ankle systolic pressure after the exercise is completed.[18] However, if the patient has true claudication and it was the basis for the initial symptoms, there will be a large drop in ankle pressure and flattening of the pulse volume recording with a very delayed recovery to the preexercise levels[19] (Fig. 3-4). True intermittent claudication cannot occur without a drop in the ankle systolic blood pressure and a diminution of the pulse volume amplitude. This is true even if the patient's walking time is less than 1 minute. What this means is that if the pressure does not fall, other causes for the leg pain must be sought.[20]

What of the circumstance in which the patient has arterial disease and also suffers from an associated condition such as spinal canal stenosis? When this occurs and when the nonvascular problem is responsible for the leg discomfort, it is this problem that usually prevents the patient from continued walking, and there is usually a disparity between the magnitude of the ankle blood pressure fall and its recovery time. For example, if a patient with true claudication is forced to stop in less than 1 minute of walking because of ischemic pain, the ankle systolic pressure often will fall to unrecordable levels and require in excess of 30 minutes of recovery. Conversely, in a patient with pseudoclaudication the pressure decrease—if any occurs—will not be of the magnitude seen with true intermittent claudication.

One or more of the above diagnostic tests may supply most of the answers to questions that may arise at the time the patient is first seen, providing enough data to confirm the initial impression and to provide the necessary information about what must be done next. The clinical presentation, along with the results of this screening procedure, will determine the course of action to follow. In most cases conservative course will be followed, the nature of which is determined by the presenting complaint. If the patient is a candidate for interventional therapy, be it angioplasty or direct arterial surgery, the next step is to proceed with arteriography. Although this is the standard practice at the moment, there will be instances in which a more complete study of the circulation with duplex scanning may provide definitive data on how to proceed.

Duplex scanning

Since duplex scanning potentially can evaluate the location and extent of disease for all levels of supply to the lower limbs, it may serve as a useful planning study for the direction of therapy.[14,21] Under what circumstances might it provide definitive data? Six circumstances are described.

1. Since angioplasty has become the standard method of treating isolated stenoses in the aortoiliac segment, being able to predict who may need the procedure would be a great help. Given these considerations, we scan patients who

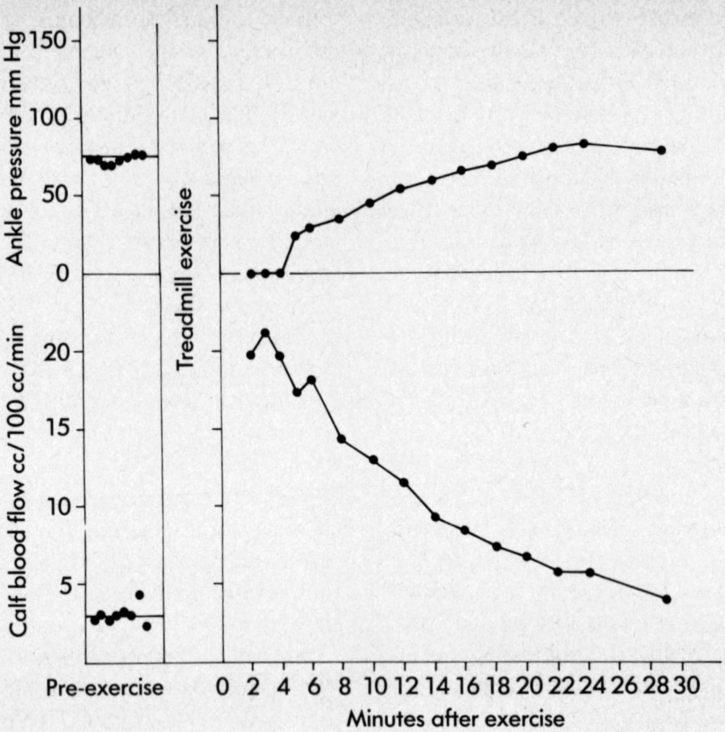

Fig. 3-4. Ankle systolic blood pressure as compared to calf blood flow in a patient with intermittent claudication. The abnormal response is characterized by a large fall in the blood pressure with a very delayed recovery time.

may well fit into this category; and if they have a stenosis, they are scheduled for angioplasty. If they are occluded, some form of direct arterial surgery is planned after arteriography has been performed. Although we continue to use preoperative arteriography to define the location and extent of the arterial disease, it is becoming clear that duplex scanning can provide functional information that is useful not only in planning therapy but in monitoring its outcome as well.

2. For patients with severe occlusive disease (A/A index of less than 0.5) it is likely there are multiple levels of disease. In this situation it is essential to define the location and extent of involvement in planning therapy. Questions always arise when there is a stenosis in the aortoiliac area combined with femoropopliteal disease. It is important to know to what extent the proximal disease contributes to the ischemia.

3. The saphenous veins of patients who will undergo femoropopliteal or femorotibial bypass grafting are scanned and measured before any procedure.[22] It is possible to define the dimensions of the vein and also to identify anomalous branches or duplications that might compromise the procedure, thus removing the uncertainty often present at the time of the operation in defining the proximal and distal sites of insertion.

4. Any patient who has had an interventional procedure, be it angioplasty or surgery, and then is seen with new complaints should be scanned with the duplex scanner.[23] This procedure will nearly always define the location and extent of the problem and permit in some cases a direct approach to the involved segment without the need for arteriography.

5. All patients with suspected aortic or peripheral aneurysms should be scanned to permit an estimate of the size and extent of the lesion. If the patient also has occlusive arterial disease, this procedure will permit locating it and estimating its extent.

6. Those patients initially seen with microemboli to the foot will benefit from a scan since it may identify the source of the embolic material. This information may then be used to direct the arteriographer to those segments in which the offending source may be found.

What information is available?

To assess the contribution of arterial lesions to the clinical picture properly, it is necessary both to localize the disease and estimate its hemodynamic significance. Ultrasonic duplex scanners combine imaging of the underlying blood vessel with the capability of estimating the velocity changes at that site by the use of a pulsed Doppler device. Although the image resolution of the modern systems has greatly improved, it is still not sufficient to permit an estimate of the degree of narrowing on the basis of the image alone. It is also necessary to measure the velocity change in an in-

Table 3-2. Comparison of duplex scanning with arteriography

Arterial segment	n	Sensitivity	Specificity	PPV*	NPV†
Aortic‡	25	1.00	1.00	1.00	1.00
Iliac	110	0.89	0.90	0.75	0.96
Common femoral	50	0.67	0.98	0.80	0.96
Superficial femoral	123	0.84	0.93	0.90	0.88
Popliteal	37	0.75	0.97	0.86	0.93
All segments	393	0.82	0.92	0.80	0.93

*PPV, Positive predictive value.
†NPV, Negative predictive value.
‡No aortic segments had >50% stenosis.

volved segment to estimate the degree of narrowing. Although the use of an absolute velocity change in centimeters per second would be helpful, there is so much variability even in healthy individuals that it is preferable to relate the velocity changes from one segment of the artery to the next as the most reliable method of documenting the extent of diameter reduction.[14,21] As the artery becomes narrowed, the velocity increase in the stenosis will increase in a predictable fashion, permitting a reasonable estimate of the degree of narrowing at the site where the velocity increase is recorded.

In documenting such changes by duplex scanning it was necessary to develop the diagnostic criteria and compare the results to those with arteriography and/or to the variability found in arteriographic estimates of the degree of stenosis. Jager, Ricketts and Strandness[14] carried out such a study and found the following criteria suitable for documentation of the status of the arterial system:

1. The normal velocity patterns in all peripheral arteries are monotonously similar with the three phases: forward flow, a prominent reverse-flow component, and a secondary late forward-flow component (see Fig. 3-3). If the velocity is recorded from a center stream site of the artery, no spectral broadening will be present.
2. When the arterial wall becomes roughened, the most prominent changes are seen in the development of spectral broadening without an increase in peak systolic velocity. The reverse flow component is preserved. These patients are labeled as having a 1% to 19% narrowing (Fig. 3-5).
3. The next category of stenosis is a 20% to 49% diameter reduction that is not hemodynamically significant at resting levels of flow. For this category an increase in the peak systolic velocity is greater than 30% but less than 100% from the preceding arterial segment, with preservation of the reverse-flow component (see Fig. 3-5).
4. For the hemodynamically significant lesions (greater than 50%) the increase in peak velocity is greater than 100% in the stenosis, with loss of reverse flow and the presence of marked spectral broadening (see Fig. 3-5).

Table 3-3. Accuracy of duplex scanning for various categories of disease compared to reading of the same film by two radiologists

Disease grade (% stenosis)	Arteriography vs duplex scanning (% agreement)	Radiologists' arteriographic reading, 1 vs 2 (% agreement)
Normal	81	68
1-19	83	58
16-49	83	57
50-95	60	70
Occlusion	94	100

5. For total occlusions there is no detectable flow within a visualized segment.

Using these criteria, the results of duplex scanning as compared to arteriography are summarized in Table 3-2. The results when two radiologists review the same films are shown in Table 3-3. The results of these studies are important in several ways, with the very high negative predictive value of particular note.[14,21] This is important because it shows that if the duplex scan predicts that a particular segment is normal "hemodynamically" (has a less than 50% stenosis), it is likely to be accurate. From an interventionist standpoint this is very important since it directs attention only to those segments that need correction. It also highlights the therapy likely to result in improvement. For example, if a stenotic lesion is found in the aorta or iliac artery, attention is immediately directed to the potential use of angioplasty, which is very good in this area for correcting the stenosis (Fig. 3-6). On the other hand, if an iliac artery is occluded, some form of bypass such as a cross-femoral graft may be indicated.

Follow-up care

Since patients with occlusive arterial disease are not cured by any form of intervention, it is only natural that noninvasive methods would be used during the follow-up

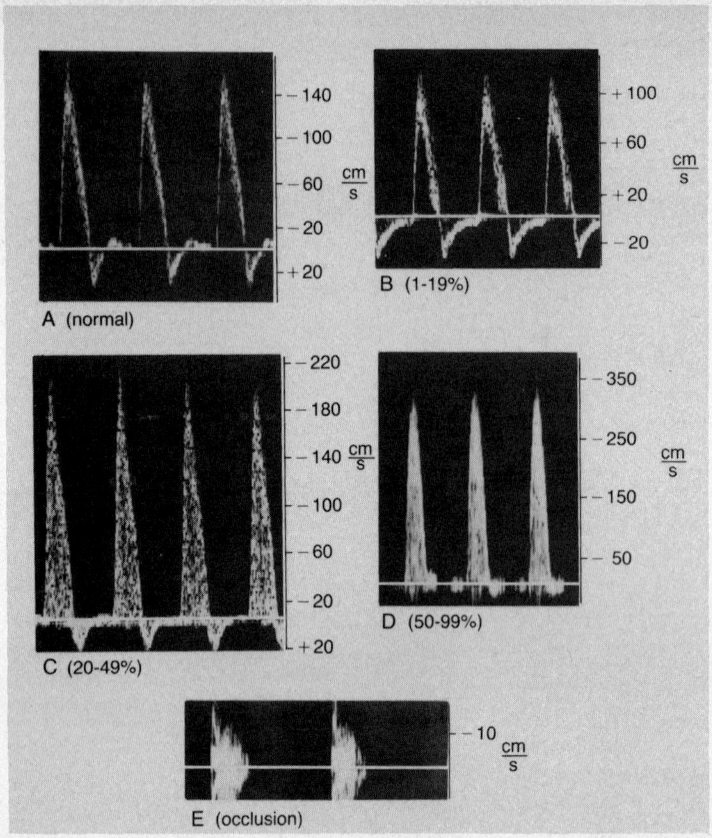

Fig. 3-5. Velocity pattern seen with varying degrees of involvement with atherosclerosis. (From Moneta GL and Strandness DE Jr: Peripheral arterial duplex scanning, J Clin Ultrasound 15:645, 1987.)

Abdominal aorta stenosis: >50%

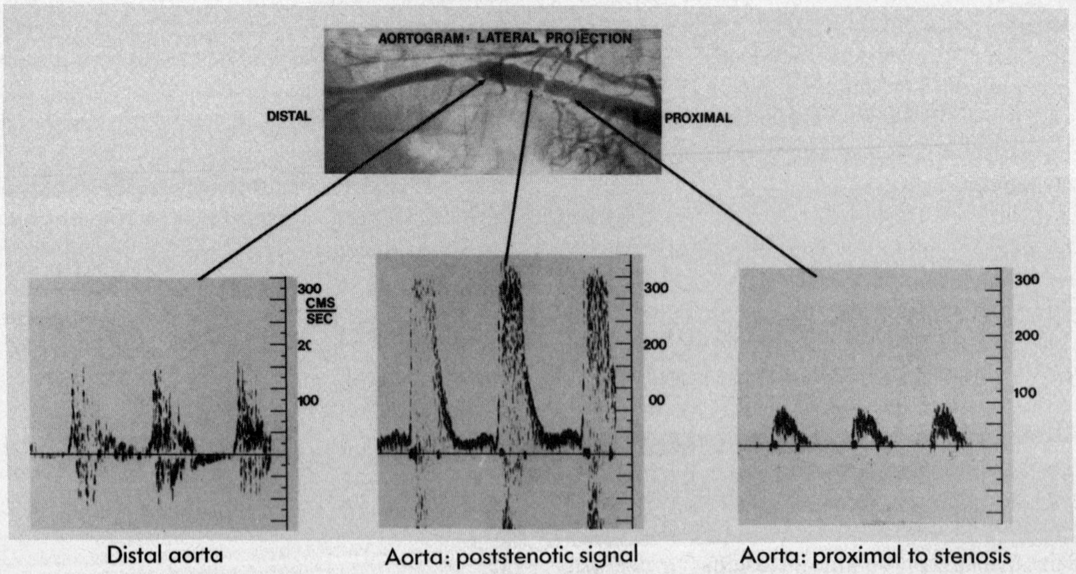

Fig. 3-6. Duplex scanning findings in a patient with a stenosis of the abdominal aorta. (From Strandness DE Jr: Duplex scanning as popliteal arterial disease. Herz: 13:372, 1988.)

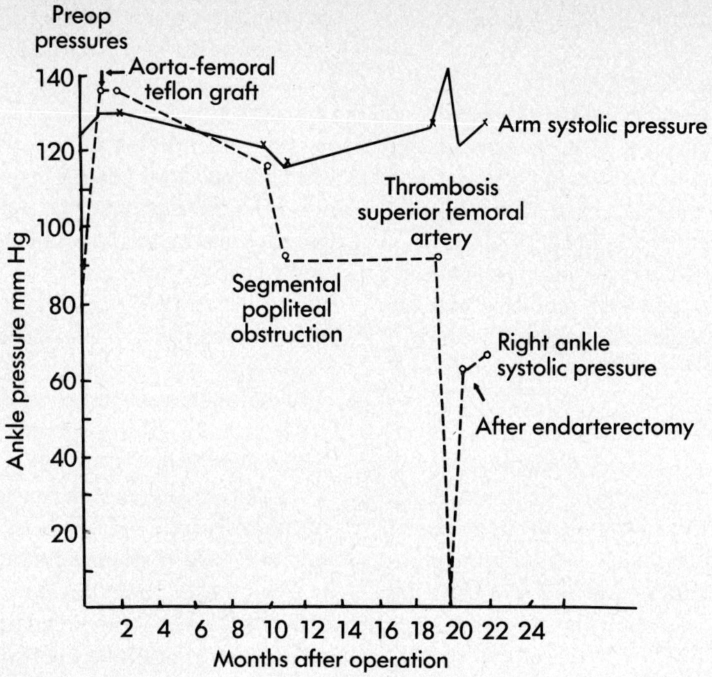

Fig. 3-7. Ankle systolic pressures recorded during a 2-year period following an aortobifemoral graft. With the development of new areas of disease, the ankle pressure decreased.

phases of a patient's care (Fig. 3-7). Those who deal with these patients have come to realize that long-term monitoring of the outcome is important both for preserving function and avoiding complications or failure of the initial reconstruction, be it by angioplasty or direct arterial surgery. Since the follow-up protocol will vary somewhat depending on the initial therapy, it is important to consider these therapies separately.

TRANSLUMINAL ANGIOPLASTY

Angioplasty achieves restoration of function by splitting the intima longitudinally adjacent to the plaque into the media and up to the adventitia, permitting the arterial lumen to increase in size.[24] If this procedure is successful, the cross-sectional area of the vessel increases, and the velocity changes across the stenotic segment will improve and in some cases return to normal. The major problem with this therapy is the development of myointimal hyperplasia, which occurs in up to 20% to 30% of the segments. The recurrence rate appears lowest for the iliac arteries and highest for the smaller peripheral arteries such as the superficial femoral and popliteal arteries. These arterial segments can be restudied early after the procedure and followed over time to monitor the long-term results.[25] If the patient becomes symptomatic, it is a simple matter to reassess the situation and determine the basis for the return in symptoms.

SAPHENOUS VEIN GRAFTS

One of the more common methods of correcting lesions involving the femoropopliteal segment is to use the greater saphenous vein either by the in situ approach or by reversing the vein. These conduits, which can provide very good long-term benefit, may develop problems—particularly during the first year—that, if detected, can be corrected before graft failure occurs. The lesions often develop at the site of valve cusps and resemble the intimal hyperplasia observed in the segments that have been dilated. If they are discovered early, they can be corrected by either simple surgical procedures or perhaps angioplasty that will ensure continued patency and function.

Since these grafts are in a subcutaneous position, it is a simple matter to monitor them by a series of noninvasive tests every 6 to 8 weeks during the first year. The methods used include the determination of the A/A index, estimation of the velocity changes along the graft with a continuous wave Doppler device, and finally, repeat duplex scanning of the entire length of the graft.

The use of the A/A index is based on the observation that when a lesion that is hemodynamically significant develops within the venous graft, the A/A index will decrease. It is well established that a fall greater than 0.15 is significant and should prompt an aggressive examination for the basis of the observed fall. In this setting it is also possible to use exercise testing to document the deterioration in graft function, but this is not a necessary routine study for most cases of graft surveillance.

Bandyk[23] in a series of excellent studies has shown that the absolute velocity within a vein graft may be predictive of outcome. If the velocity of flow in the graft is greater than 45 cm/sec, the graft can be considered not at risk and the follow-up continued. On the other hand, if the velocity is below this level and/or there is a segment of the graft in which the velocity is increased from a more proximal segment, this is indicative of a potential problem, and the patient should be further evaluated. As Bandyk has shown, if such an approach is used, long-term graft patency may be assured in most patients.

What about monitoring prosthetic arterial grafts? When these conduits fail, they do so at one of the anastomotic sites. For aortofemoral grafts it is the distal anastomosis that is the site of greatest concern since failure at the proximal end is very uncommon. For femoropopliteal grafts the problem may develop at either union, with the cause usually myointimal hyperplasia. We have not found the surveillance intervals as helpful in this case, but it is clear that follow-up with the assessment of the A/A index and the study of the anastomotic sites may detect problems before complete occlusion occurs.

ANEURYSMAL DISEASE

The most lethal vascular disorder is the abdominal aortic aneurysm that if untreated may lead to rupture and death. Even if the patient survives the initial bleeding episode to arrive at the hospital, the mortality rate will be high, in the range of 50% to 80%. Since most of these lesions are not noticed by the patient until he becomes symptomatic, it is important to define objectively the relationships between size of the aneurysm, its location, and its outcome.

What is the magnitude of the problem and how can these lesions be detected and followed? A study by Collins et al[26] screened 426 men between the ages of 65 and 74 with ultrasound to assess the prevalence of aneurysms of the abdominal aorta. An aneurysm was discovered in 5.4% of the men, with the aneurysm 4 cm or greater in size in 2.3% of them. It was found that men with evidence of occlusive arterial disease were the most likely to have lesions found on scanning. In fact, these patients accounted for 20% of the aneurysms discovered. These studies have pointed out that aneurysms are not uncommon and should be considered in any patient who is being evaluated for occlusive arterial disease.

Any patient considered at risk or who has a "palpable aorta" suggesting dilation or the presence of an aneurysm should have an ultrasound examination. As Bernstein, Harris, and Leopold[27] have shown by repeat studies, there is very little variation (2 to 3 mm) in the assessment of size when this method is used. The other option available is computed axial tomographic (CT) scanning, which appears to be more precise but should only be done when the ultrasound is deemed inadequate or inconclusive.

As noted above, the value of such a study is the determination of aneurysm size, which is important for determining which lesion should be removed. Although it is not the purpose of this chapter to discuss indications for therapy, it is clear that ultrasound is the best method for documenting changes in size over time. In the study by Bernstein, Harris, and Leopold[27] the changes in size noted during follow-up were evaluated in 110 poor-risk patients followed for a mean period of almost 4 years. The expansion rate for this group of patients was 0.4 cm/yr. In this group of patients were 46 who underwent resection because their lesions reached 6 cm or more. Thirty-six patients died of causes unrelated to the aneurysms. Six patients died of aortic rupture, with three not undergoing an operation because of serious coexisting disease. Using this method of long-term study, the mortality rate from aortic rupture was 7.5%.

We have followed this policy of using repeat ultrasound scans in patients with small aneurysms and have found it satisfactory. For those lesions greater than 4 cm we believe a follow-up interval of 3 months is satisfactory as advocated by Bernstein, Harris, and Leopold.

The problems that develop with peripheral aneurysms (femoral and popliteal) are different. These lesions rarely rupture but are known to undergo thrombosis and/or to be the site of emboli to the lower limbs.[28] Although peripheral aneurysms can occur in isolation, they are more common in patients who have aneurysms of the abdominal aorta. They can be diagnosed by both physical examination and ultrasound. However, the criteria as to size and the potential danger posed for limb survival have not been worked out. In general, the criterion for making the diagnosis has related to the dimension of the artery proximal to the suspicious area. The most frequently used guideline is that a vessel that is 1½ to 2 times the diameter of the artery immediately proximal to the suspicious area should be considered aneurysmal. Patients who are candidates for screening are those with very prominent popliteal pulses and/or any elderly patient who has sudden onset of ischemia to the limb.

EXTRACRANIAL ARTERIAL DISEASE

Because atherosclerosis is a "systemic" disorder, it is important to direct attention to those areas that may have an impact on patient management and outcome. Although stroke-related death is on the decline, it still remains the third most common cause of death in the United States. Thus in the course of the evaluation of patients with atherosclerosis it is not uncommon to find bruits in the neck that can be markers for underlying disease of the carotid bifurcation. In addition, the patients with extracranial arterial disease may develop transient ischemic attacks (TIAs) and strokes secondary to disease in the arteries of the neck.

Screening tests

A host of tests have been developed to permit assessment of the extracranial arteries. These can be divided into indirect and direct tests. The more commonly used indirect tests include those that derive their information at a point away from the carotid bulb itself. They include periorbital directional Doppler[29] and oculoplethysmography.[30,31] Both methods use information about the arterial inflow to the eye through the ophthalmic artery as an index of the hemodynamic changes that occur as the carotid artery becomes progressively narrowed. At some time in the progression of a plaque, the diameter of the artery will reach a point at which a pressure gradient will develop along with a drop in flow across the involved area. When this occurs, the pressure in the ophthalmic artery will fall, and the collateral blood supply to the ipsilateral cortex will be activated. In the case of the carotid artery, the most common input collateral artery that is easily studied is the external carotid artery and its communications with the ophthalmic artery through the medial frontal and supraorbital arteries. When the carotid artery is significantly narrowed, the direction of flow in the medial frontal and supraorbital arteries will be reversed.

The directional changes in flow induced by the tight stenoses of the carotid bulb can be detected using a direction-sensing continuous wave Doppler sensor placed over the medial frontal and supraorbital arteries[29] (Fig. 3-8). It is also possible to test the effect of temporal artery compression on the flows being recorded. Although this has been widely tested, the method has serious limitations that are readily apparent. It cannot distinguish a tight stenosis from a total occlusion and cannot be used for monitoring the progression of disease in the carotid bulb.

The oculoplethysmographic system developed by Gee[31] is an elegantly simple method that uses cups applied to the sclera of the eye that are placed under a negative pressure sufficient to stop blood flow to the eye. As the pressure in the system is gradually reduced, there will be a point at which the ocular pulsations return. It is possible to relate this pressure to that which is present in the ophthalmic artery on that side. This test, which is much like the periorbital Doppler method, is most useful in detecting those lesions that are pressure and flow reducing. It also has the problem of being unable to distinguish a tight stenosis from a total occlusion. The only advantage this method has over the use of duplex scanning is that it could depict a siphon lesion that would be missed by scanning in the neck. This is, however, a very unusual occurrence in my experience.

Although these methods have been used extensively, they have been largely superseded by the use of the direct methods of investigating not only the carotid bifurcation but also the vessels at the level of the arch and the vertebral arteries as well. More recently, with the advent of the transcranial Doppler, a new method of examining the arteries inside the skull is available.

What information is available?

When patients with suspected carotid artery disease are first seen, there is no way based on the clinical presentation alone to estimate either the location or extent of the arterial involvement. Although bruits are markers of disease of the

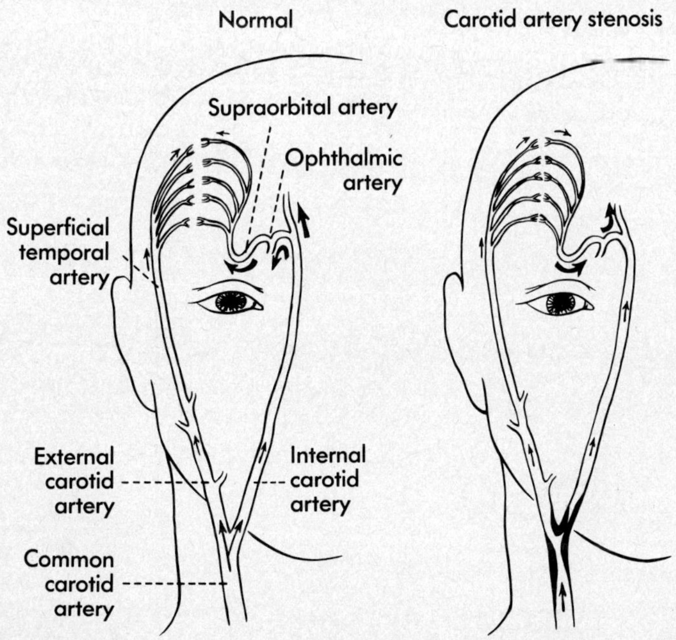

Fig. 3-8. Direction of flow in the supraorbital arteries in normal subjects and patients with a high-grade stenosis of the internal carotid artery.

bulb, they are little else. Except for arteriography, there is no way short of the use of duplex scanning to determine the degree of narrowing that is producing the noise in the neck.

Duplex scanning has been widely applied and tested in this area and has been found the best single method of screening for bifurcation disease.[32,33] It provides information about the site and extent of disease, using categories that are of clinical value. Depending on one's clinical practice and bias, it is possible to eliminate most patients from consideration for arteriography. The categories of disease that are used with minor variations from center to center are as follows:

1. *Normal*. Finding a normal carotid bulb with boundary layer separation is nearly certain evidence that the bifurcation is not the cause of either transient ischemic events and or strokes (Fig. 3-9).
2. *Minimal wall disease—1% to 15% narrowing*. This is rarely significant clinically except in the *very unusual* case in which this type of lesion may be the site of ulceration. In our experience with patients undergoing an operation for carotid artery disease only 3% of the patients had disease in this category (Fig. 3-10).
3. *16% to 49% stenosis*. These lesions are generally considered of moderate severity and are not associated with a pressure gradient or a reduction in flow. They can be the cause of TIAs and strokes, which also are not very common. In my experience only approximately 10% of patients with either a TIA or stroke will have this degree of stenosis.
4. *50% to 79% narrowing*. Once the artery is narrowed to this extent, there is a marked increase in velocity within the stenotic segment, and there may be an associated pressure drop. When this degree of stenosis is found, the lesions are more complex pathologically and can be the cause of symptoms. These lesions account for approximately 42% of patients who undergo carotid endarterectomy (see Fig. 3-10).

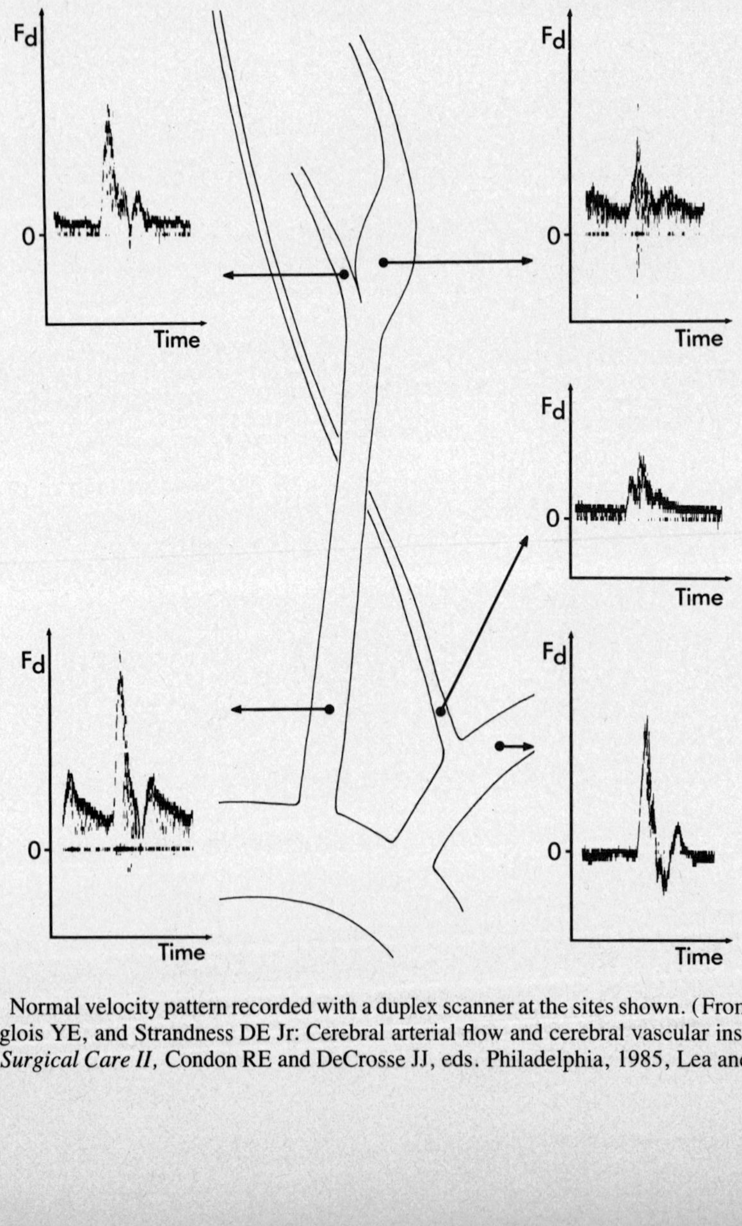

Fig. 3-9. Normal velocity pattern recorded with a duplex scanner at the sites shown. (From Roederer GO, Langlois YE, and Strandness DE Jr: Cerebral arterial flow and cerebral vascular insufficiency, Ch 12 in *Surgical Care II*, Condon RE and DeCrosse JJ, eds. Philadelphia, 1985, Lea and Febiger.)

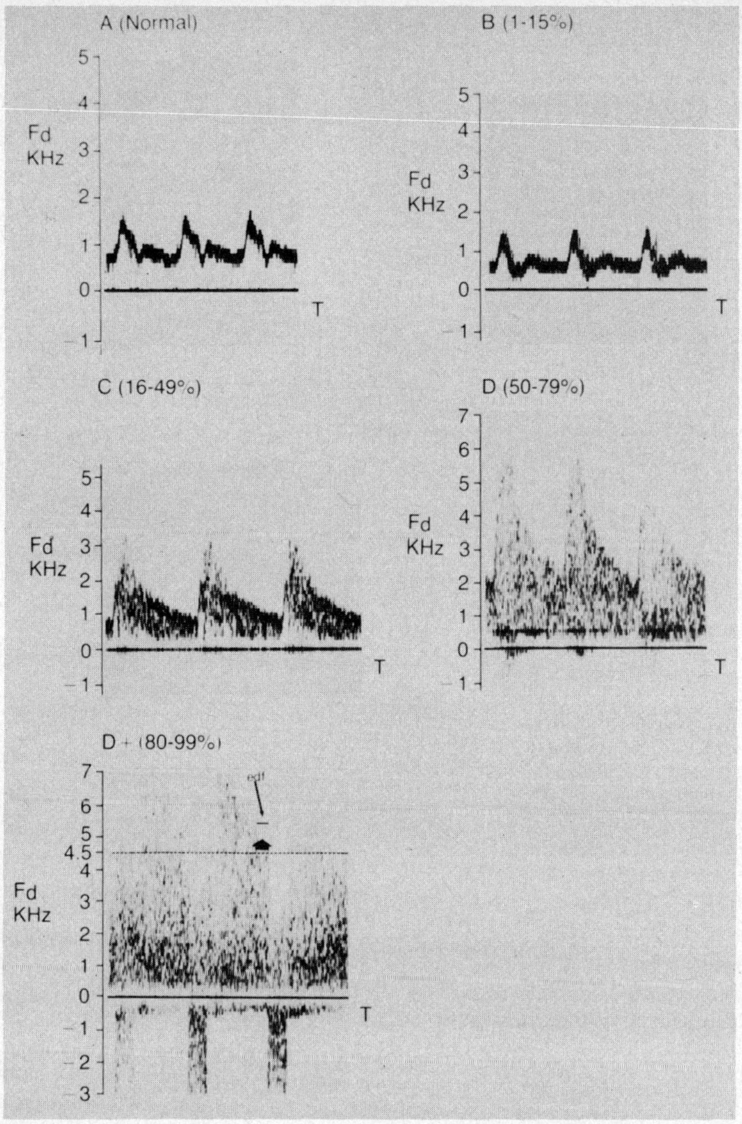

Fig. 3-10. Spectral analysis of velocity changes noted at the site of the lesion for the categories of involvement. For the 16%-49% stenosis, the main diagnostic features are a peak frequency below 4 kHz (125 cm/sec) and spectral broadening. For the 50%-79% stenosis, the peak systolic frequency is 4kHz. For the 80%-99% stenosis, the main diagnostic features are a peak systolic frequency >4kHz and an end-systolic frequency >4.5 kHz (145 cm/sec). (From Taylor DC and Strandness DE Jr: Carotid artery duplex scanning, J Clin Ultrasound 15:635, 1987.)

5. *80% to 99% stenosis*. This is often referred to as the "preocclusive" lesion because of its propensity to progress to a total occlusion of the internal carotid artery. The plaques that produce this degree of narrowing are also of the complicated variety, with loss of surface covering, necrosis, calcification, and intraplaque hemorrhage (see Fig. 3-10).
6. *Total occlusion*. The finding of a total occlusion is important because it removes the patient from consideration for surgical therapy. However, even if the artery occludes and does not lead to an event at the time of the occlusion, there is an ongoing stroke rate in the range of 5%/yr.

The type of information available through duplex scanning is important not only for planning therapy but also for serving as the baseline study for long-term follow-up (Fig. 3-11). Although there is and will continue to be some controversy about the significance of these lesions, particularly in asymptomatic patients, guidelines exist with which most investigators can agree. Those lesions that narrow the artery by less than 80% can be safely followed with a very low

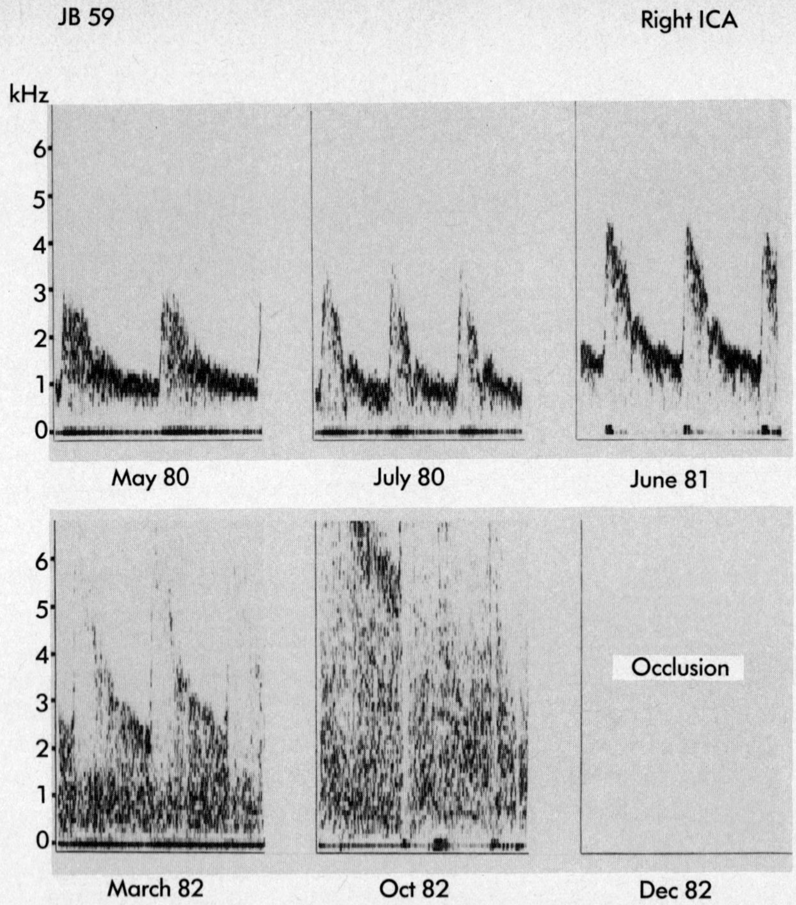

Fig. 3-11. Serial duplex velocity readings from the right internal carotid artery (ICA) in a 59-year-old white male. At the time of the first study in May 1980, the ICA was narrowed to the 16%-49% category of stenosis. (From Roederer GO et al: The natural history of carotid arterial disease in asymptomatic patients with cervical bruits. Stroke 15:605, 1984, by permission of the American Heart Association.)

incidence of ischemic events (1% to 4%/yr).[34,35] For those that narrow the artery by greater than 80% the occlusion and event rate is much higher, in the range of 5% to 10%/yr, which has led us to be more aggressive in treating this degree of involvement.

If one chooses to follow patients with carotid disease without an operation, the progression rate for a lesion going from less than 50% stenosis to more than 50% stenosis is 8%/yr.

Another major advantage of duplex scanning for the carotid circulation is for the evaluation of the patient who has undergone surgery and returns for evaluation. This evaluation can be divided into the following phases:

1. *The perioperative period—first 24 hours*. If an ischemic event occurs within this time frame, the duplex scan can be quickly done to establish patency of the reconstruction but should not be used in an attempt to define lesser degrees of involvement.
2. *The postoperative period*. Although it is possible to study patients during the early period after discharge, usually on the third hospital day, it is not wise to attempt to do a detailed examination of the bulb region until the healing process is mature and the region is stable. We have arbitrarily set this time at 3 months after the operation. After this period of time, the most common lesion that develops is myointimal hyperplasia, a process that is largely benign and not responsible for recurrent ischemic episodes.[36] Annual visits are in order to monitor the status of the carotid bulb. After the first 2 years the lesions that develop are most likely to represent new atherosclerotic plaques.

VERTEBROBASILAR INSUFFICIENCY

One of the less satisfying areas to evaluate in the vascular laboratory is ischemia of the posterior circulation. The major problems are the nonspecific nature of the patient's symptoms and the difficulty in identifying the specific arterial lesions responsible for its development. The most common syndrome is that associated with reversal of flow in the vertebral artery (the subclavian steal syndrome).[37] This is thought to occur as a result of "siphoning" blood away from the posterior fossa when there is a hemodynamically significant lesion in the ipsilateral subclavian artery. This results in reverse flow in the vertebral artery that now serves as an important collateral artery for the arm. When this syndrome was first described, it was thought that exercise of the arm on the side of the subclavian occlusion would further increase the reverse flow in the vertebral artery and lead to brainstem ischemia. However, most patients with subclavian artery stenosis and/or occlusion with reverse flow in the vertebral artery never develop symptoms either at rest or with exercise of the arm on the side of the occlusion.[38] The fully developed subclavian steal syndrome is rare.

However, it is feasible to study patients suspected of having the problem to document the presence of reverse flow in the vertebral artery. A subset of patients who have oscillatory flow (forward-reverse) in the vertebral artery are apt to be more symptomatic than those who have reverse flow at all times.[39] It is possible that the use of transcranial Doppler may help shed some light on this difficult clinical problem.

INTRACRANIAL HEMODYNAMICS

Although the skull has been considered an impenetrable barrier to the use of ultrasound, it has been shown by Aaslid, Markwaider, and Nornes[40] that it is possible to obtain velocity data from the basal cerebral arteries using 2 MHz pulsed Doppler systems to gain access to the arteries inside the skull. It appears that there are three sites that can be used to gain access to the arteries that comprise the circle of Willis: the eye, the temporal bone "window" just above the zygomatic arch, and the foramen magnum. These positions provide access to the intracranial internal carotid, the middle cerebral, and the vertebral and basilar arteries. The assumption is made that the angle of insonation of these arteries is 0 degrees. If it is assumed that the angle of insonation is 0 degrees, the maximum error that would occur if this were off by 20 degrees would be 6%. The data that can be obtained for analysis are the peak systolic velocity or the mean velocity (time-averaged maximum velocity). If an additional assumption is made that the vessel's diameter remains constant, then the method would be suitable for monitoring changes in volume flow.[41] This is an assumption that may not be correct, and one would have to define carefully the circumstances in which the measurements are being made. For example, one of the more common uses of this technique is to monitor flow in the middle cerebral artery after an episode of subarachnoid bleeding. It is well-known that cerebral vasospasm occurs, so any relationship between the velocity changes and flow to the cortex would have to take this fact into account.

What is the role of transcranial Doppler at the present time? More work will be needed to determine its place. Some of the areas in which it could be helpful are as follows:

1. *Evaluation of the circle of Willis*. In theory it is possible to monitor flow and its direction in all major components of the circle of Willis with the exception of the posterior communicating artery. It should then be possible to estimate the risk of events such as thrombosis of the internal carotid artery in terms of the likelihood that an ischemic event might occur. However, some problems have not been resolved. Although it is feasible to test the adequacy of the circle with compression of the common carotid artery, this is not the same as would occur with involvement of the internal carotid artery alone. In addition, if an ischemic event occurred because of the extension of a thrombus intracranially to block the middle cerebral artery, the effect of this event could not be predicted by transcranial Doppler. It is also possible to monitor flow in the middle cerebral artery during endarterectomy. The results are promising, but more study is needed.[42]

2. *Detection of intracranial lesions involving the middle cerebral artery*. There is no doubt that this method has the potential for discovering such lesions by virtue of the increase in velocity that occurs when a stenotic segment is located.[43] On the other hand, the absence of flow that might signify a total occlusion must be interpreted with caution. There are patients who do not have an acoustic window in the temporal bone. The problem would appear to be less severe with the vertebral and basilar arteries in which there is no problem with regard to an acoustic window.

3. *Subarachnoid hemorrhage*. The one application that has been tested and found of value is in this area. It is possible to monitor the time course of cerebral artery vasospasm by using transcranial Doppler.[44]

4. *Documentation of cerebral arterial response to carbon dioxide inhalation*. This is a potentially exciting area of research. It appears there are some patients whose vascular reactivity is severely limited, and this limitation can be uncovered by this method. Perhaps identification of these patients wil provide an idea of which patients are likely to suffer when an occlusion of the internal carotid artery occurs.[45]

5. *Evaluation of vertebrobasilar insufficiency*. As noted in an earlier section, this is one area that is very confusing and difficult to evaluate. Perhaps the ability to study directly not only the vertebral but basilar artery as well will give a better idea about the role of reverse flow in these arteries as the basis for ischemic symptoms.

Although the future for transcranial Doppler appears bright, a considerable amount of work must be done to define its role. At the present time it must still be considered an investigational method.

RENOVASCULAR HYPERTENSION

Hypertension affects approximately 10% of the U.S. population. Within this very large group of patients it has been estimated that 1% to 6% will have renal artery disease as the cause of the problem.[46] This occurs in two forms—atherosclerosis and fibromuscular hyperplasia. When atherosclerosis is the inciting disorder, it is more likely to affect people over the age of 50. The proximal renal artery is the most common site of involvement. With fibromuscular hyperplasia the involvement can be at all levels of the renal artery, but it is unusual for the orifice of the artery to be involved.[47] Since these disorders can be treated by either transluminal angioplasty or direct arterial surgery, it is important that they be detected if at all possible.

Over the years several screening methods have been tested to determine if they might be suitable for noninvasive detection of renal artery stenosis. The most common methods developed included intravenous urography and radionuclide studies. Both of these methods had unacceptably high false-positive and false-negative rates, making them unsuitable for screening purposes. The urographic and nuclear scans have a sensitivity of only approximately 70% for the diagnosis of significant renal artery stenosis.[48] They have a false-positive rate that can be as high as 20%. In addition, the screening tests are unreliable in the presence of bilateral renal artery disease, which is a common occurrence. For a screening test to be of great value it must have a very high specificity to avoid unnecessary application of invasive studies such as arteriography.[49]

Although intravenous digital subtraction arteriography was introduced as a possible method for screening purposes, it has not turned out to be a useful method. The method requires large volumes of contrast material, and the images obtained do not have the resolution necessary to permit reliable detection of most renal artery lesions.

Ultrasonic duplex scanning provides a useful alternative since it is possible to examine the renal arteries directly and to detect areas of narrowing.[50,51] It is known that when there is a fall in pressure and flow across the renal artery, the renin-angiotensin system will be activated. It has been shown experimentally and clinically that this usually occurs at the level of a 60% reduction in the diameter of the renal artery.

Patients who are candidates for this study include the following: (1) young patients with hypertension; (2) patients with rapidly accelerating hypertension; (3) those with malignant hypertension; (4) patients who have hypertension and renal failure; and (5) hypertensive patients with an abdominal bruit. The algorithm we currently use is shown in Fig. 3-12.

Ultrasonic duplex scanning studies are designed to provide the following information: (1) the status of the renal arteries from the level of the aorta to the renal hilum; (2) renal size; (3) blood flow patterns in the upper, middle, and lower poles of the kidney; and (4) information on the gross morphology of the kidney.

To obtain the maximal amount of information, it is necessary to study the patient in the fasting state—preferably

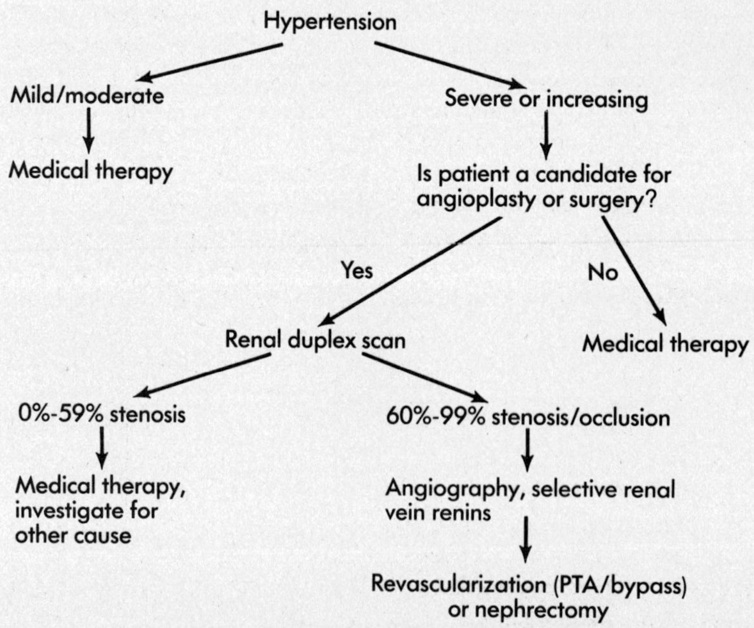

Fig. 3-12. Algorithm illustrating the proposed use of renal artery duplex scanning. (From Taylor DC et al: Duplex ultrasound scanning in the diagnosis of renal artery stenosis: a prospective study. J Vasc Surg 7:363, 1988.)

for a period of 12 hours. It is also beneficial to study the patient in the early morning before much air swallowing has occurred. Air in the bowel is one of the major problems encountered in carrying out these studies because it interferes with the transmission of ultrasound to the area of interest. When proper preparation has been done, we can study adequately approximately 90% of the patients referred for the procedure.

Although the degree of stenosis in the carotid and peripheral arteries can be characterized over a fairly wide range of categories, this is more difficult in the renal artery; largely because of the problem of following the renal artery throughout its length and knowing precisely the angle of the sound beam with the vessel. In developing this method we used the relationship between the peak systolic velocity in the renal artery compared to that in the aorta. This ratio (RAR) is normally 1:1.2. If the renal artery is narrowed by 60% or morc, this ratio exceeds 3.5 (Fig. 3-13). In patients with atherosclerosis the lesions commonly involve the orifice or the first 2 cm of the artery. In patients with fibromuscular disease the stenotic segments usually develop in the mid and distal artery.

Occlusions of the renal artery can be difficult to detect unless one is always aware of this possibility. Occlusions of the renal artery are commonly associated with a kidney less than 9 cm in length. In a series of 58 renal arteries scanned that also had arteriographic studies, total occlusions were found in five instances. This was verified by duplex scanning in four cases. In the remaining case the degree of disease was classified in the greater than 60% stenosis category.[51]

Another much more difficult problem for duplex scanning is the patient with multiple renal arteries. In the series of 58 renal arteries prospectively studied, there were four instances in which multiple arteries were present, and we were able to detect only one of them. It is certainly possible for there to be a lesion in an accessory renal artery causing hypertension, and it would be missed by this method. To date we have not encountered such a patient, but this is clearly a possibility that must be considered.

How good is such screening in detecting significant renal artery lesions? Our data suggest that with this method one can expect to obtain a sensitivity of 84%, with a specificity of 97% and an overall accuracy of 93%.[51] Is this good enough? The very high specificity is important for the use of a screening test applied to a population with a low prev-

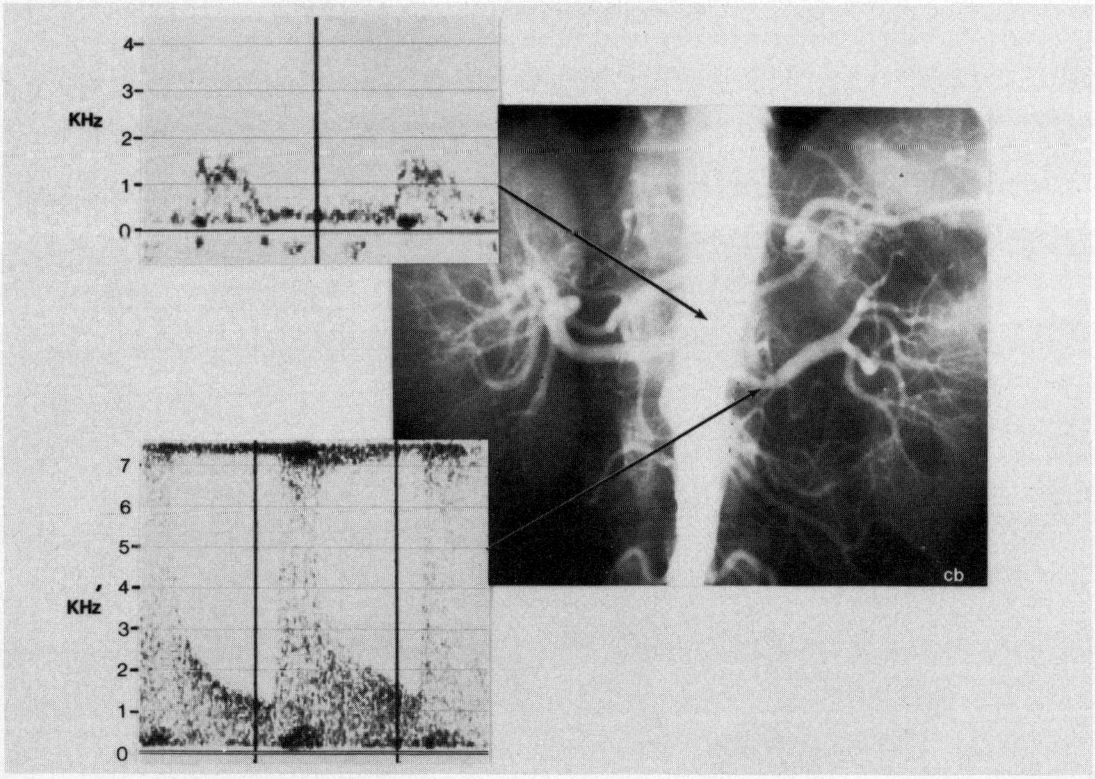

Fig. 3-13. Renal duplex scan in a patient with a >60% stenosis of the left renal artery. The renal aortic ratio was 9.4. (From Taylor DC et al: Duplex ultrasound scanning in the diagnosis of renal artery stenosis. A prospective study. J Vasc Surg 7:363, 1988.)

alence of disease such as the hypertensive population in this country. It would be unacceptable to perform unnecessary arteriograms on a large number of healthy individuals.

Follow-up studies

One of the major problems encountered in patients with renal arterial disease is the lack of suitable methods for sequential study of lesions, regardless of the treatment used. Because of this, the end point most commonly used in defining success or failure is control of the blood pressure. If the patient after transluminal angioplasty or surgery does not require drugs for therapy, it is assumed, probably rightly, that the therapy has been successful. However, most patients do not fall into this "cured" category, and assessment of the reconstructed segment is important. In addition, the largest group of patients with renal vascular disease will not have any intervention other than medical therapy. The major question that has never been answered for this group of patients is what happens to the lesions over time and in particular what effect will progression of disease have on renal function.

Once a patient with renal arterial disease has been studied successfully, the procedure can almost always be repeated to document any change that may have occurred. This is also true of those patients who have had direct intervention, be it angioplasty or surgery. It is not a difficult matter to repeat the evaluation to document the outcome both early and late. In the long-term studies we have done to date, it has been possible to document the results, thus removing any uncertainty as to outcome. Three groups of patients have been examined.[52]

1. Five patients underwent angioplasty; there was documented improvement by duplex scanning in two. Both of these patients had relief of their hypertension. In the other three patients there was no improvement in the stenotic segments revealed by duplex scanning, and in each patient the hypertension persisted. The great advantage of duplex scanning is that it can be applied immediately after the procedure to determine the status of the arterial segment. Furthermore, if at anytime later a problem with blood pressure control becomes evident, the study can be repeated.

2. In the surgical group of patients there were 10 stenotic arteries in seven patients studied after the procedure. At a mean follow-up period of 9 months, there was continued patency in eight arteries and unexpected occlusion in two bypasses (Fig. 3-14). Thus this approach has been very helpful in documenting the basis for the failure and will have increasing applications for those cases in which the bypass has been done to a small kidney. The fate of bypass grafts to small kidneys (7 cm in length or less) is an important area that needs study.

3. A most important group of patients to follow are those

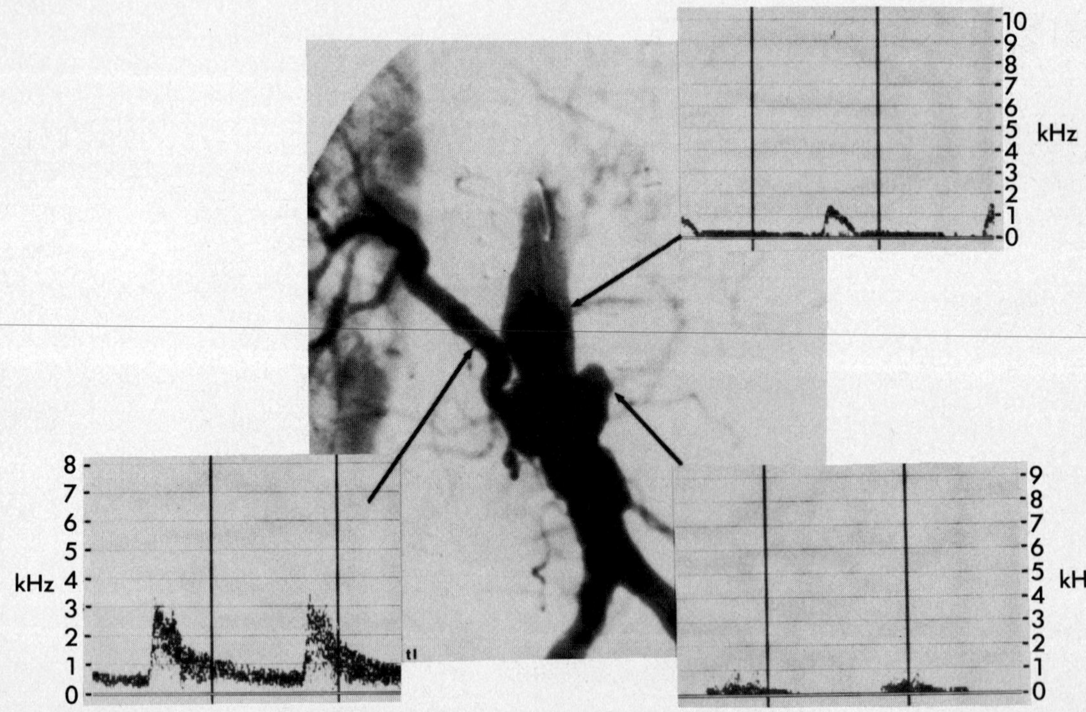

Fig. 3-14. Postoperative duplex scanning study in a patient who underwent bilateral aortorenal grafting. The graft to the left kidney was visualized, but there was no flow. (From Taylor DC, Moneta GL, and Strandness DE Jr: Follow-up of renal artery stenosis by duplex ultrasound. J Vasc Surg 9:410, 1989.)

with greater than 60% stenosis who have not had any intervention for the treatment of their lesions. We have been able to study 19 renal arteries in 15 patients during a follow-up period of 13 months. During this time none of the renal arteries went on to occlusion, but there was an average decrease in renal length of -1.0 cm, $P<0.01$. This is an important observation since it may explain the renal failure that may ultimately develop in some patients with high-grade renal arterial stenosis. It is clear that as these patients are followed for longer periods of time, some will progress to a total occlusion with its consequences.

THE TRANSPLANTED KIDNEY

Duplex scanning is also of benefit in examining the transplanted kidney, both in the early period after its placement and for the long-term. In the early postoperative period a question that frequently arises is the issue of rejection vs reversible ischemic injury.[53,54] It has been postulated that the process associated with rejection dramatically increases resistance to flow and that is in turn reflected in the pattern of the velocities detected both in the renal artery and the parenchyma of the kidney.[55] Slightly different algorithms have been used to describe this finding, but they all have taken into account the degree to which the end-diastolic frequency approaches zero. We have preferred to use the end-diastolic ratio (EDR), which is the end-diastolic velocity divided by the peak systolic velocity. The normal value for the EDR is 0.35 or less.

Other investigators have used the resistive index (RI), which is the peak systolic velocity minus the end-diastolic velocity divided by the peak systolic velocity. Both the EDR and the RI reflect the resistance to flow offered by the small vessels in the kidney. The experience with this type of analysis as a predictor of rejection remains unsettled at the moment. Fleischer et al[55] did show differences between the rejecting kidney vs controls. As the RI moved toward a value of 1.0, it appeared likely that this reflected rejection. However, Genkins, Sanflippo, and Carroll[56] showed that, although changes in the RI did reflect pathologic changes within the allograft, they did not specifically identify the cause of the transplant dysfunction. This problem will clearly require more study with more cases in which the pathologic basis for change in the RI has been documented.

One area in which duplex scanning can be of great value is in the chronic renal transplant patient who has developed hypertension or renal failure.[57] It is important to know if the renal artery supplying the patient's kidney has developed a stenotic lesion. Since the transplanted kidney is in an easily accessible location, it is a relatively simple matter to scan the renal artery from its origin to detect any areas of narrowing that may be present. This is very important since many of these narrowings may be corrected by transluminal angioplasty.

THE MESENTERIC CIRCULATION

Since atherosclerosis is a disease of branch points and bifurcations, it is not unexpected that the major suppliers to the small and large bowel, the superior and inferior mesenteric arteries, would also be affected. The other arteries of great importance to this region are the celiac and hypogastric arteries that can serve as important collateral sources when the mesenteric arteries become narrowed and occluded. In fact, the collateral potential is extremely good for this region and is the major reason that chronic lesions

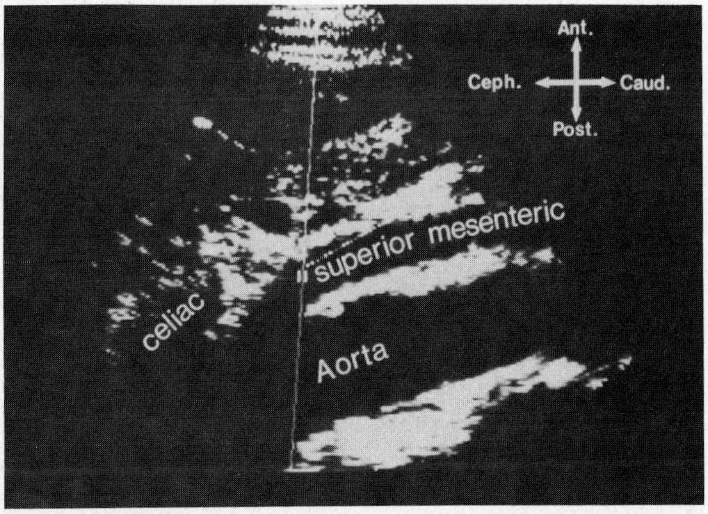

B-mode: celiac and superior mesenteric arteries
(Sample vol. in proximal superior mesenteric arteries)

Fig. 3-15. Longitudinal B-mode scan showing the aorta, the origin of the celiac and the first four centimeters of the superior mesenteric artery.

do not often lead to the development of intestinal ischemia.

The major clinical problems involving the small bowel are acute and chronic mesenteric ischemia. In acute ischemia the superior mesenteric artery becomes occluded either by emboli or by a thrombosis on a preexisting atherosclerotic plaque. When this occurs, the presentation is often dramatic, with acute and severe abdominal pain, very hyperactive bowel tones, and a nearly normal abdominal examination. If the diagnosis is not made promptly and therapy instituted quickly, bowel death rapidly ensues, and the patient will die. There is rarely time to do an ultrasound scan of the patient's abdomen to assess the inflow to the gut. In fact, such studies should be discouraged since they only delay the opportunity to correct the underlying problem.

In a patient with chronic ischemia the involvement has occurred gradually, and the clinical presentation will reflect the inability of the superior mesenteric artery to supply the blood flow needs to the gut during digestion, resulting in the syndrome commonly referred to as mesenteric angina. When this occurs, the patient when eating will develop abdominal pain that is often followed by diarrhea and progressive weight loss. Such a patient soon finds that food intake is always followed by pain, so he will markedly limit his intake. The weight loss will be profound if the lesions producing the problem are not relieved.

It is well established that the celiac, superior mesenteric, and perhaps the inferior mesenteric arteries must be involved to produce chronic mesenteric angina because the collateral supply is so rich that normal levels of blood flow, even after eating, can be provided by these alternate routes. In clinical practice the only method that has proved satisfactory in making the diagnosis is arteriography with its lateral views of the abdominal aorta to demonstrate the celiac, superior mesenteric, and inferior mesenteric arteries. Arteriography is necessary to confirm the diagnosis and is mandatory before any procedure designed to correct the situation, direct arterial surgery, or angioplasty.

Since many pain syndromes in the aging patient may suggest the diagnosis, it is only natural that duplex scanning would be used as a screening test and also as a method for monitoring the long-term results with therapy. The celiac and the superior mesenteric arteries are readily available to this modality and are relatively easy to study by virtue of their position in the upper abdomen where these vessels originate (Fig. 3-15).

The velocity patterns recorded in the normal celiac and superior mesenteric arteries reflect the resistance of the organs they supply.[58,60] The liver and spleen have low vascular resistance, similar to that of the brain and the kidneys. The low resistance means that there should always be a high mean flow level, no reverse flow, and a high end-diastolic velocity. The superior mesenteric artery supplies an organ of variable resistance with wide ranges of blood flow, depending mainly on the time of day and the relationship to eating and what the patient has ingested.[59]

In the fasting state the velocity pattern in the superior mesenteric artery is often triphasic, with a definite but brief period of reverse flow seen in late systole. The end-diastolic flow will be quite variable. However, with eating some dramatic changes occur that reflect the decrease in resistance as the small arteries and arterioles in the bowel dilate to promote the increase in flow that is needed for digestion (Fig. 3-16). This begins within 1 minute after eating, reaching a maximal level 40 minutes after the meal is completed. The magnitude of the response depends to a large degree on what has been eaten.[61] The normal range of values is shown in Tables 3-4 and 3-5.

In the six patients encountered with chronic mesenteric angina the diagnosis has been readily made on the basis of the duplex scan results alone. In each case there have been high-grade (greater than 50%) diameter-reducing lesions in both the celiac and the superior mesenteric arteries (Fig. 3-17). We have not yet seen a patient with a chronic stenosis

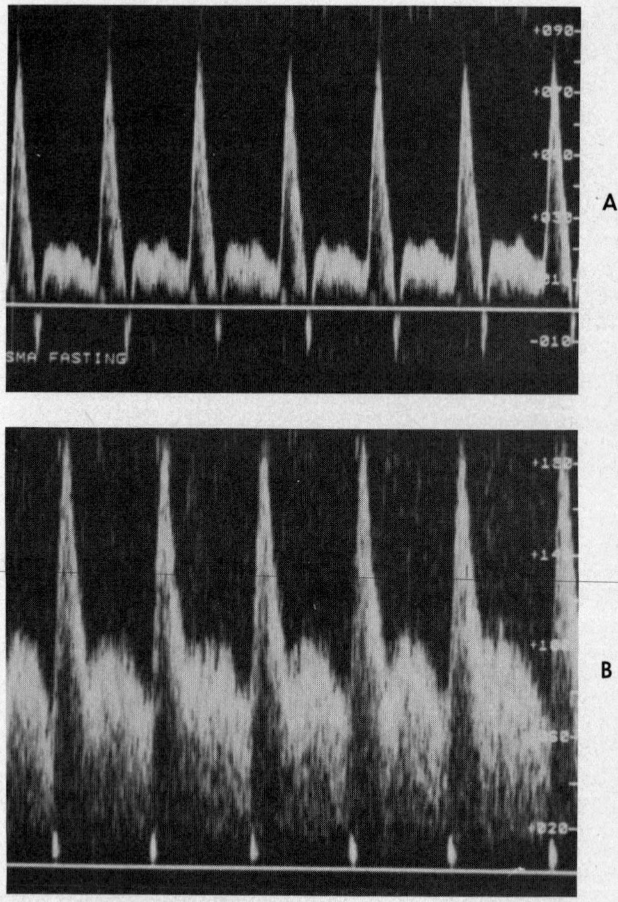

Fig. 3-16. In the fasting state **(A)** flow in the superior mesenteric shows a brief reverse flow component and a low end-diastolic velocity. After eating **(B)** there is an increase in both the peak systolic and end-diastolic velocities. (From Taylor DC and Moneta GL: Duplex ultrasound scanning of the renal and mesenteric circulation. Seminars in Vascular Surgery 1:23, 1988.)

Table 3-4. Range of values for blood flow in the celiac and superior mesenteric arteries*

Artery	Peak systolic velocity (cm/sec)	End-diastolic velocity (cm/sec)	Volume flow (ml/min)
Celiac	101 ± 3.5	33 ± 1.4	1083 ± 75
Superior mesenteric	113 ± 3.9	15 ± 1.1	538 ± 37

*Mean and standard error of the mean.

Table 3-5. Maximal percentage increases in the celiac and superior mesenteric arteries after a mixed meal*

Artery	Peak systolic velocity (cm/sec)	End-diastolic velocity (cm/sec)	Volume flow (ml/min)
Celiac	20 ± 6	24 ± 9	18 ± 4
Superior mesenteric	42 ± 4	321 ± 100	164 ± 30

*Mean and standard error of the mean.

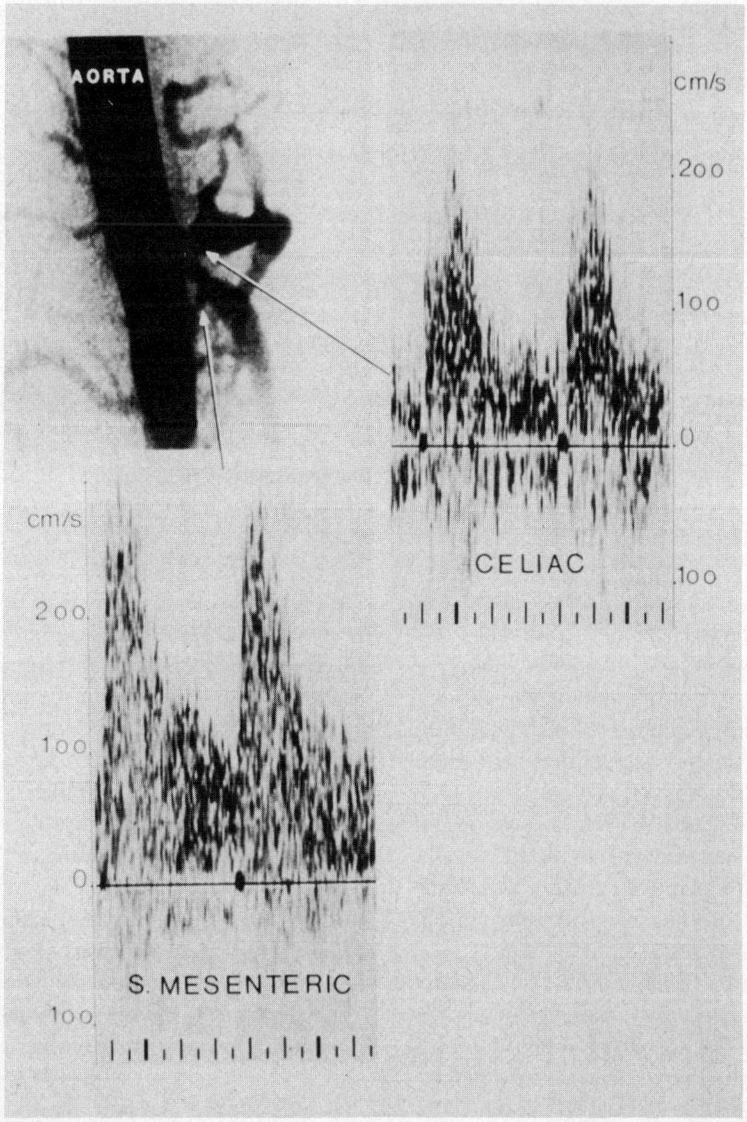

Fig. 3-17. The velocity changes seen in a patient with chronic mesenteric angina and stenoses of the celiac and superior mesenteric arteries.

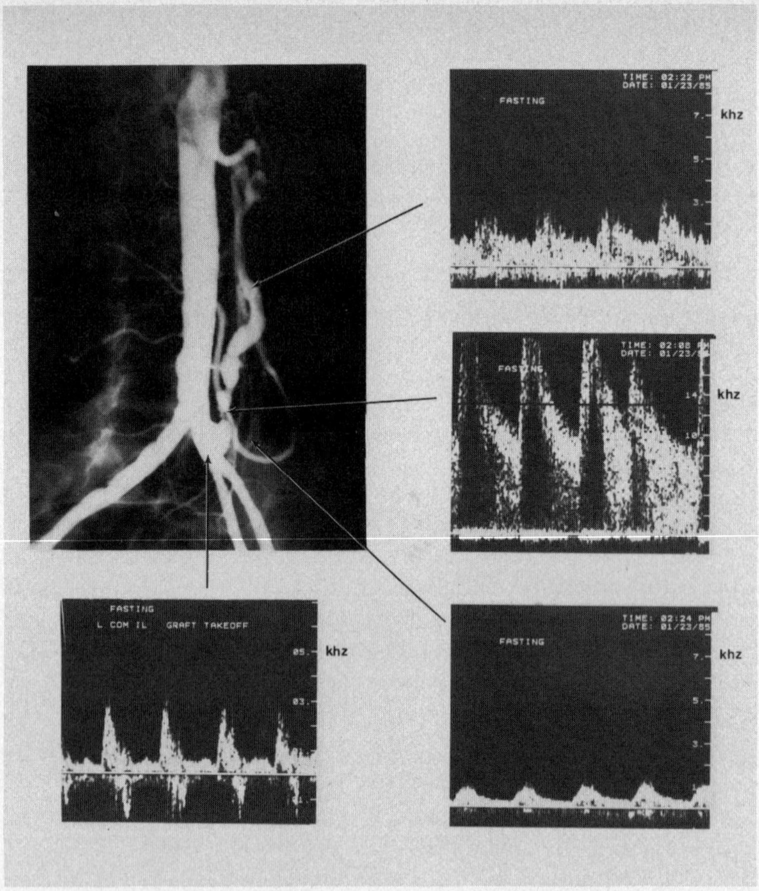

Fig. 3-18. This patient had a vein graft placed from the left common iliac artery to the superior mesenteric artery. Nine months after the operation, symptoms returned and a stenosis at the origin of the vein graft was discovered. This was treated by transluminal angioplasty.

or occlusion of the superior mesenteric artery alone who had the syndrome. We have not been able to monitor routinely the inferior mesenteric artery by duplex scanning, so it has not been possible to assess its involvement and contribution to the production of symptoms. Since the ability of the superior mesenteric artery to supply the small bowel after a meal is the primary problem, one could postulate that a test meal could in some cases be useful in determining the diagnosis. This would represent a "stress test" similar to those used to unmask disease in the coronary and lower-extremity circulation. This has not been necessary in any of the clinical cases that have been studied to date.

Another important function of the duplex studies is that they can be applied to the postoperative patient to document the results. We have found this to be very useful after angioplasty and direct arterial surgery. An example of these studies is shown in Fig. 3-18.

ACUTE VENOUS THROMBOSIS

Whereas diseases of the arterial system have dominated the attention of the American medical community, thrombosis of the deep veins with all of the potential sequelae remains a constant and ongoing problem that is not likely to diminish in numbers or importance. In fact, any patient who sustains an injury to the lower limb, be it surgical or outside the hospital, is always at risk. In addition, any patient who is hospitalized for nearly any reason is also at risk for developing the problem. A major problem that continues to face the medical profession is when to suspect the diagnosis and how to confirm it effectively. There are few areas in clinical medicine in which the need to disregard one's impression based on clinical findings can be more important. Physicians must stop trying to make a definitive diagnosis at the bedside since they will be correct only one half the time.[62] The key point to make is that if the diagnosis is entertained, it must be either established or ruled out by some objective test that has proved to be both sensitive and specific for the problem.

The one diagnostic approach that has stood the test of time is phlebography.[63] This procedure permits an objective assessment of the major deep veins at all points at which the contrast material can be found. It is usually performed by injecting contrast material in a vein on the dorsum of the foot, inserting enough volume to fill the major deep veins and follow the course of the dye to the level of the inferior vena cava. In theory this is the best possible test, but there are the following limitations: (1) the test is painful; (2) it should be done bilaterally; (3) there is always the risk of a contrast allergy occurring; (4) in a small percentage of cases (less than 10%) the dye may induce a chemical phlebitis that must be treated[64]; (5) the iliac veins and inferior vena cava will not be seen well in 20% of cases; (6) the deep femoral vein will not be seen in one half of the cases studied; (7) it is difficult to repeat the test to document changes that might have occurred; and (8) it is costly.

Because of the inaccuracy of the bedside diagnosis and the problems associated with phlebography, noninvasive methods were developed to fill this gap in the approach to this common problem. Since the 1970s a variety of methods have been developed that can satisfy the needs of the practicing community when faced with this problem. Deep venous thrombosis produces changes in flow at the site(s) of involvement, with redirection of flow through the collateral circulation that develops. It was only natural that the initial efforts would be directed at measuring these changes in flow.

Before considering the tests currently in use and their accuracy, it is necessary to review the common sites of involvement and how they affect both the clinical presentation and the methods used to detect them. Most of the knowledge about localization of deep venous thrombi has come from the studies done with the labeled fibrinogen introduced by Hobbs.[65] This method uses the injection of iodine 125–labeled fibrinogen, which is incorporated into the evolving thrombus, setting up a site of increased radioactivity that can be detected externally by scintillation detectors. These studies were designed to detect early thrombi and to permit the findings to be a marker for documenting the natural history of the disorder. This method was also used to monitor prophylactic methods designed to prevent the deep venous thrombosis from occurring.[66] These studies, which have been numerous, have shown that the site for the earliest development of thrombi is within the sinuses of the soleus muscle. If left untreated, up to 80% of the thrombi will resolve, but the remaining 20% will propagate to the deep veins of the calf and extend to the level of the popliteal vein.[67] Unfortunately, the iodine 125 test is relatively insensitive to thrombi that develop in the superficial femoral, common femoral, and iliac veins and the inferior vena cava.

One theory is that all thrombi originate in the calf and secondarily involve the more proximal deep veins. This is too simplistic a view since thrombi may develop de novo at the more proximal sites. For example, it is known that the sinuses of the venous valves are a site from which the thrombi may develop and then extend into the lumen, setting the stage for complete occlusion to occur.[66] In addition, the left iliofemoral segment is a site where there is usually compression by the right common iliac artery, producing some element of "stasis." Also, other factors that may be responsible for the development of deep venous thrombosis may predispose the patient to the development of deep venous thrombosis. It must also be recognized that the most dangerous thrombi are those that involve the large proximal veins since they can lead to the development of serious and, on occasion, fatal pulmonary emboli.[67] In this regard, thrombi that remain confined to the calf region rarely if ever result in serious and clinically evident pulmonary emboli.

Given these considerations it is important to review the current diagnostic methods and how they can be applied to the patient who is suspected of having the problem.

Continuous wave doppler

Since ultrasound penetrates the skin, it is only natural that the availability of such a method can be used to monitor the blood flow in those veins accessible to this form of energy.[68] When this modality is used alone, it cannot distinguish with certainty the vessels being interrogated. It is therefore necessary to use the companion artery to identify the vein of interest. For example, to evaluate the common femoral vein one first locates the common femoral artery as the landmark. The same applies to the other veins distal to the inguinal ligament. It is not possible to identify with certainty the iliac veins and the inferior vena cava, so one must infer on the basis of the flow patterns in the external iliac vein whether or not there is some proximal obstruction.

Below the knee it is possible to study the tibial and peroneal veins, but this has proven difficult in our laboratory because the veins are small and there are many of them, compounding the problem. There is hope that with the use of duplex scanning and color it may be possible to expedite the examination and permit a more comprehensive review of the vessels in this area.

Even with the problems of localization, several aspects of the Doppler findings are of clinical use.[69] The first is that the absence of flow from a major deep vein is certain evidence of its occlusion. This is particularly true for the proximal veins (popliteal to external iliac). Other bits of information can be obtained from veins that are patent by observing the flow patterns. Normally flow in the deep veins of the leg is very dependent on the pressure changes associated with each respiratory cycle. For example, as the diaphragm descends, the increase in intraabdominal pressure exceeds that found in the major deep veins of the leg. This results in a transient cessation in blood flow during inspiration that can normally be observed to the level of the popliteal vein. Below the knee these spontaneous flow patterns may not be detected, and one may be forced to compress the leg in an attempt to augment flow to assess patency of the venous segment. One factor that has been of assistance in documenting the presence of thrombi is to examine the velocity patterns below areas of thrombosis. It is well known both from the early studies done with continuous wave Doppler and, more recently, duplex scanning that flow in this circumstance is often continuous and not responsive to the intraabdominal pressure changes that occur with respiration.

When the Doppler method is compared with phlebography, the results are quite good. Overall the sensitivity should be in the range of 87% with a specificity of 88%.[68] The successful use of this method requires a very experienced technologist who understands both the principle of Doppler ultrasound and the physiologic basis for the changes that occur when the deep venous system becomes occluded. A major problem with the method is the subjective nature of the test and the interpretation of the results. One has to depend entirely on the skill of the person performing the test.

Venous outflow plethysmography

Since venous thrombi reduce outflow through the involved venous segment(s), it is only natural that a method be used that could assess the rate of venous outflow in the limbs. Flow—in the presence of venous occlusion—is diverted through collateral channels that have a higher resistance to flow than do the normal unobstructed veins. Thus one would expect that at least early after the onset of the event that the rate of venous emptying would be reduced. To this end, the strain-gauge method,[70,71] impedance plethysmography,[72] and air plethysmography have been used to make this measurement. All of these methods use a cuff placed around the thigh that is inflated to 50 mm Hg to impede venous outflow temporarily. During the phase of venous occlusion venous volume in the limb increases to reach a maximal level in approximately 2 minutes. When the maximal limb volume has been reached and is stabilized, the cuff is suddenly deflated, and the rate at which the venous blood is emptied is assessed. When the strain-gauge method is used, the volume change that occurs can be expressed in terms of centimeters per 100 cc of tissue per minute. The impedance and air plethysmographic methods cannot be quantitated in a similar manner but do permit a similar estimate that is related to the volume increase that occurs during cuff inflation.

Although the sensor is placed around the calf, the methods are only sensitive to the development of proximal venous thrombosis (popliteal to inferior vena cava). The methods are totally insensitive to thrombi in the calf region.

The venous outflow approach has been widely tested as a screening procedure and has been compared to phlebography. For proximal venous thrombosis the test has a sensitivity of 93% and a specificity of 94%.[72] It is accepted that this method is satisfactory as a screening method since a positive test is highly likely to be associated with acute deep venous thrombosis. A negative test can be used to withhold treatment with minimal risk of an unheralded pulmonary embolus occurring.

Although this method has been extensively tested, it does have problems of concern. It does not permit localization of the disease and cannot be reliably used as a method for documenting changes that occur with therapy. As the collateral circulation improves, venous outflow tends to normalize, and as the venous thrombi themselves begin to lyse, the vessels recanalize. Although new episodes or extension of the process will be reflected in a worsening of the venous outflow, it is not possible to define the basis for the change without some anatomic confirmation.

Another method that has been extensively applied for the detection of deep venous thrombosis is phleborheography developed by Cranley et al.[73,74] This is a segmental cuff method that permits an evaluation of the limb-volume response to standardized intermittent compression of cuffs placed at the level of the foot and lower leg. In patients with proximal venous thrombosis (popliteal to iliac veins) the limb-volume change is modified in a predictable manner. Normally when there is compression of the foot or calf, the volume of the more proximal limb segments does not change. In the presence of deep venous thrombosis with outflow obstruction, the limb volume will increase. This method has been extensively tested and compares favorably with the results of impedance and strain-gauge plethysmography.

Duplex scanning

Since duplex scanning provides both an image of the vein and the ability to assess flow, it is only natural that the method would also be applied to the venous system.[75] As the technology has improved with the availability of different transmitting frequencies and the ability to access vessels at greater depths, it has become possible to study all major veins that are the sites of venous thrombosis.

The value of this method is the combined anatomic and physiologic information that can be obtained. The imaging component is used in three ways: (1) to identify the vein of interest with certainty; (2) to identify the presence of an occluding thrombus (Fig. 3-19); and (3) to permit selective sampling of flow in the imaged vessels.

Although there have been reports of using imaging systems alone only to the level of the external iliac veins, this is not sufficient.[76] With the availability of low-frequency scan heads (2 to 3.5 MHz), one can see the entire iliac venous system and the inferior vena cava.[77] Anything less than this would constitute an inadequate examination. It is possible to study all the major veins below the inguinal ligament regularly to the level of the popliteal vein. The veins below the knee are more difficult, but with the addition of color to the system, it may be feasible to study these segments with regularity.

Imaging is used in two ways to identify the presence or absence of thrombi. Although the answers are not yet complete with regard to the echogenicity of thrombi, they apparently are most echogenic early.[78,79] As time passes, the lesion will become less echogenic. Seeing a thrombus is certain evidence that the vein is involved. However, failure

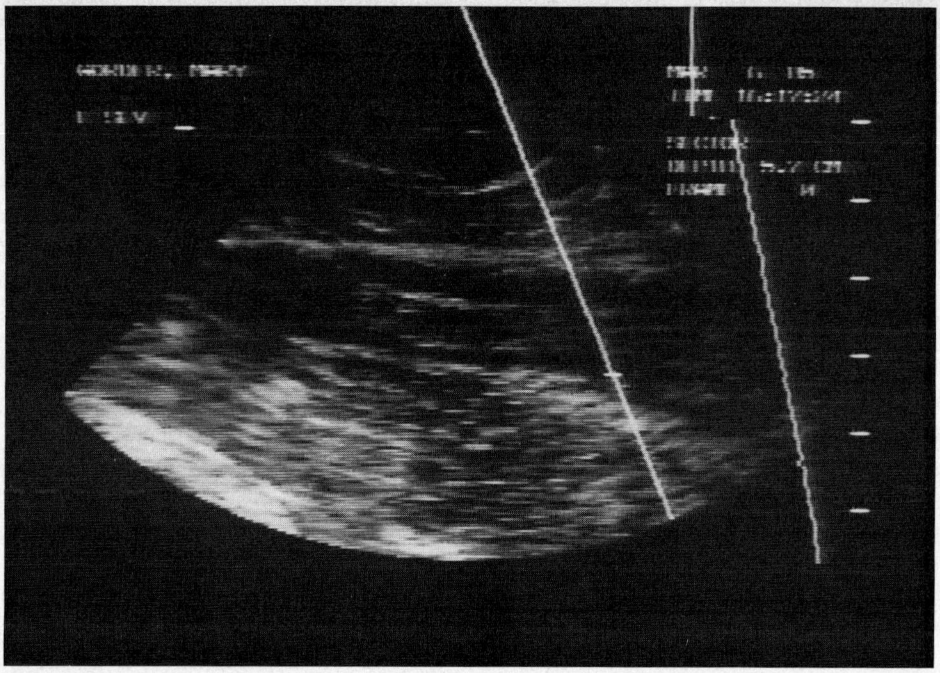

Fig. 3-19. Ultrasonic duplex scan of a superficial femoral vein showing the presence of a large thrombus.

to see a thrombus does not rule out the presence of the problem. For example, in our studies the visualization of thrombus had a positive predictive value of 95% with a negative predictive value of 50%.[77]

The other element of the imaging component that is used is the inability to compress the vein being visualized. The presumption is that a vein occluded by a thrombus will not be compressible when pressure is applied to the skin surface. Our experience is that compression is not as useful a tool as some investigators would imply, primarily because there are sites that are difficult to compress even in normal individuals. These sites include the iliac veins, the inferior vena cava, and the superficial femoral vein in the adductor canal. In our studies incompressibility had a positive predictive value of 88% with a negative predictive value of 50%.[77]

Surprisingly, the use of velocity parameters was more sensitive and specific in arriving at a diagnosis. The absence of phasicity of flow in a visualized segment had a positive predictive value of 97% and a negative predictive value of 79%. The inability to detect spontaneous flow in a venous segment had a positive predictive value of 100% and a negative predictive value of 57%. In the studies we performed, all of the false-negative cases were secondary to isolated calf vein thrombi.[77] Because of the difficulty of studying the veins of the calf, we recommend that when disease not found on the initial study is suspected in this area, the procedure should be repeated in 3 days to reassess the situation.

CHRONIC VENOUS INSUFFICIENCY

The patient who is initially seen with chronic venous problems generally falls into two categories: (1) those suspected of having primary varicose veins and (2) those whose presentation suggests the presence of underlying deep venous occlusion or valvular incompetence.[80,81] The distinction becomes important in terms of management and long-term prognosis.[82]

Patients with varicose veins as the presenting complaint generally are aware of the problem primarily in terms of the appearance of the limb, the cosmetic deformity, and the symptoms that may be associated with prolonged standing and sitting. When these patients are seen, the major question that must be answered is whether the varicose veins are secondary to defects in the superficial venous system or whether they occurred because of venous valvular incompetence of the deep veins and their communicators with the superficial system. Historically, patients with no deep venous involvement are classified into the primary category and can be treated either by the use of support hose, injection therapy, or surgical means.[80] Although these patients can be suspected because of a strong family history of the problem and no previous history of deep venous thrombosis, it is important to verify this suspicion through some noninvasive testing procedures such as screening with continuous wave Doppler or duplex scanning. Patients with varices secondary to deep venous and perforator incompetence are classified as having secondary varices.

The key issues to address in the noninvasive testing is

the patency of the deep veins and the competence of the major deep veins.[77] Competence of the deep veins is noted by the failure to induce reflux when the pressure gradient proximal to the valves is reversed by procedures such as a Valsalva maneuver, limb compression or release of the pressure in a pneumatic cuff placed around the limb.[83] The purpose is to document the status of the valves at all levels from the iliac veins to the region below the knee.

When the deep venous system has been damaged by the presence of deep venous thrombosis, there are changes occurring that explain the subsequent course of events.[84] They are as follows:

1. Production of chronic venous occlusion
2. Destruction of the venous valves at single or multiple sites
3. Lysis of the thrombi with preservation of valve function and venous patency
4. Lysis with recanalization of the involved segments but with destruction of the venous valves

The clinical problems that occur because of the above changes are well known. They include edema, pain, hyperpigmentation, and in the late stages, ulceration. In rare instances the patient may complain of pain in the involved limb that occurs with vigorous exercise and is relieved by rest.[85] We classify these patients as having *postthrombotic syndrome,* even though the more common terminology in use is *postphlebitic syndrome*. We believe this latter terminology is incorrect because it implies that the process that led to the problem had an inflammatory component, which it does not. The patient with exercise-induced leg pain secondary to chronic venous disease is termed as having *venous claudication*.

The testing procedures that might be applied are the same as those used for the patient with varicose veins except for the patient who has symptoms suggestive of venous claudication. The pathophysiology of this problem is related primarily to chronic venous obstruction and the inability of the involved limb to empty itself of the marked increase in venous volume that occurs in response to the stimulus of vigorous exercise. When this is suspected, the abnormality can be documented by carrying out measurements of venous outflow before and after a period of vigorous exercise.[86]

Another method that has been applied quite widely to assess the status of the venous valves is photoplethysmography.[87] This method uses infrared light to assess changes in the venous volume of the dermis. Its application to the study of venous disease is based on the observation that the changes in the venous volume of the dermis are similar in terms of both magnitude and time as those that occur when venous pressures are measured after a period of walking. As is well known, when a healthy individual begins to walk, there is a dramatic fall in the venous pressure measured at the level of the foot. This fall occurs with even a single step. After the walking is stopped, there is a very slow return in the pressure to the preexercise level. Although the skin blood volume change recorded with the photoplethysmograph cannot be quantitated, the directional and time-related changes can be quantitated and used as an index of venous valvular function.

The test can be performed in a variety of ways, the most widely used way has the patient sitting on the edge of a bed or examining table. The patient then dorsiflexes the foot five times, following which the changes in skin blood volume are recorded. Because it is difficult to standardize this method, we prefer to simulate exercise by inflating a pneumatic cuff to 60 mm Hg at the calf level. This inflation-deflation cycle is repeated in rapid succession five times. The variable we have found most useful is the venous recovery time.[86] This is the time required for the dermal blood volume to return to the baseline level. The normal venous recovery time in our laboratory is 24 ± 12 seconds. In patients with valvular incompetence these values are greatly shortened. If there is valvular damage, the venous recovery times are in the range of 9 seconds. This method does not permit any conclusions about the level at which the valvular incompetence is occurring. This can be sorted out to some degree by placing a tourniquet around the calf to occlude the superficial veins and then repeating the test. If the incompetence is confined to the superficial veins, the test results will normalize.

VASOSPASTIC DISORDERS

One of the more common types of patients referred to the vascular laboratory is one who, when exposed to cold, will note the development of color changes in his digits, usually the fingers but in some cases the toes as well. The clinical dilemma is to determine if the changes are of the harmless type associated with Raynaud's disease or secondary to some underlying associated disorder such as scleroderma.[88] Although the history is often useful in making this distinction, a referral to the vascular laboratory can provide useful confirmatory information concerning the status of the digital circulation. If the patient has primary Raynaud's disease, the digital arteries will be patent but hyperresponsive when exposed to cold. When the problem is secondary to an underlying disease, it is common to find the digital arteries occluded in one or more of the affected digits. This can be determined by measurement of the digit blood pressure, which can be done by the use of either strain-gauge plethysmography or photoplethysmography.[89] In addition, it is possible by examining the digit-pulse waveform to document the status of the digital vessels.[90] Normally, the digital systolic blood pressure should be greater than 80% of that recorded from the upper arm. These values are commonly seen in patients with Raynaud's disease. This gradient in pressure will not change significantly with heating.

When the digital arteries are occluded, the pressure gradient between the upper arm and the digit will widen. In addition, the shape of the digit-volume pulse will change from one with a sharp systolic peak and a dicrotic wave to one with a rounded contour in which the upslope and downslope times equalize (a damped waveform). It is also possible to study the digit blood pressure response to cooling.[89] If the patient has true cold sensitivity, the digit blood pressure will fall as the digits are cooled. This response is useful in confirming the clinical suspicion but is not helpful in defining the basis for the problem.

THORACIC OUTLET SYNDROME

When patients complain of pain, dysesthesias, and numbness in various positions of their arms, they are often referred to the vascular laboratory for screening purposes. Testing is done to assess whether or not the patient is able to diminish or completely shut off blood flow to the arm in various positions. This is done by using either a continuous wave Doppler device over the radial or brachial artery or by duplex scanning. It can also be done by checking Doppler systolic pressures or through pulse-volume recordings using the air plethysmograph. The testing is simple but does not provide any diagnostic information that cannot be obtained by a carefully performed physical examination. The problem is that there is a large number of healthy people without symptoms who can reduce or shut off blood flow in various positions of the arm. The only time the testing may be useful is when the results show no compression. Under these circumstances it is at least possible to determine that arterial compression is not the basis for the problem.

A very small number of patients will develop problems within the vessel secondary to intimal injury because of thoracic outlet compression of the subclavian artery. When this occurs, local thrombosis or embolization to the hand may take place. A duplex scan may provide some information, but in most cases an arteriogram will be needed to sort out the problem.

THE FUTURE

Although it is dangerous to attempt to predict the future of the noninvasive laboratory and its place in the field of peripheral vascular diseases, the rapid developments of the last 10 years are impressive. There has been concern about the costs of the instrumentation, particularly duplex scanning equipment, but no other diagnostic system in medicine currently offers the versatility and scope of applications that this method permits. It is remarkable to think that it is possible with this device to study every major organ system that is affected by atherosclerosis, the most common vascular disease we treat. The systems are even being modified to permit their use as a method of obtaining transcranial information—one of the new applications that is under intense study. Where will this type of study go in the future? Many of the applications of duplex scanning mentioned in this chapter are not yet in general use in the United States. The reasons are quite clear and include the following: (1) the tests in some cases require further study to document their relevance, accuracy, and cost-effectiveness in addressing the problems at hand; (2) the tests in some cases are quite time-consuming, raising the question about the costs of the procedures and the numbers of examinations that can be performed on a daily basis; (3) as the applications expand, the skills required of the technologists also increase (it is apparent that the noninvasive laboratory is only as good as the technologists who are involved); (4) the time required to train a technologist to do the entire battery of examinations is increasing because of the complexity of the testing procedures; and (5) the concern that the use of these tests does not in reality represent a saving of money for the health care delivery system but simply adds to it.

Are some of these tests performed in the noninvasive laboratory going to eliminate some of the more costly and dangerous invasive methods? The answer to this is yes if one is willing to accept certain assumptions. Some examples in which this has occurred and will continue to do so are as follows:

1. *Screening for carotid artery disease*. If one does not use a method such as duplex scanning, the only way to verify the extent of involvement in the carotid bulb is by arteriography. A concrete example of this is the asymptomatic patient with a cervical bruit. If one accepts the thesis that it is important to document the basis for the bruit and reserve arteriography only for that subset of patients with very tight lesions (greater than 80% diameter reduction), duplex scanning will remove from consideration more than 90% of the patients who present in this fashion.[34] This method represents a step forward not only for the patient but also for the costs to the health care delivery system.
2. *Diagnosis of deep venous thrombosis*. Without the availability of noninvasive testing this most common vascular disorder could be diagnosed by only one test, venography. With the extensive studies done using the Doppler and plethysmographic methods, it is clear that most patients with this problem can be spared the invasive procedure. The more recent application of duplex scanning has further reduced the need for venography.[75-77] It is certain that this will become the definitive test of the future for this problem and for the evaluation of the patient with chronic venous insufficiency.
3. *Documentation of therapeutic outcome*. In the past most therapies for vascular disease were gauged by the subjective responses of the patient and the effects noted by the physician on the status of the variables that could be evaluated on physical examinations. The mysteries surrounding this type of evaluation process are no longer a problem. The outcome for practically all therapies can now be objectively and repeatedly tested by a variety of noninvasive tests.

One area that is being slowly and cautiously examined is the possibility of eliminating arteriography before direct surgical therapy. This concept would in many circles be considered heretical given the dependence we have developed on the need to image by arteriographic means the arteries to be modified by surgical means. The areas in which this elimination might be feasible at the moment are the carotid arteries and those of the lower limbs. Given the accuracy of duplex scanning for the accurate detection and quantification of the degree of narrowing, there is no hesitancy in predicting what would be found at the time of operation. The concerns have been related to the lack of information concerning other areas that might affect the results, including the carotid siphon and inside the skull. Most intracranial abnormalities such as aneurysms, tumors, and arteriovenous malformations can be detected by CT scanning. This leaves the carotid siphon as a source of concern. However, it is currently clear that it is rare for lesions at this level to play an important role in the outcome when there is significant involvement of the carotid bulb.[91]

For reconstructions of the limb arteries the question is more difficult because of the total length of the arteries that must be surveyed and the type of information that vascular surgeons need to make judgments about the surgical approaches most likely to lead to a good outcome. On the other hand, vascular surgeons have known for many years that arteriography tends to underestimate the degree of involvement, particularly in the estimation of stenotic lesions. This is due to the fact that it is the posterior wall of the arteries that is most frequently involved and not seen well on arteriography, particularly when the views shown are not biplanar. What type of information is necessary to proceed with an interventional procedure? This can be summarized as follows:

1. *The location and hemodynamic significance of stenotic lesions, particularly in the aortoiliac and femoropopliteal segments.* Prospective studies done to compare the accuracy of duplex scanning to arteriography have shown that the duplex method is as accurate as the invasive method in defining the significance of such lesions. In fact, the variability that is found when two radiologists read the same arteriograms is at least as great as that encountered when duplex scanning is compared to the results of a single angiographer.[14]
2. *The status of the run-off vessels.* How are these vessels defined? In general, they are all the arteries distal to the point at which the reconstruction ends. For example, in the case of aortoiliac reconstructions it would be the femoropopliteal and below-the-knee arteries. For femoropopliteal and femorotibial reconstructions it is those arteries distal to the lowermost anastomosis. At the moment there is evidence that duplex scanning can be used to predict accurately the status of the femoropopliteal segments and also to assess the patency of the tibial arteries.

To test the hypothesis that the duplex scanning results can be adequate in predicting the type of reconstruction that would be needed, we provided both duplex scanning and arteriographic data, along with pertinent clinical data, to six experienced vascular surgeons in a blinded fashion to determine what the form of therapy would be.[92] The information on the location and extent of involvement was presented on anatomic charts along with an estimate of the degree of narrowing. It was clear that in most cases the duplex data were accurate enough to permit making a reasonable decision about the surgical procedure to use.

To replace arteriography with a combination of indirect tests such as obtaining ankle pressures, exercise testing, and duplex scanning represents such a departure from conventional thinking that it will require considerable study, but it is a direction that needs further investigation. We have in fact found that duplex scanning results can be sufficient for the planning of transluminal angioplasty, particularly for patients with aortoiliac disease. The finding of a hemodynamically significant stenotic lesion in this area is sufficient evidence that we can proceed with the angioplasty as the planned procedure.

Are there new technologies that may affect the role of the noninvasive laboratory and its use in the evaluation of vascular disease? The two methods that might fall into this area are CT scanning and magnetic resonance imaging (MRI). CT scanning has had its greatest impact in the evaluation of aneurysmal disease, particularly as it relates to the evaluation of thoracoabdominal lesions that are difficult to evaluate by ultrasound alone. MRI, with its potential for not only anatomic but flow information, is under intensive study.

How can MRI be of value in vascular disease evaluation? Its value can be summarized as follows:

1. *Anatomy of the vascular system.* It remains to be determined if it will be better when applied in a fashion similar to that for CT scanning.[93,94] There is evidence that the method is able to detect thrombi, but it is also true that turbulent flow may give images that are similar, making the distinction a difficult one at the moment.
2. *MRI angiography.* There is evidence that arteriograms, particularly of the thoracoabdominal vessels, can be generated that are very similar to those obtained with conventional arteriographic means.[95] Resolution with smaller arteries such as the carotid and femoropopliteal segments remains a very serious problem. The resolution currently available is similar to that seen with intravenous digital subtraction arteriography, which most clinicians find inadequate for clinical purposes. Even if it had the same resolution as standard contrast studies, we are faced with very serious logistic problems that will continue to plague the use of this method. Disregarding the costs of such systems, the demands placed on them is such that it makes MRI an impractical method at the moment. For example, it is very likely that such systems would have to be used for this purpose alone to justify their appli-

cation. The cost of the systems and the cost associated with installation and maintenance make it very unlikely that the current health care delivery system could afford such expense.

3. *Measurement of volume flow.* Such measurement with the system is possible.[96,97] In fact, prototype MRI systems designed for just this purpose are under study. At the moment attention has been directed to the lower limbs in which it appears the method may have some promise. However, before such a method is applied clinically, it must be shown that such information is of clinical value. All of the studies done in the past to examine the value of volume flow measurements have been disappointing. Whether the same type of information gathered by this new modality will be any better or any more useful is definitely open to question.
4. *Potentially, the study of the metabolic activity of skeletal muscle in the normal and ischemic state.* At the moment this is a research tool with some promise and should be pursued. Whether it will have an impact on the clinical appraisal of vascular disease remains to be demonstrated.

REFERENCES

1. Strandness DE Jr: Peripheral arterial disease: a physiological approach, Boston, 1969, Little, Brown & Co, Inc.
2. Lindbom A: Arteriosclerosis and arterial thrombosis in the lower limb. A roentgenological study, Acta Radiol Suppl 80:1, 1950.
3. McKusick VA et al: Buerger's disease: a distinct clinical and pathologic entity, JAMA 181:5, 1962.
4. Strandness DE Jr: Thromboangiitis obliterans. In Peripheral arterial disease: a physiologic approach, Boston, 1969, Little, Brown & Co, Inc.
5. Gensler SW et al: Study of vascular lesions in diabetic, nondiabetic patients, Arch Surg 9:617, 1965.
6. Strandness DE Jr, Priest RE, and Gibbons GE: A combined clinical and pathologic study of diabetic and nondiabetic peripheral arterial disease, Diabetes 13:366, 1964.
7. Winsor TA: Influence of arterial disease on the systolic blood pressure gradients of the extremity, Am J Med Sci 220:117, 1950.
8. Strandness DE Jr, McCutcheon EP, and Rushmer RF: Application of a transcutaneous Doppler flowmeter in the evaluation of occlusive arterial disease, Surg Gynecol Obstet 122:1039, 1966.
9. Carter SA: Role of pressure measurements in vascular disease. In Bernstein EF, ed.: Noninvasive diagnostic techniques in vascular disease, St Louis, 1978, The CV Mosby Co.
10. Taylor MG: Wave travel in arteries and design of the cardiovascular system. In Attinger EO, ed: Pulsatile blood flow, New York, 1964, McGraw-Hill Book Co.
11. Strandness DE Jr and Sumner DS: The effect of geometry on arterial blood flow. In Strandness DE Jr and Sumner DS, eds.: Hemodynamics for surgeons, New York, 1975, Grune & Stratton, Inc.
12. Strandness DE Jr and Bell JW: Peripheral vascular disease: diagnosis and objective evaluation using a mercury strain gauge, Am Surg 161(suppl):1-35, 1965.
13. Raines JK: Use of pulse volume recorder in peripheral arterial disease. In Bernstein EF, ed.: Noninvasive diagnostic techniques in vascular disease, ed 3, St Louis, 1985, The CV Mosby Co.
14. Jager KA, Ricketts HJ, and Strandness DE Jr: Duplex scanning for the evaluation of lower limb arterial disease. In Bernstein EF, ed.: Noninvasive diagnostic techniques in vascular disease, ed 3, St Louis, 1985, The CV Mosby Co.
15. Strandness DE Jr: Intermittent claudication. In Gifford R, ed.: Peripheral vascular disease, Philadelphia, 1971, FA Davis Co.
16. Silver RA et al: Intermittent claudication of neurospinal origin, Arch Surg 98:523, 1969.
17. Kavanaugh GJ et al: "Pseudoclaudication" syndrome produced by compression of the equina, JAMA 206:2477, 1968.
18. Stahler C and Strandness DE Jr: Ankle blood pressure response to graded treadmill exercise, Angiology 18:237, 1967.
19. Sumner DS and Strandness DE Jr: The relationship between calf blood flow and ankle blood pressure in patients with intermittent claudication, Surgery 65:763, 1969.
20. Strandness DE Jr and Zierler RE: Exercise ankle pressure measurements in arterial disease. In Bernstein EF, ed.: Noninvasive diagnostic techniques in vascular disease, ed 3, St Louis, 1985, The CV Mosby Co.
21. Kohler TR et al: Duplex scanning for diagnosis of aortoiliac and femoropopliteal disease, Circulation 5:1074, 1987.
22. Leather RP and Kupinski AM: Preoperative evaluation of the saphenous vein as a suitable graft, Semin Vasc Surg 1:51, 1988.
23. Bandyk DF: Monitoring functional patency of vascular grafts, Semin Vasc Surg 1:40, 1988.
24. Katzen BT: Percutaneous transluminal angioplasty in peripheral vascular disease. In Haimovici H et al, eds.: Vascular Surgery, ed 3, Norwalk, Conn, 1989, Appleton & Lange.
25. Yao JST: Surgical uses of pressure studies in peripheral arterial disease. In Bernstein EF, ed.: Noninvasive diagnostic techniques in vascular disease, ed 3, St Louis, 1985, The CV Mosby Co.
26. Collins J et al: Oxford screening program for abdominal aortic aneurysm in men 65-74 years, Lancet:613, 1988.
27. Bernstein EF, Harris R, and Leopold GR: Noninvasive evaluation of abdominal aortic aneurysm by ultrasonic imaging and computed tomography scanning. In Bernstein EF, ed.: Noninvasive diagnostic techniques in vascular disease, ed 3, St Louis, 1985, The CV Mosby Co.
28. Haimovici H: Peripheral arterial aneurysms. In Haimovici H et al, eds.: Vascular surgery, ed 3, Norwalk, Conn, 1989, Appleton & Lange.
29. Barnes RW et al: The Doppler cerebrovascular examination: Improved results with refinements in technique, Stroke 8:468, 1977.
30. Kartchner MM, McRae LP, and Morrison FD: Noninvasive detection and evaluation of carotid occlusive disease, Arch Surg 106:528, 1973.
31. Gee W: Carotid physiology with occular pneumoplethysmography, Stroke 5:666, 1982.
32. Langlois YE et al: Evaluation of carotid artery disease. The concordance between pulsed Doppler spectrum analysis and angiography, Ultrasound Med Biol 9:51, 1983.
33. Langlois YE, Roederer GO, and Strandness DE Jr: Ultrasonic evaluation of the carotid bifurcation, Echocardiography 4:141, 1987.
34. Roederer GO et al: The natural history of carotid arterial disease in asymptomatic patients with cervical bruits, Stroke 15:605, 1984.
35. Moneta GL et al: Operative versus nonoperative management of asymptomatic high-grade internal carotid artery stenosis: improved results with endarterectomy, Stroke 18:1005, 1987.
36. Nicholls SC et al: Carotid endarterectomy: relationship of outcome to early restenosis, J Vasc Surg 2:375, 1985.
37. Reivich M et al: Reversal of blood flow through the vertebral artery and its effects on cerebral circulation, N Engl J Med 265:878, 1961.
38. Bornstein NM and Norris JW: Subclavian steal? A harmless hemodynamic phenomenon? Lancet 2:303, 1986.
39. Nicholls SC, Koutlas T, and Strandness DE Jr: Unpublished data.
40. Aaslid R, Markwaider TM, and Nornes H: Noninvasive transcranial Doppler ultrasound recording of flow velocity in basal cerebral arteries, J Neurosurg 57:769, 1982.

41. Kirkham FJ et al: Transcranial measurement of blood velocities in the basal cerebral arteries using pulsed Doppler ultrasound: velocity as index of flow, Ultrasound Med Biol 12:15, 1986.
42. Padayachee TS et al: Monitoring middle cerebral artery blood velocity during endarterectomy, Br J Surg 73:98, 1986.
43. Hennerici M, Rautenberg W, and Schwartz A: Transcranial Doppler ultrasound for assessment of intracranial artery occlusive disorders, Surg Neurol 27:523, 1987.
44. Harders AG and Gilsbach JM: Time course of blood velocity changes related to vasospasm in the Circle of Willis measured by transcranial Doppler ultrasound, J Neurosurg 66:718, 1987.
45. Harper AM and Glass HE: Effect of alterations in the arterial carbon dioxide tension in the blood flow through the cerebral cortex at normal and low arterial blood pressures, J Neurol Neurosurg Psychiatry 28:449, 1966.
46. Gifford RW: Epidemiology and clinical manifestation of renovascular hypertension. In Stanley J, Ernst C, and Fry W, eds.: Renovascular hypertension, Philadelphia, 1984, WB Saunders Co.
47. Ernst CB: Renal artery reconstruction. In Haimovici H et al, eds.: Vascular surgery, ed 3, Norwalk, Conn, 1989, Appleton & Lange.
48. Treadway KK and Slater EE: Renovascular hypertension, Ann Rev Med 35:665, 1984.
49. Vaughan ED: Renovascular hypertension, Kidney Int 27:811, 1985.
50. Kohler TR et al: Noninvasive diagnosis of renal artery stenosis by ultrasonic duplex scanning, J Vasc Surg 4:450, 1986.
51. Taylor DC et al: Duplex scanning in the diagnosis of renal artery stenosis: a prospective evaluation, J Vasc Surg 7:363, 1988.
52. Taylor DC, Moneta GL, and Strandness DE Jr: Follow-up of renal artery stenosis by duplex ultrasound, J Vasc Surg 9:410, 1989.
53. Rigsby CM et al: Doppler signal quantitation in renal allografts. Comparison in normal and rejecting transplants, with pathologic correlation, Radiology 162:31, 1987.
54. Reinite ER et al: Evaluation of transplant renal artery blood flow by Doppler sound-spectrum analysis, Arch Surg 118:415, 1983.
55. Fleischer AC et al: Duplex Doppler sonography of renal transplants. Correlation with histopathology, J Ultrasound Med 8:89, 1989.
56. Genkins SM, Sanflippo FD, and Carroll BA: Duplex sonography of renal transplants: lack of sensitivity and specificity in establishing pathologic diagnosis, AJR 152:535, 1989.
57. Taylor DC: Evaluation of mesenteric and renal vascular disease. In Strandness DE Jr and Taylor KW, eds.: Duplex doppler ultrasound, New York, 1989, Churchill Livingstone, Inc.
58. Jager KA et al: Noninvasive diagnosis of intestinal angina, J Clin Ultrasound 12:588, 1984.
59. Nicholls SC et al: Use of hemodynamic parameters in the diagnosis of mesenteric insufficiency, J Vasc Surg 3:507, 1986.
60. Jager K et al: Measurement of mesenteric blood flow by duplex scanning, J Vasc Surg 3:462, 1986.
61. Moneta GL et al: Duplex ultrasound measurement of postprandial intestinal blood flow: effect of meal composition, Gastroenterology 95:1294, 1988.
62. Haeger K: Problem of acute deep venous thrombosis. The interpretation of symptoms and signs, Angiology 20:219, 1969.
63. Rabinov K and Paulin S: Roentgen diagnosis of venous thrombosis, Arch Surg 104:134, 1972.
64. Athanasoulis CA: Phlebography for diagnosis of deep leg vein thrombosis and pulmonary embolism, DHEW Pub (NIH) No. 76-866, Washington DC, 1975.
65. Hobbs JT: External measurement of fibrinogen uptake in experimental venous thrombosis and other pathological states, Br J Exp Pathol 43:48, 1962.
66. Nicolaides AN, Kakkar VV, and Renney JTG: Soleus sinuses and stasis, Br J Surg 58:307, 1971.
67. Kakkar VV et al: Natural history of deep vein thrombosis, Lancet 2:230, 1969.
68. Strandness DE Jr and Thiele BL: Venous thrombosis and pulmonary embolism. In Selected topics in vascular disorders, Mt Kisco, NY, 1981, Futura Publishing Co.
69. Sumner DS: Doppler evaluation of the venous circulation. In Rutherford RB, ed.: Vascular surgery, Philadelphia, 1977, WB Saunders Co.
70. Barnes RW et al: Noninvasive quantitation of maximum venous outflow in acute thrombophlebitis, Surgery 72:971, 1973.
71. Sumner DS: Strain gauge plethysmography. In Bernstein EF, ed.: Noninvasive diagnostic techniques in vascular disease, ed 3, St Louis, 1985, The CV Mosby Co.
72. Wheeler HB and Anderson FA: The diagnosis of venous thrombosis by impedance plethysmography. In Bernstein EF, ed.: Noninvasive diagnostic techniques in vascular disease, ed 3, St Louis, 1985, The CV Mosby Co.
73. Cranley JJ et al: Phleborheographic technique for diagnosing deep venous thrombosis of the lower extremities, Surg Gynecol Obstet 414:331, 1975.
74. Cranely JJ: Diagnosis of deep vein thrombosis by phleborheography. In Bernstein EF, ed.: Noninvasive diagnostic techniques in vascular disease, ed 3, St Louis, 1985, The CV Mosby Co.
75. Sullivan ED, Peter DJ, and Cranely JJ: Real-time B-mode venous ultrasound, J Vasc Surg 1:465, 1984.
76. Lensing AWA et al: Detection of deep-vein thrombosis by real-time B-mode ultrasonography, N Engl J Med 320:342, 1989.
77. Killewich LA et al: Diagnosis of deep-venous thrombosis: a prospective study comparing duplex scanning to contrast venography, Circulation 79:810, 1989.
78. Coehlo JCV et al: B-mode ultrasonography of blood clots, J Clin Ultrasound 10:323, 1982.
79. Alanen A and Kormand M: Correlation of the echogenicity and structure of clotted blood, J Ultrasound Med 4:421, 1985.
80. Strandness DE Jr and Thiele BL: Varicose veins. In Selected topics in venous disorder, Mt Kisco, NY, 1981, Futura Publishing Co, Inc.
81. Strandness DE Jr and Thiele BL: Postthrombotic venous insufficiency. In Selected topics in venous disorders, Mt Kisco, NY, 1981, Futura Publishing Co, Inc.
82. Strandness DE Jr et al: Long-term sequelae of acute venous thrombosis, JAMA 250:1289, 1983.
83. van Bemmelen PS et al: Quantitative segmental evaluation of venous valvular reflux with ultrasonic duplex scanning, J Vasc Suirg 10:425, 1990.

84. Killewich LA et al: Spontaneous lysis of deep venous thrombosis. Rate and outcome, J Vasc Surg 9:89, 1989.
85. Killewich LA et al: Pathophysiology of venous claudication, J Vasc Surg 1:507, 1984.
86. Killewich LA et al: An objective assessment of the physiologic changes in the postthrombotic syndrome, Arch Surg 120:424, 1985.
87. Flinn WR et al: The use of photoplethysmography in the assessment of chronic venous insufficiency. In Kempczinski RF, ed.: Practical noninvasive vascular diagnosis, Chicago, 1982, Year Book Medical Publishers.
88. Carter SA: Clinical problem in peripheral arterial disease: is the clinical diagnosis adequate? In Bernstein EF, ed.: Noninvasive diagnostic techniques in vascular disease, ed 3, St Louis, 1985, The CV Mosby Co.
89. Nielsen SL and Lassen NA: Finger systolic pressure in upper extremity testing for cold sensitivity (Raynaud's phenomenon). In Bernstein, EF, ed.: Noninvasive diagnostic techniques in vascular disease, ed 3, St Louis, 1985, The CV Mosby Co.
90. Thulesius O: Problems in the evaluation of hand ischemia. In Bernstein EF, ed.: Noninvasive diagnostic techniques in vascular disease, ed 3, St Louis, 1985, The CV Mosby Co.
91. Roederer GO et al: Is siphon disease important in predicting outcome of carotid endarterectomy, Arch Surg 118:1177, 1983.
92. Kohler TR et al: Can duplex scanning replace arteriography for lower extremity arterial disease? Ann Vasc Surg 4:280, 1990.
93. Kimmey MB et al: Cross-sectional imagery method: a system to compare ultrasound, computed tomography and magnetic resonance with histologic findings, Invest Radiol 22:227, 1987.
94. Hale JD et al: MR imaging of blood vessels using three-dimensional reconstruction methodology, Radiology 157, 727, 1985.
95. Herfkens RJ et al: Nuclear magnetic resonance imaging of the cardiovascular system: normal and pathologic fundings, Radiology 147:749, 1983.
96. Shimizu K et al: Visualization of moving fluid: quantitative analysis of blood flow velocity using MR imaging, Radiology 159:195, 1986.
97. Barth K et al: Visualization and measurement of flow with magnetic resonance imaging, Biomed Tech 30:12, 1985.

Chapter 4

COAGULATION, COAGULATION DISORDERS, AND ANTITHROMBOTIC THERAPY

William R. Bell
Seth D. Bilazarian

COAGULATION

Hemostasis is a physiologic process that prevents exsanguination after injury and involves the blood vessels, platelets, soluble plasma factors, protease inhibitors, and the fibrinolytic system. The first reaction to occur, or the primary response, involves vasoconstriction of a blood vessel and the formation of a platelet plug. This is a temporary measure that awaits stabilization and reinforcement from the extrinsic and intrinsic coagulation systems. This reinforcement is often referred to as the secondary response to hemostasis and results in the formation of a more stable fibrin clot. Last in this process is fibrinolysis, in which the fibrin clots are broken down or dissolved as blood vessels are repaired.

In 1905 Morawitz assembled prothrombin, thromboplastin, thrombin, fibrinogen, and fibrin into the classic theory of coagulation. The current scheme of coagulation (Fig. 4-1) outlines a cascade mechanism, proceeding through either of two pathways, the intrinsic and extrinsic systems, both of which terminate in a final common pathway. This scheme accommodates amplification and negative-feedback mechanisms, provides the coagulation process with critical sites of control, and allows for interactions with other systems.[1-8] Many of the substances currently involved in the clotting cascade (Table 4-1) have been assigned a Roman numeral (by the International Committee on Nomenclature of Blood Clotting Factors).

Extrinsic pathway of coagulation

The extrinsic pathway of coagulation is initiated when tissue factor (thromboplastin) is released from the membranes of endothelial cells after injury or insult. Tissue factor accelerates the activation of factor X in the common pathway by factor VIIa in the presence of calcium ions.

Intrinsic pathway of coagulation

The intrinsic pathway involves more protein-protein interactions and thus proceeds considerably more slowly than the extrinsic system. Intrinsic clotting initially was demonstrated in vitro by allowing plasma to clot in a glass test tube. This phenomenon is affected by the contact factors: factors XII, XI, high–molecular-weight kininogen, and prekallikrein. Hageman factor (factor XII), a sialoglycoprotein, is the plasma component affected by the high negative charge of glass. Activation is apparently accomplished without a reduction in molecular structure; however, conformational modifications are induced by in vivo activators of factor XII (e.g., collagen, endotoxin, platelet and endothelial membranes) and by ellagic acid, trypsin, or heparin. High–molecular-weight kininogen serves as a carrier protein for prekallikrein and factor XI and serves as a cofactor to orient the contact factors on negatively charged surfaces, thereby maximizing their surface interaction and activation. Whether prekallikrein and high–molecular-weight kininogen are needed to activate factor XII in vivo or are needed

Table 4-1. Plasma coagulation factors*

Factor ⟨synonym⟩	Physical and chemical properties	Site of synthesis	Biologic half-life (h)	Volume of distribution (mpv)	Concentration for hemostasis, %	Deficiency state: Prevalence cases/10^6 population	Deficiency state: IP
1 I ⟨Fibrinogen⟩	GP; mol wt, 340,000; pI, 5.5; PPTA, 25%	Liver	95-120	2.5	20	Hypofibrinogenemia[1] or afibrinogenemia, <0.5	AR
2 II ⟨Prothrombin⟩	GP, α-globulin; mol wt, 73,000; pI, 4.2; PPTA, 50%; AdB, AdK	Liver[2]	72	1.5-2.5	20	Hypoprothrombinemia, <0.5	AR
3 III ⟨Thromboplastin⟩	LP	All body tissues	—	—	—	Not reported	—
4 IV ⟨Calcium⟩	Divalent cation; mol wt, 40	—	—	—	—	—	—
5 V ⟨Proaccelerin, plasma Ac-globulin⟩	GP; mol wt, 300,000; pI, 5.3; PPTA, 50%	Liver	12-36	2	10-20	Factor V deficiency, <0.5	AR
7 VII ⟨SPCA, proconvertin⟩	GP, α-β-globulin[3]; mol wt, 48,000-100,000; PPTA, 50%; AdB, AdK	Liver[2]	4-6	2-4	10	Factor VII deficiency, <0.5	AR
8 VIII ⟨antihemophilic globulin, AHG, antihemophilic factor, AHF⟩	GP, α-β-globulin[3]; mol wt, 2,000,000[4]; PPTA, 33%	Hepatocytes	6-10[6]; 15-18[7]	1-1.5	30-40	Hemophilia A, 60-80	X-LR
VIII: VWF Ag (von Willebrand protein)	GP α-β-globulin[3]; mol wt, 30,000,000; PPTA, 33%	Vascular, endothelial cells, megakaryocytes	18-24	1-1.5	60	Von Willebrand's disease, 80-100	AD AR
9 IX ⟨Plasma thromboplastin component, PTC, Christmas factor⟩	GP, α-β-globulin[3]; mol wt, 55,000-70,000; pI, 4.50; PPTA, 50%; AdB, AdK	Liver[2]	6-10[6]; 25-30[7]	2-3	30-40	Hemophilia B (Christmas disease), 15-20	X-LR
10 X ⟨Stuart-Prower factor⟩	GP, α-globulin; mol wt, 55,000; pI, 5.5; PPTA, 50%; AdB, AdK	Liver[2]	40-50	1	10-20	Stuart-Prower deficiency, <0.5	AR
11 XI ⟨Plasma thromboplastin antecedent, PTA⟩	β- or γ-globulin; mol wt, 200,000; pI, 4-5.0; PPTA, 33%; AdK	Liver[5]	50-80	1	10-20	PTA trait, <1.0	AR[8]

12 XII (Hageman factor)	Sialo-GP; β-γ-globulin[9]; mol wt, 100,000; PPTA, 50%; AdK	Liver	50-60	—	—	Hageman trait, <1.0	AR
13 XIII (Fibrin-stabilizing factor)	α_2-globulin; mol wt, 350,000; PPTA, 33%	Liver[5]; ? megakaryocytes	95-120	1-2	1-2	Factor XIII deficiency, <0.5	AR
Protein C	GP; mol wt, 102,000; PPTA, 40%	Liver[2]	6-8	1-2	10-20	1-5	AR
Protein S	GP; mol wt, 78,000; PPTA, 40%	Endothelial cells[3]; hepatocytes[2]	42.5	1-2	10-20	<1	AR
Protein Z	GP; mol wt, 62,000; PPTA, 40%	Endothelial cells[3]; hepatocytes[2]	60	1-2	10-20	?	?

*All factors listed are present in plasma except III, and all are present in serum except for I, II, III, V, and VIII, although XIII is decreased to trace quantities. Factors I, VIII, and XIII are present in Cohn's fraction I; factors II, V, VII, IX, X, XI, and XII are present in Cohn's fraction III; and factors II, VII, IX, XI and XII are present in Cohn's fraction IV. Recently the following not previously reported factors have been detected: Fletcher (pre-kininogenin [prekallikrein]), Fitzgerald (high–molecular-weight kininogen, also designated as Williams trait, Flaujeac trait), Passovay (bleeding diathesis—prolonged partial thromboplastin time, normal known coagulation factors, autosomal dominant). Roman numerals have not yet been assigned. Factor VI is not listed because it is obsolete.

Physical and chemical properties: GP, glycoprotein; LP, lipoprotein; pI, isoelectric point; PPTA, degree of saturation of $(NH_4)_2SO_4$ solution necessary for precipitation of factor; AdK, adsorbed by Celite (infusorial earth) or kaolin or carboxymethyl cellulose (CMC); AdB, adsorbed by $BaSO_4$ or $Al(OH)_3$ or $Ca_3(PO_4)_2$. *Volume of distribution:* mpv, multiples of plasma volume, i.e., the number given, multiplied by the plasma volume, gives the total volume in which the factor is located. *Concentration for hemostasis* gives the approximate concentration required to produce hemostasis, in percent of normal concentration. *Deficiency state* is a condition in which the coagulation factor level in a given patient is below the acceptable normal level. IP, Inheritance pattern; AD, autosomal dominant; AR, autosomal recessive; X-LR, sex-linked recessive.

[1] Some pedigrees reported to have hypofibrinogenemia may be examples of dysfibrinogenemia; this condition is inherited as an autosomal dominant. [2] Synthesis is vitamin K dependent. [3] The factor migrates in an electrophoretic field between α- and β-globulins. [4] Molecular weight of procoagulant subunit is ~200,000. [5] Data are suggestive, but conclusive evidence is not yet available. [6] Initial; the shorter initial half-lives for factors VIII and IX are probably due to distribution into extravascular compartments. [7] Secondary. [8] Reported to be inherited both as an autosomal recessive and as an autosomal dominant. [9] The factor migrates in an electrophoretic field between β- and γ-globulins.

for the expression of the coagulant properties of factor XIIa is unclear. Plasmin enzymatically cleaves factor XIIa to factor XII fragments, completing the loop for regulation of factor XII activation in the kinin system (see Fig. 4-1).

Two substrates are susceptible to the actions of factor XIIa: plasminogen proactivator and factor XI, a serine protease glycoprotein. Factor XI, synthesized in the liver, is activated by factor XIIa and catalyzed by high–molecular-weight kininogen. Factor XIa converts factor IX to its activated form, factor IXa, in the presence of calcium ions. Factor IX activation can be accomplished in vitro through interactions with factor Xa, kallikrein, or the reaction product of tissue thromboplastin and factor VII. Factor VIIIa is composed of two principal parts: factor VIII:C and factor VIII:vWFAg. Factor VIII is noncovalently bound to the von Willebrand factor (f VIII:vWFAg), which is a glycoprotein that normally circulates in plasma as a series of multimers, with molecular weights ranging from 850,000 to 30,000,000 daltons. The von Willebrand factor mediates the adherence of platelets to the subendothelial collagen fibrils and the in vitro aggregation of platelets by ristocetin.

The site(s) of synthesis of factor VIII:C is believed to be the hepatocyte, whereas factor VIII:vWFAg is produced by both endothelial cells and megakaryocytes. Available data suggest that factor VIII components circulate as a noncovalently linked single molecule, but where these subunits are assembled is unknown. The association of factor VIII:vWFAg with factor VIII:C serves to stabilize the procoagulant function.

The exact function of factor VIII:C procoagulant activity in the intrinsic clotting pathway is unclear. Factor VIII appears to form a complex with factor IXa, phospholipid, and calcium ions, possibly to mediate the activation of factor X (see Fig. 4-1). Thrombin (factor IIa) is eventually elaborated in trace amounts and serves to activate factor VIII activity in plasma. When larger amounts of thrombin are produced, factor VIIIa is inactivated through the protein C system. Plasmin has also been shown to inactivate factor VIII in plasma.

Factor X activation can be accomplished by the products derived from either the intrinsic or extrinsic pathway (see Fig. 4-1). As such, it represents the beginning of the common pathway of coagulation. In vitro assays are based on the direct conversion of factor X to factor Xa by proteases such as trypsin or Russell's viper venom. Factor X (Stuart-Prower factor) is a glycoprotein with a molecular weight of 55,000 and is composed of two polypeptide chains, one heavy and one light. Activation is achieved by proteolytic cleavage of the heavy chain to yield factor Xa, a serum protease inhibited by antithrombin III–heparin complexes produced during anticoagulation. This interaction forms the rationale for using low doses of heparin to provide effective prophylaxis against thrombotic events. One microgram of the inhibitor-heparin complex can neutralize 32 units of factor Xa and thus can indirectly prevent the formation of

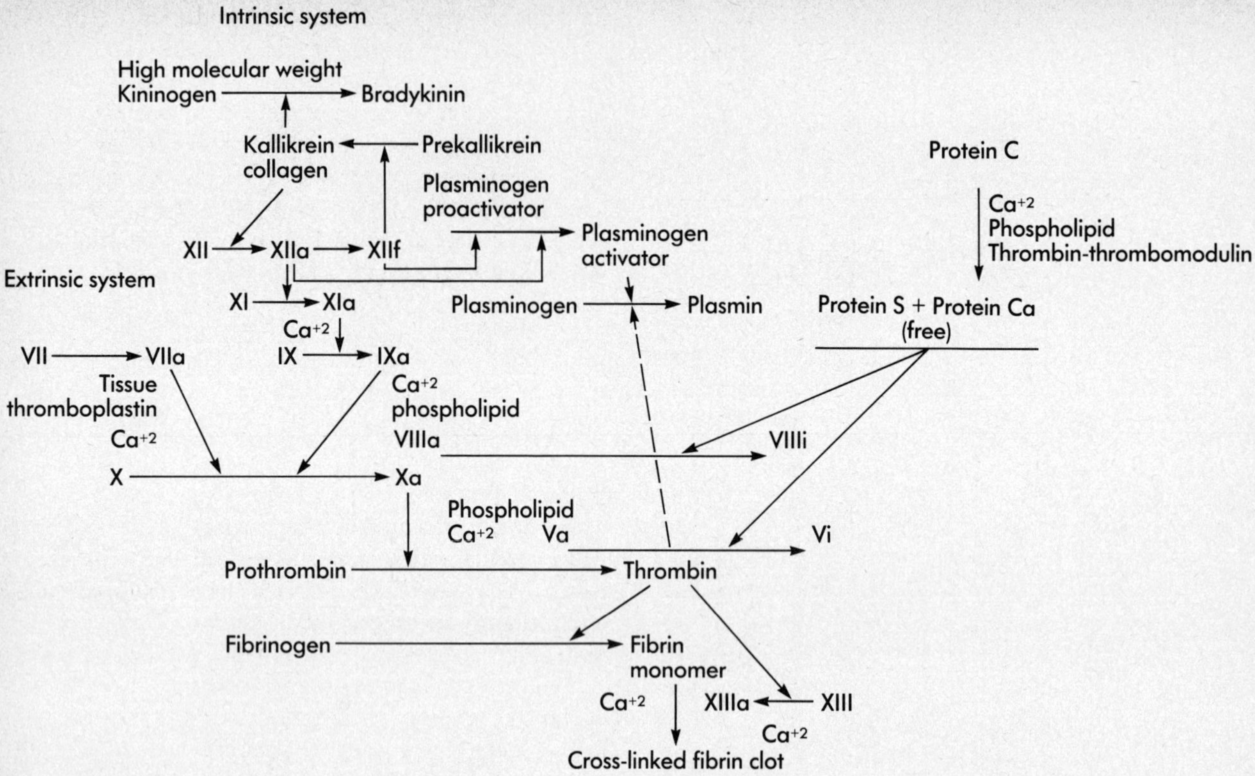

Fig. 4-1. Pathways of interaction between the components of the coagulation cascade.

1600 units of thrombin, which would otherwise be available for subsequent clot formation.

Laboratory evidence suggests that factor Xa may potentiate the activities of factors VII and IX. More importantly, factor Xa can bind to a phospholipid membrane surface where it can cleave peptides from the prothrombin molecule (factor II) in the presence of calcium ions to generate thrombin. Factor V (proaccelerin) is necessary in this reaction as a critically important procoagulant protein involved in the common pathway.

Efforts to purify and characterize factor V have been hampered by its inherent instability and lability. Factor V is found in plasma, endothelial cells, and alpha granules of platelets. With a molecular weight of approximately 300,000, this glycoprotein participates in prothrombin activation as a catalyst of factor Xa activity, possibly by increasing the affinities of factor Xa and prothrombin for the phospholipid template on which thrombin is eventually generated. Its importance can be better appreciated when one considers the effect factor V deficiency has on the prothrombin time (PT) and activated partial thromboplastin time (APTT).

Prothrombin (factor II) is a single-chain glycoprotein with a molecular weight of 73,000. When activated, the prothrombin molecule undergoes proteolytic cleavage at two sites to yield a two-chain molecule lined by a disulfide bond. This new product is thrombin. Although factor Xa alone can convert prothrombin to thrombin, the participation of phospholipid and calcium ions in the presence of factor V increases the rate of thrombin formation 100 times. Phospholipid may be instrumental in converting subsequent thrombin generation at sites where phospholipid from injured endothelial cells and adherent platelets will be available.

Thrombin, the two-chain derivative of the prothrombin molecule, has a molecular weight of approximately 37,000. Its proteolytic properties produce the conversion of fibrinogen to fibrin to produce the initial visible manifestation of coagulation, the soluble clot. In addition, thrombin influences the activity of factors II, V, VII, VIII, XIII, and plasmin. Thrombin also induces platelet aggregation and initiates activation of protein C in the presence of thrombomodulin on the endothelial cell surface.

Fibrinogen (factor I), the primary substrate of the proteolytic activity of thrombin, has a concentration in plasma of 200 to 400 mg/dl, a higher level than any other protein involved in the coagulation pathway. Fibrinogen is composed of three pairs of nonidentical disulfide-bonded polypeptide chains. These peptides are cleaved specifically by thrombin at arginine-glycine bonds to produce fibrin monomers that form the gelatin-friable fibrin clot (see Fig. 4-1).

The final phase of the coagulation cascade is stabilization

and cross-linking of soluble fibrin monomers, which are accomplished by factor XIII, fibrin-stabilizing factor (see Fig. 4-1). Factor XIII is not a serine protease. It circulates as a zymogen composed of two pairs of different polypeptide chains, designated *a* and *b*. Intact factor XIII possesses a molecular weight of approximately 350,000 and is converted to its active transglutaminase form in the presence of both calcium ions and thrombin.

Platelets

Platelet function. As noted earlier in this chapter, normal hemostasis results from a complex series of precisely integrated, interrelated reactions involving blood vessels, vascular endothelium, platelets, coagulation proteins, and the fibrinolytic system. These ever-present mechanisms become operative immediately after disruption of the blood vessel wall. Disruption may result from acute external trauma, advanced alterations in the circulating blood that directly damage endothelial cells, or the ravages of various disease processes that destroy the endothelium and the three layers of the blood vessel wall.

When the integrity of the blood vessel wall is lost, the initial change is contraction or vasoconstriction, which is mediated by nerve stimuli acting on smooth muscle. This may occur in the form of spasm or physiologic vasoconstriction. Constriction of the blood vessel lumen impedes blood flow to the site of disruption and is followed immediately by the formation of a hemostatic plug, which initially consists of masses of adherent and aggregated platelets that become enmeshed between strands of fibrin. Vasoconstriction may be enhanced by the liberation of vasoactive compounds released from activated platelets.

Disruption of the blood vessel wall also initiates changes in blood platelets involving a series of reactions designated as *adhesion* and *aggregation*.[9-11] Loss of the vascular integrity and distortion of endothelial cells results in exposure of blood to collagen and connective tissue fibers, with platelets migrating and adhering to the damaged site. This platelet adhesion is the initial event in formation of the platelet plug. The surface of the platelet, consisting of a trilaminar plasma membrane covered with acid mucopolysaccharides and glycoproteins, permits adhesion to the exposed subendothelial collagen through glycoprotein Ib and IIb/IIIa receptors and von Willebrand factor. This interaction between the platelet membrane and the endothelial cell initiates transmission of stimuli to the internal milieu of the platelet, resulting in the appearance of two phospholipase enzymes (A_2 and C) that initiate the metabolism of arachidonic acid.[12] Free arachidonic acid is converted to prostaglandin compounds, the endoperoxides PGG_2 and PGH_2, by the enzyme cyclooxygenase. These endoperoxides are spontaneously converted to thromboxane A_2 by thromboxane synthetase.

Formation of thromboxane A_2 and its secretion out of the platelet are termed the *release reaction*. This reaction results from the interaction of distinct components in the platelet cytoplasm, including granules, mitochondria, glycogen-containing particles, and a Golgi apparatus. Three types of granules (alpha, delta, and lambda) that are of particular importance in the release reaction have been identified, and each contains components that mediate the aggregation of platelets. The alpha granules contain fibrinogen, platelet factor 4, β-thromboglobulin, platelet-derived growth factor, fibronectin, and von Willebrand factor; delta granules (or dense bodies) contain calcium, adenosine diphosphate (ADP), potassium, serotonin, and catecholamines; and lambda granules (or lysosomal granules) contain cathepsin, histone, β-glucuronidase, and phosphatase. In response to stimuli initiated by the interaction of platelet and endothelial cell membranes, these granules secrete and release their contents, which amplify the message of aggregation to additional platelets in the initiation of thrombus formation.

The central component in amplification of this message is ADP.[13,14] Exposure of the platelet membrane to ADP prepares and facilitates the glycoprotein IIb-IIIa receptor to bind fibrinogen to the platelet membrane. The bound fibrinogen (from the plasma or from the alpha granule) in the presence of calcium is the essential mediator of the aggregation reaction. The release reaction is inhibited or modulated by substances that increase the concentration of, or prevent the degradation of, cyclic AMP in the platelet's internal milieu.[15] The most important of these agents is prostacyclin (PGI_2), which is synthesized by vascular endothelial cells. PGI_2 enhances the activity and production of adenylate cyclase. This agent is the most potent inhibitor of platelet aggregation and platelet plug formation that has been identified in the human body.

Platelets also participate in a facile manner in the interaction of coagulation proteins, leading to formation of fibrin. Platelets provide a lipoprotein reaction surface on which procoagulant enzymes and their respective substrates interact.[16] A receptor site for factor Xa is exposed on activated platelets, that is, platelets undergoing aggregation and the release reaction. When bound to the platelet membrane lipoprotein, factor Xa, along with factor Va, converts prothrombin (factor II) to thrombin, a potent serine protease. Thrombin initiates fibrin polymer formation from fibrinogen, thereby stabilizing and providing the network support structure of the hemostatic plug. The initiation of this localized process of solidification results from the release of four peptides from the dimeric fibrinogen molecule (two fibrinopeptides from alpha and beta chains) by the enzymatic cleavage activity of thrombin. Sequential release of these peptides yields fibrin monomers that undergo polymerization by end-to-end and side-to-side anastomotic noncovalent bonding. Although stable, this clot can be made reversibly soluble in solutions of urea and monochloroacetic acid. In the final stage of fibrin clot formation the solid lattice support structure of fibrin becomes irreversibly insoluble through the process of cross-linking. Transamidation occurs by factor XIII, a transglutaminase cross-linking enzyme that co-

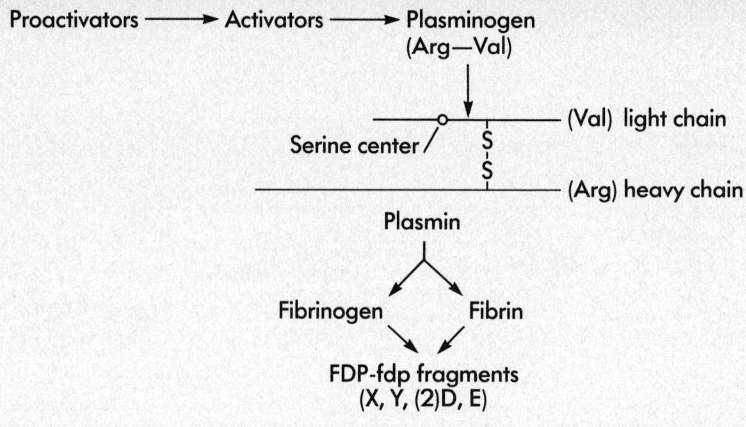

Fig. 4-2. Pathway of activation of the plasminogen-plasmin proteolytic (fibrinolytic) system.

valently links glutamyl and lysyl amino acid residues in the presence of calcium. The resultant cross-linked fibrin polymer is irreversibly insoluble and, depending on the degree of cross-linking, is resistant to the digestive degradation of plasmin. Retraction of the fibrin clot occurs and is mediated by the contractile protein thrombasthenin. When this entire process goes unchecked, as in certain pathologic states, thrombus formation and vascular obstruction begin.

The fibrinolytic system

Fibrinogen and fibrin serve as physiologic targets of plasmin, the fibrin(ogen)olytic enzyme derived from plasminogen (Fig 4-2). Complete plasminolytic degradation of fibrinogen and fibrin proceeds through three stages. The initial cleavage results in removal of peptides from the carboxyl terminal of the alpha chain of fibrinogen, resulting in the formation of fragment X. As digestion proceeds, no additional peptides from the beta chain are cleaved, resulting in a smaller fragment, Y. There follows asymmetric cleavage of the intermediate Y into the final fragments, D and E.

The mechanism of fibrinolysis homeostatically maintains intraluminal patency of blood vessels in the event of thrombus formation by counterbalancing the effects of blood coagulation. Lysis of the fibrin clot depends on the hydrolytic properties of plasmin, a nonspecific proteolytic enzyme generated by activation of the zymogen plasminogen. Naturally occurring activators of this enzyme reaction are present in the plasma and vascular endothelium and can be prepared from bacterial sources (streptokinase) and from ex vivo renal parenchymal cell cultures (urokinase) and endothelial cells by recombinant gene technology (tissue plasminogen activator). The use of exogenous fibrinolytic agents is discussed elsewhere in this text. Factor XIIa and prekallikrein (Fletcher factor) are also involved in plasminogen activation. Certain activators such as tissue plasminogen activator are probably, to a minimal extent, absorbed onto the fibrin clot surface or penetrate into its mesh but in any case remain available to plasminogen at sites where the concentration of plasmin inhibitors is low. Besides fibrin, plasmin hydrolyzes a number of other plasma proteins, including clotting factors V, VIII, and XIIa and the first component of the complement system.

Regulation mechanisms of coagulation

Coagulation factors II, VII, IX, X, and XI, as well as factors XIIa, fragments, thrombin, and plasmin, are classified as serine proteases because each possesses a serine residue at its enzymatically active site. The physiologic activities of serine proteases are modulated by endogenous circulating proteinase inhibitors, which probably form irreversible covalent complexes with the proteases and secondarily prevent the participation of the active serine sites in enzymatic reactions. The natural protease inhibitors include C1 esterase inhibitor, α-1-antitrypsin, α-1-antichymotrypsin, inter α-trypsin inhibitor, α-2-antiplasmin, α-2-macroglobulin, and antithrombin III. The influence of heparin on antithrombin III function is discussed elsewhere.

Factors II, VII, IX, and X and proteins C and S are the vitamin K–dependent clotting factors. They are synthesized in the liver along with fibrinogen, factor V, and possibly factors VIII, XI, and XIII. Vitamin K–dependent clotting factors remain nonfunctional precursors in the presence of vitamin K antagonists such as the coumarin anticoagulants. These agents block the vitamin K–dependent formation of γ-carboxylated glutamic acid residues on the amino terminal ends of the molecule. This residue normally binds calcium ions, which in turn link the clotting factors to a phospholipid template for activation. Vitamin K deficiency is difficult to achieve by dietary restriction alone; however, it may take place in combination with malabsorption or antibiotic destruction of the intestinal flora that normally synthesize vitamin K_2.

Laboratory evaluation of coagulation

Laboratory assessment of coagulation should complement a complete patient history and physical examination.

Special attention should be focused on the personal and family history. The APTT and PT add little to the evaluation of patients before surgery without clinical findings indicative of increased risk of bleeding. In evaluating patients with a coagulopathy these tests, however, are sufficiently sensitive that if both the APTT and the PT are negative, further study of the coagulation system is usually not necessary. If one or the other is positive (prolonged), attention may be focused on a limited sequence of the coagulation cascade. The utility of the APTT and PT in monitoring heparin and warfarin therapy and safety is discussed elsewhere in this chapter.

The majority of coagulation tests performed in vitro depend on the visual, mechanical, or photooptical detection of a fibrin clot. This end point requires an adequate amount of normally functioning fibrinogen. Of historical interest is the Lee-White method for measuring clotting time, an insensitive but useful bedside screening test for assessing whole-blood clotting function. Although seldom used in clinical practice today, an abnormally prolonged Lee-White clotting time reflects either a severe deficiency of coagulation factors involved in the intrinsic and common pathways or the presence of heparin or acquired endogenous circulating anticoagulants. Marked thrombocytopenia and deficiencies of factors VII and XIII do not usually affect this test. An automated whole blood assay, the activated clotting time (ACT) is particularly sensitive to heparin and is the automated version of the Lee-White clotting time for evaluating whole-blood coagulation.

Activated partial thromboplastin time (APTT). The activated partial thromboplastin time (APTT) monitors the activity of factors in the intrinsic and common pathways but is primarily used to detect deficiency of factors VIII, IX, XI, and XII. Abnormal results usually indicate that clotting factor activity is below 30% of normal values. In addition, the APTT is prolonged by heparin or by pathologically induced circulating inhibitors directed toward components of the intrinsic or common systems. This test is insensitive to platelet function and to deficiencies of factors VII and XIII. The APTT is a modification of the partial thromboplastin time (PTT) in which artificial reagents such as kaolin, micronized silica, and ellagic acid are used with phospholipid to activate the intrinsic system rapidly. The APTT is falsely prolonged when blood is sampled through a catheter containing heparin or in a patient with polycythemia, with the latter caused by a disproportionate amount of anticoagulant relative to plasma in the collecting tube.

Prothrombin time (PT). The prothrombin time (PT) measures coagulation factor activity in the extrinsic and common pathways. It reflects the activity of vitamin K–dependent factors II, VII, and X but not IX because the intrinsic pathway is bypassed. The PT may be slightly prolonged by the anticoagulant action of heparin but is significantly affected by the coumarin anticoagulants and by the adequacy of vitamin K absorption and hepatic protein synthetic capacity. An erroneous PT or APTT reading may occur when the collection tube is underfilled.

Thrombin time (TT). Thrombin time (TT) is the amount of time required to form a fibrin clot from fibrinogen after exogenous thrombin is added to plasma. This test is prolonged by fibrinogen levels depressed below 100 mg/dl; dysfibrinogenemias; substances, including heparin; certain circulating anticoagulants; and fibrinogen-fibrin degradation products that exhibit antithrombin activity. The activity of the other clotting factors does not affect TT.

Assays of specific coagulation factors. Specific in vitro assays have been developed for each of the coagulation factors. Many of these techniques are based on the ability of the test plasma to correct the clotting abnormality of substrate plasma, which is selectively deficient in the factor being evaluated. The substrate plasma is often obtained from patients with documented congenital deficiencies. Specific immunologic assays of the coagulation factors have been added to the diagnostic armamentarium.

Detection of circulating anticoagulants. Plasma samples associated with abnormalities in the screening test of coagulation function may contain circulating anticoagulants. Characteristically, abnormalities caused by clotting factor deficiencies are corrected by the addition of normal plasma to the test plasma. When plasma containing circulating inhibitors is added to normal plasma, abnormal coagulation study results persist. These changes often become more obvious after incubation of normal plasma with plasma containing the inhibitors at 37° C for 1 hour.

Interpreting results of coagulation studies. Division of the coagulation process into the intrinsic, extrinsic, and common pathways is artificial but does provide a useful approach to the definitive diagnosis of coagulation disorders. A prolonged APTT associated with a normal PT localizes the coagulation defect to the intrinsic pathway, which includes factors XII, XI, IX, and VIII, which together comprise more than 95% of all hereditary coagulopathies. Multiple deficiencies of intrinsic system factors may prolong the APTT to a significantly greater degree than does a single-factor deficiency. Deficiencies of prekallikrein (Fletcher factor), high–molecular-weight kininogen (Fitzgerald, Warren, Williams, Flaujeac, and Reid factors), and Passovoy factor also prolong the APTT. These contact phase coagulation factors are not associated with a bleeding tendency, with the exception of the Passovoy factor. Bleeding disorders characterized by prolongations of both the APTT and PT indicate deficiencies in the common pathway, factors I, II, V, or X. These abnormalities are individually identified by specific factor assays. Isolated factor VII deficiency is reflected by a normal APTT and prolonged PT. When the PT, APTT, TT, and fibrinogen concentrations are normal in a patient with a history of bleeding, factor XIII deficiency or α-2-antiplasmin deficiency must be considerd. Their activity is not detected by other screening tests and requires specific assays. Variants of von Willebrand's disease and mild factor XI deficiency rarely are associated with a normal

APTT and may fall into this laboratory category; however, specific factor procoagulant and antigen assays can confirm their absence.

COAGULATION DISORDERS

Bleeding disorders

Congenitally inherited abnormalities of coagulation usually result from the absence of a single procoagulant factor, although familial multiple-factor deficiencies have been described. These aberrations of the coagulation system result from either deficient synthesis of a glycoprotein or the synthesis of a biologically defective procoagulant protein.

Factor I deficiency

Afibrinogenemia. The congenital absence of circulating plasma fibrinogen (factor I) is an extremely rare autosomal recessive disorder often associated with consanguinity. The clinical features of this entity are manifested frequently at birth, with hemorrhage persistent from the umbilical cord or circumcision sites. Thereafter these individuals usually do not experience spontaneous hemorrhage but may bleed excessively when they experience trauma or surgery.

Laboratory findings include a very low erthyrocyte sedimentation rate, a prolonged bleeding time, and markedly abnormal PT, APTT, and TT.

Treatment of afibrinogenemia is indicated prophylactically before and during surgical procedures and therapeutically to terminate hemorrhage. This can be achieved by administering infusions of fresh frozen plasma (FFP) or cryoprecipitate.

Hypofibrinogenemia. Some individuals have persistent levels of fibrinogen in the range of 30 to 100 mg/dl. These patients may represent heterozygotes of afibrinogenemic patients, or they may represent examples of dysfibrinogenemia. The quanitity of circulating fibrinogen, if greater than 30 mg/dl, is usually adequate to produce normal coagulation studies. Very few patients have clinical symptoms, and treatment is usually not necessary.

Dysfibrinogenemia. The presence of dysfibrinogenemia is rare and is usually inherited in an autosomal dominant manner. These individuals do not usually experience clinical symptoms and are often discovered incidentally. Patients with dysfibrinogenemia are recognized because of a defective conversion of fibrinogen to fibrin. The interaction of the dysfibrinogen with thrombin may result in either a delayed release of fibrinopeptides, the inhibition of fibrin polymerization or the prevention of effective cross-linking of fibrin monomers. This abnormality is primarily reflected by a prolongation of the PT, APTT, and TT. When fibrinogen concentration is determined by a thrombin coagulable rate-dependent technique, it is severely reduced. When fibrinogen is determined by nonrate-dependent quantitative techniques or immunologically, the concentration is normal or slightly increased above normal.

Treatment with replacement therapy is rarely necessary because sufficient amounts of normal fibrinogen usually accompany the dysfibrinogen molecule.

Factor II deficiency. Hypoprothrombinemia is probably the rarest of the known coagulation disorders. Hypoprothrombinemia has been observed in association with the "lupus anticoagulant." Aprothrombinemia has not been described. Clinical hemorrhage is mild to absent. Congenital dysprothrombinemic molecules have been recognized.

In the laboratory there is modest prolongation of the PT, APTT, and TT. The bleeding time is usually normal.

In the rare instance in which therapy may be needed, FFP or purified prothrombin-complex concentrates may be used.

Factor III deficiency. Deficiency of tissue thromboplastin (factor III) has not been identified. Thromboplastin is present in abundance in several different body tissues.

Factor IV deficiency. For optimal function of the coagulation system the divalent cation calcium, factor IV, is required only in trace quantities. Before the level of calcium in the blood could be decreased sufficiently to impair function of the coagulation system, virtually all other calcium-dependent body functions would be dysfunctional and death would result.

Factor V deficiency. Deficiency of proaccelerin (factor V) is very rare and is inherited in an autosomal recessive manner. This state is associated with a variable tendency to bleed in the homozygous individual. Heterozygotes are usually asymptomatic. Combined deficiencies of factors V and VIII have been observed.

In the homozygote the PT and APTT are abnormally prolonged. The bleeding time is variably prolonged.

Treatment in the form of replacement therapy requires the use of FFP in modest amounts.

Factor VII deficiency. Deficiency of factor VII is associated with both mild bleeding tendencies and thrombosis. In the homozygous form circulating levels of factor VII activity are usually less than 10% of normal activity. Heterozygotes are for the most part asymptomatic. Deep venous thrombosis and pulmonary emboli have been reported in affected patients.

In the laboratory isolated factor VII deficiency results in a prolonged PT with normal APTT and TT. Treatment of bleeding episodes is seldom necessary but is accomplished by the infusion of FFP or the administration of purified factor VII concentrates. Anticoagulants may be used in patients with thromboembolic disease.

Factor VIII deficiency. Two hemorrhagic diseases are associated with deficiencies or abnormalities of the factor VIII molecule.[17] The one described first was classic hemophilia, or hemophilia A, in which the VIII:C portion of the factor VIII molecule is greatly decreased or absent. The second disorder is von Willebrand's disease in which there is a deficiency or abnormality of the large VIII:vWFAg portion of the factor VIII molecule. This may be the most common congenital hemorrhagic disorder recognized at the present time.

Hemophilia A. This disorder is sex-linked, is recessively inherited, and is characterized by spontaneous bleeding. Although this disorder may be clinically inactive at an early age, it generally progresses in severity and frequency with age and degree of activity. Bleeding associated with surgery or any type of trauma is common and may be severe. Its severity apparently is directly related to the degree of factor VIII deficiency. Severely affected patients (less than 1% of normal factor VIII activity) experience repeated soft-tissue hemorrhage, which may be spontaneous or result from the slightest trauma. Weight-bearing joints are frequently affected by hemorrhage that ultimately produces deforming arthritis, which often requires surgical intervention in the form of synovectomy or joint replacement. Virtually any body tissue or organ can be the site of major and devastating hemorrhage. Intracranial hemorrhage is the major cause of death from bleeding in patients with hemophilia A. This problem mandates prompt diagnosis and vigorous, aggressive treatment.

The diagnosis of hemophilia A is established in the laboratory by a prolongation of the APTT, whole blood clotting time, or reduced factor VIII:C levels. The PT, bleeding time, and TT are normal. Hemophilia may be seen in a female offspring of a female carrier and affected male, but this is a rare event. Treatment of the hemorrhage associated with hemophilia A requires prompt and adequate replacement with factor VIII. Replacement can be accomplished with the use of FFP or cryoprecipitate when modest increments in the level of factor VIII activity are required to stop the bleeding. When major bleeding in vital organs of the body occurs and factor VIII activity must be immediately increased to normal levels, factor VIII lyophilized concentrates must be used. Several different preparations are currently available. Purified factor VIII prepared by recombinant DNA techniques is currently undergoing trials and will soon be available for widespread use.

Adjunctive therapy in the treatment of hemophilia includes the antifibrinolytic agents, ε-aminocaproic acid, and transexamic acid. These agents are particularly helpful in dealing with bleeding and the performance of surgical procedures in the oral cavity.

Von Willebrand's disease. Von Willebrand's disease is characterized by spontaneous bleeding, predominantly from mucosal surfaces and the gastrointestinal tract. In females menorrhagia is particularly striking. Spontaneous hemorrhage into joints and soft tissues is rare but does occur with trauma of any type. There are at least five major types and several subtypes of this disease process.[18] The mode of inheritance for most types and subtypes is autosomal dominant, although in a few affected individuals an autosomal recessive pattern has been identified (Table 4-2).

The diagnosis of this disease in the laboratory is often complex and may require a number of different techniques. Classically, a prolonged bleeding time is present but not in all types or subtypes. The PT, TT, and whole blood clotting time are usually normal. The APTT may be prolonged, but in some individuals it may be at the upper limits of normal. The factor VIII:vWFAg is either quantitatively reduced or composed of abnormal or absent multimers on sodium dodecal sulfate gel electrophoresis. The use of platelet-aggregation studies using ristocetin, thrombin, and arachidonic acid (in various concentrations) and the quantification

Table 4-2. Types of von Willebrand's disease

	Types of von Willebrand's disease
I	Autosomal dominant VIII:C, vWF:Ag, and RCoF—reduced in plasma vWF:Ag—multimeric structure qualitatively normal vW:Ag II—reduced subtypes IB and IC identified
II	Plasma VIII:C >vWF:Ag or RCoF vWF:Ag—abnormalities of multimeric structure vWF:Ag II—variable
IIA	Autosomal dominant vWF:Ag—large and medium multimers absent in plasma and platelets RIPA—decreased
IIB	Autosomal dominant vWF:Ag—large multimers absent in plasma and normal in platelets RIPA—increased
IIC	Autosomal recessive vWF:Ag—large multimers absent in plasma and platelets vWF:Ag—multimers present are abnormal Subtypes IID-IIH—identified
III	Autosomal recessive vWF:C—markedly reduced vWF:Ag, RIPA, and RCoF—absent vWF:Ag II—absent
Pseudo-vWd	Autosomal dominant VIII:C, vWF:Ag—normal or decreased vWF:Ag—large multimers absent in plasma and present in platelets RIPA—increased and enhanced induction of thrombocytopenia GPIb—receptor is abnormal
Acquired vWd	Associated with an underlying disorder Antibody directed against vWF:Ag or RCoF may be present; frequently associated with lymphoproliferative disorders

VIII:C, Factor VIII coagulant activity; VIII:Ag (VIIIC:Ag), factor VIII coagulant antigen, the antigenic expression of VIII:C; vWF(VIII/vWF), von Willebrand factor protein; vWF:Ag(VIIIR:Ag), von Willebrand factor antigen (FVIII-related antigen); vWd, von Willebrand's disease; RIPA, ristocetin-induced platelet aggregation; RCoF, ristocetin cofactor assay, the ability of vWF to support RIPA.

of ristocetin cofactor and vWFAgII may be helpful in the identification and categorization of various subtypes of this disease.

Treatment for most types and subtypes of the disease consists of replacement of the missing or abnormal factor VIII: vWFAg with normal vWF glycoprotein. This is best achieved by the use of desmopressin acetate (DDAVP), FFP, or cryoprecipitate. DDAVP should not be used in patients with type IIB and pseudo-von Willebrand's disease because clinically significant thrombocytopenia may be induced.

Factor IX deficiency. Deficiency of factor IX (hemophilia B or Christmas disease) is transmitted as a sex-linked recessive disorder. This disease comprises a heterogenous group of disorders that clinically resembles hemophilia A. Seldom is there spontaneous bleeding in the hemophilia B patient, but severe hemorrhage, even after minimal trauma, is common.

Laboratory diagnosis of hemophilia B is characterized by a normal PT, TT, and bleeding time, with a prolonged APTT. Specific assays for factor IX reveal severely reduced activity, but levels less than 1% of normal activity are not as common as in patients with hemophilia A.

Treatment is achieved by replacement of factor IX with FFP or lyophilized factor IX concentrates.

Factor X deficiency. Congenital factor X deficiency is a rare autosomal recessive disorder that is associated with mild hemorrhagic problems. Spontaneous hemorrhage is unusual but does occur after mild to minimal physical trauma or surgery, and this deficiency state clinically resembles that caused by factor VII deficiency. Acquired factor X deficiency is more common and is observed with vitamin K deficiency, warfarin ingestion, amyloidoses, and hepatic disease.

Laboratory diagnosis is made by finding a prolonged PT, APTT, and reduced factor X level on specific assay. The TT and bleeding time are normal.

Treatment of this rare disorder is accomplished by the replacement of factor X with FFP or factor IX concentrates.

Factor XI deficiency. Deficiency of factor XI is a rare hereditary coagulation disorder that occurs predominantly in Ashkenazic Jews and has been transmitted as both an autosomal dominant and autosomal recessive disease. Spontaneous bleeding is very rare but may occur in association with mild trauma and surgery.

In the laboratory the APTT and whole blood clotting time are prolonged, whereas the PT, TT, and bleeding time are normal. Specific assay reveals a reduced level of factor XI. All studies for this deficiency state must be performed on fresh blood (plasma) collected in either siliconized glass or plastic test tubes since factor XI is activated by glass surfaces and freezing.

Treatment is provided by replacement of the missing factor XI with FFP.

Factor XII deficiency. Deficiency of factor XII is rare and is usually not associated with any hemorrhagic tendency. Mild bleeding and easy bruising have been reported in a very few patients with this autosomal recessive trait. Some affected individuals experience venous thrombosis and pulmonary emboli.

In the laboratory the PT, TT, and the bleeding time are normal, and the APTT and whole blood clotting time performed in glass tubes are prolonged. Specific factor XII assay reveals very low levels of this factor.

If treatment for bleeding is necessary, it may be accomplished by replacing factor XII with FFP. In a patient with thrombosis anticoagulants may be cautiously given.

Factor XIII deficiency. Deficiency of factor XIII is rare and may be recognized at birth because of persistent umbilical bleeding. This problem is inherited as an autosomal recessive trait. Occasionally bruising and hematoma formation may be observed. Spontaneous bleeding of any type is rare. Wound healing is defective, and wound dehiscence is common. This state should be suspected when bleeding is delayed for 24 to 72 hours after a traumatic or surgical event.

In the laboratory the standard clotting tests are all normal. A specific assay for factor XIII using clot solubility in 5M urea or 10% monochloroacetic acid is abnormal.

Treatment is provided by replacement of factor XIII with FFP, which is required in minimal quantities.

Cofactor deficiency states. Deficiency of glycoproteins such as prekallikrein (Fletcher factor), high–molecular-weight kininogen (Fitzgerald, Flaujeac, Warren, Williams, Reid factors) and Passovoy factor that act as cofactors in the coagulation cascade are rare. All of these deficiency states exhibit impressive laboratory abnormalities but, with the exception of Passovoy factor deficiency, are asymptomatic and do not require treatment.

In the laboratory these deficiency states are characterized by impressive prolongation of the APTT but normal PT, TT, whole blood clotting time, and bleeding time. Specific assays for the given factor confirm the deficiency state, with the exception of the Passovoy factor deficiency since no defect has been identified in this condition.

Treatment for hemorrhage that occurs in association with Passovoy factor defect is accomplished with FFP.

Fibrinolytic system disorders. Patients presenting with excessive activation of the fibrinolytic system may bleed and require transfusion to correct their abnormalities. One rare disorder is α-2-antiplasmin, a principal physiologic inhibitor of plasmin. Treatment for this rare disorder is administration of FFP or the use of antifibrinolytic agents.

Disorders of coagulation: thrombotic disorders

Disorders of coagulation that lead to thrombosis are sometimes classified as hypercoagulable disorders. A number of clinical conditions have been identified in which patients have been found at increased risk for thrombosis. Many of these thrombotic disorders appear to have a hereditary predisposition, whereas others may be found in patients with an underlying systemic illness.

Certain clinical findings suggest a hereditary disorder. They may include a family history of thrombosis, thrombosis at an early age, thrombosis at unusual anatomic sites, and recurrent thrombosis without apparent precipitating factors.[19]

Protein C deficiency. Protein C is a vitamin K–dependent glycoprotein-serine-protease zymogen that circulates in the blood in a proenzyme state.[20,21] In the presence of cofactor protein S, protein C selectively inactivates factors V and VIII and enhances tissue plasminogen activator by inactivating tissue plasminogen activator inhibitor. Two types of congenital protein C deficiency have been recognized. Most common is type I in which the plasma concentration of protein C is reduced in both a functional and immunologic assay. Type II protein C deficiency is characterized by a reduction in functional levels, but normal levels of protein C antigen are present. Both types are inherited as an autosomal dominant trait. Protein C–deficient patients, both heterozygotes and homozygotes, experience a high frequency of venous thromboembolism involving the peripheral veins, lungs, cerebral veins, and the venous microcirculation of soft tissues. Acquired forms of protein C deficiency are found in patients with liver disease or disseminated intravascular coagulation (DIC) or in postoperative patients.

The laboratory diagnosis is confirmed by a specific assay for protein C activity and antigen.

Treatment of this condition at the present time is prolonged anticoagulation with warfarin or one of its congeners.

Protein S deficiency. Protein S is a vitamin K–dependent plasma glycoprotein. It binds to platelets and endothelial cells, functions as a cofactor for activated protein C in a 1:1 complex, and modulates the heparin-catalyzed inhibition of thrombin by antithrombin III.[22] Plasma protein S exists in the circulating blood in two forms: as a free protein (approximately 40% of total protein S), which functions as a cofactor for activated protein C; and as a protein in a reversible complex with the complement component C4b-binding protein (approximately 60% of the total protein S), which has no cofactor activity.

Reduction in free protein S has been associated with an increased frequency of severe recurrent venous thrombosis, which may be congenital or acquired (nephrotic syndrome, warfarin therapy, pregnancy, antiphospholipid syndrome, and DIC). Interestingly, this problem has been observed in patients with normal protein C levels.

The laboratory diagnosis is made by specific assay for free protein S.

Treatment of this condition is prolonged anticoagulation.

Antithrombin III deficiency. Deficiency of antithrombin III in congenital or acquired states is associated with an increased frequency in recurrent venous and arterial thrombosis.[23] Antithrombin-III deficiency is inherited in an autosomal dominant manner, with a reported prevalence of 1:2000 to 1:500 in the general population. This glycoprotein, which is synthesized in the liver and endothelial cells, functions as a cofactor that enhances the anticoagulant properties of heparin and also exerts inhibitory activity against the serine proteases, factors IIa, IXa, Xa, XIa, XIIa, and plasmin.

Three types of deficiency of antithrombin III have been described. Type I, or classic deficiency, is characterized by a pure quantitative defect. Type II is a qualitative defect, and type III is both a quantitative and qualitative defect. An acquired form may occur in patients with the nephrotic syndrome or severe liver disease or in patients receiving estrogen therapy.

The laboratory diagnosis of antithrombin-III deficiency is made by specific assay.

Treatment is prolonged anticoagulation with warfarin, although antithrombin-III concentrates are currently undergoing further investigational studies.

Heparin cofactor II. Heparin cofactor II is a serine protease inhibitor initially described in 1974. It is synthesized in the liver and inhibits thrombin activity by forming a covalent complex with this enzyme. There have been a few case reports of thrombosis associated with heparin cofactor deficiency, but a definite causal relationship has not been established.[24,25]

Disorders of the fibrinolytic system. The fibrinolytic system comprises the inactive zymogen plasminogen, active enzyme plasmin, plasminogen activators (both endogenous and exogenous), and plasminogen activator inhibitors.[26] Excessive activation of the fibrinolytic system may result in bleeding, whereas decreased fibrinolytic activity may lead to thrombosis.[27-29] Congenital and acquired disorders of the fibrinolytic system are well described. Patients with either qualitative or quantitative abnormalities of plasminogen have been reported to have recurrent venous thrombosis. Abnormalities involving both endogenous plasminogen activators and plasminogen activator inhibitors are also known to predispose patients to thrombotic events. Acquired states are seen in postoperative patients, patients with liver disease, patients taking birth control pills or during pregnancy, and patients with sepsis or DIC.

Treatment of the disorders of the fibrinolytic system leading to thrombosis includes prolonged warfarin administration.

Lupus anticoagulant. Lupus anticoagulants are often identified during routine laboratory evaluation by the presence of a prolonged APTT and, at times, an associated prolonged PT. Unlike patients with other disorders in which these laboratory tests are prolonged, these patients are more frequently associated with thrombotic problems than with bleeding problems.[30]

Clinically, patients with the lupus anticoagulant are initially seen with arterial or venous thrombosis. Venous thrombotic complications include deep venous thrombosis, renal or hepatic vein thrombosis, or pulmonary embolism.

Arterial events most often involve the cerebral vessels and may be seen as transient ischemic attacks (TIAs), cerebrovascular accidents, or amaurosis fugax. Obstetric complications include recurrent abortions and deep venous thrombosis. Thrombocytopenia, livedo reticularis, migraine headaches, chorea, and pulmonary hypertension are also reportedly associated with this disorder.

The term *lupus anticoagulant* is probably a misnomer. Most patients do not have systemic lupus erythematosus. More recently, the term *antiphospholipid syndrome* has been introduced by authors to clarify this entity.[31] Antiphospholipid antibodies include the lupus anticoagulant, antibodies to cardiolipin, and antibodies causing a false-positive test for syphilis.

Treatment generally consists of long-term anticoagulation, although aspirin, plasmapheresis, and immunosuppressive agents have been used.

Disseminated intravascular coagulation. DIC is also known as consumptive thrombohemorrhagic disorder or consumptive coagulopathy. DIC may lead to disorders of the coagulation system, including bleeding and thrombosis.[32] Unchecked activation of both the coagulation and fibrinolytic systems leading to widespread deposition of fibrin in small blood vessels is characteristic. DIC is seen in a number of clinical settings. It may be associated with obstetric emergencies such as abruptio placentae, the dead fetus syndrome, or placenta previa. In addition, it is well described as occurring in patients with either gram-negative or gram-positive sepsis, leukemia, incompatible blood transfusions, burns, aneurysms, and head injuries.

The diagnosis is often clinical. Laboratory findings include a dropping platelet count, decrease in fibrinogen levels, or a peripheral blood smear demonstrating a microangiopathic hemolytic anemia. High titers of fibrin-split products or an elevation in the D-dimer test are also seen.

Treatment is aimed at correcting the underlying disorder. Antithrombotic agents such as heparin are often helpful in blocking thrombotic occlusion of the microcirculation. Transfusion of FFP, cryoprecipitate, red blood cells, and platelets may be of benefit if the underlying defect is hemorrhage.

DIC presenting either as a manifestation of dissecting aortic aneurysms or other aneurysms is well described. Patients may be initially seen with mild bruising or bleeding. Laboratory abnormalities include a prolonged PT, thrombocytopenia, hypofibrinogenemia, and increased fibrin and fibrinogen degradation products. The cause of the DIC may be damage to the subendothelium, with subsequent activation of the intrinsic pathway. Treatment consists of correcting hemostasis, surgical repair, and the search for any additional aneurysms that may potentiate the DIC.[32]

Trousseau's syndrome: chronic DIC. A chronic form of DIC associated with underlying malignancies, better known as Trousseau's syndrome, is also well recognized.[33,34] Patients are first seen with superficial phlebitis and venous or arterial thrombosis. Bleeding is a less commonly recognized complication of this disorder. Patients may also have nonbacterial thrombotic endocarditis, and secondary neurologic manifestations include stroke and diffuse metabolic encephalopathy. Thrombotic events often precede the diagnosis of the underlying malignancy. Tumors commonly recognized include adenocarcinoma of the gastrointestinal tract (pancreas, stomach) and of the lung, prostate and breast. Therapy is aimed at diagnosing and treating the underlying malignancy. Heparin is the treatment of choice for venous and arterial thrombotic events, which are recurrent in most of these patients. Warfarin anticoagulation is not helpful in some patients with Trousseau's syndrome.

ANTITHROMBOTIC THERAPY

Anticoagulants are substances that retard coagulation of blood. The indication for their use in patients with peripheral vascular diseases is common but is controversial in patients with some vascular diseases.[35]

Two main categories of anticoagulants are in common clinical use, heparin and the coumarin-indanedione derivatives. The response of different individuals to the administration of both categories of these anticoagulants is variable; consequently, the dosage must be carefully adjusted. The usual dosage of anticoagulants is 300 to 500 U/kg/day by continuous infusion for heparin and 2.5 to 10 mg/day for oral maintenance with warfarin sodium. Therapeutic goals are discussed later in this chapter, but an adequate therapeutic level is selected that provides the maximal depression of coagulation without an increased risk for serious hemorrhage. The clinician must be aware that deficiencies of coagulation factors and thrombocytopenia render the patient particularly sensitive to anticoagulants. In these instances the usual doses may induce severe hemorrhage.

Contraindications to anticoagulants

Anticoagulants are absolutely contraindicated in patients with an active hemorrhagic diathesis, in those who are allergic to the agents, and in those patients undergoing surgery of the central nervous system or the eye. Relative contraindications to heparin and the coumarin-indanedione derivatives include gastrointestinal ulceration, severe hypertension (diastolic greater than 130 mm Hg), a past history of cerebral hemorrhage, inadequate cooperation of the patient, or the absence of adequate laboratory facilities. Anticoagulants must be used with caution in patients with pericarditis, bacterial endocarditis, liver disease, steatorrhea, or malnutrition. Because they cross the placenta, the coumarin-indanedione agents are contraindicated during pregnancy and at the time of delivery. These oral agents are secreted in breast milk and should not be given to nursing mothers.

Heparin

Despite the more recent introduction of thrombolytic therapy, heparin remains the mainstay in treatment for thromboembolic disorders. Heparin is the most universally used, parenterally administered anticoagulant. It is a heterogenous mixture of sulfided mucopolysaccharides, having the highest anionic charge density recognized in living organisms.[36] Heparin interferes with coagulation at several steps in the coagulation scheme. It has been documented to inhibit the action of thrombin on fibrinogen; to inhibit many of the early stages of the cascade, including activation of factors VIII, IX, and X; and to interfere with the action of thrombin on platelets. The mechanism of the action of heparin is attributed to its ability to complex with an α_2-globulin (heparin cofactor, antithrombin III) and in such combination to augment the inhibitory capacity of this endogenous agent. Heparin does not depress the production of any coagulation factors. In addition, heparin possesses anticomplement activity, is capable of releasing histaminase, and has lipemia-clearing activity resulting from the release of lipoprotein lipase. Heparin does not cross the placenta and is not secreted in breast milk.

Monitoring heparin therapy. The therapeutic antithrombotic dosage of heparin is best monitored by measurement of the APTT or PTT. A control APTT should be measured before the start of therapy. The dosage of heparin should be adjusted to maintain the APTT at 1½ to 2½ times the control value. Because the action of heparin can be altered by several drugs (antihistamines, ascorbic acid, EDTA, hyaluronidase, hydroxyzine, penicillin, phenothiazines, tetracycline) and heparin can also disturb the action of several drugs (oral anticoagulants), the clinician must be aware of these interrelationships. Whenever heparin is used, a flow sheet should be used to monitor the following on a daily basis: the date, patient's weight, hour of administration, agent (name, source, type), dosage per 24 hours, and results of the APTT or PTT and urine and stool tests for occult blood. Other tests may be used to monitor heparin therapy, including the Lee-White clotting time, the activated thrombin time, thrombin time, and heparin levels; however, these tests are not without their limitations and availability.

Administration. Aqueous heparin must be given intravenously (continuously or intermittently) or subcutaneously. It is best administered through an intravenous infusion using a constant infusion pump. Subcutaneous administration may cause erratic absorption, vessel puncture, bleeding, and discomfort and is a less desirable route. The subcutaneous route can be used if careful monitoring of intravenous infusions is not available or if intravenous infusion interferes with ambulation.

Intravenous route, continuous infusion, or intermittent route. A loading dose of 5000 to 10,000 units given slowly over 10 to 15 minutes should be administered intravenously, and immediately following this, the constant infusion should be started (heparin 15 to 20 U/kg/hr). An APTT should be checked 6 hours later and repeated until a satisfactory APTT is obtained. The intravenous route using intermittent infusion has been associated with more bleeding complications and is seldom used today.

Subcutaneous route. When the subcutaneous route is used, the approximate dosage and schedule is 10,000 to 25,000 U every 6 to 12 hours. The APTT should be measured 3 to 4 hours after the first dose, and subsequent doses should be adjusted to provide the desired prolongation. Thereafter, the APTT should be measured every 12 hours or just before administration of heparin to determine a possible cumulative effect. Heparin has been combined with agents such as gelatin, Pitkin's menstrum, peanut oil, and beeswax in an attempt to delay absorption and produce a more sustained effect. Use of these preparations is not recommended because of varying rates of absorption, high frequency of local reactions, other undesirable side effects, and the difficulty of reversing the anticoagulant effect with specific antidotes. The use of low-dose subcutaneous heparin (5000 U every 8 to 12 hours) for most patients requiring deep venous thrombosis prophylaxis is well established, but this regimen has not been effective in patients who have had major joint surgery.

Hemorrhagic complications. Hemorrhage is the most commonly encountered complication of treatment with any of the anticoagulants. The incidence of serious hemorrhage fortunately is low and may be proportionate to the intensity of the regimen used. Fatalities have been reported, and moderate hemorrhage such as hematuria, ecchymosis, hematomas, epistaxis, and melena occurs in 10% to 33% of patients.[37-40]

Bleeding may involve any organ system, but certain types of hemorrhage deserve special mention. Hemopericardium occurs in some patients with myocardial infarction, and anticoagulant therapy may increase this tendency. Bleeding from the gastrointestinal tract may develop. The term *anticoagulant ileus* has been used to describe obstructions of the small or large bowel caused by hemorrhages into the abdominal wall, peritoneal cavity, mesentery, or wall of the bowel. Bleeding from the gastrointestinal, genitourinary, or respiratory tracts during anticoagulant therapy may indicate the presence of previously unrecognized lesions and warrant further investigation. Physicians should be especially alert to the possible development of a subdural hematoma after head injury in patients receiving anticoagulants. Adrenal corticol insufficiency resulting from bilateral adrenal hemorrhage has been described.[41,42] The occurrence of bleeding at the sites of intramuscular or subcutaneous injections of heparin has been mentioned.

Patients receiving heparin should have daily physical examinations to detect abnormal bleeding and should have tests of urine and stool for occult blood. Unusual care is required in performance of venipuncture, and prolonged pressure should be applied to these sites. Invasive procedures, including arterial punctures, lumbar punctures, thoacentesis, paracentesis, and subcutaneous and intramuscular injections, should not be performed on patients receiving anticoagulants. An exception is the use of invasive procedures such as catheterization required for the management of a patient with a pulmonary embolism, acute myocardial infarction, or unstable angina.

Other complications. Reactions to heparin other than hemorrhage are rare. Hypersensitivity and anaphylactoid reactions have ranged from mild fever, urticaria, rhinitis, and conjunctivitis to sudden severe hypertension, respiratory distress, and chest pain. Hyperkalemia, hypoaldosteronism, elevation in transaminases, and transient alopecia have also been reported.

The syndrome of heparin-associated thrombocytopenia and thrombosis can be devastating. Although most patients with this disorder are asymptomatic, some will develop thrombotic complications, including acute arterial thrombosis leading to myocardial infarction, cerebrovascular accidents, limb ischemia, and death (Fig. 4-3). The overall incidence of heparin-associated thrombocytopenia is not well known but has been reported as low as 1% and as high as 30% in patients receiving heparin.[43,44] Heparin-associated thrombocytopenia with thrombosis, however, occurs less frequently, and its incidence is reported as approximately 1% to 2%.[45]

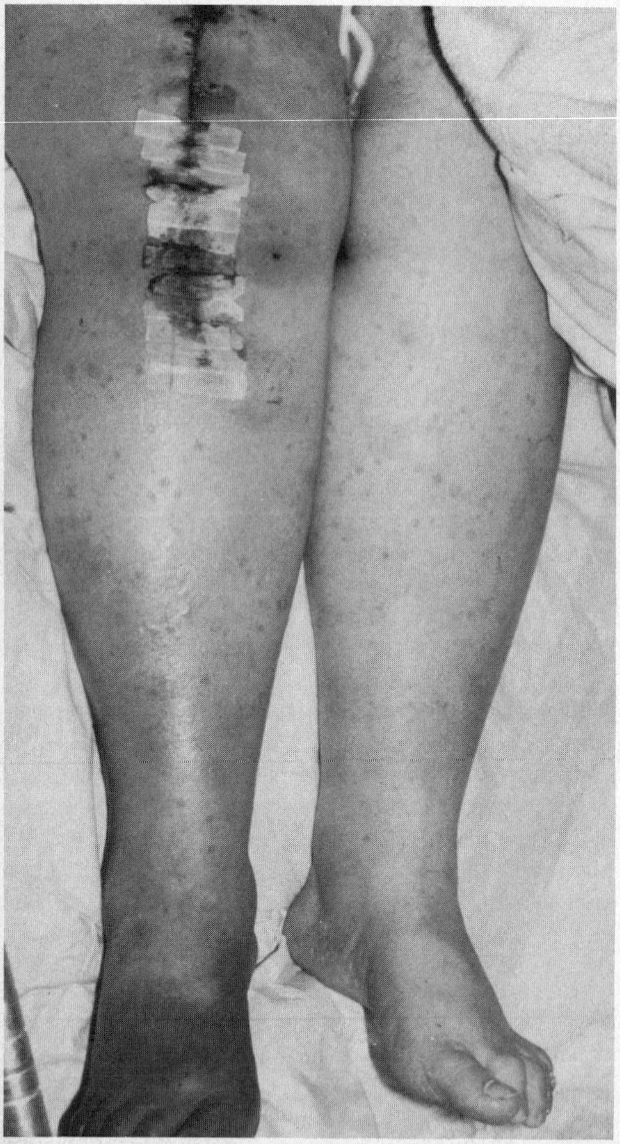

Fig. 4-3. Heparin associated thrombocytopenia and thrombosis. Patient underwent a total knee replacement and postoperatively developed an acute deep vein thrombosis. While on heparin she developed an acute arterial occlusion, thrombocytopenia and a positive test for heparin associated antibody.

Thrombocytopenia typically begins 5 to 10 days after the initiation of heparin therapy. The diagnosis should be suspected whenever the platelet count starts to drop from the baseline in patients receiving heparin, although generally it is not considered until this count reaches 100,000 or below. The diagnosis may be difficult to make since patients are often seriously ill and are taking numerous other medications that can predispose to thrombocytopenia.

Most laboratory tests for heparin-associated thrombocytopenia lack sensitivity and specificity, and not all facilities are able to perform those tests that are available. The most commonly used test involves platelet aggregometry, but a negative test result using this method does not exclude the diagnosis. Sheridan, Carter, and Kelton[46] have adapted this method by measuring heparin-dependent platelet release at two different heparin concentrations, with reported increased sensitivity for their test.

Patients with heparin-associated thrombocytopenia or heparin-associated thrombocytopenia with thrombosis are often seriously ill and need some form of antithrombotic therapy. Some have advocated switching from a bovine heparin preparation to a porcine heparin preparation.[47] Use of low–molecular-weight heparin has also been advocated; however, it is generally not commercially available.[48] Warfarin (Coumadin) is an acceptable anticoagulant, but it takes several days to become effective. During this delay the patient is unprotected and at risk for further thromboembolic events. Antiplatelet agents such as aspirin and dipyridamole have been used during this delay period, although their efficacy has been questioned.[49] An investigational drug, ILOPROST,* has also been used and has been shown effective in treating patients with heparin-associated thrombocytopenia who are undergoing open heart surgery. However, it also has adverse side effects that make its application for extended periods of time impractical.[50] Other agents available include the thrombolytic agents such as streptokinase, urokinase, or tissue plasminogen activator. Ancrod is another potential agent for therapy, but it is not commercially available in the United States. The use of an umbrella or filter placement in the inferior or superior vena

*Berlex Laboratories Inc., Cedar Knolls, NJ.

cava may be beneficial and should be considered in individuals with lower- or upper-extremity deep venous thrombosis.

Osteoporosis has been reported in patients who receive heparin for extended periods of time (more than 9 months).[51] It appears related to the dose and duration of therapy. Vertebral fractures of the thoracic and lumbar spine are the most frequently seen complications.

Antidotes. Several antidotes reverse the anticoagulant effect of heparin, including protamine sulfate, hexadimethine bromide (polybrene), clupein, polylysine, toluidine blue, fuchsin, and tryptophan. The antidote that is most frequently recommended and most commonly used is protamine sulfate. The size of the dose administered depends on the amount of heparin present and on the time and route of the last dose of heparin. The recommended dose is 1.0 mg for every 100 U (USP) of heparin present in the body. It should be administered slowly, intravenously, and at a rate not greater than 5 mg/min. No single injection of protamine sulfate should exceed 50 mg. The antiheparin effects last approximately 2 hours. An APTT should be checked approximately 15 minutes after the administration of protamine sulfate and before additional doses are given. Some heparin effect may reappear after a single dose of protamine sulfate, especially if a large dose of heparin was administered subcutaneously shortly before the injection of protamine. Transfusions of blood, plasma, or other blood products are not antidotes against heparin, although they are of value in replacement therapy after hemorrhage.

Low–molecular-weight heparin (LMWH). Low–molecular-weight heparin (LMWH) and heparinoids are currently being used for the management of venous and arterial disease. These agents reportedly have maximal antithrombotic activity and very little hemorrhagic risk when compared to standardized heparin.[52] Their reduced hemorrhagic effect is believed related to their decreased effect on collagen-induced platelet aggregation, and the anticoagulant effect appears related to its ability to inhibit factor Xa, thrombin, and antithrombin III.[53]

Multicenter studies using low–molecular-weight heparin in the prevention of postsurgical thrombosis and in the treatment of peripheral arterial disease and prosthetic graft occlusion show exciting promise.[54]

Coumarin-indanedione anticoagulants

A large variety of coumarin-indanedione derivatives are commonly used as anticoagulants.[55] These agents do not inhibit the rate of clotting when added to blood in vitro. When administered in vivo, they impair coagulation by altering the biologic function (clotting activity) of the end product of the vitamin K–mediated hepatic synthesis of factors II, VII, IX, and X. Normal levels (measured by immunologic techniques) of these factors are present during the administration of the coumarin-indanedione agents. Although the synthesis of factors II, VII, IX, and X are not depressed by these vitamin K antagonists, their functional properties are altered. This defect has been identified and is caused by the absence of the second carboxyl group on the carbon of glutamic acid.

The coumarin-indanedione anticoagulants have certain pharmacologic actions other than those related to coagulation. They include enhancement of uric acid excretion in the urine and a rise in serum transaminase and lactic dehydrogenase activity. Some patients who receive coumarin derivatives may excrete orange or reddish-colored urine because of a metabolic breakdown product that gives this color in an alkaline medium. This is not of clinical significance.

Control of dosage. The one-stage prothrombin test devised by Quick is the most widely used test to monitor the effect of the coumarin anticoagulants. After the administration of these agents the coagulant activity of the vitamin K–dependent factors decreases in the following sequence: VII, IX, X, and II. The order in which they disappear corresponds to the intravascular biologic half-life of these factors. The one-stage PT is influenced by changes in three of these factors (II, VII, and X), but there is close parallelism in the levels of factors VII and IX with the coumarin derivatives during therapy. Thus the one-stage PT is considered a reliable method for use in monitoring the effect and in guiding the dosage of the coumarin anticoagulants. Because heparin can also affect the one-stage PT, a control PT should be obtained before the institution of either warfarin or heparin. In recent years the goal in using coumarin anticoagulants was to maintain the PT at a level 1.5 to 2 times normal. More recent recommendations have concluded that a ratio of 1.25 to 1.5 times control is acceptable treatment.[56]

Administration. The coumarin-indanedione derivatives are attractive because they can be administered orally. Some of these agents, for example, warfarin, can also be administered intravenously. The coumarin derivatives are preferred to the chemically similar indanedione derivatives because in clinical practice they produce fewer adverse side effects. The approximate dosage schedule for bishydroxycoumarin, warfarin, and one of the indanedione derivatives is shown in Table 4-3. The old technique for initiating therapy used a loading dose of one of the coumarin derivatives (for example, warfarin, 25 to 35 mg) after obtaining a control PT. Approximately 36 hours later a PT was determined, and a daily maintenance dose, usually 5 to 10 mg, was selected. The newer technique, and the one preferred, is based on the observation that a loading dose produces a rapid fall in factor VII activity before other factors' activities are depressed. Some investigators point out that even though there is prolongation of the PT, antithrombotic protection is not present until factor X activity is also reduced.[57] Therefore the recommendation has been made that no loading dose be given and smaller daily doses (warfarin, 10 to 15 mg) be given when therapy is initiated. Reaching the desired

Table 4-3. Anticoagulants: representative agents

Class	Generic name	Chemical	Trade name	Routes of administration	Usual dose in adults (units)		Usual onset of peak activity	Dosage monitored by measurement of	Antidote
Heparin	Heparin sodium*	Sulfate containing mucopolysaccharide	Heparin Sodium Liquaemin Sodium Lipo-Hepin Panheprin	IV Continuous	300-500 U/kg/24 hr		1-2 hr	APTT	Protamine sulfate
				Intermittent	50-100 U/kg/q 4 hr		<30 min	APTT	
				Subcutaneous	10,000-25,000 U		4-6 hr	APTT	
					Initial (mg/24 hr)	Maintenance (mg/24 hr)			
Coumarin	Bishydroxycoumarin	3,3′-methylene-bis (4-hydroxycoumarin)	Dicumarol	PO	200-400	25-100	1.5-3 days	PT	Vitamin K and/or Transfusion of blood, or plasma fractions containing the vitamin K–dependent clotting factors
	Warfarin sodium	3-(α-Acetonylbenzyl)-4-hydroxycoumarin	Coumadin Panwarfin	PO or IV	10-15	2.5-10	1-2 days		
Indanedione	Anisindione	2-phenyl-1, 3 indanedione	Miradon	PO	300	25-250	1-2 days		

*1 mg of crystalline standard heparin sodium is equivalent to 100 USP U or 130 IU of heparin.

therapeutic prolongation of the PT often requires 4 or 5 days when the second method is used. A reasonably stable maintenance dose can be achieved within 5 to 15 days. Once it has been achieved, the PT can be checked at progressively longer intervals—from daily while hospitalized to weekly as an outpatient. Clinical experience suggests that no longer than 2 to 3 weeks should pass without a PT check for the duration of therapy.

Therapy with heparin and warfarin may be initiated simultaneously. Although heparin can somewhat alter the PT, it can be reliably used as a measure of coumarin's effect on most patients receiving continuous intravenous heparin.

A rebound phenomenon has been reported to follow the cessation of oral anticoagulant therapy occasionally.[58] The precise nature of the rebound phenomenon has not been defined. Some physicians believe that further thromboembolic episodes are more likely to occur at this time, and they recommend a gradual reduction in dosage over several days rather than abrupt discontinuation. The biologic half-life of these agents varies from 40 to 75 hours, however, and with such a gradual disappearance from the body, additional efforts to taper the dose are probably unnecessary.

Factors influencing dosage. A genetically determined hereditary (autosomal dominant) resistance to the anticoagulant effects of the coumarin-indanedione derivatives has been reported, although there have been no complications associated with this resistance.[59]

Disorders that interfere with the availability, absorption, or utilization of vitamin K such as malnutrition, gastrointestinal disorders, sprue, and cystic fibrosis and antibiotics that alter intestinal bacterial flora, biliary obstruction, or liver disease increase the sensitivity to the coumarin-indanedione derivatives.

Hypermetabolic states, excessive intake of alcohol, and congestive heart failure may also increase susceptibility to these anticoagulants. Females are more sensitive than males, and dose requirements may decrease with advancing age.

Concomitant administration of many other drugs may either potentiate or decrease the patient's response to these agents. A partial list of these drugs is presented in the accompanying box. The PT of patients receiving oral anticoagulants and any of these drugs must be monitored frequently. The simultaneous administration of other drugs may necessitate frequent alterations in the dose of the anticoagulant, either to maintain therapeutic effectiveness or to prevent potential bleeding disasters.

Complications. As with heparin, the most common untoward reaction to the coumarin-indanedione anticoagulants is hemorrhage. This complication has been discussed extensively earlier in this chapter. Other reactions are rare but include rashes, atheromatous embolization, and skin necrosis. Nausea, vomiting, and diarrhea also occur. Other less common side effects are listed in the box on p. 88.

The association of purple toes and coumarin is well described.[60] Initially believed to be an idiosyncratic reaction, it is now known to be caused by atheroemboli and cholesterol crystals that break loose from ulcerated atherosclerotic plaques and migrate distally.

Warfarin necrosis is reported to occur in less than 1% of patients receiving oral anticoagulant therapy.[61] It generally is initially seen as a sudden, localized, painful skin lesion characterized by an initial erythematous or hemorrhagic appearance. This later develops into gangrenous necrosis (Fig. 4-4). Lesions usually develop between days 3 and 6 of therapy, appear more often in women, and are found more

Some drugs that affect the response to coumarin-indanedione anticoagulants

Drugs that may potentiate anticoagulant effects

- Pyrazolane compounds
  - Phenylbutazone (Butazolidin)
  - Oxyphenbutazone (Tandearil)
- Antihyperlipidemic agents
  - Clofibrate (Atromid-S)
  - Dextrothyroxine (Choloxin)
- Anabolic steroids
  - Methandrostenolene (Dianabol)
  - Norethandrolone (Nilevar)
  - Oxymetholone (Adroyd)
  - Nandrolone decanoate (Deca-Durabolin)
- Muscle relaxants
  - Phenyramidol (Analexin)
- Salicylates—in large doses
- Quinine, quinidine, cimetidine, amiodarone
- Sulfonamides and antibiotics (moxalactam)
- Disulfiram (Antabuse), mineral oil, glucagon

Drugs that may decrease anticoagulant effects

- Sedatives and hypnotics
  - Barbiturates
  - Glutethimide (Doriden)
  - Ethchlorvynol (Placidyl)
- Griseofulvin (Fulvicin, Grifulvin, Grisactin)
- Rifampin (Rimactane)
- Mercurial diuretics and some thiazides
- Multivitamins containing vitamin K
- Tranquilizers
  - Meprobamate (Miltown, Equanil)
  - Haloperidol (Haldol)

Drugs that do not alter anticoagulant effects

- Diazepam (Valium)
- Chloridazepoxide (Librium)
- Chlorothiazide (Diuril) in standard doses
- Flurazepam (Dalmane)
- Tolmetin (Tolectin)

Medication inactivated by warfarin

- Cyclosporine

Coumarin-indanedione anticoagulants: untoward reactions

Hemorrhage
Skin lesions—rashes, necrosis, petechiae, purpura, exfoliation
Syndrome of purple toes
Nausea, vomiting, diarrhea
Leukopenia
Thrombocytopenia
Agranulocytosis
Eosinophilia
Pyrexia
Hepatic damage, hepatitis, jaundice
Stomatitis, sore throat
Nephropathy
Alopecia
Resistance

commonly in areas of increased subcutaneous fat, including the breasts, buttocks, thighs, and calves. The cause of this entity is not clear, although some patients have been observed to have decreased levels of protein C. Treatment is aimed at recognizing and discontinuing the medication immediately. Anticoagulation with another antithrombotic agent is then recommended.

The use of oral anticoagulants is not recommended during pregnancy because they cross the placental barrier and may lead to warfarin embryopathy syndrome, which is characterized by nasal hypoplasia and skeletal abnormalities. Other reported complications of warfarin use during pregnancy include agenesis of the corpus callosum, optic atrophy, spontaneous abortions, and central nervous system bleeding.

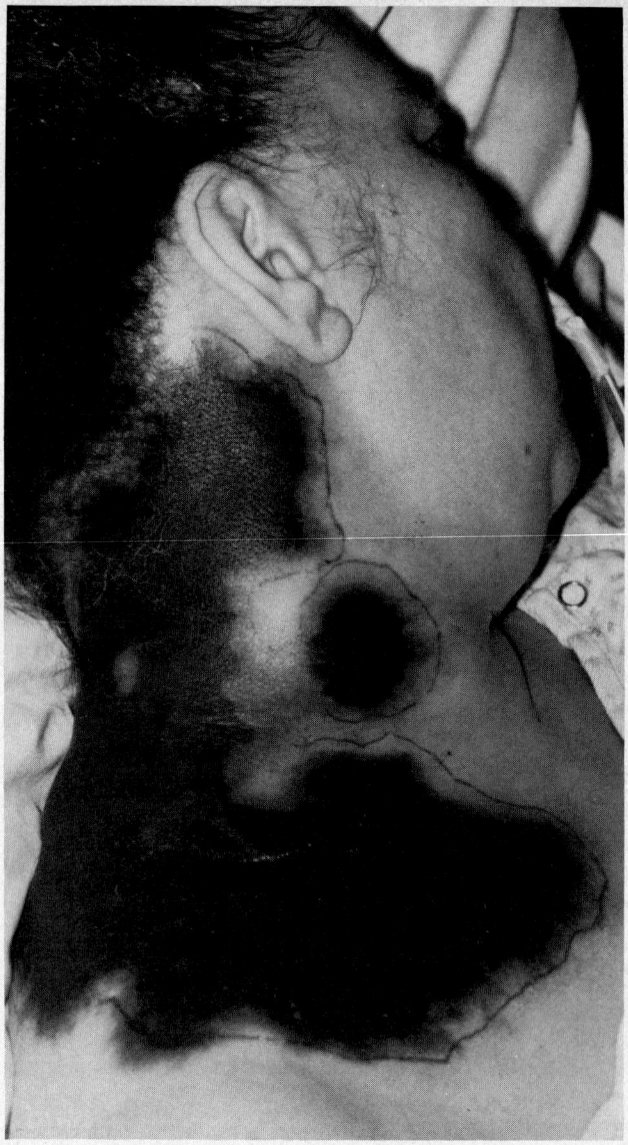

Fig. 4-4. Warfarin skin necrosis. This patient was treated for an acute deep vein thrombosis. She developed cutaneous purpura and soft tissue necrosis while on warfarin therapy.

Antidotes. The anticoagulant effects of coumarin-indanedione derivatives can be reversed by administration of vitamin K_1, which is a naturally occurring, oil-soluble, 3-phytyl derivative of 2-methyl-1,4-naphthoquinone (vitamin K). Certain synthetic water-soluble vitamin K preparations such as menadione and hykinone, which are not 3-phytyl derivatives, are much less effective and should not be relied on as antagonists. The oil-soluble preparation of vitamin K_1 (Mephyton) should be administered intravenously at a rate not faster than 5 mg/min. The water-soluble analog of vitamin K_1 (AquaMEPHYTON) is an effective antagonist and can be administered intravenously or orally, depending on the rapidity of effect that is desired. The subcutaneous and intramuscular routes can also be used but are less desirable because of variable absorption and local hematomas. The dose of vitamin K_1 depends on the amount and time of the last dose of anticoagulant and the urgency of the situation. In patients with life-threatening hemorrhage, if the dose of anticoagulant was not excessively large, 25 to 50 mg of vitamin K_1 given intravenously usually will produce a therapeutic effect within 4 hours, and within 12 to 24 hours the PT will have returned to control values. Such large doses of vitamin K_1 may make the patient resistant to subsequent doses of anticoagulants for several days. Smaller doses (5 to 10 mg) of vitamin K_1 are given if the indications for its use are less urgent. The rise in serum transaminases and lactic dehydrogenase activity and the antithyroid activity produced by these agents are not reversed by any vitamin K preparation. The clotting factors that are functionally altered by these anticoagulants are stable during storage and are present in acid-citrate-dextrose or citrate-phosphate-dextrose bank blood and FFP. Transfusions of blood or plasma can act as antagonists to the coumarin-indanedione anticoagulants. A plasma fraction concentrate containing factors II, VII, IX, and X (Konyne, Proplex) is an effective antagonist. Because of the significant recognized risk of transmitting hepatitis through these concentrates, their use is not recommended unless a life-threatening emergency is present.

Fibrinolytic therapy

The use of fibrinolytic or thrombolytic agents has added a new dimension to the treatment of peripheral vascular disease. The agents streptokinase, urokinase, and tissue plasminogen activator are well known to the physician who deals with thromboembolic disorders. These agents and others are discussed in the chapter dealing with fibrinolytic therapy (Chapter 5). The antifibrinolytic agents, including ϵ-aminocaproic acid and transexamic acid, are discussed below.

Antifibrinolytic therapy

The degree of hemorrhage in many different disease processes is directly related to the excessive activity of the plasminogen-plasmin proteolytic enzyme system. Control of this process is frequently helpful in managing the underlying disease.[62] In patients with hemophilia A or B and von Willebrand's disease hemorrhage in the oropharynx is augmented by numerous enzymes present in the mouth. In patients with non–immune- and immune-mediated severe thrombocytopenia a significant percentage of blood loss from cutaneous and mucous membranes is promoted by the activity of the fibrinolytic system. Similar observations have been made in patients with bleeding associated with ulcerative colitis, genitourinary tract bleeding associated with prostatic surgery, and diseases or mechanical devices altering uterine endothelium.

Although several agents can effectively inhibit the fibrinolytic system, two are currently commercially available: ϵ-aminocaproic acid (ϵ-ACA) and trans-4 (aminoethyl) cyclohexane carboxylic acid (AMCA). Both of these lysine analogs inhibit the plasminogen system by altering the configuration of the plasminogen molecule in a manner that prevents plasmin formation. Considerable clinical experience exists with the use of ϵ-ACA. This agent may be given by mouth in tablet or elixir form and intravenously. The initial dose is 5 g, followed by a maintenance dose of 1 to 2 g every 4 to 8 hours. A total dose of 30 g per day must not be exceeded. When ϵ-ACA is used in the above-mentioned situations, controlled studies have demonstrated that patients with congenital factor deficiencies require significantly less or no factor replacement therapy for dental procedures. Patients with severe thrombocytopenia may experience a reduction in bleeding despite no increase in the platelet count.[63] In some instances uterine or urinary tract bleeding can be controlled with these agents. A potential risk in using these agents is the induction of thrombus formation. Thus before administration of either antifibrinolytic agent, the absence of DIC and Trousseau's syndrome must be demonstrated.

Antiplatelet agents

Recent studies have indicated possible efficacy of agents that inhibit platelet aggregation and release in the prophylactic treatment of thrombotic disease. The three agents that have been studied in large numbers of patients are aspirin, dipyridamole, and sulfinpyrazone. All of these agents are given orally. The clinical indications for their use is different for each drug. At present the evidence suggests that aspirin may be helpful in prophylaxis against TIAs; the other antiplatelet agents are not useful.[64] Although some preliminary studies suggest that antiplatelet agents may be useful in treating ischemic heart disease and myocardial infarction, their long-term value in reducing the incidence or mortality rate remains unproven. Sulfinpyrazone may be useful in reducing the frequency of thrombotic occlusions in arteriovenous communications.[65] Prevention of thromboembolism in patients with prosthetic devices, particularly heart valves, may be possible by combining one or more of the three antiplatelet agents with oral anticoagulation therapy.[66] The problem with drug interactions, however, requires thoughtful consideration and careful monitoring. The value of the antiplatelet agents in the prevention of venous thrombosis is controversial, with more negative than positive results reported.[67,68]

The beneficial effect of aspirin in treating both TIAs and venous thrombosis after hip surgery was demonstrated in males but not in females.[61,69] Although some studies have demonstrated a favorable effect of the antiplatelet agents in some diseases, no studies have established an unequivocal benefit of any antithrombotic agent. It is clear that additional studies are needed.

Aspirin (acetylsalicylic acid). Aspirin's therapeutic benefit in vascular disease has been attributed to its effect on platelet-platelet and platelet-vascular endothelial interactions. Aspirin induces a functional defect in platelets, demonstrable clinically as a prolongation of the bleeding time. Through acetylation of the enzyme cyclooxygenase by aspirin, the synthesis of thromboxane A_2 is eliminated, preventing the induction of platelet aggregation by ADP release. The appropriate aspirin dose to achieve a thromboxane A_2–prostacyclin balance is not clear. Even 1 mg given by mouth every fourth day eventually equally inhibits both thromboxane A_2 and prostacyclin. Thus in studies reporting benefit when aspirin is taken in doses of several hundred milligrams per day, the aspirin is working by a mechanism as yet not understood.[70]

Dipyridamole. The principle mechanisms by which dipyridamole inhibits platelet function are as follows: (1) inhibition of adenosine uptake and metabolism resulting in increased concentration at the platelet-vascular interface; (2) inhibition of platelet phosphodiesterase, increasing cyclic AMP and potentiating platelet-inhibiting actions of prostacyclin; (3) stimulation of eicosanoid release by vascular endothelium; and (4) augmentation of the platelet-inhibiting effect of aspirin through pharmacokinetic interactions. The use of dipyridamole and aspirin in the prevention of occlusion in obliterative arterial disease in the lower limbs has been reported in a randomized, placebo-controlled trial.[71]

It remains unclear whether dipyridamole alone or in combination with aspirin can alter the progression of peripheral vascular insufficiency from arteriosclerosis, but combination therapy is commonplace and is recommended for patients having prosthetic or saphenous vein bypass grafts or for patients at the time of angioplasty.[72] It must be pointed out that in every study in which this combination has been evaluated and compared with the use of aspirin alone, the results clearly demonstrate that the effect of aspirin alone is equal to the combination of aspirin plus dipyridamole.[73] Further, extensive review of all published data on dipyridamole discretely points out that this agent has not been identified as efficacious in the treatment of any illness known.[73]

REFERENCES

1. Blake CCF, Harlos K, and Holland SK: Exam and domain evaluation in the proenzymes of blood coagulation and fibrinolysis, Cold Spring Harbor Symp Quant Biol; 52:925-931, 1987.
2. Chock PB, Rhee SG, and Stadtman ER: Interconvertible enzyme cascades in cellular regulation, Annu Rev Biochem 49:813-843, 1980.
3. Davie EW: The proteins of blood coagulation: their domains and evolution, Chem Scripta 26B:241-245, 1986.
4. Doolittle RF and Feng DF: Reconstructing the evolution of vertebrate blood coagulation from a consideration of the amino acid sequences of clotting proteins, Cold Spring Harbor Symp Quant Biol 52:869-874, 1987.
5. Furie B and Furie BC: The molecular basis of blood coagulation, Cell 53:505-518, 1988.
6. Jackson CM and Nemerson Y: Blood coagulation, Annu Rev Biochem, 49:765-811, 1980.
7. Mason RG and Saba HI: Normal and abnormal hemostasis—an integrated view, Am J Pathol 92:775-812, 1978.
8. Murano G: A basic outline of blood coagulation, Semin Thromb Hemost 6:140-162, 1980.
9. Day HJ and Rao AK: Evaluation of platelet function, Semin Hematol 23:89-101, 1986.
10. Rao AK and Holmsen H: Congenital disorders of platelet function, Semin Hematol 23:102-118, 1986.
11. Zucker MB: The functioning of blood platelets, Sci Am 242: 86-103, 1980.
12. Shittil SJ and Bennett JS: Platelets and their membranes in hemostasis: physiology and pathophysiology, Ann Intern Med 94:108-118, 1980.
13. Colman RW: Platelet activation: role of an ADP receptor, Semin Hematol 23:119-128, 1986.
14. George JN, Nurden AT and Phillips DR: Platelet membrane glycoproteins, New York, 1985, Plenum Press.
15. Phillips DR and Shuman MA: Biochemistry of platelets, New York, 1986, Academic Press.
16. Kroll MH and Schafer AI: Biochemical mechanisms of platelet activation, Blood 74:1181-1195, 1989.
17. Lawn RM and Vehar GA: The molecular genetics of hemophilia, Sci Am 254:48-54, 1986.
18. Zimmerman TS and Ruggeri ZM: von Willebrand disease, Hum Pathol 18:140-152, 1987.
19. Schafer AI: The hypercoagulable states, Ann Intern Med 102:814-828, 1985.
20. Clouse LH and Comp PC: The regulation of hemostasis: the protein C system, N Engl J Med 314:1298-1304, 1986.
21. Esmon CT: The regulation of natural anticoagulant pathways, Science 235:1348-1352, 1987.
22. Engesser L et al: Hereditary protein S deficiency: Clinical manifestations, Ann Intern Med 106:677-682, 1987.
23. Rosenberg RD: Role of antithrombin III in coagulation disorders: state of the art review, Am J Med 87:3B, 1989.
24. Sie P et al: Constitutional heparin cofactor II deficiency associated with recurrent thrombosis, Lancet 2:414-416, 1985.
25. Tran TH, Marbert GA, and Duckert F: Association of hereditary heparin cofactor II deficiency with thrombosis, Lancet 2:413-414, 1985.
26. Patthy L: Evolution of the proteases of blood coagulation and fibrinolysis by assembly from modules, Cell 41:657-663, 1985.
27. Francis CW and Marder VJ: Physiologic regulation and pathologic disorders of fibrinolysis, Hum Pathol 18:263-274, 1987.
28. Marder VJ and Bell WR: Fibrinolytic therapy. In Colman RW et al eds.: Hemostasis and Thrombosis, ed 2, Philadelphia, 1987, JB Lippincott Co.
29. Francis JL: Fibrinogen, fibrin stabilisation and fibrinolysis, chemical and biochemical aspects, London, 1988, Ellis Horwood Publishers.
30. Coull BM and Godnight SH: Antiphospholipid antibodies, prethrombotic states, and stroke, Curr Concepts Cerebrovasc Disc Stroke 25:13-18, 1990.
31. Simon LS: Antiphospholipid syndrome, N Engl J Med 322:754-769, 1990.
32. Bell WR: Disseminated intravascular coagulation, Johns Hopkins Med J 146:289-299, 1980.
33. Bell WR et al: Trousseau's syndrome: devastating coagulopathy in the absence of heparin, Am J Med 79:423-430, 1975.
34. Sack GH, Levin J, and Bell WR: Trousseau's syndrome and other manifestations of chronic disseminated coagulopathy in patients with neoplasms, Medicine 56:1-37, 1977.
35. Stemerman MB: Hemostasis, thrombosis and atherogenesis, Atherosclerosis Rev 6:105-146, 1979.
36. Rosenberg RD: The heparin-antithrombin system: natural anticoagulant mechanism. In Colman RW et al, eds.: Hemostasis and thrombosis, ed 2, Philadelphia, 1987, JB Lippincott Co.
37. Pitney WR, Pettit JE, and Armstrong L: Control of heparin therapy, Br Med J 4:139-141, 1970.
38. Coon WW and Willis PW: Hemorrhagic complications of anticoagulant therapy, Arch Intern Med 133:386-342, 1974.
39. Glazier RL and Crowell EB: Randomized prospective trial of continuous vs. intermittent heparin therapy, JAMA 236:1365-1367, 1976.
40. Levine MN, Raskob G, and Hirsh J: Hemorrhagic complications of long-term anticoagulation therapy, Chest 89:2, 16S-25S, 1986.
41. Case records of the Massachusetts General Hospital (case 49-1989), N Engl J Med 321:1595-1603, 1989.
42. Liu L, Haskin ME, and Rose LI: Diagnosis of bilateral adrenocortical hemorrhage by computed tomography, Ann Intern Med 97:720-721, 1982.

43. Bell WR et al: Thrombocytopenia occurring during the administration of heparin, Ann Intern Med 85:155-160, 1975.
44. King DJ and Kelton JG: Heparin-associated thrombocytopenia, Ann Intern Med 100:535-540, 1984.
45. Becker PS and Miller VT: Heparin-induced thrombocytopenia, Stroke 20:1449-1459, 1989.
46. Sheridan D, Carter C, and Kelton JG: A diagnostic test for heparin-induced thrombocytopenia, Blood 67:27-30, 1989.
47. Bell WR and Royall RM: Heparin-associated thrombocytopenia: a comparison of three heparin preparations, N Engl J Med 303:902-907, 1980.
48. Leroy J et al: Treatment of heparin-associated thrombocytopenia and thrombosis with low molecular weight heparin (CY216), Semin Thromb Hemost 11:326-329, 1985.
49. Miller ML: Heparin-induced thrombocytopenia, Cleve Clin J Med 56:483-490,1989.
50. Kraenzler EJ and Starr NJ: Heparin associated thrombocytopenia: management of patients for open heart surgery. Case reports, Anesthesiology 69:964-967, 1988.
51. Deswiet M et al: Prolonged heparin therapy in pregnancy causes bone demineralization, Br J Obstet Gynaecol 90:1129-1134, 1983.
52. Carter CJ et al: The relationship between the hemorrhagic and antithrombotic properties of low molecular weight heparin in rabbitts, Blood 59:1239-1245, 1982.
53. Cade JF et al: A comparison of the antithrombotic and hemorrhagic effects of low molecular weight heparin fraction: the influence of the method of preparation, Thromb Res 35:613-625, 1984.
54. Hass S and Blumel G: An objective evaluation of the clinical potential of low molecular weight heparins in prevention of thromboembolism, Semin Thromb Hemost 15:424-434, 1989.
55. O'Rielly RA: Vitamin K antagonists. In Colman RW et al, eds.: Hemostasis and thrombosis, ed 2, Philadelphia, 1987, JB Lippincott Co.
56. Hirsh J, Poller L, and Deykin D: Optimal therapeutic range for oral anticoagulants, Chest 95(suppl):5S-11S, 1989.
57. Wessler S and Gitel SN: Warfarin from bedside to bench, N Engl J Med 311:645-652, 1984.
58. Sise HS et al: The risk of interrupting long-term anticoagulant treatment: a rebound hypercoagulable state following hemorrhage, Circulation 24:1137-1142, 1961.
59. Alving BM, Strickler MP, and Knight RD: Hereditary warfarin resistance, Arch Intern Med 145:499-501, 1985.
60. Feder W and Auerbach R: "Purple toes": an uncommon sequelae of oral coumarin therapy, Ann Intern Med 55:911-917, 1961.
61. Cole MS, Minifee PK, and Wolma FJ: Coumarin necrosis—a review of the literature, Surgery 103:271-277, 1988.
62. Ogsto D: Current status of antifibrinolytic drugs, Blood Rev 3:1-4, 1989.
63. Bartholomew JR, Salgia R, and Bell WR: Control of bleeding in patients with immune and nonimmune thrombocytopenia with aminocaproic acid, Arch Intern Med 149:1959-1961, 1989.
64. The Coumadin Cooperative Study Group: A randomized trial of aspirin and sulfinpyrazone in threatened stroke, N Engl J Med 299:53-59, 1978.
65. Kaegi A et al: The role of sulfinpyrazone in the prevention of arteriovenous thrombosis, Circulation 52:497-499, 1975.
66. Dale J et al: Prevention of arterial thromboembolism with acetylsalicylic acid: a controlled clinical study in patients with aortic ball valves, Am Heart J 94:101-111, 1977.
67. O'Brien JR and Butterfield WJH: Aspirin in the prevention of thrombosis, Am Heart J 86:711-712, 1973.
68. Hume M et al: Prevention of postoperative thrombosis by aspirin, Am J Surg 133:420-422, 1977.
69. Harris WH et al: Aspirin prophylaxis of venous thromboembolism after total hip replacement, N Engl J Med 297:1246-1249, 1977.
70. Lekstrom J and Bell WR: Utility of aspirin in prevention of thrombosis, Medicine, 1990 (in press).
71. Hess H, Mietaschik A, and Deichsel G: Drug induced inhibition of platelet function delays progression of peripheral occlusive arterial disease: a prospective double-blind arteriographically controlled trial, Lancet 1:416-419, 1985.
72. Mayer JE Jr et al: Influence of aspirin and dipyridamole on patency of coronary artery bypass grafts, Ann Thorac Surg 31:204-210, 1981.
73. Fitzgerald GA: Dipyridamole, N Engl J Med 316:1247-1257, 1987.

Chapter 5

FIBRINOLYSIS AND FIBRINOLYTIC THERAPY

Robert A. Graor

BACKGROUND

The fibrinolytic system and thrombolytic therapy have recently been subjects of renewed and intense interest, sparked by a better understanding of the pathophysiology of the cardiovascular system and the balance between thrombus formation and fibrinolysis. Although this renewed interest in fibrinolysis makes it appear that understanding of the fibrinolytic system is relatively new, in 1838 Denis described the dissolution of fibrin in solutions of neutral salts. In 1893 Dastre made the important additional observation that fibrin was digested when it was incubated with serum; he named this process *fibrinolysis*.[1]

In experiments whose implications were generally ignored, Gratia, in 1921, noted that staphylococcal extracts induced lysis of a thrombus. In 1933 Tillett and Garner reported that bacteria-free filtrates of cultures of β-hemolytic streptococci contained a substance that rapidly dissolved clotted plasma, or fibrin.[2] They named this agent *streptococcal fibrinolysin*. Milstone soon discovered that streptococcal fibrinolysin's activity depended on a substance in plasma that was later identified by Kaplan and that proved to be plasminogen, the agent that is easily converted to plasmin.[3,4] In 1945 Christensen named the streptococcal derivative *streptokinase*.[5] Thus began the study of exogenous fibrinolytic agents, a field that would rapidly expand.

All exogenous fibrinolytic proteins activate plasmin. Plasmin is an enzyme of broad specificity, which digests not only fibrin but also other plasma proteins, including fibrinogen, other clotting factors, components of the complement system, and the kallikrein and kinin systems.

The fibrinolytic-thrombolytic agents initiate the mechanisms for removing pathologic intravascular fibrin deposits that cannot be dissolved by spontaneous lysis and for restoring vascular patency as rapidly as possible to retard tissue damage. From their observation that hemolytic streptococcal filtrates liquefy human plasma clots, Johnson and Tillett demonstrated the efficacy of streptokinase by showing that it lysed an experimentally induced thrombus in the marginal veins of rabbits.[6] In 1959 Johnson and McCarty showed that streptokinase lysed artificially induced thrombi in human volunteers. These findings stimulated the clinical use of fibrinolysis.[7]

Coincident with the development of fibrinolytic agents came the understanding that thrombi play a critical role in pathologic arterial or venous obstruction and, ultimately, in organ damage.

The fibrin clot formed in a physiologic process of hemostasis is normally controlled by the fibrinolytic system through the activation of plasminogen to plasmin. This process not only provides the mechanism for removing the fibrin when the need for the hemostatic barrier has been passed but also limits the extension of the fibrin clot. Thus the fibrinolytic system serves both as a regulator of hemostasis as well as a significant intermediary mechanism in a variety of pathologic lesions.

COMPONENTS OF THE FIBRINOLYTIC SYSTEM

Plasminogen

Central to understanding the role of the fibrinolytic system in thrombosis is the concept that a physiologic clot contains not only the factors responsible for clot formation but also the components and inhibitors of the fibrinolytic system (Table 5-1). The core of the fibrinolytic system is plasminogen, which is the zymogen precursor of the proteolytic enzyme, plasmin (Fig. 5-1).[8,9] Plasminogen activators cannot liquefy clots by themselves. Clot liquefaction

Table 5-1. Components of the fibrinolytic system

Plasminogen	Proenzyme form of the fibrinolytic enzyme
Plasmin	Active fibrinolytic enzyme
Streptokinase	Streptococcal protein that activates the fibrinolytic system in human plasma indirectly
Urokinase	Plasminogen activator isolated from urine or kidney cell cultures, consisting of two polypeptide chains; different from t-PA
Tissue-type plasminogen activator (t-PA)	Enzyme present in tissues that converts plasminogen to plasmin; identical or similar to blood plasminogen activator and vascular plasminogen activator
Single-chain urokinase-type plasminogen activator (scu-PA)	Enzyme present in blood and urine, related to urokinase but consisting of a single-chain M_r54,000 polypeptide
α_2-Antiplasmin	Specific fast-reacting plasmin inhibitor in human plasma
Plasminogen activator inhibitor-1 (PAI-1)	Fast-acting inhibitor of t-PA (and urokinase) in blood and secreted by endothelial cells
Plasminogen activator inhibitor-2 (PAI-2)	Fast-acting inhibitor of urokinase and t-PA isolated from placenta and present in blood in late pregnancy
Plasminogen activator inhibitor-3 (PAI-3)	Inhibitor of urokinase and thrombin, present in plasma and urine, stimulated by heparin

occurs as a result of the activation of plasminogen through the conversion of plasminogen to plasmin.

Plasminogen (single chain) ———————> Plasmin (double chain)
↑
Activator cleavage
arginine$_{560}$—valine bond

Human plasminogen is a single-chain glycoprotein synthesized by the liver.[10] The plasminogen molecule contains 790 amino acid residues, 25 disulfide bridges, and 5 homologous triple-loop "kringles."[11-13] The kringles contain binding sites that mediate the binding of fibrinogen to substrates such as fibrin. When bound to fibrin, plasminogen is more easily converted to plasmin, and the effect of plasmin is relatively localized to the adjacent fibrin.

Two forms of plasminogen have been purified from human plasma and differ in the composition of their NH_2-terminals. One type, containing a glutamic acid, is termed *Glu-plasminogen* and the other, containing mostly lysine in this position is termed *Lys-plasminogen*. Glu-plasminogen is the native form and Lys-plasminogen results from limited proteolysis of the Glu-plasminogen form.[14-18]

Plasminogen activators

Plasminogen can be activated to form plasmin through one of three pathways: (1) the *contact system* (Hageman factor and kallikrein)—dependent pathway, (2) the *tissue plasminogen activator (t-PA) pathway,* and (3) the *urokinase-dependent pathway* (Fig. 5-2).[16,18-21]

The contact system-dependent pathway is of less interest clinically and will not be examined in depth in this chapter. This pathway depends on the contact system of coagulation and is blocked by C1 esterase inhibitor.[19]

The t-PA pathway has received much attention recently.[21] It consists of t-PA and a fast-acting inhibitor of t-PA called *plasminogen activator inhibitor* (PAI).[22,23] Identified in several tissues, including endothelium, t-PA can be released from the endothelium by a number of substances, including thrombin, epinephrine, bradykinin, histamine, acetylcholine, platelet activating factor, and an analog of vasopressin, DDAVP.[24] Exercise and venous occlusion will also induce its release.

t-PA is a serine protease that hydrolyses several tripeptide substrates.[21] When t-PA is present during the formation of fibrin clots, it has a high affinity for fibrin-bound plasminogen and does not influence the catalytic efficiency of the enzyme.[25,26] Fibrin essentially increases the local plasminogen concentration by creating an additional interaction between t-PA and its substrate. The high affinity of t-PA for plasminogen in the presence of fibrin thus efficiently activates the fibrin-bound plasminogen on the fibrin clot.[27]

In the urokinase-dependent pathway urokinase converts plasminogen directly to plasmin.[28-30] Urokinase is initially synthesized as an inactive single-chain protein, called *prourokinase* (pro-UK), or a single-chain, urokinase-like plasminogen activator (scu-PA). Pro-UK is a normal component of plasma, and the conversion of pro-UK to urokinase is mediated by plasmin, an effect that may be stimulated or enhanced by heparin.

Inhibitors of plasminogen activity

Two types of inhibitors inhibit both plasmin (antiplasmins) and the activation of plasminogen (antiactivators).[31] The major plasmin inhibitor, α_2-antiplasmin, and several other inhibitors of t-PA and urokinase have recently been identified. A fast-acting inhibitor of t-PA and urokinase is relatively well characterized. Slower-acting inhibitors include α_2-macroglobulin and α_1-antitrypsin. The pharmacologic effects of exogenously administered plasminogen activators depend on the initial concentration of α_2-macroglobulin and, more importantly, of α_2-antiplasmin. When the plasminogen activator inhibitors are depleted, a systemic lytic state is invoked and fibrinogen and fibrin are consumed.[31]

$$\text{Plasmin} + \alpha_2\text{-antiplasmin} \underset{k_{-5}}{\overset{k_5}{\rightleftharpoons}} [\text{Plasmin} \cdot \alpha_2\text{-antiplasmin}]$$

$$[\text{Plasmin} \cdot \alpha_2\text{-antiplasmin}] \xrightarrow{k_6} \text{Inactive fragments}$$

$$\text{Plasmin} + \text{fibrinogen} \underset{k_{-7}}{\overset{k_7}{\rightleftharpoons}} [\text{Plasmin} \cdot \text{fibrinogen}]$$

$$[\text{Plasmin} \cdot \text{fibrinogen}] \xrightarrow{k_8} \text{Plasmin} + \text{fibrinogen degradation products}$$

$$\text{Plasmin} + \alpha_2\text{-macroglobulin} \xrightarrow{k_9} [\text{Plasmin} \cdot \alpha_2\text{-macroglobulin}]$$

Fig. 5-1. Reactions involving plasmin in the circulation. Brackets surrounding two constituents joined by a dot symbolize a complex; k_x and k_{-x} refer to forward and reverse rate constants, respectively. (From Tiefenbrunn AJ et al, Circulation 73:1291, 1986.)

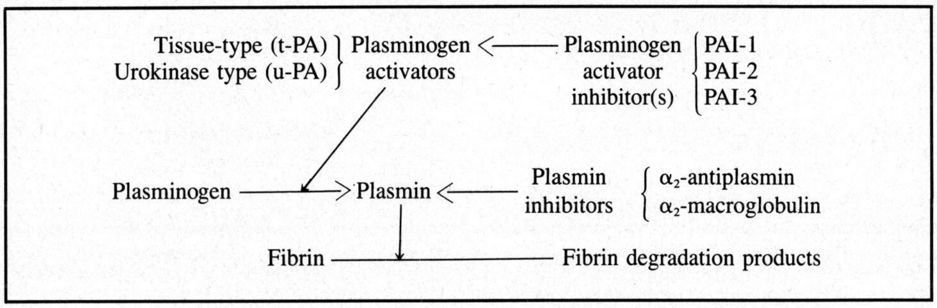

Fig. 5-2. Schematic representation of the fibrinolytic system.

Fibrinogen and fibrin

Two other major components of the fibrinolytic system, as well as the clotting system, are fibrinogen and fibrin. Both substances are digested by plasmin in a predictable manner and yield known and measurable products (Fig. 5-3).[32,33] Fibrinogen is composed of three pairs of polypeptide chains, including the α-, β-, and γ-chains linked by disulfide bonds.[34,35] The fibrinogen molecule is divided into four regions: (1) the carboxy terminal (D region) domain, (2) the central amino terminal (E region) domain, (3) the α-helical connecting coil, and (4) the polar α-chain appendages.[34-37] Thrombin (factor II) mediates the conversion of fibrinogen to fibrin by sequential cleavage at the amino terminal ends of the α- and β-chains. This cleavage generates fibrinopeptides A and B (FpA, FpB).[38,39]

Fibrin monomers, produced after the removal of FpA and FpB, remain in solution and will circulate in blood as long as they constitute a small fraction of the total fibrinogen concentration. Plasmin will sequentially cleave fibrinogen, yielding early split products called the X and Y fragments and late split products called the D and E fragments.[39-42] Plasmin first cleaves the α-chain at the carboxy terminal end, corresponding to the polar appendages. Next, the β-chain is cleaved at the amino terminal end, producing a fragment termed B-$\beta_{1\text{-}42}$ and a large residual fragment called fragment X. The B-$\beta_{1\text{-}42}$ fragment indicates the action of plasmin on fibrinogen (primary fibrinogenolysis), and it can be measured using enzyme-linked immunosorbent assay (ELISA). Fragment X is further degraded to fragments Y and D. The Y fragment is then split into D and E fragments, which are resistant to plasmin digestion. The D and E fragments are measured in commercially available latex agglutination fibrin split-product assays.

The products from the degradation of fibrin by plasmin vary by whether or not the fibrin clot has been stabilized by factor XIIIa.[41,42] If plasmin acts on uncrossed-linked fibrin, the split-products will be similar to those produced during fibrin degradation. Plasmin digestion of a crosslinked clot yields a wide variety of unique fragments, both higher and lower in molecular weight than fibrinogen.[31] One of these is a small peptide, B-$\beta_{15\text{-}42}$, which is a product of plasmin proteolysis of the β chain after thrombin cleavage of the fibrinopeptide B. Another unique fragment termed D-dimer is a dimer composed of γ-chain, crosslinked D domains of adjacent fibrin molecules. Elevated levels of either B-$\beta_{15\text{-}42}$ or D-dimer indicate the action of plasmin on an unstabilized fibrin clot.

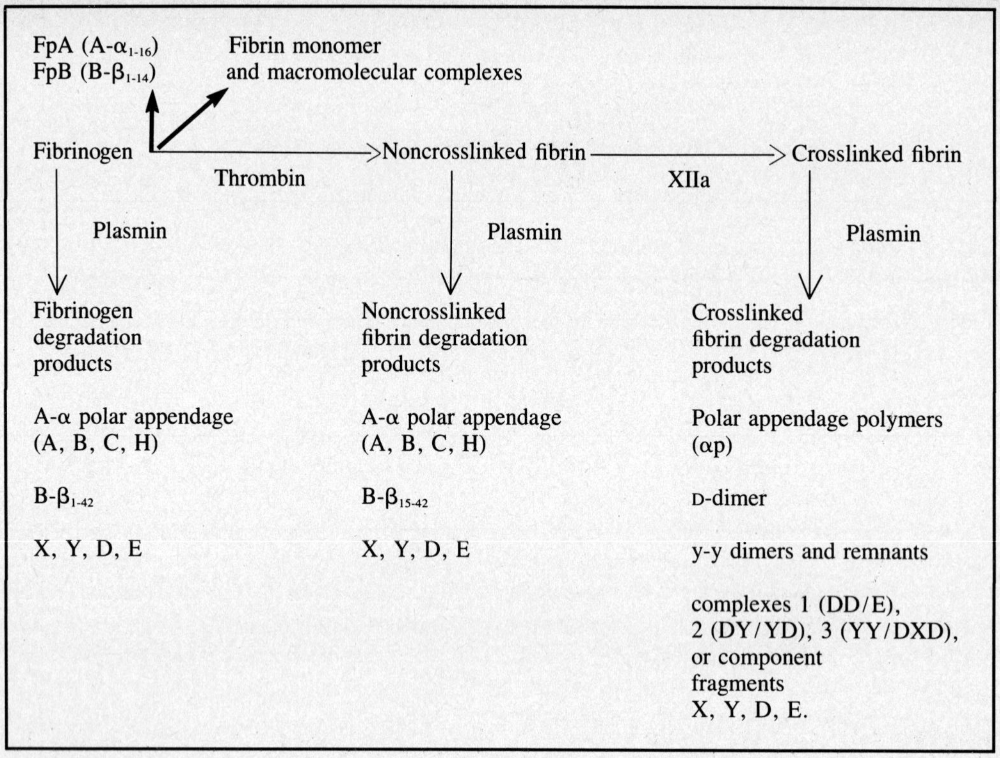

Fig. 5-3. Schematic representation of fibrinogen conversion to fibrin and its degradation process. The degradation products can be measured in the plasma.

BIOLOGIC PLASMINOGEN ACTIVATORS

Streptokinase

In 1933 Tillett and Garner observed that β-hemolytic streptococci filtrate liquefied human plasma clots.[2] The filtrate was later named *streptokinase*. Its mechanism of action is complex and requires a combination of human plasminogen and streptokinase in a 1:1 molar complex.[43,44] Once the streptokinase-plasminogen complex has been formed, the activator complex proceeds by cleavage of a single arginyl-valine peptide bond, and the streptokinase-plasminogen complex is gradually converted to streptokinase-plasmin complex, which is also an activator. Therefore this streptokinase molecule has no direct enzymatic activity. All assay studies first involve the formation of the activator complex.

Because streptokinase is derived from Lancefield classification group C strains of β-hemolytic streptococcal material, it is antigenic in humans, and because most humans have been exposed to streptococcal infections, streptokinase antibodies are present in most patients.[45] Therefore when streptokinase is infused into humans, enough potential activator must be given to neutralize the circulating antibody before a "lytic state" can be achieved. Alternatively, and more commonly, a standardized loading dose that is adequate to overcome circulating antibodies in 97% of the population, followed by an hourly maintenance dose, may be used. The loading dose necessary to overcome the antibodies varies from 250,000 to 600,000 units. The bolus infusion is followed by a 100,000 unit per hour maintenance dose in most cases.

Anisoylated streptokinase plasminogen activator

Anisoylated plasminogen streptokinase activator complex (APSAC) is a plasminogen streptokinase complex in which an anisoyl group covers the site of activation and completes the structure of a molecule that is fibrin-specific without producing the thrombolytic effect until it has undergone deacylation in vivo.[46,47] Essentially, this drug represents a plasminogen streptokinase complex with a protective cover over the activation point. This complex allows the thrombolytic activity to be maintained for several hours after a single intravenous bolus without continuing infusion.[46] Once deacylated in plasma, APSAC's biologic half-life in humans is about 100 minutes after an intravenous infusion.

Urokinase

Urokinase is a plasminogen activator that was initially isolated from human urine and later from tissue.[17,18,48-50] Urokinase directly activates plasminogen, unlike streptokinase, without forming an intermediate complex. Urokinase is a double-chain molecule held together by disulfide bonds. Two forms of urokinase exist, and little is known about the possible clinical benefits or advantages of one form compared with another.[48,51] Activation of plasmin in purified systems has shown differences in the Michaelis constant and the catalytic rate constant of urokinase forms.[52]

The current recommended dosage for urokinase is 4400 IU/kg/hr with a bolus infusion over 10 minutes of the same hourly dose for the treatment of deep vein thrombosis and pulmonary embolism. Peripheral arterial infusion doses are 2000 to 6000 units per minute, infused directly into the clot. Different dosage regimens of urokinase have been used with varying success. Several investigators have found no antibody formation after treatment with urokinase, which distinguishes it substantially from streptokinase.[53]

Single-chain urokinase activator (scu-PA)

The scu-PA molecule is a single-chain glycoprotein precursor of high molecular weight urokinase, secreted by human embryonic kidney cells, plasma and in cell culture.[54-58] In vitro, in the absence of fibrin, scu-PA causes no significant activation or fibrinolysis. However, in the presence of fibrin or fibrin-degradation products, scu-PA is unmasked and results in a high clot affinity or in clot selectivity. It apparently does not activate plasminogen in plasma in the absence of a fibrin clot because of the presence of a competitive inhibitor.[59,60] Fibrin neutralizes the competitive inhibition, although this process does not seem to occur via a specific binding of scu-PA to fibrin.[60]

Recombinant tissue-type plasminogen activator (rt-PA)

Tissue plasminogen activator, a serine proteinase that converts plasminogen to plasmin, is identical to vascular and blood plasminogen activators. Originally described by Pennica, t-PA was later purified and characterized by Rijken and Collen.[61,62] The primary structures of high molecular weight urokinase and t-PA have a high degree of homology, except t-PA contains a unique 43-residue amino acid region. This amino acid sequence is not found on urokinase and is homologous with the finger domains responsible for the fibrin affinity of fibronectin.[63]

The notion that t-PA in blood originates from vascular endothelial cells is supported by the finding that cultured endothelial cells secrete plasminogen activator, which may be either t-PA or urokinase-like.[64,65] Increased levels of plasminogen activator found after exercise or venous occlusion are immunologically related to t-PA.[66]

During the formation of fibrin clots, t-PA and plasminogen absorb to a fibrin clot, yielding a ternary complex. This complex results in the ability of fibrin to increase the local concentration of plasminogen by creating an additional interaction between t-PA and plasminogen.[21] In the absence of fibrin, t-PA is a poor enzyme, but the presence of fibrin strikingly enhances the activation rate of plasminogen. This enhancement explains an increased affinity of fibrin-bound t-PA for plasminogen but does not fully explain why systemic activity is apparent during t-PA administration.

These target-specific thrombolytic agents, or high-fibrin-affinity thrombolytic agents, have been called the "second generation" of fibrinolytic agents. The rationale for promoting second-generation agents is that only local fibrinolysis occurs in a reduced or noninduced systemic fibrinolysis. It is clear that systemic activation of the fibrinolytic system occurs with these agents, thereby indicating that although fibrin affinity is of value in producing potent clot lysis, it does not provide protection from fibrinogenolysis.[31,67]

The way these new agents act biochemically is that they bind specifically to fibrin and, when bound on the fibrin surface, efficiently convert the plasminogen bound to the fibrin to plasmin. The plasmin, already bound to fibrin, is partially protected from inactivation by circulating α_2-antiplasmin.[68] Initial clinical studies on acute myocardial infarction found that the second-generation agents were highly successful in inducing lysis of the thrombi and in initiating reperfusion to the ischemic myocardium.[69-71] Data from these studies established that these newer agents induced systemic fibrinolysis, but to a lesser degree than the first-generation agent, streptokinase. Unfortunately, the second-generation agents have not decreased the undesirable side effects of bleeding. If these agents are target-specific or fibrin-specific (i.e., the plasminogen-plasmin system is activated only at the site of the thrombus), there will be no systemic fibrinolysis.

The bleeding that occurs during fibrin-specific thrombolysis may be explained by the fact that bleeding associated with thrombolytic therapy most often occurs at invaded arterial or venous sites. The major component of the seal that forms at the invaded sites is fibrin, identical to the fibrin of the pathologic thrombus. Thus all target-specific or fibrin specific agents should activate the plasminogen associated with the pathologic fibrin as well as that associated with the physiologic fibrin.

LABORATORY MONITORING OF FIBRINOLYSIS

Laboratory tests can evaluate either specific or global markers of thrombolytic activity. Four types of tests have been used: (1) global tests of the fibrinolytic pathway, (2) measurement of specific components of the pathway, (3) markers of lytic activity, and (4) tests to predict rethrombosis following lytic therapy (see box on p. 98).

Simulations of serial changes in plasma constituents during infusion of a thrombolytic agent are shown in Fig. 5-4. Once α_2-antiplasmin is consumed, fibrinogenolysis occurs and FDPs (fibrin[ogen] degradation products) are elaborated in the circulation.

Before initiating thrombolytic therapy, screening or baseline tests should identify patients predisposed to an adverse outcome. We recommend obtaining a thrombin time, a complete blood count, and a fibrinogen evaluation. These tests provide reference data from which comparisons can be made.

To stop the fibrinolysis in the blood sample, we place the sample in ice immediately after venipuncture and cen-

Laboratory evaluation of the fibrinolytic pathway

Global tests of the fibrinolytic pathway

Whole blood clot lysis
Plasma clot lysis
Euglobulin clot lysis
Fibrin plate lysis
^{125}I-labeled fibrin clot lysis
Thromboelastography

Measurement of specific components of the pathway

Tissue plasminogen activator
Plasminogen activator inhibitor
Plasminogen
α_2-Plasmin inhibitor
Plasmin-α_2-plasmin inhibitor complexes

Markers of lytic activity

Fibrinogen
Fibrin(ogen) degradation products
D-dimer
B-$\beta_{1\text{-}42}$, B-$\beta_{15\text{-}42}$

Tests of rethrombosis potential following lytic therapy

Fibrinopeptide A
Soluble fibrin

trifuge it at 4° C. Plasma samples should then be frozen at −70° C. The rapid separation of plasma from red cells and the immediate freezing avoids spurious low plasminogen levels that result from its activation in vitro by the plasminogen activator in the sample. In addition, to obtain an accurate measurement of fibrinogen, the blood should be collected in sodium citrate that has been supplemented with fibrinolytic inhibitors, such as aprotinin and ε-aminocaproic acid. These inhibitors are sometimes insufficient to prevent in vitro fibrinogenolysis in the presence of high circulating plasma concentrations of thrombolytic drugs.

Tests to evaluate the global fibrinolytic pathway include whole blood clot-lysis time, but this test is too insensitive to be of much value during fibrinolysis. Whole blood clot-lysis may be accurately evaluated by using a thromboelastograph. This test indicates the presence of lytic activity within an hour or two.

The euglobulin clot-lysis time is a test based on the precipitation of fibrinogen, plasmin, and factors drawn from solution by acidification and the reduction of ionic strength. After thrombin clots the resolubilized precipitate, the end point is the time required for clot lysis to occur, which is normally 3 to 4 hours but may be as short as several minutes during systemic fibrinogenolysis.

Measuring the components of the fibrinolytic pathway includes introducing chromogenic and fluorogenic substrates to measure the functional levels of plasminogen,

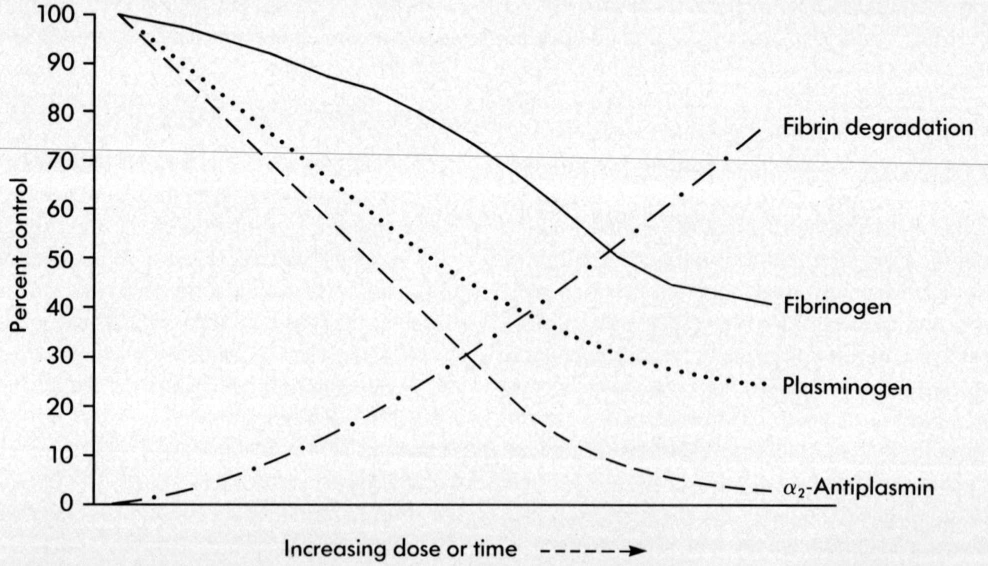

Fig. 5-4. This graph demonstrates a simulation of serial changes in the plasma constituents of the fibrinolytic system during infusion of a thrombolytic agent at variable doses and time. Once α_2-antiplasmin has been consumed, plasmin produces fibrinogenolysis and the expression of fibrin degradation products. Variable changes in each of these constituents can occur based on the amount of thrombolytic agent delivered or the time and duration of the infusion.

α_2-antiplasmin, t-PA, urokinase, and plasminogen activators. In patients infused with thrombolytic agents, these components of the fibrinolytic pathway will decrease in direct proportion to the extent of the fibrinolytic state.

Depletion of plasma fibrinogen has been used as an indirect marker of the "lytic state" as well as a marker of clinical safety during thrombolytic infusions. Correlations between the degree of fibrinogen depletion and the risk of bleeding have not been reported.[72]

Fibrinogen may be measured with thrombin-clotting, precipitation, or immunologic techniques. Thrombin time based on a clotting rate assay is preferred to precipitation or immunologic measurements.

The thrombin-clotting, or Clauss fibrinogen, technique is based on the rate of fibrin formation and not on the amount of protein in the final clot. The amount of protein in the clot may be assessed by chemical assay, weight measurement, or ultraviolet absorption.

Precipitation techniques are based on either heat or salt methods and take advantage of the fact that fibrinogen is one of the least soluble plasma proteins. Precipitation techniques are claimed to be less affected by fibrin degradation products and are therefore supposed to be more accurate. The extent to which these claims are true probably depends on the types of fibrin degradation products, the type of lytic agent, and the accuracy with which fibrin degradation products are quantified.

Immunologic methods include a variety of procedures, including latex agglutination, immunodiffusion, immunoelectrophoresis, radioimmunoassay, and nephelometry. Spuriously low values may result from the presence of high levels of fibrin degradation or defective fibrin polymerization.

Until recently, fibrin degradation products have been limited because the antibodies could not distinguish between degradation products of fibrin and those of fibrinogen. Split products of fibrin would be evidence of secondary or physiologic fibrinolysis, which accompanies disseminated anticoagulation, the postoperative state, and deep-vein or peripheral-arterial thromboembolism. Split products of fibrinogen, however, would be evidence of primary fibrinogenolysis, a condition in which pathologic proteolytic activity is directed at circulating fibrinogen.

Antibodies specific to fibrin degradation products are now available. One that has been extensively investigated and is now available for clinical laboratory use recognizes the D domains of fibrin after they have been cross-linked by factor XIII and digested by plasmin. This test, the D-dimer, can be performed either as a latex agglutination procedure or as a more sensitive ELISA technique. Other antibodies to fibrin degradation products are available but have been used less in clinical laboratories. Plasma degradation of fibrin yields the β-chain peptide, B-$\beta_{15\text{-}42}$, whereas degradation of fibrinogen yields B-$\beta_{1\text{-}42}$. Because these fragments are measured by ELISA, the technique is extremely sensitive. Elevated levels of both the 1-42 and 15-42 fragments during lytic therapy suggests that both fibrin clot and circulating fibrinogen are being degraded. Elevated levels of B-$\beta_{15\text{-}42}$, following cessation of rt-PA administration and long after rt-PA has cleared from the circulation, suggest sustained clot lysis from the incorporation of rt-PA into the clot. This sustained lysis effect is less apparent with streptokinase. The D-dimer and B-$\beta_{15\text{-}42}$ fractions are elevated higher and longer with rt-PA than with streptokinase, suggesting that fibrinolysis with rt-PA is more intense and persistent.

Clinical applications of laboratory tests

The clinical use of laboratory evaluations during thrombolysis is controversial but, in general, could potentially be applied in the management of patients in three ways: (1) to detect and monitor the presence of the fibrinolytic state, (2) to predict clinical events (i.e., reperfusion or reocclusion), and (3) to control the clinical course following thrombolysis (see box on p. 98). Unfortunately, changes in the constituents of the fibrinolytic system do not correlate with bleeding complications, and therefore laboratory monitoring has not been effective in predicting complications. Bleeding is likely to be the result of the physiologic clots lysing in the same fashion as the pathologic clots. The physiologic clots occur at areas of previous arterial or venous invasion or at a site of pathologic change, such as a stroke. If there is a nidus that could potentially bleed, there is little justification or predictive ability in measuring plasma constituents of the fibrinolytic system.

In our experience, the fibrinogen measurement is valuable if clinical decisions need to be made with regard to an ongoing bleeding complication. Fibrinogen levels do not predict bleeding; they only allow the clinician to act appropriately if bleeding should occur, to determine whether fibrinogen needs to be transfused to achieve hemostasis.

Platelets and thrombolytic agents

Platelets contribute to normal hemostasis by adhering to subendothelial surfaces after blood vessels have been damaged and then amassing additional platelets at the site.[73,74] These two processes, termed *adhesion* and *aggregation,* can activate the coagulation mechanism, resulting in the deposition of fibrin. In some pathologic conditions, thrombogenic surfaces, such as ruptured atherosclerotic plaque, are the initial site of platelet deposition and, if this deposition remains unmodulated, larger aggregates can develop, resulting in the occlusion or embolization of platelet fibrin.[75,76] This platelet adhesion is mediated by a number of platelet surface receptors with a high affinity for adhesive glycoproteins found in the subendothelium and in pathologic lesions.[77,78] The surface receptors most responsible for platelet activity are the glycoprotein IIb-IIIa-complex receptors. Platelet aggregation is mediated exclusively by platelet glycoprotein IIb and IIIa receptors.

In vitro studies have shown that platelets can enhance the generation of plasmin, inhibit the generation of plasmin, and neutralize active plasmin. It is thus not surprising that both profibrinolytic and antifibrinolytic effects have been described.[79,80]

Tissue plasminogen activator and single-chain urokinase plasminogen activator are present on platelet surfaces, but the functional status of these activators remains unclear.[81,82] Platelets can also bind plasminogen directly to their surface under usual conditions, and this binding can be augmented approximately fivefold if thrombin converts platelet-associated fibrinogen to fibrin.[83] Miles and Plow have demonstrated that platelet glycoproteins IIb and IIIa are involved in the binding mechanisms.[84] These data suggest that plasminogen can be localized on or near platelets by several means. High concentrations of plasmin can potentially be generated in their vicinity. Supporting these data is the fact that both the fibrinolysis of clots and the activation of plasminogen by t-PA are enhanced in the presence of platelets.[83-86]

Platelets also contain the potent plasminogen activator inhibitor, PAI-1, and the rapid-acting α_2-antiplasmin in their granules.[86-88] The release of these substances after platelet activation could therefore limit thrombolysis. Platelets are also responsible for releasing cross-linking proteins, notably factor XIII, and have the ability to cross link α_2-antiplasmin to fibrin, inhibiting fibrinolysis.[89]

Although in vitro studies show that platelets have profibrinolytic and antifibrinolytic properties, their correlation to in vivo thrombolysis is unclear. The ability of the platelet to function will likely differ under various conditions. Some in vivo data suggest that platelet-rich thrombi are particularly resistant to thrombolysis, raising the possibility that at least some patients whose arteries have thrombosed and have an unusually rich platelet thrombus may be resistant to clot lysis.[79,90]

Plasminogen activation can have profound and opposing effects on platelet function. Both platelet activation and inhibition have been identified in in vitro systems, and preliminary evidence suggests that both effects may be expressed in vivo as well. Activation and inhibition times appear to differ in such a way that platelet activation dominates immediately after the administration of a thrombolytic agent and platelet inhibition appears later.[91,92] Both streptokinase and rt-PA activate platelets within minutes of administration as judged by increased levels of urinary metabolites of thromboxane A_2 and enhanced platelet aggregation.[93] On the basis of elevations of fibrinopeptide A levels, thrombolytic therapy might also result in regeneration of thrombin, a potent platelet activator and a stimulus for thromboxane production.[94] Fibrinopeptide A is a highly nonspecific marker for thrombin activity, and rt-PA can cleave fibrinopeptide A directly from fibrinogen, indicating that it may not be resulting from platelet activation.[95] Regardless of the mechanism by which thrombolytic agents can cause activation, such activation does occur and can contribute to reocclusion or perhaps resistance to clot lysis. The interaction between thrombolytic agents and the activation of platelets is important because if this activation is a clinical obstacle, then thrombolytic agents may be designed to prohibit platelet activation.

An impressive number of mechanisms have been proposed by which thrombolytic therapy may inhibit platelet function. Prominent among these mechanisms is the pharmacologic inhibition of platelet arachidonic acid metabolism and platelet aggregation by low-dose plasmin, especially when combined with prostacyclin and selective lysis of the fibrinogen bound to the platelet surface, which disaggregates the platelets.[96] Although only a few early experimental and clinical studies indicated that thrombolytic therapy with streptokinase prolonged bleeding time and inhibited platelet function, the bleeding time has not been evaluated routinely in more recent major trials of thrombolytic therapy.[97,98]

Gimple et al recently reported that patients receiving rt-PA had significantly prolonged bleeding times when tested approximately 1.5 hours following the infusion.[99] If these data are consistent for all thrombolytic agents, the hemorrhagic complications of fibrinolytic therapy may be related, at least in part, to platelet dysfunction and an existing nidus for bleeding. Although this hypothesis may seem obvious, it is important because most thinking has focused on systemic fibrinogenolysis as the main cause of hemorrhage. Additional information to corroborate these ideas comes from tests for coagulation, including those designed to assess systemic lysis of fibrin and fibrinogen that have no value in estimating the risk of hemorrhage. Tissue plasminogen activator, which produces less systemic fibrinogenolysis than streptokinase or urokinase, produces comparable rates of serious bleeding, indicating a possible alternate primary reason for hemorrhage and implicating platelet inhibition as a possible influencing factor.[92,100,101]

Several clinical studies have examined the use of antiplatelet agents in patients undergoing thrombolytic therapy.[102-104] The most comprehensive data came from the second international study of infarct survival (ISIS-2) in which 17,187 patients who were suspected on clinical grounds of having myocardial infarction were given placebo, streptokinase, aspirin, or streptokinase plus aspirin.[105] This study showed that both aspirin and streptokinase reduced mortality during the first 35 days after treatment and that the combination of aspirin and streptokinase was considerably more effective than either agent alone. The short-term benefits were sustained at 2 years. The risk of minor hemorrhage increased slightly with aspirin and increased greatly with streptokinase when compared with the placebo group. Adding aspirin to streptokinase further increased the risk, but not significantly. The number of major bleeding complications did not increase in the aspirin group, but it did increase in the streptokinase group. Adding aspirin to streptokinase had little effect on the actual number of major bleeding complications. The risk of both major and minor hemorrhagic complications tended to correlate with the clinician's intention at the beginning of the patient's hospitalization to use heparin therapy, suggesting that concomitant heparin therapy may be an important determinant in hemorrhagic risk in this group of patients.

The dreaded complication of intracranial bleeding was also examined in the ISIS-2 trial. Although the streptokinase-treated groups had more cerebral hemorrhages on the first day of therapy, this rate decreased after day 1 until the number of strokes in these two groups was lower than the number in the placebo group. The group taking only aspirin did not have an increased incidence of hemorrhagic strokes on day 1 and had the lowest stroke rate of all.

Previous studies have found an extremely high risk of thromboembolic stroke after acute myocardial infarction that correlates with the extent of the infarction.[106,107] Therefore antiplatelet and thrombolytic therapy may reduce this risk by reducing the extent of infarction, inhibiting the thromboembolic process itself, or both. In contrast to the ISIS-2 study, a recent preliminary report from the Phase I Thrombolysis in Myocardial Infarction (TIMI) group found no

Table 5-2. Total mortality reduction, total bleeding complications, and CNS bleeding in myocardial infarction trials

Study Agent Dose (duration)	Mortality reduction in thrombolysis groups	Total hemorrhage Events/no. of patients (% frequency)	CNS hemorrhage Events/no. of patients (% frequency)
TIMI phase 1 (110)*	NE		
SK 1,500,000 U (60 min)		46/147 (31)	0
rt-PA 80 mg (180 min)		47/143 (33)	0
TIMI II B (111)*	NE		
rt-PA 100 mg (180 min)		21/47 (44)	15(0.5)
ISAM (112)†	NE		
SK 1,500,000 U (60 min)		51/859 (5)	4/859 (0.4)
Placebo		13/882 (1)	1/882 (0.1)
GISSI (113)†	Yes		
SK 1,500,000 U (60 min)		207/5860 (3)	10/5860 (0.1)
AIMS (114)†	Yes		
APSAC 30 U (5 min)		25/502 (5)	2/502 (0.3)
Placebo		9/502 (1)	5/502 (1.0)
ISIS-2 (105)†	Yes		
SK 1,500,000 U (60 min)		171/4300 (3)	2/4300 (0.04)
SK 1,500,000 U (60 min) with ASPIRIN/160 mg/day (30 days)		191/4292 (4)	5/4295 (0.12)
Aspirin 160 mg/day (30 days)		124/4295 (2)	5/4295 (0.12)
Placebo		44/4300 (1)	0/4300 (0)
GAUS (115)†	NE		
UK 3,000,000 U (90 min)		27/121 (22)	0
rt-PA 70 mg (90 min)		24/124 (19)	1

NE, Not a designated end point.
* With intervention.
† Without intervention.

significant differences in the rate of reperfusion 18 to 48 hours after rt-PA therapy in a group given aspirin, compared with the group not given aspirin. The high rate of reperfusion in the control group, however, weakened the statistical analysis on the number of patients studied.[108]

COMPLICATIONS OF THROMBOLYTIC THERAPY

Concomitant with the introduction of second-generation fibrin-specific thrombolytic agents was the prediction that they would activate the human fibrinolytic system only at the site of the thrombus and not induce systemic fibrinolysis. The rationale for this prediction was the belief that systemic activation of the fibrinolytic system was associated with, and was the causative factor for, the bleeding observed during treatment with these agents. The best comparison of the effects of first- and second-generation agents on bleeding complications is among patients with acute myocardial infarction. Although some studies fail to mention bleeding complications, and others overestimate it, there remains considerable disagreement as to what constitutes a significant or major bleeding complication. It is fair to conclude that the incidence of bleeding complications with the second-generation agents is *not* lower but is comparable to that of first-generation agents.

Bleeding complications associated with thrombolytic therapy have been known since the first clinical trials were conducted in the late 1960s. According to the Food and Drug Administration, during the first 5 years after streptokinase and urokinase became commercially available, the bleeding frequency in patients receiving thrombolytic agents for pulmonary emboli, venous thrombosis, and arterial thromboemboli was between 5% and 7%.[109] The frequency of bleeding with urokinase and streptokinase in this period was no different from the frequency observed for heparin anticoagulation.

The data from thrombolytic therapy trials for acute myocardial infarction support some interesting conclusions (Table 5-2).[100-115] The frequency of bleeding associated with the "newer agents," rt-PA and APSAC, is not less than that observed for the first-generation agents, streptokinase and urokinase. The most frequent location for bleeding during thrombolytic therapy is unequivocally where an invasive procedure is performed at the time of, or adjacent to, thrombolytic therapy. On the other hand, the most grave complication associated with thrombolytic infusions is intracranial bleeding, and this complication does not appear to occur more frequently with any one thrombolytic agent.

Despite what some believe to be the case, earlier and recent data establish that there is no correlation with the circulating blood levels of fibrinogen, plasminogen, or fibrin degradation products and the frequency of bleeding.[70,72] These proteins correlate with the degree of systemic activation and, in our opinion, the fibrinogen level is valuable only when a potential nidus results in a bleeding complication. Then, the fibrinogen level is important in determining whether hemostasis can be achieved at the levels in that individual patient. Conceivably, more fibrin-selective thrombolytic agents may have a higher affinity for the fibrin in the physiologic plug and could, perhaps, aggravate bleeding complications. This aggravation has not been established to date. Thus the degree or the lack of systemic fibrinolysis is not related to the problem of bleeding in any situation.

An additional factor that may be important to the process of bleeding complications is thrombocytopenia, which has been observed in association with rt-PA infusions but not with SK or UK.[73-85] Other factors that may play a role in bleeding associated with thrombolytic therapy include an increase in the activation of the complement system with increases in C3a, C4a, and C5a.[78]

CLINICAL APPLICATION OF THROMBOLYTIC THERAPY

The clinical application of thrombolysis is, in part, based on the fact that anticoagulant therapy cannot remove thrombi—it can only prevent thrombus propagation. Fibrinolytic agents not only prevent formation of the thrombus, but also provide a rapid return of the normal physiologic and hemodynamic states and possibly prevent the late sequelae of the disease and organ damage. These agents should be considered as adjuncts to anticoagulation therapy or surgical treatment, and decisions regarding their use should be governed by a knowledge of the disease state, alternate therapies, and experience with the use of the agents and their administration.

The promise of thrombolysis was recognized in the late 1950s, but its use has diffused slowly. The slow acceptance of this therapy is the result of the lack of definitive knowledge of its efficacy and of the risks of the associated invasive procedures, including the perception that bleeding is common.

Table 5-3 summarizes the agents currently available for clinical thrombolysis, their physical characteristics, their clinical indications as reported in thc literature, and the preferred route of administration.

To simplify the clinical use of thrombolytic agents, it is convenient to divide their therapeutic use into four major categories (1) acute myocardial infarction, (2) thromboembolic venous disease, (3) peripheral arterial occlusive disease, and (4) other conditions.

Thrombolytic therapy for myocardial infarction

Perhaps the most well-studied indication for a thrombolytic agent is acute myocardial infarction.[105,113,114,116] Intravenous thrombolytic therapy has become the cornerstone of treatment of patients with acute myocardial infarction. Data generated from the trials listed in Fig. 5-5[105,113,114,116] have proven that early intervention with an intravenous thrombolytic agent can significantly reduce the mortality associated with myocardial infarction. An increasing amount of evidence confirms that thrombolysis can restore patency to an occluded coronary artery and thus can decrease

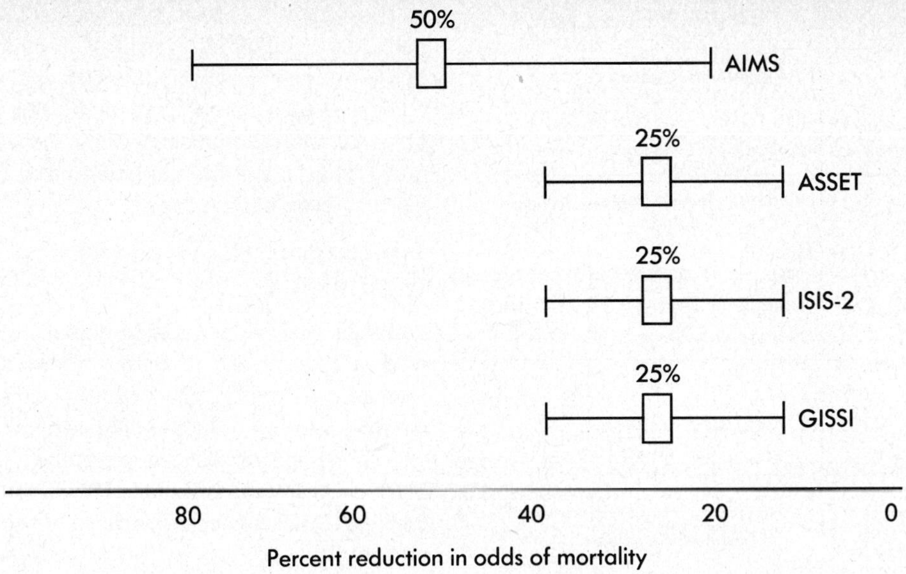

Fig. 5-5. Percent reduction in odds of mortality within 30 days for patients randomized within 6 hours of the onset of chest pain to thrombolysis or a control group. Mortality rates in the treated groups were 6.4% in AIMS. This represents approximately 50% odds reduction in AIMS and 25% reduction in ASSET, ISIS II, and GISSI, but the 95% confidence intervals of the studies overlap.

infarct expansion and left ventricular volume and improve left ventricular remodeling after the infarction.[110-116]

Numerous other conditions related to acute myocardial infarction are undergoing trials with thrombolytic treatment. These conditions include unstable angina, occluded coronary artery bypass grafts, and opening of chronically occluded coronary arteries.[117-121] Thrombolytic agents are also being investigated for their effects when given before, during, and after angioplasty.

Thrombolytic therapy for deep vein thrombosis

Thrombolytic therapy for acute venous thrombosis is controversial, although physicians agree that a thrombus in the deep venous system results in severe sequelae and that the elimination of the thrombus is beneficial. The decision to use thrombolysis in selected patients with deep vein thrombosis and pulmonary embolism is clouded by poorly conducted studies in which patients were included at differing times after the onset of symptoms, with incomplete follow-up studies, follow-up studies that ignored the influence of intercurrent events, and the lack of objective hemodynamic testing. Rapid advances in noninvasive vascular technology will soon allow more complete, accurate, and repetitive evaluations of the deep venous system.

Table 5-4 lists several studies in which patients with a deep vein thrombosis were treated with thrombolysis and the results were evaluated by venography.[122-135] Selection bias may be important when evaluating these pooled studies, but clearly the concern about bleeding complications in the treatment of thromboembolic disorders has been exaggerated, especially with deep vein thrombosis.

Table 5-3. Pharmacologic and clinical features of thrombolytic preparations*

	Agent				
Features	**SK**	**APSAC**	**UK**	**scu-PA**	**rt-PA single chain**
Half-life (min)	23	90	16	7	5
Fibrin enhancement	1+	1+	2+	4+	3+
Plasma proteolytic state	4+	4+	3+	2+	1+
Bleeding complications	4+	4+	4+	4+	4+
Allergic side effects	Yes	Yes	No	No	No
Antigenicity	Yes	Yes	No	NK	NK

*The clinical data were derived mostly from reported experience with current intravenous dosages in the treatment of acute myocardial infarction; 0 is none and 4+ is highest.
SK, Streptokinase.
APSAC, Acylated plasminogen-streptokinase activator complex.
UK, Urokinase.
scu-PA, Recombinant single-chain urokinase plasminogen activator.
rt-PA, Recombination tissue-type plasminogen activator.

Table 5-4. Heparin vs lytic therapy for DVT[122-135]: 14 studies

Degree of lysis	**Lytic therapy n = 322**	**Heparin n = 271**
None/worse	32% (104)	82% (222)
Partial	21% (68)	12% (32)
Sig./complete	47% (150)	6% (17)

Table 5-5. Heparin vs lytic therapy for proximal DVT

Author	Length of follow-up	Therapy	Long-term results: Symptoms (%) Severe	Moderate	None
Arnesen, Hoiseth, and Ly,[133] 1982	6.5 yr	Heparin	17	50	33
		SK	0	24	76
Elliot et al,[132] 1979	1.6 yr	Heparin	24	66	10
		SK	9	36	55

Table 5-6. Heparin vs lytic therapy for DVT[134]

Venous hemodynamic assessment	Therapeutic response: Clot lysed (n = 12)	Not lysed (n = 28)	*P*-value
PPG-$T_{1/2}$			
Mann-Whitney	12.2 ± 4.1	5.0 ± 2.3	<0.001
Foot volumetry			
$T_{1/2}$	11.1 ± 5.8	4.7 ± 2.6	<0.001

Table 5-7. Major bleeding complications in patients treated for DVT[137]

Therapy	Total patients	Percent major bleeding
Heparin	146	9
Streptokinase	654	14
t-PA	14	7
Urokinase	132	0.8

The importance of thrombolytic therapy for the treatment of deep vein thrombosis is in the long-term results, that is, in preventing venous insufficiency. Tables 5-5 and 5-6 present results of patients with significant or complete clearance of DVT by thrombolytic therapy in the long-term as measured by venographic and clinical data.[132-134] Although not all patients experienced complete thrombolysis or a normal phlebogram, a higher percentage in the thrombolytic treated group were asymptomatic for venous insufficiency.

The bleeding complication rate for streptokinase is higher than that for urokinase. In a study done at the Cleveland Clinic, a very low major bleeding rate was observed for urokinase (0.0%) compared to streptokinase-treated patients (17%) ($P < 0.01$).[136] Pilla and Comerota reported major bleeding complications in pooled patient groups (Table 5-7).[137]

A common concern—the incidence of fatal or major pulmonary emboli as a result of thrombolytic treatment of DVT—is also reviewed by Pilla and Comerota.[137] They compared each therapy and found that pulmonary emboli occurred more commonly in the heparin-treated patients (10%) than in the thrombolytic-treated patients (5%). This has also been our experience.

THROMBOLYTIC THERAPY FOR PULMONARY EMBOLI

When massive pulmonary embolism occurs, aggressive medical therapy, including thrombolysis, may be necessary to reduce mortality. The definition of massive pulmonary emboli varies according to the patient's underlying medical conditions and the size of the emboli. In trials of thrombolytic therapy the National Heart, Lung, and Blood Institute (NHLBI) defined massive pulmonary emboli as "significant filling defects in two or more pulmonary lobar arteries." This definition implied involvement of at least 40% of the pulmonary arterial tree. Other definitions require anatomic involvement of 40% to 50% or more of the pulmonary vasculature. With underlying cardiopulmonary disease, significantly smaller pulmonary emboli may result in the consequences that are commonly seen with an anatomically defined massive pulmonary emboli.

A hemodynamic, rather than an anatomic, stratification of the patient's condition is clearly the most reliable indicator of prognosis, but not necessarily the most obvious clinically at the onset of massive pulmonary emboli. In addition, a relatively high percentage of patients sustain great permanent derangement of their pulmonary vasculature if the thrombus does not resolve.[138] Chronic thromboembolic pulmonary hypertension can be a devastating disease, but it is potentially preventable with thrombolytic agents.

In autopsy studies of fatal emboli, whether death occurs suddenly or more slowly, only half of the clots meet the anatomic definition of massive pulmonary emboli. Often the fatal embolus is relatively small; however, it is poorly tolerated because of an underlying disease, such as congestive heart failure, chronic lung disease, or a history of pulmonary emboli. Mortality, even among patients with an anatomically massive pulmonary embolism, is low if patients have adequate pulmonary circulation reserve. Patients who do have adequate pulmonary circulation reserve often are stable with relatively large emboli, and therefore the clinician treats them with conventional therapy (anticoagulation). These patients are at considerable risk of suffering the consequences of chronic thromboembolic pulmonary hypertension if recurrent emboli occur or if the anticoagulation results in incomplete resolution of the emboli.

The rationale for employing thrombolysis in pulmonary emboli is described in Chapter 25. Briefly, thrombolysis relieves the obstruction to pulmonary artery flow and thus improves right ventricular function, reduces pulmonary artery pressure, and allows pulmonary tissue reperfusion. This

Table 5-8. Summary of pulmonary embolus comparative trials of heparin and thrombolytic treatment

Study	No. of patients	Treatment allocation	Outcome
Tibbutt et al[141]	32	Random: 15 heparin, 17 thrombolytic	Improved right heart pressures and anatomy in thrombolytic group
Hirsh et al[142]	27	Nonrandom: 10 heparin, 17 streptokinase	Hemodynamic and anatomic improvement in thrombolytic group
Miller et al[143]	23	Nonrandom: 9 heparin, 14 thrombolytic	Anatomic improvement in thrombolytic group
Ly et al[144]	25	Random/nonrandom: 11 heparin, 14 thrombolytic	Anatomic improvement statistically better in thrombolytic group
Phase I UPET*[145]	160	Random: 78 heparin, 82 urokinase	Improved hemodynamic and anatomic response in urokinase group
Goldhaber et al[147]	30	Nonrandom: 30 t-PA historic heparin control group	Substantial qualitative and quantitative improvement in t-PA group compared to historic control group treated with heparin

*Urokinase Pulmonary Embolism Trial.

therapy avoids a continuous afterload increase to the right ventricle and the associated morbidity. By accelerating the reversal of right heart failure, thrombolysis might reduce the mortality rate from pulmonary embolism, the risk of thrombotic venous insufficiency, and the source for potential further or recurrent pulmonary emboli. Thereby, thrombolytic therapy may also reduce the frequency of chronic pulmonary hypertension caused by recurrent or single massive pulmonary embolism.[139]

The Food and Drug Administration approved the use of urokinase and streptokinase for pulmonary embolism in 1977 and rt-PA for the same indication in 1990. Nonetheless, thrombolytic agents have been used in less than 10% of patients with acute pulmonary emboli. During a recent 1-year period, 44 clinical centers in the United States reviewed 2539 patient charts and determined that 53.5% of patients could have been treated with thrombolytic agents, more than anticipated.[140]

Table 5-8 reviews the published pulmonary embolism trials in which patients were treated with heparin or thrombolytic agents. Unfortunately, efforts to define the proper role for thrombolytic therapy in treating pulmonary embolism may have to be based on little clinical data. Although all studies found more pronounced anatomic and physiologic improvement in patients treated with thrombolytic agents, no study could associate these findings with improvements in mortality or any other clinical conditions. Limitations of sample size and relatively low mortality rates among control subjects greatly limit the power of these clinical studies to show an improvement in mortality.

Survival rates may be considerably improved as a result of a specific therapy, but such a benefit may not yet have been demonstrated in these small studies. The largest study, sponsored by the NHLBI, the Urokinase Pulmonary Embolism Trial (UPET), randomly selected 160 patients for heparin or urokinase treatment.[145] The urokinase patients had statistically greater anatomic improvement and comparatively more rapid resolution of hemodynamic abnormalities. The differences were most striking during the first few days of treatment and narrowed with time to the point where, within 5 to 7 days, the benefit of thrombolytic therapy could no longer be seen.

A subsequent cooperative study, the Urokinase, Streptokinase Pulmonary Embolism Trial (USPET) had an identical design to the UPET and compared 12 hours of urokinase with 24 hours of streptokinase in a total of 167 patients.[146] Urokinase appeared to act more quickly, especially in patients with anatomically large emboli, and both thrombolytic agents appeared to have a greater favorable impact on pulmonary hemodynamics. Mortality was equal in the three groups and was reported as 7% to 9% at 2 weeks and 10% to 15% at 6 weeks.

Goldhaber et al reported the results of the treatment of pulmonary emboli with rt-PA in 30 patients.[147] They demonstrated that 28 of 30 patients had angiographic evidence of clot lysis with qualitative and quantitative improvement on pulmonary arteriography. A statistically significant decrease in pulmonary artery pressure occurred in the rt-PA treated patients. In addition, these investigators demonstrated that right ventricular dysfunction and tricuspid regurgitation improved dramatically and rapidly after rt-PA therapy. Our experience using rt-PA or urokinase for pulmonary emboli parallels that of Goldhaber et al.

Thrombolytic therapy for peripheral arterial disease

A patient may have a history of intermittent claudication that suddenly worsens, leading to rest pain (progressive atherosclerosis obliterans with thrombosis in situ), or sudden onset of pain, pallor, pulselessness, paresthesias, or paralysis (acute arterial emboli or thrombosed bypass graft). The classic teaching has been that thrombectomy, embolectomy, and surgical revascularization are the treatments of choice for acute or chronic arterial ischemia. In the last 10 years,

Table 5-9. Pooled data on the use of streptokinase, urokinase, and t-PA in the treatment of peripheral arterial occlusions

Drug	No. of infusions	Duration of infusion (hr)	Successful thrombolysis (%)	Major complications (%)
Streptokinase	474	40	316 (67)	88 (19)
Author and study				
Dotter, Rosch, and Seaman, 1974[152]				
Katzen and van Breda, 1981[155]				
Totty et al, 1982[156]				
Berni et al, 1983[157]				
Mori et al, 1983[158]				
Becker et al, 1983[159]				
Katzen et al, 1984[160]				
Wolfson, Kumpe, and Rutherford, 1984[161]				
van Breda et al, 1984[162]				
Kakkasseril et al, 1985[163]				
Graor et al, 1985[164]				
Belkin et al, 1986[165]				
van Breda, Katzen, and Deutsch, 1987[166]				
Koltun et al, 1987[167]				
Urokinase	162	30	130 (81)	19 (12)
Author and study				
McNamara and Fischer, 1985[153]				
Belkin et al, 1986[165]				
van Breda, Katzen, and Deutsch, 1987[166]				
Koltun et al, 1987[167]				
t-PA	55	4.7	51 (93)	4 (7.2)
Author and study				
Graor et al, 1986[168]				

there have been many studies that support the use of intraarterial thrombolytic therapy in the management of patients with peripheral arterial occlusions.

As early as 1959 Fletcher, Alkjaersig, and Sherry administered IV streptokinase to patients with peripheral arterial occlusions and demonstrated thrombolysis.[148] During the next 15 years there were more reports describing the use of IV streptokinase for arterial disease. Successful thrombolysis occurred in approximately 55% of these early studies with extraordinarily high bleeding complications and a 7% fatality rate in one series.

In the 1960s several reports described intraarterial administration of thrombolytic agents for acute occlusions of the superficial femoral and popliteal arteries.[148-153] This intraarterial technique led to a rapid proliferation of the medical literature for the treatment of peripheral arterial occlusions with an intraarterial method.

The technique of administration was further defined by McNamara et al, and their data suggested that urokinase produced a higher degree of efficacy and a lower complication rate.[153,154]

Summarized in Table 5-9 is a selection of the most recent reports of the various thrombolytic agents in the treatment of peripheral arterial occlusions. In these reports evaluation of success and complications could be objectively established. From these studies it is clear that the success rate with urokinase or rt-PA has been greater than in those reports using streptokinase. In addition the complication rates are substantially reduced with both urokinase and rt-PA. Based on the volume of data available in the current literature, urokinase has been used most commonly for peripheral arterial occlusion.

There has been much interest in the use of thrombolytic agents in the last 20 years. We have progressed from IV infusions of high doses of streptokinase to direct intraarterial infusions of streptokinase, urokinase, or rt-PA. Urokinase and rt-PA appear to lyse clot in a shorter period of time with fewer bleeding complications. Thrombolytic agents are useful adjuncts to surgery and percutaneous transluminal angioplasty. They allow lysis of small distal runoff vessels, decreasing outflow resistance and enabling the native artery or bypass graft to remain open. They also further define the anatomy so that the angiographer, internist, and surgeon can select a rational and elective form of therapy after thrombolysis. However, there have been no prospective, randomized, or double-blind controlled trials comparing the use of individual thrombolytic agents or comparing thrombolysis against surgery. These studies are needed to further define the appropriate role for thrombolysis and peripheral arterial occlusive disease.

SUMMARY

Great advances in the use of thrombolytic therapy have occurred in recent years. The better understanding of the fibrinolytic system and the extensive use of thrombolytic agents in clinical vascular disease have provided useful data to improve patient selection and provide better therapy for patients with occlusive vascular disease.

REFERENCES

1. Dastre A: Fibrinolyse dans le sang, Arch Physiol Norm Path (Paris) 5:661, 1893.
2. Tillett WS and Garner RL: The fibrinolytic activity of hemolytic streptococci, J Exp Med 58:485, 1933.
3. Milstone H: A factor in normal human blood which participates in streptococcal fibrinolysis, J Immunol 42:109, 1941.
4. Kaplan MH: Nature and role of the lytic factor in hemolytic streptococcal fibrinolysis, Proc Soc Exp Biol Med (NY) 57:40, 1944.
5. Christensen LR: Streptococcal fibrinolysis: a proteolytic reaction due to a serum enzyme activated by streptococcal fibrinolysis, J Gen Physiol 28:363, 1945.
6. Johnson AJ and Tillett WS: Lysis in rabbits of intravascular blood clots by the streptococcal fibrinolytic system (streptokinase), J Exp Med 95:449, 1952.
7. Johnson AJ and McCarty WR: The lysis of artificially induced intravascular clots in man by intravenous infusions of streptokinase, J Clin Invest 39:426, 1959.
8. Troll W and Sherry S: The activation of human plasminogen by streptokinase, J Biol Chem 213:881, 1955.
9. Davies MC, Englert ME, and DeRenzo EC: Interaction of streptokinase and human plasminogen. I. Combining of streptokinase and plasminogen observed in the ultracentrifuge under a variety of experimental conditions, J Biol Chem 239:2651, 1964.
10. Maturen AJ and Barnhart MI: Cell loci and plasminogen antigen. Proceedings of the twenty third Wayne State Symposium on Blood, Detroit, 1975 (abstract).
11. Paoni NF and Castellino FJ: Isolation of a low-molecular weight form of plasminogen, Biochem Biophys Res Commun 65:757, 1975.
12. Sottrup-Jensen L et al: The primary structure of human plasminogen: isolation of two lysine-binding fragments and one "mini"-plasminogen (M_w, 38,000) by elastase-catalyzed specific limited proteolysis. In Davidson JF et al, eds: Progress in chemical fibrinolysis and thrombolysis, vol 3, New York, 1978, Raven Press.
13. Dayhoff MO: Atlas of protein sequence and structure, vol 5 (suppl 3), Silver Spring, Md, 1978, The National Biomedical Research Foundation.
14. Kwaan HC, Lo R, and McFadzean AJS: On the production of plasma fibrinolytic activity within veins, Clin Sci 16:241, 1957.
15. Robbins KC and Summaria L: Plasminogen and plasmin. In Lorand L, ed: Methods in enzymology, New York, 1976, Academic Press.
16. Wiman B and Wallen P: Activation of human plasminogen by an insoluble derivative of urokinase: structural changes of plasminogen in the course of activation to plasmin and demonstration of a possible intermediate compound, Eur J Biochem 36:25, 1973.
17. Kwaan HC: Fibrinolytic proteins. In Coleman RW et al, eds: Hemostasis and thrombosis, Philadelphia, 1982, JB Lippincott Co.
18. Bernik MB and Kwaan HC: Plasminogen activator activity in cultures from human tissues: an immunological land histochemical study, J Clin Invest 48:1740, 1969.
19. Kaplan AP and Austen KF: Activation and control mechanism of Hageman factor-dependent pathways of coagulation, fibrinolysis and kinin generation and their contribution to the inflammatory response, J Allergy Clin Immunol 56:491, 1975.
20. Marder VJ et al: Changes in the plasminogen-plasmin fibrinolytic system during urokinase therapy: comparison of tissue culture urokinase with urinary source urokinase in patients with pulmonary embolism, J Lab Clin Med 92:721, 1978.
21. Hoylaerts M et al: Kinetics of the activation of plasminogen by human tissue plasminogen activator, J Biol Chem 257:2912, 1982.
22. Collen D: Identification and some properties of a new fast-reacting plasmin inhibitor in human plasma, Eur J Biochem 69:209-216, 1976.
23. Moroi M and Aoki N: Isolation and characterization of α_2-plasmin inhibitor from human plasma: a novel proteinase inhibitor which inhibits activator-induced clot lysis, J Biol Chem 251:5956, 1976.
24. Todd AS: The blood vessel wall and fibrinolytic activity. In Johnson SA and Guest MM, eds: Dynamics of thrombus formation and dissolution, Philadelphia, 1961, JB Lippincott Co.
25. Ranby M: Studies on the kinetics of plasminogen activation by tissue plasminogen activator, Biochem Biophys Acta 704:461, 1982.
26. Zamarron C, Lijnen HR, and Collen D: Kinetics of the activation of plasminogen by natural and recombinant tissue-type plasminogen activator, J Biol Chem 259:2080, 1984.
27. Suenson E, Lutzen O, and Thorsen S: Initial plasmin-degradation of fibrin as the basis of a positive feedback mechanism in fibrinolysis, Eur J Biochem 140:513, 1984.
28. Lijnen HR et al: Activation of plasminogen by pro-urokinase. I. Mechanism, J Biol Chem 261:1253, 1986.
29. Collen D et al: Activation of plasminogen by pro-urokinase. II. Kinetics, J Biol Chem 261:1259, 1986.
30. Holmes WE et al: Cloning and expression of the gene for pro-urokinase in *Escherichia coli,* Biotechnology 3:923, 1985.
31. Tiefenbrunn AJ et al: Pharmacodynamics of tissue-type plasminogen activator characterized by computer-assisted simulation, Circulation 73:1291, 1986.
32. Marder VJ and Budzynski AZ: The structure of the fibrinogen degradation products. In Spaet T, ed: Progress in hemostasis and thrombosis, New York, 1974, Grune & Stratton.
33. Gaffney PJ: The biochemistry of fibrinogen and fibrin degradation products. In Ogston D and Bennett B, eds: Haemostasis: biochemistry, physiology and pathology, London, 1977, John Wiley & Sons.
34. Doolittle RF: Fibrinogen and fibrin. In Bloom A and Thomas DP, eds: Haemostasis and thrombosis, London, 1981, Churchill Livingstone, Inc.
35. Doolittle RF et al: The amino acid sequence of the α-chain of human fibrinogen, Nature 280:464, 1979.
36. Marder VJ, Shulman NR, and Carroll WR: The importance of intermediate degradation products of fibrinogen in fibrinolytic hemorrhage, Trans Assoc Am Physicians 53:156, 1967.
37. Marder VJ, Shulman NR, and Carroll WR: High molecular weight derivatives of human fibrinogen produced by plasmin. I. Physicochemical and immunological characterization, J Biol Chem 244:2111, 1969.
38. Shainoff JR and Page IH: Cofibrins and fibrin-intermediates as modificators of thrombin activity, in vivo, Circ Res 8:1013, 1960.
39. Shainoff JR and Dardik BN: Fibrinopeptide B and aggregation of fibrinogen, Science 204:200, 1979.
40. Nussenzweig V et al: Les produits de degradation du fibrinogene humain par la plasmine. I. Separation et proprietes physicochimiques, Ann Inst Pasteur Immunol 100:377, 1961.
41. Pizzo SV et al: The effect of plasmin on the subunit structure of human fibrin, J Biol Chem 248:4574, 1973.
42. Francis CW, Marder VJ, and Martin SE: Plasmic degradation of crosslinked fibrin. I. Structural analysis of the particulate clot and identification of new macromolecular soluble complexes, Blood 56:456, 1980.
43. Kosow DP: Kinetic mechanism of the activation of human plasminogen by streptokinase, Biochemistry 14:4459, 1975.
44. Gonzales-Gronow M, Siefring GE Jr, and Castellino FJ: Mechanism of activation of human plasminogen by the activator complex, streptokinase-plasmin, J Biol Chem 253:1090, 1978.
45. Mullertz S and Lassen M: An activator system in blood indispensable

for the formation of plasmin by streptokinase, Proc Soc Exp Biol Med 82:264, 1953.

46. Been M et al: Clinical effects and kinetic properties of intravenous APSAC—anisoylated plasminogen-streptokinase activator complex (BRL 26921) in acute myocardial infarction, Int J Cardiol 11:53, 1986.
47. Anderson JL: Development and evaluation of anisoylated plasminogen streptokinase activator complex (APSAC) as a second generation thrombolytic agent, J Am Coll Cardiol 10:22B, 1987.
48. White WF, Barlow GH, and Mozen MM: The isolation and characterization of plasminogen activators (urokinase) from human urine, Biochemistry 5:2160, 1966.
49. Gunzler WA et al: Structural relationship between human high and low molecular mass urokinase, Hoppe Seyler's Z Physiol Chem 363:133, 1982.
50. Heyneker HL, Holmes WE, and Vehar GA: Preparation of functional human urokinase proteins, European Patent Office, Munich, Federal Republic of Germany, 1983.
51. Duckert F: Urokinase. In Markwardt F, ed: Fibrinolytics and antifibrinolytics, New York, 1983, Springer-Verlag.
52. Sobel BE, Gross RW, and Robison AK: Thrombolysis, clot selectivity, and kinetics, Circulation 70:160, 1984.
53. Barlow GH et al: Production of plasminogen activator by tissue culture techniques. In Paoletti R and Sherry S, eds: Thrombosis and urokinase, London, 1977, Academic Press.
54. Bernik MB: Increased plasminogen activator (urokinase) in tissue culture after fibrin deposition, J Clin Invest 52:823, 1973.
55. Nolan C et al: Plasminogen activator from human embryonic kidney cell cultures: evidence for a proactivator, Biochem Biophys Acta 496:384, 1977.
56. Stump DC, Thienpont M, and Collen D: Urokinase-related proteins in human urine. Isolation and characterization of single-chain urokinase (pro-urokinase) and urokinase-inhibitor complex, J Biol Chem 261:1267, 1986.
57. Kasai S et al: Proteolytic cleavage of single-chain pro-urokinase induces conformational change which follows activation of the zymogen and reduction of its high affinity for fibrin, J Biol Chem 260:12377, 1985.
58. Stump DC, Lijnen HR, and Collen D: Purification and characterization of single-chain urokinase-type plasminogen activator (scu-PA) from human cell cultures, J Biol Chem 261:1274, 1986.
59. Lijnen HR, Zamarron C, and Collen D: Characterization of the high-affinity interaction between human plasminogen and pro-urokinase, Eur J Biochem 150:141, 1985.
60. Zamarron C et al: Biological and thrombolytic properties of proenzyme and active forms of urokinase. I. Fibrinolytic and fibrinogenolytic properties in human plasma in vitro of urokinase obtained from human urine or by recombinant DNA technology, Thromb Haemost 52:19, 1984.
61. Pennica D et al: Cloning and expression of human tissue-type plasminogen activator cDNA in *E. coli*, Nature (London) 301:214, 1983.
62. Rijken DC and Collen D: Purification and characterization of the plasminogen activator secreted by human melanoma cells in culture, J Biol Chem 256:7035, 1981.
63. Banyai L, Varadi A, and Patthy L: Common evolutionary origin of the fibrin-binding structures of fibronectin and tissue-type plasminogen activator, FEBS Lett 163:37, 1983.
64. Loskutoff DJ and Edgington T: Synthesis of a fibrinolytic activator and inhibitor by endothelial cells, Proc Natl Acad Sci USA 74:3903, 1977.
65. Levin EG and Loskutoff DJ: Cultured bovine endothelial cells produce both urokinase and tissue-type plasminogen activators, J Cell Biol 94:631, 1983.
66. Rijken DC, Wijngaards G, and Welbergen J: Relationship between tissue plasminogen activator and the activators in blood and vascular wall, Thromb Res 18:815, 1980.
67. Graor RA et al: Peripheral artery and bypass graft thrombolysis with recombinant human tissue-type plasminogen activator, Circulation 72(suppl III): III-15, 1985 (abstract).
68. Chmielewska J, Ranby M, and Wiman B: Evidence for a rapid inhibitor to tissue plasminogen activator in plasma, Thromb Res 31:427, 1983.
69. Verstraete M et al: Randomized trial of intravenous recombinant tissue-type plasminogen activator versus streptokinase in acute myocardial infarction, Lancet 1:842, 1985.
70. TIMI Study Group: The Thrombolysis in Myocardial Infarction (TIMI) Trial, N Engl J Med 312:932, 1985.
71. Topol EJ, Bell WP, and Weisfeldt ML: Coronary thrombolysis with recombinant tissue-type plasminogen activator: a hematologic and pharmacologic study, Ann Intern Med 103:837, 1985.
72. Marder VJ and Bell WR: Fibrinolytic therapy in hemostasis and thrombosis. In Colman RW, et al, eds: Philadelphia, 1987, JB Lippincott Co.
73. Leonard EF, Turitto VT, and Vroman L, eds: Blood in contact with natural and artificial surfaces, Ann NY Acad Sci 516:1, 1987.
74. Walsh PN: Platelet-mediated coagulant protein interactions in hemostasis, Semin Hematol 22:178, 1985.
75. Falk E: Unstable angina with fatal outcome: dynamic coronary thrombosis leading to infarction and/or sudden death—autopsy evidence of recurrent mural thrombosis with peripheral embolization culminating in total vascular occlusion, Circulation 71:699, 1985.
76. Fuster V, Steele PM, and Chesebro JH: Role of platelets and thrombosis in coronary atherosclerotic disease and sudden death, J Am Coll Cardiol 5(suppl):175B, 1985.
77. Coller BS et al: Collagen-platelet interactions: evidence for a direct interaction of collagen with platelet GPIa/IIa and an indirect interaction with platelet GPIIb/IIIa mediated by adhesive proteins, Blood 74:182, 1989.
78. Plow EF and Ginsberg MH: Cellular adhesion: GPIIb-IIIa as a prototypic adhesion receptor, Prog Hemost Thromb 9:117, 1989.
79. Thorsen S, Brakman P, and Astrup T: Influence of platelets on fibrinolysis: a critical review. In Ambrole JL, ed: Hematologic reviews, vol 3, New York, 1972, Marcel Dekker.
80. Joist JH: Platelets and fibrinolysis, Thromb Haemost 38:955, 1977.
81. Jeanneau C and Sultan Y: Tissue plasminogen activator in human megakaryocytes and platelets: immunocytochemical localization, immunoblotting and zymographic analysis, Thromb Haemost 59:529, 1988.
82. Park S et al: Demonstration of single chain urokinase-type plasminogen activator on human platelet membrane, Blood 73:1421, 1989.
83. Miles LA et al: Plasminogen interacts with human platelets through two distinct mechanisms, J Clin Invest 77:2001, 1986.
84. Miles LA and Plow EF: Binding and activation of plasminogen on the platelet surface, J Biol Chem 260:4303, 1985.
85. Stricker RB et al: Activation of plasminogen by tissue plasminogen activator on normal and thrombasthenic platelets: effects on surface proteins and platelet aggregation, Blood 68:275, 1986.
86. Erickson LA, Ginsberg MH, and Loskutoff DJ: Detection and partial characterization of an inhibitor of plasminogen activator in human platelets, J Clin Invest 74:1465, 1984.
87. Kruithof EK, Tran-Thang C, and Bachmann F: Studies on the release of plasminogen activator inhibitor from human platelets, Thromb Haemost 55:201, 1986.
88. Plow EF and Collen D: The presence and release of α_2-antiplasmin from human platelets, Blood 58:1069, 1981.
89. Sakata Y and Aoki N: Significance of cross-linking of α_2-plasmin inhibitor to fibrin in inhibition of fibrinolysis and in hemostasis, J Clin Invest 69:536, 1982.
90. Jang I-K et al: Differential sensitivity of erythrocyte-rich and platelet-rich arterial thrombi to lysis with recombinant tissue-type plasminogen activator: a possible explanation for resistance to coronary thrombolysis, Circulation 79:920, 1989.

91. Rudd MA et al: Temporal effects of tissue plasminogen activator infusion on platelet aggregation ex vivo, Blood 72(suppl I):374A, 1988 (abstract).
92. Loscalzo J: Platelets and thrombolysis, J Vasc Med Biol 1:4, 213, 1989.
93. Fitzgerald DJ et al: Marked platelet activation in vivo after intravenous streptokinase in patients with acute myocardial infarction, Circulation 77:142, 1988.
94. Eisenberg PR, Sherman LA, and Jaffe AS: Paradoxic elevation of fibrinopeptide A after streptokinase: evidence for continued thrombosis despite intense fibrinolysis, J Am Coll Cardiol 10:527, 1987.
95. Weitz JI et al: Human tissue-type plasminogen activator releases fibrinopeptides A and B from fibrinogen, J Clin Invest 82:1700, 1988.
96. Schafer AI et al: Synergistic inhibition of platelet activation by plasmin and prostaglandin I_2, Blood 69:1504, 1987.
97. Kowalski E, Kopec M, and Wegrzynowicz A: Influence of fibrinogen degradation products (FDP) on platelet aggregation, adhesiveness and viscous metamorphosis, Thromb Diath Haemorrh 10:406, 1963.
98. Cronberg S: Effect of fibrinolysis on adhesion and aggregation of human platelets, Thromb Diath Haemorrh 19:474, 1968.
99. Gimple LW et al: Correlation between template bleeding times and spontaneous bleeding during treatment of acute myocardial infarction with recombinant tissue-type plasminogen activator, Circulation 80:581, 1989.
100. Rao AK et al: Thrombolysis in Myocardial Infarction (TIMI) Trial, Phase I: hemorrhagic manifestations and changes in plasma fibrinogen and the fibrinolytic system in patients treated with recombinant tissue plasminogen activator and streptokinase, J Am Coll Cardiol 11:1, 1988.
101. Califf RM et al: Hemorrhagic complications associated with the use of intravenous tissue plasminogen activator in treatment of acute myocardial infarction, Am J Med 85:353, 1988.
102. Topol EJ et al: A randomized, placebo-controlled trial of intravenous recombinant tissue-type plasminogen activator and emergency coronary angioplasty in patients with acute myocardial infarction, Circulation 75:420, 1987.
103. White HD et al: Effect of intravenous streptokinase as compared with that of tissue plasminogen activator on left ventricular function after first myocardial infarction, N Engl J Med 320:817, 1989.
104. Van de Werf F: Lessons from the European cooperative recombinant tissue plasminogen activator (rt-PA) versus placebo trial, J Am Coll Cardiol 12(suppl A):14A, 1988.
105. ISIS-2 (Second International Study of Infarct Survival) Collaborative Group: Randomized trial of intravenous streptokinase, oral aspirin, both, or neither among 17,187 cases of suspected acute myocardial infarction: ISIS-2, Lancet 2:349, 1988.
106. Thompson PL and Robinson JS: Stroke after acute myocardial infarction: relation to infarct size, Br Med J 2:457, 1978.
107. Puletti M et al: Cerebrovascular accidents in acute myocardial infarction, Ital J Neurol Sci 8:245, 1987.
108. Robertson TL et al: Aspirin, rt-PA, and reperfusion in AMI: a TIMI observational study, Circulation 78(suppl II)II-128, 1988 (abstract).
109. Sherry S, Bell WR, and Duchert FH: Thrombolytic therapy in thrombosis: a National Institute Health Consensus Development Conference, Ann Intern Med 93:141, 1980.
110. Chesebro JH et al: Thrombolysis in myocardial infarction (TIMI) trial, Phase I: A comparison between intravenous tissue plasminogen activator and intravenous streptokinase, Circulation 76(1):142, 1987.
111. The TIMI Research Group: Comparison of invasive and conservative strategies after treatment with rt-PA in acute myocardial infarction, N Engl J Med 320:618, 1989.
112. The ISAM Study Group: A prospective trial of intravenous streptokinase in acute myocardial infarction (ISAM): mortality, morbidity, and infarct size at 21 days, N Engl J Med 314:1465, 1986.
113. Gruppo italiano per lo studio della streptochinasi nelp'infarto miocardico (GISSI): Effectiveness of intravenous thrombolytic treatment in acute infarction, Lancet 1:397, 1986.
114. AIMS Trial Study Group: Effect of intravenous APSAC on mortality after acute myocardial infarction: preliminary report of a placebo-controlled clinical trial, Lancet 1:545, 1988.
115. Neuhaus KL and GAUS Study Group: Thrombolysis in acute myocardial infarction: results of the German Activator-Urokinase Study, Circulation 76:IV, 1987.
116. Trial of tissue plasminogen activator for mortality reduction in acute myocardial infarction, Anglo-Scandinavian study of early thrombolysis (ASSET), Lancet, September 3, 525-530, 1988.
117. Gotoh K et al: The role of intracoronary thrombus in unstable angina: angiographic assessment and thrombolytic therapy during ongoing anginal attacks, Circulation 77:526, 1988.
118. Schrieber T et al: Urokinase plus heparin versus aspirin in unstable angina and non-Q wave myocardial infarction, Am J Cardiol 64:840, 1989.
119. Ambrose JA and Hjemdahl-Monsen CE: Arteriographic anatomy and mechanisms of myocardiol ischemia in unstable angina, J Am Coll Cardiol 9:1397, 1987.
120. Hartmann J et al: Prolonged infusion of urokinase for chronically occluded aorto-coronary bypass grafts, Am J Cardiol 61:189, 1986.
121. Rentrop P et al: Recanalization of an acutely occluded aorto-coronary bypass by intragraft fibrinolysis, Circulation 62:1123, 1980.
122. Gormsen J: Thrombolytic therapy of acute phlebothrombosis. In Heimeyer V, ed: Therapeutische and Experimentelle Fibrinolyse, Stuttgart, 1969, KF Schattauer Verlag.
123. Browse NL, Thomas ML, and Pim HP: Streptokinase and deep vein thrombosis, Br Med J 3:307, 1967.
124. Robertson BR, Nilsson IM, and Nylander G: Value of streptokinase and heparin in therapy of acute deep vein thrombosis, Acta Chir Scan 134:203, 1968.
125. Robertson BR, Nilsson IM, and Nylander G: Thrombolytic effect of streptokinase as evaluated phlebography of deep venous thrombi of the leg, Acta Chir Scan 136:173, 1970.
126. Kakkar VV et al: Treatment of deep vein thrombosis: a trial of heparin, streptokinase and arvin, Br Med J 1:806, 1969.
127. Tsapogas MJ et al: Controlled study of thrombolytic therapy in deep vein thrombosis, Surgery 74:973, 1973.
128. Duckert F et al: Treatment of deep vein thrombosis with streptokinase, Br Med J 1:479, 1975.
129. Rosch JJ et al: Healing of deep vein thrombosis: venographic findings in a randomized study comparing streptokinase and heparin, AJR 127:533, 1976.
130. Marder VJ, Soulen RL, and Atichartakarn V: Quantitative venographic assessment of deep vein thrombosis in the evaluation of streptokinase and heparin therapy, J Lab Clin Med 89:1018, 1977.
131. Watz R and Savidge GF: Rapid thrombolysis and preservation of venous valvular function in high deep vein thrombosis, Acta Med Scand 205:293, 1979.
132. Elliot MS et al: A comparative randomized trial of heparin versus streptokinase in the treatment of acute proximal venous thrombosis: an interim report of a prospective trial, Br J Surg 66:838, 1979.
133. Arnesen H, Hoiseth A, and Ly B: Streptokinase or heparin in the treatment of deep vein thrombosis: follow-up results of a prospective study, Acta Med Scand 211:65, 1982.
134. Jeffrey P, Immelman E, and Amoore J: Treatment of deep vein thrombosis with heparin or streptokinase: long-term venous function assessment. Proceedings of the Second International Vascular Symposium, London, 1986 (abstract no. S20.3).
135. Kakkar VV and Lawrence D: Hemodynamic and clinical assessment after therapy for acute deep vein thrombosis, Am J Surg 150:54, 1985.
136. Graor RA et al: Comparison of cost effectiveness of streptokinase and urokinase in the treatment of deep vein thrombosis, Ann Vasc Surg 1:524, 1987.
137. Pilla T and Comerota AJ: Basic data related to thrombolytic therapy for venous thrombosis, Ann Vasc Surg 3:81, Jan 1989.

138. Korn D et al: Pulmonary arterial bands and webs: an unrecognized manifestation of organized pulmonary emboli, Am J Pathol 40:129, 1962.
139. Sharma GVRK, Burleson VA, and Sasahara AA: Effective thrombolytic therapy on pulmonary capillary blood volume in patients with pulmonary embolism, N Engl J Med 303:842, 1980.
140. Terrin M et al: Selection of patients with acute pulmonary embolism for thrombolytic therapy: thrombolysis in pulmonary embolism (TIPE) patient survey, Chest 95:279S, 1989.
141. Tibbutt DA et al: Comparison by controlled clinical trial of streptokinase and heparin in the treatment of life-threatening pulmonary embolism, Br Med J 1:343, 1974.
142. Hirsh J et al: Comparison of the effects of streptokinase and heparin in the early rate of resolution of major pulmonary embolism, Can Med Assoc J 104:485, 1971.
143. Miller GAH et al: Comparison of streptokinase and heparin in the treatment of isolated acute massive pulmonary embolism, Br Med J 2:681, 1971.
144. Ly B et al: Controlled clinical trial of streptokinase and heparin in the treatment of major pulmonary embolism, Acta Med Scand 203:465, 1978.
145. Urokinase Pulmonary Embolism Trial Study Group: Phase I results, JAMA 214:2163, 1970.
146. Urokinase Pulmonary Embolism Trial Study Group: Urokinase-streptokinase embolism trial: phase II results, JAMA 229:1606, 1974.
147. Goldhaber SZ et al: Acute pulmonary embolism treated with tissue plasminogen activator, Lancet 2:886, 1986.
148. Fletcher AP, Alkjaersig N, and Sherry S: Maintenance of a sustained fibrinolytic state in man: induction and effects, J Clin Invest 38:1096, 1959.
149. Cotton LT, Flute PT, and Tsapogas MJC: Popliteal artery thrombosis treated with streptokinase, Lancet 2:1081, 1962.
150. Hirsh J et al: Thrombosis in a patient with chronic thrombocytopenia: successful treatment with intra-arterial infusion of streptokinase, Med J Aust 2:1304, 1969.
151. McNicol GP and Douglas AS: Treatment of peripheral vascular occlusion by streptokinase perfusion, Scand J Clin Lab Invest 16(suppl 78):23, 1964.
152. Dotter CT, Rosch J, and Seaman AJ: Selective clot lysis with low dose streptokinase, Radiology 111:31, 1974.
153. McNamara TO and Fischer JR: Thrombolysis of peripheral, arterial and graft occlusions: improved results using high dose urokinase, AJR 144:769, 1985.
154. McNamara TO and Bomberger RA: Factors affecting initial and 6 month patency rates after intra-arterial thrombolysis with high dose urokinase, Am J Surg 152:709, 1986.
155. Katzen BT and van Breda A: Low dose streptokinase in the treatment of arterial occlusions, AJR 36:1171, 1981.
156. Totty WG et al: Low dose intravascular fibrinolytic therapy, Radiology 143:59, 1982.
157. Berni GA et al: Streptokinase treatment of acute arterial occlusion, Ann Surg 198:185, 1983.
158. Mori KW et al: Selective streptokinase infusion: clinical and laboratory correlates, Radiology 148:677, 1983.
159. Becker GJ et al: Low dose fibrinolytic therapy: results and new concepts, Radiology 148:663, 1983.
160. Katzen BT et al: Low dose fibrinolysis in peripheral vascular disease, J Vasc Surg 1:718, 1984.
161. Wolfson RH, Kumpe DA, and Rutherford RB: Role of intra-arterial streptokinase in the treatment of arterial thromboembolism, Arch Surg 119:697, 1984.
162. van Breda A et al: Local thrombolysis in the treatment of arterial graft occlusions, J Vasc Surg 1:103, 1984.
163. Kakkasseril JS et al: Efficacy of low dose streptokinase in acute arterial occlusions and graft thrombosis, Arch Surg 120:427, 1985.
164. Graor RA et al: Local thrombolysis in the treatment of thrombosed arteries, bypass grafts and arteriovenous fistulae, J Vasc Surg 2:406, 1985.
165. Belkin M et al: Intra-arterial fibrinolytic therapy: efficacy of streptokinase vs. urokinase, Arch Surg 121:769, 1986.
166. van Breda A, Katzen BT, and Deutsch AF: Urokinase vs streptokinase in local thrombolysis, Radiology 165:109, 1987.
167. Koltun WA et al: Thrombolysis in the treatment of peripheral arterial vascular occlusions, Arch Surg 122:901, 1987.
168. Graor RA et al: Thrombolysis with recombinant human tissue type plasminogen activators in patients with peripheral artery and bypass graft thrombosis, Circulation 74(suppl I):I-15-I-20, 1986.

Chapter 6

INTERVENTIONAL TREATMENT OF PERIPHERAL VASCULAR DISEASE

Robert A. Graor
Bruce H. Gray

In the past 10 years the treatment of cardiovascular disease has changed greatly. Technologic advances have fueled an interest in interventional therapy for peripheral vascular disease. Percutaneous techniques, such as balloon angioplasty, laser angioplasty, atherectomy, stent therapy, thrombolytic therapy, and ultrasound ablation methods, have been used with increasing frequency. These methods have been aided by an equal advancement of diagnostic and monitoring techniques such as duplex ultrasound, intravascular ultrasound, intravascular angioscopy, and digital angiography. The use of these procedures is often coordinated with surgical treatments and should be viewed as alternatives for the patient with peripheral arterial disease. Either approach, nonsurgical intervention or surgical treatment, has its own costs, risks, and potential benefits.

Surgical options are less attractive than nonsurgical options because of the high prevalence of cardiovascular disease and the expense associated with medical and surgical treatment. In response, a perceived cost savings for nonsurgical treatments has fostered their development. Both nonsurgical intervention and surgery palliate symptoms—they do not treat the primary disease, atherosclerosis. Meanwhile, sophisticated research is addressing the genetic and biochemical aspects of atherosclerosis in hopes of developing specific treatments to resolve or prevent this disabling and sometimes fatal process.

HISTORICAL DEVELOPMENT OF TRANSLUMINAL TREATMENTS

Percutaneous transluminal angioplasty (PTA) with balloon catheters was introduced in Europe by Gruntzig and Hopff in 1974, and in the United States in 1979 by Gruntzig and Kumpe.[1,2] Valuable earlier experience was reported by Zeitler, Porstmann, and Van Andel et al.[3-8] By 1980 enough experience had accumulated to justify the use of PTA in the treatment of atherosclerotic peripheral vascular disease.[9-12] Although Dotter and Judkins first reported an intraarterial dilating technique in 1964, they did not use a coaxial balloon system but rather the "Dotter" technique to progressively enlarge the lumen of the artery by using intraarterial dilating sounds.[13] This first report by Dotter predicted that catheter-directed treatments would make a marked impact on the future treatment of peripheral vascular disease (Fig. 6-1).

Although early skepticism regarding PTA was voiced by the surgical community, it has become more widely accepted in recent years. Despite numerous reports involving hundreds of patients, there is still some uncertainty about the long-term results of PTA and about its role in the treatment of lesions of specific arterial segments in patients with different degrees of ischemia of the lower extremity. This uncertainty is caused in large part by the lack of standardized reporting, which is critical for accurate evaluation and application of these techniques.[14,15] These procedures are less expensive than standard surgical procedures, but durability remains the major question at present.

PATHOPHYSIOLOGY OF PTA

Mechanism of balloon angioplasty

Dotter and Judkins, in their original description, and later Gruntzig and Kumpe, attributed the mechanism of dilation and balloon angioplasty to redistribution and compression of intimal atherosclerotic plaque.[2,13] The balloon inflation was thought to compress the atherosclerotic plaque components against the arterial wall, thereby producing a larger

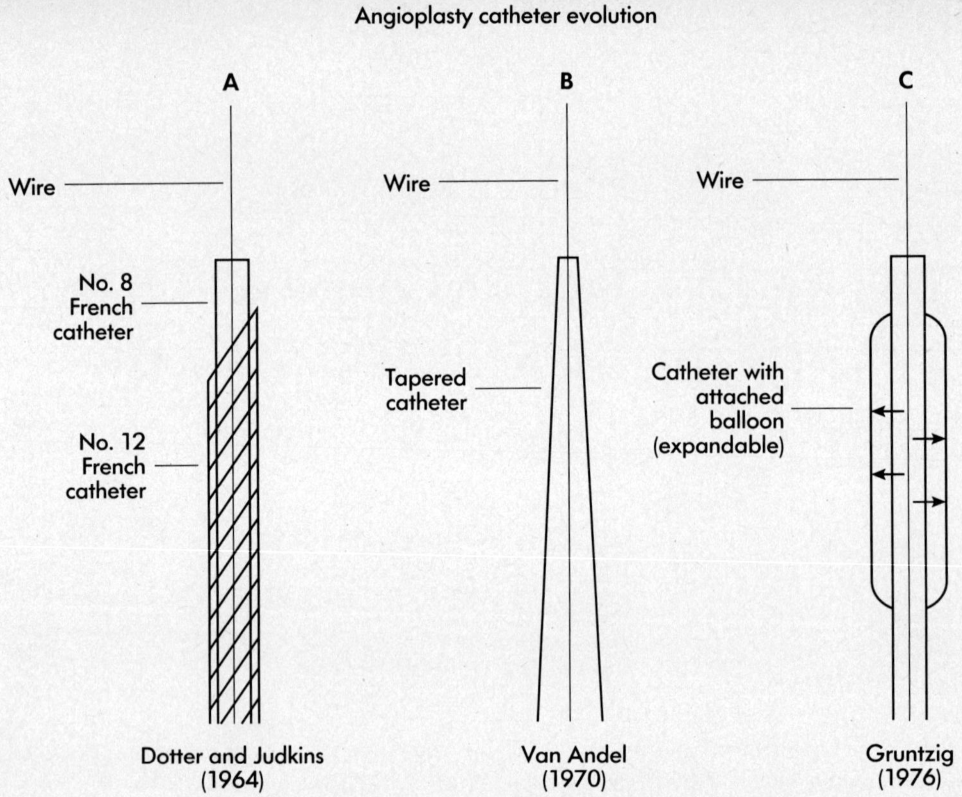

Fig. 6-1. Dotter and Judkins, Van Andel, and Gruntzig angioplasty catheters. **A,** Dotter and Judkins first introduced the no. 8 French catheter into the artery, after which a no. 12 French beveled catheter was passed over the smaller catheter, producing axial force or the "snowplow" effect on the treated artery. **B,** Van Andel used catheters of increasing diameter in a sequential fashion to minimize axial force and generate more radial force. **C,** Gruntzig developed an expandable balloon catheter technique that could generate high radial force with a substantially lower profile.

vessel lumen. Although this appeared logical, the majority of atherosclerotic plaque in human arteries is composed of dense fibrocollagenous tissue with varying degrees of calcific deposits and much smaller amounts of intracellular and extracellular lipid. Thus it appears unlikely that plaque compression plays a major role in human artery angioplasty dilation.

The reason for using PTA is to remodel the stenotic or occlusive atherosclerotic plaque. Various techniques and instruments have been developed to alter the shape or the size of the obstructing lesion by displacing plaque or thrombi or both by cracking or breaking the plaque or by stretching a portion of the vessel wall to enlarge the lumen.

Experimental animal models with vessel-induced injury and high-cholesterol diets create atherosclerotic lesions but, unfortunately, these lesions are composed mainly of lipid-laden foam cells without dense collagen or calcific deposits. Therefore this model is not applicable to humans. Data from angioplasty results in experimental models, human necropsy studies, and human vessels examined after successful angioplasty suggest that the major mechanism of angioplasty is "breaking, cracking, splitting, or fracturing" of the atherosclerotic plaque.[16,20,25] These plaque fractures or breaks extend from the lumen for variable depths into the plaque and provide a means for improving vessel patency by creating additional channels or avenues for blood flow. The healing process at the angioplasty site itself may increase or decrease luminal size.[28] An increase is the desired outcome, and a decrease is labeled "restenosis."

Another mechanism of artery dilation is the stretching of the plaque-free wall segments of eccentric atherosclerotic lesions.[29-32] Inflation of the angioplasty balloon across eccentric plaque lesions may distend or stretch the normal wall segment and produce little or no damage to the plaque on the remaining portions of the arterial wall. Stretching this plaque-free wall segment will result initially in an increase in arterial diameter, but the gradual relaxation of this overstretched segment reduces the lumen toward the predilation state several weeks later. This relaxation may be another explanation for early restenosis after initially successful dilation.[31,32] For arteries with eccentric-type plaque, the stretching of the plaque-free wall segment may be a frequent mechanism of clinically successful early angioplasty.

The last mechanism for balloon angioplasty resulting in an increase in luminal dimensions is a combination of vessel

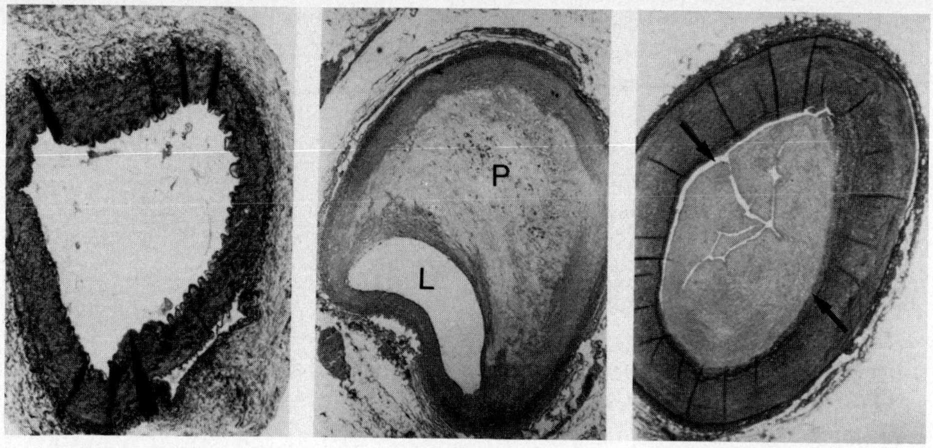

Fig. 6-2. Histologic cross sections of arterial specimens. **A,** Normal artery with intima, media, and adventitia. **B,** Eccentric atherosclerotic plaque (*P,* plaque; *L,* lumen). **C,** Marked intimal hyperplasia *(between arrows)* after balloon catheter induced trauma.

stretching with minimal or mild plaque compression. In this situation an oversized angioplasty balloon may stretch the entire arterial segment that is concentrically narrowed by fibrocollagenous plaque. Although this overstretching technique has been highly successful, it has been plagued with two major problems at the angioplasty site that will be discussed later in this chapter: (1) early or abrupt closure and (2) late closure or restenosis.

The morphologic and histologic observations following balloon dilation are somewhat limited but do provide clues about the actual mechanism of action of dilation. The observations appear to be best divided into two categories: (1) acute changes (within 30 days) after balloon angioplasty and (2) late changes (more than 30 days) after balloon angioplasty.

Acute morphologic changes of PTA

Early morphologic changes in arteries less than 30 days after dilation have been reported by several investigators.[16-23] Block et al reported that in balloon-dilated coronary arteries the fracturing of atherosclerotic plaque in some patients resulted in deep splits into the media.[16] In virtually all patients with adequate dilation, "a crack, tear, fracture, or break" appears in the plaque and occurs in variable degrees of medial penetration, but adventitial disruption was not observed.[18,24] Waller et al reported in necropsy studies of coronary artery dilation that intimal-medial tears were common, and intramural hemorrhage was also present.[23] In a necropsy study Mizuno, Jurita, and Imazeki described serially sectioned arteries at a balloon angioplasty site and observed intimal and medial splitting that led to arterial dissection.[20] Soward, Essed, and Serruys reported plaque splitting, medial dissection, and lifting atherosclerotic plaque from the medial layer at the site of the balloon angioplasty.[25] La Delia et al recently reported histologic findings in the left anterior descending coronary artery of a patient who underwent angioplasty and streptokinase therapy for an evolving acute myocardial infarction.[26] They observed atherosclerotic plaque cleavage, subintimal leukocyte infiltrations, and medial and adventitial fractures.

Late morphologic changes of PTA

Late changes observed in human arteries after PTA may be divided into two categories: (1) no morphologic evidence of previous angioplasty injury and (2) intimal fibrous proliferation (Fig. 6-2).

Waller et al reported no morphologic or histologic changes at the site of angioplasty in three men who died suddenly after coronary angioplasty.[17,19,21] At necropsy the balloon angioplasty site was significantly narrowed (75% to 95%) in cross section as a result of fibrous atherosclerotic plaque, but each site was free of thrombi and intramural hemorrhage. Histologic assessment of the atherosclerotic plaque in the areas of previous angioplasty, when compared with other areas of atherosclerotic plaque in the same artery or arteries in the same patient, disclosed no distinctive morphologic differences.

Essed, Brand, and Becker were the first to report intimal fibrous proliferation at the site of a coronary angioplasty[27] (see Fig. 6-2). Cross sections of the dilated artery showed evidence of previous disruption of the media with extensive proximal and distal dissection. A large intimal crack with a partial flap created false channels in the artery. After 5 months fibrocellular proliferation surrounded portions of the atherosclerotic plaque, in addition to the area of previous plaque fracture, producing a severely narrowed artery. Austin et al observed a late angioplasty site that appeared to have distinct layers, an outer layer composed of hypocellular connective tissue with cholesterol clefts and an inner layer composed of smooth muscle cells, fibroblasts, and a basophilic interstitial matrix.[22] The outer atherosclerotic plaque layer contained gaps that were presumed to be evidence of previous angioplasty. These gaps were filled with cellular proliferation of the inner layer. In all cases the initial underlying atherosclerotic plaque was still clearly identified, and the luminal channels created by angioplasty were filled with fibrocellular tissue, which coated the denuded media.

Thus at the angioplasty site, after angiographically successful balloon dilation, distinctive lesions may be seen. Most commonly, a concentric fibrocellular proliferation is observed that is distinctly different from underlying atherosclerotic plaque. The absence of morphologic signs of previous angioplasty should not be interpreted as an acceleration of underlying atherosclerotic plaque.

Abrupt closure of PTA

Abrupt closure of PTA occurs at a peripheral artery angioplasty site in fewer than 5% of patients treated with balloon angioplasty.[33] Clinical explanations for abrupt closure include spasm, localized thrombus formation, and dissection.[33-37]

Acute vessel occlusion from a folded or curled large intimal flap probably accounts for the majority of abrupt closures. This morphologic finding may correspond with the category of dissection in that a large intimal flap is created by an extensive intimal-medial dissection plane.

Acute closure may also be produced by abrupt relaxation of the overstretched, disease-free wall of an eccentric plaque. The arterial media of the disease-free segment contains smooth muscle cells that can react to various stimuli, including balloon dilation.

Fibrin-platelet thrombi frequently layer the angioplasty site, but the occurrence of occlusive thrombi at the site of balloon angioplasty is not common.[17,19] Although thrombi may be associated with large, curled intimal flaps, the primary mechanism of abrupt closure is the flow obstructing the intimal-medial flap.

Subintimal hemorrhage from traumatic balloon injury of atherosclerotic plaque is also a possible cause for abrupt closure. Subintimal or intraplaque bleeding may acutely expand the plaque and severely narrow or occlude the angioplasty site.

Treatment of the abrupt closure has included repeat balloon angioplasty with prolonged inflations, the infusion of thrombolytic agents, intraarterial stents, thermal welding laser angioplasty, and atherectomy devices to remove the large intimal flaps, thrombi, or other obstructing lesions.

Late closure (restenosis) after PTA

The major problem with balloon angioplasty has been restenosis. The frequency of clinical restenosis ranges from 15% to 75%, depending on the size and location of the artery and the definition of restenosis. Multiple clinical, angiographic, technical, and pharmacologic factors have been analyzed to determine their role in promoting restenosis. Despite the large number of factors evaluated, studies disagree on the individual significance of many factors and concur on the significance of a few.[38-40]

The most widely accepted theory for the development of restenosis is that fibrocellular intimal proliferation results in response to the damaged endothelium and media of the vessels.[22,27,41,42] Balloon angioplasty is the likely initiating stimulus for this restenosis. Fibrous intimal proliferation may be precipitated by the release of thromboxane A_2, which leads to platelet deposition, release of platelet-derived growth factors (PDGF), and fibroblast and endothelial growth factors.[42] This process results in migration, proliferation, and alteration of smooth muscle cells from the media, resulting in fibrocellular tissue accumulation. The fibrocellular coating narrows the vessel lumen.

Other mechanisms that have been implicated in late luminal narrowing at the angioplasty site include the gradual elastic recoil of an overstretched, disease-free wall; the return to the predilation state of the stretched concentric lesion; and progression of the atherosclerotic plaque. Plaque progression appears to be an unlikely cause in the 2 to 4 months after angioplasty, but it may be responsible for late recurrences.

Waller, Pinkerton, and Foster reported the effects of balloon angioplasty on the adjacent nondilated vessel wall.[41] Their histologic observations noted an accelerated stenotic lesion occurring just proximal to the previously dilated lesion. The tissue was described as fibrocellular, which was histologically identical to that observed at the site of the balloon angioplasty. The acceleration of the fibrocellular tissue proliferation at this site may be caused by several mechanisms, including intimal injury from the catheter or retrograde extension of the fibrocellular tissue from the adjacent site without arterial wall injury.[29,43]

Two reports on 344 patients studied angiographically within 1 year after a coronary dilation, in which specific attention was given to the arterial segments adjacent to the balloon angioplasty, found only four patients (1%) with accelerated changes in the adjacent artery segments.[43,44] Therefore accelerated changes proximal or distal to the balloon dilation are unusual and when they do occur, may result from the aforementioned mechanisms.

Effects of thermal balloon angioplasty

Thermal balloon angioplasty remodels the stenotic atherosclerotic vessel lesion with various energy sources, including laser, radio frequency, chemical, or ultrasound to produce thermal injury on adjacent plaque.

In general, laser balloon angioplasty has the traditional features of balloon angioplasty followed by laser irradiation or thermal remodeling of the atherosclerotic plaque-lined artery during the final balloon dilation. The laser energy is transmitted through an ultrathin central fiber to the balloon, where it enters the adjacent wall and plaque as heat. Animal and cadaver studies indicate that thermal balloon angioplasty decreases vessel elasticity at the dilation site, and that the heat molds the arterial segment to the size and shape of the inflated angioplasty balloon.[45-49] In addition to the acute effects of remolding, the thermal effects on the underlying media may destroy smooth muscle cells that may be involved in the late restenosis process.

Lee et al recently evaluated radio frequency as an alternate energy source for balloon thermal angioplasty.[49] Radio frequency combined with angioplasty balloon inflation effectively mold the atherosclerotic plaque within the vessel. In general, however, regardless of the source of the thermal energy, thermal balloon angioplasty has a high restenosis rate and, to date, has not proven to be very useful.

Laser therapy to remove tissues has included hot-tip probes and pulsed lasers of various energy spectra. Histologic studies of vascular tissue after continuous-wave laser therapy show a cone-shaped crater surrounded by concentric zones of protein denaturation and tissue vacuolization.[50] The resulting charred endothelial surface is not desirable and has led to high restenosis rates.[51-55]

Laser research has now concentrated on ablating tissue by limiting the thermal injury. The two most common methods to achieve this goal are a modified tip for the delivery system of continuous-wave lasers and the use of pulsed lasers. Other newer systems include fluorescence spectroscopy, which identifies tissue before laser treatment and thereby allows the energy delivered to the tissue to be modified for the type of tissue involved.

Atherectomy

New cutting instruments can now incise vascular obstructions. A prototype of such instruments is the Simpson AtheroCath,* an atherectomy instrument that consists of a high-speed, circular cutting blade that can excise plaque when pressed against the diseased portion of the wall with an inflated balloon[56-61] (Fig. 6-3). Other atherectomy instruments use pulverization techniques to recanalize the artery.[62-64] Only the Simpson device, however, retains tissue samples that can be removed from the catheter and examined microscopically, thereby providing unique, important information.

Atherectomy is an exciting new mechanical technique for treating primary and restenotic lesions. A major advantage of atherectomy is that the tissue debulking may reduce the rate of restenosis. Exposure of large segments of medial smooth muscle may predispose atherectomy sites to intimal proliferation and restenosis. These concerns are under investigation. Better guidance methods will likely be developed to remove tissue more precisely.

Catheter technology

Several generations of interventional catheters have evolved primarily from improvement on the profile or diameter of the balloon and its inflation characteristics (see Fig. 6-1). Compliance, profile, and trackability are the major functional characteristics of catheters.

*Devices for Vascular Intervention, Inc., Redwood City, California.

A

B

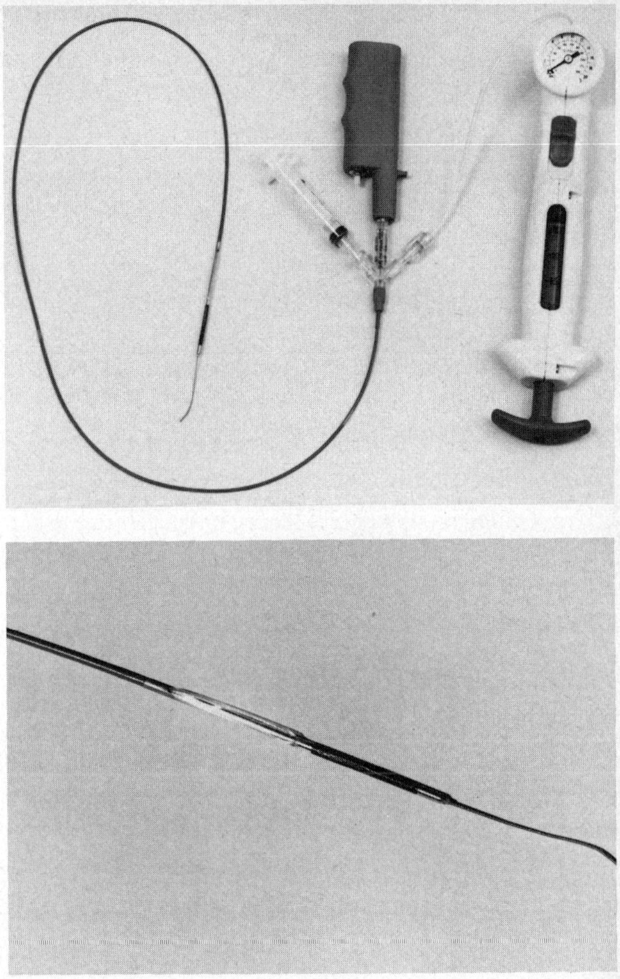

Fig. 6-3. Simpson AtheroCath. **A,** A directional atherectomy catheter with pressure manometer, battery-powered motor drive, and flush port. **B,** The catheter has a leading fixed wire, collection chamber, and cutting chamber with an eccentrically placed expandable balloon.

Catheter compliance

Compliance is the change in the balloon diameter per unit change in pressure ($\Delta D/\Delta P$). Gruntzig's original balloons, as well as all the early PTA balloons, were made of polyvinyl chloride, a relatively compliant balloon material.[65,66] Since these early catheters were introduced, much less compliant polyethylene and polyurethane materials have become available. Polyvinyl chloride balloons tend to increase in diameter with increasing pressure.[66,67] Overstretching the balloon results in maldistribution of dilating forces, frequently resulting in balloon rupture, overdilation, and, less commonly, vessel rupture during angioplasty.[68,69]

The most important cause of vessel rupture during balloon angioplasty is overdistention of the vessel. The simplest way to prevent this is to use a balloon of noncompliant material and to select the appropriate size. Balloons currently available maintain constant, or nearly constant, balloon diameters, ensuring that the dilating force increases linearly with the inflation pressure.[70]

Catheter profile

Profile, another important characteristic, is best described as the cross-sectional diameter of the catheter. Low-profile balloons are balloons on thin catheters with balloon materials that wrap nicely around the catheter itself. Low-profile balloons help minimize entry site complications and aid in negotiating and crossing severely stenotic lesions. The lower the profile, the smaller the shaft of the catheter. Low-profile balloons are now as small as 2 mm in diameter. Along with the small balloon, these catheters can also be accurately positioned by a central guide wire.

Catheter trackability

Trackability refers to the tendency of the catheter to follow a wire placed in the desired position without disturbing that position or pulling the wire back. This characteristic depends on the axial (along the length) components of the catheter and the technical capability of the operator.

These same three characteristics also apply to atherectomy catheters and laser-assisted balloon angioplasty systems.

RESULTS OF PERIPHERAL ARTERIAL INTERVENTION

The majority of data on peripheral arterial interventions are from balloon angioplasty studies. Although early results of PTA appeared to be comparable with those of surgery, the reports often did not address the rate of acute failure, and follow-up studies were brief. More recent studies with observations from 1 to 5 years after the procedures revealed less optimistic patency rates.

A prospective, randomized, cooperative study has compared PTA to surgery in patients who had lesions amenable to either therapy.[71] Although PTA had a higher technical failure rate (immediate failure 15.5%, technical failure 7.8%, and no mortality) compared to surgery (immediate failure 7.1%, no technical failures, and operative mortality 0.8%) the results of successful PTA and reconstructive surgery were comparable for up to 3 years.

Clinical variables proposed as predictors of good PTA results include the site of occlusion and the absence of diabetes, as well as several more controversial variables such as the length of lesion, runoff artery patency, indications for PTA, severity of the lesion (stenosis vs occlusion), and the degree of ischemia (see the accompanying box).

Clinical variables that are predictors of good PTA outcome

- Larger, high flow arteries
- Stenotic lesions less than 7 cm in length
- Short segment occlusion less than 3 cm or occlusions pretreated with thrombolysis, producing a patent but stenotic artery
- Nonostial lesion
- Concentric plaques
- Lesions without a polypoid morphology
- Nondiabetic
- Symptoms of claudication rather than ischemic rest pain or gangrene

Complications of PTA have been inconsistently reported. Some studies listed all hematomas as complications, yielding complication rates as high as 20%, whereas others listed only complications requiring surgical interventions, yielding rates of 2% to 3%. The reporting of complications should be standardized and perhaps should include those that lengthen hospital stay or that require surgery or blood transfusions.[72] Examples of common and consistently reported complications associated with balloon angioplasty reported by Gardiner et al[72] are shown in Tables 6-1 and 6-2. Of these 453 patients 54% had surgery or treatment that prolonged the hospital stay.

Aortic and iliac PTA

Atherosclerotic stenosis of the distal aorta that is focal and concentric has been successfully treated with PTA. Although these lesions are unusual and the published experience is small, technical success rates are high and complications are low (Fig. 6-4). The combined results of three published series revealed that 48 of 52 patients had technically successful PTA with an 83% patency rate at a mean follow-up period of 13 months.[73-75] Three patients had a second PTA during the follow-up period. Three major complications occurred: (1) distal emboli in one patient, (2) pseudoaneurysm formation in another, and (3) thrombosis of the common femoral artery in a third.

For dilation of iliac artery stenosis, immediate success rates range from 79% to 93%, and from 70% to 80% of the treated vessels are patent at 2 to 3 years (Table 6-3).[8,12,76-85] The clinical indications for PTA in these arterial segments have ranged from claudication to limb salvage for impending gangrene (Fig. 6-5). More than 95% of all PTAs in this group are technically successful.

Because of these results, PTA is probably the procedure of choice for segmental stenosis in the aortoiliac arterial segments.[84,86] Aortoiliac bypass grafting is associated with a considerably higher morbidity and mortality (2% to 14%). In most series serious complications during and following PTA occurred in less than 2% of patients.[72]

The safety and patency rates of iliac PTA, when compared with those of surgical reconstruction, make PTA an attractive treatment. Despite these data PTA best serves only those patients who have segmental disease, that is, disease not extending from the aorta into the iliac arteries. In some series suitable candidates for PTA represented only 0.5% to 5% of patients seen for lower-extremity ischemia. Our experience suggests a similar figure—about 5% to 8% of such

Table 6-1. Types of angioplasty site complications in 453 dilations

Location of lesion	Thrombosis	Guide wire dissection	Angioplasty dissection	Embolus	Rupture
Renal artery	1 (1)	3 (2)	2 (2)*	2	2
Common iliac artery	2 (2)	1 (0)	2 (1)*	3	0
External iliac artery, common femoral artery	1 (1)	2 (1)	1 (0)	1	0
Superficial femoral artery	2 (1)	2 (2)	1 (0)	1	0
Popliteal artery and distal branches	2 (2)	3 (1)	0	0	0
Other (profunda femoral artery)	1 (1)	0	0	0	0

Numbers in parentheses indicate cases resulting in luminal obstruction.
*Transient.

Table 6-2. Other complications of angioplasty in 352 patients

Complication	No. of cases (%)	Required surgery
Puncture site (total)	20 (6)	4 (1)
Hematoma	16 (4)	1
False aneurysm	1 (0.3)	1
Thrombus	3 (1)	2
Renal failure	3 (1)	1*
Fatalities	1 (0.3)	1

*Patient required dialysis after suffering thrombosis of single, remaining renal artery.

Table 6-3. Results from selected studies of iliac angioplasty

Referenced studies	Total no. patients	Technical success rate	2-year patency rate	5-year patency rate
8, 12, 76-85, 89	1337	93.3%	82.3%	71%

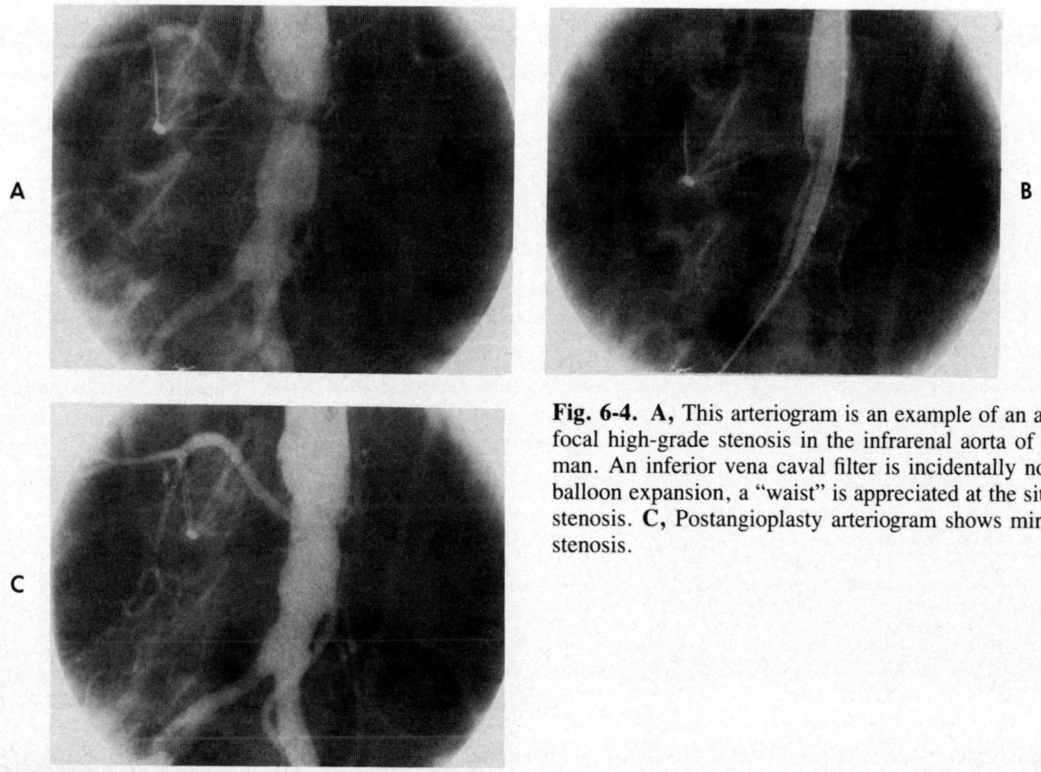

Fig. 6-4. A, This arteriogram is an example of an atherosclerotic focal high-grade stenosis in the infrarenal aorta of a 43-year-old man. An inferior vena caval filter is incidentally noted. **B,** With balloon expansion, a "waist" is appreciated at the site of maximal stenosis. **C,** Postangioplasty arteriogram shows minimal residual stenosis.

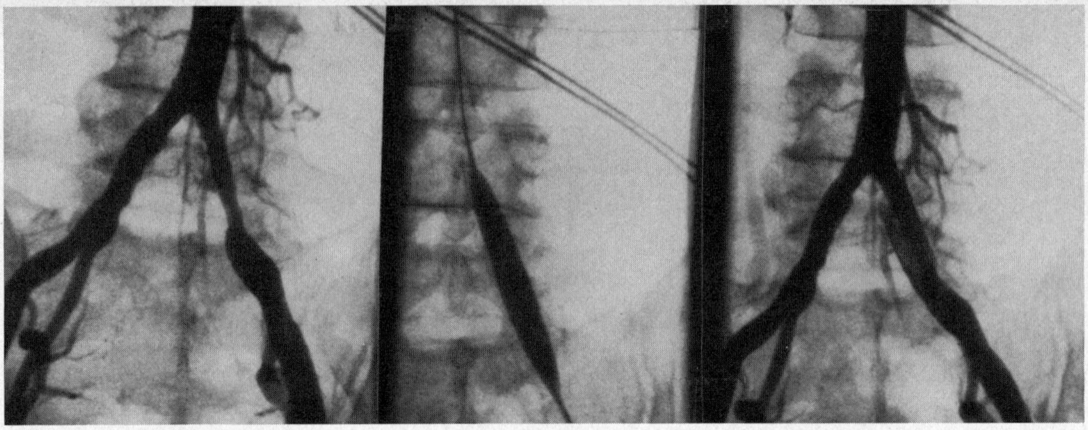

Fig. 6-5. Arteriogram of the distal abdominal aorta and iliac arteries. **A,** Stenosis of the left common iliac artery with poststenotic dilation. **B,** Full angioplasty balloon inflation across the stenosis. **C,** After angioplasty, a widely patent common iliac artery PTA with good flow and a typical local dissection is apparent.

patients are candidates for PTA. One additional advantage of PTA over surgery for iliac disease is the cost savings associated with the low complication rates and short hospital stays (usually 1 or 2 days).

Femoropopliteal PTA

Pooled data from studies reporting initial or technical results in 1426 patients with femoropopliteal PTA show mean 2- and 4-year patency rates of 89% and 67% respectively (Table 6-4).* A two-year patency rate for 622 patients with stenotic lesions is 84%, whereas for 191 patients with occluded femoropopliteal arteries it is 57%.

A study by Martin et al compared PTA to saphenous vein bypass grafts during the same time interval but not in a prospective, randomized fashion.[90] Therefore lesions treated with the two methods were not necessarily equivalent. Despite these study flaws initial patency rates (76% for both groups) and 2-year patency rates (57% for PTA and 56% for bypass grafts) were the same. However, the two procedures cannot be assumed to be equivalent based solely on these data.

Blair et al conducted a retrospective study comparing the results of PTA with those of infrainguinal bypass procedures in patients with critical limb ischemia.[91] Of the 54 patients, 39 (72%) initially improved after PTA, but only 18% had improved Doppler studies at the 2-year follow-up examination. Despite these poor results, the limb salvage rate was 78%. In the surgical group the 2-year patency rate was 68%, and limb salvage was 90%. In this study 2-year patency for bypass grafts was statistically better ($P < 0.001$) than PTA results, but no significant difference was noted for limb salvage. The PTA group had more subsequent procedures

*References 2, 12, 33, 79, 80, 82-85, 87-89.

Table 6-4. Results of femoropopliteal angioplasty

Referenced studies	Total no. patients	Initial success rate	2-year patency rate	4-year patency rate
2, 12, 33, 79, 80, 82-85, 87-89	1426	89%	71.5%	67%

than the surgery group ($P < 0.01$). These data support the contention that bypass grafting is more durable than PTA when limb salvage is the indication for the procedure.

In a similar study of patients with severe ischemia, Glover et al reported a limb salvage rate of 71% when PTA was combined with bypass procedures, but only a 34% limb salvage for PTA alone.[92] In contrast, Wilson et al compared PTA to surgery in a randomized trial and concluded that each treatment produced similar durable results.[71] An important difference of this study was that 60% of the patients had claudication as their initial symptom, and therefore the severity of disease in this group was probably less.

Zeitler reported that of 437 patients with occluded superficial femoral arteries, 73% had an initially good response to PTA, and 60% of the arteries remained patent at 2 years.[93] Waltman et al reported successful PTA outcome in 87% of stenoses and 76% of occlusions.[77] Johnston, Colapinto, and Baird reported a 60% cumulative patency rate at 1 year for stenoses and a 40% rate for occlusions.[84]

Overall, the rate of nonfatal complications associated with PTA in this region is believed to be less than 5%, and the rate of serious complications is believed to be less than 1%. Mortality has been reported to be less than 0.4%. This is a low mortality rate compared with a surgical mortality rate of 2% to 4% for femoropopliteal or femorotibial bypass grafting.[72]

Infrapopliteal PTA

Table 6-5 shows the combined results of infrapopliteal PTA. PTA in the infrapopliteal region is generally performed in conjunction with proximal PTA rather than by itself. Better patency rates in recent studies are the result of improvements in balloon catheters and adjunctive medications.[94,95]

Renal artery PTA

PTA has been used to treat hypertension and renal failure associated with renal artery stenosis. Establishing the diagnosis of renal artery stenosis is difficult at times, but still essential. Several authors have suggested approaches to confirm that the diagnosis (hypertension, renal failure, or both) is associated with the renal artery lesion.[96-99] Better medications for the treatment of renal vascular hypertension are now available and have decreased the need for renal artery PTA for renal artery stenosis. Good blood pressure control does not prevent the progression of renal artery stenosis, and therefore serial measurements of renal function should be obtained. If the blood pressure cannot be adequately controlled, if the side effects of blood pressure medications

Table 6-5. Results of infrapopliteal PTA: the combined result of two studies

Authors	No. patients	Initial success rate	2-year patency rate
Schwarten and Cutcliff[94]	126	94%	NA
Brown et al[95]			

NA, Not available.

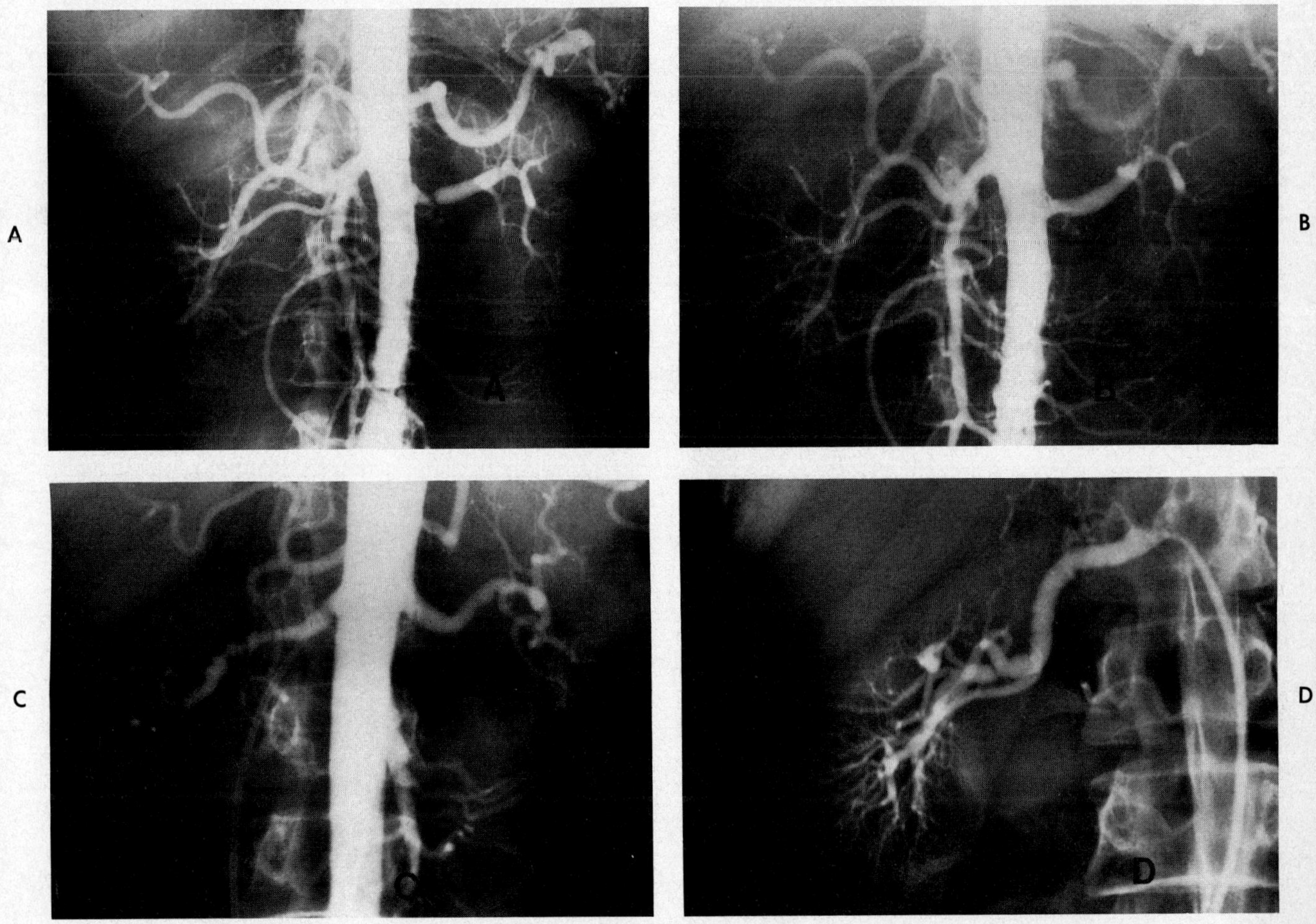

Fig. 6-6. A, Arteriogram of visceral aorta demonstrating a tight atherosclerotic stenosis of the left renal artery. **B,** Arteriogram post-angioplasty of left renal artery. **C,** Arteriogram demonstrating right renal artery stenosis secondary to fibromuscular dysplasia. **D,** Same right renal artery as in **C,** post-angioplasty.

prevent their use, or if renal function should deteriorate, then steps should be taken to improve renal blood flow.

Knowledge of the natural history of renal artery diseases is limited. Studies by Meaney, Dustan, and McCormack and Schreiber, Pohl, and Novick found that in patients with atherosclerotic renal artery disease, progression occurred in 39% and 44%, respectively.[97,98] In the latter study 39% of renal artery lesions with stenosis of 75% to 99% on the initial angiogram were eventually occluded. Fibromuscular renal artery disease seems to progress less often. In the former study fibromuscular disease of the arteries progressed in only 16% of patients who were less than 40 years of age and in no patients who were more than 40 years of age.

Atherosclerotic disease must be distinguished from fibromuscular disease because of the difference in its response to PTA. Fibromuscular disease responds more readily to PTA and is the treatment of choice (see Table 6-6) (Fig. 6-6).

Results of PTA for atherosclerotic lesions are shown in Table 6-6.[100-113] Atherosclerotic lesions can be divided into two types: (1) those involving the orifice of the renal artery at the aortic wall and (2) those involving the renal artery distal to the orifice. Lesions involving the orifice of the renal artery do not respond to balloon dilation, in contrast to lesions distal to the orifice. Failure of an orificial lesion to respond to PTA is thought to result from the plaque originating in the aorta and encroaching on the ostium of the renal artery.

PTA for renal transplant patients has also been successful. Hypertension in this group of patients may be the result of graft renal artery stenosis or allograft rejection.

Complications of renal artery PTA are similar to all other PTA-associated complications, with a few exceptions. Renal artery rupture, acute occlusion secondary to dissection or thrombosis, embolization, and perforation are rare (less than 1%) complications. More common complications include renal failure (acute and usually transient) resulting from contrast media or from transient ischemia (less than 5%).

The studies of renal artery PTA should be reviewed with caution. Successful control of blood pressure and preservation of renal function can only be established with adequate follow-up study and objective testing. Many of the published reports do not provide adequate information in this regard.

Subclavian and innominate artery PTA

The fear of embolic complications dampened enthusiasm for PTA in the subclavian and innominate arteries until recently. Pooled data from studies reporting the results of PTA in 423 patients are shown in Table 6-7.[114-120] Initial success was seen in 92% of the patients. The recurrence rate was between 20% and 25% at 12 to 26 months. Embolic complications occurred in 2% to 4% of patients, usually in the hand or arm but occasionally in the brain.

Vertebral artery PTA

The data are insufficient to suggest a role for PTA in the vertebral-basilar system. In a series reported by Courtheoux et al, 26 PTAs in 24 patients were successful in 24 attempts.[121] Resolution of symptoms occurred in 21 of the 24 patients. Symptoms were not well described in this paper, and complications occurred in two patients. One patient

Table 6-6. Initial and late clinical follow-up studies of renal artery PTA

		Clinical improvement ASO (%)/FMD (%)		
Study	**No. patients treated**	**Initial**	**1 Yr**	**2 Yr**
Cicuto et al[100]	43	83/NA	NA	NA
Colapinto et al[101]	68	85/NA	NA	81/NA
Geyskes et al[102]	70	85/NA	81/NA	NA/95
Ingrisch, Hegels, and Frey[103]	64	94/NA	NA	81/NA
Katzen, Chang, and Knox[104]	17	94/NA	NA	75/NA
Lohr et al[105]	128	63/NA	NA	NA
Mahler et al[106]	40	NA	NA	69/NA
Martin et al[107]	100	88/NA	70/NA	NA/85
Martin et al[108]	108	93/NA	NA	70/NA
Miller et al[109]	63	93/NA	87/NA	NA/100
Richter, Kronert, and Zeitler[110]	61	92/NA	67/NA	NA
Schwarten[111]	173	93/NA	NA	82/NA
Sos et al[112]	101	78/NA	69/NA	NA/82
Tegtmeyer, Kellum, and Ayes[113]	109	93/NA	NA	75/100
TOTALS*	1145	87	74	76/92

ASO, Atherosclerosis.
FMD, Fibromuscular disease.
NA, Not available.
*Total percent expressed as weighted mean.

experienced temporary blindness, and another had thrombosis of the vertebral artery.

Carotid artery PTA

Despite the great concern for embolization, PTA has often been used to open stenotic carotid arteries (Table 6-8).[114-126] Some interventionists would recommend PTA of the carotid in the following situations:

1. For smooth, concentric, nonulcerated atherosclerotic lesions
2. For lesions involving the proximal common carotid artery, the common carotid bifurcation, and the intracranial carotid artery
3. For fibromuscular lesions

The risks and rate of restenosis for carotid endarterectomy are low, and the treatment of carotid disease has become somewhat controversial. Thus it is difficult to state clearly the indications for PTA as opposed to surgical repair. More data with better follow-up study are required before recommending this procedure over carotid endarterectomy.

Table 6-7. Subclavian and innominate artery PTA: data from more than 400 procedures

Series	No. patients/ no. arteries	Initial technical success (%)	Recurrence	Follow-up	Complication (no. and type)
Theron, Melancon, and Ethier[116]	42/42	42/42 (100)	?	?	?
Motarjeme et al[114]	22/23	16/22 (73)	?	5 yr	0
Wilms et al[124]	22/23	21/23 (91)	0	25 mo	1 axillary occlusion 1 digital embolus
Ringelstein and Zeumer[125]	12/12	12/12 (100)	1	?	1 digital embolus (transient)
Vitek, Raymon, and Oh[119]	15/15	15/15 (100)	?	?	1 hematoma 1 brachial embolus
Burke et al[126]	27/30	28/30 (93)	6	37 mo	1 left hemiparesis 1 digital embolus (transient)
Kachel et al[118]	21/21	21/21 (100)	?	?	1 left arm paresis (transient)
Tournade et al[123]	24/24	24/24 (100)	3	12-18 mo	0
Pavone et al[115]	83/83	76/83 (91)	?	?	1 CNS complication
Mathias[122]	72/72	68/72 (93)	?	?	?
TOTALS	340/345	323/345 (94)			2.6%

Table 6-8. Carotid artery PTA for ischemic cerebral symptoms: results summarized

Series	No. patients/ no. arteries	Disease	Initial technical success	Recurrence*	Follow-up period	Complications (no. and type)
Motarjeme et al[114]	10/10	ASO	10	?	?	1 temporary blindness
Pavone et al[115]	15/15	?	15	?	?	1 CNS
Theron, Melancon, and Ethier[116]	40/40	ASO	?	?	?	1 permanent blindness (postsurgical stenosis)
Tsai et al[117]	34/34	28 ASO 5 FMD 1 Takayasu	27	0	3 mo-4 yr	1 hematoma
Kachel et al[118] (ICA)	24/24	ASO	22	?	?	1 transient paresis
(CCA)	2/2	ASO	2			
Vitek, Raymon, and Oh[119] (ECA)	19/19	ASO	19	?	?	?
Galichia et al[120]	6/6	ASO	100	?	?	0
TOTALS	165		≈ 85%			≈ 3.6%

ASO, Atherosclerosis.
FMD, Fibromuscular disease.
ICA, Internal carotid artery.
ECA, External carotid artery.
CCA, Common carotid artery.
*Clinical recurrence of symptoms and signs.

Table 6-9. Miscellaneous applications of PTA and laser

Author	Type of laser	No. patients	Success early (%)/late (%)	Follow-up period (mo)
Sanborn[131]	LTBA*	124	93/72	6
Katzen[132]	Excimer	22	90/NA	NA
Nordstrom[133]	Argon	34	/68	9
Leon[134] and Geschwind[135]	Pulsed-Dye	35 (29 lesions treated)	72/NA	NA
Geschwind[55]	LTBA*	555	82-100/74	18
Abela and Seeger[136]	LTBA*	49	82/50	6

*Laser assisted balloon angioplasty.

Table 6-10. Results of PTA for hemodialysis access legions

Study	No. patients	Patency		
		3 Months	1 Year	2 Years
Hunter[152]	45	82%	NA	NA
Glanz[153]	84	78%	52%	38%

NA, Not available.

Miscellaneous applications of PTA

PTA for other arterial and venous locations have been reported with varying degrees of success. These miscellaneous applications are shown in Tables 6-9 and 6-10.

ATHERECTOMY

Directional

Atherectomy for peripheral vascular disease has only recently emerged as an alternative to PTA. The first such device to be approved by the FDA is the Simpson Peripheral AtheroCath* (Fig. 6-7). The AtheroCath consists of a cylinder that is opened throughout a portion of its circumference and fitted with a fixed terminal guide wire. A circular cutter that rotates at 2000 rpm is enclosed within the cylinder. The cylinder is positioned within a stenotic segment, and after the cutter is withdrawn into the proximal end of the cylinder housing, an eccentric balloon is inflated. The housing is thus fixed against the atheroma and the rotating cutter advanced so that the excised material is impacted into a storage compartment in the tip of the housing for subsequent withdrawal (see Fig. 6-3). This technique is advantageous because the risks of peripheral emboli and intimal dissection are minimized. An initial experience with 27 patients has been reported wherein 51 stenotic lesions requiring 131 passes were treated with a mean reduction in luminal stenosis from 79% to 22%.[127] This initial experience has now been expanded to include 136 lesions in 61 patients, which provided an initial successful result in 87%. In 30 of these individuals follow-up angiography at 6 months demonstrated significant recurrent stenosis in the majority of patients (52%). If the stenotic lesion was initially reduced to less than 30% residual stenosis, the recurrent stenosis rate was only 18%.[56]

Results from our series at the Cleveland Clinic are particularly encouraging for the superficial femoral and popliteal arteries (see Fig. 6-11).[59] We studied 162 patients successfully treated with directional atherectomy alone or in combination with thrombolysis with urokinase and evaluated the factors influencing patency. Patients were divided into two groups, labeled simple and complex. The patients in the simple group had short segmental occlusions or stenotic lesions and a 100% patency rate in 30 days and an 88.4% patency rate at 24 months following atherectomy. The complex group had greater than 5 cm occlusions and exhibited a 96.8% patency rate at 30 days and a 73.1% patency rate at 24 months. Univariate predictors of patency included biphasic or triphasic Doppler flow following atherectomy, a good angiographic cosmetic appearance after atherectomy, demonstrating less than 20% residual stenosis, and urokinase pretreatment ($P < 0.05$). Nine major complications (5.5%) occurred, including one acute myocardial infarction resulting in death. The other major complications were bleeding at the catheter site.

In our experience directional atherectomy has been an effective treatment for symptomatic peripheral arterial occlusive disease. It allows selective plaque debulking and histologic evaluation of the material extracted from primary stenotic lesions and restenotic lesions.

Rotational

The second atherectomy device to be approved by the FDA is the Kensey catheter,* which employs two entirely different mechanisms to affect both atherectomy and dilation. First a tip secured to a central drive shaft housed with a no. 8 flexible French catheter rotates at speeds up to 100,000 rpm and results in pulverization of the atheroma into microparticles. The second mechanism consists of a powered infusion system that spins a radial jet of fluid against the wall from the rotating tip. This not only dilates the lumen but also centers the tip and provides cooling. The advantages of this catheter include its efficacy in vessels

*Devices for Vascular Intervention, Inc., Redwood City, California.

*Theratek, Inc.

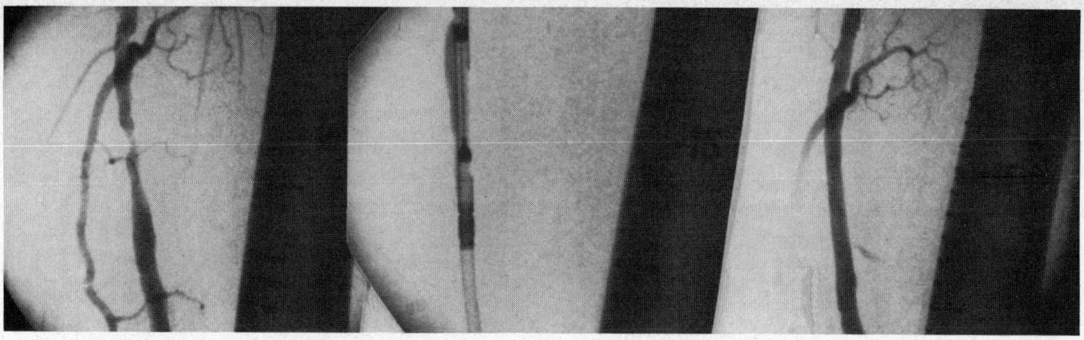

A B C

Fig. 6-7. Directional atherectomy of left superficial femoral artery atherosclerotic stenosis at Hunter's canal. **A,** Simpson AtheroCath before atherectomy. **B,** During atherectomy. **C,** After atherectomy.

totally occluded by either atheroma or thrombus. The catheter is positioned only once within the artery and is advanced steadily until the desired result is achieved. There is currently no guide wire, and the risk of perforation is higher than with other devices.

The fate and consequences of the pulverized material remain uncertain but have no apparent clinical impact beyond the occasional distal embolus. Initial experimental results indicate this material may indeed produce microinfarctions, but none were of clinical significance in canine models.

In a collective experience of over 100 patients in whom this catheter has been used, only 1 clinically significant distal embolus has been observed.

A representative preliminary clinical experience has been reported in a group of 20 patients undergoing transluminal atherectomy of the superficial femoral artery.[62,128] The lesions ranged from complete occlusion to a limited 2 cm stenotic segment. Claudication was the primary indication in 15 extremities while severe rest pain or tissue necrosis was present in 8. All procedures were carried out using a regional anesthetic in the operating room with open technique and fluoroscopic control. The catheter was successfully passed in 14 of the 20 patients, and 11 of those underwent adjunctive transluminal percutaneous balloon angioplasty of the residual lumen, following initial catheter passage. Of the nine unsuccessful passages, perforation occurred in eight, only one of which required suture repair. In the 14 patients with initial success, the ankle-brachial index remained higher than preoperative determinations, with a mean follow-up period of 6 months. According to a recent update, however, the 1-year cumulative patency rate appears to be 37%. The peripheral applications for this device, currently named the *Trac-Wright system** are under continual development, and several design modifications are in progress. The catheter has been made more flexible; a guide wire has been incorporated; and a smaller caliber, no. 5 French configuration will soon be available.

The third atherectomy catheter currently under investigation is the Rotoblator device, which consists of a burr secured to a central drive shaft capable of rotating at speeds of up to 200,000 rpm.[129] The rotating tip consists of a brass burr into which diamond chips have been embedded and ranges in size from 1.75 to 6.0 mm in diameter. The turbine mechanism is powered by compressed air, which also pumps cooling solution to the tip. The system employs a central guide wire that can be independently manipulated and over which the burr is advanced. In theory soft viscoelastic tissue is deflected by the tip, while hard, fixed atheromatous tissue allows the diamond chips to engage. The primary advantage of using this device is a reduced incidence of perforation. It is not, however, as effective in the setting of totally occluded vessels and still results in microembolization of pulverized particles. As is true with the previous devices, the incidence of restenosis appears to be significant. Of the nine patients initially treated in the UCLA experience, four developed significant restenosis within 6 months.[64] This restenosis rate appears to be somewhat higher than that recently reported by Ginsberg et al who documented successful results in 19 of 21 atherectomized vessels.[130] After 5 months the restenosis rate was a minimal 10%.

The Bard rotary atherectomy device* consists of a cylindrical cutting tip affixed to a flexible catheter that rotates at speeds of up to 1500 rpm and is advanced through a lesion over an augered guide wire. The auger on the guide wire allows retrieval of the incised atheromatous material through the central portion of the catheter. The prime advantages of this catheter appear to be related to its low rotational speeds and reduced heat generation, minimal tendency for perforation because of its being guided by a central wire, and the fact that the atheromatous debris is actually removed. The device may not, however, be as efficacious

*Dow Corning Wright, Arlington, Tennessee.

*Bard, Inc.

for totally occluded vessels. Preliminary clinical trials are ongoing under an Investigational Device Exemption.

A fifth device, the TEC System, has recently been approved for use in the peripheral vasculature and is manufactured by Interventional Technologies, Inc. The conical cutting tip passes over a central guide wire, and debris is constantly aspirated, reducing the chances for microembolization. The incidence of perforation appears quite low at present, and more complete follow-up data are awaited. The TEC peripheral atherectomy system has been used in 93 patients with 143 lesions in 12 clinical centers thus far. As is true with most series, the majority of lesions treated were located in the superficial femoral artery. The initial reported success rate of 92% required adjunctive balloon angioplasty for 35 lesions. The TEC system was able to reduce the degree of arterial stenosis by a mean of 59%. Six-month follow-up data are available in 57 of the 107 cases, but no consistent angiographic follow-up data are available.

Provided the hazards of perforation and distal embolization, which are associated to some extent with all atherectomy devices, are minimized, the overall long-term efficacy will depend on the fate of the atherectomized luminal surface left behind. It seems unlikely in the small-vessel caliber setting that sustained patency will result without some adjunctive pharmacologic control of the fibrous intimal hyperplastic response. Well-controlled prospective studies are much needed to define the role of these devices in the management of peripheral vascular disease.

Developments resulting from this information should make directional and rotational atherectomy more applicable. The concept of tissue debulking is theoretically more appealing than the process of balloon angioplasty.

LASER ANGIOPLASTY

Laser angioplasty results have not been encouraging. Table 6-9 lists the results in selected studies using different types of laser-assisted recanalization of peripheral arteries.[55,131-136] A significant effort is underway to develop better laser products. The fascination of laser light in medicine has generated a large demand among physicians and consumers. In some cases there are overwhelming financial incentives to make this technology work, and therefore frequently it is used as a marketing tool to attract patients. Unfortunately, the primary concept that lasers can ablate atherosclerotic plaque and therefore improve patency has yet to be proven.

ANGIOSCOPY AND INTRAARTERIAL ULTRASOUND

New and useful information can be obtained from these developing imaging devices (Figs. 6-8 and 6-9). Angioscopic images of the luminal morphology add information not seen on arteriograms.[137-139]

The intraarterial ultrasound instruments generate highly accurate cross-sectional images of the arterial wall and can depict the separate layers and the composition of these layers.[140-143] Features, such as plaque localization (concentric vs eccentric); discrimination of plaque characteristics (the presence of calcium; fatty vs fibrous composition); and evaluation of integrity of luminal surfaces (presence of fissures or dissection) can be determined with this technique.

PHARMACOLOGIC ADJUNCTIVE THERAPY TO PTA, ATHERECTOMY, AND LASER ANGIOPLASTY

Physicians administering interventional therapy need to be familiar with pharmacologic agents that alter platelet aggregation and with the thrombotic processes that occur during catheterization. These can cause reocclusion and may promote restenosis and need to be treated specifically. Moreover, elastic recoil resulting in vessel spasm and vasoconstriction can also contribute to the failure of a procedure and needs appropriate pharmacologic therapy.

Mechanical injury and distortion induced by balloon or other catheter manipulation may lead to significant platelet and clotting activation. This is probably the most important mechanism of acute postangioplasty occlusion. Recent angioscopic studies following angioplasty have confirmed the presence of mural thrombus at the site of balloon dilation.[144] Because thrombus formation appears to be important to the genesis of intraprocedural and postprocedural complications, the mechanism of thrombus formation in such settings needs to be briefly discussed.

Antiplatelet therapy

During experimental observations, when superficial endothelial cells are injured, platelets adhere to the subendothelial structures until a single- or double-platelet layer covers the exposed injury site. This process depends on the interaction between platelet membrane receptors; adhesive glycoproteins; and the substrate formed by collagen, subendothelial microfibrils, and other proteins.[145] One of the platelet membrane receptors, the glycoprotein Ib, serves as a binding site for the von Willebrand factor, particularly at high shear rates, and is necessary for the initial contact of platelets with the subendothelial surface. Glycoprotein Ia binds subendothelial collagen, particularly at low shear rates and may also be important in platelet adhesion. The third platelet membrane receptor, the glycoprotein IIb-IIIa, not only binds fibrinogen during platelet aggregation but also is important in the process of adhesion by serving as an additional binding site for the von Willebrand factor. The process of platelet adhesion to the damaged vascular wall is important in thrombotic occlusion and also may contribute to intimal hyperplasia and restenosis through the release of mitogens from platelets.

If platelet aggregation following angioplasty is allowed to go unmodified, thrombus would form along the luminal surface. Therefore limiting platelet aggregation is important in preventing both early closure and long-term restenosis.

A

B

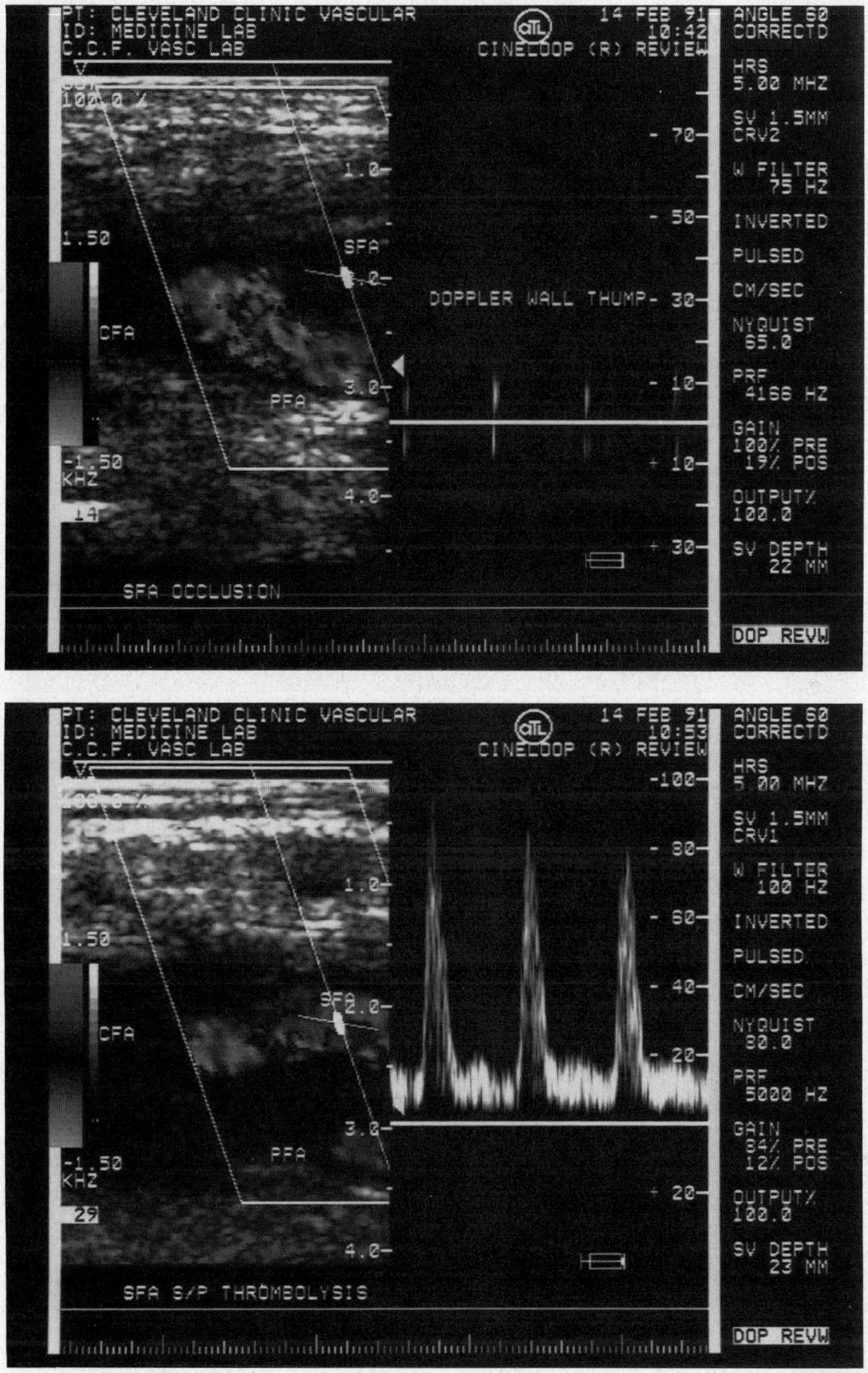

Fig. 6-8. Duplex ultrasound evaluation of superficial femoral artery occlusion. **A,** Doppler wall thump characteristic of occlusion without flow. **B,** After thrombolysis of superficial femoral artery occlusion, demonstrating flow.

A

B

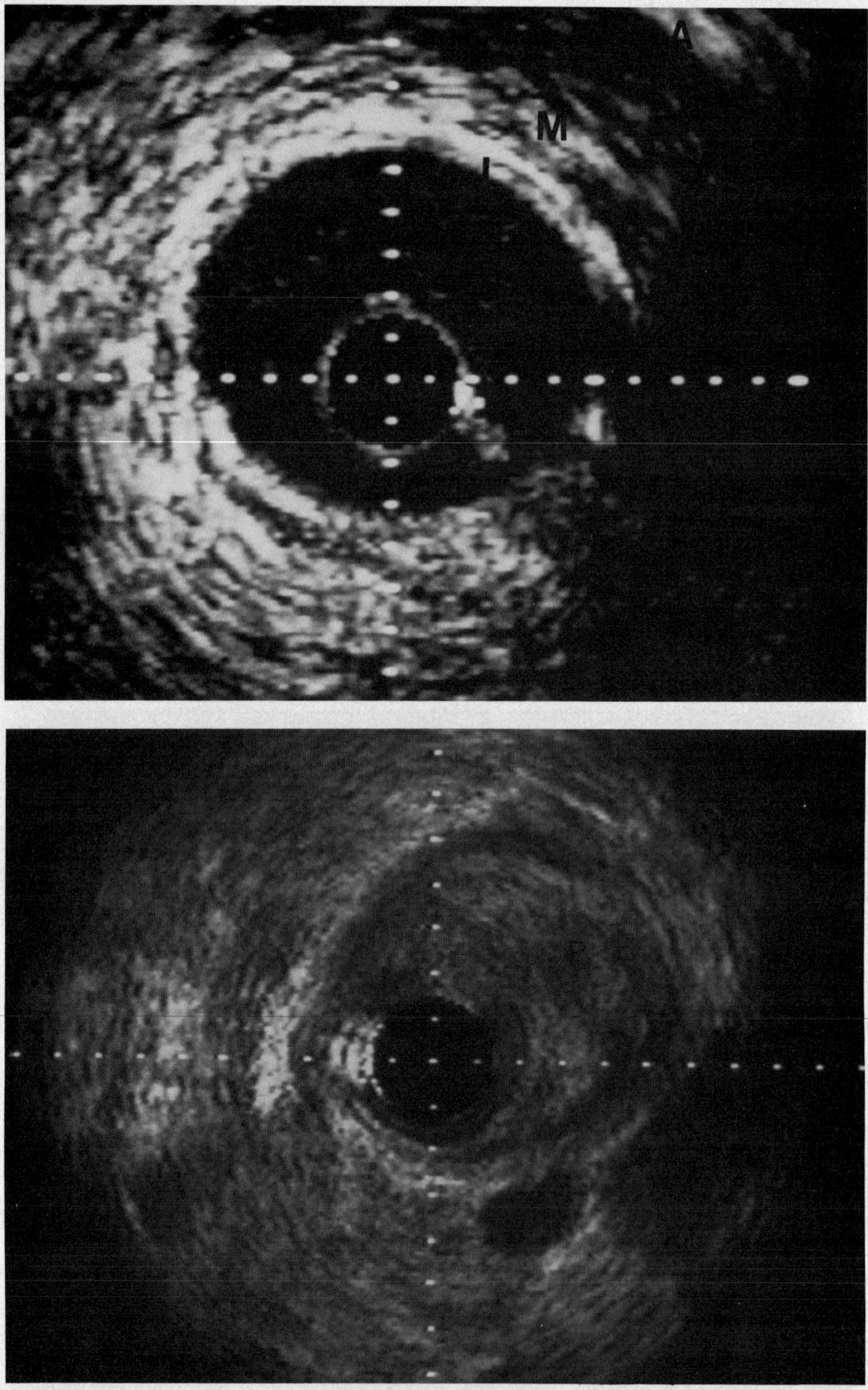

Fig. 6-9. Intravascular ultrasound images of **(A)** normal arterial wall (*I*, intima; *M*, media; *A*, adventitia); **(B)** eccentric atherosclerotic plaque *(P)*; and **(C)** intimal flap *(F)* after balloon angioplasty.

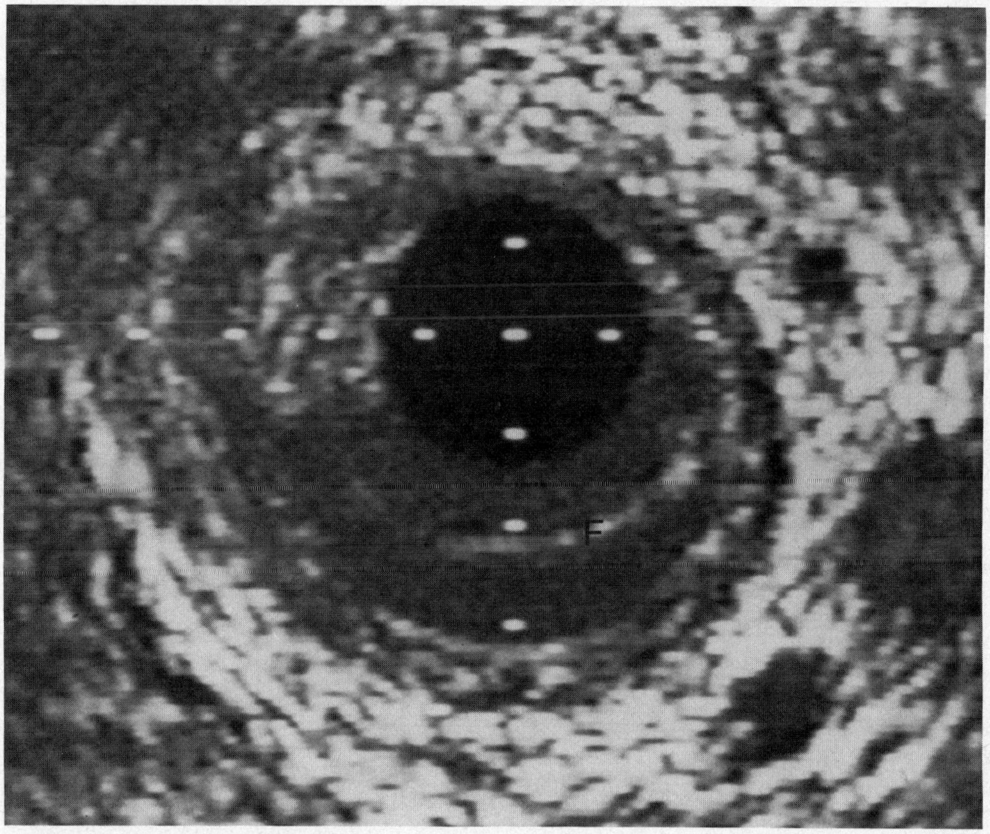

C

Fig. 6-9, cont'd. For legend see opposite page.

In both platelets and endothelial cells, the metabolism of prostaglandin endoperoxides has a profound regulatory impact on the process of platelet aggregation and accretion. In platelets arachidonic acid is mobilized from cell membranes by the action of enzyme phospholipase A_2. This mobilization also occurs in endothelial cells. Cyclooxygenase, present in both types of cells, converts arachidonate to endoperoxides. In endothelial cells endoperoxides are converted by the action of prostacyclin synthase to prostacyclin. Prostacyclin prevents platelet aggregation, disaggregates platelet clumps, and is a potent vasodilator. In platelets endoperoxides are converted by the action of thromboxane synthetase to thromboxane A_2. Thromboxane A_2 induces platelet aggregation and constricts arterial smooth muscle. Although thromboxane A_2 has a short half-life and is rapidly metabolized to thromboxane B_2, its extremely potent effects in the immediate environment demand that it be inhibited during angioplasty or other catheter-directed therapy.

Aspirin is a nonspecific inhibitor of cyclooxygenase. In small doses it can cause acetylation of cyclooxygenase and can reduce thromboxane A_2, thereby producing a favorable prostacyclin predominance and an unfavorable environment for thromboxane A_2. Therefore the desired effect of decreased platelet activation and aggregation occurs as a result of aspirin therapy.

In the experimental model of angioplasty, platelet thrombus deposition has been reduced with aspirin, aspirin plus dipyridamole, and other experimental platelet inhibitors. No benefit has been achieved with sulfinpyrazone or dipyridamole alone.[146] Therefore the result of these trials indicates that aspirin or aspirin plus dipyridamole, but not dipyridamole alone, is effective. Early evidence suggests that the drug ticlopidine is also an effective antiplatelet agent.[147]

Anticoagulation

Heparin anticoagulation is generally used during interventional procedures to prevent thrombosis from indwelling sheaths, catheters, or guide wires. It is also used to prevent thrombosis from balloon inflation during standard balloon angioplasty. Occasionally, it is helpful in the prevention of thrombosis during angioplasty or catheter-induced vasospasm, which can be severe and prolonged and can produce thrombus.

Other antithrombin proteins are being studied. The saliva from a leech produces a protein called *hirudin*. Hirudin has the unique ability to bind irreversibly at the thrombin-active site and can readily penetrate a clot. Heparin cannot penetrate the clot and only works on soluble, circulating thrombin.

Vasodilators

Spasm caused by the release of vasoactive substances by aggregating platelets or endothelium-derived cyclooxygenase products has been demonstrated in experimental angioplasty.[148] In addition, loss of endothelium-derived relaxing factor in areas of endothelial damage may predispose the arterial segment to vasoconstriction. Therefore vasoconstriction may contribute not only to early occlusion but also to late stenosis, as suggested by recent data.[149]

Calcium channel blockers, especially nifedipine, block the movement of calcium into the cytoplasm through calcium channels. In so doing, these drugs inhibit the formation of calcium complexes that normally increase actin and myosin interaction and therefore smooth muscle contraction. Administering calcium channel blockers before PTA is helpful in preventing this vasospastic phenomenon.[150,151]

Nitroglycerin dilates both arterial and venous smooth muscle. Its principal action in preventing peripheral arterial smooth muscle constriction is stimulated by an increase in cyclic guanosine monophosphate. This stimulation leads to dephosphorylation of myosin and muscular relaxation. The marked venodilating effect of nitroglycerin decreases venous return and therefore left ventricular systolic and diastolic pressure.

During interventional procedures nitroglycerin is valuable because it is a rapid-acting arterial dilator that may be injected directly into the vessel undergoing angioplasty. Nitroglycerin is largely inactivated on a first-pass through the liver and therefore should be given continuously if it is to be used as a vasodilator during angioplasty. An infusion of 20 μg to 100 μg per hour will generally produce the desired vasodilation.

GENERAL PRINCIPLES OF CATHETER INTERVENTION

For balloon angioplasty the ideal morphologic indication is a single, short stenotic segment in medium- to large-size vessels. Other indications include multiple discrete stenoses and short occlusions. Long-segment stenotic or occluded segments in smaller vessels may be treated with angioplasty, but less successfully. Similar limitations and indications may apply for laser-assisted angioplasty. Data to identify the most appropriate lesions for atherectomy are not available, although the lesions most appropriate are probably the same as those for balloon angioplasty.

In many cases long-segment occlusions can be transformed to short-segment stenotic lesions by intraarterial thrombolysis (Fig. 6-10). Management of the thrombotic component of any occlusion must be considered before angioplasty or atherectomy is performed because it may reduce the length of the occlusion and thus improve initial success and late patency.

Ulcerated atherosclerotic lesions may be associated with distal embolization, or the "blue toe" syndrome. PTA has successfully managed this syndrome. Atherectomy would probably be equally effective in treating patients with this syndrome.

CONCLUSION

PTA is an established method of revascularization in a variety of medical conditions. It is performed for specific morphologic and clinical indications. The role of PTA in

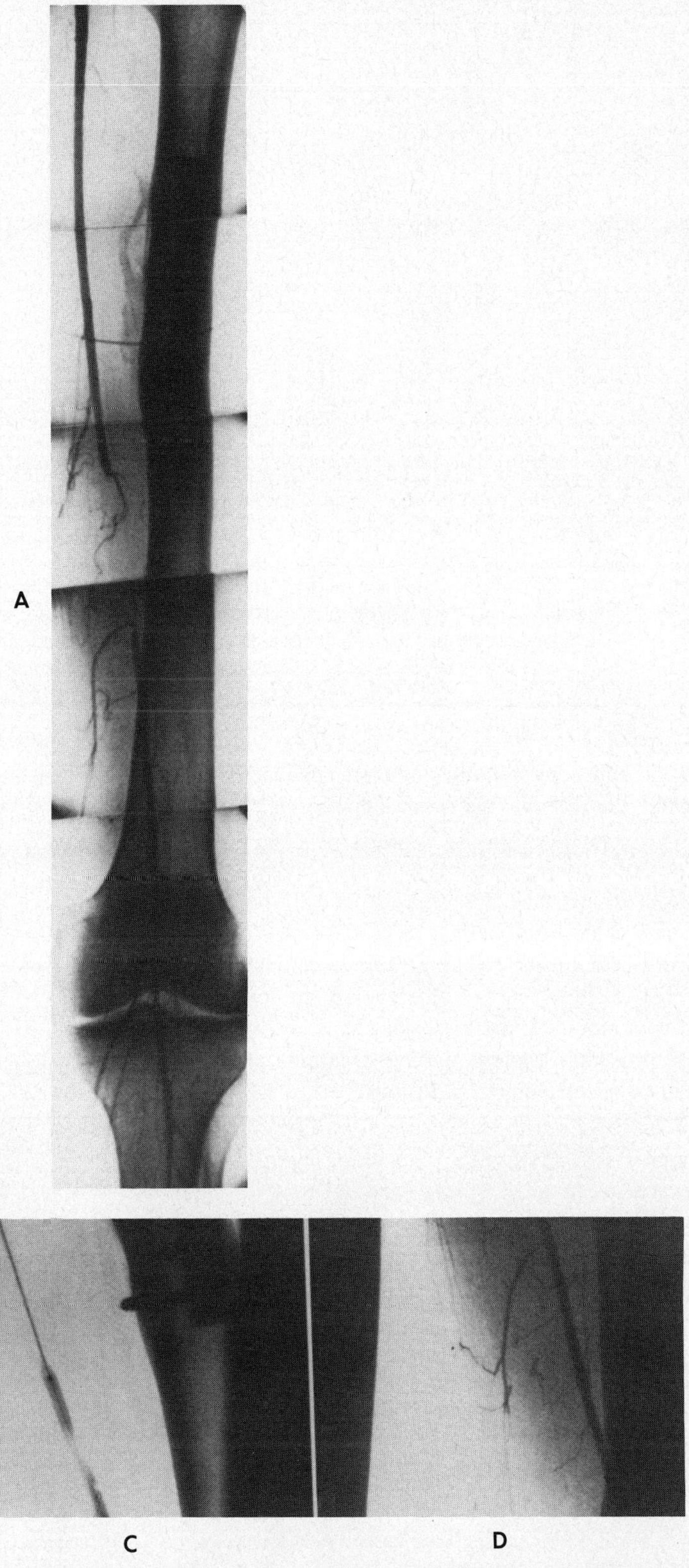

Fig. 6-10. A, Arteriogram of the left superficial femoral artery with a 6 cm occlusion at Hunter's canal. **B,** Arteriogram with use of an intraarterial catheter after 24 hours of thrombolysis. Note resolution of occluded segment into a patent but stenotic artery. **C,** Balloon angioplasty of residual atherosclerotic stenosis. **D,** Postangioplasty arteriogram showing resolution of stenosis.

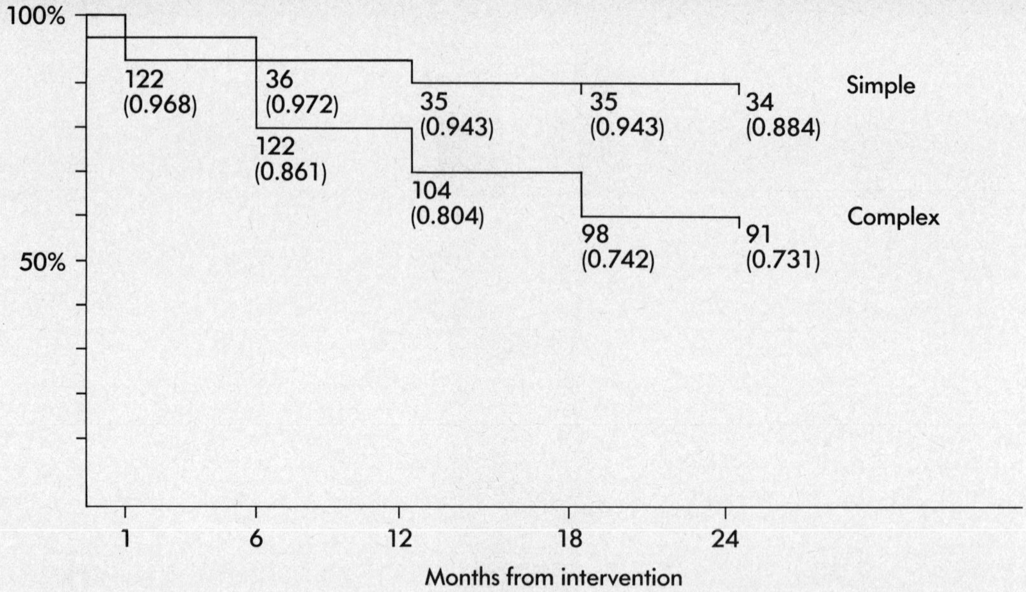

Fig. 6-11. Directional atherectomy for occlusive peripheral vascular disease. Life table analysis of patency rates for atherectomy of superficial femoral artery and popliteal/tibial arteries at the Cleveland Clinic in 162 patients treated with directional atherectomy.

treating carotid and vertebral atherosclerotic disease is uncertain, despite the fact that the overwhelming majority of these arteries are morphologically suitable for PTA.

Serious complications associated with angioplasty or atherectomy occur in less than 5% of cases. Of PTA patients, 2% to 3% have complications that require surgery or that prolong or alter the hospital course. The morbidity, mortality, and cost of angioplasty or atherectomy are low. The discomfort is minor and the postprocedural recovery is rapid. These procedures appear to have a definite place in the treatment of occlusive arterial lesions.

REFERENCES

1. Gruntzig A and Hopff H: Percutane Rekanlisation chronisch arterieller Verschlusse mit einem neuen Dilationskatheter, Dtsch Med Wochenschr 99:2502, 1974.
2. Gruntzig A and Kumpe DA: Technique of percutaneous angioplasty with Gruntzig balloon catheter, AJR 132:547, 1979.
3. Zeitler E and Muller R: Erste Ergebnisse mit der Katheterrekanalisation nach Dotter bei arterieller Verschlusskrankheit, Roe Fo 111 33:345, 1969.
4. Zeitler E: Results of percutaneous transluminal angioplasty, Radiology 146:57, 1983.
5. Zeitler E, Schoop W, and Zahnow W: The treatment of occlusive arterial disease by transluminal catheter angioplasty, Radiology 99:19, 1971.
6. Porstmann W and Wierny L: Intravasale Rekanalisation inoperabler arterieller Obliterationen, Zentralbl Chir 92,26:1586, 1968.
7. Van Andel GJ: Transluminale angioplastiek volgens Dotter, Ned Tijdschr Geneeskd 119:343, 1975.
8. Van Andel GJ et al: PTA of the iliac artery: long-term results, Radiology 156:321, 1985.
9. Velasquez G et al: Nonsurgical aortoplasty in the Leriche syndrome, Radiology 134:359, 1980.
10. Grollman JH, Del Vicario M, and Mittal AK: Percutaneous transluminal abdominal aortic angioplasty, AJR 134:1053, 1980.
11. Tegtmeyer CJ, Wellons HA, and Thompson RN: Balloon dilation of the abdominal aorta, JAMA 244:2636, 1980.
12. Kumpe DA: Percutaneous dilation of an abdominal aortic stenosis: three-balloon-catheter technique, Radiology 141:536, 1981.
13. Dotter CT and Judkins MP: Transluminal treatment of atherosclerotic obstruction: description of a new technique and a preliminary report of its application, Circulation 30:654, 1964.
14. Council on Scientific Affairs (Council Report): Percutaneous transluminal angioplasty, JAMA 251:764, 1984.
15. Rutherford RB, Patt A, and Kumpe DA: The current role of percutaneous angioplasty. In Greehalgh RM, Jamieson CW, and Nicoloaides NA, eds: Vascular surgery: issues in current practice, London, 1986, Grune & Stratton, Inc.
16. Block PC et al: Morphology after transluminal angioplasty in human beings, N Engl J Med 305:382, 1981.
17. Waller BF: Early and late morphologic changes in human coronary arteries after percutaneous transluminal coronary angioplasty, Clin Cardiol 6:363, 1983.
18. Waller BF, Dillon JC, and Cowley MH: Plaque hematoma and coronary dissection with percutaneous transluminal angioplasty (PTCA) of severly stenotic lesion: morphologic coronary observations in 5 men within 30 days of PTCA, Circulation 68(suppl III):111, 1983 (abstract).
19. Waller BF et al: Status of the major coronary arteries 80 to 150 days after percutaneous transluminal coronary angioplasty: analysis of 5 necropsy patients, Am J Cardiol 5:403, 1983.
20. Mizuno K, Jurita A, and Imazeki N: Pathologic findings after percutaneous transluminal coronary angioplasty, Br Heart J 52:588, 1984.
21. Waller BF et al: Early and late morphologic changes in major epicardial coronary arteries after percutaneous transluminal coronary angioplasty, Am J Cardiol 53:42C, 1984.
22. Austin GE et al: Intimal proliferation of smooth muscle cells as an explanation for recurrent coronary artery stenosis after percutaneous transluminal coronary angioplasty, J Am Coll Cardiol 6:369, 1985.

23. Waller BF et al: Status of the myocardium and infarct-related coronary artery in 19 necropsy patients with acute recanalization using pharmacologic, mechanical or combined types of reperfusion therapy, J Am Coll Cardiol 9:785, 1987.
24. Waller FB: Pathology of transluminal balloon angioplasty used in the treatment of coronary heart disease, Hum Pathol 18:476, 1987.
25. Soward AL, Essed CE, and Serruys PW: Coronary arterial findings after accidental death immediately after successful percutaneous transluminal coronary angioplasty, Am J Cardiol 56:794, 1985.
26. La Delia V et al: Coronary histology after percutaneous transluminal coronary angioplasty, Tex Heart Inst J 15:113, 1988.
27. Essed CD, Brand MVD, and Becker AE: Transluminal coronary angioplasty and early restenosis, Br Heart J 49:393, 1983.
28. Levine S et al: Coronary angioplasty: clinical and angiographic follow-up, Am J Cardiol 55:673, 1985.
29. Vlodaver Z and Edwards JE: Pathology of coronary atherosclerosis, Prog Cardiovasc Dis 14:256, 1971.
30. Saner HE et al: The disease-free wall in coronary atherosclerosis: its relation to degree of obstruction, J Am Coll Cardiol 6:1096, 1985.
31. Waller BF: Coronary luminal shape and the arc of disease-free wall: morphologic observations and clinical relevance, J Am Coll Cardiol 6:1100, 1985.
32. Waller BF: The eccentric coronary atherosclerotic plaque: morphologic observations and clinical relevance, Clin Cardiol 12:14, 1989.
33. Casarella WJ: Noncoronary angioplasty, Curr Probl Cardiol 11:138, 1986.
34. LeVeen RF, Wolf GL, and Biery D: Angioplasty induced vasospasm in rabbit model: mechanisms and treatment, Invest Radiol 20:938, 1985.
35. Needleman P, Coor PB, and Johnson EM Jr: Drugs used for the treatment of angina: organic nitrates, calcium channel blockers, and β-adrenergic antagonists. In Gilman AG et al, eds: The pharmacological basis of therapeutics, ed 7, New York, 1985, MacMillan Publishing Co.
36. Simpfendorfer C et al. Frequency, management, and follow-up of patients with acute coronary occlusions after percutaneous coronary angioplasty, Am J Cardiol 59:267, 1987.
37. Sinclair IN et al: Predictors, therapeutic options and long term out come of abrupt reclosure, Am J Cardiol 61:615, 1988.
38. Myler RM et al: Recurrence after coronary angioplasty, Cathet Cardiovasc Diagn 13:77, 1987.
39. Zollikofer CL et al: Acute and long-term effects of massive balloon dilation on the aortic wall and vasa vasorum, Radiology 164:145, 1987.
40. Cragg AH et al: The vasa vasorum and angioplasty, Radiology 148:75, 1983.
41. Waller BF, Pinkerton CA, and Foster LN: Morphologic evidence of accelerated left main coronary artery stenosis: a late complication of percutaneous transluminal balloon angioplasty of the proximal left anterior descending coronary artery, J Am Coll Cardiol 9:1019, 1987.
42. Fuster V et al: Platelet-inhibitor drugs' role in coronary artery disease, Prog Cardiovasc Dis 29:325, 1987.
43. Slack JD and Pinkerton CA: Subacute left main coronary stenosis: an unusual but serious complication of percutaneous transluminal angioplasty, Angiology 36:130, 1983.
44. Graf RH and Verani MS: Left main coronary artery stenosis: a possible complication of transluminal coronary angioplasty, Cathet Cardiovasc Diagn 10:163, 1984.
45. Spears JR: Percutaneous transluminal coronary angioplasty restenosis: potential prevention with laser balloon angioplasty, Am J Cardiol 60:61B, 1987.
46. Jenkins RD et al: Laser balloon angioplasty vs balloon angioplasty in normal iliac arteries, Circulation 76(suppl IV):IV-47, 1987 (abstract).
47. Sinclair IN: Effect of laser balloon angioplasty on normal dog coronary arteries in vivo, J Am Coll Cardiol 11:108A, 1988 (abstract).
48. Jenkins RD et al: Laser balloon angioplasty: effect of exposure duration on shear strength of welded layers of postmortem human aorta, Circulation 76(suppl IV):IV-46, 1987 (abstract).
49. Lee BL et al: Thermal compression and molding or atherosclerotic vascular tissue with use of radiofrequency energy: implication for radiofrequency balloon angioplasty, J Am Coll Cardiol 13:1167, 1989.
50. Forrester JS, Litvack F, and Grundfest W: Vaporization of atheroma in man: the role of lasers in the era of balloon angioplasty, Int J Cardiol 20:1, 1988.
51. Sanborn TA: Laser angioplasty: What has been learned from experimental studies and clinical trials? Circulation 78:769, 1988.
52. Sanborn TA et al: Angiographic and histologic follow-up of laser angioplasty with a laser probe, J Am Coll Cardiol 5:408, 1985 (abstract).
53. Cumberland DC et al: Percutaneous laser thermal angioplasty: initial clinical results with a laser probe in a total peripheral artery occlusion, Lancet 1:457, 1986.
54. McCowan TC et al: Laser thermal angioplasty for the treatment of obstruction of the distal superficial femoral or popliteal arteries, AJR 150:1169, 1988.
55. Geschwind HJ et al: Laser angioplasty of arterial stenoses, Cardiovasc Intervent Radiol 9:313, 1986.
56. Simpson JB et al: Transluminal atherectomy for occlusive peripheral vascular disease, Am J Cardiol 61:965, 1988.
57. Dorros G et al: Angiographic follow-up and clinical outcome of 126 patients after percutaneous directional atherectomy (Simpson AtheroCath) for occlusive peripheral vascular disease, Cathet Cardiovasc Diagn 22:79, 1991.
58. Hoffing B et al: Percutaneous atherectomy in iliac, femoral and popliteal arteries, Klin Wochenschr 65:528, 1987.
59. Graor RA and Whitlow PL: Transluminal atherectomy for occlusive peripheral vascular disease, J Am Coll Cardiol 6:1551, 1990.
60. Simpson JB et al: Transluminal atherectomy for occlusive peripheral vascular disease. Am J Cardiol 61:965, 1988.
61. Schwarten DE et al: Simpson catheter for percutaneous transluminal removal of atheroma, AJR 150:799, 1988.
62. Kensey KR et al: Recanalization of obstructed arteries with a flexible, rotating tip catheter, Radiology 165:387, 1987.
63. Hansen DD et al: Rotational atherectomy in atherosclerotic rabbit iliac arteries, Am Heart J 115:160, 1988.
64. Ahn SS et al: Removal of focal atheramatous lesions by angioscopically guided high-speed rotary atherectomy: preliminary experimental observations, J Vasc Surg 7:292, 1988.
65. Gruntzig A and Hopff M: Perkutane rekanalisation chronischer arterieller verschlusse mit einen neuer dilationskatheter: modification der Dotter-technik, Dtsch Med Wocheschr 99:2502, 1974.
66. Abele JE: Balloon catheters and transluminal dilatation: technical considerations, AJR 135:901, 1980.
67. Gerlock AJ, Regen DM, and Shaff MI: An examination of the physical characteristics leading to angioplasty balloon rupture, Radiology 144:421, 1982.
68. Simonetti G et al: Iliac artery rupture: a complication of transluminal angioplasty, AJR, 140:989, 1983.
69. Zollikofer CL et al: The relation between arterial and balloon rupture in experimental angioplasty, AJR 144:777, 1985.
70. Zollikofer CL et al: Mechanism of transluminal angioplasty. In Castaneda-Zuniga WR and Tadavarthy SM, eds: Interventional Radiology, Baltimore, 1988, Williams & Wilkins.
71. Wilson SE et al: Percutaneous transluminal angioplasty versus operation for peripheral arteriosclerosis, J Vasc Surg 9:1, 1989.
72. Gardiner GA et al: Complications of transluminal angioplasty, Radiology 159:201, 1986.
73. Heeney D et al: Transluminal angioplasty of the abdominal aorta, Radiology 148:81, 1983.
74. Charlebois N, Saint-Georges G, and Hudon G: Percutaneous transluminal angioplasty of the lower abdominal aorta, AJR 146:369, 1986.

75. Tegtmeyer CJ et al: Percutaneous transluminal angioplasty in the region of the aortic bifurcation: the two-balloon technique with results and long-term follow up study, Radiology 157:661, 1985.
76. Katzen BT: Percutaneous transluminal angioplasty for arterial disease of the lower extremities, AJR 142:23, 1984.
77. Waltman AC et al: Transluminal angioplasty of the iliac and femoropopliteal arteries: current status, Arch.Surg 117:1218, 1982.
78. Schwarten DE: Aortic, iliac and peripheral arterial angioplasty. In Castaneda-Zuniga WR and Tadavarthy SM, eds: Baltimore, 1988, Williams & Wilkins.
79. Ring EJ et al: Percutaneous recanalization of common iliac artery occlusions: an unacceptable complication rate? AJR 139:587, 1982.
80. Colapinto RF, Harries-Jones EP, and Johnston KW: Percutaneous transluminal angioplasty of peripheral vascular disease: a two-year experience, Cardiovasc Intervent Radiol 3:213, 1980.
81. Spence R et al: Long-term results of transluminal angioplasty of the iliac and femoral arteries, Arch Surg 116:1377, 1981.
82. Gallino A et al: Percutaneous transluminal angioplasty of the arteries of the lower limbs: a 5-year follow-up, Circulation 70:619, 1984.
83. Hewes RC et al: Long-term results of superficial femoral artery angioplasty, AJR 146:1025, 1986.
84. Johnston KW, Colapinto RF, and Baird RJ: Transluminal dilation: an alternative? Arch Surg 117:1604, 1982.
85. Graor RA et al: Percutaneous transluminal angioplasty: review of iliac and femoral dilations at the Cleveland Clinic, Cleve Clin Quart 51:149, 1984.
86. Johnson KW: A surgeon's view of peripheral arterial transluminal dilation. In Bergan J, ed: Arterial surgery, New York, 1984, Churchill Livingstone, Inc.
87. Greenfield AJ: Femoral, popliteal, and tibial arteries: percutaneous transluminal angioplasty, AJR 135:927, 1980.
88. Krepel VM et al: Percutaneous transluminal angioplasty of the femoropopliteal artery: initial and long-term results, Radiology 156:325, 1985.
89. Rooke TW et al: Percutaneous transluminal angioplasty in the lower extremities: a 5-year experience, Mayo Clin Proc 62:85, 1987.
90. Martin EC et al: Angioplasty for femoral artery occlusion: comparison with surgery, AJR 137:915, 1981.
91. Blair JM et al: Percutaneous transluminal angioplasty versus surgery for limb-threatening ischemia, J Vasc Surg 9:698, 1989.
92. Glover LJ et al: Balloon catheter dilation for limb salvage, Arch Surg 118:557, 1983.
93. Zeitler E: Percutaneous dilation and recanalization of iliac and femoral arteries, Cardiovasc Intervent Radiol 3:207, 1980.
94. Schwarten DE and Cutcliff WB: Arterial occlusive disease below the knee: treatment with percutaneous transluminal angioplasty performed with low profile catheters and steerable guide wires, Radiology 169:71, 1988.
95. Brown KT et al: Percutaneous transluminal angioplasty of infrapopliteal vessels: preliminary results and technical considerations, Radiology 169:75, 1988.
96. Tegtmeyer CJ: Renal angioplasty: technique and patient selection (abstract). Program of the 13th Annual Meeting on Diagnostic Angiography and Interventional Radiology of the Society of Cardiovascular and Interventional Radiology. Reston, VA: Society of Cardiovascular and Interventional Radiology, pp 58-68, 1986.
97. Meaney TF, Dustan HP, and McCormack LJ: Natural history of renal artery disease, Radiology 91:881, 1968.
98. Schreiber MJ, Pohl MA, and Novick AC: The natural history of atherosclerotic and fibrous renal artery disease, Urol Clin North Am 11:383, 1984.
99. Dean RH et al: Renovascular hypertension: anatomic and renal function changes during drug therapy, Arch Surg 116:1408, 1981.
100. Cicuto KP et al: Renal artery stenosis: anatomic classification for percutaneous transluminal angioplasty, AJR 137:599, 1981.
101. Colapinto RF et al: Percutaneous transluminal dilatation of the renal artery: follow-up studies on renovascular hypertension, AJR 139:727, 1982.
102. Geyskes GG et al: Follow-up study of 70 patients with renal artery stenosis treated by percutaneous transluminal dilatation, Br Med J [Clin Res] 287:333, 1983.
103. Ingrisch H, Hegels T, and Frey KW: Angiographic control of renal artery stenoses 6 months following percutaneous transluminal angioplasty, Cardiovasc Intervent Radiol 5:249, 1982.
104. Katzen BT, Chang J, and Knox WG: Percutaneous transluminal angioplasty with the Gruntzig balloon catheter: a review of 70 cases, Arch Surg 114:1389, 1979.
105. Lohr E et al: Renal angioplasty: experiences with 94 patients, Urol Radiol 4:211, 1982.
106. Mahler F et al: Long-term results of percutaneous transluminal angioplasty for renovascular hypertension using the coaxial catheter technique in patients with atherosclerosis and fibromuscular dysplasia. In Dotter CT et al, eds: Percutaneous transluminal angioplasty: technique, early and late results. New York, 1983, Springer Publishing Co, Inc.
107. Martin E et al: Renal angioplasty for hypertension: predictive factors for long-term success, AJR 137:921, 1981.
108. Martin LG et al: Percutaneous angioplasty in clinical management of renovascular hypertension: initial and long-term results, Radiology 155:629, 1985.
109. Miller GA et al: Percutaneous transluminal angioplasty vs. surgery for renovascular hypertension, AJR 144:447, 1985.
110. Richter EI, Kronert E, and Zeitler E: Technique, indications, complications, and results of percutaneous transluminal artery diltation. In Dotter CT et al, eds: Percutaneous transluminal angioplasty: technique, early and late results, New York, 1983, Springer Publishing Co, Inc.
111. Schwarten DE: Percutaneous transluminal renal angioplasty, Urol Radiol 2:193, 1981.
112. Sos TA et al: Percutaneous transluminal renal angioplasty in renovascular hypertension due to atheroma or fibromuscular dysplasia, N Engl J Med 309:274, 1983.
113. Tegtmeyer CJ, Kellum CD, and Ayes C: Percutaneous transluminal angioplasty of the renal artery: results and long-term follow-up, Radiology 153:77, 1984.
114. Motarjeme A et al: Percutaneous transluminal angioplasty for treatment for subclavian steal, Radiology 155:611, 1985.
115. Pavone P et al: PTA of subclavian artery: comparative study with surgical procedures (abstract). Program of the Cardiovascular and Interventional Radiology Society of Europe, Porto Cervo, Sardinia, Italy, May 27, 1987, pp. 85-86.
116. Theron J, Melancon D, and Ethier R: "Pre" subclavian steal syndromes and their treatment by angioplasty: hemodynamic classification of subclavian artery stenoses, Neuroradiology 27:265, 1985.
117. Tsai FY et al: Percutaneous transluminal angioplasty of the carotid artery, AJNR 7:349, 1986.
118. Kachel R et al: Percutaneous transluminal angioplasty (dilatation) of carotid, vertebral, and innominate artery stenoses, Cardiovasc Intervent Radiol 10:142, 1987.
119. Vitek JJ, Raymon BC, and Oh SJ: Innominate artery angioplasty. AJNR 5:113, 1984.
120. Galichia JP et al: Subclavian artery stenosis treated by transluminal angioplasty: six cases, Cardiovasc Intervent Radiol 6:78, 1983.
121. Courtheoux P et al: Transcutaneous angioplasty of vertebral artery atheromatous ostial stricture, Neuroradiology 27:259, 1985.
122. Mathias K: Catheter treatment of cerebrovascular disease (abstract). Program of the Cardiovascular and Interventional Radiology Society of Europe, Porto Cervo, Sardinia, Italy, May 27, 1987, pp. 84-85.
123. Tournade A et al: Percutaneous transluminal angioplasty of the vertebral and subclavian arteries: an angiographic-velocimetry comparison, J Neuroradiol 13:95, 1986.

124. Wilms G et al: Percutaneous transluminal angioplasty of the subclavian artery: early and late results, Cardiovasc Intervent Radiol 10:123, 1987.
125. Ringelstein EB and Zeumer H: Delayed reversal of vertebral artery blood flow following percutaneous transluminal angioplasty for subclavian steal syndrome, Neuroradiology 26:189, 1984.
126. Burke DR et al: Percutaneous transluminal angioplasty of subclavian arteries, Radiology 164:699, 1987.
127. Simpson JB et al: Transluminal atherectomy: initial clinical results in 27 patients, Circulation 74(suppl 2):203, 1986 (abstract).
128. Snyder SO Jr et al: Kensey catheter: early results with a transluminal endarterectomy tool, J Vasc Surg 8:541, 1988.
129. Ahn SS: The rotablator: high speed rotary atherectomy. In WS Moore, and SS Ahn, eds: Endovascular surgery, Philadelphia, 1989, WB Saunders Co.
130. Ginsberg R et al: Transluminal rotational atherectomy: clinical experience in 20 patients, Circulation (suppl II):II-415, 1988 (abstract).
131. Sanborn TA: Laser thermal angioplasty. In White RA and Grundfest WS, eds: Lasers in cardiovascular disease, Chicago, 1987, Year Book Medical Publishers, Inc.
132. Katzen BT et al: Initial experience with an excimer in peripheral lesions, Circulation 78:2, 1988.
133. Nordstrom LA et al: Laser angioplasty: controlled delivery of argon laser energy, Radiology 167:463, 1988.
134. Leon MB et al: Human arterial surface fluorescence: atherosclerotic plaque identification and effects of laser atheroma ablation, J Am Coll Cardiol 12:94, 1988.
135. Geschwind HJ et al: Percutaneous pulsed laser angioplasty with atheroma detection in humans, J Am Coll Cardiol 11:49A, 1988.
136. Abela GS and Seeger JM: Laser angioplasty: clinical experience. Presented at the Cardiovascular Plenary Session of the Lasers in Medicine and Surgery Meeting, Dallas, April 27, 1988.
137. White GH et al: Intraoperative video angioscopy compared with arteriography during peripheral vascular operations, J Vasc Surgery 6:488, 1987.
138. Grundfest WS et al: Delineation of peripheral and coronary detail by introperative angioscopy, Ann Surg 202:394, 1985.
139. Mehigan JT and Olcott C: Video angioscopy as an alternative to intraoperative arteriography, Am J Surg 152:139, 1986.
140. Isner JM et al: Percutaneous intravascular US as adjunct to catheter-based interventions: preliminary experience in patients with peripheral vascular disease, Radiology 175:61, 1990.
141. Yock PG et al: Real-time, two-dimensional catheter ultrasound: a new technique for high resolution intravascular imaging, J Am Coll Cardiol 2:130A, 1988 (abstract).
142. Pandian N et al: In vivo ultrasound angioscopy in humans and animals: intraluminal imaging of blood vessels using a new catheter-based high resolution ultrasound probe, Circulation 78:II-22, 1988.
143. Yock P et al: Intravascular two-dimensional catheter ultrasound: initial clinical studies, Circulation 78:II-20, 1988 (abstract).
144. Uchida Y et al: Angioscopic observation of the coronary luminal changes induced by percutaneous transluminal coronary angioplasty, Am Heart J 117:769, 1989.
145. Fuster V et al: Insights into the pathogenesis of acute ischemic syndromes, Circulation 77:1213, 1988.
146. Steele PP, Chesebro JH, and Fuster V: The natural history of arterial balloon angioplasty in pigs and intervention with platelet-inhibitor therapy: implications for clinical trials, Clin Res 32(suppl):209A, 1984 (abstract).
147. White CW et al: Antiplatelet agents are effective in reducing the immediate complications of PTCA: results form the ticlopidine multicenter trial, Circulation 76(suppl):IV-400, 1987 (abstract).
148. Fischell TA et al: Endothelium-dependent arterial vasoconstriction after balloon angioplasty, Circulation 79:899, 1989.
149. Bertrand ME et al: Relation to restenosis after percutaneous transluminal coronary angioplasty to vasomotion of the dilated coronary arterial segment, Am J Cardiol 63:277, 1989.
150. Faxon DP et al: Effect of nifedipine on restenosis following experimental angioplasty, Circulation 70(suppl):II-175, 1984 (abstract).
151. Corcos T et al: Failure of diltiazem to prevent restenosis after PTCA, Am Heart J 109:926, 1985.
152. Hunter DW et al: Failing arteriovenous dialysis fistulas: evaluation and treatment, Radiology 152:631, 1984.
153. Glanz S et al: The role of percutaneous angioplasty in the management of chronic hemodialysis fistulas, Ann Surg 206:777, 1987.

Part II

ARTERIAL DISEASES

Chapter 7

PATHOGENESIS OF ATHEROSCLEROSIS

Guy M. Chisolm
Paul E. DiCorleto
L. Allen Ehrhart
Paul L. Fox
Henry F. Hoff
Richard E. Morton

CHARACTERISTICS OF ATHEROSCLEROTIC DISEASE IN HUMANS

Atherosclerosis is a disease with both degenerative and regenerative characteristics that initially affects the tunica intima of major arteries in man. In general, atherosclerosis leads to luminal narrowing of the affected artery and ischemia of the end organ. Atherosclerosis can lead to sufficient narrowing of the lumen at the iliac bifurcation and origins of the iliac arteries to induce ischemia of the lower limbs. Extensive atherosclerosis in the aorta that has progressed to involve the tunica media can result in dissecting aneurysms. In muscular arteries such as the coronary or cranial arteries stenosis caused by atherosclerosis can result in myocardial infarction or cerebral infarction (stroke), respectively.

Extending from the media to the endothelium, the intima of an artery comprises an internal elastic lamina and an acellular layer rich in connective tissue, especially proteoglycans. Intimal thickening, either focal or diffuse, occurs throughout the aortic, coronary, and carotid arteries in adult humans. Intimal thickening first develops during fetal life, steadily growing during puberty, and is considered a physiologic rather than pathologic event since it can be present without any development of atherosclerosis. However, advanced and clinically relevant atherosclerotic lesions consistently develop at anatomic sites that exhibit intimal thickening.

The initial atherosclerotic lesion is believed to be the fatty-streak lesion. When sufficiently large, these lesions can be observed grossly as yellow elevations of the intimal surface. In the thoracic aorta they can be seen as yellow stripes running parallel to the vessel axis adjacent to the branches of the intercostal arteries (Fig. 7-1). Smaller fatty streaks can be seen grossly only after staining the artery with lipid stains. Microscopically, cross sections of fatty streaks are characterized by an abundance of cells filled with vacuoles that contain predominantly cholesteryl esters (Fig. 7-2). These cells have been termed *foam cells* because of their foamy appearance. Foam cells are usually observed in the intima close to the lumen immediately underlying the endothelium. Fatty streaks initially appear in the first decade of life in the aorta, in the second decade in coronary arteries, and in the third decade in cerebral arteries.

The more advanced form of atherosclerotic lesion is called the fibrous plaque, which appears grossly as a raised, pearly white region of varied size (Fig. 7-3). Some pathologists refer to fibrous lesions having a major lipid component as fibrofatty plaques. Fibrous plaques are usually composed of two distinct parts. One is a large region referred to as the necrotic core, which is frequently but not exclusively at the base of the lesion near the internal elastic lamina (Fig. 7-4). The core is composed of abundant extracellular lipid and extensive cell debris (Fig. 7-5). The second region is the fibrotic cap, which often comprises the largest portion of the atherosclerotic lesion (Fig. 7-6). The cap consists of numerous connective tissue components, especially collagen, surrounding smooth muscle cells. When these cells are

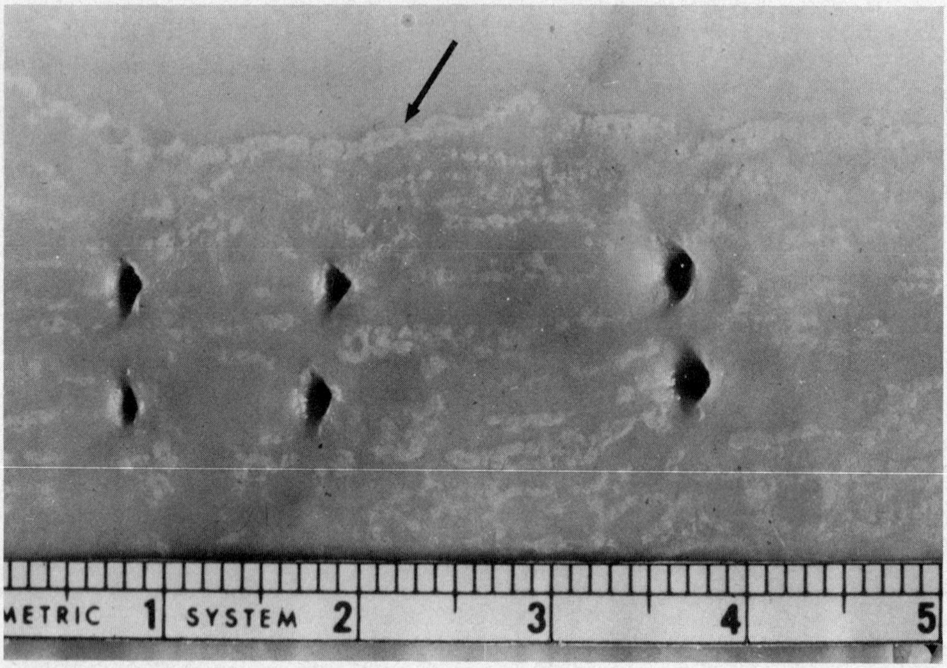

Fig. 7-1. Gross specimen of a human thoracic aorta, showing raised fatty streaks *(arrow)* running parallel to orifices of intercostal arteries.

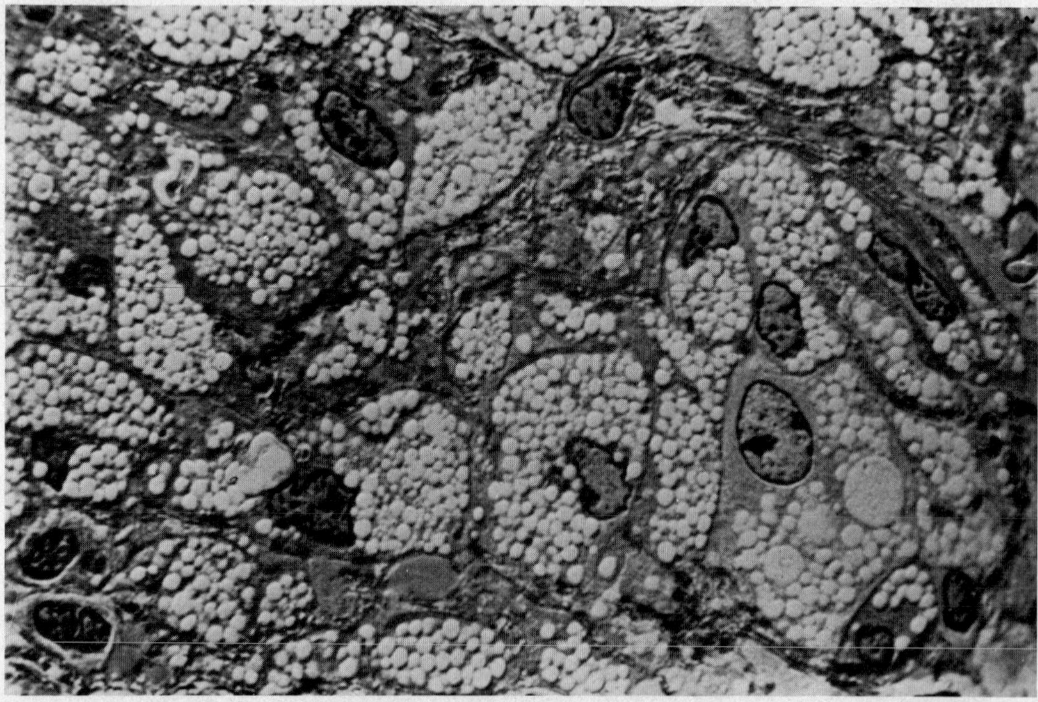

Fig. 7-2. Light micrograph of cross section of a fatty streak from a human cerebral artery, illustrating close packing of round foam cells. Interference contrast microscopy was used.

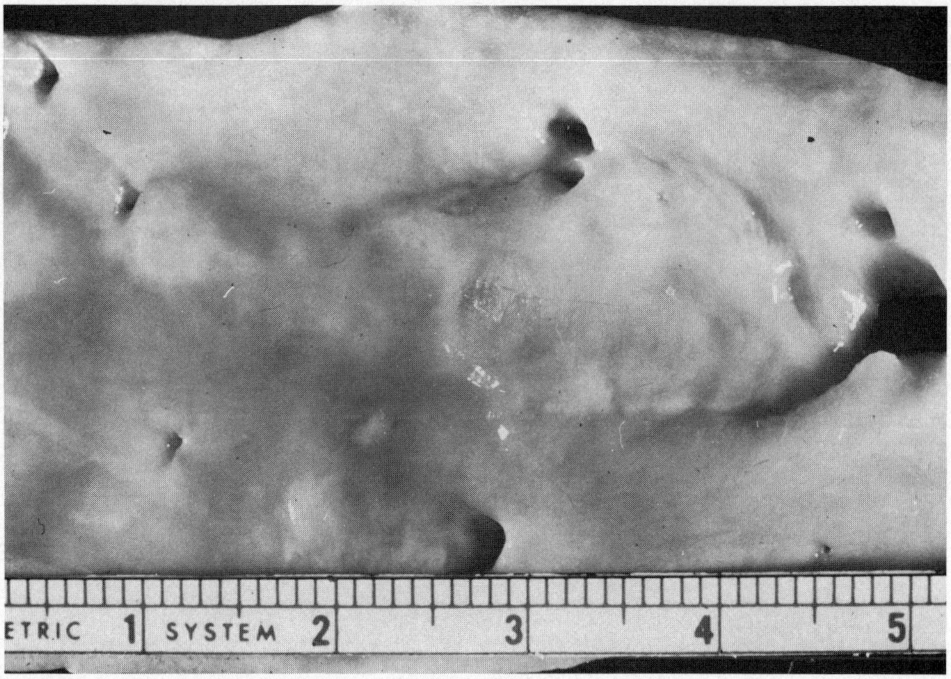

Fig. 7-3. Gross specimen of a fibrous plaque, showing a slightly raised, pearly-white lesion.

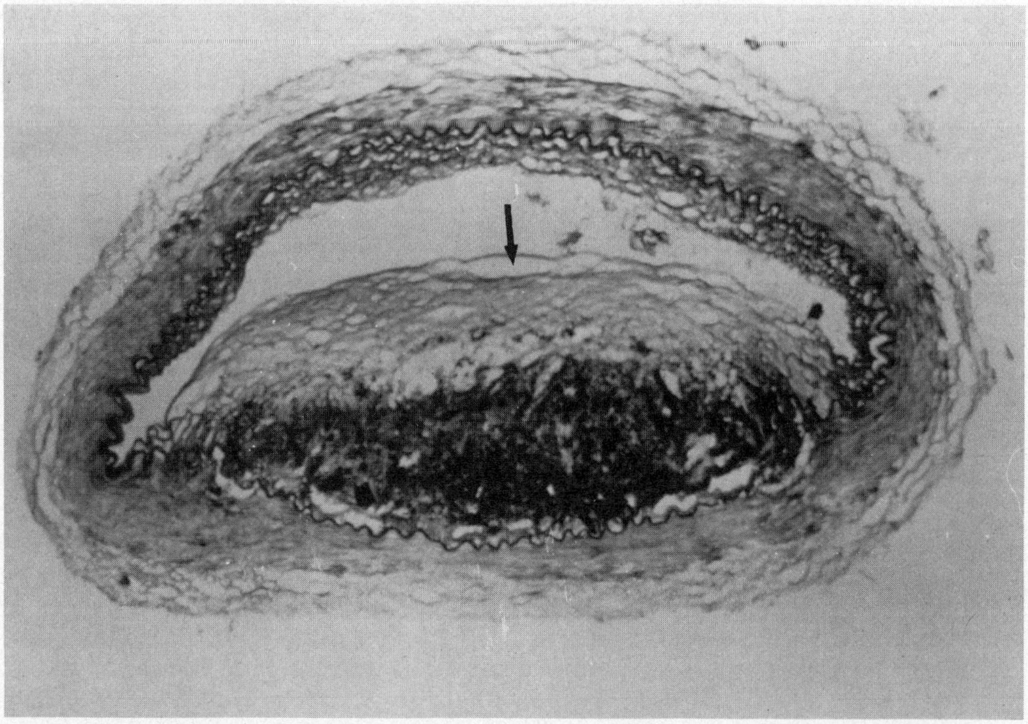

Fig. 7-4. Light micrograph of cross section of a fibrous plaque in a cerebral artery, demonstrating the eccentric location of the lesion and how the lesion compromises the lumen of the vessel. The lesion is composed of a necrotic core filled with lipid (stained black) and a fibrous cap *(arrow)*.

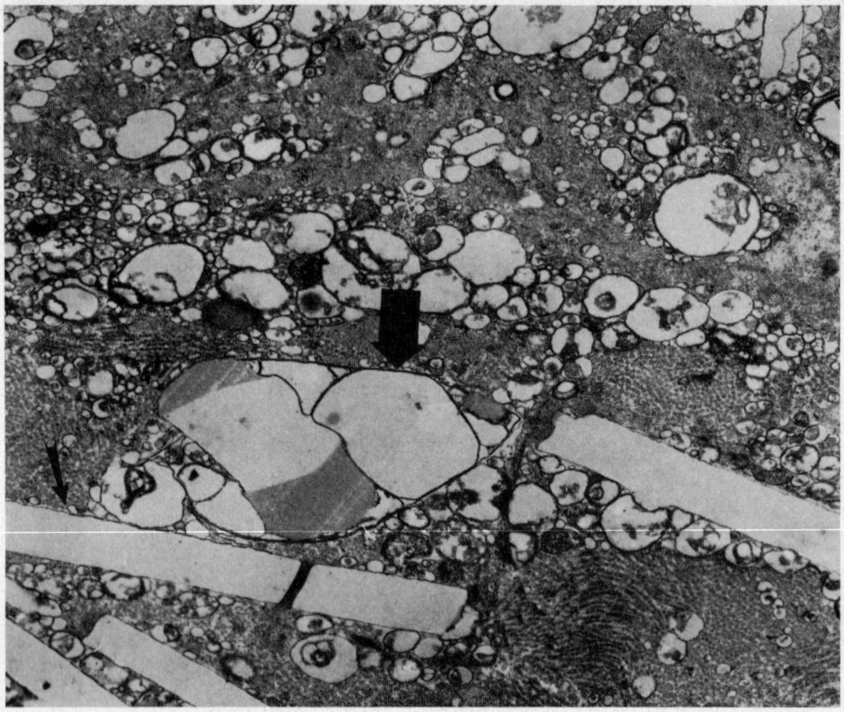

Fig. 7-5. Electron micrograph of the necrotic core of a fibrous plaque lesion. Note the cholesterol crystals *(small arrow)* and the extracellular lipid droplets *(large arrow)* embedded in a matrix of collagen.

Fig. 7-6. Light micrograph of fibrous plaque in a human aorta, illustrating the fibromuscular cap *(arrow)* filled with smooth muscle cells (nuclei are stained black). Beneath the cap is the necrotic core, which is stained positive for lipid.

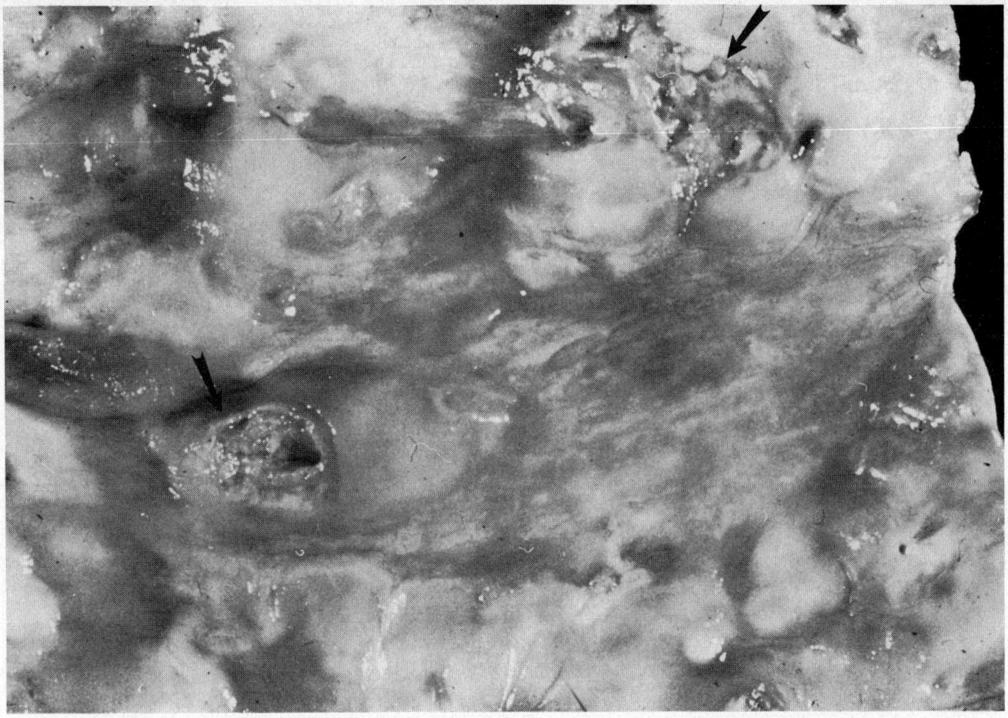

Fig. 7-7. Gross specimen of a human abdominal aorta, illustrating several ulcerated lesions *(arrows).*

present in abundance, this part of the lesion is referred to as a fibromuscular cap, whereas when few cells are present, the term *fibrous* or *fibrotic cap* is usually used. The term *atherosclerosis* reflects the two major components of the atherosclerotic lesion, that is, *athero* from the Greek word for gruel, corresponding to the necrotic debris at the base of the plaque, and *sclerosis,* from the Greek word for hard, corresponding to the fibrotic cap. In coronary arteries fibrous plaques may also begin to appear in the second decade of life. Numerous studies have indicated an association between the surface area occupied by fibrous plaques in the coronary arteries and subsequent myocardial infarction several decades later. No such association exists between fatty streaks and clinical manifestations. Indeed, fatty streaks present in children at several anatomic sites such as the aortic arch and thoracic aorta may disappear later in life. However, in the coronary and cranial arteries the early fatty streaks and the late fibrous plaques occur at similar anatomic sites. In addition, there are lesions that appear to represent transitions between these two types of lesions. These findings strongly suggest that fatty streaks are precursors of fibrous plaques.

The term *complicated lesion* is used to identify a wide variety of advanced atherosclerotic lesions that exhibit characteristics not consistently found in the classic fibrous plaque. One form of complicated lesion, for example, is the ulcerated lesion, which appears grossly as an open wound with an uneven surface more darkly colored than the surrounding intimal surface (Fig. 7-7). This lesion is believed formed by the rupture of the fibrous cap (Fig. 7-8), allowing direct interaction between the lipid and cell debris of the necrotic core and blood. This usually occurs when the cap above a large necrotic core filled with cholesterol crystals is very thin (Fig. 7-9). Because of the thrombogenic nature of many of the plaque components in the core, such an event leads to mural thrombus formation. If this event occurs in a lesion that has already led to severe narrowing of the lumen, thrombus formation can completely occlude the vessel, resulting in myocardial infarction when occurring in the coronary circulation or stroke when occurring in the extra-intracranial circulation. Recent studies using angioscopy have demonstrated a direct association between the appearance of such ulcerated lesions in coronary arteries and the clinical symptoms of unstable angina.[1] It is believed that rupture of the fibrous cap occurs at specific sites when the size of the necrotic core greatly exceeds that of the fibrous cap; lumen pressure then breaks the thin and fragile cap.

Another occasional feature of complicated lesions is the invasion of networks of capillaries derived from both the vasa vasorum of the adventitia and new capillary sprouts originating from the lumen (Fig. 7-10). Hemorrhage occurring in the necrotic core as a result of the rupture of capillaries is frequently observed in ulcerated lesions.

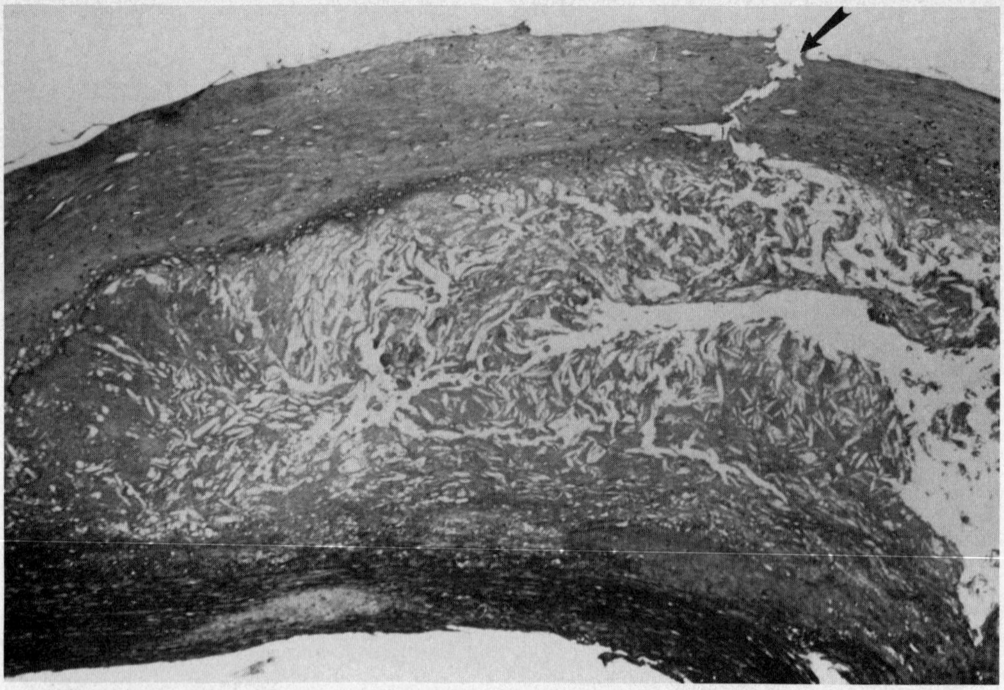

Fig. 7-8. Light microscopy of cross section of a human aortic plaque, illustrating a crack in the fibrous cap *(arrow)*.

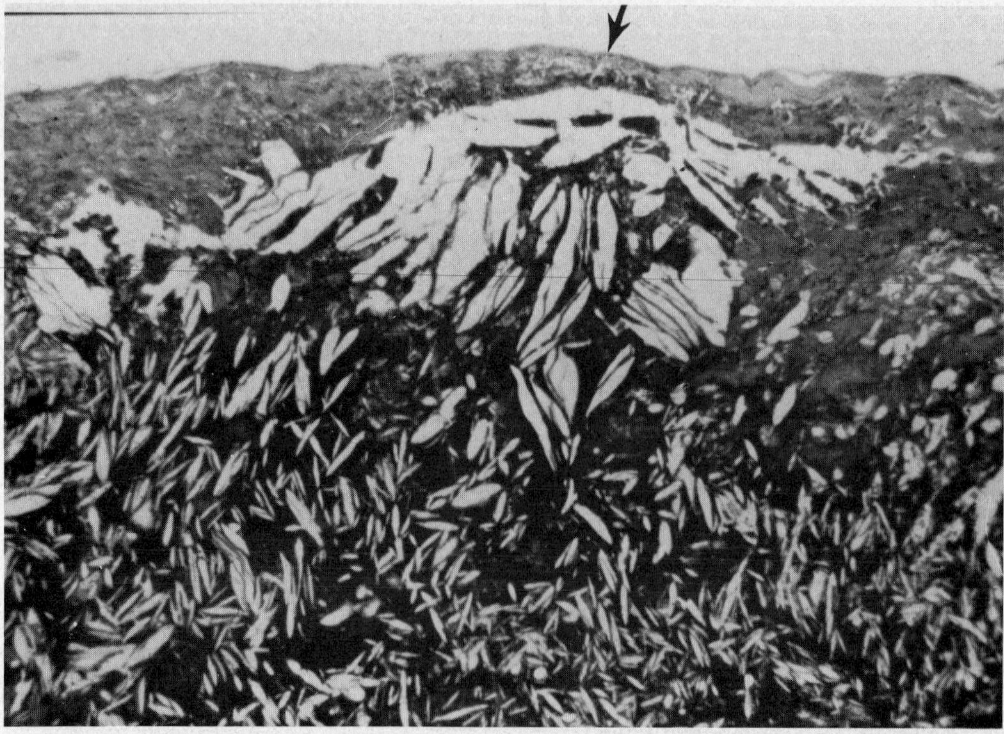

Fig. 7-9. Light microscopy of cross section of a human aortic fibrous plaque, showing how thin the fibrous cap can be at specific sites *(arrow)*. Such areas are prone to rupture.

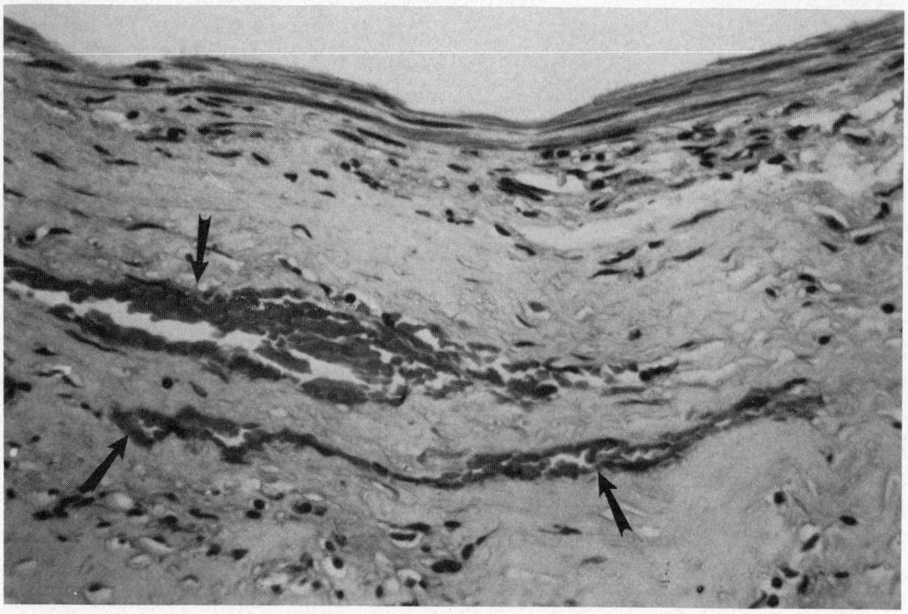

Fig. 7-10. Light micrograph of cross section of a complicated lesion, showing several capillaries filled with red blood cells *(arrows)*.

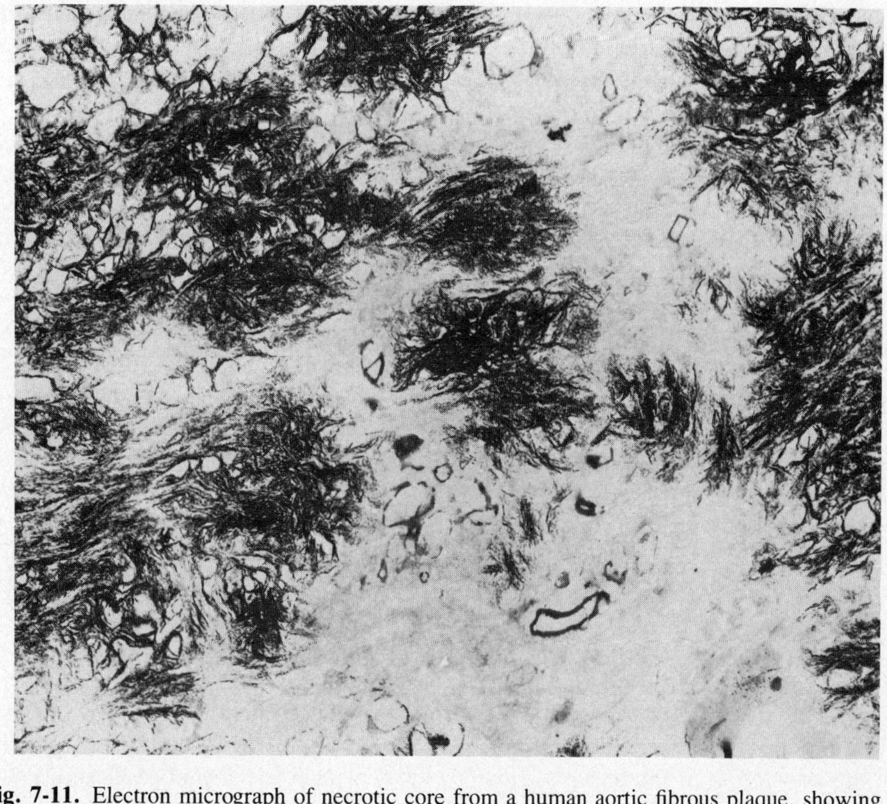

Fig. 7-11. Electron micrograph of necrotic core from a human aortic fibrous plaque, showing an area of calcification. Spicules of calcium apatite crystals *(dark structures)* can be seen throughout this area.

One of the most common characteristics of advanced, complicated lesions is the appearance of calcium in the form of apatite crystals in atherosclerotic lesions (Fig. 7-11), giving such lesions their characteristic brittleness. The phrase commonly used by the lay public, "hardening of the arteries," describes this lesion calcification.

THEORIES OF ATHEROGENESIS

Lipid hypothesis

Even several decades ago descriptive pathology and animal experimentation allowed researchers to propose the sequence of events that occurs during the development of the atherosclerotic lesion. It was established early, for example, that the fatty-streak lesion is characterized by the accumulation of lipids,[2] primarily cholesterol, in its esterified form.[3,4] Moreover, the smaller (and presumably newer) the lesion, the greater is the fraction of lipid that is intracellular. Since both fatty streaks and fibrous plaques are characterized by the presence of cholesterol, primarily intracellular in fatty streaks and extracellular in fibrous plaques, it is understandable that much research has focused on how and why cholesterol accumulates. Virchow's early theory of atherogenesis[5] included the infiltration of lipids from the plasma into arterial walls. Further refinements of the lipid hypothesis have been made over the years.[6,7] It is currently believed that the primary source of lesion cholesterol is plasma low density lipoprotein (LDL) that preferentially accumulates in the arterial intima. This accumulation may be the result of one or more of the following: (1) alterations in the permeability of the arterial intima to LDL; (2) increases in interstitial space in the intima; (3) poorer metabolism of LDL by vascular cells; (4) impeded transport of LDL from the intima to the media; (5) increased plasma LDL concentrations; or (6) specific binding of LDL to connective tissue components in the arterial intima. These factors are discussed in more detail in later sections. Studies of human arteries and studies of animals placed on high cholesterol diets have clearly established that the lower density lipoproteins accumulate to substantial levels in the tunica intima even before lesions develop.[8,9] In fact, the primary site of such accumulation is the acellular zone close to the lumen within the thickened intima.[10] The wealth of studies in humans and experimental animal models demonstrating a direct association between diets rich in cholesterol and/or saturated fats, elevations in plasma LDL levels, and accelerated atherosclerosis have established high plasma cholesterol, specifically elevated plasma LDL concentration, as a major risk factor for atherosclerosis and its clinical sequelae, myocardial infarction and stroke.

Another event believed to play a critical role in atherogenesis is the binding of blood monocytes to the endothelial lining at specific arterial sites and the subsequent diapedesis of these monocytes into the thickened intima to become tissue macrophages.[11] In experimental animals fed cholesterol early lesion development is preceded by an abundance of mononuclear cells, which have been identified as chiefly monocyte-derived macrophages.[11] More than a century ago, Virchow[5] proposed that there was an inflammatory component to the atherosclerotic process that was responsible for the recruitment of white blood cells into the intima.

The second critical event after monocyte infiltration is the engorgement of these cells with lipid to become the foam cells characteristic of the early fatty-streak lesion.[2] Many believe the mechanism of foam cell formation involves the accumulation of lipid from interstitial LDL. LDL oxidation[12,13] and LDL associated with proteoglycans[14] are among the proposed ways in which LDL might be altered to become a substrate for uptake by macrophages. Whether or not removal by macrophages of accumulated LDL or other forms of lipid is beneficial may depend on the degree of cholesterol accumulation that has occurred. One could envisage that if the accumulation of cholesterol in the form of LDL is minor, the macrophage could readily remove this material, playing a role analogous to removing foreign material such as bacteria from a tissue. One can further speculate that in Western societies in which diet-induced levels of plasma LDL are high and intimal LDL is proportionately elevated, the removal mechanism is overloaded. Since a characteristic of the transition from the "benign" fatty streak (which does not always develop into advanced lesions) to the clinically significant fibrous plaque is the lysis of many of these foam cells and the deposition of the intracellular cholesteryl ester droplets into the extracellular space, the hypothesized "overloading of the system" may be a critical event.

Hemodynamic hypothesis

Fatty streaks and fibrous plaques develop at specific anatomic sites of the vasculature. Likewise, the binding of blood monocytes to endothelium and the accumulation of LDL in the thickened intima of normal arteries are found to be focal. A theory of atherogenesis that attempts to explain the focal nature of the atherosclerotic process is the hemodynamic theory proposed in the 1950s by several investigators. It was theorized that hydrostatic and shear forces were primarily responsible for lesion development. The fact that atherosclerosis is accelerated in patients with hypertension suggests a role for increased hydrostatic pressure in vascular disease. In addition, altered and/or fluctuating shear, including both turbulent flow and relatively stagnant flow, was shown as present at anatomic sites at which lesions preferentially develop such as at arterial branching sites. The association between altered shear forces and preferential lesion development is widely accepted as important in understanding lesion development. It is still not known how altered shear actually affects atherogenesis. Hemodynamics may change endothelial permeability to LDL or induce endothelial binding sites for monocyte adhesion, or it may alter other vascular processes.[15]

Fibrin incrustation hypothesis

In the nineteenth century Rokitansky proposed the fibrin incrustation theory of atherosclerosis to explain the growth of atherosclerotic lesions. The theory stated that fibrinogen is converted to fibrin on the intimal surface of large arteries to form a thrombus. The thrombus then becomes organized and tissuelike. In the fifties Duguid and his colleagues continued to be strong proponents of this theory.[16] Duguid and others have demonstrated that thrombi on the surface of atherosclerotic lesions can become incorporated into the vessel wall over time and thereby increase the size of the lesion.[16] However, these are events that occur at late stages in the development of advanced, complicated lesions. The data supporting this mechanism as an initial event in atherogenesis are weak. The amount of cholesterol derived from the platelets and plasma present in an organized thrombus is far too small to explain the accumulation of cholesterol usually seen in an atherosclerotic plaque. The frequently seen layered appearance of advanced plaques in cross section is more likely attributable to transient periods of rapid intimal smooth muscle cell hyperplasia and connective tissue deposition rather than to the organization of thrombi.

Although the incrustation theory has not received much support in recent years, it has focused attention on the important role of the arterial endothelium in coagulation and thrombotic events. Recent studies have demonstrated an intricate balance between the production by endothelium of pro- and anti-coagulation factors, which are discussed below. Thus, although mural thrombus formation, its organization, and its incorporation into the intima of large arteries are not believed initial events in atherogenesis, they can occur as late and clinically significant events.

Nonspecific mesenchymal hypothesis

Atherosclerosis consists of both degenerative and regenerative events. Most of the steps involved with cholesterol accumulation can be considered part of the degenerative process. The two major regenerative events in atherogenesis are the proliferation of smooth muscle cells in the tunica intima and the subsequent production by these cells of connective tissue elements. Chief among these elements are proteoglycans, considered by some to be responsible for the trapping of infiltrated LDL,[14] and collagen, which represents the major space-filling component of an advanced atherosclerotic lesion. Hauss, Junge-Hulsing, and Hollanden[17] proposed that the migration of smooth muscle cells (mesenchymal cells) from the tunica media to the tunica intima, their proliferation, and the production of connective tissue comprised a nonspecific reaction of the artery wall to a wide array of irritating stimuli, hence the name nonspecific mesenchymal theory of atherogenesis. Many of the reactions were thought parallel, if not identical, to wound healing. This theory attempted to explain why physical factors such as shear stress and chemical factors such as vasoactive agents appeared to induce the same sequence of events in the vessel wall.

Response-to-injury hypothesis

During the past two decades much has been learned about how cells respond to various stimuli. In particular, a plethora of factors secreted by cells (cytokines) that dramatically affect the function of neighboring cells has been identified. This has led to a refinement of the earlier nonspecific mesenchymal theory to one in which specific factors are proposed as responsible for the wound-healing reactions. In the early seventies Ross and Glomset[18] proposed the response-to-injury theory of atherogenesis. Originally, they proposed that different forms of injury (physical or chemical) induced frank denudation of the endothelial lining, leading to platelet adherence to the denuded areas of the arterial intima. Subsequent release of a growth factor, termed *platelet-derived growth factor* (PDGF), triggered the movement of smooth muscle cells from the media to the intima and their subsequent proliferation. This theory may be correct in specific situations in which the endothelium has been mechanically removed such as in balloon catheter injuries (experimental or during percutaneous transluminal coronary or peripheral artery angioplasty), or it may apply in later stages of lesion development. However, during the early stages endothelial denudation is considered a rare event as is discussed in the next section. More recent versions of the response-to-injury hypothesis have stressed the role of paracrine, or local, cell–derived factors provoked by vascular injury in the development of the atherosclerotic plaque.[19]

SEQUENCE OF EVENTS IN THE DEVELOPMENT OF THE ATHEROSCLEROTIC PLAQUE

Endothelial cell activation and the initiation of atherogenesis

The response-to-injury hypothesis has influenced the recent thoughts and experimental directions of vascular cell biologists and pathologists interested in atherogenesis. In the original model[18] described above the sole "function" of the endothelial cell in the disease process was its susceptibility to injury, leading to cell death and sloughing. Investigations in many laboratories during the past decade have failed to produce evidence that frank denudation of endothelium occurs as an early event in atherogenesis. Only in advanced atherosclerotic plaques have regions of vessel wall lacking intact endothelium been identified morphologically. The presence of an intact endothelium over lesion-prone areas of artery suggests the possibility of an active role for the endothelial cell in atherogenesis. Injury to the endothelium may shorten the endothelial cell's lifetime and cause increased endothelial cell turnover in specific regions of the artery. This injury may, in turn, lead to the expression of genes that are suppressed under physiologic rather than pathologic conditions. An activated state of an endothelial cell may exist in which these cells (1) express binding sites for monocytes and perhaps secrete monocyte activators, (2) secrete oxygen-free radicals that can modify nearby LDL, and (3) synthesize and secrete a PDGF-like protein and/or other mitogens and chemoattractants for medial smooth muscle cells.

Current knowledge about the identity of the triggering agent(s) that causes endothelial cell injury or activation in vivo is extremely limited. Multiple candidates have been under study for years, including hemodynamic factors, chemical toxicity (cholesterol or its oxidized derivatives), immunologic injury (immune complexes), viral infection, cigarette smoking, and indirect mediators such as tumor necrosis factor that are generated in the vessel wall in response to one of the above stimuli. In animal models a single intervention such as high dietary cholesterol generates a predictable atherosclerotic response in specific regions of the vasculature, but whether this is due directly to increased plasma cholesterol level or to a secondary initiating factor remains unknown.

Several functions of the normal healthy endothelium can be referred to as anti-atherogenic. The most noted of these functions is the ability of the endothelium to produce potent anticoagulant substances such as the prostanoid, prostacyclin. Second, it has been demonstrated in cell culture experiments that under certain conditions the endothelial cell produces molecules that inhibit the proliferation of smooth muscle cells. Third, the endothelium represents a permeability barrier and a signal transducer responding to substances in the serum so that the milieu of the intimal and medial cells can be affected directly by substances transported or generated by the endothelium. The endothelial cell functions that help maintain vessel wall homeostasis may be altered in the initiating steps of atherogenesis.

The activated endothelium may represent a procoagulant rather than anticoagulant surface. It has been demonstrated in cell culture that endothelial cells respond to such activators as the cytokine interleukin-1 or the bacterial wall product lipopolysaccharide by expressing high levels of procoagulant activity. Whether such an event occurs in early atherogenesis is not known; however, the conversion of the endothelium to a thrombogenic surface could lead to the sequelae of the response-to-injury hypothesis even in the absence of frank denudation of endothelial cell. The same sequelae would occur if the endothelial cell were triggered to produce smooth muscle cell growth factors rather than growth inhibitors. This possibility is discussed later in this chapter.

Adhesion of monocytes to the endothelium

The monocyte-derived macrophage has been implicated as a participant in several aspects of atherosclerotic plaque development. Macrophages evolve into foam cells through unregulated ingestion of lipid. They also have the capacity to produce growth factor(s) for vascular smooth muscle cells to generate cytotoxic factors for neighboring cells, leading to necrosis. The initial event in the interaction of a monocyte with the vessel wall is its attachment to the endothelium. The adherence of mononuclear cells to the endothelial cells of large vessels during the early stages of experimentally induced atherosclerosis has been observed in multiple animal models.[11,20] In each of these systems a distinctly focal adhesion of monocytes was observed as an early event after cholesterol feeding. The mechanism by which hypercholesterolemia causes increased adherence of monocytes to the endothelium and the reason why monocytes adhere to specific regions of the vessel wall remain unknown.

The cell surface molecules involved in the binding of leukocytes to the endothelium have been the object of much recent study, although more progress has been made in characterizing neutrophil- and lymphocyte-binding proteins than monocyte-binding proteins. Several leukocyte surface proteins have been identified that appear to mediate adherence to endothelium.[21] The literature on endothelial cell proteins involved in leukocyte adhesion is much less extensive. Bevilacqua et al[22] have used two monoclonal antibodies to identify a transiently expressed surface protein, endothelial-leukocyte adhesion molecule (ELAM 1), on endothelial cells stimulated with interleukin-1 or tumor necrosis factor. This cell surface antigen, which plays a role in neutrophil-endothelium recognition and possibly monocyte-endothelial cell binding, has been cloned and sequenced and apparently is a member of a family of cell surface molecules that are expressed during inflammation.

Experiments with cultured endothelial cells have led to several conclusions about monocyte adhesion that appear applicable to multiple species and to multiple vascular beds. First, the expression of monocyte-binding sites on the endothelial cell surface is low under "control" or "physiologic" conditions, that is, when the endothelial cells are confluent, quiescent, and unstimulated by exogenous agents. Second, when treated with specific exogenous agents or when stimulated to migrate and divide in response to an in vitro "wound," endothelial cells exhibit a greatly increased ability to bind monocytes. Third, although the above-mentioned stimulators also induce increased neutrophil adhesion to endothelial cells, the cell surface binding sites on the endothelial cells apparently are specific for one or the other of these two leukocytes.[23] Thus monocyte and neutrophil adhesion to endothelial cells may be regulated through distinct pathways and induced differentially by certain as yet undefined exogenous agents. Many important questions remain unanswered regarding the mechanism of specific, transient adhesion of blood-borne monocytes to the endothelium in vivo. Further investigation is required to define the intracellular signalling pathways and gene expression that are necessary for the appearance of monocyte-binding sites on the endothelial cell surface.

Lipoprotein involvement in atherogenesis

Much of the research pertaining to atherosclerosis and much of the focus in the treatment of atherosclerotic patients are related to the known link between the development of the disease and plasma concentrations of cholesterol or certain of the lipoproteins.[24-30] Total plasma cholesterol is related closely enough to coronary disease in humans that epidemiologic studies predict a monotonic increase in the risk of coronary events with increases in total plasma cholesterol above approximately 170 to 200 mg/dl. This, of course, is an oversimplification since the LDL cholesterol level is a very strong predictor of atherosclerosis, whereas the high density lipoprotein (HDL) cholesterol level is an inverse correlate of the disease. It is therefore useful to review briefly the lipoprotein categories. The roles they are believed to play in vascular diseases are related to their composition and, thereby, their effects on cells and tissues.[31]

The major classes of plasma lipoproteins are chylomicrons, very low density lipoprotein (VLDL), LDL, intermediate density lipoprotein (IDL), and HDL. The chylomicrons are produced in gut epithelial cells and traverse the mesenteric lymph to the thoracic duct where they enter the bloodstream. The chylomicron core consists chiefly of triglycerides and secondarily of cholesteryl esters, which are synthesized by the epithelium from dietary fatty acids and cholesterol. Once in the bloodstream, chylomicrons are referred to as chylomicron remnants since their catabolism begins immediately by the action of endothelium-associated lipoprotein lipase, which breaks down the triglycerides. The liberated fatty acids are resynthesized to triglycerides in adipose tissue for storage. The remnant is ultimately removed from the bloodstream through specific receptors on hepatic cells. In healthy humans chylomicrons are cleared from the bloodstream within several hours after a fatty meal and are not appreciably present in the plasma after 12 hours of fasting. VLDL is synthesized by the liver and its principal function is the transport of cholesterol and triglycerides from the liver to other tissues, including adipose tissue. Although smaller than chylomicrons, VLDL has a similar composition with a predominance of triglyceride. Smaller yet, and with less triglyceride, is LDL, which can be considered the final metabolic breakdown product of the VLDL remnant. In healthy humans LDL carries most of the cholesterol present in fasting plasma. Approximately 70% of LDL cholesterol is carried in esterified form; the balance is free cholesterol. Twenty percent of the mass of this lipoprotein particle is a single protein, apolipoprotein B.

HDL has the highest proportion of protein comprising its mass. The protein component is a composite of several apolipoproteins, the major ones of which are designated apolipoproteins A-1 and A-2. The various apolipoproteins of HDL influence specific metabolic activities, for example, apolipoprotein A-2 plays a regulatory role in the action of hepatic lipase. HDL is believed to function in "reverse cholesterol transport," the movement of cholesterol from peripheral tissues to the liver. Consistent with such a beneficial role are epidemiologic data that show a correlation between less risk of atherosclerosis and the concentration of HDL cholesterol in plasma. HDL is synthesized in the liver and in gut epithelium and is ultimately removed from the circulation by the liver.

Animal studies of dietary-induced elevations in lipoproteins that lead to the development of atherosclerosis, the epidemiologic data in humans, and the studies showing atherosclerosis regression in both humans and primates following chronic, substantial reductions in plasma cholesterol have led to the conclusion that lipoproteins can cause atherosclerosis. Identification of the mechanism(s) by which LDL or related lipoproteins can induce the documented cellular events that take place in the disease is lacking. Native, or "normal," LDL does not lead to foam cell formation when it is incubated with macrophages or vascular smooth muscle cells in cell culture, yet these two cell types are known to be the precursors of intimal foam cells in vivo. Typically, when animals are fed cholesterol, a distinct lipoprotein particle appears in plasma in concentrations related to the amount of cholesterol (and other fats) substituted in the diet. This lipoprotein is unlike the normally occurring lipoproteins and has been named β-VLDL since on electrophoresis of plasma proteins this particle migrates in the beta band along with LDL, yet it co-isolates with VLDL in the ultracentrifuge separation of plasma lipoproteins. β-VLDL can lead to cholesteryl ester accumulation in macrophages and is therefore considered an atherogenic particle; however, it is present in human plasma only in rare circumstances (type III hypercholesterolemia), and its presence certainly cannot explain the widespread incidence of this disease in humans in Western cultures.

It has been proposed that atherosclerosis is worsened by adverse interactions between arterial cells and lipoproteins after a modification of the lipoprotein.[12,13,19] The pathologic lipoprotein may be produced in a modified form as suggested by the demonstration that an LDL–related lipoprotein called Lp(a) exists in human plasma, and its concentration, in general, correlates, with atherosclerosis risk.[32] In addition, however, there are suggestions that normal LDL can be modified, for example, by oxidation caused by reactions with free radicals. Oxidation of LDL alters many cellular interactions with the lipoprotein, including causing an enhanced, unregulated uptake by macrophages.

In 1973 Drs. Michael S. Brown and Joseph L. Goldstein discovered the cellular receptor for LDL. They and others have since characterized the cellular pathway by which LDL can regulate cellular cholesterol metabolism through this receptor.[33] The interaction of LDL with its cellular receptor leads to the inhibition of cellular synthesis of cholesterol by the cholesterol that enters the cell on LDL. In addition, the cell becomes down regulated with respect to the expression of the receptor. The importance of these discoveries is far-reaching. Genetic defects in the receptor are now known to occur in humans in heterozygous and homozygous forms, with frequencies of approximately 1:500 and 1:1 million, respectively. Receptor defects result in the impaired removal of chylomicrons, VLDL, and LDL from plasma, allowing LDL cholesterol levels to increase. In general, heterozygotes have plasma-cholesterol concentrations of approximately two to four times normal and develop clinical atherosclerosis between ages 30 and 60; homozygotes have plasma-cholesterol levels six to 10 times normal and typically suffer myocardial infarction between the ages of 18 months and 25 years.

This fundamental work, which led to the award of the 1985 Nobel Prize in Medicine and Physiology to Drs. Brown and Goldstein, has furthered the knowledge of cholesterol regulation and lipoprotein metabolism. It has also led to new therapies for patients at risk for atherosclerosis, one of which, for example, lowers plasma cholesterol through suppression of HMG CoA reductase, the rate-limiting enzymatic step in cellular synthesis of cholesterol. Although their work revealed an important mechanism by which LDL can reach high plasma concentrations, it did not provide answers to questions relating to how these high LDL levels lead to atherosclerosis.

The LDL receptor is not the only binding site at which lipoproteins can interact with cells. Binding of HDL to specific plasma membrane sites has been documented and in part characterized. The binding of HDL to cultured cells can be increased by loading the cells with cholesterol. Under these circumstances the HDL, which is not internalized with its receptor, departs the cell surface after having removed some free cholesterol from the cell. The interaction of HDL with its receptor appears to stimulate the movement of cholesterol from internal pools to the plasma membrane.

A third class of lipoprotein receptor has been identified that is expressed on macrophages and endothelial cells but not on vascular smooth muscle cells.[34] This receptor recognizes certain forms of modified LDL and is referred to as either the scavenger receptor or the *acetyl-LDL receptor,* named after its recognition of LDL that has been chemically modified by acetylation. LDL modified chemically or by oxidation is recognized by this class of receptor, and the receptor-ligand interaction leads to the internalization and degradation of the altered lipoprotein. Unlike the LDL receptor activity, however, the cholesterol liberated intracellularly from the lipoprotein degradation does not result in down regulation of the receptor. Rather, excess cholesterol is esterified and accumulates in the macrophage. Numerous studies have focused on identifying the possible in vivo ligand of this interesting receptor class, and at least two have been proposed: malondialdehyde-modified LDL and oxidatively modified LDL. These are not mutually exclusive entities since malondialdehyde, in addition to being produced by stimulated platelets, is also one of hundreds of compounds produced during LDL oxidation.

In recent decades numerous studies of the pathology of arterial lesions of humans and of experimental animals have revealed that apolipoprotein B accumulates in very high concentrations in the interstitial spaces. Although the interstitial fluid and lymphatic concentrations of plasma proteins are generally estimated at 10% to 30% of their plasma concentrations, estimates of LDL concentrations in lesions, as calculated from immunochemical quantification of apolipoprotein B, rival or exceed those of plasma.[8,9] The localization of LDL as demonstrated by immunofluorescence studies is primarily in the intima among foam cells in fatty-streak lesions (Fig. 7-12), at the intimal-medial border in transitional lesions (e.g., fatty-streak to fibrous plaque [Fig. 7-13]), and in the necrotic core of advanced fibrous plaques (Fig. 7-14).

The interstitial intimal accumulation of plasma lipoproteins is the result of numerous processes, any of which may yet be shown to play an important controlling role. Mediating these processes are (1) the ability of the endothelium to regulate the traffic of these large plasma molecules; (2) the sieving properties of the internal elastic lamina, which separates the intimal, or disease-prone, part of the arterial wall from the media, which becomes involved in the later stages of the disease; (3) the capabilities for degradation of the lipoprotein by smooth muscle cells that may be residing in the intima; and (4) the capacity for binding of lipoprotein by extracellular connective tissue components. In the case of the accumulation of LDL a few comments pertinent to the relative roles of these processes can be made. The LDL concentration that maximally suppresses LDL receptor expression on these cells is approximately 25 μg LDL cholesterol/ml. In humans plasma LDL cholesterol is typically 900 μg/ml. Even if the normal, intimal interstitial concentration of LDL were 10% of that of plasma, it would be three to four times that necessary for LDL receptor down regulation. Thus removal and degradation of LDL locally by arterial smooth muscle cells in the intima may be quantitatively unimportant.

LDL is known to bind to certain connective tissue substances. Large proteoglycans of the interstitial space and their glycosaminoglycan subunits co-localize with LDL in the grossly normal intima and in fatty streaks (Figs. 7-15 and 7-16). They also bind LDL under conditions believed to pertain in vivo. In addition, both collagen and elastin bind LDL and certain lipids carried by LDL. Thus sequestration of certain lipoproteins by connective tissue may be an important contributor to the extracellular lipid accumulation of arterial lesions. In addition, certain of the complexes formed between lipoproteins and connective tissue proteins may be taken up by macrophages and may contribute to foam cell formation.

The role of endothelial permeability to LDL as it relates to the control of lipoprotein accumulation has been discussed earlier in this chapter; however, another barrier to macromolecular transport is the internal elastic lamina. Little is known about its capabilities in regulating the passage of lipoproteins through to the smooth muscle cell–rich media other than the observation that in early experimental atherosclerosis relatively little lipoprotein accumulates in the interstitial spaces of the media. The effects of high levels of intimal interstitial lipoprotein on the permeability prop-

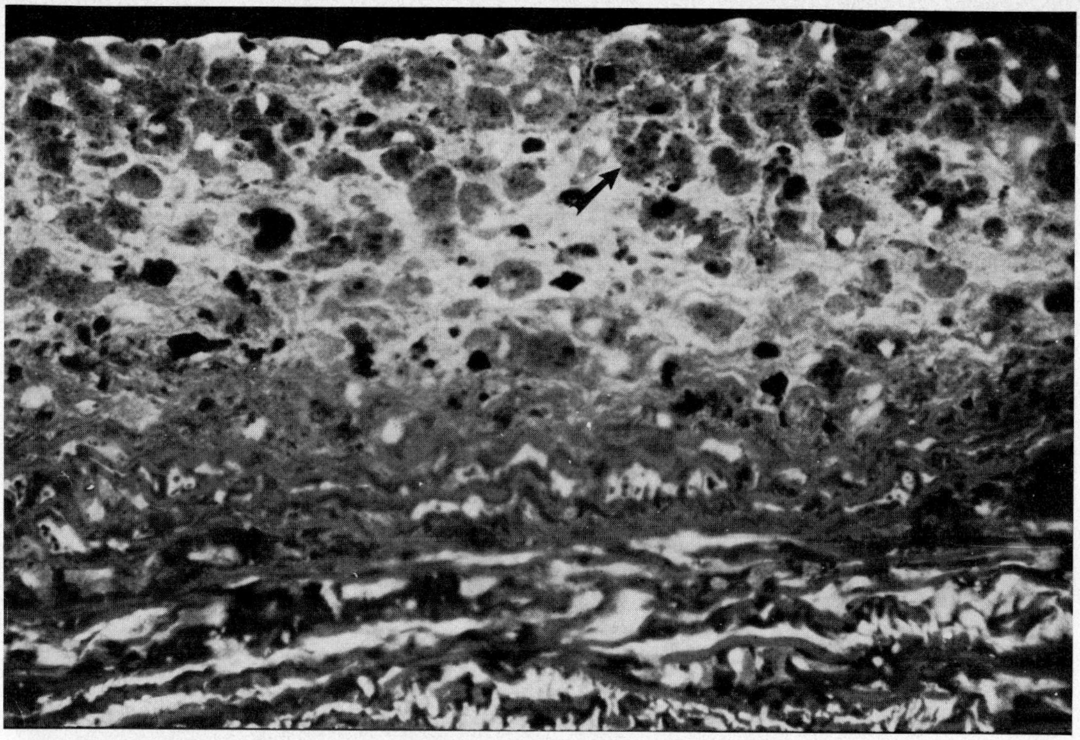

Fig. 7-12. Immunofluorescence localization of LDL *(white)* in cross section of a fatty streak from the aorta of a hypercholesterolemic swine. LDL can be seen in the spaces between foam cells *(arrow)*. Dark field microscopy has been used.

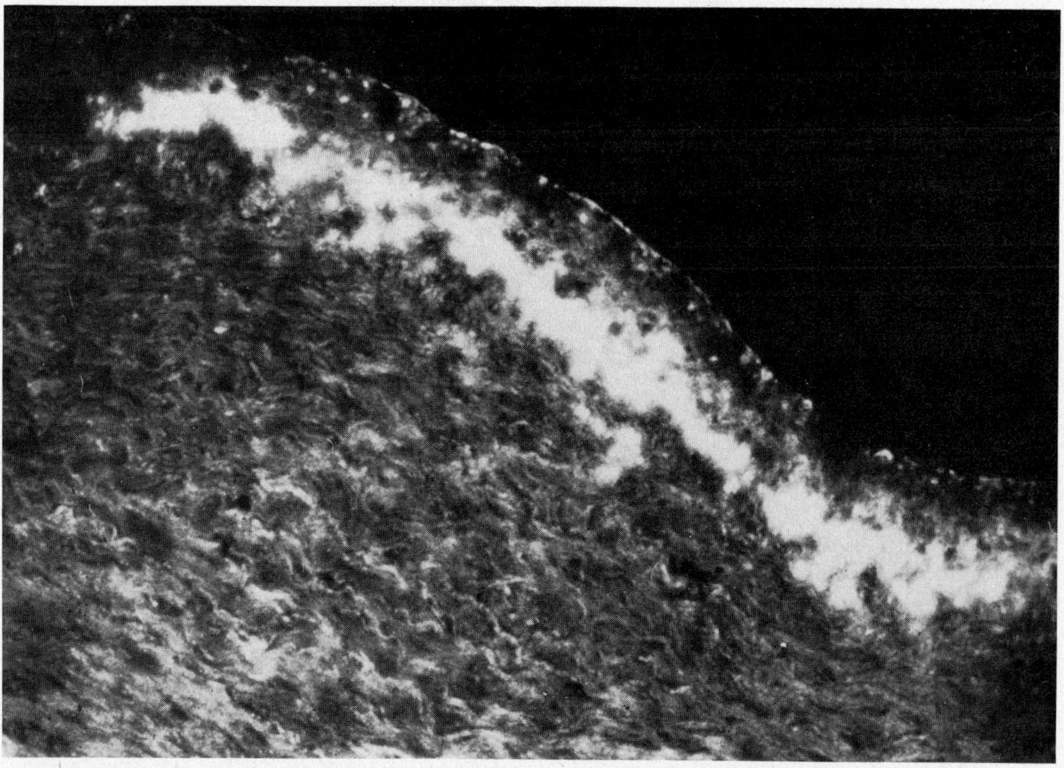

Fig. 7-13. Immunofluorescent staining of LDL *(white)* at the intimal-medial border in cross section of a coronary artery lesion from a hypercholesterolemic swine.

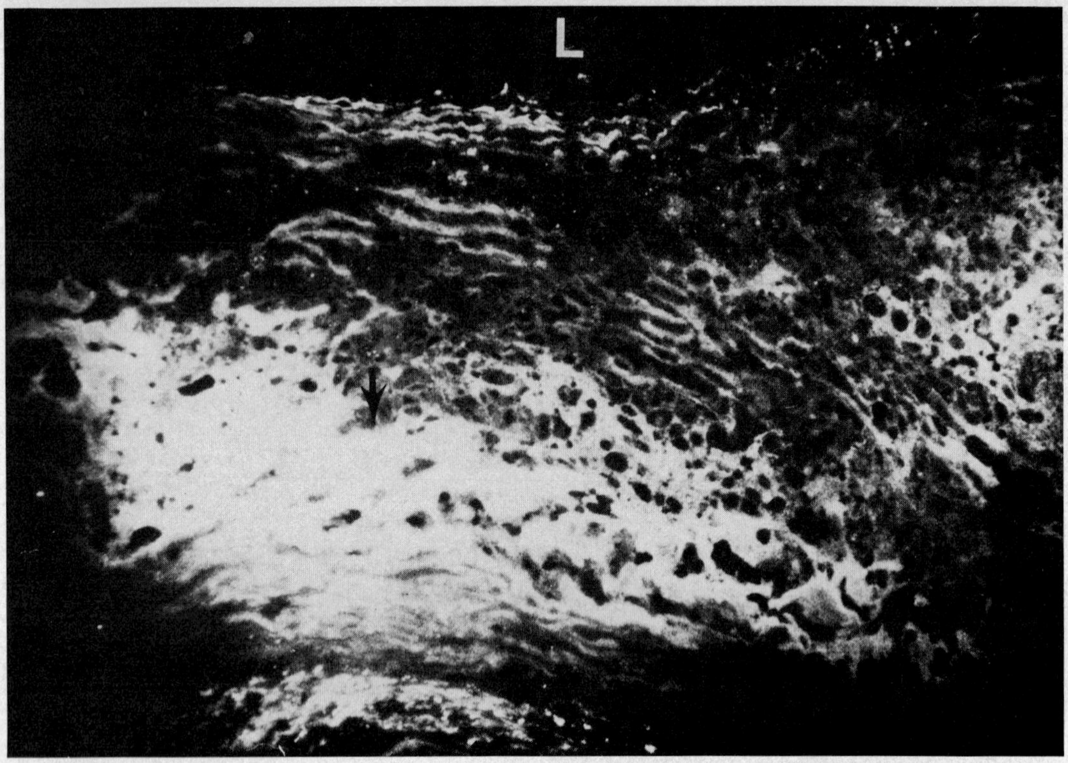

Fig. 7-14. Immunofluorescence localization of LDL *(white)*, primarily in the necrotic core *(arrow)* but focally in the fibrotic cap, of a fibrous plaque in a human coronary artery. *L*, lumen.

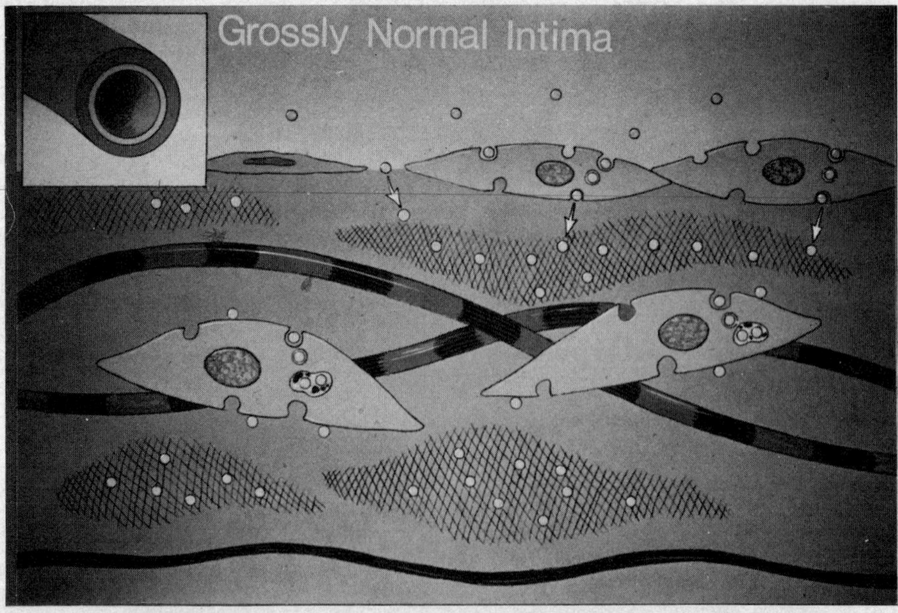

Fig. 7-15. Schematic representation of the deposition of LDL *(spheres)* in the grossly normal intima caused by trapping by glycosaminoglycans in intimal proteoglycans *(crosshatched area)*.

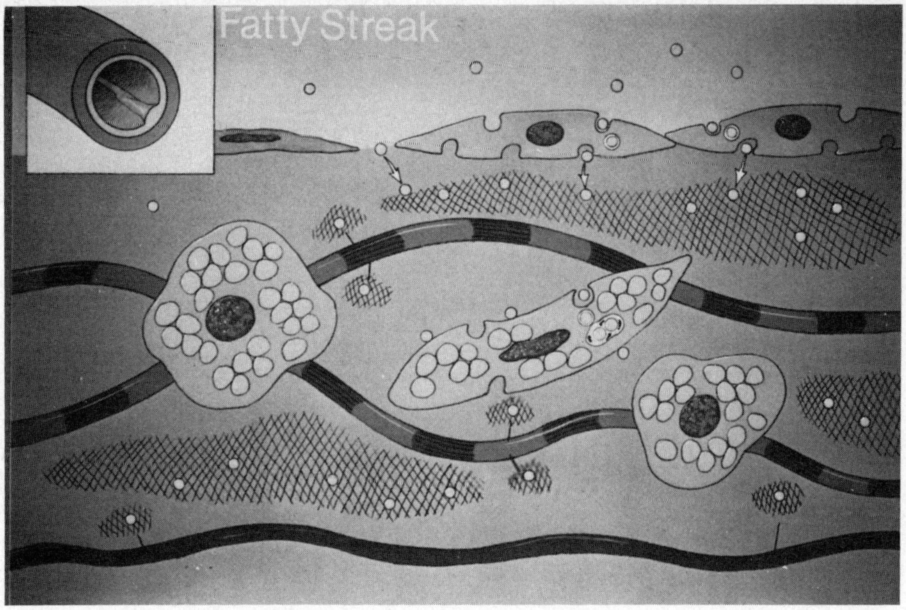

Fig. 7-16. Schematic representation of the deposition of LDL *(spheres)* in fatty-streak lesions. The lipid-laden cells (foam cells) are formed by the uptake of LDL accumulating in the extracellular space bound to proteoglycans *(crosshatched section)*.

erties of the internal elastic lamina are not known.

Despite the association between plasma LDL concentration and increased risk of atherosclerosis, the interactions of normal LDL, even in high concentrations, with various cells grown in culture apparently do not exhibit properties typically associated with atherosclerosis. For example, LDL does not lead to foam cell formation on incubation with macrophages, and it does not injure endothelium. On the other hand, certain forms of modified LDL, briefly mentioned previously, do in fact have these properties, leading to speculation that the involvement of LDL (or VLDL) in atherosclerosis is secondary to lipoprotein modification. Both acetylated LDL and malondialdehyde-modified LDL interact with the scavenger receptor on macrophages and lead to cholesterol ester accumulation similar to that believed to take place during foam cell formation. Although it is difficult to rationalize acetylation of LDL in vivo, malondialdehyde can be produced in vivo from polyunsaturated fatty acids (e.g., during platelet stimulation), leading to speculation that a malondialdehyde-modified form of LDL may be possible in vivo. In experimental atherosclerotic lesions antibodies recognizing malondialdehyde-linked protein have been shown to co-localize in part with antibodies recognizing LDL.

LDL modified by oxidation is a chemoattractant for monocytes, can injure endothelial cells, and is recognized by the scavenger receptor. Vascular cells in culture can oxidize LDL. This indirect evidence and the demonstration that antibodies recognize in lesions various lipid-oxidation products linked to LDL or other proteins have led to proposals that LDL oxidation may occur in vivo and worsen the course of atherosclerosis.

Another variant of LDL known to occur in humans that has been studied in relationship to atherosclerosis is Lp(a). Lp(a) is a macromolecular complex of LDL with apolipoprotein (a), a protein structurally homologous to plasminogen. Plasminogen is a naturally occurring serine protease that is a component of the body's fibrinolytic system; however, unlike plasminogen, apolipoprotein (a) cannot be converted to an active protease form. A number of studies have linked plasma levels of Lp(a) to premature coronary disease in humans. Coupled with high plasma LDL concentrations, Lp(a) increases atherosclerosis risk to several times that predicted for high LDL alone. This has led to speculation that Lp(a) and the genetic aberration contributing to its production can hasten the development of arterial lesions. The mechanism by which this modified lipoprotein may be involved in the disease is not known.

That lipoproteins can play a causal role in atherosclerosis is no longer considered in doubt by the vast majority of physicians and scientists worldwide. The mechanisms by which lipoproteins interact with cells to injure them or disturb their metabolism and thereby lead to fatty-streak formation and other complications are only poorly understood. Research focusing on the interactions between vascular cells and lipoproteins suggests that certain steps in the mechanisms of these interactions offer opportunities to intervene in the processes that lead to vascular pathology.

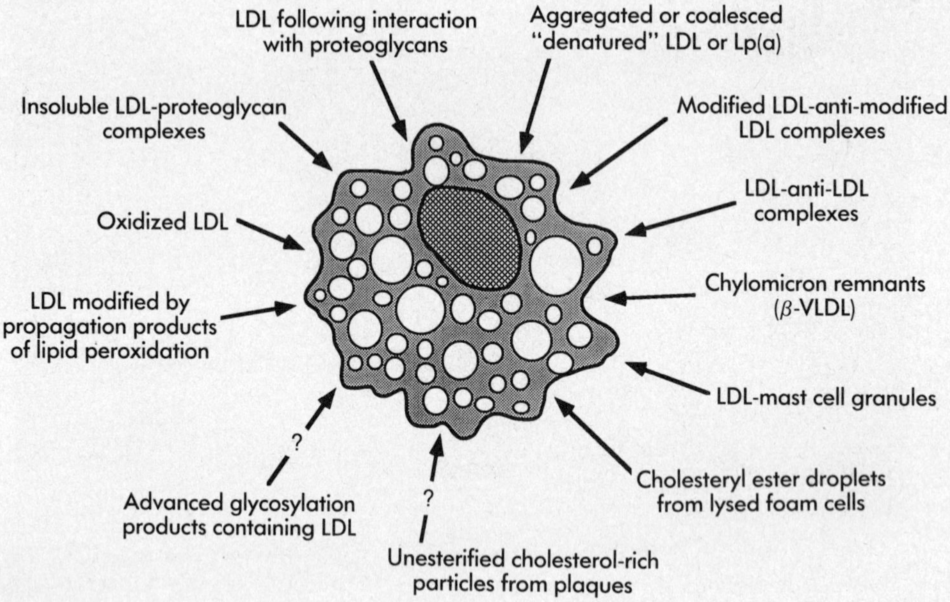

Fig. 7-17. Schematic representation of the large number of cholesterol-rich substrates that can be taken up by tissue macrophages, leading to the formation of foam cells.

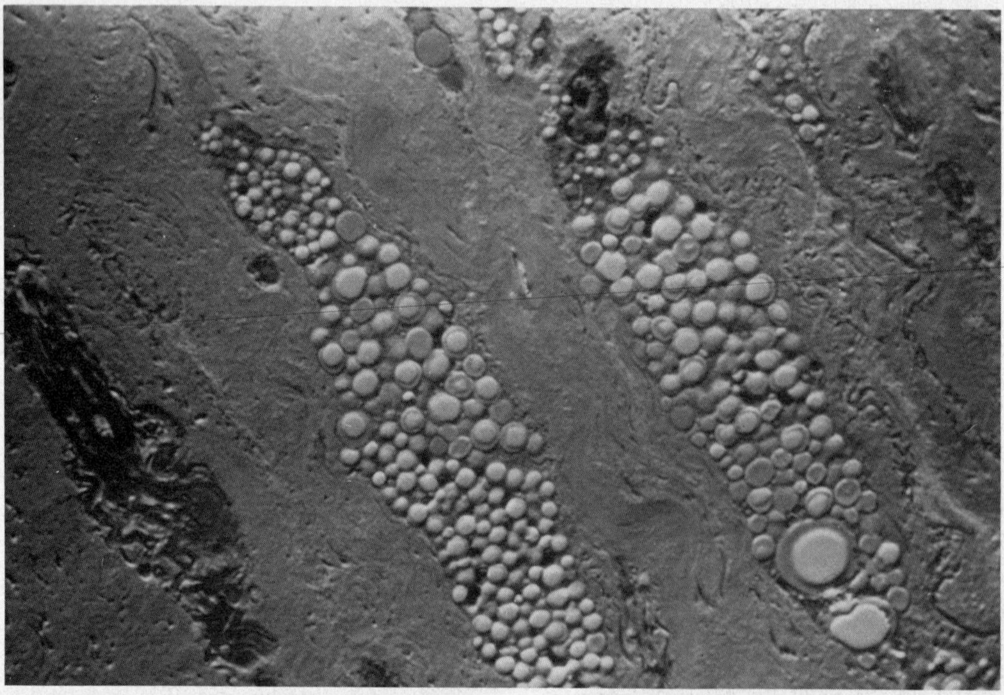

Fig. 7-18. Light micrograph of cross section of a fatty streak in a human cerebral artery, illustrating two spindle-shaped, lipid-laden foam cells believed derived from smooth muscle cells. Interference contrast microscopy was used.

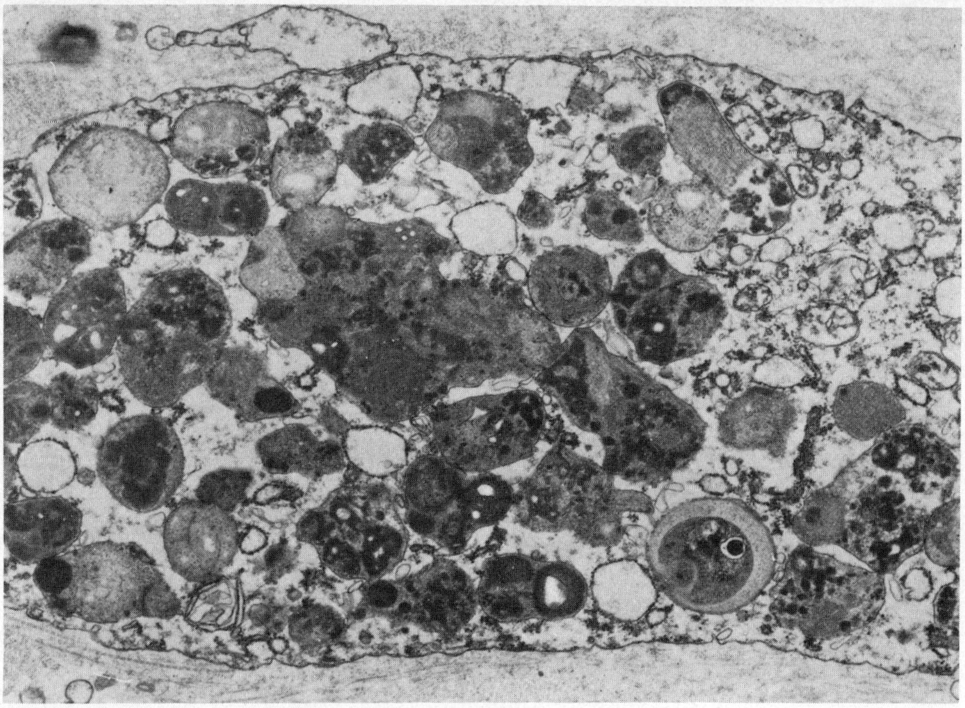

Fig. 7-19. Electron micrograph of a foam cell, showing numerous lipid inclusions of different densities.

Evolution of the fatty streak lesion—foam cell development

The foam cell is characteristic of the early fatty-streak lesion in man. Most of the foam cells are derived from tissue monocyte-macrophages[11] as a result of avid uptake of modified LDL that has accumulated in the interstitial space of the grossly normal intima of large arteries. Some of the mechanisms believed responsible for lipid loading of cells in these early lesions are discussed in this section. Since many of the mechanisms are currently under investigation, they must be considered speculative.

Fig. 7-17 illustrates the myriad of cholesterol-rich substrates that induce lipid loading of macrophages in cell culture. This mechanism may also be responsible for lipid loading of smooth muscle cells (Fig. 7-18). As observed by electron microscopy, lipid-laden cells in lesions contain a heterogeneous array of electron-dense inclusions believed to represent internalized lipoproteins at various stages of processing (Fig. 7-19).

As discussed in the previous section, LDL modification (e.g., by oxidation) may lead to enhanced recognition of the lipoprotein by the scavenger receptor on macrophages. Oxidation may also result in aggregation of LDL.[35] The aggregates that are formed are avidly taken up by macrophages in culture by a process called phagocytosis in which extensions of the cell membrane surround the aggregates and engulf them. In this manner large amounts of the modified LDL can be taken up by cells in a short time. This mechanism also leads to lipid loading of macrophages since it, too, is not regulated by intracellular cholesterol. Consistent with this concept, some of the LDL contained in atherosclerotic lesions is recognized by scavenger receptors on macrophages, and some is aggregated and could be internalized by phagocytosis (Fig. 7-20).

LDL forms soluble and insoluble complexes with glycosaminoglycans contained within proteoglycans extracted from human aortic intima from both grossly normal sites and atherosclerotic lesions.[14] Such complexes are avidly taken up by macrophages in culture. The mechanism of macrophage uptake of these insoluble complexes apparently is the same as for aggregated LDL after oxidation (i.e., by phagocytosis). The previously mentioned lipoprotein, Lp(a), also accumulates in human atherosclerotic lesions. It, too, forms insoluble complexes in vitro with arterial proteoglycans, and these complexes are avidly phagocytosed by macrophages in culture. This may explain why Lp(a) is considered an independent risk factor for atherosclerosis.

Two major forms of cholesterol are found in the extracellular space of atherosclerotic lesions in addition to that found on lipoproteins. One is the cholesteryl ester–rich droplets believed derived from lysed foam cells and therefore rich in cholesteryl oleate. The other is a particle rich

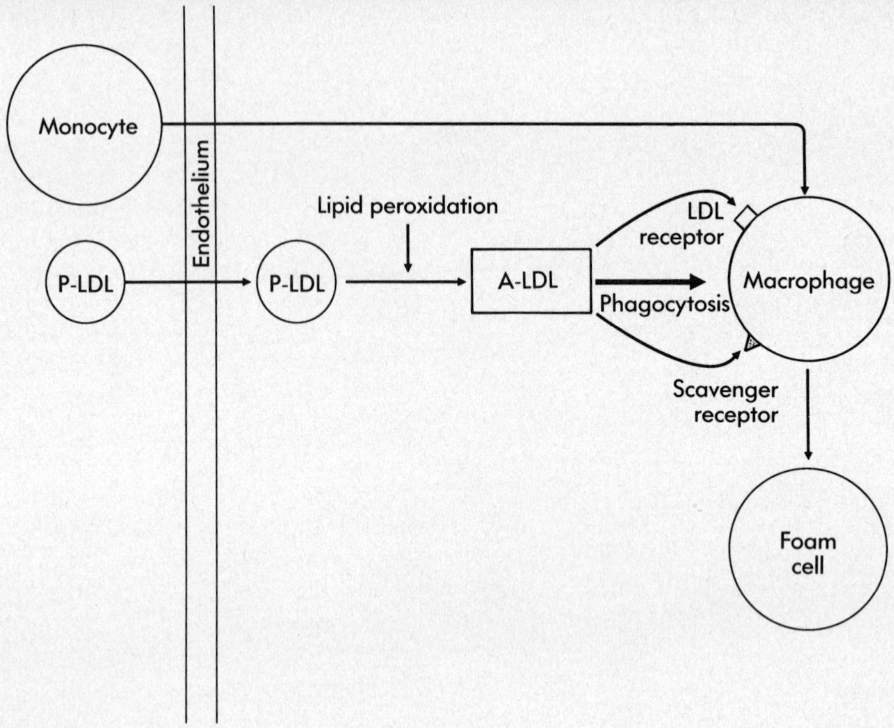

Fig. 7-20. Depiction of one mechanism by which plasma LDL *(P-LDL)* that accumulates in atherosclerotic lesions may become modified, normally by lipid peroxidation. We call this modified form of LDL, *A-LDL*. This modification in turn can lead to enhanced uptake of A-LDL by macrophages, resulting in foam cell formation (e.g., by phagocytosis or uptake through the scavenger receptor).

in both free cholesterol and cholesteryl linoleates believed derived directly from LDL without any intracellular processing. The exact etiology of this particle is not certain, but it could be derived from modification of LDL by specific lipolytic enzymes in the extracellular space that could hydrolyze the LDL cholesteryl esters to form a particle rich in unesterified cholesterol. Recent data suggest that both types of particles can be internalized by macrophages, again contributing to the lipid loading of these cells. Uptake of cell debris (e.g., cell membranes) by macrophages may also contribute. It is likely that these latter mechanisms play a greater role in the development of advanced atherosclerotic lesions from a fatty streak. Fig. 7-20 schematically illustrates some of the mechanisms that have been proposed by which macrophages become lipid laden.

Although most foam cells in early fatty-streak lesions are presumed to represent monocyte-macrophages, in somewhat more advanced lesions vascular smooth muscle cells also become lipid laden (see Fig. 7-18). The mechanisms by which smooth muscle cells become lipid laden is still not clear in that, in contrast to macrophages, smooth muscle cells do not express scavenger receptors and they are not generally considered phagocytes. However, recent studies have demonstrated that smooth muscle cells in culture avidly take up lipid droplets derived from lysed, lipid-laden macrophages, suggesting that phagocytosis of cell debris by smooth muscle cells may be a mechanism by which smooth muscle cells become foam cells.[36]

Intimal hyperplasia of smooth muscle cells

Smooth muscle cells are not homogeneously distributed through the distinct layers of the normal and atherosclerotic arteries. In the healthy artery smooth muscle cells are absent in the outermost, adventitial layer (containing primarily fibroblasts and connective tissue) but are the major cellular component of the medial layer. Their relative abundance in the media does not significantly change during development. Only a few smooth muscle cells are present in the intimal layer of the infant artery, but a gradual accumulation of intimal cells occurs during normal development. In the diseased artery smooth muscle cells comprise a significant component of the early fatty-streak lesion (although perhaps secondary to macrophages), but they are the predominant cellular component of the fibrotic plaque (see Fig. 7-6).

Growth factors (or mitogens) are hormonelike proteins that bind to specific receptors on target cells, initiating a cascade of events that result in cell replication. Cultured smooth muscle cells possess receptors for, and are stimulated to divide by, PDGF. In addition, PDGF can act as a chemoattractant for smooth muscle cells, and a scenario can easily be imagined in which arterial cells situated near the lumen of the vessel secrete growth factors into the media, thereby stimulating both migration of smooth muscle cells into the intima and proliferation of intimal cells. During the last decade attention has been focused both on the function of PDGF and on possible sources of PDGF in the arterial wall. Much of the understanding of the regulation of production of PDGF from vascular cells is derived from in vitro studies. The endothelial cell was the first vascular cell (other than the platelet) shown to secrete PDGF.[37] Endothelial cells cultured from all major vessels and from all species examined to date secrete PDGF into their medium. The process is constitutive, that is, exogenous stimulation of the cells is not required; however, there is evidence that factors related to arterial injury further stimulate the release of the growth factor. Certain members of the coagulation cascade, including thrombin and factor Xa, increase the rate of synthesis of PDGF by cultured endothelial cells by up to tenfold. In addition, several agents that mortally injure cultured bovine aortic endothelial cells, including bacterial lipopolysaccharide, cause the release of a large burst of PDGF, presumably from dying cells.

Evidence that endothelial cells are involved in smooth muscle cell proliferation in vivo is largely circumstantial. Intimal proliferation takes place even in the presence of an intact endothelium, suggesting that exogenous factors such as platelet products may not be required. Furthermore, intimal hyperplasia in many circumstances correlates with regions of endothelialization, for example, at the anastomoses of synthetic vascular grafts. Direct in vivo measurements of growth factor production by endothelial cells or other vascular cells are not easily accomplished because of technical problems. However, the transcriptional activity of the genes encoding growth factors can be measured in freshly isolated tissue. Barrett et al[38] have shown that the expression of PDGF B-chain mRNA (one of the two polypeptides forming human PDGF) was at least tenfold lower in endothelium freshly scraped from blood vessels than in the comparable cultured endothelial cell. Furthermore, Barrett and Benditt[39] have shown that PDGF B-chain mRNA was present in fivefold greater amounts in human carotid artery lesions than in a healthy artery (although the responsible cell type was not specifically identified). These results raise the possibility that endothelial cells may be "activated," either as a response to pathologic stimuli in vivo or simply by the transition from the physiologic state in vivo to the foreign in vitro condition. If this is the case, studies of the conditions that inactivate cultured endothelial cells (i.e., lead to the reduction of growth factor production) may give insights into the physiologic conditions required to maintain endothelial cells in the inactive state. Certain modified lipoproteins, including LDL that has been modified by oxidation, reduce the rate of synthesis of PDGF by cultured endothelial cells by at least 70%, whereas unaltered LDL does not decrease PDGF production.[40]

Vascular cells other than endothelial cells may also synthesize and secrete growth factors into the arterial wall. Several laboratories have shown that human peripheral blood monocytes, activated in vitro by bacterial lipopolysaccharide or by immune complexes, secrete PDGF. In addition, smooth muscle cells themselves, under certain circumstances, secrete growth factors. Smooth muscle cells cultured from the aorta of rat pups secrete significantly more PDGF than smooth muscle cells isolated from adult rats, suggesting that a normal function of PDGF may be related to blood vessel development. (Cultured smooth muscle cells derived from the intima of mechanically injured rat arteries also produce more PDGF than medial smooth muscle cells from uninjured arteries.) This concept is supported by a study reported by Wilcox et al[41] in which the method of in situ hybridization histochemistry is used to determine the in vivo location and identity of cells in atherosclerotic lesions expressing the genes for the A chain and the B chain of PDGF. Endothelial cells and intimal smooth muscle cells express both gene transcripts, but medial smooth muscle cells and macrophages show little of either. These results suggest that smooth muscle cell–derived growth factors may stimulate their own growth in an autocrine fashion similar to the mechanism postulated for the uncontrolled cell proliferation of certain tumors.

Several parallels exist between atherosclerotic lesions and tumors. The B chain of human PDGF is homologous to the protein product of the v-*sis* oncogene, a tumor-causing gene derived from the simian sarcoma virus. Furthermore, many transformed cells (tumor forming) in culture express the genes for one or both of the PDGF chains and also secrete PDGF into their medium. Finally, the morphologic similarity of atherosclerotic lesions to uterine smooth muscle tumors led Benditt and Benditt[42] to propose that their underlying causes are also related. According to their "monoclonal" hypothesis, atherosclerotic lesions are derived from a single or, at most, a few mutated smooth muscle cells that, like tumor cells, proliferate in an unregulated fashion. Evidence supporting this hypothesis is found in the lesions of individuals who are heterozygous for both allogenic forms of glucose 6-phosphate dehydrogenase, in which only one allele is found in each lesion. This hypothesis, if correct, does not necessarily exclude a role for vessel injury or for growth factor secretion by nearby cells, but it does specify a distinct smooth muscle cell alteration as a critical event in the formation of atherosclerotic lesions.

Certainly other factors besides PDGF contribute to the proliferation of arterial smooth muscle cells. Other growth factors may be involved, including fibroblast growth factors, transforming growth factors (which, depending on the target cell and various conditions, may stimulate or inhibit cell proliferation), and macrophage-derived cytokines. The physical structure and chemical composition of the extracellular matrix are known to regulate smooth muscle cells growth in vitro and are likely to play a key role in the vessel wall as well. Finally, the lipids present in the extracellular environment are likely to influence smooth muscle cells' function and growth rate.

Identifying inhibitors of smooth muscle cell proliferation is of considerable importance considering the possible therapeutic avenues such molecules could open. The structure of these inhibitors may shed light on the underlying mechanisms regulating smooth muscle cell growth in the vessel wall. Castellot et al[43] have reported that cultured endothelial cells produce and secrete a heparin-like molecule that inhibits smooth muscle cell proliferation in vitro. Other investigators have subsequently shown that heparin infusion inhibits the proliferative response of smooth muscle cells to balloon injury of the rat carotid. Recent studies have suggested that there may be therapeutically useful, nonanticoagulant fractions of heparin that inhibit smooth muscle cell growth in this model. Powell et al[44] have shown that cilazapril and other angiotensin-coverting enzyme inhibitors reduce intimal thickening in rat carotid arteries subject to balloon catheterization, suggesting an alternate therapeutic approach. Another potential inhibitor of arterial smooth muscle cell proliferation is the omega-3–rich lipids in fish oil. The cardiovascular benefits of fish and fish oils are suggested from numerous epidemiologic studies involving Greenland Eskimos and other fish-eating populations. These studies in humans have been supported by studies in animal models that showed that fish oils reduce intimal thickening in rhesus monkeys, in hyperlipidemic swine, and in vein grafts implanted into dogs. The mechanism of action of fish oils is not known, but effects on lipid lowering (especially triglycerides) and on platelet function have been reported. A recent report shows that fish oils inhibit the production of PDGF by vascular endothelial cells and suggests that this may account for the decreased hyperplasia reported by others.[45]

Synthesis and composition of the extracellular matrix in atherosclerotic lesion formation

One of the hallmarks of atherosclerosis is the gradual accumulation of an elaborate extracellular matrix in the arterial intima. This material, consisting mainly of collagen, glycoproteins, and proteoglycans, is synthesized by cells residing in the thickened intimal layer of the atherosclerotic vessel. Although the accumulation of collagen is generally regarded as a later event in the pathogenesis of atherosclerosis, usually associated with the development of the fibrous plaque, the synthesis and deposition of excessive collagen and other matrix components begins earlier.

Arteries of newborns are composed of an intima, which consists of a monolayer of endothelial cells covering an internal elastic lamina, a medial layer, in which the only cell is the smooth muscle cell, and the adventitia, in which fibroblasts are the predominant cell. As discussed in the preceding section, intimal thickening is an early event in atherosclerosis characterized by the proliferation of smooth muscle cells that have migrated from the media. These cells continue to proliferate as the lesion grows, but it is not certain that continued proliferation is a prerequisite for excessive matrix accumulation. In fact, a dissociation between active proliferation of smooth muscle cells and excessive production of extracellular matrix has been observed. Clowes et al[46] subjected rat carotid arteries to abrasive endothelial denudation by balloon catheter. Platelet deposition occurred within minutes of endothelial cell removal and stabilized within 24 hours, after which smooth muscle cells started to synthesize DNA as regeneration of the endothelium began. Migration of the proliferating, medial smooth muscle cells into the intima began at 4 days, and proliferation continued in the intima. The mass of smooth muscle cells increased to a maximum at 4 weeks. Intimal thickening, however, continued for another 8 to 12 weeks. The increase in thickness and mass of the intima during this time was due completely to additional accumulation of extracellular matrix synthesized by resident smooth muscle cells that were no longer proliferating. The chain of events seen in this experimental model may be relevant to the pathogenesis of restenosis that follows percutaneous transluminal coronary angioplasty. Restenosis is frequently accompanied by additional intimal hyperplasia, hypertrophy, and deposition of extracellular matrix components, resulting in fibrotic and complicated lesions that are even more occlusive than those seen before angioplasty. It thus appears that regardless of whether the artery is in the early or later stages of atherosclerotic lesion formation, the predominant cell, if not the only cell, responsible for synthesis of extracellular collagen and other glycoproteins is the smooth muscle cell.

Although smooth muscle cells are thought responsible for the bulk of extracellular matrix production in the atherosclerotic intima, these cells are probably not the same as smooth muscle cells of the normal media. It has been proposed that there are two different phenotypes of arterial smooth muscle cells.[47] Medial smooth muscle cells are characterized as being in the "contractile" state and are filled with myofilaments. These cells are responsible for the normal contraction of arterial tissue and produce only a maintenance level of connective tissue components. The other phenotype is represented by smooth muscle cells that have been induced to migrate into the intima where they proliferate and exist in a "synthetic" state. These cells synthesize large amounts of extracellular matrix and contain increased levels of cytoplasmic rough endoplasmic reticulum, Golgi apparatus, and free ribosomes with very few filament bundles. Thus cells in atherosclerotic lesions that are producing excessive quantities of matrix most likely originated as medial smooth muscle cells but may no longer have all the characteristics of normal smooth muscle cells.

Other cellular components of human atherosclerotic plaques are macrophages and lymphocytes, but it is unlikely that they contribute significantly to the matrix components known to accumulate in developing lesions. The presence of various leukocytic cells in different types of lesions, however, suggests a strong potential for these cells to influence the composition of arterial matrix molecules by several mechanisms. Production of a variety of cytokines and other mediators of the inflammatory process together with the secretion of collagenases could profoundly affect the synthesis and accumulation of matrix components by resident smooth muscle cells.

Monocyte-derived macrophages have been shown to be present in the fatty-streak or fibrofatty lesions, as well as in the advanced or complicated plaques.[48,49] Human arterial tissue taken from aortic, carotid, and femoral vessels showed two types of plaques beyond the fatty-streak stage, both of which contained extracellular connective tissue. The first type consisted of an elevated fibrous plaque without a necrotic core. The second was composed of a fibrous cap surrounding an atheromatous core. The fibrous plaque and the fibrous cap both contained collagen and elastin. In the lipid core of the complicated lesion 60% of the cells were monocyte-derived macrophages, whereas in the overlying fibrous cap they represented 24% of the total cells.

The presence of macrophages in lesions suggests that atherosclerosis can be considered an inflammatory response. In most tissues inflammation is often accompanied by a proliferation of fibroblasts, which is then followed by deposition of collagen and other extracellular matrix components. This sequence of events is analogous to the proliferation and subsequent matrix deposition in atherosclerotic arteries. In addition to smooth muscle cells and macrophages, T lymphocytes account for nearly 20% of the cells in fibrous caps.[49] The presence of T cells together with activated macrophages in lesions also suggests the possibility of a cell-mediated, delayed type hypersensitivity form of immune response.[50] Activated T cells produce a variety of proteins, including interferon gamma, which is known to inhibit smooth muscle cell proliferation. This cytokine also inhibits collagen synthesis at the level of mRNA synthesis and may be responsible for reducing the elastin content of the tissue by increasing elastase activity. Smooth muscle cells, macrophages, and lymphocytes together produce a variety of growth factors, cytokines, and matrix protein hydrolytic enzymes. The coexistence of these cells in varying proportions in different types of lesions emphasizes the potential for regulation of extracellular matrix synthesis and remodeling as atherosclerotic plaques progress.

The macromolecular composition of the extracellular matrix of normal arteries and of atherosclerotic arteries consists of the fibrous proteins, collagen, and elastin, together with other glycoproteins and various glycosaminoglycans and proteoglycans. During development of atherosclerosis compositional changes occur in the absolute and relative concentrations of several of these macromolecules, and they may have profound influences on the structure and metabolism of the arterial wall. Some of the known alterations in the synthesis, degradation, and accumulation of these components are discussed below.

Proteoglycans are composed of glycosaminoglycans, or polymers of amino sugars, previously referred to as *mucopolysaccharides,* which are linked to specific core proteins. One of the major types of proteoglycans in the arterial wall is the chondroitin sulfate/dermatan sulfate (CS/DS) proteoglycan. This proteoglycan is increased with the progression of atherosclerosis.[14] CS/DS proteoglycan is reported to associate with collagen and to sequester apolipoprotein B–containing lipoproteins, which would contribute to the trapping and deposition of LDL cholesterol in the intima[14] (see Figs. 7-15 and 7-16).

The major structural components of all blood vessels are collagen and elastin. Collagen fibrils are the structures that provide the tensile strength throughout the entire cardiovascular system. Regulation of arterial smooth muscle cell collagen production is not well understood. Studies in which collagen synthesis was determined in isolated atherosclerotic arteries or in vivo concluded that one of the mechanisms responsible for the increased arterial collagen in atherosclerosis was an increase in the rate at which arterial collagen was synthesized.[50,51] This increase was significantly greater than that seen for noncollagen protein synthesis and was specific for arterial tissue. Whether a decrease in rates of arterial collagen degradation also accompanies the onset of atherosclerosis is not known.

These and other investigations established that arterial smooth muscle cells exhibit increased rates of collagen synthesis in response to changes taking place even in the relatively early stages of atherosclerosis in which lesion formation has not progressed beyond the fatty-streak stage. Types I and III collagen account for approximately 90% of all blood vessel collagen, with less than 10% contributed by type V collagen and much smaller quantities by types IV, VI, and VIII.[53] Changes in the distribution or proportions of the various types of collagen that occur in atherosclerosis have been difficult to assess, but the relative percentages of types I and III in intimal plaques do not seem to differ from that of the unaffected medial layer.

Elastin is the other major fibrous protein component of blood vessels. In the aortic arch and thoracic aorta elastin is present in larger quantities than collagen. In the abdominal aorta and in smaller blood vessels collagen becomes the predominant fibrous structural protein. Although elastin is seen in developing plaques in humans and in experimental atherosclerosis, it does not accumulate as collagen does. It is interesting that elastin synthesis apparently is increased in arteries of atherosclerotic rabbits to the same extent as collagen synthesis when measured in isolated segments of thoracic aorta.[51] Increased production of elastin in the arterial intima thus apparently is offset by increased degradation. Elastin concentration does not increase, and many of the elastin fibers in lesions are fragmented.

REGRESSION OF ATHEROSCLEROTIC LESIONS

The regression of atherosclerotic lesions ideally reflects a return of the vascular wall to the prelesion or normal state. However, in practice this ideal is rarely observed. The extent to which regression occurs has been documented in a number of animal models and in humans.[54-63] Regression in humans is discussed in detail in Chapter 8. Animal models of atherosclerosis have been invaluable in understanding the mechanisms of lesion development; however, these models rarely adequately replicate the severe lesions that typify advanced human atherosclerosis, perhaps because human atherosclerotic lesions evolve slowly over decades, whereas animal models of this disease are developed in months to several years and are usually elicited by excessive elevations in blood cholesterol. Nevertheless, experimental models of atherosclerosis in rabbits, swine, and nonhuman primates do replicate many of the morphologic features of human atherosclerotic lesions, thus permitting a study of their potential for regression and the mechanisms involved.

Collectively, the data obtained from regression studies in animal models have identified several important properties of the regression process.[58-61] Notably, regression is a common feature of lesions in both peripheral artery and coronary artery beds. Within these lesions most of the morphologic and biochemical alterations noted in atherosclerotic lesions are reversible, including the normalization of vascular wall cholesterol content by the removal or resolution of intracellular and extracellular lipid deposits, a reduction in smooth muscle cell number, the loss of necrotic material, and the repair of endothelial cell damage. Important exceptions to this trend are the connective tissue, particularly collagen, and calcium components of the atherosclerotic lesion, which usually increase during regression. Consistent with these conclusions, the extent to which lesion regression occurs is directly dependent on the severity of the initial lesion. Uncomplicated fatty-streak lesions induced by cholesterol feeding completely regress when the induction stimulus is removed and the animals are returned to a normal diet. More complicated lesions such as fibrofatty lesions diminish markedly but never reach the prelesion state even after an extended regression period. Advanced, humanlike lesions regress only partially, often resulting in a highly fibrous lesion that is only slightly smaller in size than the original.

The cellular and biochemical mechanisms responsible for regression are poorly understood. The primary initial step in the regression of all lesions apparently is the loss of cholesteryl esters, resulting in a marked reduction in the number of foam cells. Evidence exists to support at least three mechanisms of foam cell regression: (1) cell death; (2) the egress of lipid-laden macrophages from the lesion into the circulation from which they are cleared; and (3) removal from intact foam cells of cholesterol, which is subsequently cleared from the extracellular space by effective cholesterol acceptors such as HDL. This latter process, referred to as *reverse cholesterol transport,* may explain why elevations in plasma HDL levels are correlated with enhanced lesion regression.[54,62] Secondary to foam cell loss, a reduction in smooth muscle cell number appears related to a normalization of cell division rates,[59] and the resolution of the necrotic debris of the lesion suggests that cell death stops and that adequate scavenger mechanisms exist to resolve large amounts of material when the input side of the equation is terminated. The mechanisms underlying the enhanced collagen production during the regression of fibrous lesions are unclear; however, it appears that this induction is dependent on the initial stimulation of collagen synthesis in the developing lesion.[61] The increase in fibrous lesion collagen content during regression is problematic in the return of vasodilation capacity. In some instances vessel stiffness decreases to near-normal levels with regression[55]; in other studies the increased fibrosis prevents the regression of vasodilation capacity, even when luminal diameter markedly improves.[63]

Thus, based on animal studies, it is understandable why the complicated lesions of advanced human atherosclerosis are slow to regress and require aggressive lipid-lowering therapy. The fact that the most easily resolved component of lesions, foam cells, represents a relatively small part of the advanced lesion, coupled with the propensity for collagen to accumulate in the resolving lesion appears to impair effective lesion regression. These findings underscore the importance of reducing recognized risk factors for atherosclerotic lesion development in asymptomatic individuals.

REFERENCES

1. Falk E: Unstable angina with fatal outcome: dynamic coronary thrombosis leading to infarction and/or sudden death, Circulation 71:699, 1985.
2. McGill HC Jr: Fatty streaks in the coronary arteries and aorta, Lab Invest 28:560, 1968.
3. Adams CWM: Vascular histochemistry, Chicago, 1967, Year Book Medical Publishers, Inc.
4. St Clair RW: Pathogenesis of the atherosclerotic lesion; current concepts of cellular and biochemical events. In *Recent advances in arterial disease: atherosclerosis, hypertension, and vasospasms,* New York, 1986, Alan R Liss, Inc.
5. Virchow R: Gesammte Abhandlung zu wissenschafltiche, Medizin 550:458, 1856.
6. Page IH: Atherosclerosis: an introduction, Circulation 10:1, 1954.
7. Gofman JW and Young W: The filtration concept of atherosclerosis and serum lipids in the diagnosis of atherosclerosis. In Sandler M and Bourne GH, eds: Atherosclerosis and its origins, New York, 1963, Academic Press, Inc.
8. Smith EB and Slater RS: Relationship between low density lipoproteins in aortic intima and serum lipid levels, Lancet 1:463, 1972.
9. Hoff HF, Gaubatz JW, and Gotto AM: ApoB concentration in the normal human aorta, Biochem Biophys Res Commun 85:1424, 1979.

10. Yamauchi E and Hoff HF: Apolipoprotein B accumulation and development of foam cell lesions in coronary arteries of hypercholesterolemic swine, Lab Invest 51:325, 1984.
11. Gerrity RG: The role of the monocyte in atherogenesis I. Transition of blood-borne monocytes into foam cells in fatty lesions, Am J Pathol 103:181, 1981.
12. Steinberg D et al: Beyond cholesterol. Modifications of low density cholesterol that increase its atherogenicity, N Engl J Med 320:915, 1989.
13. Jurgens G et al: Modification of human serum low density lipoprotein by oxidation—characterization and pathophysiological implications, Chem Phys Lipids 45:315, 1987.
14. Berenson GS et al: Carbohydrate-protein macromolecules and arterial wall integrity—a role in atherosclerosis, Exp Mol Path 4:267, 1984.
15. Davies PF et al: Influence of hemodynamic forces on vascular endothelial function, J Clin Invest 73:1121, 1984.
16. Duguid JB: Thrombosis as a factor in the pathogenesis of coronary atherosclerosis, J Pathol Bacteriol 58:207, 1946.
17. Hauss WH, Junge-Hulsing G, and Hollanden HJ: Changes in metabolism of connective tissue associated with aging and arterio- or atherosclerosis, J Atherosclerosis Res 6:50, 1962.
18. Ross R and Glomset JA: The pathogenesis of atherosclerosis, N Engl J Med 295:369-377, 420-425, 1976.
19. Ross R: The pathogenesis of atherosclerosis—an update, N Engl J Med 314:488, 1986.
20. Taylor RG and Lewis JC: Endothelial cell proliferation and monocyte adhesion to atherosclerotic lesions in white carneau pigeons, Am J Pathol 125:152, 1986.
21. Lewinsohn DM, Bargatze RF, and Butcher EC: Leukocyte-endothelial cell recognition: evidence of a common molecular mechanism shared by neutrophils, lymphocytes and other leukocytes, J Immunol 138:4313, 1983.
22. Bevilacqua MP et al: Endothelial leukocyte adhesion molecule 1: an inducible receptor for neurophils related to complement regulatory proteins and lectins, Science 243:1160, 1989.
23. DiCorleto PE and de la Motte CA: Thrombin causes increased monocytic cell adhesion to endothelial cells through a protein kinase C–dependent pathway, Biochem J 264:71, 1989.
24. The Lipid Research Clinics Program: The lipid research clinics coronary prevention trial results. I. Reduction in incidence of coronary heart disease, JAMA 251:351, 1984.
25. The Lipid Research Clinics Program: The lipid research clinics coronary primary prevention trial results. II. The relationship of reduction in incidence of coronary heart disease to cholesterol lowering, JAMA 251:365, 1984.
26. Castelli WP et al: Incidence of coronary heart disease and lipoprotein cholesterol levels: the Framingham Study, JAMA 256:2835, 1986.
27. Multiple Risk Factor Intervention Trial Research Group: Multiple Risk Factor Intervention Trial: risk factor changes and mortality results, JAMA 248:1465, 1982.
28. Report of the National Cholesterol Education Program Expert Panel on detection, evaluation, and treatment of high blood cholesterol in adults, Arch Intern Med 148:36, 1988.
29. Stamler J, Wentworth D, and Neaton JD: Is relationship between serum cholesterol and risk of premature death from coronary heart disease continuous and graded? Findings in 365,222 primary screenees of the Multiple Risk Factor Intervention Trial (MRFIT), JAMA 256:2823, 1986.
30. Schaefer DJ and Levy RI: Pathogenesis and management of lipoprotein disorders, N Engl J Med 312:1300, 1985.
31. Mahley RW et al: Plasma lipoproteins: apolipoprotein structure and function, J Lipid Res 25:1277, 1984.
32. Utermann G: The mysteries of lipoprotein(a), Science 246:904, 1989.
33. Brown MS and Goldstein JL: A receptor-mediated pathway for cholesterol homeostasis, Science 232:34, 1986.
34. Brown MS and Goldstein JL: Lipoprotein metabolism in the macrophage: implications for cholesterol deposition in atherosclerosis, Ann Rev Biochem 52:223, 1983.
35. Hoff HF et al: Modification of LDL with 4-hydroxynonenal induces uptake of LDL by macrophages, Arteriosclerosis 9:538, 1989.
36. Wolfbauer G et al: Development of the smooth muscle foam cell: uptake of macrophage lipid inclusions, Proc Natl Acad Sci USA 83:7760, 1986.
37. DiCorleto PE and Bowen-Pope DF: Cultured endothelial cells produce a platelet-derived growth factor-like protein, Proc Natl Acad Sci USA 80:1919, 1983.
38. Barrett TB et al: Expression of the *sis* gene by endothelial cells in culture and in vivo, Proc Natl Acad Sci USA 81:6772-6774, 1984.
39. Barrett TB and Benditt EP: *sis* (platelet-derived growth factor B chain) gene transcript levels are elevated in human atherosclerotic lesions compared to normal artery, Proc Natl Acad Sci USA 84:1099, 1987.
40. Fox PL, Chisolm G, and DiCorleto P: Lipoprotein-mediated inhibition of endothelial cell production of platelet-derived growth factor-like protein depends on free radical lipid peroxidation, J Biol Chem 262:6045, 1987.
41. Wilcox JN et al: Platelet-derived growth factor mRNA detection in human atherosclerotic plaques by in situ hybridization, J Clin Invest 82:1134, 1988.
42. Benditt EP and Benditt JM: Evidence for a monoclonal origin of human atherosclerotic plaques, Proc Natl Acad Sci USA 70:1753, 1973.
43. Castellot JJ Jr et al: Cultured endothelial cells produce a heparinlike inhibitor of smooth muscle cell growth, J Cell Biol 90:372, 1981.
44. Powell JS et al: Inhibitors of angiotensin-converting enzyme prevent myointimal proliferation after vascular injury, Science 245:186, 1989.
45. Fox PL and DiCorleto PE: Fish oils inhibit endothelial cell production of platelet-derived growth factor-like protein, Science 241:453, 1988.
46. Clowes AW et al: Regulation of smooth muscle cell growth in injured artery, J Cardiovasc Pharmacol 14(suppl 6):S12, 1989.
47. Campbell GR and Campbell JH: Smooth muscle phenotypic changes in arterial wall homeostasis: implications for the pathogenesis of atherosclerosis, Exp Mol Pathol 42:139-162, 1985.
48. Gown AM, Tsukada T, and Ross R: Human atherosclerosis. II. Immunocytochemical analysis of the cellular composition of human atherosclerotic lesions, Am J Pathol 125:191, 1986.
49. Hansson GK et al: Immune mechanisms in atherosclerosis, Arteriosclerosis 9:567, 1989.
50. Munro JM and Cotran RS: The pathogenesis of atherosclerosis: atherogenesis and inflammation, Lab Invest 58:249, 1988.
51. Ehrhart LA and Holderbaum D: Aortic collagen, elastin and nonfibrous protein synthesis in rabbits fed cholesterol and peanut oil, Atherosclerosis 37:423, 1980.
52. Opsahl WP, DeLuca DJ, and Ehrhart LA: Accelerated rates of collagen synthesis in atherosclerotic arteries quantified in vivo, Arteriosclerosis 7:470, 1986.
53. Mayne R: Collagenous proteins of blood vessels, Arteriosclerosis 6:585, 1986.
54. Malinow MR: Atherosclerosis: progression, regression, and resolution, Am Heart J 108:1523, 1984.
55. Blankenhorn DH: Regression of atherosclerosis: dietary and pharmacologic approach, Can J Cardiol 5:206, 1989.
56. Blankenhorn DH: Prevention or reversal of atherosclerosis: review of current evidence, Am J Cardiol 63:38H, 1989.
57. Glueck CJ: Role of risk factor management in progression and regres-

sion of coronary and femoral artery atherosclerosis, Am J Cardiol 57:35G, 1986.
58. St Clair RW: Atherosclerosis regression in animal models: current concepts of cellular and biochemical mechanisms, Prog Cardiovasc Dis 26:109, 1983.
59. Kim DN et al: The "turning off" of excessive cell replicative activity in advanced atherosclerotic lesions of swine by a regression diet, Atherosclerosis 71:131, 1988.
60. Hollander W et al: Changes in the connective tissue proteins, glycosaminoglycans and calcium in the arteries of the cynomolgus monkey during atherosclerotic induction and regression, Atherosclerosis 51:89, 1984.
61. Langner RO and Bement CL: Lesion regression and protein synthesis in rabbits after removal of dietary cholesterol, Arteriosclerosis 5:74, 1985.
62. Kashyap ML: Basic considerations in the reversal of atherosclerosis: significance of high-density lipoprotein in stimulating reverse cholesterol transport, Am J Cardiol 63:56H, 1989.
63. Armstrong ML et al: Hemodynamic sequelae of regression of experimental atherosclerosis, J Clin Invest 71:104, 1983.

Chapter 8

DIAGNOSIS AND TREATMENT OF LIPID DISTURBANCES

Jeffrey W. Olin
Michael D. Cressman
Byron J. Hoogwerf
Cheryl E. Weinstein

In the last 10 years results of several epidemiologic studies have been published and have confirmed the observation that increased serum total cholesterol or low density lipoprotein cholesterol (LDL-C) levels and decreased high density lipoprotein cholesterol (HDL-C) levels are strongly associated with the development of complications resulting from atherosclerotic vascular disease. In addition, several controlled clinical trials have demonstrated that lowering serum cholesterol levels decreases the risk of developing coronary heart disease (CHD). There is also considerable interest in the possibility that aggressive LDL-C reduction may cause regression of atherosclerosis. Because of the interest in the role of lipoproteins in the pathogenesis of atherosclerosis, this chapter discusses the epidemiologic evidence linking blood lipids to atherosclerotic vascular disease, evidence that cholesterol-lowering therapy decreases cardiovascular morbidity and mortality rates, and the role that lipids play in the progression and regression of atherosclerosis. This discussion is followed by reviews of lipoprotein metabolism and clinical aspects of various lipid and lipoprotein disorders, including the treatment of these conditions.

ROLE OF BLOOD LIPIDS IN PATHOGENESIS OF ATHEROSCLEROTIC VASCULAR DISEASE

The Framingham Study was one of the first epidemiologic studies demonstrating a strong association between total blood cholesterol (TC) levels and the development of cardiovascular disease.[1] The 8-year probability of developing CHD was directly related to the level of TC even when the TC values were still within the "normal" range. The Framingham data also showed that CHD risk at any cholesterol level was highly dependent on the presence or absence of other cardiovascular risk factors (glucose intolerance, hypertension, cigarette smoking, electrocardiographic [ECG] evidence of left ventricular hypertrophy). The risk was substantially increased in patients with multiple risk factors. In 4374 Framingham participants less than 50 years old, Anderson, Castelli, and Levy[2] noted that for each 10 mg/dl increment in TC there was a 9% increase in cardiovascular mortality.[2]

Six-year follow-up data were obtained in the Multiple Risk Factor Intervention Trial (MRFIT) from more than 350,000 middle-aged men who had no history of atherosclerotic coronary artery disease.[3] There was strong correlation between the TC level at screening and the 6-year coronary heart disease death rates (Table 8-1). This relationship was continuous and graded. In agreement with the Framingham Study data cigarette smoking and/or increased blood pressure substantially increased the CHD mortality rate at any given TC level. The relationship between TC level and stroke mortality rate was also examined during the 6-year MRFIT follow-up.[4] A significant positive correlation ($P = .007$) between nonhemorrhagic stroke and TC level was found using a proportional hazards regression analysis controlling for age, cigarette smoking, diastolic blood pressure, and race or ethnic group. In a recent review Tell, Crouse, and Furberg[5] reported that a positive relationship between elevated blood lipid and lipoprotein levels and clinical evidence of cerebrovascular atherosclerosis was apparent in 23 of 26 studies reviewed. An association between increased TC levels and decreased HDL-C levels and the

Table 8-1. MRFIT: 6-year coronary mortality rate

		CHD Mortality		
Quintile	Serum cholesterol (mg/dl [mmol/L])	Number of deaths	Rate per 1000	Relative risk
1	≤181 (≤4.68)	196	3.2	1.0
2	182-202 (4.71-5.22)	288	4.2	1.29
3	203-220 (5.25-5.69)	395	5.6	1.73
4	221-244 (5.72-6.31)	533	7.1	2.21
5	≥245 (≥6.34)	846	11.1	3.42

(From Stamler J, Wentworth D, and Neaton JD: JAMA 256:2823-2828, 1986. Copyright 1986, American Medical Association.)

development of peripheral arterial atherosclerotic disease was also noted in the Lipid Research Clinics Program Prevalence Study.[6]

Although most of the early epidemiologic studies focused on the relationship between TC and the risk of atherosclerosis, it has become apparent that separation of cholesterol-containing lipoproteins into different lipoprotein fractions improves the predictive power of this risk assessment. For example, LDL-C levels have been shown superior to TC levels in predicting CHD risk.[7] A very strong inverse relationship between HDL-C levels and CHD risk has also been reported.[8,9] The risk is particularly great when HDL-C levels are below 35 mg/dl. It has been suggested that HDL-C is the single most important predictor of cardiovascular morbidity and mortality, particularly in individuals 50 years of age or older.

In the Framingham Study (after 12 years of follow-up) myocardial infarction occurred in six times as many patients in the lowest quartile of HDL-C distribution (HDL-C <46 mg/dl) compared to those in the highest HDL-C quartile (HDL-C ≥67 mg/dl).[10] For this reason screening with TC levels may be inadequate in predicting cardiovascular risk since some high-risk individuals with normal TC levels may have low HDL-C levels and escape detection.[11] Although reduction of TC and LDL-C have been shown to decrease CHD risk (see below), no trials have adequately shown that raising HDL-C levels decreases CHD risk in patients with TC levels below 200 mg/dl.[12] However, the magnitude of risk reduction in gemfibrozil-treated patients in the Helsinki Heart Study[13] was greater than the risk reduction observed in the cholestyramine-treated participants of the Lipid Research Clinics Coronary Primary Prevention Trial (LRC-CPPT)[14,15] even though gemfibrozil and cholestyramine produced similar effects on LDL-C levels. Since the study groups were similar, this difference may be due to the 10% increase in HDL-C levels that occurred in patients treated with gemfibrozil in the Helsinki Heart Study. No change in HDL-C levels was noted in the cholestyramine-treated group of the LRC-CPPT.

Plasma triglycerides and cardiovascular disease

Whether triglycerides are an independent risk factor for cardiovascular disease is a matter of continued controversy. A recent analysis of Framingham data addressed this issue. Fasting very low density lipoprotein cholesterol (VLDL-C) levels were directly related to overall cardiovascular mortality, and the relationship was stronger for VLDL-C than for TC or LDL-C levels. The association remained significant on multivariate Cox regression analysis after adjustment for TC and LDL-C.[16] Hypertriglyceridemia is often shown associated with increased cardiovascular risk when analyzed by univariate statistical techniques. However, when the influence of obesity, diabetes mellitus, and other lipoprotein factors are included in multivariate analyses, triglyceride or VLDL-C levels have not been shown to influence risk independently. This issue has recently been reviewed by Austin.[17]

EVIDENCE THAT CHOLESTEROL-LOWERING THERAPY REDUCES CARDIOVASCULAR RISK

A number of well-controlled clinical trials have been designed to determine the effects of lipid-lowering therapy on cardiovascular morbidity and mortality. Only the most important studies are discussed below.

Primary prevention trials

Lipid Research Clinics Coronary Primary Prevention Trial.[14,15,18] The LRC-CPPT was a randomized, placebo-controlled double-blind multicenter trial designed to test the effectiveness of cholesterol-lowering therapy in reducing the risk of developing CHD. Enrolled in this study were 3806 middle-aged men (35 to 59 years at entry) with plasma cholesterol levels greater than or equal to 265 mg/dl and LDL-C levels greater than or equal to 190 mg/dl. Participants had no clinical evidence of atherosclerotic heart disease at entry. All participants were advised to follow a cholesterol-lowering diet and were randomly assigned to treatment with a placebo (n = 1900) or the bile acid binding resin cholestyramine (n = 1906) at a dose of 24 g/day. Patients were followed 7 to 10 years (mean, 7.4 years). Definite CHD death plus definite nonfatal myocardial infarction were the primary end points. There was a 19% reduction in these primary end points in the cholestyramine group vs the placebo group, $P < 0.05$ (Fig. 8-1). CHD death and nonfatal myocardial infarction were reduced by 24% and 19%, respectively, in the cholestyramine vs placebo groups. There were also a 25% reduction in the development of positive exercise tests, a 20% reduction in angina pectoris, a 21% reduction in coronary artery bypass surgery, and a 15% reduction in intermittent claudication in the group receiving cholestyramine compared to the group receiving a placebo. All-cause mortality, however, was no different in the two groups. The trial was not designed to show a difference in all-cause mortality, and the absence of a dif-

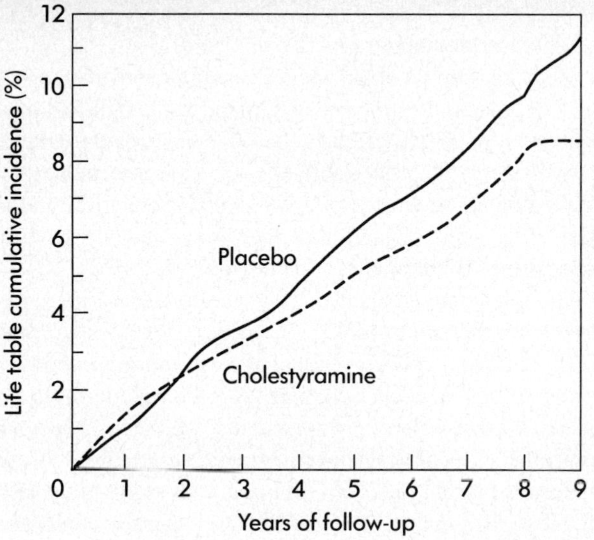

Fig. 8-1. Life-table cumulative incidence of primary end points in treatment groups computed by Kaplan-Meier method. (From Lipid Research Clinics Program, JAMA 251:365, 1984.)

ference was due to an increased number of accidental and violent deaths in the cholestyramine group compared to the placebo group. Not all participants in the trial took full doses of cholestyramine. Approximately 50% of the cholestyramine-treated patients ingested 20 to 24 g of cholestyramine per day; approximately 25% took 8 g or less. The relationship between the total dose of cholestyramine taken and the reduction in TC and LDL-C levels was significant. Using a Cox proportional hazards model, a significant relationship between the reduction in LDL-C and the reduction in CHD risk was demonstrated.[19] For every 1% reduction in the TC level, there was a 2% reduction in CHD risk. Although there were not differences in mean HDL-C levels at baseline or after treatment in the cholestyramine group vs the placebo group, some patients did demonstrate an increase in HDL-C. In these patients there was a 5.5% decrease in CHD risk for each 1 mg/dl increment in HDL-C.[18]

The Helsinki Heart Study.[13] The Helsinki Heart Study was a randomized, double-blind, 5-year primary prevention trial comparing a placebo with the fibric acid derivative gemfibrozil (600 mg twice daily) in 4081 middle-aged men (40 to 55 years). In contrast to cholestyramine, which only lowers TC and LDL-C levels, gemfibrozil lowers TC, triglycerides, and LDL-C and VLDL-C levels. Gemfibrozil also increases HDL-C levels. There were similar changes in TC and LDL-C in the gemfibrozil-treated patients as in the cholestyramine-treated LRC-CPPT patients. In the Helsinki Heart Study gemfibrozil produced a 9% decrease in TC, an 8% decrease in LDL-C, and a 10% increase in HDL-C. Participants with the lowest HDL-C levels at entry had the greatest increase in HDL-C during gemfibrozil treatment. Trigylceride levels were reduced by approximately 35% in the gemfibrozil-treated group.

The life-table curves for primary end points in the Helsinki Heart Study were almost identical to those of the LRC-CPPT. There was a 34% reduction in the incidence of fatal and nonfatal myocardial infarction and cardiac death in the gemfibrozil-treated groups vs the placebo group. Nonfatal myocardial infarction was reduced by 37%, whereas CHD mortality was reduced by 26%. As in the LRC-CPPT, the overall mortality rate was no different between the placebo group and the gemfibrozil group in the Helsinki Heart Study. An increased incidence of accidental and violent deaths occurred in gemfibrozil-treated patients vs placebo-treated patients in this trial. Although this may have been a chance occurrence, it is bothersome that accidental and violent deaths occurred more frequently in the treated group in this study and in the LRC-CPPT. The relationship between serum cholesterol level and the risk of death from violence or accidents has been examined in a cohort of 1580 Finnish men, and no correlation was found.[20]

As previously stated, for every 1% reduction in TC or LDL-C levels, there was a 2% decrease in CHD risk in the LRC-CPPT. In the Helsinki Heart Study for every 1% decrease in TC or LDL-C levels there was approximately a 3.8% reduction in fatal and nonfatal myocardial infarction and cardiac death in the gemfibrozil group. The more favorable effect of gemfibrozil compared to cholestyramine may be attributed to the rise in HDL-C levels observed in the gemfibrozil group. However, gemfibrozil also reduced triglyceride levels and may also have produced favorable effects on the composition of other atherogenic lipoproteins.

Secondary prevention trials

Coronary Drug Project. [21,22] The Coronary Drug Project (CDP) assessed the effect of various drugs in 8341 men with a history of myocardial infarction. Although conjugated estrogens, clofibrate, or dextrothyroxine sodium showed no benefit compared to a placebo, patients treated with nicotinic acid demonstrated a reduced incidence of nonfatal myocardial infarction and an 11% decrease in all-cause mortality after 15 years of follow-up ($P = .0004$). Interestingly, this favorable effect was not apparent after 6 years of follow-up when the formal CDP ended and drug therapy was discontinued. Although the exact cause of this late benefit of niacin is not clear, it has been suggested that the drug either prevented mild non–life-threatening myocardial infarction early or reduced progression of coronary atherosclerosis during the period of niacin administration. Theoretically, these effects could reduce the rate of later ischemic complications. Perhaps additional similar benefits will be seen in the LRC-CPPT and Helsinki Heart Study participants with a longer period of follow-up.

Leiden Intervention Trial.[23] This study assessed the

effects of marked cholesterol-lowering therapy on the progression of coronary artery disease in 39 patients with stable angina pectoris. Every patient had at least 50% narrowing of one coronary artery proven by coronary arteriography. All patients were treated with a vegetarian diet that contained a high polyunsaturated to saturated fat ratio (P/S) and less than 100 mg of dietary cholesterol per day. Repeat coronary arteriography was performed 24 months later.

Coronary disease progressed in 21 of 39 patients, and there was no progression in 18 patients (46%). Progression of atherosclerosis correlated with the TC:HDL-C ratio ($r = 0.50$, $P = .001$) but not with other cardiovascular risk factors. There was no progression of atherosclerosis in any patient who had a TC:HDL-C ratio of less than 6.9.

Cholesterol Lowering Atherosclerosis Study[24]

In this angiographic trial a group of highly motivated patients with CHD who had undergone coronary artery bypass graft surgery were randomized to receive either colestipol hydrochloride (30 g/day) and niacin (3 to 12 g/day) or placebo treatment. Both groups were advised to follow a low-fat diet. This trial was designed to determine the effect of cholesterol-lowering therapy on coronary bypass grafts and native coronary arteries. All patients had initial TC levels of 185 to 350 mg/dl and had undergone coronary artery bypass surgery at least 3 months before entry into the study. Coronary arteriography was performed at the beginning of the study and after 2 years of treatment. A complex system of coronary lesion analysis was used to obtain a global score for each film in the pair of coronary arteriograms obtained from an individual patient. Although this visual system of lesion analysis has limitations, the investigators took great care to minimize observer bias. The treated patients demonstrated marked improvement in TC (246 mg/dl to 180 mg/dl), triglycerides (151 mg/dl to 110 mg/dl), LDL-C (171 mg/dl to 97 mg/dl), and HDL-C (46 mg/dl to 60 mg/dl) levels. This represents a decrease in TC and LDL-C levels of 26% and 43%, respectively. In addition, HDL-C increased 37%, an effect almost certainly due to niacin. There were no major changes in any lipid parameter in the placebo group.

More patients in the placebo-treated group showed progression of atherosclerosis in their native coronary arteries or saphenous vein bypass grafts when compared to those receiving colestipol and niacin (61% vs 39%). This difference is statistically significant ($P < .001$). Regression of atherosclerosis occurred in 16% of the drug-treated patients compared to 2% of the placebo group. This study demonstrated the following: (1) TC and LDL-C levels can be significantly reduced with combination drug therapy, and (2) stabilization and perhaps even regression of atherosclerosis may occur in some aggressively treated patients. The number of treated patients with evidence of significant lesion regression was small, and the visual assessment of these lesions when before and after angiograms are compared may be biased. This issue may be clarified when computerized quantitation of angiograms is completed.

Recently Brown et al[25] showed that patients treated with lovastatin and colestipol or niacin and colestipol had more regression of atherosclerosis than patients treated with colestipol alone. The favorable angiographic effects were directly related to the degree of LDL-C reduction and/or HDL-C increase. In addition, there were fewer cardiovascular events in the lovastatin-colestipol group ($P < .05$) and niacin-colestipol group ($P < .006$) compared to the colestipol monotherapy group.

In summary, we currently have an enormous body of epidemiologic evidence linking blood cholesterol to the cause of atherosclerotic vascular disease, data from well-controlled clinical trials documenting that reducing elevated cholesterol levels reduces CHD risk, and suggestions from recent studies that cholesterol-lowering therapy can reduce the progression or even induce regression of advanced atherosclerotic lesions.

The scope of the problem regarding elevated cholesterol among adults in the United States is enormous. Sempos et al[26] estimated that approximately 41% of adults should have lipoprotein analysis after initial measurement of TC. Additionally, other investigators estimate that 36% of all adults age 20 to 74 years require advice and medical intervention for high blood cholesterol levels. This translates into approximately 64 million Americans who are candidates for cholesterol-lowering therapy.

LIPOPROTEIN METABOLISM

Cholesterol and triglycerides are transported in the blood in complexes called lipoproteins. The plasma lipoproteins contain a core of water-insoluble lipids (cholesterol esters and triglycerides) surrounded by a coat containing a small amount of unesterified cholesterol, phospholipids, and specialized proteins referred to as apoproteins (apo).[27] Lipoproteins are mainly synthesized in intestinal cells and hepatocytes but are modified considerably in the circulation by lipolytic enzymes and transfer of several lipoprotein components between the various plasma lipoproteins. Thus they are extremely heterogeneous structures. Classically, the plasma lipoproteins are separated into five major classes: (1) chylomicrons, (2) very low density lipoproteins (VLDL), (3) intermediate density lipoproteins (IDL), (4) low density lipoproteins (LDL), and (5) high density lipoproteins (HDL). This separation is based on their flotation density (d), which is determined by ultracentrifugation (Table 8-2). Clinically, the dyslipoproteinemias are often classified on the basis of the concentration of these major lipoprotein classes. Alternatively, a genotypic classification can be used if the disorder appears to have a genetic basis.[28]

Chylomicrons are large triglyceride-rich lipoproteins ($d < 1.006$ g/ml) that are synthesized in intestinal cells. Chylomicrons transport dietary fats through the lymphatics to the systemic circulation. Triglycerides are removed from chylomicrons by lipoprotein lipase, which is located on the luminal side of endothelial cells in adipose tissue and muscle (Fig. 8-2). Remnants of these particles are rapidly removed by the liver. In healthy individuals chylomicrons are no longer present in blood a few hours after a meal.

The liver secretes VLDLs (d <1.006 g/ml) that are similar to chylomicrons but contain a large apoprotein called ApoB-100 (subsequently referred to as apoB). Each VLDL particle contains one apoB molecule, but the triglyceride content of specific VLDLs varies widely. VLDLs are converted to VLDL remnants through lipoprotein lipase–stimulated removal of triglycerides from these particles. Some of these particles reside in the IDL range (d, 1.006 to 1.019 g/ml) and are removed by hepatic LDL receptors, which avidly bind the apoE on the IDL particle. Others are converted to LDLs (d, 1.019 to 1.063 g/ml). However, the precise mechanisms responsible for conversion of IDLs to LDLs are not known.

LDLs, the major atherogenic lipoproteins, contain apoB as their sole apoprotein. In general, two thirds of the TC is carried in LDLs. Although factors regulating LDL synthetic rate are poorly understood, considerable progress in understanding LDL catabolism has been made in recent years. Goldstein and Brown[29] characterized an LDL receptor–me-

Table 8-2. Classification of plasma lipoproteins

Lipoprotein	Source	Major density (g/ml)	Apoproteins	Lipids
Chylomicrons	Intestine	<1.006	B-48, E, C, A-I, A-II, A-IV	TG >C
VLDL	Liver	<1.006	B-100, E, C	TG >C
IDL	VLDL	1.006-1.019	B-100, E	TG = C
LDL	IDL	1.019-1.063	B-100	C >TG
HDL	Liver, intestine	1.063-1.21	A-I, A-II, C, E	C >TG

TG, Triglycerides.
C, Cholesterol.

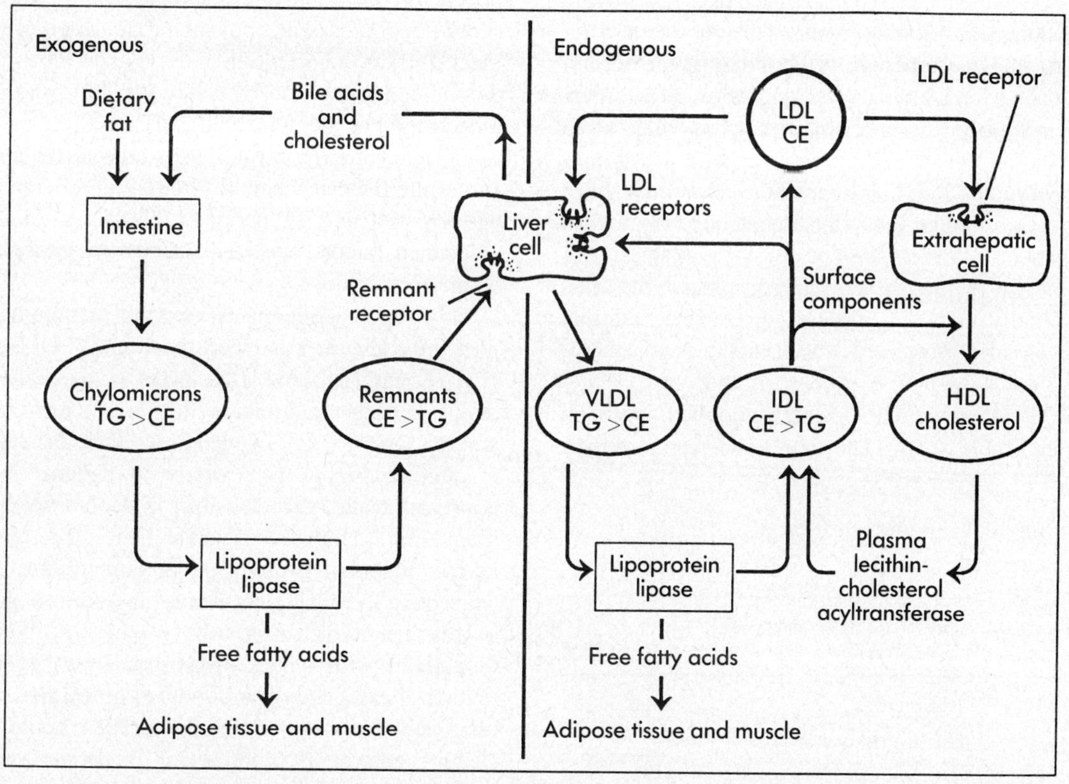

Fig. 8-2. Endogenous and exogenous metabolism of lipoproteins, emphasizing the importance of lipoprotein lipase in chylomicron and VLDL metabolism and of liver cell and extrahepatic cell specific receptors in LDL metabolism. (From Goldstein JL and Brown MS: Hosp Pract 20:35, 1985.)

diated process (referred to as receptor-mediated endocytosis) that is tightly coupled to the regulation of intracellular cholesterol synthesis. It has become apparent that a complex interaction exists between LDL receptor–mediated removal of plasma LDL, recycling of LDL receptor protein into the cell membrane, synthesis of intracellular cholesterol, regulation of new LDL receptor synthesis, and conversion of intracellular cholesterol to bile acids. This interaction maintains the intracellular cholesterol concentration at a constant level. The number and activity of LDL receptors apparently is particularly important in regulating plasma LDL concentration.[30]

The intestine and liver also synthesize HDLs that seem to be involved in "reverse cholesterol transport." Conceptually, this is a process by which HDLs (d, 1.063 to 1.21 g/ml) transport cholesterol from extrahepatic tissues. HDLs exchange a variety of structural components (lipids and apoproteins) with other lipoproteins.[31] Certain HDLs may be removed by the liver, although the routes of HDL catabolism have not been completely characterized. Apoproteins A-1 and A-2 are the major HDL apoproteins.

PHENOTYPIC CLASSIFICATION OF THE DYSLIPOPROTEINEMIAS

Fredrickson, Levy, and Lees[32] developed a classification scheme based on the concentration of the major lipoprotein classes. Although this phenotypic approach does not provide information about specific abnormalities of apoprotein structure, lipolytic enzyme function, or lipoprotein-receptor activity, it is useful for the clinical classification of disorders of lipoprotein metabolism and is particularly helpful when drug treatment is considered. Several genetic syndromes (e.g., heterozygous familial hypercholesterolemia) have been identified, although laboratory techniques to confirm presumed genetic disorders are not always available.[33] For these reasons we review the Fredrickson phenotypic classification initially and then discuss some of the familial dyslipoproteinemias associated with a high risk of atherosclerosis.

There are five major Fredrickson phenotypic lipoprotein abnormalities (Table 8-3).[32] The type I and type V hyperlipidemias are characterized by fasting chylomicronemia. In type I, the least common Fredrickson phenotype, concentrations of the other lipoproteins (VLDL, IDL, LDL) are usually decreased. The familial form generally is identified in the first decade of life and is due to a marked reduction in lipoprotein lipase activity.[34] Episodes of eruptive xanthomas and/or pancreatitis dominate the clinical picture. The risk of developing premature atherosclerosis is probably not increased. Affected individuals have fasting triglyceride levels greater than or equal to 1500 mg/dl, and triglyceride levels greater than 10,000 mg/dl are not unusual. Chilled plasma from type I patients contains a creamy layer above clear plasma. Treatment requires severe dietary fat restriction, although medium chain triglycerides can be added to the diet since they are not transported in chylomicrons. This lipoprotein disorder is not amenable to lipid-lowering drug therapy.

Table 8-3. Fredrickson classification of dysliproproteinemias

Lipoprotein phenotype	Elevated lipoprotein fraction	Frequency
I	Chylomicrons	Rare
IIa	LDL	Common
IIb	LDL and VLDL	Common
III	IDL	Rare
IV	VLDL	Common
V	Chylomicrons and VLDL	Uncommon

In patients with type V hyperlipidemia there is fasting chylomicronemia with severe hypertriglyceridemia. Patients also have elevated VLDL levels.[35] With this disorder chilled plasma contains a creamy layer and a milky layer. Since VLDLs carry some cholesterol, fasting triglyceride and cholesterol levels are usually both increased. LDL and HDL levels are usually reduced. As is true in patients with type I hyperlipidemia, the clinical picture in patients with type V hyperlipidemia is dominated by eruptive xanthomas and pancreatitis. Carbohydrate intolerance, obesity, hyperuricemia, and excess alcohol intake are often present. Treatment consists of correction of these underlying medical conditions and institution of a low fat, low calorie diet. Administration of nicotinic acid and/or a fibric acid derivative is indicated if triglyceride levels are greater than 500 mg/dl despite these measures. The risk of atherosclerosis may be increased slightly, although this increase may be due to associated factors such as diabetes mellitus, hyperinsulinemia, or obesity.

Hypertriglyceridemia is also the predominant lipid abnormality in type IV hyperlipidemia. VLDL levels are increased, and LDL and HDL levels are generally below normal.[36] Fasting chylomicronemia is not present. TC levels may be low, normal, or increased. Type IV hyperlipidemia is quite common, particularly in patients with obesity, poorly controlled diabetes, excess alcohol intake, or chronic renal failure. High carbohydrate diets and certain drugs such as the diuretics, β-blockers, or isotretinoin can cause or exacerbate hypertriglyceridemia. In addition, genetic forms of this phenotypic disorder have been identified. Treatment of patients with type IV hyperlipidemia begins with correction of associated conditions. A moderately low fat diet, restricted in calories when appropriate, should be initiated. "Tight" control of blood sugar in patients with diabetes mellitus should be emphasized. The omega-3 fatty acids contained in fatty fish may reduce triglyceride levels, but many of the fish oil capsules contain a considerable amount of calories and cholesterol.[37] A paradoxic rise in LDL-C may occur. In addition, hyperglycemia has been noted in previously well-controlled diabetics who take large doses of the fish oils. Nicotinic acid and the fibric acid derivatives are the most useful triglyceride-lowering drugs (see section, "Pharmacologic Treatment of Lipid Disorders"). The HMG CoA reductase inhibitors and probucol are relatively ineffective in treating type IV hyperlipidemia. The bile acid sequestrants may exacerbate preexisting hypertriglyceridemia.

Type III hyperlipidemia is an uncommon disorder caused by the presence of a structurally abnormal apoE that does not bind to the LDL receptor.[38] ApoE exists in three isoforms (apoE-2, apoE-3, apoE-4) and six genotypes: E-2/2, E-2/3, E-2/4, E-3/3, E-3/4, and E-4/4. The E-2/2 genotype is present in approximately 1% percent of the population and most commonly is associated with type III hyperlipidemia. Since the apoE-2 isoform does not bind to the LDL receptor, chylomicron remnants and IDLs can both accumulate in the circulation, particularly when obesity, diabetes mellitus, or hypothyroidism are present. In patients with type III hyperlipidemia the plasma cholesterol and triglycride levels are elevated to a similar degree. Palmar and tuberous xanthomas may occur, and these patients have a significantly increased risk of atherosclerosis. Dietary treatment (saturated fat restriction, weight loss) may be quite effective. Nicotinic acid, the fibric acid derivatives, and the HMG CoA reductase inhibitors have been used when drug therapy is needed.

The type II hyperlipidemias are characterized by either an isolated elevation of LDL (type IIa) or a combined increase in LDL and VLDL (type IIb). The current approach to reduce the incidence of atherosclerotic vascular disease depends primarily on the detection and treatment of patients with elevated LDL levels. Plasma LDL levels are under the influence of a variety of environmental and genetic factors. The high saturated fat diet habitually consumed in the United States is believed to contribute to the high prevalence of mild elevations of LDL-C seen in a subset of the population. In contrast, it has become apparent that genetic factors also play a major role in regulating plasma LDL levels. The most obvious example is the twofold to threefold elevation of LDL levels seen in patients with heterozygous familial hypercholesterolemia, a relatively common disease with an autosomal dominant mode of inheritance.[39] Several other genetic disorders such as the familial combined hyperlipidemia syndrome, the hyperapobetalipoproteinemia syndrome, and a syndrome characterized by elevated levels of lipoprotein (a) (Lp[a]), a plasminogen-like glycoprotein covalently bound to apoB in an LDL-like lipoprotein, have been described.[40] It seems likely that a spectrum of defects in the genetic control of lipoprotein synthesis, apoprotein structure, and LDL receptor defects will be characterized in the next few years.

GENETIC DYSLIPIDEMIAS ASSOCIATED WITH ATHEROSCLEROSIS

Familial hypercholesterolemia

This is the prototype of the genetic dyslipidemia that is due to a single gene defect that results in failure to produce functionally active cell-surface receptors that normally bind apoB in LDLs.[39] The heterozygous form of familial hypercholesterolemia is present in approximately 0.2% of the U.S. population. The disease is transmitted as an autosomal dominant trait. Individuals who inherit one normal and one abnormal gene (heterozygote) have only one half the normal number of LDL receptors and a twofold to threefold increase in circulating LDL-C (usually in the 250 to 400 mg/dl range) (Fig. 8-3). Tendon xanthomas and overt CHD are frequent in the third or fourth decade of life. Patients with the rare homozygous form of the disease have no functioning LDL receptors and develop massive hypercholesterolemia, accelerated atherosclerosis, and death in the first to third decades. Five percent of patients with myocardial infarction below the age of 55 to 60 years have familial hypercholesterolemia.[41]

Although LDL receptor assays in fibroblasts and peripheral blood lymphocytes can be used to confirm the presence of the LDL receptor defect in patients with heterozygous familial hypercholesterolemia,[34] these tests are usually not necessary to establish the diagnosis since the patient often has the triad of (1) tendinous xanthomas, (2) LDL-C levels greater than 250 mg/dl, and (3) a family history of severe hypercholesterolemia and/or premature CHD in approximately 50% of the patient's first degree relatives.

It is important to screen relatives of patients with familial hypercholesterolemia for lipid abnormalities. With affected adult relatives, teenagers' serum total cholesterol will nearly always exceed 250 mg/dl. The elevation in LDL-C is apparent at birth (and should be two to three times the level of a normal neonate). In adults adequate treatment often requires diet, a bile acid sequestrant, and an HMG CoA reductase inhibitor. Some patients require three or four drugs. Although lovastatin and the other HMG CoA reductase inhibitors are not currently recommended as the first step in drug therapy for patients with elevated LDL-C levels, an argument can be made for initiating therapy with one of these agents in patients with heterozygous familial hypercholesterolemia.

Familial combined hyperlipidemia

Goldstein et al[42] proposed this designation, familial combined hyperlipidemia (FCHL), to characterize families exhibiting multiple lipoprotein phenotypes (IIa, IIb, IV, and occasionally V). These investigators originally suggested that an autosomal dominant mode of inheritance was present in this syndrome as it is in familial hypercholesterolemia. Unfortunately, there is no unique marker for this syndrome, thus impairing the ability to determine its prevalence or

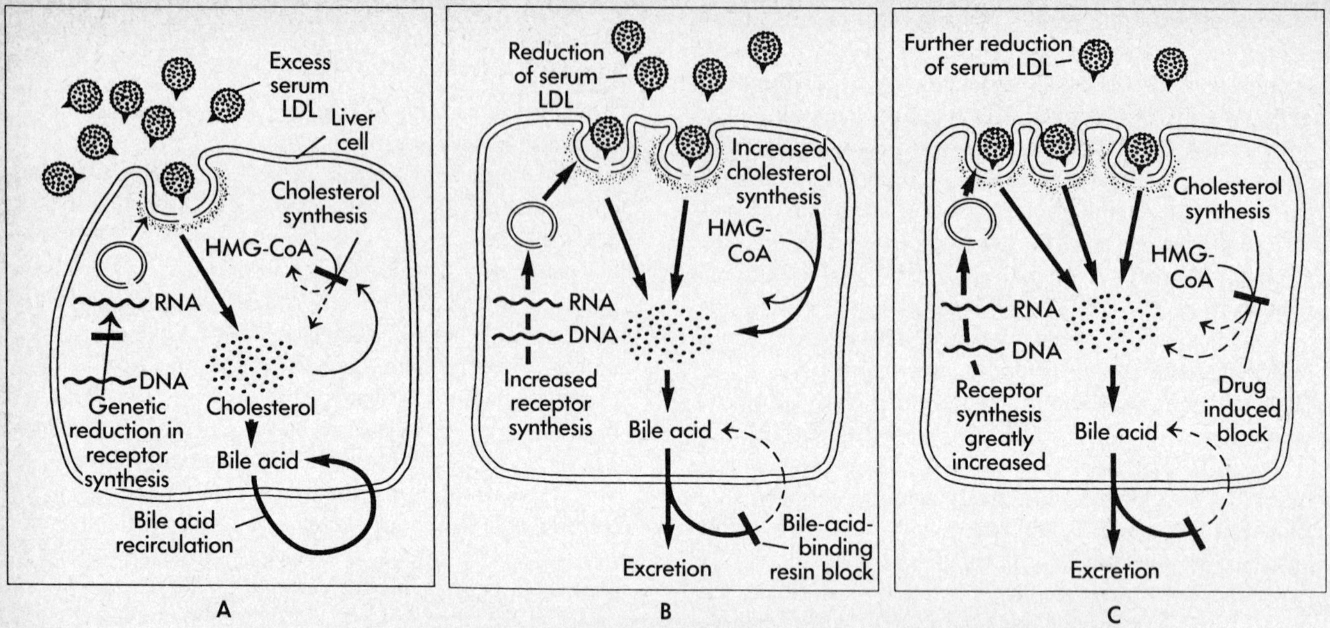

Fig. 8-3. Liver cells in heterozygote familial hypercholesterolemia, **A,** produce only half the normal number of LDL receptors. As a result, LDL accumulates in serum. Treatment with a resin that binds bile acids, **B,** reduces intracellular cholesterol slightly and thereby up regulates receptor synthesis and lowers serum LDL; however, the effect is partially offset by increased cholesterol synthesis. Addition of a drug that blocks this process, **C,** up regulates receptor formation still further and produces near-normal LDL serum levels. (From Goldstein JL and Brown MS: Hosp Pract 20:35, 1985.)

mode of inheritance precisely. The diagnosis depends on finding elevated levels of cholesterol and triglycerides in affected patients and their first degree relatives. Multiple lipoprotein phenotypes are often observed in a single patient. In addition to the abnormalities of lipoprotein concentration, the composition of lipoproteins is often abnormal, and there is an increased risk of premature CHD in these families.[43] Ten percent of patients less than 60 years old with myocardial infarction have FCHL.

The LDL fraction often contains a wide range of LDL particle size and a high number of small, dense LDL particles with a relative reduction in cholesterol. The concentration of apoB in whole plasma is often increased, but the LDL-C level may be normal. The situation is analogous to the hyperapobetalipoproteinemia syndrome described by Sniderman et al.[44] Perhaps these structural abnormalities contribute to the high risk of premature CHD noted in patients with this syndrome.

The nature of the metabolic defect(s) leading to FCHL is not clear. Several lines of evidence suggest that there is an increased hepatic apoB synthetic rate.[45] This could lead to simultaneous overproduction of LDL. However, the fractional catabolic rate of LDL tends to be high so that LDL levels, and particularly LDL-C levels, may not be increased. Thus in patients with FCHL there apparently is overproduction of apoB-containing lipoproteins, many of which are small, dense, and possibly highly atherogenic.

It seems prudent to recommend a diet moderately low in saturated fat and cholesterol and low in calories if the patient is obese. However, weight reduction may cause a paradoxic rise in LDL-C when triglycerides are reduced in patients with this syndrome. Nicotinic acid seems the most logical drug to use since it reduces synthesis of all of the apoB-containing lipoproteins, increases lipoprotein lipase activity, and raises HDL-C. Bile acid sequestrants can be added to nicotinic acid if LDL-C levels remain high. The bile acid sequestrants or lovastatin have been given in combination with gemfibrozil as well.[46]

Lipoprotein(a)

Lipoprotein(a), or Lp(a), is an atherogenic lipoprotein structurally related to LDL.[40] The lipid composition of Lp(a) and LDL is similar, and both of these cholesterol-rich lipoproteins contain apoB. The presence of a glycoprotein, apo(a), that is covalently bound to apoB in the Lp(a) accounts for the immunologic properties of Lp(a) and its higher density when compared to LDL. Apo(a) may be responsible for the markedly reduced binding of Lp(a) by the hepatic LDL receptor. Lp(a) apparently is synthesized by the liver, but its route of catabolism is not known.[47] Serum Lp(a) does not appear to interact with other lipoproteins, and Lp(a) levels do not correlate with other lipoprotein levels.

Lp(a) levels apparently are primarily under genetic control, with different Lp(a) glycoprotein phenotypes related to serum Lp(a) concentrations.[40] The Lp(a) glycoprotein phenotypes associated with the highest Lp(a) levels are relatively uncommon in the population so that the frequency of distribution of Lp(a) levels is highly skewed, with higher frequencies of low Lp(a) values. This skewed distribution of Lp(a) levels has been observed in all Caucasian populations studied. Hoefler et al[48] found that approximately 15% of 1486 white men had Lp(a) levels greater than 25 mg/dl, which are associated with approximately a two and one-half higher risk of myocardial infarction.[48] Similar conclusions were reached by Kostner et al.[49] At this time, few laboratories routinely measure serum Lp(a) levels, but there is interest in including this assay in patients with significant atherosclerosis and no apparent risk factors. Lp(a) levels are not affected by diet, and the only drugs known to reduce Lp(a) levels are neomyocin and nicotinic acid.[50]

Familial hypoalphalipoproteinemia

Most of the current knowledge about the relationship between HDLs and atherosclerosis is derived from studies relying on measurement of cholesterol in HDLs (HDL-C). These studies have generally shown that patients with HDL-C in the lowest decile of the HDL-C distribution have a high risk of atherosclerosis. This correlates with an HDL-C level of approximately 35 mg/dl or less. A variety of factors such as physical activity, diet composition, triglyceride levels, estrogen levels, and smoking habits influences HDL-C levels, but it appears that genetic factors play a major role in the etiology of low HDL levels in 50% of these individuals.[31] This syndrome seems to be inherited in an autosomal dominant mode and is characterized by premature atherosclerosis without corneal opacifications or xanthomas. It is estimated that as many as one third of patients with premature CHD have this syndrome. There is no specific way to establish this genotypic diagnosis; the presence of HDL-C levels less than 35 mg/dl in a patient and in approximately 50% of his relatives is suggestive. This is particularly true if obesity, diabetes mellitus, or hypertriglyceridemia is not present.

Several rare genetic HDL deficiency states have been identified, including familial lechithin, cholesterol acyltransferase deficiency, fish eye disease, Tangier disease, and several syndromes caused by the presence of apoA-1 mutations. Corneal opacifications are often present in these uncommon disorders. A detailed discussion of these syndromes is beyond the scope of this text but may be found in the comprehensive review edited by Angel and Frohlich.[51]

EVALUATION OF THE PATIENT WITH HYPERLIPIDEMIA

The principal goals of the evaluation of the patient with a presumed or documented dyslipoproteinemia are to (1) confirm the presence of the lipoprotein disorder, (2) assess the patient's overall state of health, (3) evaluate and treat other cardiovascular risk factors, (4) detect the presence of atherosclerotic vascular disease, and (5) rule out secondary causes of dyslipoproteinemia. Detection of abnormalities in lipoprotein metabolism may result from cholesterol screening programs or during patient contact with a physician in the office setting.

SECONDARY DYSLIPIDEMIAS

In addition to the primary hyperlipidemias many other factors and diseases can influence serum lipoprotein metabolism, producing a secondary dyslipoproteinemia.[52] The common causes of secondary dyslipoproteinemias are shown in the accompanying box.

In the Lipid Research Clinics Prevalence Study, less than 10% of the dyslipoproteinemias could be attributed to other diseases on the basis of laboratory abnormalities.[53] However, if obesity, alcohol use, medications, or menopause are included, the prevalence of secondary forms is considerably higher. The importance of identifying secondary causes of dyslipoproteinemia is that alteration of the secondary factor may ameliorate the lipid disorder. In patients with primary lipid and lipoprotein abnormalities, secondary factors may exacerbate the lipid abnormalities.

Obesity is commonly associated with hypercholesterolemia, hypertriglyceridemia, and low HDL-C levels. Hypertriglyceridemia and low HDL-C are particularly common and, when detected, should prompt a careful assessment of glucose metabolism. Weight reduction may alleviate the lipid disorder, reduce fasting blood glucose levels, correct hyperinsulinemia, and decrease blood pressure. Of particular importance is upper body (android) obesity. It is as-

Causes of secondary dyslipoproteinemia

Common

Obesity
Ethanol use
Diabetes mellitus
Hypothyroidism
Obstructive liver disease
Chronic renal failure
Nephrotic syndrome
Medication (β-blockers, diuretics, isotretinoin, etretinate, cyclosporine A, progesterones, estrogens, corticosteroids)
Menopause

Uncommon

Cushing's syndrome
Pancreatitis
Dysgammaglobulinemia
Glycogen storage disease
Acute intermittent porphyria

sociated with a waist:hip ratio greater than 0.85 and is associated with increased cardiovascular risk.[54,55] Alcohol consumption contributes to obesity and also may adversely affect lipoprotein metabolism, leading to elevations in triglycerides and VLDL levels even in the absence of obesity. Alcohol also may contribute to the development of hypertension and may worsen glucose tolerance.

The CHD mortality rate is two to four times higher in diabetics than in nondiabetics and is the main cause of death in patients with noninsulin dependent diabetes mellitus (NIDDM) and insulin dependent diabetes mellitus (IDDM). The relative risk of cardiovascular death in diabetic vs nondiabetic individuals was 2.1 for men and 4.9 for women in the Framingham Study.[56] Even mild abnormalities of glucose metabolism increased the risk of CHD mortality. Lipid disorders may contribute to the increased risk of atherosclerosis in diabetics. As noted previously, there is controversy regarding the role of high plasma triglyceride levels (the most common lipid abnormality in patients with diabetes) and CHD. The low HDL-C levels frequently observed in these patients may contribute to this risk. Alterations in metabolism of VLDLs and LDLs may cause certain lipoproteins to be particularly atherogenic. For example, hypertriglyceridemia may be a marker for the presence of increased levels of VLDL remnants or may be associated with small, dense LDLs. Massive hypertriglyceridemia and chylomicronemia with eruptive xanthomas, lipemia retinalis, and chronic abdominal pain or pancreatitis can occur in patients with poorly controlled diabetes. In treating the dyslipidemia of diabetes, achievement of ideal body weight and control of blood sugar with diet, oral hypoglycemics, and/or insulin often correct the underlying lipid disturbance. Lipid-lowering drug therapy should be used when good diabetic control alone is not effective.[57]

In patients with hypothyroidism TC, VLDL-C, and LDL-C may all be increased.[52,58,59] There are increased synthesis and decreased catabolism of LDL. The association of elevated cholesterol with hypothyroidism has been recognized for many years and was used as an aid to the diagnosis of hypothyroidism in the past. Patients with "subclinical hypothyroidism" (elevated thyroid-stimulating hormone levels with normal thyroxine levels) may also develop hypercholesterolemia.[59] Treatment of hypothyroidism with thyroid replacement usually improves or corrects the underlying lipid abnormality.

A variety of abnormalities of lipoprotein concentration and/or composition occurs in patients with chronic renal failure.[60,61] Hypertriglyceridemia and low HDL-C levels are the most frequently observed abnormalities. It is not certain if the abnormalities in lipoprotein metabolism contribute to the development of progression of atherosclerosis in these patients. Marked hypercholesterolemia frequently occurs in patients with nephrotic syndrome.[60] Overproduction of apoB-containing lipoproteins by the liver apparently is the major cause of these abnormalities. There is considerable controversy about the role of the dyslipoproteinemia of nephrotic syndrome in the development of atherosclerosis.

Certain drugs (see Table 8-5) may adversely affect blood lipids and lipoproteins. In some patients β-blockers (except those with both α- and β-blocking activity or those with intrinsic sympathomimetic activity)[62] and diuretics may increase triglycerides and decrease HDL-C. Isotretinoin[63] and etretinate may cause marked hypertriglyceridemia and modest increases in TC and LDL-C. Progestins may increase LDL-C and decrease HDL-C, and some progestins may reverse the beneficial effect of postmenopausal estrogen replacement on HDL-C.[64] Several studies suggest a beneficial effect of postmenopausal estrogen therapy on HDL-C levels and cardiovascular mortality.[65,66] Estrogens may also elevate triglycerides in some patients. Corticosteroids may also have an adverse effect on blood lipids.

A detailed discussion of other causes of secondary hyperlipidemia is beyond the scope of this text.

The most useful laboratory tests that should be included in the evaluation of patients with hypercholesterolemia or other lipoprotein abnormalities include measurement of (1) fasting blood glucose, (2) thyroid-stimulating hormone, (3) alkaline phosphatase, (4) serum creatinine, (5) serum albumin, and (6) urinalysis. Most of the secondary dyslipoproteinemias will be detected with these relatively inexpensive tests.

EYE AND SKIN MANIFESTATIONS OF HYPERLIPIDEMIAS

During the physical examination several ocular and cutaneous abnormalities may suggest the presence of an abnormality of lipoprotein metabolism or suggest a specific genotypic or phenotypic dyslipidemic state. Xanthomas (yellow to gray plaques on the eyelids and periorbital skin) and corneal arcus (a light gray pigment deposition in the periphery of the cornea) are seen with increased frequency with aging and may be associated with presence of hypercholesterolemia. In the Lipid Research Clinics Program Prevalence Study xanthomas were noted in approximately 1% of the 8998 study participants, and corneal arcus was present in approximately 20%.[67] Corneal arcus was more common in blacks than whites and more prevalent in men than in women. The presence of xanthomas and corneal arcus was associated with an increased risk for developing ischemic heart disease, particularly in men less than 49 years of age, but it was not associated with manifestations of peripheral arterial disease. The clinical findings of xanthomas or corneal arcus, especially in younger patients, should serve as a reminder to assess lipid status and other cardiovascular risk factors.

Lipemia retinalis, which is a salmon or creamy coloration of the retinal blood vessels, occurs with marked elevation of triglycerides to greater than 2500 mg/dl. These patients usually have fasting hyperchylomicronemia and a phenotype V dyslipoproteinemia.

Cutaneous markers for lipoprotein disorders are associated with both primary and secondary lipid disorders.[68] Deposition of lipids, lipoproteins, and their remnants in tissues close to the surface of the body causes xanthomas of various types. Recognition of these physical findings should lead to a complete lipoprotein evaluation and may allow the physician to recognize specific disease states. The type of lesion frequently correlates with the types of lipid or lipoproteins that are elevated.

Tendon xanthomas are firm to hard subcutaneous nodules with normal-appearing overlying skin that can be moved over the nodules easily. These xanthomas are often noted as a swelling or prominence in the Achilles tendon or on the extensor tendons of the digits. Tendon xanthomas strongly suggest the presence of familial hypercholesterolemia. Two unusual disorders produce tendon xanthomas because of accumulation of other steroid molecules: (1) cerebrotendinous xanthomatosis is a disorder of bile acid metabolism; and (2) β-sitosterolemia is due to accumulation of plant sterols. Both of these conditions are rare and are associated with an increased risk for the development of atherosclerosis.

Eruptive xanthomas are reddish-yellow, 1 to 4 mm dermal papules that are somewhat acneiform in appearance and develop rapidly in crops or showers. They tend to form on the extensor surface of the hands, arms, knees, and buttocks. They can also arise on the flexor creases, the face, or in areas of trauma. Acutely they may be quite pruritic and tender. Eruptive xanthomas usually occur in patients with hyperchylomicronemia from primary or secondary causes. They tend to resolve rapidly with treatment of the lipid disorder.

Tuberoeruptive and tuberous xanthomas appear on the elbows, knees, and buttocks and less commonly in other areas. The tuberous form is nodular and noninflammatory. The tuberoeruptive xanthomas have an inflammatory component that begins as dermal papules. They are most commonly seen in association with familial dysbetablipoproteinemia (type III) or heterozygous familial hypercholesterolemia.

Planar xanthomas may be diffuse or well-circumscribed noninflammatory dermal macules or plaques. Intertriginous xanthomas are slightly raised yellow plaques with a cobblestone-like surface seen in the finger web spaces and sometimes in the axillary antecubital and popliteal fossae. They are pathognomonic for homozygous familial hypercholesterolemia.

Palmar crease xanthomas (xanthoma palmeris striatum) are identified as a yellow-to-orange discoloration in the creases of the palms and fingers that is very easily overlooked. They are pathognomonic of familial dysbetalipoproteinemia (type III).

SCREENING OF LIPID ABNORMALITIES

On the basis of the Framingham Study, MRFIT, and other[1-3] population-based epidemiologic studies, one may identify most patients at increased risk by measuring total serum cholesterol. In most people the major contributor to the total serum cholesterol value is LDL-C. Total concentrations of cholesterol in the blood are not markedly affected by ingestion of a meal. Therefore, fasting is not required when TC levels are used as a screening tool. This observation and the low cost of total serum cholesterol measurements are major advantages.

However, there are several major limitations of screening people using only a TC determination, including the following: (1) variability of cholesterol measurements: (2) failure to detect potentially significant dyslipidemias such as low HDL-C; (3) failure to discriminate high levels of HDL-C; and (4) variability of non-fasting cholesterol as a result of changes in chylomicrons or VLDL-C concentration.

The quality and reproducibility of cholesterol determinations are quite variable. The use of automated methods or fingerstick determinations of capillary cholesterol is common but may have coefficients of variation as wide as 10%. Consequently, a TC determination of 230 mg/dl might be as low as 207 mg/dl or as high as 253 mg/dl. These values may have different implications for further evaluation and treatment. In fact, management decisions should only be made using precise measurements on multiple tests.

The evidence that low HDL-C is associated with increased risk for atherosclerotic vascular disease is quite convincing,[8,10] and, in fact, there is suggestive evidence that raising HDL-C may reduce the risk for CHD events.[13,25] In 125 consecutive patients with lower-extremity arteriosclerosis obliterans at our institution, 48% of patients had low HDL-C, and 28% of the entire group had TC less than 200 mg/dl.[69] Anderson et al[11] showed that the prevalence of HDL-C less than 35 mg/dl was 14% in men and 4% in women with TC levels less than 200 mg/dl in a screened working population.

Not all elevations of TC are associated with an increased risk of CHD. This is true for a subgroup of people with high HDL-C levels and includes many women—especially premenopausal women and postmenopausal women receiving estrogen therapy. According to Framingham data, a person with an LDL-C level of 100 mg/dl and an HDL-C level of 25 has a higher risk for the development of CHD (relative risk, 1.2) than a person with an LDL-C level of 220 and HDL-C level of 80 (relative risk, 0.3).[70] Frequently, undue anxiety is generated by the use of high TC levels alone, and such persons may initiate unnecessarily restrictive diets and inappropriate over-the-counter medications; in some cases physicians who treat on the basis of TC alone may initiate the use of lipid-lowering drugs.

Each of these problems has been addressed in the report of the National Cholesterol Education Program (NCEP) expert panel on Detection, Evaluation and Treatment of High Blood Cholesterol in Adults.[71] The NCEP guidelines suggest that all adults over 20 years of age have a random TC determination. For all persons whose TC is greater than 200 mg/dl, a repeat TC measurement should be obtained. If the TC remains greater than 200 mg/dl on repeat measurement, a complete lipid profile should be performed. Treatment

Table 8-4. Treatment decisions based on LDL-cholesterol

Type of treatment	Initiation level (mg/dl)	Minimal goal (mg/dl)
Dietary		
Without CHD *or* two other risk factors	≥160	<160
With CHD *or* two other risk factors	≥130	<130
Drug		
Without CHD or two other risk factors	≥190	<160
With CHD or two other risk factors	≥160	<130

(From The Expert Panel: Arch Inter Med 148: 36-69, 1988.)

decisions are then made based on LDL-C levels and the patient's overall cardiovascular risk (Table 8-4). CHD risk factors are male sex, family history of premature CHD, cigarette smoking, hypertension, low HDL-C (<35 mg/dl), diabetes mellitus, or severe obesity (≥30% overweight). Patients with known CHD or other vascular disease and those with two or more of these risk factors are considered as "high risk." The role of HDL-C levels in screening and therapeutic decisions has been the subject of considerable debate. This issue was addressed in a subsequent publication from the NCEP Working Group on HDL.[72] The Working Group concluded that HDL-C levels should not be used for screening based on several factors. First, the evidence that low HDL-C levels substantially increase the risk for CHD when cholesterol levels are below 200 is inconclusive. Second, the cost and complexity of screening would be increased if routine HDL-C levels were obtained. Finally, HDL-C determinations are somewhat complex and subject to considerable error. In fact, some commonly used methods systematically underestimate true HDL-C concentrations. Concerns also were raised about the difficulty of raising HDL-C levels and the relative paucity of data from intervention trials supporting such a strategy. Clinical trials using interventions to elevate HDL-C also produced significant reduction in LDL-C and triglyceride levels. The clinical implications of HDL-C were recently reviewed by Gordon and Rifkind.[12]

DIETARY TREATMENT OF LIPID DISTURBANCES

The initial steps to lower cholesterol involve dietary intervention. Useful dietary guidelines are outlined in the NCEP report.[71] For obese persons the first goal is to reduce calories to achieve desirable body weight. The next major step is to reduce the total fat intake in the diet to 30% or less of the total calories. Since saturated fat contributes more substantially to elevations of LDL-C than polyunsaturated or monounsaturated fat, the total saturated fat intake should be reduced to 10%. Saturated fat intake should be reduced to less than 7% of total calories for persons whose cholesterol levels are not reduced to target levels with the 10% saturated fat ingestion level. The most common sources of saturated fat in the American diet are hamburger meat, other red meats, fried foods, and dairy products, including milk and cheese. Increasing the quantity of fish and poultry and changing the nature of dairy products to skim milk and nonfat cheese may help bring the diet into conformity with these recommendations for saturated fat intake. The third major goal is to reduce the amount of cholesterol intake to less than 300 mg/day (or 100 mg/1000 kcal/day).This usually occurs if saturated fat intake is reduced. Common sources of cholesterol include egg yolks, organ meats, shell fish, and animal meats. Increasing dietary fiber, especially soluble fiber such as that found in oats, lentils, and beans has a beneficial effect on lipid levels. Additional dietary recommendations include the restriction of ethanol ingestion, especially in obese patients for whom it is a source of "empty" calories and in persons with elevated triglyceride levels. There is a suggestion that increasing the quantity of monounsaturated fats in the diet to 10% of the total calories (with an increase in total fat to 35% of total calories) may have a beneficial effect on lipid profiles by increasing the HDL-C levels. Oat bran or psyllium hydrophilic mucilloid may be helpful in further lowering TC and LDL-C.

Fast foods, snack foods, and restaurant dining account for a large amount of the increased fat intake in the United States. The commonly used vegetable oils in the fast food industry and in many snack foods include coconut oil, palm oil, and palm kernel oil. These oils contain a large amount of saturated fats. Their widespread use is the result of stability with storage and heating as well as general palatability. Furthermore, many restaurants use butters and sauces containing saturated fats to enhance the flavor of their meals. Persons on cholesterol-lowering diets must be instructed in these more subtle forms of fat intake in conjunction with overall proper nutrition instruction. Dietary counseling by a registered dietitian is recommended for all patients who do not have a satisfactory dietary response to physician counseling alone. Table 8-4 provides useful guidelines for treatment based on LDL-C.

PHARMACOLOGIC TREATMENT OF LIPID DISORDERS (Table 8-5)

Specific pharmacologic therapy generally includes the use of five major drug groups as well as a number of other drugs.

Nicotinic acid[73-76] is a very effective drug for lowering VLDL-C and LDL-C and is an effective agent to raise HDL-C. It is inexpensive and readily available. Major limiting factors include symptomatic flushing, which can be managed by starting at relatively low doses and increasing the

Table 8-5. Drugs that lower blood lipids

Drug	Affect on lipoproteins	Mechanism of action	Dose	Side effects
Nicotinic acid (Niacin)	↓↓ VLDL ↓↓ LDL ↑↑↑ HDL	Inhibits lipoprotein synthesis Inhibits apolipoprotein B synthesis	1500-6000 mg/day	Flushing Itching Gastrointestinal intolerance Hepatic toxicity Gout Glucose intolerance
Gemfibrozil (Lopid)	↓↓↓ VLDL ↓ LDL ↑↑ HDL	Inhibits lipoprotein synthesis Increases lipoprotein lipase activity	600 mg bid	Gastrointestinal intolerance Myositis (rare)
Bile acid resins Cholestyramine (Questran) Colestipol (Colestid)	→↑ VLDL ↓↓ LDL →HDL	Increases clearance of cholesterol by binding bile acids Increases LDL receptor; mediates catabolism of LDL cholesterol	4-8 g tid 5-10 g tid	Gastrointestinal bloating and constipation Increased triglycerides
HMG CoA reductase inhibitors Lovastatin (Mevacor)	↓ VLDL ↓↓↓ LDL ↑ HDL	Inhibits the rate-limiting enzyme in cholesterol synthesis Inhibits apolipoprotein B synthesis Increases LDL receptor–mediated catabolism of LDL cholesterol	20 mg qd up to 40 bid	Gastrointestinal intolerance Liver toxicity Myositis
Probucol (Lorelco)	→ VLDL ↓ LDL ↓↓ HDL	Inhibits oxidation of LDL cholesterol Increases nonreceptor-mediated low density lipoprotein catabolism	250-500 bid	Gastrointestinal intolerance Prolongation of QT interval

dose over a period of weeks. In general, 1.5 g/day is an effective dose in many patients, although higher doses (3 to 6 g) are commonly recommended, especially if the goal is to increase HDL-C substantially. The incidence of flushing is high but tends to remit if doses are limited to less than 2 g/day. Flushing may be reduced by taking the nicotinic acid in conjunction with food, by avoiding ingestion with hot liquids, or by taking an aspirin tablet 1 hour before ingesting nicotinic acid. Other side effects include gastrointestinal side effects and hepatic toxicity (the latter may be worse with the timed-release preparations).[75,76] Liver enzymes should be measured periodically. Nicotinic acid also causes insulin resistance and therefore may raise blood glucose. Significant blood glucose elevations are relatively uncommon in nondiabetic patients, and the effect on insulin dosage in type I diabetic patients is modest. A major concern is for those patients who have evidence of impaired glucose tolerance (i.e., type II diabetic patients). Nicotinic acid should not be used in patients with active peptic ulcer disease or acute gout. It is useful in treating all types of lipid disturbances except when chylomicrons are elevated.

The *fibric acid derivatives*[73,74,77-80] are characterized by the capability to lower VLDL-C. As demonstrated in the Helsinki Heart Study, they may also lower LDL-C. They also raise HDL-C. In many patients with marked elevations of triglycerides (i.e., VLDL), lowering of VLDL is associated with increased levels of LDL. The exact impact of this on the risk for patients with CHD is as yet unknown. Currently available drugs include clofibrate, which has been associated with an increased risk for gallstones and malignancies and is now very rarely used, and gemfibrozil, which has been available for a shorter period of time, has not been associated with these abnormalities, and is generally well tolerated. These drugs may rarely be associated with myositis, especially when given in high doses or when combined with lovastatin. Fenofibrate, an experimental drug in the United States, may be available in the near future. This class of drugs may be used in patients with endogenous hypertriglyceridemia, familial combined hyperlipidemia, dysbetalipoproteinemia, and polygenic hypercholesterolemia. They are useful in treating type V hyperlipidemia.[81]

The *bile acid binding resins*[73,74,82,83] include cholestyramine and colestipol. Their major effect is to lower LDL-C. The resins bind bile acids in the gut and increase cholesterol secretion into the bile, thus helping to clear cholesterol from the body. The major side effects are associated with gastrointestinal bloating and constipation, which limit compliance in many patients. With continued use, the incidence of side effects seems to reduce. In patients with a predisposition to elevations of VLDL, these levels may be made worse by the resins.[83] In addition, the resins may bind other drugs such as coumarin (Coumadin), L-thyroxine, and thiazides. Recent reports suggest that they delay the absorption of β-blockers; however, it is not clear whether they have an impact on the integrated effect of such drugs. These agents are useful first-line drugs to treat increases in LDL-C. They have no significant effect on HDL-C.

The fourth major category of drugs comprises the *HMG CoA reductase inhibitors*.[84-90] They work most effectively to lower LDL-C. There is limited effect on lowering VLDL-C and increasing HDL-C. The mechanism of action is to block HMG CoA reductase, which is the rate-limiting enzyme of cholesterol synthesis in the liver. This reduction in cholesterol synthesis causes a decrease in intracellular cholesterol stores, with a corresponding increase in the hepatic LDL receptor numbers, which helps to lower plasma LDL-C concentration. The HMG CoA reductase inhibitors comprise the most effective drug class for patients with heterozygous familial hypercholesterolemia. They are generally well tolerated with a low incidence of side effects. Because of concerns about hepatic toxicity that may occur late, patients taking these medications need their liver enzymes (aspartate transaminase or alanine transaminase) checked every 6 weeks for at least the first 15 months. Slight elevations occur in approximately 3% of people, although they do not always necessitate discontinuing the drugs. When the liver enzymes increase to greater than three times normal, the medication should be stopped. There apparently is an increased risk for lens opacities in animals receiving large doses of this medication. Baseline and annual ophthalmologic examinations to check for cataracts are recommended for humans who are placed on these drugs; however, there is no direct evidence that cataracts form in humans as a result of the HMG CoA reductase inhibitors. Another side effect is myositis. The risk for myositis apparently increases when these drugs are used in conjunction with cyclosporine A, nicotinic acid, or gemfibrozil. HMG CoA reductase inhibitors should be discontinued when patients are in the hospital because the incidence of rhabdomyolysis is increased in those undergoing surgery.

These agents are the most effective and the best tolerated of all drugs available to lower blood lipids. They are also

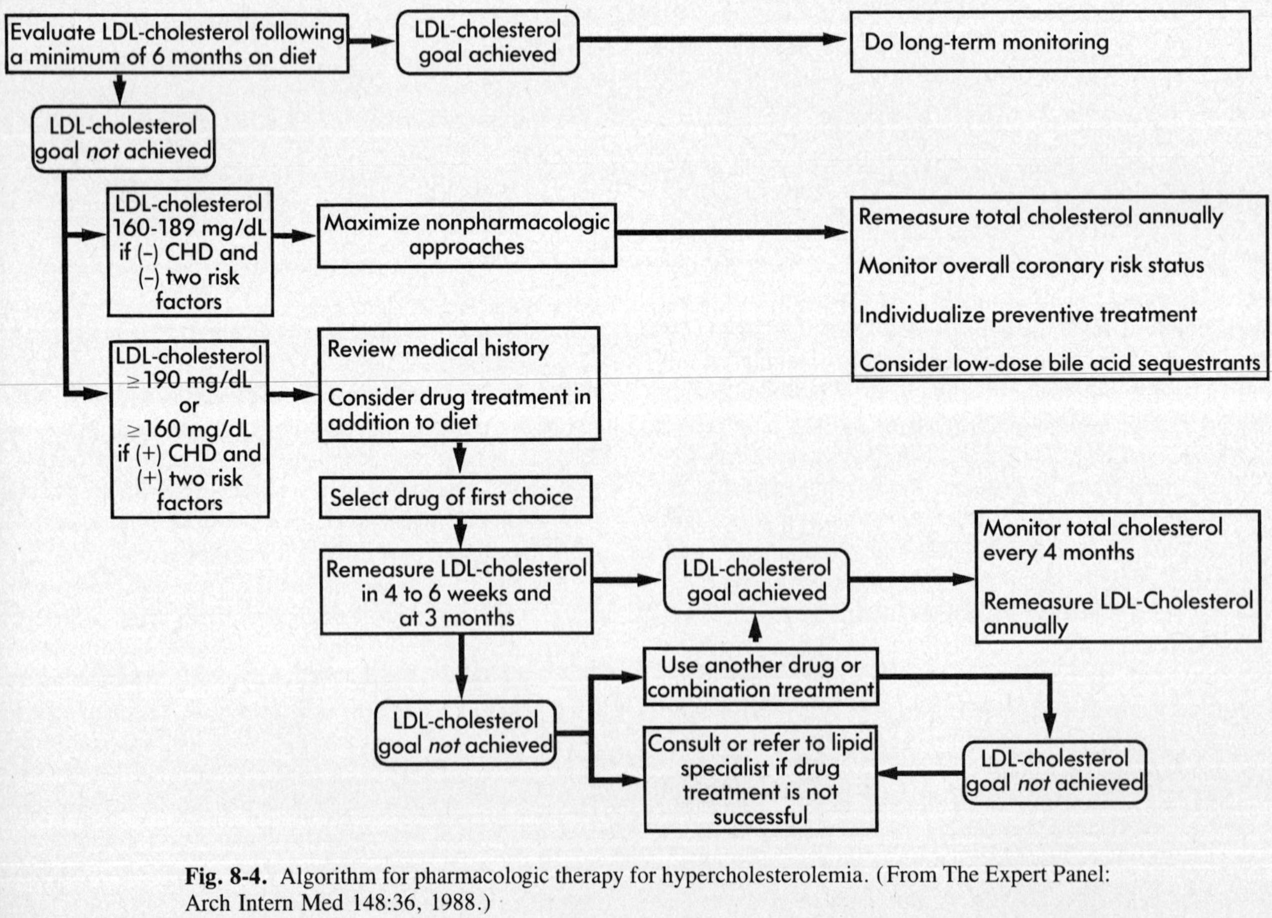

Fig. 8-4. Algorithm for pharmacologic therapy for hypercholesterolemia. (From The Expert Panel: Arch Intern Med 148:36, 1988.)

the most expensive, limiting their use as a first-line drug. They should be used for patients with heterozygous familial hyperlipidemia, in combination with other drugs when necessary, or in patients who cannot tolerate other cholesterol-lowering agents. A number of new HMG CoA reductase inhibitors will be on the market in the near future.

Probucol[73,74] is a very commonly used drug that lowers both LDL-C and HDL-C. It has not been tested in any major clinical trial, so its efficacy, considering it can reduce HDL-C, as an agent to lower CHD is unproven. It is very effective in lowering cholesterol in animal models, and xanthomas may regress in some patients. It is a potent antioxidant, and this may be its main beneficial effect since oxidized LDL-C is a very potent stimulator of foam cell production, an early step in the formation of the atherosclerotic plaque. Many investigators have some hesitancy about its use in view of all the epidemiologic data that have demonstrated an association of low HDL-C and increased risk for atherosclerotic vascular disease. Side effects include gastrointestinal side effects and a tendency to prolong the QT interval on an ECG. Probucol should be used cautiously in patients receiving therapy to increase the QT interval or with a history of cardiac arrhythmias.

Other agents may be used in selected circumstances to lower cholesterol. They include L-thyroxine for patients with hypothyroidism (marked elevations of cholesterol may occur with hypothyroidism) and sulfonylureas or insulin to achieve rigorous control of blood sugar in patients with elevations of VLDL-C and reductions of HDL-C and estrogens, which may elevate HDL-C. D-thyroxine, neomycin, and psyllium hydrophilic mucilloid have also been used in selected circumstances.

Omega-3 fatty acids[37,91] (i.e., eicosapentaenoic acid and docosahexaenoic acid) may be used as a third-line agent to lower triglycerides in patients who cannot tolerate gemfibrozil or nicotinic acid. They should probably be avoided in patients with NIDDM because of the potential to worsen glycemic control. Fish oil capsules are not recommended for use in the treatment of hypercholesterolemia.

Combinations of drugs may be particularly effective when the drugs work by different mechanisms of action and have major effects on different lipids and lipoproteins.[46] For example, nicotinic acid and the bile acid binding resins form a very effective combination in a number of clinical trials.[24,25] There are accumulating trials on the use of HMG CoA reductase inhibitors and bile acid binding resins,[25,87] particularly for patients with familial heterozygote hypercholesterolemia. Furthermore, many lipid experts find that using low doses of more than one agent frequently reduces the side effect profile and increases the efficacy. Hence, there is a trend away from using full doses of a single medication before moving to another medication. A useful algorithm for following patients receiving medication for lipid disturbances is shown in Fig. 8-4.

REFERENCES

1. Kannel WB, Castelli WP, and Gordon T: Cholesterol in the prediction of atherosclerotic disease. New perspectives based on the Framingham Study, Ann Intern Med 90:85, 1979.
2. Anderson KM, Castelli WP, and Levy D: Cholesterol and mortality—30 years of follow-up from the Framingham Study, JAMA 257:2176, 1987.
3. Stamler J, Wentworth D, and Neaton JD: Is the relationship between the serum cholesterol and risk of premature death from coronary heart disease continuous and graded? Findings in 356,222 primary screenees of the Multiple Risk Factor Intervention Trial (MRFIT), JAMA 256:2823, 1986.
4. Iso H et al: Serum cholesterol levels and 6 year mortality from stroke in 350,977 men screened for the Multiple Risk Factor Intervention Trial, N Engl J Med 320:904, 1989.
5. Tell GS, Crouse JR, and Furberg CD: Relation between blood lipids, lipoproteins and cerebrovascular atherosclerosis. A review, Stroke 19:423, 1988.
6. Pomrehn P et al: The association of dyslipoproteinemia with symptoms and signs of peripheral arterial disease. The Lipid Research Clinics Program Prevalence Study, Circulation 73(suppl I):I100, 1986.
7. Kannel WB, Gordon T, and Castelli WP: Role of lipids and lipoprotein fractions in assessing atherogenesis. The Framingham Study, Prog Lipid Res 20:339, 1981.
8. Gordon T et al: High density lipoprotein as a protective factor against coronary heart disease. The Framingham Study, Am J Med 62:707, 1977.
9. Castelli WB et al: The incidence of coronary heart disease and lipoprotein cholesterol levels: The Framingham Study, JAMA 256:2835, 1986.
10. Abbott RD et al: High density lipoprotein cholesterol, total cholesterol screening, and myocardial infarction. The Framingham Study, Arteriosclerosis 8:207, 1988.
11. Anderson AJ et al: The prevalence of low HDL cholesterol levels in three groups of patients with cholesterol less than 200 mg/dl, Circulation 80(suppl II):II538, 1989 (abstract).
12. Gordon DJ and Rifkind BM: High density lipoprotein—the clinical implications of recent studies, N Engl J Med 321:1311, 1989.
13. Frick MH et al: Helsinki Heart Study: Primary-Prevention Trial with gemfibrozil in middle aged men with dyslipidemia, N Engl J Med 317:1237, 1987.
14. Lipid Research Clinics Program: The Lipid Research Clinics Coronary Primary Prevention Trial results. I. Reduction in incidence of coronary heart disease, JAMA 251:351, 1984.
15. Lipid Research Clinics Program: The Lipid Research Clinics Coronary Primary Prevention Trial results. II. The relationship of reduction in incidence of coronary heart disease to cholesterol lowering, JAMA 251:365, 1984.
16. Anderson KM et al: Non-fasting VLDL and long-term cardiovascular disease mortality. The Framingham Study, CVD Epidemiol News Lett 41:30, 1987.
17. Austin MA: Plasma triglyceride as a risk factor for coronary heart disease: the epidemiologic evidence and beyond, Am J Epidemiol 129:249, 1989.
18. Gordon DJ et al: High density lipoprotein cholesterol and coronary heart disease in hypercholesterolemic men: The Lipid Research Clinics Coronary Primary Prevention Trial, Circulation 74:1217-1225, 1986.
19. Rifkind BM: Clinical trials in cholesterol lowering, Atherosclerosis Rev 18:59, 1988.
20. Pekkanen J et al: Serum cholesterol and risk of accidental or violent death in a 25-year follow-up, Arch Intern Med 149:1589, 1989.
21. Levy RI et al: The influence of changes in lipid values induced by cholestyramine and diet on progression of coronary artery disease: results of the NHLBI Type II Coronary Intervention Study, Circulation 69:325, 1984.

22. Canner PL: Fifteen year mortality in coronary drug project patients: long-term benefit with niacin, J Am Coll Cardiol 8:1245, 1986.
23. Arntzenius AC et al: Diet, lipoproteins, and the progression of coronary atherosclerosis. The Leiden Intervention Trial, N Engl J Med 312:805, 1985.
24. Blankenhorn DH et al: Beneficial effects of combined colestipol-niacin therapy on coronary atherosclerosis and coronary venous bypass grafts, JAMA 257:3233, 1987.
25. Brown BG et al: Niacin or lovastatin combined with colestipol, regress coronary atherosclerosis and prevent clinical events in men with elevated apolipoprotein B, Circulation 80(suppl II):II266, 1989 (abstract).
26. Sempos C et al: The prevalence of high blood cholesterol levels among adults in the United States, JAMA 262:45, 1989.
27. Schaefer EJ and Levy RI: Pathogenesis and management of lipoprotein disorders, N Engl J Med 312:1300, 1985.
28. Goldstein JL and Brown MS: Familial hypercholesterolemia: a genetic receptor disease, Hosp Pract 20:35, 1985.
29. Goldstein JL and Brown MS: The LDL receptor locus and the genetics of familial hypercholesterolemia, Annu Rev Genet 13:259, 1979.
30. Slater HR et al: Contribution of the receptor pathway to low density lipoprotein catabolism in humans. New methods for quantitation, Arteriosclerosis 4:604, 1984.
31. Krauss RM: Regulation of high density lipoprotein levels, Med Clin North Am 66:403, 1982.
32. Fredrickson DS, Levy RI, and Lees RS: Fat transport in lipoproteins—an integral approach to mechanisms and disorders, N Engl J Med 276:32-44, 94-103, 148-156, 215-226, 273-281, 1967.
33. Cuthbert JA et al: Detection of familial hypercholesterolemia by assaying functional low-density–lipoprotein receptors on lymphocytes, N Engl J Med 314:879, 1986.
34. Glueck CJ, Levy RI, and Fredrickson DS: Norethindrone acetate, postheparin lipolytic activity, and plasma triglycerides in familial Types I, III, IV and V hyperlipoproteinemia, Ann Intern Med 75:345, 1971.
35. Brunzell JD and Bierman EL: Chylomicronemia syndrome, Med Clin North Am 66:455, 1982.
36. Kissebah AH et al: The mechanism of action of clofibrate and tetranicotinoylfructose (Bradilan) on the kinetics of plasma free fatty acid and triglyceride transport in Type IV and Type V hypertriglyceridemia, Eur J Clin Invest 4:163, 1974.
37. Phillipson BE et al: The reduction of plasma lipids, lipoproteins and apoproteins in hypertriglyceridemic patients by dietary fish oils, N Engl J Med 312:1210, 1985.
38. Davignon J, Gregg RE, and Sing CF: Apolipoprotein E polymorphism and arteriosclerois, Arteriosclerosis 8:1, 1988.
39. Goldstein JL and Brown MS: Hyperlipidemia in coronary heart disease: a biochemical genetic approach, J Lab Clin Med 108:174, 1986.
40. Utermann G et al: LP(a) glycoprotein phenotypes. Inheritance and relation to LP(a)-lipoprotein concentrations in plasma, J Clin Invest 80:458, 1987.
41. Hazzard WR et al: Hyperlipidemia in coronary heart disease. III. Evaluation of lipoprotein phenotypes of 156 genetically survived survivors of myocardial infarction, J Clin Invest 52:1569, 1973.
42. Goldstein JL et al: Hyperlipidemia in coronary heart disease. II. Genetic analysis of lipid levels in 176 families and delineation of a new inherited disorder, combined hyperlipidemia, J Clin Invest 52:1544, 1973.
43. Grundy SM, Chait A, and Brunzell JD: Familial combined hyperlipidemia workshop, Arteriosclerosis 7:203, 1987.
44. Sniderman AS et al: Association of coronary atherosclerosis with hyperapobetalipoproteinemia (increased protein but normal cholesterol levels in human plasma low density [beta] lipoproteins), Proc Natl Acad Sci USA 77:604, 1980.
45. Kissebah AH, Alfarsi S, and Evans DJ: Low density lipoprotein metabolism in familial combined hyperlipidemia. Mechanism of the multiple lipoprotein phenotypic expression, Arteriosclerosis 4:614, 1984.
46. East C, Bilheimer DW, and Grundy SM: Combination drug therapy for familial combined hyperlipidemia, Ann Intern Med 109:25, 1988.
47. Krempler S et al: Turnover of lipoprotein(a) in man, J Clin Invest 65:1483, 1980.
48. Hoefler G et al: Lipoprotein Lp(a). A risk factor for myocardial infarction, Arteriosclerosis 8:398, 1988.
49. Kostner GM et al: Lipoprotein Lp(a) and the risk for myocardial infarction, Atherosclerosis 38:51, 1981.
50. Gurakar A et al: Levels of lipoprotein Lp(a) decline with neomycin and niacin treatment, Atherosclerosis 57:293, 1985.
51. Schaefer EJ et al: Genetic high density lipoprotein deficiency states in atherosclerosis. In Angel A and Frolich J, eds: Lipoprotein deficiency syndromes, New York, 1986, Plenum Press.
52. LaRosa JC: Secondary hyperlipoproteinemia. In Rifkin BM and Levy RI, eds: Hyperlipidemia: prognosis and therapy, New York, 1977, Grune & Stratton, Inc.
53. Wallace RS: The Lipid Research Clinics Program Prevalence Study. Alterations in clinical chemistry levels associated with dyslipoproteinemias, Circulation 73(suppl I):I62, 1986.
54. Peiris AN et al: Adiposity, fat distribution and cardiovascular risk, Ann Intern Med 110:677, 1989.
55. Kaplan NM: The deadly quartet. Upper-body obesity, glucose intolerance, hypertriglyceridemia and hypertension, Arch Intern Med 149:1514, 1989.
56. Kannel WB and McGee DL: Diabetes and cardiovascular disease. The Framingham Study, JAMA 241:2035, 1979.
57. Dunn FL: Treatment of lipid disorders in diabetes mellitus, Med Clin North Am 72:1379, 1988.
58. O'Reilly DSTJ: Hypercholesterolaemia and thyroid hormone status, J Endocrinol 118:349, 1988.
59. Althans BU et al: LDL/HDL–changes in subclinical hypothyroidism: possible risk factors for coronary heart disease, Clin Endocrinol 28:157, 1988.
60. Wheeler DC, Varghese Z, and Moorhead JF: Hyperlipidemia in nephrotic syndrome, Am J Nephrol 9(suppl I):78, 1989.
61. Grundy SM: Management of hyperlipidemia of kidney disease, Kidney Int 37:847, 1990.
62. Disler LJ, Joffe BI, and Seftel HC: Massive hypertriglyceridemia associated with atenolol, Am J Med 85:586, 1988.
63. Bershad S et al: Changes in plasma lipids and lipoproteins during Isotretinoin therapy for acne, N Engl J Med 313:981, 1985.
64. Hirvonen E, Malkonen M, and Manninen V: Effects of different progestogens on lipoproteins during post-menopausal replacement therapy, N Engl J Med 304:560, 1981.
65. Bush TC et al: Cardiovascular mortality and noncontraceptive use of estrogens in women: results from the Lipid Research Clinic Program Follow-Up Study, Circulation 75:1102, 1987.
66. Stampfer MJ et al: A prospective of post-menopausal estrogen therapy and coronary heart disease, N Engl J Med 313:1044, 1985.
67. Segal P et al: The association of dyslipoproteinemia with corneal arcus and xanthelasma. The Lipid Research Clinic Program Prevalence Study, Circulation 73(suppl I):I108, 1986.
68. Cruz PD, East C, and Bergstresser PR: Dermal, subcutaneous and tendon xanthomas: diagnostic markers for specific lipoprotein disorders, J Am Acad Dermatol 19:95, 1988.
69. Olin JW et al: Lipid and lipoprotein abnormalities in patients with atherosclerotic lower extremity vascular disease, Arteriosclerosis 8:A581, 1988.
70. Kannel W: Lipids, diabetes, and coronary heart disease: insights from the Framingham Study, Am Heart J 110:1100, 1985.

71. The Expert Panel: Report of the National Cholesterol Education Program Expert Panel on Detection, Evaluation and Treatment of High Blood Cholesterol in Adults, Arch Intern Med 148:36, 1988.
72. Grundy SM et al: The place of HDL cholesterol and cholesterol management. A perspective from the National Cholesterol Education Program, Arch Intern Med 149:505, 1989.
73. Illingworth DR: Lipid-lowering drugs: an overview of indications and optimum therapeutic use, Drugs 33:259, 1987.
74. Hunninghake DB: Pharmacologic therapy for the hyperlipidemic patient, Am J Med 74(suppl 5A):19, 1983.
75. Knopp RH et al: Contrasting effects of unmodified and time-release forms of niacin on lipoproteins and hyperlipidemic subjects: clues to mechanism of action, Metabolism 34:642, 1985.
76. Mullin GE, Greenson JK, and Mitchell MC: Fulminant hepatic failure after ingestion of sustained-release nicotinic acid, Ann Intern Med 111:253, 1989.
77. Samuel J: Effects of gemfibrozil on serum lipids, Am J Med 74(suppl 5A):23, 1983.
78. Gustafson A: Clofibrate and related compounds in hyperlipoproteinemia: review, Postgrad Med J 51(suppl 8):66, 1975.
79. Grundy SM and Vega GL: Fibric acids: effects on lipids and lipoprotein metabolism, Am J Med 83(suppl 5B):9, 1987.
80. Brown WV et al: Effects of fenofibrate on plasma lipids: double-blind, multicenter study in patients with Type IIA or IIB hyperlipidemia, Atherosclerosis 6:670, 1986.
81. Leaf DA et al: The hypolipidemic effects of gemfibrozil in Type V hyperlipidemia. A double-blind crossover study, JAMA 262:3154, 1989.
82. Heel RC et al: Colestipol: a review of its pharmacological properties and therapeutic efficacy in patients with hypercholesterolemia, Drugs 91:161, 1980.
83. Crouse JR: Hypertriglyceridemia: a contraindication to the use of bile acid binding resins, Am J Med 83:243, 1987.
84. Grundy SM: Drug therapy: HMG-CoA reductase inhibitors for the treatment of hypercholesterolemia, N Engl J Med 319:24, 1988.
85. Cressman MD et al: HMG-CoA reductase inhibitors: a new approach to the management of hypercholesterolemia, Cleve Clin J Med 55:93, 1988.
86. Hoeg JM and Brewer HB: Three-hydroxy-three-methylgluteryl-coenzyme A reductase inhibitors in the treatment of hypercholesterolemia, JAMA 258:3532, 1987.
87. The Lovastatin Study Group III: A multicenter comparison of lovastatin and cholestyramine therapy for severe primary hypercholesterolemia, JAMA 260:359, 1988.
88. The Lovastatin Study Group II: The therapeutic response to lovastatin (Mevinolin) in nonfamilial hypercholesterolemia. A multicenter study, JAMA 256:2829, 1986.
89. Illingworth DR: Mevinolin (lovastatin) plus colestipol in therapy for severe heterozygous familial hypercholesterolemia: a multicenter trial, Ann Intern Med 104:598, 1984.
90. Havel RJ et al: Lovastatin (Mevinolin) in the treatment of heterozygous familial hypercholesterolemia: a multicenter study, Ann Intern Med 107:609, 1987.
91. Herold PM and Kinsella JE: Fish oil consumption and decreased risk of cardiovascular disease: a comparison of findings from animal and human feeding trials, Am J Clin Nutr 43:566, 1986.

Chapter 9

ATHEROSCLEROSIS OF THE AORTA AND LOWER EXTREMITY ARTERIES

Leonard P. Krajewski
Jeffrey W. Olin

HISTORICAL PERSPECTIVES

Arteriosclerosis obliterans (ASO) of the aorta and lower extremities may involve the abdominal aorta and/or its major branches to both lower extremities. Atherosclerosis of the lower extremities occurs in various "patterns of disease."[1] These patterns may affect local segments of the arterial anatomy, or they may occur in combinations of multiple segments.[2] Recognition of the pattern of disease is extremely useful for a plan of management, whether that involves medical treatment, nonsurgical intervention, or surgical reconstruction.

The modern era of direct arterial repair of lower extremity occlusive vascular disease began in the early 1950s. The pioneering experiments in 1906 by Carrel and Guthrie[3,4] using vascular suture demonstrated that direct arterial reconstruction was technically feasible. During the first half of this century, the techniques of arteriography, blood transfusion, anesthetic management, anticoagulation, and antibiotics were developed and led to the ability to perform successful vascular reconstruction.[5] Before the early 1950s arterial grafting with venous replacements was occasionally reported. It was not until 1949 that Kunlin[6] reported a successful femoropopliteal bypass using reversed greater saphenous vein. In 1950 Oudot[7] replaced the aortoiliac bifurcation with an arterial homograft.

These two landmark reports started a new era of arterial reconstruction for lower extremity occlusive disease. Before this time lumbar sympathectomy and arteriectomy, as advocated by Leriche, were the only other recognized methods of surgical treatment. The technique of thromboendarterectomy had been introduced in 1947 when Jao Cid Dos Santos and his father Reynaldo[8] extended their interest in arterial embolectomy to perform "desobliteration" of the iliofemoral and subclavian-axillary segments. This technique was soon extended to the abdominal aorta and other peripheral arteries.[9] In the early 1950s the techniques of endarterectomy and vein bypass caught on rapidly and were used at a number of medical centers in the United States. Within a few years, fabric prostheses were created and used successfully as arterial replacements.[10] Extensive endarterectomy gradually fell into disfavor compared with either venous bypass grafts for femoropopliteal disease or Dacron prostheses for aorto-iliac-femoral reconstructions. During the 1950s and into the 1960s most lower extremity bypass reconstructions were performed to the above-knee popliteal artery and less commonly to the below-knee popliteal artery. A few reports of bypasses to tibial vessels were published in the early-to-mid 1960s, but it was not until the 1970s that larger series with acceptable results were reported.[11-13]

Interest in the use of the saphenous vein in a "nonreversed" position for lower extremity bypass reconstruction spread gradually.[14] However, this method proved to be very tedious and time-consuming because of the difficulty of reliable valve disruption. After Leather, Powers, and Karmody[15] reintroduced the "in situ" method for saphenous vein bypass in 1979, widespread interest in more distal tibial bypass occurred. In the United States, Leather et al developed new techniques and instrumentation that made valve disruption easier and more reproducible. Since then, the in situ method has become the preferred technique for infrapopliteal bypass by many surgeons when the ipsilateral saphenous vein is available, whereas Dacron replacement grafts remain the preferred method for aorto-iliac-femoral reconstructions.

INCIDENCE AND PREVALENCE

Information is sparse about the prevalence and incidence of ASO of the lower extremities in the general population. The most common initial symptom is intermittent claudication. In a literature review Dormandy et al[16] found that about 1.5% of men under 49 years and 5% of men over 50 years developed intermittent claudication during their lifetime. However, the incidence of asymptomatic arterial disease is much higher. Women have an incidence similar to that reported by Dormandy for men, but onset usually occurs later by 10 years, and the disease generally follows a more benign course. Only about 25% of patients progress to the point of requiring reconstructive surgery and less than 5% require a major amputation.

The onset of symptomatic disease usually occurs between 50 and 70 years of age. When lower extremity atherosclerosis does become symptomatic in patients under 50 years old, it generally follows a particularly virulent course. A study by McCready, Vincent, and Schwartz[17] identified 25 patients under the age of 40 years who required peripheral vascular reconstruction. All were heavy cigarette smokers. Interestingly, the ratio of men to women was approximately equal. All of these patients also had a strong family history of atherosclerotic disease, but only two of the men were diabetic. In this group of patients the incidence of repeat operations for both femoropopliteal and aortofemoral occlusive disease was very high. These data are contradicted in one study by Evans, Hayes, and Vermillion[18] who showed no significant difference in limb salvage/graft patency or mortality between younger and older patients. Further studies are necessary to resolve this controversy about ASO in individuals under 50 years of age.

ASSOCIATION OF ASO WITH CORONARY ARTERY DISEASE

During the past decade it has become increasingly clear that the presence of aortic and lower extremity ASO itself is a significant risk factor for death caused by myocardial infarction and stroke. When compared with the general population of comparable age, men with chronic leg ischemia have a mortality rate 2 to 3 times higher after 5 years. Approximately 50% of deaths are caused by myocardial infarction, 15% by stroke, and 10% by vascular disease in the abdomen. In only 25% is the principal cause of death unrelated to the circulation. Virtually no information is available on the incidence of nonfatal myocardial infarction or stroke in patients with lower extremity ASO. Population-based studies and follow-up studies of surgically treated patients indicate that for those individuals with lower extremity occlusive vascular disease the mortality rate at 5 years is approximately 30%, at 10 years 50%, and at 15 years 70%. An overall 10-year decline in life expectancy is seen in patients with lower extremity ASO.[19] The strong association of peripheral atherosclerosis with coronary artery disease is discussed in detail in Chapter 10.

RISK FACTORS AND ATHEROSCLEROSIS

The specific cause of atherosclerotic arterial plaque is a subject of intense research. Many important risk factors may be involved in the development of atherosclerosis. The cellular and biochemical events leading to the development of an atherosclerotic plaque are probably similar whether the plaque occurs in the coronary arteries or in the peripheral arterial circulation. These traditional risk factors include age and sex, presence of hypertension, diabetes, elevated total and LDL cholesterol levels, decreased HDL cholesterol levels, smoking, obesity, sedentary life-style, a family history of vascular disease, and genetic factors. In recent years other potential risk factors such as altered platelet function, abnormal levels of fibrinogen and fibrinolytic activity, hyperinsulinemia, and the activity of prostaglandins as a reflection of endothelial cell function have received increasing attention. These risk factors are discussed in detail in Chapters 7, 8, and 16.

Diabetes mellitus remains a significant risk factor in the development of lower extremity ASO. The Framingham study[20] demonstrated that any degree of impaired glucose tolerance was associated with an increased risk of ASO. Glycosuria increased the relative risk of ASO to 3.5% among men and to 8.6% among women. If diabetes, impaired glucose tolerance, or glycosuria is present, the incidence of ASO is equal in men and women. In individuals who have diabetes mellitus and lower extremity ASO, the severity and extent of disease are greater. Patients with diabetes mellitus have a higher incidence of below-knee disease, a similar incidence of femoropopliteal disease, and a lower incidence of aortoiliac disease than their nondiabetic counterparts.

In the Framingham study[20] hypertension imposed a threefold increased risk of intermittent claudication during a follow-up period of 26 years. No reports have been published on the effect of antihypertensive treatment on the course of clinically evident lower extremity occlusive disease. Nevertheless, control of hypertension is considered an important factor in lowering overall cardiovascular risk.

It has been estimated that cigarette smoking is directly related to about 325,000 to 350,000 deaths annually in the United States. Approximately 37% of the male population and 29% of the female population older than 17 years smoke.[21] In the Framingham study[20] cigarette smoking doubled the risk of lower extremity ASO for both men and women. Risk also increased in proportion to the number of cigarettes smoked per day. A population-based study of unselected persons in Finland[22] indicated that men who smoked and who had symptoms of intermittent claudication were at a remarkably high risk of death during their follow-up study, compared with nonsmokers. The risk of death was

15% for age-adjusted male smokers who were studied for 5 years. Cigarette smoking is also strongly associated with advanced lower extremity ASO in patients under 50 years of age. Jonason and Ringquist[23] found that in patients who quit smoking after they developed intermittent claudication, none progressed to rest pain as opposed to those who continued to smoke. Patients who stopped smoking had fewer amputations, fewer myocardial infarctions, less rest pain, and lived twice as long as those who continued to smoke.

While the risk of cardiac death from cigarette smoking seems to be related to the number of cigarettes smoked in a dose-response fashion, abstinence from smoking may reduce the risk of death from coronary artery disease by 50% after 2 years of cessation with a further reduction of risk to nonsmokers after 20 years of cessation.[24] Excluding patients with diabetes, nonsmokers comprise only 1% of all patients with intermittent claudication.[25] The risk of claudication is nine times greater for smokers than for nonsmokers.[26] Evidence also suggests that smoking significantly contributes to femoropopliteal and aortic graft failure.[27]

In spite of a great deal of basic research the precise mechanism by which cigarette smoking causes atherosclerosis remains undefined. Cigarette smoking has been implicated as a factor in lowering HDL cholesterol levels, altering platelet function, directly injuring endothelial cells, causing proliferation of arterial smooth muscle cells, and altering circulatory neuropharmacology. In addition, because cigarette smoking increases carboxyhemoglobin levels in the blood, it therefore decreases the oxygen carrying capacity of red blood cells. It stimulates the sympathetic nervous system and therefore increases heart rate, blood pressure, stroke volume, and cardiac output. Any or all of these mechanisms may play a significant role in the development of atherosclerotic lesions.[21]

The habit of cigarette smoking has recently been accepted as a recognized medical disorder described as tobacco dependency disorder (TDD). It is defined by Pollin[28] as the "inability to discontinue smoking despite awareness of its medical consequences." It is difficult to persuade smokers who have ASO to give up their smoking habit. Physicians should strongly recommend the cessation of smoking to all of their patients, not only those with clinically significant vascular disease.

The relationship between hemostatic factors and atherosclerosis has been of interest in recent years. Thrombosis in a region of severe ASO is the final event that may precipitate more severe symptoms or signs, such as ischemic rest pain, focal gangrene, or ischemic ulceration. Abnormalities of regulating proteins, circulating lupus-like anticoagulant, and altered platelet reactivity have been identified in patients with peripheral ASO.[29] When present, these blood coagulation abnormalities may lead to early failure of arterial reconstruction. Hemorrheologic factors, such as increases in blood viscosity, elevated hematocrit, and elevated fibrinogen levels, may also influence the success of reconstruction in patients with ASO.[30]

PATHOPHYSIOLOGY

The pathology of atherosclerosis is discussed in detail in Chapter 7.

Atherosclerotic plaque tends to occur on the posterior aspect of the lower extremity arteries. As the plaque develops it may involve the artery circumferentially in certain areas. Atherosclerosis is most often involved at the origin of arteries or at sites of arterial bifurcation, but other areas of local involvement include the distal superficial femoral artery at Hunter's canal. The superficial femoral artery itself is often diffusely involved with occlusive disease (Fig. 9-1). As the obstructing plaque accumulates, thrombus may be deposited on the obstructing lesion as well as on the adjacent arterial wall. Eventually, blood flow will be so impaired that the artery will thrombose.

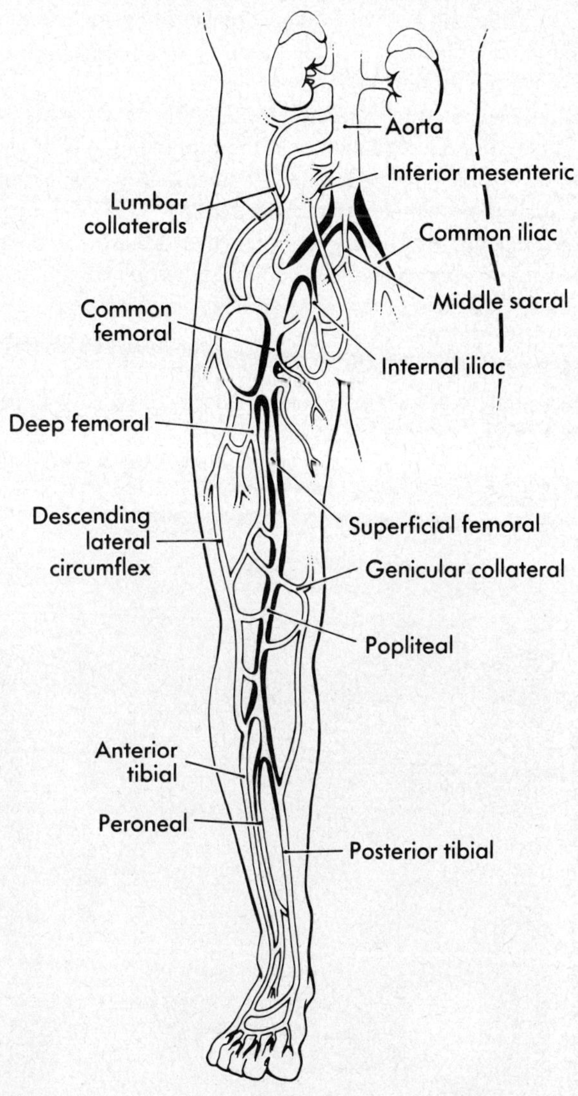

Fig. 9-1. Common sites of atherosclerosis *(shown in black)* in the aorta and lower extremities.

As atherosclerosis progresses, segmental occlusion of the arterial supply to the lower extremities develops, and nutritive blood flow to the extremities is impaired. Tissues distal to the obstruction experience ischemia, although the degree of ischemia depends on the location and extent of the occlusive process and the development of collateral channels. The most common symptom is intermittent claudication of the calf, which is most often related to occlusion of the superficial femoral artery. This process usually is initiated at Hunter's canal and gradually extends to involve occlusion of the entire superficial femoral artery. Blood flow to distal tissues is usually maintained through collateral channels. In most cases the process is so gradual that collateral pathways develop that adequately maintain viability of more distal tissue. If occlusion occurs more abruptly (i.e., emboli), then the onset of acute symptoms may be more dramatic.

The collateral pathways that often develop to maintain distal circulation include the lumbar aortic branches or internal iliac system in relationship to common iliac occlusion, the circumflex femoral vessels in relationship to common femoral occlusion, and the profunda femoris system in relationship to superficial femoral artery occlusion. The geniculate collaterals around the knee also perform a vital collateral function when occlusive disease more extensively involves both the superficial femoral and popliteal arteries. The extent of development in these collateral beds may be quite dramatic when the occlusive process progresses slowly (Fig. 9-2). In fact, patients may be symptomatic only when walking long distances or when walking briskly.

The more severe manifestations of lower extremity occlusive disease, such as pain at rest, gangrene, or ischemic ulceration, usually occur when the collateral pathways are inadequate to provide enough oxygen to maintain tissue viability. In these individuals the obstructive process usually involves multiple levels or compromise of the main trunk of the collateral bed. Collateral circulation in diabetic patients is often not as well developed as in nondiabetic patients. Occasionally, distal embolization or thrombosis in situ of the distal vascular bed may acutely compromise the viability of more distal ischemic tissues. Frequently, some minor degree of external trauma will be an initiating factor for a more serious ischemic lesion. If arterial blood flow has been compromised sufficiently, even minor degrees of trauma may lead to the development of gangrene or ischemic ulceration. At this point the individual often seeks medical consultation for arterial insufficiency.

CLINICAL MANIFESTATIONS

The symptoms of atherosclerotic occlusive disease of the lower extremities usually are of gradual onset. The individual may often be unaware of subtle symptoms. In fact, the extent of disease may be quite severe and involve multiple arterial segments before the patient becomes aware that a problem exists. Most often, the symptoms are so insidious and gradual in their progress that they may be brought to medical attention only at a far advanced stage. Some evidence also suggests that milder symptoms may remain stable for many years.[20,31] At times, however, acute occlusion (thrombosis in situ) superimposed on preexisting disease may make the problem acutely apparent.

A

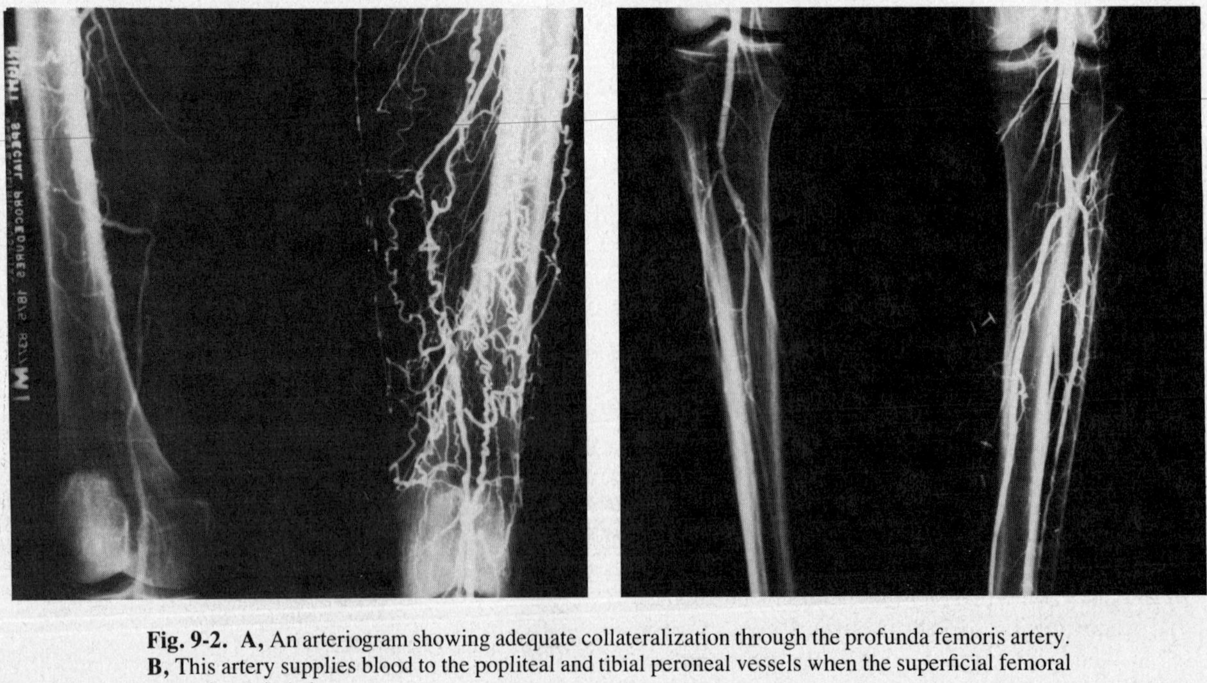

B

Fig. 9-2. **A,** An arteriogram showing adequate collateralization through the profunda femoris artery. **B,** This artery supplies blood to the popliteal and tibial peroneal vessels when the superficial femoral artery is occluded.

Intermittent claudication

The primary symptom of lower extremity occlusive disease is intermittent claudication. Its onset is usually gradual and often unrecognized by many older adults who may attribute their symptoms to arthritis or simply to aging. Intermittent claudication is usually described as an aching sensation associated with walking. This discomfort occurs in a muscle group distal to an arterial obstruction. Most characteristically, it occurs in the calf as a result of superficial femoral artery obstruction. The specific location of the obstruction is commonly at "Hunter's canal" in the distal thigh. Intermittent claudication may also occur in the thigh, hip, and buttock if the obstruction involves the aortofemoral segment or internal iliac arteries. Intermittent claudication rarely may be felt in the foot alone. If multilevel occlusive disease is present, the most distal muscle group is affected first, followed by more proximal muscle groups if the patient continues to walk. An exception to this general rule may occur in an individual who has mainly proximal occlusive disease that involves the common and internal iliac arteries. This individual may experience hip or buttock claudication only. The aching or cramplike sensation of intermittent claudication is progressive as the individual exercises, but it diminishes rapidly with rest.

Intermittent claudication has been associated with progression to more severe symptoms in only 25% to 30% of cases.[31-35] However, actual progression, when measured by noninvasive testing, is more common and occurs in 41% to 52% of affected individuals.[36-38] Intermittent claudication is also a marker for more diffuse atherosclerosis. Therefore the afflicted individual should be examined carefully for signs of disease in the carotid or coronary arteries since these manifestations are more life threatening. Intermittent claudication is usually unilateral at its onset. It may appear as a bilateral symptom in those individuals who have occlusion of the distal abdominal aorta. More commonly, one leg is affected first, followed by the onset of similar symptoms in the opposite lower extremity.

Once intermittent claudication has been identified as a symptom of atherosclerotic occlusive disease, the patient may recognize that it has been present for years, in a lesser degree. If questioned carefully, the individual usually can identify the approximate time when the symptoms started. Most patients also can provide an accurate description of their walking distance before claudication occurs. The onset of symptoms usually occurs when the patient walks between one half and two city blocks at a normal pace on level ground. Walking up a grade or at increased speed brings on the discomfort more quickly. In most patients the symptoms are consistent and reproducible. In those who are poor observers, the treadmill exercise test is an excellent means of determining their functional disability. Some individuals describe the ability to "walk through" their symptoms. These individuals usually have a well-developed collateral circulation and will adjust their walking pace to compensate for the degree of arterial insufficiency. In addition, walking exercise will often result in "conditioning" of the affected muscle bed that permits the individual to walk demonstrably greater distances even though the segmental arterial pressures and pulse waveforms may not change appreciably on follow-up treadmill testing. True claudication must be differentiated from pseudoclaudication (neurogenic claudication) caused by lumbar canal stenosis or disk disease.[39,40] This differentiation can usually be made on the basis of the patient's history and physical examination (Table 9-1). Since many patients with pseudoclaudication have concomitant ASO, lower extremity pulses may be diminished or absent. The patient's history is quite important in determining which disease is actually responsible for the symptoms.

Table 9-1. Differentiating true claudication from pseudoclaudication

	Intermittent claudication	Pseudoclaudication
Character of discomfort	Cramping, tightness, tiredness	Same or tingling, weakness, clumsiness
Location of discomfort	Buttock, hip, thigh, calf, foot	Same
Exercise induced	Yes	Yes or no
Distance to claudication	Same each time	Variable
Occurs with standing	No	Yes
Relief	Stop walking	Often must sit or change body positions

Rest pain

Progession to critical ischemia is evidenced by the onset of rest pain and at 5 years will occur in approximately 24% of those who experience intermittent claudication.[38] Pain at rest characteristically occurs at night when the patient lies supine. Usually described as a dull aching sensation in the toes or forefoot, this sensation may awaken the patient from sleep and cause him or her to hang the foot over the side of the bed or get up and walk around for relief. As the symptom persists, the individual may start to sleep in a chair with the legs dependent. This often results in a moderate degree of lower extremity edema. The affected foot usually demonstrates dependent rubor.[41] In patients who have rest pain the degree of arterial insufficiency is severe and usually involves multiple arterial segments.

Ischemic ulceration and gangrene

If an individual is able to tolerate ischemic pain at rest, eventually ischemic necrosis between two toes ("kissing ulcer") may occur. Dry gangrene or ulcerations (Fig. 9-3)

A

B

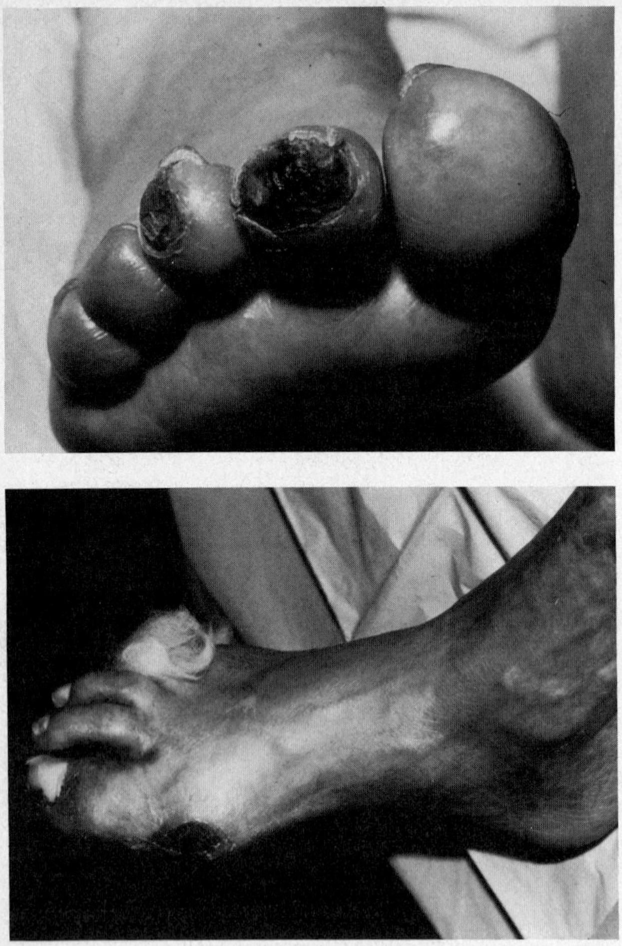

Fig. 9-3. Typical ischemic ulcer caused by arteriosclerosis obliterans. These ulcers occur distally **(A)** or over pressure points **(B)** where trauma is more likely. The base is dry and necrotic and does not contain healthy granulation tissue.

may also begin at the tips of the toes or over pressure points and is common after minor trauma such as nail trimming. By the time tissue necrosis occurs, the individual's ability to walk is usually severely limited. However, only about 5% of patients who develop intermittent claudication will progress to eventual amputation because of limb ischemia.[37]

Ischemic neuropathy

If ischemia is severe and longstanding, an individual may develop pain along the distribution of a peripheral sensory nerve. This pain, referred to as *ischemic monomelic neuropathy*,[42] may occur in the absence of ulceration or gangrene and is often described as a sensation of numbness, deadness, or burning. Ischemic neuropathy may occur after acute arterial thrombosis and subsequent revascularization, particularly if the ischemia has been quite prolonged. This type of pain is very difficult to treat and may persist indefinitely in some individuals.

Disuse atrophy

Patients with severe arterial insufficiency who are sedentary and nonambulatory may experience considerable loss of muscle mass in the lower extremity and foot. Occasionally, their complaint of pain in the limb is out of proportion to the findings on segmental blood pressure measurements. These individuals may experience pain on simple palpation of the calf or thigh muscles, and osteoporosis may be demonstrated on plain x-ray films of the limb. This condition of disuse phenomenon, or reflex sympathetic dystrophy, is discussed in detail in Chapter 29. This condition may also cause problems for rehabilitation after lower extremity arterial reconstruction. A supervised course of physical therapy may be needed to rehabilitate the postoperative patient when the disuse syndrome is present.

Other sensory disturbances

Many individuals with arterial insufficiency describe cold sensitivity of the feet, often complaining that they have had cold feet for many years. On some occasions, they may have injured the skin if they used a heating pad in an attempt to warm the feet. Other individuals complain of a numb or dead sensation in the toes and forefoot, while others experience a tingling or prickling sensation. A burning type of discomfort that involves the plantar aspect of the feet is usually associated with diabetes. This complaint, which may occur even in the presence of adequate arterial circulation, is likely to be related to peripheral diabetic neuropathy. Diabetic patients with impaired sensation may develop traumatic ulceration over the plantar metatarsal heads, which are referred to as *neurotrophic ulcers* (Chapter 38). Foot sepsis may occur if secondary infection supervenes. The infection may become aggressive even though the patient may not be aware of it, and if unrecognized, the degree of infection may preclude salvage of an otherwise viable foot.

Muscular weakness and joint stiffness

In situations of severe arterial insufficiency, muscle weakness inevitably occurs because of the limited degree of ambulation and associated atrophy. As previously noted under *Disuse atrophy,* this condition may be associated with pain. Muscle pain may persist even after revascularization and considerable rehabilitation may be required to restore muscle mass and normal function. In situations of acute and prolonged arterial insufficiency, entire muscle groups become infarcted. This condition is most common in the anterior compartment syndrome.

Joint stiffness and flexion contractures at the hip and knee may occur as a result of chronic arterial insufficiency, since many individuals will keep the hip and knee flexed in an effort to relieve pain. These contractures may be difficult to treat after successful revascularization or amputation. Physical therapy should be recommended to maintain joint mobility and muscle strength for individuals with severe arterial insufficiency.

PHYSICAL EXAMINATION

The combination of a careful history and physical examination should lead the experienced clinician to an accurate diagnosis of the anatomic location and severity of arterial occlusive disease. However, in patients with relatively mild occlusive disease, the physical diagnostic findings may be minimal.

It is helpful to compare one lower extremity with the other, because one limb is usually affected more severely than the other. Simultaneous visual examination of both lower extremities will also allow the physician to evaluate the color and skin nutrition of both lower extremities. Physical findings such as gangrene, ulceration, edema, and atrophy will all be readily apparent. The skin should be examined for dryness and cracking. The distribution of hair growth is a poor indicator of arterial insufficiency since it may decrease normally with advancing age. When both legs and feet are examined and compared with each other, a temperature difference may often be evident. The limb with severely impaired circulation may feel cool, and often an obvious area of demarcation in temperature is present.

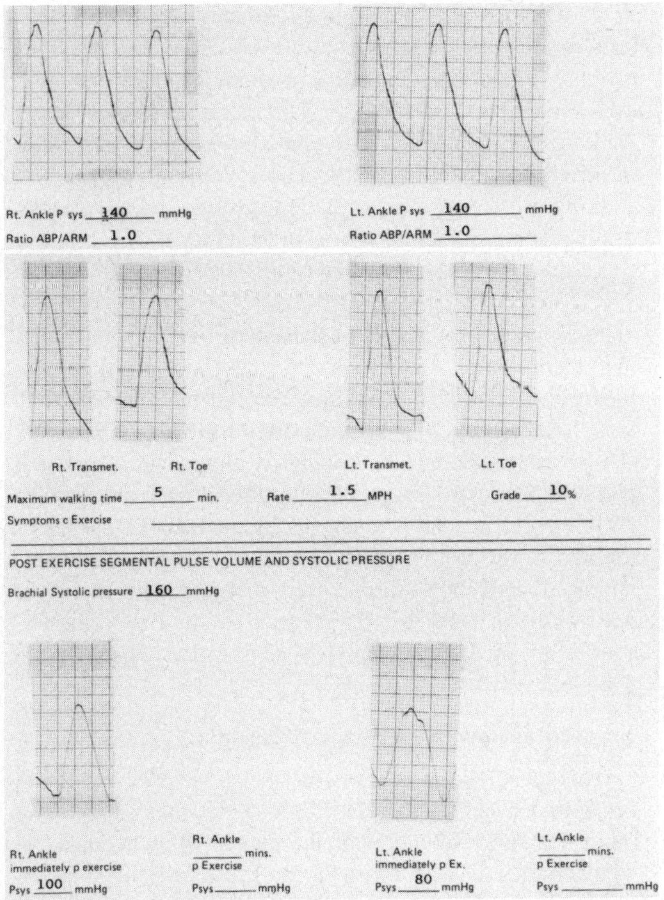

Fig. 9-4. Pulse volume recordings and Doppler blood pressures were normal at rest. The ankle/arm blood pressure ratio was 1.0 bilaterally. The patient walked for 5 minutes on the treadmill and developed bilateral calf claudication. After excercise, the arm blood pressure increased to 160 mm Hg, and the ankle blood pressure decreased to 80 mm Hg on the left and to 100 mm Hg on the right, indicating the presence of underlying arterial occlusive disease.

Palpation of the arterial pulses at the femoral, popliteal, posterior tibial, and dorsalis pedis areas is one of the most important clinical diagnostic maneuvers (see Chapter 2). A systematic approach should be used to examine the relative strength and quality of the arterial pulsation. Initial examination of the blood pressure in both upper extremities and the palpation of both radial pulses will generally provide a baseline evaluation for comparison with lower extremity pulses. Lower extremity pulsation should be compared in a stepwise fashion beginning with the femoral areas bilaterally. The popliteal, posterior tibial, and dorsalis pedis pulses of both limbs should be compared with each other, and both of these should be compared with the quality of the radial pulsation. The pulses should be graded as normal, diminished, or absent. It is important to recognize that some individuals may have nonpalpable dorsalis pedis pulses with essentially normal lower extremity arterial perfusion. This is most often the result of an anomaly of the below-knee arterial anatomy.[43] Patients with significant ASO may demonstrate pallor on elevation and rubor on dependency. Occasionally, patients with typical complaints of intermittent claudication may have palpable pedal pulses at rest. A brief period of walking exercise and reexamination may be required to determine if the pulses disappear and if segmental blood pressure decreases with exercise (Figs. 9-4 and 9-5).

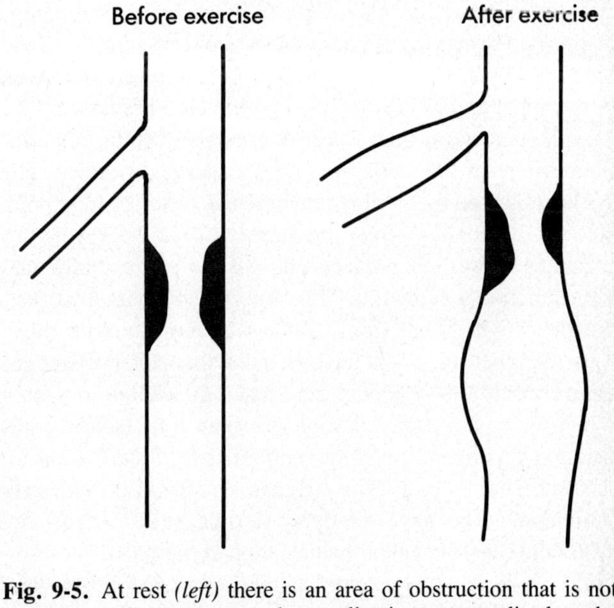

Fig. 9-5. At rest *(left)* there is an area of obstruction that is not severe enough to cause an abnormality in pressure distal to the obstruction. Therefore the pulses and blood pressure at rest are normal. Exercise increases the metabolic demand to the muscles. However, the obstruction only allows oxygen to be delivered at a fixed rate. In an attempt to compensate, more blood is shunted in the collateral vessels proximal to the obstruction. The vessels distal to the obstruction dilate so less blood is delivered to dilated segments of the distal vessels and the pressure decreases.

A sensory examination is also very helpful. Diabetics particularly will demonstrate impaired sensation for vibration, pain, and light touch, even though they may not have severe arterial insufficiency. Also, individuals with ischemic neuropathy often have impaired sensation, and at times hyperesthesia is present.

LABORATORY STUDIES

During the past decade the use of noninvasive methods of circulatory assessment has increased dramatically (see Chapter 3). Techniques range from simple measurement of the ankle/brachial systolic blood pressure index to the use of MRI to measure arterial blood flow. While the recording of ankle/brachial systolic blood pressure index provides some information at the bedside, segmental Doppler systolic blood pressures and pulse waveform analysis by plethysmography provide more objective information about the level and severity of occlusive disease. Arteriography is the definitive examination when interventional or surgical treatment is being considered.

Doppler ankle/brachial index (ABI)

The simplest vascular laboratory test for lower extremity circulation is the ankle/brachial systolic blood pressure index (ABI). The equipment is inexpensive and consists of an ordinary blood pressure cuff and a Doppler ultrasonic velocity detector. The blood pressure cuff is placed over both brachial areas and inflated above systolic pressure. Resumption of blood flow is detected with the Doppler probe over the radial artery. If there is a discrepancy in the readings of the two arms, the higher of the two arm systolic blood pressures is used. Next, the blood pressure cuff is moved to the ankle and inflated above systolic blood pressure. The Doppler detector is then placed alternately over the posterior tibial artery at the ankle and the dorsalis pedis artery. The ABI is obtained by dividing the brachial systolic blood pressure by the ankle systolic pressure.

Under most circumstances the ABI correlates quite well with functional symptoms.[44] In a normal individual at rest, the index will range from 0.9 to 1.3. Patients with intermittent claudication will have an index that generally ranges from 0.35 to 0.9. Patients experiencing ischemic rest pain will usually have an index of less than 0.4. Ischemic ulceration or impending gangrene is usually found when indexes are below 0.25. The ABI can also be used to identify individuals who have relatively normal pulses at rest but who complain of typical caludication symptoms. These individuals should be exercised and the ankle systolic pressure index measured following exercise (Fig. 9-4). If there is no significant drop in the ankle systolic pressure index following exercise, the cause of their symptoms is something other than ASO. Measurement of ABI can also be used as a convenient means of observing patients who have had bypass reconstructions. The level of improvement following the reconstruction can be compared with future measurements during follow-up visits. This method of surveillance may detect functional deterioration of the bypass before limb-threatening occlusion occurs.

Absolute systolic pressures may also provide information about the expectation of healing. For example, a foot wound or below-knee amputation is unlikely to heal if the ankle systolic pressure is less than 65 mm Hg in nondiabetics and less than 90 mm Hg in diabetics.[45] The absolute ankle pressure may be erroneous in diabetics with calcified, noncompressible arteries. In this situation pulse waveform analysis is needed to accurately evaluate the circulation.

Segmental pressures

Segmental pressures can be measured by placing blood pressure cuffs at the high thigh, calf, and ankle level to determine the level of occlusive disease. This examination is usually performed in combination with segmental volume plethysmography or analysis of Doppler-derived pulse waveforms. Vascular stress testing with walking exercise or reactive hyperemia produces increased arterial blood flow in an extremity and can be used to unmask subcritical stenoses or marginally significant stenotic lesions. Treadmill exercise provides a functional evaluation of the patient's symptoms. Standard stress measurements are used, such as walking at 1.5 mph on a 10% grade for 5 minutes. The time of onset of symptoms is recorded as well as the maximum walking time. Postexercise ankle pressures and recovery at 2 minutes after exercise are recorded (Fig. 9-4).

Segmental volume plethysmography

Pulse waveform analysis can be performed with a system that incorporates mercury strain gauges or the pneumoplethysmograph (Pulse Volume Recorder, Life Sciences, Inc., Greenwich, CT). We prefer the Pulse Volume Recorder (PVR) as the method of evaluation along with segmental pressure measurements and treadmill walking exercise. The PVR waveforms can be analyzed by qualitative analysis of the waveform profile, or PVR category criteria. A combination of segmental limb pressure measurements and PVR waveform analysis has been accurate to the 97th percentile in predicting the level and extent of occlusive disease.[46]

Transcutaneous oxygen measurement

This technique assesses tissue metabolism as a function of perfusion and is therefore thought by many to yield a more accurate evaluation of the degree of ischemia. Absolute values may be used (TC Po_2) or a calf/brachial Po_2 index can be calculated.[47] Studies have suggested that this method can be predictive of the success of ulcer healing or the ability to heal an amputation site.

Duplex ultrasonography

Recently duplex ultrasonography has been extended to the evaluation of lower extremity arterial occlusive disease. This method can assess both arterial anatomy and physiology. By spectral analysis it evaluates the hemodynamic effect of localized stenoses. Measurements of velocity profiles can be compared before and after interventional procedures such as atherectomy and balloon dilation, or following bypass reconstructions. However, tibial vessels cannot yet be reliably evaluated with this technique.

Positron emission tomography (PET)

By means of positron emission tomography (PET) specifically labeled tracers can be localized and quantified without the need for tissue destruction.[48] The positron is an elementary particle of antimatter. Several synthetic radioactive isotopes decay by positron emission. When a positron travels through tissues, it quickly encounters an electron. When these two particles collide, the positron-electron pair is completely annihilated. This reaction gives off two 511 KeV γ-rays traveling in opposite directions, which are then detected by the scanner.

The value of PET is that it can make absolute measurements in vivo of regional, physiologic, and biochemical processes rather than in its use as an imaging technique. The use of PET in the study of vascular disease appears valuable in the evaluation of regional blood flow, regional oxygen extraction ratio, and local metabolic rate for oxygen. Major substrates of interest in vascular disease are fatty acids and glucose. The metabolic rates for both can be determined with PET.

The brain has been more extensively studied than any other tissue. In the brain PET appears capable of distinguishing ischemic from infarcted tissue. In the periphery PET has not been studied as extensively. One can speculate that it might eventually be able to predict healing of ischemic ulcers or amputations. It may also provide a physiologic indication for revascularization. For the present PET is an interesting research tool. Whether it will evolve into a cost-effective, valuable clinical tool remains to be determined.

Magnetic resonance imaging (MRI)

MRI has been studied somewhat more extensively than PET[49,50] for its use in the peripheral circulation. With MRI blood flow velocity can be estimated, and a contrast medium is not needed to enhance the images obtained. Images can be obtained in transverse, sagittal, and coronal planes. Moreover, the technique has no known harmful effects. The patient under study is placed in a magnetic field and subjected to millisecond bursts of high-frequency energy that alters the alignment of nuclei in the magnetic field and thus creates a condition of "excitement." When bursts of radio frequency energy stop, the nuclei "relax" and realign in the magnetic field. This relaxation is associated with the emission of radio frequency energy that can be detected and analyzed by two-dimensional Fourier reconstruction to produce an image.

The disadvantages of MRI are its limited resolution (1.0 to 1.5 cm slice thickness) and its high cost. Patients with pacemakers, metallic heart valves, or intracerebral metallic clips should not be evaluated by MRI, although patients with metal joint prostheses have been safely evaluated. While images of major intraabdominal arteries and veins are easily obtained, images of smaller, more peripheral arteries have more limited definition and spatial resolution. The capability of MRI to characterize blood flow may prove useful in assessing hemodynamics in vivo, but further research for both MRI and PET is needed before they will become practical clinical tools for evaluating vascular disease.

Blood chemistry studies

Several chemistry studies should be considered for every patient undergoing evaluation of lower extremity atherosclerosis. If a fasting blood glucose is elevated, an HbA_{1c} should be measured to assess diabetic control. A complete lipid profile should also be obtained after a 12-hour fast (see Chapter 8). A complete blood count and a kidney and liver profile should be performed as well. Some individuals with ASO, particularly those who smoke, have a high hematocrit value, which may contribute to increased blood viscosity and possibly arterial thrombosis. Some evidence suggests that fibrinogen levels may also be significantly elevated in smokers who have vascular disease and that this elevation may be a contributing factor in thrombosis.[51]

Cardiac testing

Long-term survival in patients with lower extremity atherosclerosis is directly related to their underlying cardiac status.[52,53] All patients seen for initial evaluation should have a 12-lead electrocardiogram. Since a history of myocardial infarction or electrocardiographic evidence of myocardial infarction places the individual in a higher risk category for future cardiac events, this information is important for prognosis. If an interventional procedure or surgical reconstruction is considered, cardiac stress testing is advisable. If the patient cannot exercise, a dipyridamole thallium or PET scan may be performed. If the patient has clinical symptoms of angina pectoris or resting electrocardiographic evidence of ischemia, cardiac catheterization may also be indicated.

Plain x-ray films

In the presence of digital gangrene or ischemic ulceration, plain x-ray films of the foot may help detect underlying osteomyelitis or deep soft tissue infection. Patients with diabetes and individuals with chronic renal failure may have severe diffuse calcification of the leg and foot arteries. Diabetics who have neurotrophic ulcers may have underlying osteomyelitis with relatively little external evidence of chronic infection. Thus the radiograph may help determine whether other conservative or more aggressive treatment is indicated, including the possibility of amputation as primary treatment for the involved digit.

Arteriography

With the advent of reliable noninvasive vascular laboratory testing, arteriography is no longer necessary unless interventional or surgical treatment is being considered. Ad-

A

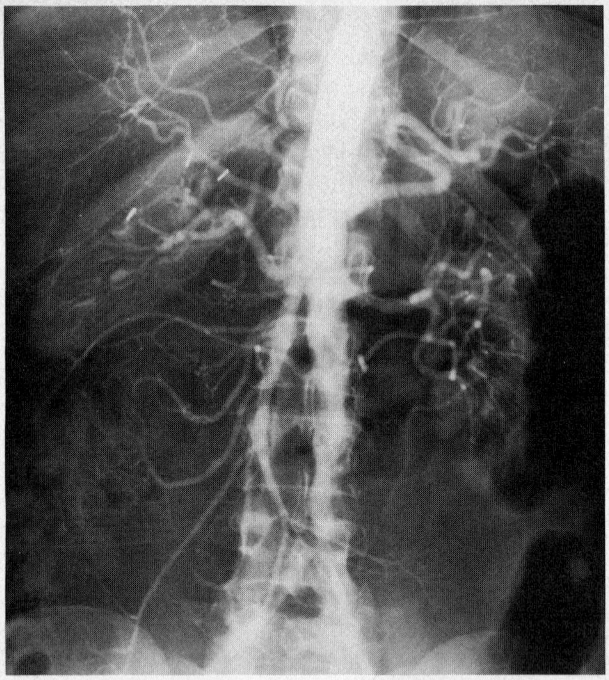

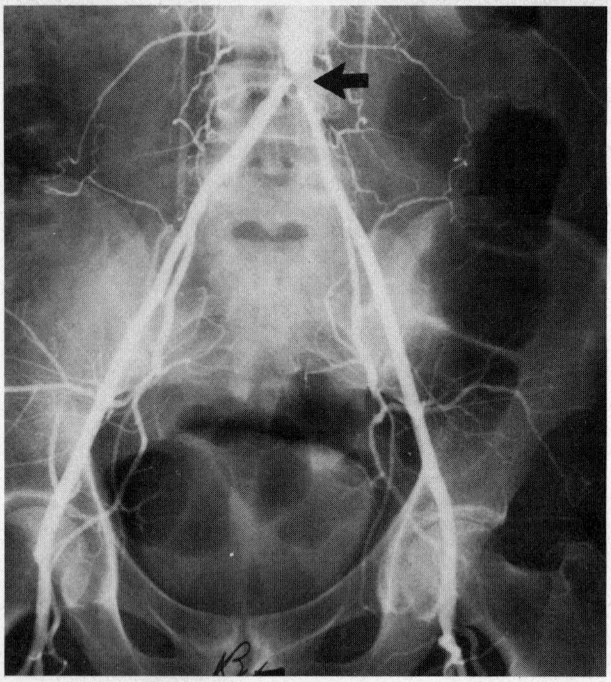

B

C

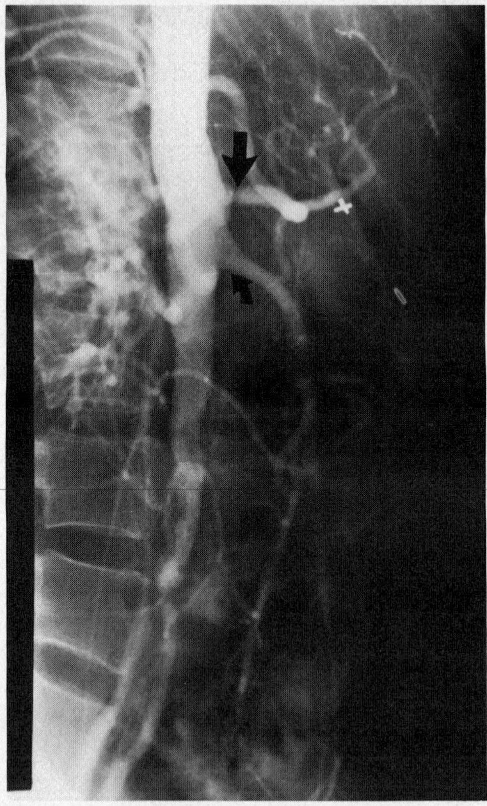

Fig. 9-6. Aortogram (anteroposterior and lateral view) with runoffs. **A,** The intraabdominal portion of the aorta is shown. Corresponding anatomy can be compared with Fig. 9-1. **B,** Severe atherosclerosis in the distal aorta *(arrow)* and proximal common iliac arteries. **C,** Lateral view of the aorta demonstrating the origins of the celiac artery *(large arrow)* and superior mesenteric artery *(small arrow)*. **D,** The common femoral, superficial femoral, and profunda femoris are shown and are normal. **E,** Normal superficial femoral and popliteal arteries. **F,** Tibial peroneal vessels are shown in this view. The posterior tibial artery in the left leg is occluded *(arrow)*. **G,** Anterior and posterior tibial arteries are patent into the right foot.

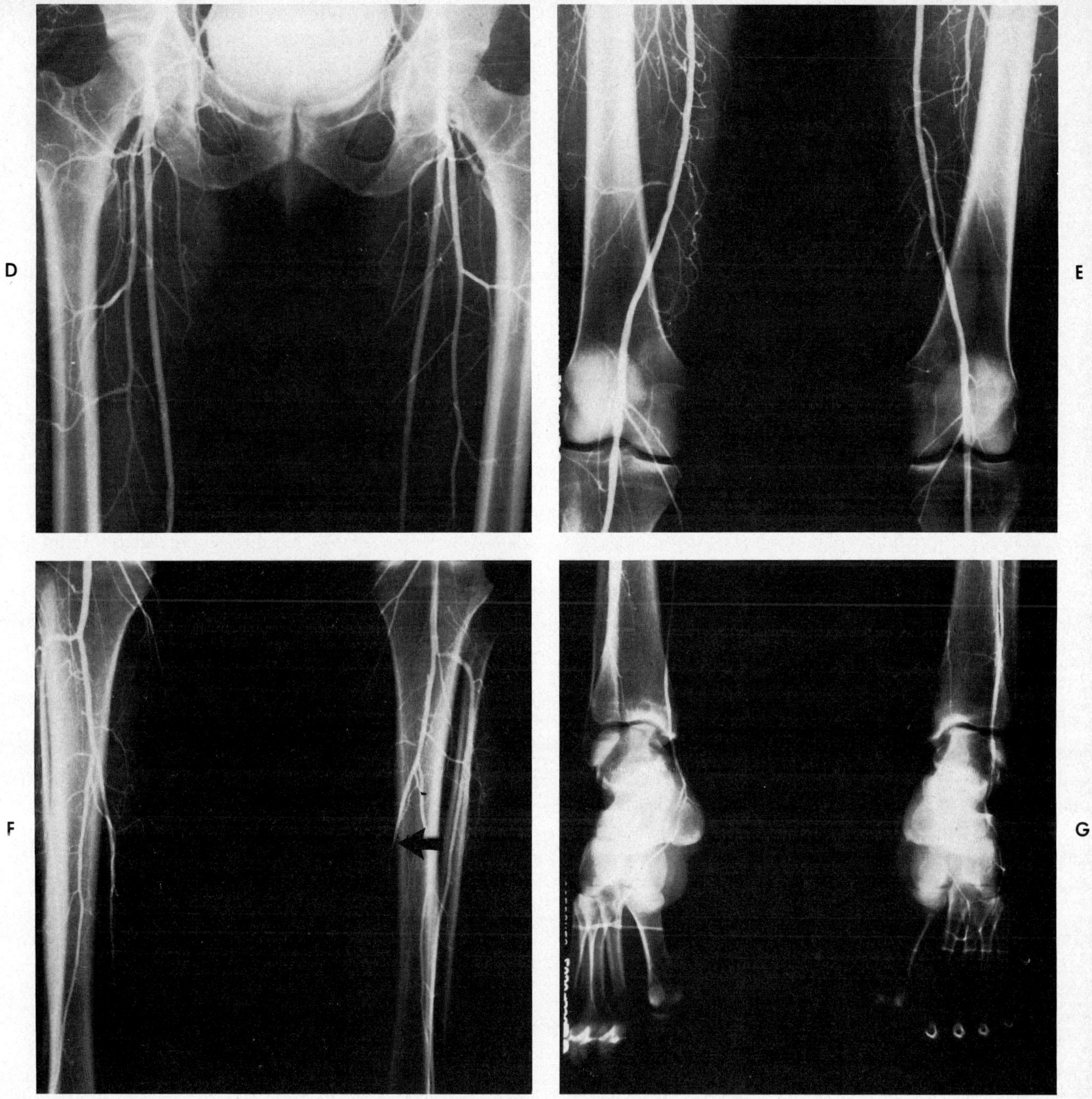

Fig. 9-6, cont'd. For legend see opposite page.

equate information can be obtained from the patient's clinical history, physical diagnosis, and noninvasive testing to assess the level and extent of occlusive vascular disease. Clear guidelines have been developed to determine when more aggressive treatment is indicated. If interventional or surgical treatment is being considered, complete arteriography of the abdominal aorta and run-off vessels in both lower extremities should be performed. In the past aortograms were frequently performed using the translumbar percutaneous approach, and lower extremity arteriograms were obtained by direct femoral artery puncture. More recently, radiologists trained in the subspecialty of cerebrovascular and peripheral arteriography are readily available in most larger hospitals. Generally, these studies are now performed using a transfemoral Seldinger catheter approach.[54] With the aid of fluoroscopic control, flexible guidewires, preformed catheters, and power injection of contrast, detailed and complete studies can be obtained (Fig. 9-6). The development of equipment with moving tables and the use of digital subtraction fluoroscopy has increased the versatility of radiographic studies. Complete studies, including the pedal arch of the foot, should be obtained. Oblique views may

Differential diagnosis in patients with a history suggestive of intermittent claudication

1. Atherosclerosis
2. Thromboangiitis obliterans (see Chapter 19)
3. Takayasu's arteritis (see Chapter 20)
4. Giant cell arteritis (see Chapter 20)
5. Arterial embolism (see Chapter 12)
6. Chronic pernio (see Chapter 33)
7. Popliteal artery entrapment syndrome (see Chapter 22)
8. Fibromuscular dysplasia (see Chapter 22)
9. Ergotamine use and abuse
10. Phlegmasia cerulea dolens (venous gangrene) (see Chapter 24)
11. Cystic adventitial disease of the popliteal artery (see Chapter 22)
12. Atheromatous emboli (see Chapter 11)
13. Lumbar canal stenosis and lumbar disk disease
14. Degenerative joint disease of the hip and back

also be needed to define certain areas such as the iliac or femoral bifurcation. Intraoperative arteriography still has an important role in distal lower extremity bypass reconstruction.[55]

Diagnosis

To establish the diagnosis of atherosclerosis of the extremities, it is necessary to combine the information obtained by a careful clinical history, physical examination, and noninvasive vascular laboratory testing. Intermittent claudication is a classic symptom, and when clearly described by a reliable observer, it is strongly indicative of vascular disease. Associated risk factors such as hypertension, diabetes, and cigarette smoking are commonly present in patients with symptoms of intermittent claudication, ischemic rest pain, or digital gangrene. A clinician who is experienced in the evaluation of peripheral vascular disease will usually recognize when some aspect of the history, physical examination, or laboratory findings do not fit the picture of peripheral ASO. Several other vascular and nonvascular conditions may simulate symptoms of atherosclerosis. These differential diagnoses are discussed in detail in other chapters and are summarized in the accompanying box.

PROGNOSIS

The clinical course for the patient with lower extremity atherosclerosis depends on many factors. The extent or pattern of disease and the initial symptoms are major determinants. The need for surgical intervention or the risk of limb loss will differ for patients with intermittent claudication from those with ischemic rest pain or tissue necrosis. Among patients with intermittent claudication who seek medical attention, the likelihood of surgical intervention is approximately 25% to 30%.[16] However, in large epidemiologic studies, which include patients not seeking medical advice, the likelihood that these patients will require surgical treatment is 10%. Similarly, the likelihood of eventual amputation is approximately 5% in surgical series vs 1.6% to 1.8% in general epidemiologic studies. Therefore the need for surgical intervention or the risk of limb loss because of severe arterial insufficiency varies from case to case. It is usually not possible to predict whether any one patient with recent onset claudication will need surgical treatment eventually or whether loss of a limb will occur.

Perhaps more important for individuals with lower extremity occlusive disease is the prevalence of coronary and cerebrovascular disease. Numerous studies have recognized a high associated incidence of coronary occlusive disease (see Chapter 10) although the incidence depends on the means of investigation. Those studies using only clinical history or electrocardiograph abnormalities show a prevalence of approximately 40% to 60%, while the presence of coronary atherosclerosis may be as high as 90% in those patients studied arteriographically.[56] The major concern is detecting the presence of life-threatening disease. From the information available, approximately 30% of patients with lower extremity occlusive disease may have potentially life-threatening coronary atherosclerosis. The prevalence of associated cerebrovascular disease is lower than that of coronary atherosclerosis, but it also depends on the means of screening. Various studies suggest that the incidence of cerebrovascular disease ranges from 10% to 15%.[16]

The long-term prognosis may be significantly affected by other factors such as continued cigarette smoking. In one study cigarette smokers who continued to smoke for up to 11 years after diagnosis had a three times greater mortality than those who stopped smoking when their disease was diagnosed.[22,23] The presence of diabetes mellitus is also a poor prognostic indicator. Long-term survival among patients with associated diabetes mellitus was 35% lower than it was among nondiabetic patients.[57]

MEDICAL TREATMENT

Medical management of patients with lower extremity occlusive vascular disease is generally advocated for those with intermittent claudication (see the box on p. 191). In contrast, surgical treatment has usually been reserved for patients who develop limb-threatening ischemia with ischemic rest pain, tissue necrosis, or life-style disabling claudication.

Since cigarette smoking is so highly correlated with the presence of ASO and its progression, the cessation of smoking is strongly recommended. It is the single most important measure that may prevent the progression of atherosclerosis. Patients who are able to stop smoking successfully have been shown to improve their treadmill walking distance, compared with those who continued to smoke.[58] It has also been demonstrated that long-term graft patency in both the aortofemoral and femoral popliteal locations is adversely

Conservative treatment of patients with arteriosclerosis obliterans of the lower extremities

1. Discontinue smoking tobacco in all forms
2. Engage in a regular walking program
3. Put the bed in a vascular position (reverse Trendelenburg) for patients with rest pain or ischemic ulcers that will not heal
4. Foot care
   a. Daily inspection of the feet
   b. Careful trimming of the toenails
   c. Avoid trauma or injury to the feet
   d. Keep skin in good condition, i.e., use a lanolin-based cream 2 to 4 times per day
   e. Treat underlying tinea infection
   f. Wear properly fitting soft shoes or orthotics
   g. Wear protective foam or wool boots, and use lamb's wool between the toes to prevent pressure (kissing) ulcers
5. Trial of pentoxifylline

affected by continued cigarette smoking.[59,60] Every effort should be made to offer assistance to individual patients in their efforts to stop smoking completely. Numerous programs are available for guidance and assistance in stopping this addictive behavior.

Aggressive management of lipoprotein abnormalities should be undertaken as recommended in Chapter 8. Reasonable evidence now exists that regression of atherosclerosis may occur in some patients who follow a program of aggressive risk factor modification.[61,62]

Associated blood clotting disorders such as protein C, protein S, and antithrombin III deficiency have all been identified in more recent years.[63] Other blood clotting disorders have also been recognized, such as hyperaggregable platelet dysfunction, lupus anticoagulant, and abnormal plasminogen activator inhibitor levels. Since heparin is so frequently used to treat acute lower extremity ischemia, heparin-associated antibodies may also occur and promote thrombosis rather than the desired therapeutic effect of anticoagulation. When these conditions are identified as coexisting with peripheral atherosclerosis, the use of long-term anticoagulant therapy for patients with ASO may be considered. Although anticoagulant therapy has not demonstrated a significant improvement in either the amputation rate or long-term survival, recent reports have shown that it may improve the patency rate of infragenicular prosthetic bypass reconstructions.[64,65]

The use of vasodilating drugs has been popular in the past, although no convincing studies support their use.[66] More recently, pentoxifylline (Trental) has been introduced, and it is effective in some patients when combined with conditioning exercise. A multicenter, prospective randomized study in the United States has supported its use[67] (Table 9-2). However, others have questioned whether it provides sufficient benefit over conditioning exercise alone to warrant its general use in patients with intermittent claudication.[68,69] Pentoxifylline is reported to act by reducing blood viscosity and enhancing oxygen delivery to the muscle of the affected limb. The dose of pentoxifylline is 400 mg three times a day. Only about 20% of patients who take pentoxifylline will subjectively note improvement. The major side effect of gastrointestinal intolerance can be avoided if the medication is taken with meals.

Table 9-2. Pentoxifylline in arteriosclerosis obliterans

	Initial claudicating distance (meters)		Actual claudicating distance (meters)	
	Pentoxifylline (n=42)	Placebo (n=40)	Pentoxifylline (n=42)	Placebo (n=40)
Baseline	111	117	172	181
Week 24	195	180	268	250
Percent increase	59	36	38	25

(Modified from Porter JM et al: Am Heart J 104:66, 1982.)

Other pharmacologic agents such as ketanserin and L-carnitine have been investigated for their potential usefulness in the treatment of intermittent claudication, but thus far they have not been clearly demonstrated to be effective.[70,71] Intraarterial infusions of prostaglandin have been suggested to be beneficial in patients with advanced lower extremity arterial insufficiency.[72,73] However, a multicenter randomized trial by Schuler et al[74] failed to demonstrate effectiveness when prostaglandin was administered intravenously. In another study Cronenwett et al[75] infused prostacyclin intravenously to treat ischemic ulcers and rest pain, but no objective improvement was noted. Thus the search continues for an effective pharmacologic agent to treat lower extremity arteriosclerosis obliterans.

Conventional conservative therapy advocates the use of graded lower extremity conditioning exercises. Skinner and Strandness[76] demonstrated that a physical training program of repeated walking exercise improved resting limb blood flow, reduced the onset of claudication symptoms, and increased maximal walking time. Others have confirmed the same results. These studies support the traditional recommendation that daily walking exercise is beneficial to patients with intermittent claudication, although the precise mechanism by which a walking program improves symptoms is controversial. It probably involves a combination of "training effect" and an increase in the collateral blood supply to the extremity. Many patients can increase their walking distance four-to eightfold with a walking program, and most can avoid surgery if they exercise regularly and stop smoking. Caution is indicated, however, if the individual has symptoms of angina pectoris, chronic congestive heart failure, or severe chronic pulmonary disease.

Patients with lower extremity occlusive disease should also be instructed in regular foot care. They should wash their feet daily and dry the skin carefully. Creams containing lanolin should also be used to maintain skin moisture. The patient should be cautioned against careless trimming of ingrown toenails and warned about the potential for tissue injury from careless nail clipping. Patients should also wear comfortable, well-fitting shoes, especially during walking exercise. Many individuals will benefit from custom-fitted orthotic devices. Heating pads or hot water soaks should not be used, since sensation may be impaired, especially in diabetics. Thermal trauma may lead to irreversible skin loss even if revascularization is undertaken. For some individuals who have advanced lower extremity ischemia, placing the individual's bed in the reverse Trendelenburg position will help alleviate rest pain or night pain caused by arterial insufficiency. Protective boots of lamb's wool or other materials sometimes help patients who frequently complain of cold feet.

INTERVENTIONAL THERAPY

During the 1980s an entirely new field of treatment for atherosclerotic vascular disease called *interventional therapy* arose. It uses catheter-directed techniques. Interventional treatment is discussed in detail in Chapter 6.

SURGICAL TREATMENT

Preoperative considerations

Surgical treatment of lower extremity atherosclerosis may be elective or mandatory. When an individual is threatened with limb loss caused by arterial insufficiency, surgical therapy is indicated. Once a decision for operative intervention has been made, a surgeon's clinical judgment will determine the optimal procedure that has the expectation of the best possible outcome for the individual patient. Surgical judgment is often as important as technical skill in surgical treatment of patients with atherosclerosis.

For a patient who develops intermittent claudication as the primary symptom, surgical treatment is usually elective. In this circumstance, the patient and the immediate family should be informed completely about treatment alternatives, whether medical, surgical, or nonsurgical intervention. The physician must determine how severely the patient is disabled by the claudication. For example, an elderly individual with a sedentary life-style and the recent onset of 2 to 3 block claudication would usually require only a physical examination and noninvasive vascular testing to determine the degree of arterial insufficiency. If additional medical risk factors are present, the most appropriate treatment for this individual would be conservative medical management. On the other hand, if the individual is employed and supporting a family or retired and actively pursuing recreational interests such as golf, tennis, or travel, the same symptoms may be intolerable. In these circumstances, a decision to pursue surgical treatment is considered elective. It is the obligation of the treating physician to obtain additional information about the extent of disease, including the level of involvement and the anticipated surgical procedure required to alleviate the symptoms. In addition, the patient should understand the potential risks involved relative to the anticipated benefit.

In patients with lower extremity atherosclerosis, the most critical risk factor is the presence of coronary artery disease.[77] Patients needing vascular surgery for leg ASO who underwent preliminary coronary bypass had a 30% higher 5-year survival rate than a comparable group who did not have myocardial revascularization in the presence of severe correctable disease.[78] The use of coronary arteriography for preoperative assessment of cardiac disease is discussed in Chapter 10. If significant coronary artery disease is present and cannot be corrected, some alternative less stressful operative intervention may be considered such as axillofemoral or femoral-femoral bypass reconstruction rather than an intraabdominal aortobifemoral procedure. Other important medical risks also need to be considered, such as the presence of chronic pulmonary disease, renal insufficiency, poorly controlled hypertension, and uncontrolled diabetes mellitus. Age alone is usually not a contraindication to surgical treatment.

When surgical treatment is considered for lower extremity atherosclerosis, a complete arteriographic study of the abdominal aorta and lower extremity arteries is mandatory (Fig. 9-6). Lateral or oblique views of selected areas such as the iliac and profunda femoris vessels may be necessary. Digital subtraction arteriography is useful in certain situations in which severe multilevel disease is present.[79] However, in our practice at the Cleveland Clinic, we have found that standard arteriographic studies with delayed views or selective injections are preferable to digital subtraction studies in the lower extremities.

Preoperative preparation

Once the preliminary preoperative studies have been performed and a decision has been made to proceed with surgical treatment, the patient should be prepared medically. A review of the patient's medications is important. If the individual has been under treatment with daily aspirin for its antiplatelet effect, this medication should be stopped at least 1 week before aortic reconstruction. Although aspirin does not cause a measurable effect on blood coagulation, many surgeons find increased bleeding and delayed clotting in retroperitoneal dissection. In addition, if the patient has been taking diuretics for antihypertensive management, the total body potassium may be depleted; these patients should receive replacement therapy to avoid cardiac complications. For individuals with known coronary artery disease, perioperative transcutaneous or intravenous nitrates may also be beneficial. Assessment of pulmonary function with screening spirometry and cessation of cigarette smoking, if only for a few days, may be extremely helpful in the mobilization of pulmonary secretions. Preoperative respiratory therapy with bronchodilators may be helpful for some individuals with chronic pulmonary disease. Adequate hydration is also important, particularly in patients who may have marginal renal function and have recently undergone contrast arteriographic studies. In those who have known impairment of ventricular contractility, preoperative assessment in the intensive care unit with Swan-Ganz placement and hemodynamic evaluation may be useful.

Prophylactic antibiotics are recommended by most vascular surgeons when the use of a prosthetic vascular conduit is anticipated. *Staphylococcus*, *Streptococcus*, and *E. coli* are the most common organisms associated with perioperative wound infections and major complications of graft infection. Therefore most surgeons commonly employ a cephalosporin that is effective against these organisms.

Each hospital should also be aware of the most common flora present in its own operating rooms and intensive care units. Most institutions do surveillance testing with antibiotic sensitivities to the organism most commonly encountered in a particular environment. Ideally, selection of antibiotic prophylaxis should be based on this information for individual institutions.

Most aortic reconstructions require transfusion of at least two or three units of blood during or immediately after the surgical procedure. Although the risk of hepatitis and acquired immunodeficiency syndrome is very low from the transfusion of anonymous donor-banked blood, some institutions have developed a program of predonation of autologous blood that will be used during major aortic reconstructive operations. Most surgeons also employ a blood recovery system and retransfuse autologous packed red blood cells during major aortic reconstructions.[80] Rarely is there sufficient blood loss during femoropopliteal reconstructions alone to require the use of autotransfusion devices. However, for reoperations, predonation of autologous blood is also a reasonable consideration.

Lumbar sympathectomy

Surgical lumbar sympathectomy has been employed as treatment for lower extremity occlusive disease since the concept was advocated by Leriche in 1913.[81] Diez elaborated on the technique and included the use of ganglionectomy along with periarterial sympathectomy.[82] In 1925 Adson and Brown first used lumbar sympathectomy in the United States for the treatment of Raynaud's disease.[83] For the next three decades sympathectomy was the only surgical alternative to amputation for the treatment of lower extremity occlusive disease. Even after direct reconstructive procedures were introduced in the early 1950s, surgical sympathectomy was used either as sole treatment for patients with distal, tibial occlusive disease or as an adjunct for reconstructive procedures.

The effectiveness of sympathectomy has always been controversial. Although laboratory studies have demonstrated that sympathectomy can increase total limb blood flow in normal subjects, no convincing clinical studies have demonstrated improved limb blood flow in patients with arterial occlusive disease. Experimental studies by Rutherford and Valenta[84] and Cronenwett and Lindenauer[85] have shown that most of the increased blood flow following sympathectomy involves redistribution to the skin rather than to muscle. These studies support the impression that sympathectomy does not relieve symptoms of intermittent claudication or rest pain. However, sympathectomy may be useful in patients who have ischemic skin ulceration related to arterial insufficiency and local trauma. Clinical studies by Persson, Anderson, and Padberry[86] and Walker and Johnston[87] suggested that patients with ischemic rest pain or ulceration may be reasonable candidates for lumbar sympathectomy if they have an ABI of greater than 0.30, if the symptoms are limited to the forefoot, and if sensory neuropathy is absent. Yao and Bergan[88] reported in 1973 that more than 90% of patients who had an ABI lower than 0.35 failed to experience symptomatic relief from lumbar sympathectomy alone. Diabetic patients with sensory neuropathy are particularly unresponsive to the effects of lumbar sympathectomy for ischemic foot lesions.

The use of lumbar sympathectomy as an adjunct to surgical reconstruction has gradually declined among vascular surgeons. The resurgence of interest in the use of in situ saphenous vein bypass to distal tibial and pedal vessels and the use of reversed veins to similar distal arteries in recent years has resulted in revascularization of many extremities that were previously considered "nonoperable." The success of these distal arterial reconstructions has consequently reduced the use of sympathectomy. Some surgeons continue to use lumbar sympathectomy in association with aortic reconstruction when there is evidence of digital ischemia from atheroembolization or in the presence of severe multilevel disease. However, no conclusive evidence supports the persistence of this practice.[89] Sympathectomy may be useful in the treatment of causalgia, Buerger's disease, frostbite or digital ischemia if a trial of percutaneous lumbar sympathectic blocks demonstrates a positive response. Chemical sympathectomy with a phenol or alcohol injection has also been advocated by some,[90] and it may be as effective as surgical sympathectomy when performed by an experienced physician.

Aorto-Iliac-femoral reconstruction

Patients with the onset of calf claudication followed by thigh and hip claudication commonly have multisegment disease involving the aortoiliac region and superficial femoral arteries. Patients with pain at rest or ischemic necrosis of the feet will often have diffuse multisegment disease involving the aortoiliac region, femoropopliteal segment, as well as tibial occlusive disease. Isolated aortoiliac occlusive disease, when associated with impotence in men and with diminished femoral pulses, is often referred to as *Leriche's syndrome*. While originally described by Leriche as complete aortic occlusion at the bifurcation of the iliac arteries, this term has come to be applied loosely to patients who have stenotic lesions in the aortoiliac segment.

If atherosclerosis affects the patient at multiple segments, the proximal segments are generally treated initially if their occlusive lesions have hemodynamic consequences. Current methods of noninvasive testing that measure segmental pressures as well as intraarterial pressure measurements at the time of the arteriographic study may help define the significance of arteriographically demonstrated lesions. Patients with proximal atherosclerosis often manifest symptoms of hip, buttock, and thigh claudication.

The first aortic reconstructive operations performed in the early 1950s used cadaver homograft replacements.[7] Within a short time the technique of thromboendarterectomy was also applied to atherosclerotic lesions of the aortoiliac segment.[9] At the same time, Dacron fabric prostheses were constructed that were found to be adequate replacements for occluded vessels in the aortoiliac and femoral segments.[10] The use of homografts has gradually been abandoned because of the deterioration of the conduit by aneurysm formation. However, thromboendarterectomy is still a useful technique for patients who have localized disease, particularly in younger individuals with disease confined to the aortic bifurcation.[91] A syndrome in young women who smoke has been described, and this technique may be particularly well suited to them.[92]

For the most part Dacron graft replacement has become the standard reconstructive method for most patients with aortoiliac and femoral occlusive disease, although there are still some controversial aspects. Controversies include the method of proximal anastomosis (i.e., end-end vs end-side) and the type of prosthesis (i.e., knitted vs woven material and standard vs velour construction). Another area of controversy concerns the use of adjunctive lumbar sympathectomy. Without any substantive data to indicate that lumbar sympathectomy improves long-term graft patency, the trend in recent years has been to forego this additional procedure unless there is severe multilevel occlusive disease with ischemic superficial skin lesions on the foot or ischemic pain at rest. Controversy also exists over whether the optimal approach to the aorta is a transabdominal midline incision or retroperitoneal exposure through the flank.[93] Most vascular surgeons continue to use a transabdominal midline approach. Since different approaches may have specific benefits for selected patients, the vascular surgeon should be familiar with a wide variety of repair techniques.

For aortofemoral reconstruction it is important to be aware of the blood supply to the left side of the colon.[94] The arteriogram will often demonstrate whether the inferior mesenteric artery is occluded or patent and whether prominent collateral circulation exists between the inferior mesenteric bed and the superior mesenteric artery distribution. If an end-end proximal aortic-to-graft anastomosis is constructed and there is significant external iliac occlusive disease, some alternative means may be needed to maintain perfusion to the internal iliac arteries or inferior mesenteric artery. This can be accomplished by reimplantation of the inferior mesenteric artery or branched Dacron limbs to the internal iliac or common iliac arteries when the main reconstruction extends to the common femoral arteries bilaterally. Frequently, substantial disease is present in the common femoral arteries that may extend a short distance into the profunda femoris or superficial femoral origin. A localized femoral endarterectomy may be needed to make sure there is adequate outflow for the proximal reconstruction. This procedure is even more important if combined segment disease is present with significant stenosis or segmental occlusions of the superficial femoral artery.[95]

Other alternatives exist for the treatment of aortoiliac occlusive disease. These include axillofemoral-femoral reconstruction or femoral-femoral bypass if unilateral iliac occlusive disease is present. In general, these alternative forms of reconstruction are used for the medically high-risk individual in cases where a transabdominal procedure would place the patient at substantial risk. They are particularly useful for patients who have nonreconstructible coronary disease or severe pulmonary disease. However, these alternative forms of reconstruction are not as durable as an anatomic aortoiliac or aortofemoral reconstruction.[96] A more recent alternative to bypass reconstruction is the catheter-directed interventional techniques such as balloon dilation, atherectomy, or intravascular stent placement. Further long-term study may determine whether these interventional procedures have the same durability as bypass graft reconstructions.

Profunda femoris reconstruction

In 1961 Morris et al[97] as well as Leeds and Gilfillan[98] recognized the importance of the profunda femoris artery in lower extremity perfusion. The concept of profunda femoris reconstruction was later emphasized by Martin, Bernhard, and others.[2,99,100] The profunda femoris or deep femoral artery serves as a bridge or major collateral pathway between the aortofemoral segment and the femoropopliteal segment when the superficial femoral artery is occluded. Therefore the profunda femoris artery plays an important role in both "inflow" and "outflow" lower extremity reconstructions. Maintenance of profunda femoris blood flow is always an objective of lower extremity revascularization when the superficial femoral artery is occluded. In many situations, the Dacron prosthesis may be extended down onto the profunda femoris for a short distance to provide unobstructed outflow. In femoropopliteal reconstruction it is important to assess whether a profundaplasty may be needed to maintain this collateral pathway. This adjunct to femoropopliteal reconstruction may help maintain limb viability if the femoropopliteal or tibial bypass subsequently becomes occluded.

For a time there was considerable interest in profunda reconstruction as an isolated procedure for limb salvage. However, further study has indicated that while profunda reconstruction alone may help to relieve symptoms of intermittent claudication, it is often insufficient to heal ischemic necrosis of the foot or to relieve rest pain when critical ischemia is present.[101] Therefore profunda reconstruction is most often an adjunct to either an "inflow" aortofemoral procedure or to "outflow" femoropopliteal reconstruction. At times if disease in the profunda femoris is quite extensive, a procedure referred to as "extended profundaplasty" may be required to preserve its function.[102,103] This condition is particularly common in patients with associated diabetes mellitus.

Profundaplasty alone, as an isolated procedure for limb salvage, should be considered in highly selected patients. Boren et al[101] have advocated the use of a profunda-popliteal collateral index as a means of providing an objective criterion for success. Limb salvage may be expected in 91% of those limbs that have an index of less than 0.19. Calculation of the index may be influenced by the presence of iliac inflow disease and should not be relied on as the only criterion for performing profundaplasty. Profundaplasty should also be considered for those patients who have "nonreconstructible" disease before a major amputation is undertaken, since the level of amputation may be reduced from above-knee to below-knee in some patients.[103]

Femoropopliteal and femorotibial reconstruction

The first successful surgical reconstructions for lower extremity vascular disease were femoropopliteal bypass operations using a reversed greater saphenous vein. Early experience confirmed that the saphenous vein was a reliable conduit.[104] For the most part bypasses were performed to the above-knee or below-knee popliteal artery, whereas reversed vein bypass to tibial arteries were less commonly performed. In the United States it was not until 1979 that a large well-analyzed series was reported.[105] At the same time some surgeons felt that the use of the reversed saphenous vein had reached the limits of its effectiveness for surgical treatment of femoropopliteal disease.[106] Leather, Powers, and Karmody[15] reintroduced the use of the saphenous vein in situ as a conduit for femoropopliteal and tibial reconstruction. The resurgence of interest in this technique, as well as many of their adjuncts to the in situ technique, have helped spur the advancement of bypass reconstruction to more distal tibial vessels. During the 1980s the in situ method of saphenous vein bypass reconstruction has received a great deal of attention. Although many surgeons feel that this method represents a distinct advancement in reconstructive technique, others maintain that similar results can be obtained with reverse saphenous vein to tibial vessels.[107]

Several different prosthetic conduits have been used for femoropopliteal reconstruction. These include Dacron, bovine heterografts, umbilical vein, polytetrafluoroethylene (PTFE), and composites of Dacron-PTFE. Unfortunately, these prosthetic materials are unable to achieve the same primary patency rates as autogenous vein for bypass reconstructions to the below-knee popliteal and tibial arteries. The development of a suitable arterial substitute for small caliber arteries has been frustratingly slow during the past two decades. Carefully controlled studies demonstrated that PTFE has comparable patency rates to the above-knee popliteal artery as a reversed saphenous vein. However, the primary patency drops off dramatically in bypasses to the below-knee popliteal artery or individual tibial vessels.[108] Attempts have been made to improve the results of prosthetic grafting by means of composite or sequential use with saphenous vein for the below-knee portion of the bypass.[109] Attempts to coat the lumen of the PTFE bypass with endothelial cells have also been studied. To date none of these methods has substantially improved the patency of prosthetic material in distal bypass reconstructions. Extensive femoropopliteal thromboendarterectomy was also used for a time. These methods consisted of both closed and semiopen techniques with and without vein or Dacron patch angioplasty.[110,111] However, the experience over time was that these reconstructed femoropopliteal arteries eventually reoccluded as a result of myointimal hyperplasia.

In more recent years interventional techniques using laser heated probes to recanalize occluded femoropopliteal arteries have been attempted. Once the arteries have been recanalized, catheter-directed balloons are used to dilate the stenotic artery. The results of these interventional techniques have been inferior to results from bypass reconstruction for extensive disease involving the femoropopliteal segments.[112]

The indications for bypass reconstruction of the femoropopliteal and femoral tibial segments are generally more stringent than for aortofemoral reconstruction. Intermittent claudication is an acceptable indication if the patient's walking distance is extremely limited. Some differentiation is necessary about the extent of femoropopliteal disease. If an above-knee bypass can be performed with either the saphenous vein or a prosthetic conduit and distal runoff is unimpaired, the results of surgical treatment are quite acceptable, that is, 70% to 80% 5-year graft patency. However, when reconstruction requires bypass to the below-knee popliteal or individual tibial arteries, the results may not be durable enough (40% to 50% 5-year patency) to justify reconstruction in the presence of intermittent claudication as the sole symptom. In patients with more extensive lower extremity occlusive disease, ischemic pain at rest or tissue necrosis that threatens limb viability are more acceptable indications for operation. Most centers have reserved distal tibial bypass reconstruction for patients with limb-threatening ischemia. The results of more recent reports indicate that bypass to individual tibial arteries is comparable to bypass to the below-knee popliteal artery if either an in situ or reversed saphenous vein graft is used.[113,114,130]

Many subtle technical variations have been reported for

Table 9-3. Published results of femoropopliteal and femorotibial bypass grafts

Author	No. of bypasses	Graft material	Location of bypass	1-year Patency (%)	1-year Limb salvage (%)	5-year* Patency (%)	5-year* Limb salvage (%)
DeWeese and Rob[52] (1977)	113	Vein	Popliteal (above- and below-knee)	65		59	
Reichle et al[105] (1979)	474	Vein and Dacron	Popliteal (above- and below-knee)		67.6		59.7
		Vein	Tibial/peroneal		53.9		46.9
Harris et al[116] (1984)	70	Vein	Popliteal and tibial/peroneal	85		68	85
Weaver et al[115] (1987)	29	Vein	Tibial/peroneal	72			
Veith et al[108] (1986)	522	Vein	Proximal popliteal	80		61	75
			distal popliteal	84		76	76
			tibial/peroneal	75		49	57
		PTFE	Proximal popliteal	80		38	70
			distal popliteal	84		54	70
			tibial/peroneal	56		12	61
Leather et al[130] (1988)	725	Vein (in situ)	Distal popliteal	90.8		78.5	
			tibial/peroneal	91.7		74.3	
Taylor, Edwards, and Porter[114] (1990)	516	Vein	Proximal popliteal	86.6		76.6	
			distal popliteal	92		80.2	90.2
			tibial/peroneal	81.2		69.1	

*Four-year patency/limb salvage data for Veith et al.[108]

femoropopliteal and femorotibial reconstruction. When a sufficient length of autogenous greater saphenous vein is unavailable, other sources of autogenous conduit have been suggested such as the lesser saphenous or cephalic veins and endarterectomized superficial femoral artery.[115-118] Other combinations of autogenous and prosthetic material have been recommended as have the use of sequential bypasses. Alternative inflow sites such as the profunda femoris artery or distal superficial artery have been suggested when the length of vein is inadequate for distal bypass reconstruction. Another reported variation in technique is the use of short tibial-to-tibial vein interposition bypasses.[119] These innovative techniques have resulted in successful bypass reconstructions to the posterior tibial and dorsalis pedis arteries below the malleoli.

Most series report significant attrition of bypass patency during the first 1 to 2 years of follow-up study. Table 9-3 lists the results of reported series for femoropopliteal and femorotibial reconstructions. Some investigators have reported that if distal bypass reconstructions are observed carefully postoperatively, failing bypasses can be identified, and timely intervention may be able to salvage a failing bypass.[120,121] However, secondary reconstructions in the lower extremity bypass are significantly less successful than primary reconstruction (50% patency at 1 year in most series). In more recent years noninvasive techniques provide a convenient method of objective follow-up. Rutherford et al have recommended a standard scheme of reporting of lower extremity bypass reconstruction so that series from different institutions can be compared.[122] Standardized reporting should lead to more accurate comparisons of surgical techniques and graft materials among published series. Continued refinements of surgical technique, graft materials, and objective means of assessment should lead to improvements and salvage of lower extremities afflicted with arterial insufficiency.

Amputation

The treatment of lower extremity occlusive disease may, at times, require amputation of a limb. Lalka and Malone[123] stated that "the purpose of amputation surgery is to remove gangrenous, necrotic, or infected tissue; relieve pain; obtain primary healing of the most distal amputation possible; and achieve maximal rehabilitation after amputation. These goals can only be met by careful preoperative evaluation and aggressive preparation of patients for surgery." Amputation of a limb is an emotional issue for patients. Some individuals will go to great lengths to avoid major amputation, often enduring many attempts at revascularization or extended periods of intense pain in an effort to avoid an inevitable amputation. The physician should view amputation as an alternative treatment option for selected patients with the long-term goal of functional rehabilitation.

Amputations are characterized as primary or secondary, depending on whether they are undertaken as definitive surgical treatment for lower extremity ischemia or whether they follow a previous attempt at revascularization. Primary amputation vs revascularization for patients with limb-threatening ischemia is a controversial issue. Methods to assess the possibility of limb salvage by revascularization as opposed to the need for definitive amputation include Doppler ankle systolic pressures, pulse volume waveform measurements, skin temperature measurements, laser Doppler velocity measurements, xenon-133 skin blood flow measurements, fluorescein dye injections, transcutaneous oxygen measurements, and transcutaneous carbon dioxide measurements. After analysis of these and other methods, the final decision about whether to pursue primary amputation or revascularization depends on the surgeon's clinical judgment. The surgeon's decision also includes personal experience and subjective factors such as the patient's potential for rehabilitation and willingness to accept amputation as the recommended definitive treatment. Other issues in this decision making process include the patient's general medical condition and history of myocardial infarction, previous stroke, chronic organic brain syndrome, and chronic renal insufficiency.

Secondary amputations are those that follow a previous vascular reconstructive procedure. The decision to perform a secondary amputation depends on the type and location of previous vascular reconstruction, the number of repeated attempts at maintaining bypass graft patency, the type of bypass employed in femoral distal reconstructions, such as vein or PTFE, and the presence of coexisting factors such as sepsis.

Amputation may be required for acute, as opposed to chronic, limb-threatening conditions. Acute or urgent amputations are often required for those patients who have such extensive tissue necrosis that salvage of a viable foot is not possible. Ischemia accompanied by extensive soft tissue infection with signs of systemic sepsis is another indication for urgent amputation, often found in patients with coexistent diabetes mellitus. Many surgeons prefer a guillotine amputation at the ankle level as an initial procedure to eliminate the source of sepsis rather than definitive below-knee amputation when extensive sepsis is present.[124] The patient can be treated for several days with antibiotics and surgical drainage to allow time for the infection to subside. Diabetes mellitus has been associated with more than 50% of major amputations in patients with lower extremity occlusive disease.[125] Secondary amputation may also be considered for the patient who has intractable ischemic rest pain following occlusion of previous bypass reconstruction.

Minor amputations of individual toes, or transmetatarsal amputation, may be necessary in some individuals who undergo a reconstructive procedure. In general, revascularization will improve perfusion sufficiently to heal local amputation of toes or amputations in the midfoot region. If more than two digits are involved with fixed gangrenous changes that preclude conservative management, a full transmetatarsal amputation is usually preferable to individual toe amputation. Patients tolerate transmetatarsal amputation quite well without functional disability. They will often benefit from the use of a custom-fitted, toe-filling orthotic for the shoe.

Major amputation involves below-knee amputation through the midcalf or above-knee amputation in the distal thigh. Standard techniques have been described elsewhere in surgical texts. Although the Syme's amputation technique (through the ankle) has been advocated by some as an acceptable alternative to below-knee amputation, in general we have found that this technique has very limited applicability. Because of recent advances in prosthetic design and patient rehabilitation therapy, below-knee amputees should have excellent functional recovery.

Perioperative mortality from amputation ranges from 9% to 15%, depending on the patient's age and associated risk factors.[126] The same risk factors are present for patients who require amputation as for those who are candidates for lower extremity revascularization. In general, the risk might be expected to be even higher because many of these individuals have advanced nonreconstructible occlusive disease. Survival of amputees has been reported to be only approximately 30% at 5 years for major amputations.[127]

Rehabilitation therapy for patients who are able to retain the knee joint is so superior to above-knee amputation that a conservative approach should be used before a major amputation is undertaken. In some cases the level of amputation may be reduced by revascularization.[128] For example, some patients may require only below-knee amputation if a proximal reconstruction in the aortoiliac segment or above-knee femoropopliteal bypass is undertaken. In addition, profundaplasty alone may aid in maintaining a below-knee level of amputation in selected cases.

Amputations through the knee and hip joints do not usually offer any advantage over standard below-knee or above-knee amputations. Knee disarticulation is an alternative as a means of débridement when acute infection involves the leg above the ankle. Hip disarticulation is usually reserved for those individuals who have extensive ischemia that extends proximally in the thigh and precludes an above-knee amputation through the femur. Functional rehabilitation in patients with hip disarticulation is usually poor.

More than half of patients who undergo lower extremity amputation have coexisting diabetes mellitus. Diabetics often develop a sensory neuropathy that leads to bony changes in the foot and to neurotrophic ulceration over bony prominences. These individuals may develop extensive foot sepsis with little awareness of pain or discomfort. If arterial circulation to the foot is preserved, their condition often responds dramatically to aggressive surgical drainage and antimicrobial therapy. Occasionally, excision of an involved metatarsal head may be required to allow the foot lesion to heal. If sepsis can be controlled locally, and if arterial perfusion is adequate, foot salvage is often possible.[129]

It is extremely important that amputees receive physical therapy or supervised rehabilitation. Some patients may require transfer to a specific inpatient rehabilitation facility if their progress during in-hospital convalescence is not adequate. Various prosthetic options are available. Prosthetics may be fitted immediately to allow the patient to begin walking soon after surgery. In some patients with vascular disease who have delayed wound healing, prosthetic fitting should be delayed for 2 to 3 months until the amputation site has healed completely. An experienced prosthetist is very important to help the patient achieve the proper fitting and adjustment of the artificial limb. A close working relationship between the physician, prosthetist, physical therapist, and patient is important for the long-term recovery of the patient with vascular disease who requires an amputation.

REFERENCES

1. Darling RC et al: Aortoiliac reconstruction, Surg Clin North Am 59:565, 1979.
2. Samson RH, Scher LA, and Veith FJ: Combined segment arterial disease, Surgery 97:385, 1985.
3. Carrel A and Guthrie CC: Results of biterminal transplantation of veins, Am J Med Sci 132:415, 1906.
4. Carrel A and Guthrie CC: Unilateral and biterminal venous transplantation, Surg Gynecol Obstet 2:266, 1906.
5. Dale WA: The beginnings of vascular surgery, Surgery 76:849, 1974.
6. Kunlin J: Le traitement de l'arterite obliterante par la greffe veneuse, Arch Mal Coeur 42:371, 1949.
7. Oudot J: La greffe vasculaire dans les thromboses du carrefour aortigue, Presse Med 59:234, 1951.
8. Dos Santos JC: Sur la desobstruction des thromboses arterielles anciennes, Mem Acad Chir 73:409, 1947.
9. Wylie EJ: Thromboendarterectomy for arteriosclerotic thrombosis of major arteries, Surgery 23:275, 1952.
10. Blakemore A and Voorhees AB: The use of tubes constructed from Vinyon-N cloth in bridging arterial defects: experimental and clinical, Ann Surg 140:324, 1954.
11. Imparato AM et al: The results of tibial artery reconstruction procedures, Surg Gynecol Obstet 138:33, 1974.
12. Maini BS and Mannick JA: Effect of arterial reconstruction on limb salvage: a ten year apprisal, Arch Surg 113:1297, 1978.
13. Reichle FA et al: Long-term results of 474 arterial reconstructions for severely ischemic limbs: a 14 year follow-up, Surgery 85:93, 1979.
14. Hall V: The great saphenous vein used in-situ as an arterial shunt after extirpation of the vein valves, Surgery 51:492, 1962.
15. Leather RP, Powers SR, and Karmody AM: A reapprisal of the in-situ saphenous vein arterial bypass and its use in limb salvage, Surgery 86:453, 1979.
16. Dormandy J et al: Fate of the patient with chronic leg ischemia, J Cardiovasc Surg 30:50, 1989.
17. McCready RA, Vincent AE, and Schwartz RW: Atherosclerosis in the young: a virulent disease, Surgery 96:863, 1984.
18. Evans WE, Hayes JP, and Vermillion BD: Atherosclerosis in the younger patient: results of surgical management, Am J Surg 154:225, 1987.
19. Coffman JD: Intermittent claudication: not so benign, Am Heart J 112:1127, 1986.
20. Kannel WB and McGee DL: Update on some epidemiologic features of intermittent claudication: the Framingham study, J Am Geriatr Soc 33:13, 1985.
21. Couch NP: On the arterial consequences of smoking, J Vasc Surg 3:807, 1986.
22. Reunanen AL, Takkunen H, and Aromaa A: Prevalence of intermittent claudication and its effect on mortality, Acta Med Scand 211:249, 1982.
23. Jonason T and Ringquist I: Factors of prognostic importance for subsequent rest pain in patients with intermittent claudication, Acta Med Scand 218:27, 1985.
24. Kannel WB: Update on the role of cigarette smoking in coronary heart disease, Am Heart J 101:319, 1981.
25. Thomas M: Smoking and vascular surgery, Br J Surg 68:601, 1981.
26. Hughson WG, Mann JI, and Garrod A: Intermittent claudication: prevalence and risk factors, Br Med J 1:1379, 1978.
27. Myers KA et al: The effect of smoking on the late patency of arterial reconstructions in the legs, Br J Surg 65:267, 1978.
28. Pollin W: The role of the addictive process as a key step in causation of all tobacco related diseases, JAMA 252:2874, 1984.
29. Eldrup-Jorgenson J et al: Hypercoagulable states and lower limb ischemia in young adults, J Vasc Surg 9:334, 1989.
30. Ciuffetti G et al: The hemorrheological role of cellular factors in peripheral vascular disease, VASA 17:168, 1988.
31. McAllister FF: The fate of patients with intermittent claudication managed non-operatively, Am J Surg 132:593, 1976.
32. Juergens JL, Barker NW, and Hines EA: Arteriosclerosis obliterans: a review of 520 cases with special reference to pathologic and prognostic factors, Circulation 21:188, 1960.
33. Bloor K: Natural history of arteriosclerosis of the lower extremities, Ann R Coll Surg Engl 28:36, 1961.
34. Boyd AM: The natural course of arteriosclerosis of the lower extremities, Proc R Soc Med 55:591, 1962.
35. Kannel WB and Shurteff O: The natural history of arteriosclerosis obliterans, Cardiovasc Clin 3:37, 1971.
36. Strandness DE and Stahler C: Arteriosclerosis obliterans: manner and rate of progression, JAMA 196:1, 1966.
37. Cronenwett JL, Warner KG, and Zelenock GB: Intermittent claudication: current results of non-operative management, Arch Surg 119:430, 1984.
38. Rosenbloom MS et al: Risk factors affecting the natural history of intermittent claudication, Arch Surg 123:867, 1988.
39. Castronuevo JJ and Flanigan DP: Pseudoclaudication of neurospinal origin, Vasc Diag Ther 5:21, 1984.
40. Stephens MM, O'Connell D, and McManus F: Neurogenic claudication (spinal stenosis), Ir Med J 77:235, 1984.
41. Kozol RA et al: Dependent rubor as a predictor of limb risk in patients with claudication, Arch Surg 119:932, 1984.
42. Wilbourn AJ et al: Ischemic monomelic neuropathy, Neurology 33:447, 1983.
43. Kim D, Orron DE, and Skillman JJ: Surgical significance of popliteal arterial variants and a unified angiographic classification, Ann Surg 210:776, 1989.
44. Yao JST: Hemodynamic studies in peripheral arterial disease, Br J Surg 57:761, 1970.
45. Hodgson KJ and Sumner DS: Noninvasive assessment of lower extremity arterial disease, Ann Vasc Surg 2:174, 1988.
46. Rutherford RB, Lowenstein DH, and Klein MF: Combining segmental systolic pressures and plethysmography to diagnose arterial disease of the legs, Am J Surg 138:211, 1979.
47. Kram HB, Appel PL, and Shoemaker WC: Multisensor transcutaneous oximetric mapping to predict below knee amputation wound healing: use of a critical Po_2, J Vasc Surg 9:796, 1989.
48. Cone JB: Positron emission tomography: new analytic tool for vascular disease, J Vasc Surg 2:360, 1985.
49. Rhodes RS and Cohen AM: Magnetic resonance imaging and spectroscopy in the study of cardiovascular disease, J Vasc Surg 2:354, 1985.
50. Mitchell DG and Carabasi A: Vascular applications of magnetic resonance imaging, Ann Vasc Surg 3:400, 1989.
51. Dientfass L: Elevation of blood viscosity, aggregation of red cells, hematocrit values and fibrinogen levels in cigarette smokers, Med J Aust 1:617, 1975.
52. DeWeese JA and Rob CG: Autogenous venous grafts ten years later, Surgery 82:775, 1977.

53. Hertzer NR et al: Late results of coronary bypass in patients presenting with lower extremity ischemia: the Cleveland Clinic Study, Ann Vasc Surg 1:411, 1986.
54. Seldinger S: Catheter replacement of the needle in percutaneous arteriography, Acta Radiol 39:368, 1953.
55. Dardik I et al: Routine intraoperative angiography: an essential adjunct in vascular surgery, Arch Surg 110:184, 1975.
56. Hertzer NR et al: Coronary artery disease in peripheral vascular patients: a classification of 1000 coronary angiograms and results of surgical management, Ann Surg 199:223, 1984.
57. Hertzer NR et al: Late results of coronary bypass in patients with peripheral vascular disease. II. Five year survival according to sex, hypertension and diabetes, Cleve Clin J Med 54:15, 1987.
58. Quick CRG and Cotton LT: The measured effect of stopping smoking on claudication, Br J Surg 69(suppl):24, 1982.
59. Robicsek F et al: The effect of continued cigarette smoking on the patency of synthetic vascular grafts in Leriche syndrome, J Thorac Cardiovasc Surg 70:107, 1975.
60. Greenhalgh RM et al: Smoking and arterial reconstruction, Br J Surg 68:605, 1981.
61. Brown BG et al: Regression of coronary artery disease as a result of intensive lipid-lowering therapy in men with high levels of apolipoprotein B, N Engl J Med 323:1289, 1990.
62. Blankenhorn DH et al: Beneficial effects of combined colestipol-Niacin therapy on coronary atherosclerosis and coronary venous bypass grafts, JAMA 257:3233, 1987.
63. Rick ME: Protein C and Protein S: vitamin K dependent inhibitors of blood coagulation, JAMA 263:701, 1990.
64. Flinn WR et al: Improved long-term patency of infragenicular polytetrafluoroethylene bypass grafts, J Vasc Surg 7:685, 1988.
65. Baxter BR et al: Prospective assessment of antithrombotic therapy following primary below knee prosthetic bypass, Paper presented at the meeting of the Society for Vascular Surgery, Los Angeles, June 1990.
66. Coffman JD: Vasodilator drugs in peripheral vascular disease, N Engl J Med 300:713, 1979.
67. Porter J et al: Pentoxifylline efficacy in the treatment of intermittent claudication: multicenter controlled double blind trial with objective assessment of chronic occlusive arterial disease patients, Am Heart J 104:66, 1982.
68. Green RM and McNamara J: The effects of pentoxifylline on patients with intermittent claudication, J Vasc Surg 7:356, 1988.
69. Halperin JL, Rothlauf EB, and Von Polnitz A: Limb hemodynamic effects of pentoxifylline in patients with intermittent claudiation, J Vasc Med Biol 1:294, 1989.
70. Prevention of Atherosclerotic Complications with Ketanserin Trial Group: Prevention of atherosclerotic complications: controlled trial of Ketanserin, Br Med J 298:424, 1989.
71. Brevetti G et al: Increases in walking distance in patients with peripheral vascular disease treated with L-Carnitine: a double-blind, crossover study, Therapy and Prevention 77:767, 1988.
72. Carlson LA and Erikksson I: Femoral artery infusion of prostaglandin E in severe peripheral vascular disease, Lancet 1:155, 1976.
73. Gruss JD et al: Conservative treatment of inoperable arterial occlusion of the lower extremities with intraarterial prostaglandin E_1, Br J Surg 69(suppl II):II-103, 1982.
74. Schuler JJ et al: The efficacy of prostaglandin E_1 (PGE_1), in the treatment of lower extremity ischemic ulcers secondary to peripheral vascular occlusive disease: results of a prospective, randomized, double-blind, multicenter clinical trial, J Vasc Surg 1:160, 1984.
75. Cronenwett JL et al: Prostacyclin treatment of ischemic ulcers and rest pain in unreconstructable peripheral arterial occlusive disease, Surgery 100:369, 1986.
76. Skinner JS and Strandness DE Jr: Exercise and intermittent claudication. II. Effect of physical training, Circulation 36:23, 1967.
77. Hertzer NR: Fatal myocardial infarction following lower extremity revascularization, Ann Surg 193:492, 1981.
78. Hertzer NR et al: Late results of coronary bypass in patients with peripheral vascular disease. I. Five year survival according to age and clinical cardiac status, Cleve Clin Quart 53:133, 1986.
79. Blakeman BM, Littody FN, and Baker WH: Intra-arterial digital subtraction angiography as a method to study peripheral vascular disease, J Vasc Surg 4:168, 1986.
80. O'Hara PJ et al: Intraoperative autotransfusion during abdominal aortic reconstruction, Am J Surg 145:214, 1983.
81. Ewing M: The history of lumbar sympathectomy, Surgery 70:791, 1971.
82. Diez J: Un neuro metodo de simpatectomia perferica para el tratamiento de affecionas trofilas y gangrenosas de las miembrios, Med Soc Cir Buenos Aires 8:10, 1924.
83. Adson AW and Brown CE: Treatment of Raynaud's disease by lumbar ramisection and ganglionectomy and perivascular sympathectomy neurectomy of the common iliacs, JAMA 84:1908, 1925.
84. Rutherford RB and Valenta J: Extremity blood flow and distribution: the effect of arterial occlusion, sympathectomy and exercise, Surgery 69:332, 1971.
85. Cronenwett JL and Lindenauer SM: Hemodynamic effects of sympathectomy in ischemic canine hind limbs, Surgery 87:417, 1980.
86. Persson AV, Anderson LA, and Padberry FT Jr: Selection of patients for lumbar sympathectomy, Surg Clin North Am 65:393, 1985.
87. Walker PM and Johnston KW: Predicting the success of sympathectomy: a retrospective study using discriminant function and multiple regression analysis, Surgery 87:216, 1980.
88. Yao JST and Bergan JJ: Predictability of vascular reactivity relative to sympathetic ablation, Arch Surg 107:767, 1973.
89. Satiani B et al: Prospective randomized study of concomitant lumbar sympathectomy with aortoiliac reconstruction, Am J Surg 143:755, 1982.
90. Walker PM et al: Phenol sympathectomy for vascular occlusive disease, Surg Gynecol Obstet 146:741, 1978.
91. Naylor AR, Ah-See AK, and Engeset J: Aortoiliac endarterectomy: an eleven year review, Br J Surg 77:190, 1990.
92. Costantino MJ, Smith RB III, and Perdue GD: Segmental aortic occlusion: an unusual lesion found in menopausal women, Surgery 114:318, 1979
93. Sicard GA et al: Comparison between the transabdominal and retroperitoneal approach for reconstruction of the infrarenal aorta, J Vasc Surg 5:19, 1987.
94. Ernst CB: Prevention of intestinal ischemia following abdominal aortic reconstruction, Surgery 93:102, 1983.
95. Martinez BD, Hertzer NR, and Beven EG: Influence of distal arterial occlusive disease on prognosis following aorto-bi-femoral bypass, Surgery 88:795, 1980.
96. Rutherford RB, Patt A, and Pierce WH: Extra-anatomic bypass: a closer view, J Vasc Surg 5:437, 1987.
97. Morris GC Jr et al: Surgical importance of profunda femoris artery: analysis of 102 cases with combined aortoiliac and femoropopliteal occlusive disease treated by revascularization of the deep femoral artery, Arch Surg 82:52, 1961.
98. Leeds FH and Gilfillan RS: Revascularization of the ischemic limb: importance of the profunda femoris artery, Surgery 82:25, 1961.
99. Martin P, Renwick S, and Stephenson CL: On the surgery of the profunda femoris artery, Br J Surg 55:539, 1968.
100. Bernhard VM, Ray LI, and Militello JP: The role of angioplasty of the profunda femoris artery in revascularization of the ischemic limb, Surg Gynecol Obstet 142:840, 1976.
101. Boren CH et al: Profunda popliteal collateral index: a guide to successful profundaplasty, Arch Surg 115:1366, 1980.
102. David TE and Drezner AD: Extended profundaplasty for limb salvage, Surgery 84:758, 1978.
103. Edwards WH et al: Extended profundaplasty to minimize pelvic and distal tissue loss, Ann Surg 211:694, 1990.

104. Dale WA, DeWeese JA, and Scott JM: Autogenous venous shunt grafts, Surgery 46:145, 1959.
105. Reichle FA et al: Long-term results of 474 arterial reconstructions for severely ischemic limbs: a fourteen year follow-up, Surgery 85:93, 1979.
106. Szilagyi DE et al: Autogenous vein graft in femoropopliteal atherosclerosis: the limits of its effectiveness, Surgery 86:836, 1979.
107. Taylor LM Jr et al: Reversed vein bypass to infrapopliteal arteries: modern results are superior to or equivalent to in-situ bypass for patency and vein utilization, Ann Surg 205:90, 1987.
108. Veith FJ et al: Six-year prospective multicenter randomized comparison of autologous saphenous vein and expanded polytetrafluoroethylene grafts in infrainguinal arterial reconstructions, J Vasc Surg 3:104, 1986.
109. DeLaurentis DA and Friedman P: Sequential femoropopliteal bypasses: another approach to the inadequate saphenous vein problem, Surgery 71:400, 1972.
110. Edwards WS: Composite reconstruction of the femoral artery with saphenous vein after endarterectomy, Surg Gynecol Obstet 111:651, 1960.
111. Sobel I et al: Gas endarterectomy, Surgery 59:517, 1961.
112. Seeger JM et al: Initial results of laser recanalization in lower extremity arterial reconstruction, J Vasc Surg 9:10, 1989.
113. Rafferty TD et al: A metropolitan experience with infrainguinal revascularization: operative risk and late results in Northern Ohio, J Vasc Surg 6:365, 1987.
114. Taylor LM, Edwards JM, and Porter JM: Present status of reversed vein bypass grafting: five year results of a modern series, J Vasc Surg 11:193, 1990.
115. Weaver FA et al: The lesser saphenous vein: autogenous tissue for lower extremity revascularization, J Vasc Surg 5:687, 1987.
116. Harris RW et al: Successful long-term limb salvage using cephalic vein bypass grafts, Ann Surg 200:785, 1984.
117. Balshi JD et al: The use of arm veins for infrainguinal bypass in end-stage peripheral vascular disease, Arch Surg 124:1078, 1989.
118. Mukherjee D, Schickler WJ, and Inahara T: The superficial femoral artery as a conduit: an alternative to prosthetic material, J Vasc Surg 2:739, 1985.
119. Veith FJ et al: Tibiotibial vein bypass grafts: a new operation for limb salvage, J Vasc Surg 2:552, 1985.
120. Bandyk DF et al: Monitoring functional patency of in-situ saphenous vein bypasses: the impact of a surveillance protocol and elective revision, J Vasc Surg 9:286, 1989.
121. Green RM et al: Comparison of infrainguinal graft surveillance techniques, J Vasc Surg 11:207, 1990.
122. Rutherford RB et al: Suggested standards for reports dealing with lower extremity ischemia, J Vasc Surg 4:80, 1986.
123. Lalka SG and Malone JM: Patient evaluation and preparation for amputation. In Rutherford RB, ed: Vascular surgery, Philadelphia, 1989, WB Saunders Co.
124. McIntyre KE Jr et al: Guillotine amputation in the treatment of nonsalvagable lower extremity infections, Arch Surg 119:450, 1984.
125. Malone JM and Goldstone J: Lower extremity amputation. In Moore WS, ed: Vascular surgery: a comprehensive review, New York, 1986, Grune & Stratton.
126. Plecha FR et al: The early results of vascular surgery in patients 75 years of age and older: an analysis of 3259 cases, J Vasc Surg 2:769, 1985.
127. Couch NP et al: Natural history of the leg amputee, Am J Surg 133:469, 1977.
128. Johansen K et al: Improvement of amputation level by lower extremity revascularization, Surg Gynecol Obstet 153:707, 1981.
129. Martin JD et al: Radical treatment of mal perforans in diabetic patients with arterial insufficiency, J Vasc Surg 12:264, 1990.
130. Leather RP et al: Resurrection of the in situ saphenous vein bypass, Ann Surg 208:435, 1988.

Chapter 10

CORONARY ARTERY DISEASE ASSOCIATED WITH PERIPHERAL VASCULAR DISEASE

Robert A. Graor
Patrick Whitlow

It has long been known that atherosclerosis, the principal cause of death in western civilization, is a progressive disease that generally begins in childhood and has clinical manifestations in middle and late adulthood. It is a multifactorial process, which, when advanced, involves multiple biologic processes and foci. Therefore it is not surprising that most patients who have aneurysmal or occlusive peripheral vascular disease may also have extensive coronary artery disease. For this reason, myocardial ischemia is the most common adverse outcome associated with patients with peripheral vascular disease. Accordingly, cardiovascular risk assessment is a fundamental component of the evaluation of patients being treated for peripheral vascular disease.

In recent years several studies have evaluated the significance of coronary disease in patients with peripheral vascular disease (Table 10-1).[1-8] The complications of associated coronary artery disease include myocardial infarction, arrhythmia, and congestive heart failure, and these have always been the leading causes of early and late death among patients who require peripheral vascular reconstruction.

Coincident with the understanding that coronary disease is prominent among these patients, the development of safer and more effective coronary artery bypass surgery and percutaneous catheter-directed therapies have allowed more treatment options to be available to a greater number of patients. The conventional history and standard ECG now should be supplemented with objective exercise stress test-

Table 10-1. Incidence of fatal and nonfatal cardiac complications* after peripheral vascular surgery

Preoperative assessment for CAD*	All perioperative cardiac events† (%)	References
Based on clinical evidence		
Absent (3858 patients)		1-6
Range	0-16	
Mean	7.1	
Present (784 patients)		
Range	4.9-42	
Mean	11	
Noninvasive cardiac testing		
Normal (206 patients)		4,5,7,8
Range	0-16	
Mean	6.3	
Positive (200 patients)		
Range	15-69	
Mean	33	

*CAD, Coronary artery disease.
†Myocardial infarction, life-threatening arrhythmia, or congestive heart failure.

ing, radionuclide myocardial imaging, or cardiac catheterization to document the presence of functional coronary artery disease.

Ideally, a noninvasive diagnostic modality, which is capable of reproducibly and accurately identifying preoperative coronary artery disease, would facilitate a triage of high-risk patients to coronary angiography, preoperative coronary revascularization, or aggressive perioperative medical therapy. Unfortunately, this diagnostic modality does not exist.

PREVALENCE OF CORONARY ARTERY DISEASE IN PATIENTS WITH PERIPHERAL VASCULAR DISEASE

The data from the Framingham heart study have suggested that the risk of coronary artery disease in patients with peripheral atherosclerosis is 2.4 times greater in men and 1.4 times greater in women than an age- and sex-matched population.[9] This epidemiologic study has been confirmed by angiographic studies, which clearly demonstrate the prevalence and severity of the coexistence of coronary artery disease with peripheral atherosclerosis.[10-12] It is interesting and important to note that the prevalence of coronary disease, proven by coronary arteriography, is often higher in patients with peripheral vascular disease than in other groups using clinical evidence of coronary disease. These data are shown in Table 10-2.[2-5,8,10-35]

A separation of three major peripheral vascular disease conditions and a comparison of coronary disease prevalence according to the disease state is shown in Table 10-2. These data indicate that patients with abdominal aortic aneurysms have the highest rate compared to those patients with occlusive PVD (lower extremity and carotid occlusive disease) of associated coronary artery disease (65% abdominal aortic aneurysms vs 57% to 60% for other occlusive vascular disease). These rates are significantly greater than those of the normal age-matched population.

In a study done by Hertzer et al 1000 consecutive patients with peripheral arterial disease were evaluated with coronary arteriography.[11] Coronary artery disease was clinically suspected in 52% of 263 patients with abdominal aortic aneurysm, in 56% of 381 patients with lower extremity ischemia, and in 57% of 169 patients with cerebrovascular disease. Overall, only 18% of these patients were found to have normal coronary arteries. These data indicate that occult or asymptomatic coronary disease was present in a large number of patients. Severe, correctable, three-vessel coronary disease, thought to represent the highest risk group, was found in 25% of the patients studied. Severe inoperable coronary artery disease or severely impaired left ventricular function was present in only 6% of patients. Of great interest was that severe coronary artery disease (both correctable and inoperable) was present in 35% of patients with abdominal aortic aneurysm, in 32% of patients with cerebrovascular disease, and in 28% of patients with lower extremity ischemia. This study also emphasized the high incidence of severe three-vessel coronary disease in patients of all age groups and specifically in 22% of patients younger than 50 years of age, in 24% of patients between 50 and 59 years of age, in 30% of patients between 60 and 69 years of age, and in 41% of patients older than 70 years of age.

Several years before the data of Hertzer et al Tomatis, Fireens, and Verbrugge studied 100 patients who submitted to coronary angiography before vascular surgery.[12] They

Table 10-2. Prevalence of associated coronary disease in peripheral vascular patients

	Peripheral vascular disease				
Clinical features	**Abdominal aortic aneurysms (%)**	**Carotid artery disease (%)**	**Lower extremity ischemia (%)**	**General vascular series (%)**	**References**
Clinical evidence of coronary disease					
Patients evaluated	4263	989	2797	718	2, 3, 10, 11, 18-31
% with CAD					
Range	31-70	24-66	22-58	19-62	
Mean	47	56	41	53	
Coronary disease by objective cardiac testing					
Patients evaluated		133		1083	4, 5, 8, 32-34
% with CAD					
Range		25-58		17-47	
Mean		38		21	
Serious coronary disease by angiography					
Patients evaluated	375	295	453	1000	10-12
% with CAD					
Range	58-82		56-57		
Mean	65	59	57	60	

found severe coronary artery disease to be present in 47% of those with aortoiliac occlusive disease, in 48% of those with femoropopliteal occlusive disease, and in 75% of those with abdominal aortic aneurysms.

SURVIVAL OF PATIENTS WITH PERIPHERAL VASCULAR DISEASE

The prevalence of coronary artery disease in patients with peripheral vascular disease is significant and has been shown to be a major determinant of early and late mortality after arterial reconstruction. In several recent publications coronary artery disease was found to be responsible for early mortality in 41% to 61% and for late mortality in 52% to 55% of patient deaths following peripheral vascular reconstruction (Table 10-3).*

Crawford et al reviewed their extensive experience with aortic replacement for either aneurysmal or occlusive disease of the aortic bifurcation and found that an actuarial 5-year survival rate was 84% to 89% for patients who had no other complicating features, 59% for those with hypertension, 55% for those with diabetes, and 54% for patients who had traditional clinical indications of coronary artery disease.[16,17] Campbell, Hoar, and Wheelock reported that the incidence of fatal cardiac events far exceeded the late stroke rate after carotid endarterectomy and that cardiac deaths were three times more common in diabetics (38%) than in nondiabetics (14%) during comparable periods of observation.[39]

These data are generally consistent with previous studies from The Cleveland Clinic.† Cumulative 5-year survival for patients suspected to have coronary artery disease by standard criteria was 15% less after extracranial vascular procedures, 20% less after lower extremity revascularization,

*References 2, 3, 13, 14, 16, 17, 19, 20-27, 29, 31, 32, 34-39, 42.
†References 2, 3, 11, 18, 31, 32, 37, 38, 43, 44.

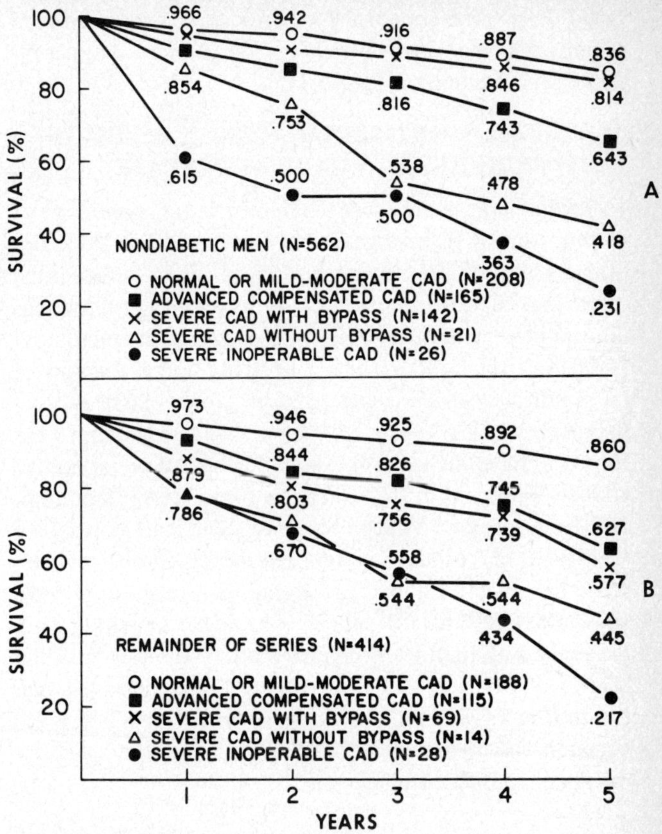

Fig. 10-1. The cumulative 5-year survival in a single series by cohorts. **A**, Nondiabetic men. **B**, All other patients with peripheral vascular disease undergoing vascular surgery. All patients had preoperative cardiac arteriography. Survival after coronary bypass was superior ($P = 0.0002$) to that for similar patients with uncorrected or inoperable coronary artery disease as well as survival in women or diabetics ($P = 0.003$). (From Hertzer NR et al: Late results of coronary bypass in patients with peripheral vascular disease. II. Five-year survival according to sex, hypertension and diabetes, Cleve Clin J Med 54:15, 1987.)

Table 10-3. Early and late mortality of vascular surgical patients

	Vascular surgical territory			
Mortality	**Abdominal aortic (%)**	**Carotid artery (%)**	**Lower extremity (%)**	**References**
Overall (mean)				
Early (30 days)	4.6	1.6	3.3	1-3, 11, 13-17, 19, 20, 22-25, 29, 31, 34, 35, 37, 38
Late (5 years)	32	24	32	
Deaths caused by coronary artery disease				
Early	56	41	61	
Late	53	55	52	
Overall mortality in patients with previous coronary bypass surgery				
Early	0.4	2.6	0.6	8, 37-42
Late	28	16	28	

and 27% less after aortic aneurysm resection, compared with patients who had insignificant coronary artery disease by conventional criteria (Fig. 10-1).[43]

ASSESSMENT OF CARDIAC RISK IN PATIENTS WITH PERIPHERAL VASCULAR DISEASE

Several large studies have examined factors predictive of coronary artery disease generated from the medical history (Table 10-4).[1,45-50] Age; sex; history of angina, myocardial infarction, diabetes, smoking, and hypertension were significant predictors of coronary disease in a large ambulatory population referred to Duke University for evaluation of chest pain and cardiac catheterization.[45] In this study a subset of patients being evaluated before vascular surgery were shown to have the same factors predictive of perioperative cardiac events, with the exception of male sex, smoking, and hypertension. The presence of claudication was not predictive of coronary artery disease or cardiac events. Nonetheless, the catheterization data of Hertzer et al have shown that 56% of 381 patients with lower extremity limb ischemia had significant coronary artery disease, and the studies of Pryor et al and Hertzer et al demonstrated that the resting ECG with significant Q waves or ST-T wave changes was predictive of both coronary disease and perioperative cardiac complications.[38,45]

Table 10-4. Coronary artery disease predictors

	Ambulatory	Preoperative		
Clinical variable	**Pryor***	**Cooperman†**	**Cutler‡**	**Eagle§**
n =	3627	566	116	200
Typical angina	0.0001		NS	.003
History of MI	0.0001	0.0001	NS	.03
Male sex	0.0001			NS
Age ≥ 70	0.0001			.06
Diabetes	0.001			.03
CHF	NS	0.0001	NS	.05
Smoking	0.001			NS
Hypertension	0.05			NS
PVD				NS
ECG changes				
Q waves	0.0001	0.0001	NS	.002
ST changes	0.0001			.01
PVCs	NS	0.009		NS

* Based on data from Pryor DB et al: Estimating the likelihood of significant coronary artery disease, Am J Med 75:771, 1983.

† Based on data from Cooperman M et al: Cardiovascular risk factors in patients with peripheral vascular disease, Surgery 84:505, 1978.

‡ Based on data from Cutler et al: Applicability and interpretation of electrocardiographic stress testing in patients with peripheral vascular disease, Am J Surg 141:501, 1981.

§Eagle KA et al: Combining clinical and thallium data optimizes preoperative assessment of cardiac risk before major vascular surgery, Ann Int Med 110:859, 1989.

Cooperman et al used multivariant analysis to show that previous myocardial infarction, congestive heart failure, previous cerebrovascular accident, arrhythmias, and abnormal ECGs are significantly associated with increased mortality when the patient is undergoing peripheral vascular surgical procedures.[1] When two or more risk factors were combined, the likelihood of complications increased dramatically. In a study by Jamieson et al clinical coronary artery disease, previous peripheral vascular disease surgery, or diabetes were risk factors that influenced late mortality significantly.[20] When none of the risk factors was present preoperatively, the late mortality from cardiac causes was 3.8% following peripheral vascular reconstruction. If one or more risk factors were present, the late mortality was 20.6% (clinical coronary artery disease 16%, peripheral vascular surgery 21%, diabetes 29%, and two of the above 33%). The actuarial freedom from cardiac death at 5 years for the high-risk group was 71 ± 17.7%, compared with 96 ± 4.4% for the low-risk group.

Various methods for estimating perioperative cardiac risk in patients having noncardiac surgery have been described, but it appears that the clinical markers that correlate with postoperative myocardial infarction or cardiac death include ECG evidence of past myocardial infarction, a history of angina pectoris, hypertension, diabetes, cerebrovascular accident, congestive heart failure, and cardiac arrhythmias. Additional markers described have included advanced age and abnormal baseline ECGs. Data from Eagle et al support the association of hightened perioperative risk factors for patients with many of these clinical features.[46] They describe five clinical factors—advanced age, Q waves on ECG, diabetes mellitus, a history of ventricular arrhythmias, and a history of angina as independent correlates of postoperative cardiac events (see Table 10-4). Although not tested in the Eagle et al study, it would be reasonable to assume that these risk factors would also be significant in those patients not undergoing surgery for peripheral vascular disease.

Goldman identified nine clinical features that correlated with an increased cardiac risk and developed a risk index that could be used to estimate the overall likelihood of major postoperative cardiac events in any given patient.[48] Goldman's criteria were later validated and slightly modified by Detsky et al.[49] Detsky et al added a category for angina pectoris and for any history of pulmonary edema. While these indexes provide general estimates of risk for a general population of surgical patients, they are less effective in estimating risk in a more homogeneous, high-risk subgroup of patients such as those undergoing major peripheral vascular reconstruction. Eagle et al compared their risk factor analysis with the modified Goldman criteria and found a univariate correlation with increased risk; however, in a multivariate analysis, the Goldman criteria were not independent correlates of adverse outcome (Table 10-5).[46,48]

Table 10-5. Comparison of patients with and without postoperative myocardial infarction or cardiac death after vascular surgery

Variable	Postoperative infarction or cardiac death (n = 15) (%)	No postoperative infarction or cardiac death (n = 185) (%)	*P* value
Clinical variables			
Age > 70 years	6(40)	64(34)	NS*
History of angina	9(60)	49(26)	0.01
Q wave(s) on ECG	8(53)	32(17)	0.002
History of MI	6(40)	40(22)	0.21
History of heart failure	5(33)	14(8)	0.0001
Diabetes mellitus	6(40)	30(16)	0.02
S_3 gallop	2(13)	0(0)	0.0003
History of ventricular ectopy	0(0)	11(6)	NS
Goldman index	6.0(3.33 to 8.67)†	5.0(4.36 to 5.64)†	NS
Modified Goldman index	5.7(2.09 to 9.31)†	4.1(3.41 to 4.79)†	NS
Dipyridamole-thallium test variable			
Chest pain during test	3(20)	30(16)	NS
Ischemic ECG changes	9(60)	36(19)	0.0003
Fixed thallium defect	8(53)	59(32)	0.09
Redistribution of thallium	13(87)	69(37)	0.0002

*NS, Not significant; $P \geq 0.30$.
†Modified from Eagle KA et al: Combining clinical and thallium data optimizes preoperative assessment of cardiac risk before major vascular surgery, Ann Int Med 110:859, 1989.

INDICATORS OF CARDIAC RISK IN PATIENTS WITH PERIPHERAL VASCULAR DISEASE

Disease prevalence strongly influences the predictive accuracy of any test. Assuming a 50% coronary artery disease prevalence in the peripheral vascular disease population, the predictive accuracy of a 95% sensitive and 95% specific test would be 95%. Ideally, a highly specific and sensitive test would provide useful information regarding the need for further evaluation of the preoperative vascular patient.

Noninvasive evaluation for coronary artery disease in patients with peripheral vascular disease

History and physical examination. Coronary artery disease may be suspected by the presence of a history of stable angina pectoris, unstable angina pectoris, atypical chest discomfort, dyspnea as an anginal equivalent, previous myocardial infarction, or a history of a positive stress test. A history and physical examination may identify a group of patients who have had a noticeable history of coronary disease, but it does not exclude all patients with asymptomatic severe coronary disease and is not sensitive enough to identify mild to moderate asymptomatic coronary disease. Even in the absence of symptoms, the presence of cardiovascular risk factors such as hypertension, hypercholesterolemia, diabetes, smoking, a familial atherosclerotic history, history of myocardial infarction, or vascular disease elsewhere should prompt minimally noninvasive investigation for silent myocardial ischemia even in the most active patients. Table 10-5 describes the influence of risk factors from the history and physical examination and their influence on cardiac ischemic events and mortality.

Electrocardiogram testing. In several reviews Q waves on a resting ECG are described as major risk factors for significant coronary disease.[1,45-47,51,52] Krueger, Kannel, and Cupples reviewed the ability of ECG to predict sudden death in patients in the Framingham study.[52] They showed that in patients with known coronary artery disease, especially those with ECG evidence of myocardial infarction, interventricular block, left ventricular hypertrophy, or tachycardia were at higher risk of sudden death. Kannel et al further emphasized the importance of nonspecific ST-T wave ECG abnormalities in predicting sudden death and suggested that patients with such abnormalities deserve further investigation.[51] In the Framingham study premature ventricular beats seem to have no independent influence on predicting sudden death. However, in survivors of acute myocardial infarction, ventricular ectopic activity is an independent predictor of total mortality. ST depression, cardiomegaly, and prior history of myocardial infarction separates survivors of acute myocardial infarction into four risk groups, with mortality rates as follows: three criteria—36%, two criteria—19%, one criterion—12%, and no criteria—5%. Table 10-4 demonstrates the significance of ECG findings and their ability to predict coronary artery disease.[1,45-47]

Exercise ECG testing. ECG stress testing has been used for many years to detect coronary artery disease in patients with chest pain syndromes. For the average individual, the sensitivity, specificity, and predictive value for ST segment depression in two studies were 64%, 85%, and 90%, respectively.[53,54] In comparison the same values in an asymptomatic population without associated peripheral vascular disease were 61%, 92%, and 28%, respectively.[53,54] Thus the standard exercise stress test ST segment response is highly predictive of the presence of coronary artery disease in patients with a high prevalence who are able to exercise maximally, but is significantly limited in patients with low disease probability and in patients who are unable to exercise to 80% of their predicted maximal heart rate (Table 10-6).[8,55]

Therefore treadmill exercise tests are helpful in patients who are capable of performing the test adequately. Unfortunately, exercise testing is less feasible in patients who have intermittent claudication. Gage et al evaluated 50 peripheral vascular disease patients with exercise treadmill testing and found 25 (50%) had an abnormal response, 13 (26%) had a normal response, and 12 (24%) performed inadequately because of shortness of breath or claudication.[56]

In a series of 130 patients undergoing treadmill or arm ergometric electrocardiographic stress testing before vascular surgical procedures, Cutler et al found an impressive correlation between exercise-induced ischemia and subsequent cardiac events.[47] They reported the results of 100 patients with peripheral arterial occlusive disease and the incidence of postoperative myocardial infarction and death. Of the patients exercising to more than 75% of their maximal predicted heart rate, those with normal findings on exercise and electrocardiogram had no cardiac mortality or postoperative myocardial infarction. Those patients with ischemic electrocardiographic response had a 4.3% incidence of nonfatal myocardial infarction. A high-risk group was identified in those who exercised to less than 75% of maximal predicted heart rate and had ischemic electrocardiographic changes. In this subgroup the incidence of perioperative infarction was 25.9%, and overall cardiac mortality was 18.5%. McCabe et al also reported collaborative data that positive treadmill exercise tolerance predicted postoperative cardiac events.[57]

The advantages of exercise testing include its relatively low cost and its wide applicability since most hospitals have exercise laboratories that can readily perform and interpret stress electrocardiograms. The limiting factor, however, is the ability of the peripheral vascular disease patient to exercise adequately to simulate an increase in cardiac output and myocardial oxygen consumption demand that will occur during the surgical procedure. Other factors that may influence the exercise test outcome include the frequent use of β-blocking agents and calcium channel blocking agents, which may limit the heart rate response during exercise and the diagnostic utility of the exercise test. Furthermore, digitalis and diuretics can cause falsely positive ST segment changes in the exercise electrocardiogram.

Table 10-6. Comparisons of standard exercise criteria and presence of CAD in patients with and without left main or three-vessel CAD*

Variable	Left main or three-vessel CAD: Present (n = 215)	Left main or three-vessel CAD: Absent (n = 466)
Exercise angina	50%	37%
ST ↓ > 1.5 mm	47%	18%
Downsloping ST ↓	43%	14%
Exercise EF†	0.46	0.55
Peak RPP‡	16,562	20,400
All $P < 0.001$		

* Based on data from Gibbons RJ et al: Noninvasive identification of severe coronary artery disease using exercise radionuclide angiography, J Am Coll Cardiol 11:28, 1988.

† Ejection fraction.

‡ Rate pressure product.

Thallium exercise electrocardiography

Thallium exercise electrocardiography is based on the principle that thallium-201 distributes uniformly through the normally perfused left ventricular myocardium. Established, old infarcts appear as cold spots. During myocardial ischemia, such as that induced by exercise, an underperfused area is not exposed to the same quantity of isotope as normally perfused myocardium and is also detected as a cold spot. Subsequently, when another image is obtained at rest, the cold spot disappears, provided the myocardial ischemia is reversible. This thallium redistribution, as a result of exercise, is a marker for relative hypoperfusion of viable myocardium, whereas a persistent defect suggests that an established infarct is present. Thallium redistribution is a strong predictor of future myocardial infarction.[58-61]

To summarize, regions that are perfused normally at rest but exhibit reduced perfusion during exercise represent ischemic zones, while perfusion defects seen both at rest and during exercise usually represent zones of scar, most commonly from previous infarction. Abnormal perfusion during stress in patients with transient ischemia is caused by a heterogeneous increase in myocardial blood flow. In patients with coronary artery disease, the increase in blood flow to the myocardium distal to a hemodynamically significant arterial stenosis is less than normal and may in fact be absent. There is an inverse relationship between the increase in flow and the percentage of coronary artery stenosis once the lumen is narrowed by approximately 30% to 50%. Thus the difference between the absolute quantity of radiotracer available for uptake by myocardial cells beyond arterial obstruction and the quantity available in beds supplied by normal coronary arteries is maximal during exercise. Since myocardial thallium clearance is high, the relative differences in regional myocardial blood flow will be reflected in disproportionate concentrations of regional myocardial radioactivity on the scans.

The accuracy of thallium stress testing is lower in patients who are on β-blocker therapy and who fail to achieve a maximum heart rate of at least 110 beats per minute. The specificity of the test is lower in women because of breast attenuation of thallium counts. Myocardial perfusion studies with thallium should be used to complement exercise electrocardiography, and the use of thallium imaging adds to the sensitivity, specificity, and predictive value of the exercise test. The exercise ECG should be obtained first, before the perfusion study.

In patients with peripheral vascular disease a common cause of uninterpretable exercise ECG is failure to achieve 85% of predicted maximal heart rate with no ST segment changes. The sensitivity and specificity of thallium-201 imaging in patients who achieve a maximum heart rate of only 100 to 110 beats per minute are approximately the same as for patients who are able to achieve an adequate heart rate response.[59,61]

The major problem with exercise thallium stressing is associated with the inability of peripheral vascular disease patients to exercise and achieve adequate heart rate responses. Patients with abdominal aortic aneurysms or carotid artery disease may be able to participate in the standard exercise protocol, and therefore thallium stress testing is available and highly accurate in this group. For those patients who cannot exercise adequately, dipyridamole stress thallium testing may be of value.

Dipyridamole may be used to increase coronary blood flow and has several advantages over the exercise test in patients with limited exercise capability.[62,63] Perfusion imaging can be performed after intravenous or oral administration of dipyridamole, a potent coronary vasodilator that produces little clinical evidence of myocardial ischemia. Accuracy in detecting coronary artery disease is comparable to that of standard exercise testing with an improvement in image quality.[62,64] An accurate scan to detect coronary artery disease requires an intense vasodilatory stimulus to maximize regional blood flow abnormalities and an imaging agent whose uptake is directly proportional to the flow rate. Dipyridamole produces coronary vasodilation to a greater degree than that produced by exercise but without a concomitant increase in myocardial oxygen consumption.

Dipyridamole is thought to exert its action by increasing cellular concentrations of adenosine. The uptake of thallium-201 by the heart is linearly related to the blood flow except at peak flow rates. During this test, dipyridamole is intravenously administered over a 4-minute period followed by the injection of thallium-201. Scans are obtained immediately following thallium administration and 3 hours later. The sensitivity of this test may be enhanced by low-level exercise following dipyridamole administration or by a second injection of thallium. Side effects are common but rarely life threatening. About 30% of patients will experience chest pain. Adverse reactions are reversible with the intravenous administration of aminophylline, which competes for the adenosine receptors. Interpretation of defects following dipyridamole injection is identical to that achieved during exercise stress thallium imaging. Results of dipyridamole thallium stress testing are demonstrated in Tables 10-6 and 10-7.[4,32,65-68] The presence of thallium-201 redistribution was associated with an average risk of 22% for a perioperative myocardial infarction and an 8% risk of cardiac death. A report on a series of 150 patients in the Massachusetts General Hospital demonstrated that in 28 patients with a positive scan who were further evaluated with coronary angiography, hemodynamically significant three-vessel coronary artery disease was present in 17 patients and two-vessel disease in another 11 patients.[62]

Several potential sources of error occur in both dipyridamole as well as in standard thallium stress testing. These tests depend on thallium-201 to be well perfused in nonischemic zones and ischemic myocardium to be underper-

Table 10-7. Dipyridamole-thallium scintigraphy as a predictor of cardiac events after aortic surgery

		Perioperative MI		Fatal MI	
Author	Number of patients	Pos. scan (%)	Neg. scan (%)	Pos. scan (%)	Neg. scan (%)
Boucher et al[4]	48	25	0	6	0
Cutler and Leppo[62]	118	23	1.3	0	0
Eagle et al[65]	61	22	0	11	0
Sachs et al[66]	46	21	0	7	0
Fletcher et al[67]	17	14	0	0	0
Weighted average	290 (Total)	22	0.5	8.1	0

From Leppo J et al: Noninvasive evaluation of cardiac risk before elective vascular surgery, J Am Coll Cardiol 9:269, 1987.
MI, Myocardial infarction.

fused. If there is uniformly poor thallium uptake because of global myocardial ischemia, the image may be mistakenly interpreted as a normal scan. A falsely normal test can also occur if there is a very slow redistribution of the isotope on the 3-hour scan. A second injection of thallium and a third scan may identify the area in question as severely ischemic rather than infarcted tissue. False positive scans may occur from soft tissue attenuation because of overlying breast tissue, from left ventricular hypertrophy, or from variations in coronary anatomy.

For patients who cannot exercise, dipyridamole-thallium stress testing can provide objective information about the presence and severity of coronary artery disease. Intravenous dipyridamole has recently been approved for general use by the Food and Drug Administration.

Follow-up of studies of 293 patients undergoing exercise thallium imaging and cardiac catheterization for evaluation of chest pain demonstrated a significantly better 6-year survival in patients without exercise-induced ST depression ($P = 0.02$).[68] Similarly, there was a significant difference in the 7-year survival of patients who experience typical angina during exercise treadmill testing compared with patients without pain on the treadmill.[69] Of 681 patients studied at the University of Virginia, left main or three-vessel coronary disease was present in 215 patients who exhibited more exercise chest pain (50% vs 37%), ST segment depression greater than 1.5 mm (47% vs 18%), downsloping ST segment depression (43% vs 14%), and a lower exercise fraction (0.46 vs 0.55 EF units), and peak rate pressure product (16,562 vs 20,400) compared with patients without this type of severe coronary disease.[55] (See Table 10-6.) Based on these studies, patients with ST segment depression and exercise-induced chest pain are more likely to have extensive coronary artery disease, which may shorten their life span. Patients with a positive exercise test response should be considered candidates for coronary arteriography before any major vascular surgical procedure or, for that matter, in any patient with peripheral vascular disease regardless of the plan for reconstructive surgery.

Exercise testing may be combined with a functional measurement of left ventricular performance such as multiple gated blood pool acquisition scanning (MUGA) or two-dimensional echocardiography.[70] The change in resting ejection fraction with exercise correlates strongly with the presence or absence of significant coronary artery disease. An ejection fraction decrease of greater than or equal to 5% during exercise, although nonspecific, is usually predictive of cardiovascular pathology. In addition to coronary artery disease, this response is also observed in patients with significant valvular and hypertensive heart disease. The appearance of exercise-induced wall motion abnormalities, specifically new hypokinesis, akinesis, or dyskinesis, strongly suggests the presence of regional hypoperfusion resulting from coronary artery disease. Apical wall motion abnormalities may occur in cardiomyopathy and valvular heart disease.

Exercise echocardiography may demonstrate the appearance of new exercise-induced regional wall motion abnormalities and improve the sensitivity for the detection of significant coronary artery disease over the exercise ECG response without any loss of specificity. Diagnostic accuracy for detection of one-vessel coronary disease is 81% and for multivessel disease 93% in combined studies.[71,72] The technique is operator dependent and requires considerable technical expertise to be useful. As with the exercise ST segment response, its accuracy depends on achieving maximal exercise stress with immediate postexercise evaluation of wall motion. As in the case of preexisting ST segment abnormalities, the sensitivity is reduced in patients with preexisting wall motion abnormalities before exercise stress. This procedure has its major advantage in its relatively low cost, no radiation exposure, reproducibility, and rapid patient processing. A positive exercise echocardiographic response is highly predictive ($P < 0.001$) of an adverse 7-year prognosis when compared with patients with a negative response.[71,72]

The presence of multiple segmental wall motion abnormalities on a MUGA or echocardiographic stress study is strongly suggestive of extensive coronary artery disease.[7,73,74] The prediction of extensive coronary artery disease can also be made in this type of patient using standard echocardiographic techniques. If the patient exhibits a history of previous congestive heart failure, one may deduce that coronary disease is highly likely. An exercise ejection fraction of less than 50% is associated with a significant decrease in myocardial infarction–free survival over the subsequent 2 years.[56] Exercise ejection fraction of greater than 50% has a greater than 95% 2-year event-free survival. Event free survival in patients with an exercise ejection fraction of 20% to 50% falls dramatically to the range of 55%. A significant proportion of normal persons over 60 years of age and one third of all women demonstrate an abnormal decrease in exercise left ventricular ejection fraction. Subjects with a resting ejection fraction in excess of 75% may not display a normal 5% or greater increase in ejection fraction during exercise. Also normal subjects receiving calcium or β-blocking drugs may have no increase in ejection fraction.

Ambulatory ECG monitoring. Considerable interest has been generated in recent years regarding the syndrome of silent myocardial ischemia.[75-77] In patients with a low probability of disease, one cannot justify routine recording of an ambulatory ECG for detection of ischemic ST segment shifts. False positive ST segment shifts can occur in this population, and the appropriate cost-benefit ratio is difficult to demonstrate. Although it is known that approximately 4% of asymptomatic middle-aged men have significant coronary artery stenosis, the percentage of these patients with silent ischemia remains unknown. The asymptomatic patient with significant coronary artery disease demonstrated by ambulatory ECG monitoring has a low annual mortality but an increased cardiac morbidity. No data exist on mass screening with ambulatory ECG monitoring, although selective screening in patients with multiple cardiac risk factors or co-existing peripheral vascular disease may prove useful.

Special equipment is required to actively reproduce ischemic ST segment depression during ambulatory ECG monitoring. Men over 40 years of age with two or more coronary artery disease risk factors or the presence of severe peripheral vascular disease, women over 55 years of age with two or more coronary artery disease risk factors, and patients at high risk for premature coronary disease, such as patients with peripheral vascular disease, are appropriate candidates for ambulatory ECG monitoring. When ambulatory ECG monitoring is performed in a high-risk population, greater than or equal to 2 mm of ST segment depression and the presence of greater than or equal to six episodes of ischemia per day are considered high-risk criteria associated with adverse outcomes.[77]

Raby et al performed a prospective study of 176 patients who subsequently underwent vascular surgery.[78] Thirty two patients (18%) demonstrated ischemic ST segment depression during ambulatory monitoring performed preoperatively. Thirteen patients (7%) had major postoperative cardiac events, including fatal and nonfatal myocardial infarction, unstable angina, and ischemia-related pulmonary edema. Of these 13 patients, while only 12 had evidence of ischemia during ambulatory monitoring, one event occurred in a patient with no ischemic ST segment depression during monitoring. This study concluded that the absence of myocardial ischemia during ambulatory monitoring is predictive of a low risk of postoperative cardiac event.

Ouyang et al performed ambulatory monitoring preoperatively, intraoperatively, and postoperatively in patients who underwent vascular surgical procedures.[79] Fifteen patients (63%) demonstrated postoperative myocardial ischemia during ambulatory monitoring. Of these patients, three had ischemia during the preoperative recordings and five had ischemia intraoperatively. Eight of the 15 patients with postoperative myocardial ischemia had a cardiac event, including myocardial infarction, congestive heart failure, or a new onset of unstable angina.

CARDIAC CATHETERIZATION AND MANAGEMENT OF ASSOCIATED CORONARY DISEASE IN PATIENTS WITH PERIPHERAL VASCULAR DISEASE

As mentioned, during the past two decades several large series have demonstrated that coronary artery disease can seriously limit late survival following successful peripheral vascular reconstruction. Since coronary artery disease is the leading cause of both perioperative and late mortality in patients undergoing peripheral vascular surgery, a variety of strategies have been presented to diagnose and aid in the management of these patients. Routine screening of patients, using coronary arteriography in patients with peripheral vascular disease, is probably not warranted, despite the high prevalence of coronary artery disease in this population. Most specialists caring for patients with peripheral vascular disease would suggest a thallium exercise test or dipyridamole-thallium stress testing for all patients before peripheral vascular reconstructive surgery.[55] Those patients with a positive outcome of the noninvasive study should undergo coronary angiography before surgical intervention.

Thallium-201 redistribution, exercise-induced angina, and electrocardiographic ST segment depression have been shown to correlate with the increased likelihood of perioperative cardiac events.[45-49,58,62,80-82] However, many patients considered for vascular surgery are unable to exercise adequately because of claudication and other peripheral ischemic problems. Eagle et al have demonstrated that in a group of 200 patients, 116 (58%) were severely limited by claudication or other physical problems.[46] For this reason dipyridamole-thallium imaging has been recommended.

The correct approach to managing such patients with peripheral vascular disease continues to be debated. We and others have argued for the consideration of coronary angiography in all patients with clear-cut evidence of thallium redistribution or with adequate clinical criteria (angina, ECG evidence of previous myocardial infarction, congestive heart failure) to suggest a high incidence of significant coronary artery disease. Several nonrandomized and uncontrolled studies have suggested that coronary artery bypass surgery done before peripheral vascular surgery can reduce the likelihood of myocardial infarction and cardiac death after surgical reconstruction.[8,20,38-40,43] Unfortunately, patients with peripheral vascular disease are often poor risks for coronary artery bypass surgery because of advanced age, severe multivessel disease, reduced left ventricular function from one or more previous myocardial infarctions, and other factors. The operative mortality for coronary bypass surgery in these patients probably exceeds 5%.[11] Therefore in some patients the short-term risk of cardiac catheterization and coronary revascularization may actually exceed the potential risk reduction to be achieved by successful coronary artery bypass surgery.[83]

The role of percutaneous transluminal coronary angioplasty (PTCA) in the treatment of significant coronary disease in patients with peripheral vascular disease is not well defined. Data are not available to indicate the risk of PTCA, the outcome, or its influence on 5-year survival in patients with severe peripheral vascular disease. It is likely that PTCA in patients with peripheral vascular disease does not carry the same significant risk as coronary artery bypass surgery.

We believe that the best approach to patients with peripheral vascular disease is to appropriately investigate the status of their coronary artery disease regardless of the planned treatment for their peripheral vascular disease. In the nonoperative group, thallium stress testing, dipyridamole thallium stress testing, or other available modalities that are noninvasive would be selected as the optimal screening test. Under two conditions coronary arteriography should be done. The first condition is if the patient develops significant clinical risk factors such as angina, prior myocardial infarction on ECG, or a demonstration of silent ischemia. The second condition would be if the patient has a positive noninvasive study. In either of these situations, cardiac catheterization should be elected.

INDICATIONS FOR CORONARY ARTERY REVASCULARIZATION IN PATIENTS WITH PERIPHERAL VASCULAR DISEASE

Although several authors have suggested that coronary artery revascularization should be performed in patients with significant coronary artery disease before vascular surgery, no prospective, randomized trials have taken place to address this issue. The premise is that coronary revascularization will either reduce the risk associated with the vascular surgical procedure or reduce the late morbidity and mortality associated with coronary artery disease in this group of patients or both. Data shown in Table 10-3 are derived from retrospective reviews of vascular surgical patients who had had successful coronary artery revascularization before vascular surgery. Most of these trials fail to report the morbidity and mortality of noninvasive cardiac testing, cardiac catheterization, and myocardial revascularization (Table 10-8). Therefore, at this point, it is not possible to recommend a general policy in which all patients with significant coronary artery disease undergo prophylactic myocardial revascularization before vascular surgical procedures. There may be selected groups where this policy would apply.[43]

Pending the outcomes of prospective randomized trials, patient selection must be individualized for those who are at greatest risk for myocardial infarction or death or both. Such individuals can be inferred from several prospective, randomized trials conducted in patients with coronary artery disease including the Veterans Administration Coronary Artery Bypass Surgery Cooperative Study Group, the European Coronary Surgery Study Group, and the Coronary Artery Surgery Study.[87-91] These studies demonstrated that patients with left main coronary artery disease and those with three-vessel coronary disease and impaired left ventricular function survive longer if myocardial revascularization is performed than if they are treated medically. In addition, patients with Class III or Class IV angina (Canadian Heart Association classification) refractory to medical management might also be considered candidates for prophylactic myocardial revascularization before peripheral vascular surgery.

Nevertheless, other cooperative surveys have suggested that the expectations of coronary bypass may be compromised in candidates who have systemic atherosclerosis and other concurrent illnesses.[11,83] The results of the Coronary Artery Surgery Study in patients over 65 years of age demonstrated a 5-year survival rate of 71% for those having two or more related medical disorders compared with 89% for a subset, in which coronary artery disease was an isolated finding. The European Coronary Surgery Study Group calculated that the 5-year mortality after bypass in patients who also had peripheral vascular disease was 11%, while those without peripheral vascular disease had an 8% mortality. The most revealing data in the randomized European Coronary Surgery Study Group, however, concerned the outcome of nonoperative cardiac management. When myocardial revascularization was not performed, late survival was only 66% among entrants with associated peripheral vascular disease compared with 85% in all others.

Hertzer et al reported that following 8 years of critical review, nondiabetic men appear to have the most to gain from a comprehensive approach for the treatment of associated coronary artery disease preceding peripheral vascular reconstruction (see Fig. 10-1).[38] Despite the early mortality from coronary artery bypass itself (4.9%), a factor reflecting the age of the candidate more than any other consideration, nondiabetic men in this series with severe coronary artery

Table 10-8. Complication rates of diagnostic tests for CAD detection

Author	Year	No. of patients	Death (%)	Major complications (%)
Coronary angiography				
Soc Card Angio, Kennedy[84]	1989	53,581	0.14	0.14
Exercise testing				
Rochimis, Blackburn[85]	1971	170,000	1.0	2.4
American Medical Association[86]	1981	90,000	0.3	1.3

disease who received myocardial revascularization had few fatal complications at the time of arterial procedures (0.7%), a low risk for cardiac death within the subsequent 5 years (6.3%), and a cumulative survival that was virtually identical to that of patients with only trivial coronary artery disease (81%). Superiority of late results in this subset was statistically significant and may encourage others who have been reluctant to pursue even selective coronary angiography to do so. It is also likely that this improved outcome in this subselected group of patients also holds true for all other patients, yet the difference is not seen statistically because of the size of the cohorts.

SUMMARY

It is our present policy to perform a careful clinical evaluation on all patients scheduled for vascular surgery as well as on those with vascular disease who are not undergoing surgical revascularization. The clinical evaluation includes a history and physical examination from which risk factors for cardiac disease can be obtained. It is our opinion that all patients with peripheral vascular disease should undergo noninvasive screening. The relative specificity and sensitivity of noninvasive tests has been determined, and the positive predictive value is high in this group of patients. These noninvasive studies would include exercise tolerance testing, dipyridamole-thallium imaging, or some other form of noninvasive testing available at the respective institutions.

If the screening test suggests a high risk for a subsequent coronary event, or if the patient has angina pectoris or has had a prior myocardial infarction, coronary arteriography should be performed and appropriate revascularization or medical treatment should be instituted.

REFERENCES

1. Cooperman M et al: Cardiovascular risk factors in patients with peripheral vascular disease, Surgery 84:505, 1978.
2. Hertzer NR: Fatal myocardial infarction following abdominal aortic aneurysm resection: three hundred forty-three patients followed six to eleven years postoperatively, Ann Surg 192:667, 1980.
3. Hertzer NR: Fatal myocardial infarction following lower extremity revascularization: two hundred seventy-three patients followed six to eleven postoperative years, Ann Surg 193:492, 1981.
4. Boucher CA et al: Determination of cardiac risk by dipyridamole thallium imaging before peripheral vascular surgery, N Engl J Med 312:389, 1985.
5. Von Knorring J and Lepantalo M: Prediction of perioperative cardiac complications by electrocardiographic monitoring during treadmill exercise testing before peripheral vascular surgery, Surgery 99:610, 1986.
6. Riles TS, Kopelman I, and Imparato AM: Myocardial infarction following carotid endarterectomy: a review of 683 operations, Surgery 85:249, 1978.
7. Pasternack PF et al: The value of radionuclide angiography as a predictor of perioperative myocardial infarction in patients undergoing abdominal aortic aneurysm resection, J Vasc Surg 1:320, 1984.
8. Arous EG and Baum PL: The ischemic exercise test in patients with peripheral vascular disease: implications for management, Arch Surg 119:780, 1984.
9. Dawber TR, Moore FE, and Mann GV: Measuring the risk of coronary heart disease in adult population groups II: coronary heart disease in the Framingham study, Am J Public Health 47:4, 1957.
10. Blombery PA et al: The role of coronary artery disease in complications of abdominal aortic aneurysm surgery, Surgery 101:150, 1986.
11. Hertzer NR et al: Coronary artery disease in peripheral vascular patients: a classification of 1000 coronary angiograms and results of surgical management, Ann Surg 199:223, 1984.
12. Tomatis LS, Fireens EE, and Verbrugge GP: Evaluation of surgical risk in peripheral vascular disease by coronary arteriography: a series of 100 cases, Surgery 71:429, 1972.
13. Whittemore AD et al: Aortic aneurysm repair: Reduced operative mortality associated with maintenance of optimal cardiac performance, Ann Surg 192:414, 1980.
14. Bouchard JP et al: Carotid endarterectomy: survival rates of 227 patients, Can Med Assoc J 113:949, 1975.
15. Brown OW et al: Abdominal aortic aneurysm and coronary artery disease: a reassessment, Arch Surg 116:1484, 1981.
16. Crawford ES et al: Aortoiliac occlusive disease: factors influencing survival and function following reconstructive operation over a twenty-five-year period, Surgery 90:1055, 1981.
17. Crawford ES et al: Infrarenal abdominal aortic aneurysm: factors influencing survival after operation performed over a 25-year period, Ann Surg 193:699, 1981.
18. Diehl JT et al: Complications of abdominal aortic reconstruction: an analysis of perioperative risk factors in 557 patients, Ann Surg 197:49, 1983.
19. Hollier LH et al: Late survival after abdominal aortic aneurysm repair: influence of coronary artery disease, J Vasc Surg 1:290, 1984.
20. Jamieson WRE et al: Influence of ischemic heart disease on early and late mortality after surgery for peripheral occlusive vascular disease, Circulation 66:I-92, 1982.
21. Kallero KS et al: Arteriosclerosis in popliteal artery trifurcation as a predictor for myocardial infarction after arterial reconstructive operation, Surg Gynecol Obstet 159:133, 1984
22. Kallero KS et al: Late mortality and morbidity after arterial reconstruction: the influence of arteriosclerosis in popliteal artery trifurcation, J Vasc Surg 2:541, 1985.
23. Malone JM, Moore WS, and Goldstone J: Life expectancy following aortofemoral arterial grafting, Surgery 81:551, 1977.
24. Reigel MM et al: Late survival in abdominal aortic aneurysm patients: the role of selective myocardial revascularization on the basis of clinical symptoms, J Vasc Surg 5:222, 1987.
25. Ruby ST et al: Coronary artery disease in patients requiring abdominal aortic aneurysm repair: selective use of a combined operation, Ann Surg 201:758, 1985.
26. DeWeese JA and Rob CG: Autogenous venous bypass grafts five years later, Ann Surg 174:346, 1971.
27. DeWeese JA et al: Results of carotid endarterectomies for transient ischemic attacks: five years later, Ann Surg 178:258, 1973.
28. Hicks GL et al: Survival improvement following aortic aneurysm resection, Ann Surg 181:863, 1975.
29. Szilagyi DE et al: Autogenous vein grafting in femoropopliteal atherosclerosis: the limits of its effectiveness, Surgery 86:836, 1979.
30. Yeager RA et al: Application of clinically valid cardiac risk factors to aortic aneurysm surgery, Arch Surg 121:278, 1986.
31. Martinez BD, Hertzer NR, and Beven EG: Influence of distal arterial occlusive disease on prognosis following aortobifemoral bypass, Surgery 88:795, 1980.
32. Hertzer NR and Arison R: Cumulative stroke and survival ten years after carotid endarterectomy, J Vasc Surg 2:661, 1985.
33. Dipasquale G et al: Cerebral ischemia and asymptomatic coronary artery disease: a prospective study of 83 patients, Stroke 17:1098, 1986.
34. Soreide O et al: Abdominal aortic aneurysms: survival analysis of four hundred thirty-four patients, Surgery 91:188, 1982.

35. Thompson JE, Austin DJ, and Patman RD: Carotid endarterectomy for cerebrovascular insufficiency: long-term results in 592 patients followed up to thirteen years, Ann Surg 172:663, 1970.
36. Lord RSA: Late survival after carotid endarterectomy for transient ischemic attacks, J Vasc Surg 1:512, 1984.
37. Hertzer NR et al: Late results of coronary bypass in patients presenting with infrarenal aortic aneurysms: The Cleveland Clinic Study, Ann Surg 205:360, 1987.
38. Hertzer NR et al: Late results of coronary bypass in patients presenting with lower extremity ischemia: The Cleveland Clinic Study, Ann Vasc Surg 1:411, 1986.
39. Campbell DR, Hoar CS, and Wheelock FC Jr: Carotid artery surgery in diabetic patients, Arch Surg 119:1405, 1984.
40. Ennix CL Jr et al: Improved results of carotid endarterectomy in patients with symptomatic coronary disease: an analysis of 1,546 consecutive carotid operations, Stroke 10:122, 1979.
41. O'Donnell TF Jr et al: The impact of coronary artery disease on carotid endarterectomy, Ann Surg 198:705, 1983.
42. Reul GJ Jr et al: The effect of coronary bypass on the outcome of peripheral vascular operations in 1093 patients, J Vasc Surg 3:788, 1986.
43. Hertzer NR et al: Late results of coronary bypass in patients with peripheral vascular disease. II. Five-year survival according to sex, hypertension, and diabetes, Cleve Clin J Med 54:15, 1987.
44. Hertzer NR et al: The risk of vascular surgery in a metropolitan community: With observations on surgeon experience and hospital size, J Vasc Surg 1:13, 1984.
45. Pryor DB et al: Estimating the likelihood of significant coronary artery disease, Am J Med 75:771, 1983.
46. Eagle KA et al: Combining clinical and thallium data optimizes preoperative assessment of cardiac risk before major vascular surgery, Ann Int Med 110:859, 1989.
47. Cutler BS et al: Applicability and interpretation of electrocardiographic stress testing in patients with peripheral vascular disease, Am J Surg 141:501, 1981.
48. Goldman L: Assessment of the patient with known or suspected ischaemic heart disease for non-cardiac surgery, Br J Anaesth 61:38, 1988.
49. Detsky AS et al: Predicting cardiac complications in patients undergoing noncardiac surgery, J Gen Intern Med 1:211, 1986.
50. Von Knorring JP: Postoperative myocardial infarction: a prospective study in a risk group of surgical patients, Surgery 90:55, 1981.
51. Kannel WB et al: Nonspecific electrocardiographic abnormality as a predictor of coronary heart disease: The Framingham Study, Am Heart J 113:370, 1987.
52. Krueger BE, Kannel WB, and Cupples LA: Electrocardiographic precursors of sudden unexpected death: The Framingham Study. (Monograph No. 2: Recognition, Pathogenesis, and Management Options in Silent Coronary Artery Disease, Part II), Circulation 75 (suppl II):22, 1987.
53. Ellestad MH et al: Stress testing: clinical application and predictive capacity, Prog Cardiovasc Dis 21:431, 1979.
54. Redwood et al: Whither the ST segment during exercise? Circulation 54:703, 1976 (editorial).
55. Gibbons RJ et al: Noninvasive identification of severe coronary artery disease using exercise radionuclide angiography, J Am Coll Cardiol 11:28, 1988.
56. Gage AA et al: Assessment of cardiac risk in surgical patients, Arch Surg 112:1488, 1977.
57. McCabe CJ et al: The value of electrocardiogram monitoring during treadmill testing for peripheral vascular disease, Surgery 89:183, 1981.
58. Ritchie JL et al: Myocardial imaging with thallium-201: a multicenter study in patients with angina pectoris or acute myocardial infarction, Am J Cardiol 42:345, 1978.
59. Verani MS et al: Sensitivity and specificity of thallium-201 perfusion scintigrams under exercise in the diagnosis of coronary artery disease, J Nucl Med 19:773, 1978.
60. Ritchie JL et al: Myocardial imaging with thallium-201 at rest and during exercise: comparison with coronary arteriography and resting and stress electrocardiography, Circulation 56:66, 1977.
61. Botvinick EH et al: Thallium-201 myocardial perfusion scintigraphy for the clinical clarification of normal, abnormal, and equivocal electrocardiographic stress tests, Am J Cardiol 41:43, 1978.
62. Cutler BS and Leppo JA: Dipyridamole thallium 201 scintigraphy to detect coronary artery disease before abdominal aortic surgery, J Vasc Surg 5:91, 1987.
63. Francisco DA et al: Tomographic thallium-201 myocardial perfusion scintigrams after maximal coronary artery vasodilation with intravenous dipyridamole, Circulation 66:370, 1982.
64. Josephson MA et al: Noninvasive detection and localization of coronary stenoses in patients: comparison of resting dipyridamole and exercise thallium-201 myocardial perfusion imaging, Am Heart J 103:1008, 1982.
65. Eagle KA et al: Dipyridamole-thallium scanning in patients undergoing vascular surgery: Optimizing preoperative evaluation of cardiac risk, JAMA 257:2185, 1987.
66. Sachs RN et al: Assessment by dipyridamole-thallium-201 myocardial scintigraphy of coronary risk before peripheral vascular surgery, Surgery 103:584, 1988.
67. Fletcher JP et al: Dipyridamole-thallium scan for screening of coronary artery disease prior to vascular surgery, J Cardiovasc Surg 29:666, 1988.
68. Kaul S et al: Superiority of quantitative exercise thallium-201 variables in determining long-term prognosis in ambulatory patients with chest pain: a comparison with cardiac catheterization, J Am Coll Cardiol, 12:25, 1988.
69. Kaul S et al: Prognostic utility of the exercise thallium-201 test in ambulatory patients with chest pain: comparison with cardiac catheterization, Circulation 77:745, 1988.
70. Borer JS et al: Assessment of ventricular function by radionuclide angiography: applications and results, Cardiology 71:1339, 1984.
71. Armstrong WF: Exercise echocardiography: ready, willing and able, J Am Coll Cardiol 11:1359, 1988.
72. Bairey et al: Exercise echocardiography: ready or not? J Am Coll Cardiol 11:1355, 1988.
73. Kazmers A, Cerqueira MD, and Zierler RE: The role of preoperative radionuclide ejection fraction in direct abdominal aortic aneurysm repair, J Vasc Surg 8:128, 1988.
74. Pasternack PF et al: The value of the radionuclide angiogram in the prediction of perioperative myocardial infarction in patients undergoing lower extremity revascularization procedures, Circulation 72(suppl II):II-13, 1985.
75. Crawford MH et al: Limitations of continuous ambulatory ECG monitoring for detecting coronary artery disease, Ann Int Med 89:1, 1987.
76. Epstein S et al: Myocardial ischemia: silent or symptomatic? N Engl J Med 318:1038, 1988.
77. Schang SJ et al: Transient asymptomatic ST-segment depression during daily activity, Am J Cardiol 39:396, 1977.
78. Raby KE et al: Correlation between preoperative ischemia and major cardiac events after peripheral vascular surgery, N Engl J Med 321:1296, 1989.
79. Ouyang P et al: Frequency and significance of early postoperative silent myocardial ischemia in patients having peripheral vascular surgery, Am J Cardiol 64:1113, 1989.
80. Leppo J et al: Noninvasive evaluation of cardiac risk before elective vascular surgery, J Am Coll Cardiol 9:269, 1987.
81. McPhail NV et al: The use of preoperative exercise testing to predict cardiac complications after arterial reconstruction, J Vasc Surg 7:60, 1988.

82. McPhail NV et al: A comparison of dipyridamole-thallium imaging and exercise testing in the prediction of postoperative cardiac complications in patients requiring arterial reconstruction, J Vasc Surg 10:51, 1989.
83. Coley CM et al: Decision analysis for preoperative cardiac risk evaluation before vascular surgery, Clin Res 35:342A, 1987.
84. Kennedy JW: Complications associated with cardiac catheterization and angiography, Cathet Cardiovasc Diagn 8:5, 1982.
85. Rochimis P and Blackburn H: Exercise tests: a survey of procedures, safety and litigation experience in approximately 170,000 tests, JAMA 217:1061, 1971.
86. Council on Scientific Affairs, American Medical Association: Indications and contraindications for exercise testing, JAMA 246:1015, 1981.
87. The Veterans Administration Coronary Artery Bypass Surgery Cooperative Study Group: eleven-year survival in the Veterans Administration randomized trial of coronary bypass surgery for stable angina, N Engl J Med 311:1333, 1984.
88. European Coronary Surgery Study Group: Prospective randomized study of coronary artery bypass surgery in stable angina pectoris, Lancet 2:491, 1980.
89. Varnauskas E and the European Coronary Surgery Study Group: Twelve-year follow-up survival in the randomized European coronary surgery study, N Engl J Med 319:332, 1988.
90. CASS Principal Investigators and Their Associates: Coronary Artery Surgery Study (CASS): a randomized trial of coronary artery bypass surgery—survival data, Circulation 68:939, 1983.
91. Passamani E et al: A randomized trial of coronary artery bypass surgery: survival of patients with a low ejection fraction, N Engl J Med 312:1665, 1985.

Chapter 11

ATHEROMATOUS EMBOLIZATION

John R. Bartholomew
Jeffrey W. Olin

The atheromatous embolization syndrome has received little attention in most major medical textbooks. It is a frequently misdiagnosed and unrecognized disorder but one that may lead to significant morbidity and mortality. Even the term "atheromatous embolization" is confusing to many clinicians.

Two different types of atheroemboli may lead to this syndrome. Some investigators refer to this as a noncardiac embolization of one or more large atheromatous plaques that contain red blood cells, fibrin, platelet aggregates, and cholesterol crystals. These are often called macroemboli. Others refer to the atheromatous embolization syndrome as a showering of multiple smaller cholesterol crystals or fibrin platelet aggregates. This is called microembolization or cholesterol embolization. Both macroemboli and microemboli originate from ulcerated atherosclerotic plaques of the major arteries. In this chapter the term *atheromatous embolization* will refer to both types.

Atheromatous embolization syndrome, initially believed to be little more than a curiosity to pathologists, is now being encountered more commonly.[1,2] It may appear in a variety of ways, and physicians in many different specialties see patients with atheromatous embolization. A misunderstanding of this disorder and failure to recognize it exposes patients to undue risk, since the diagnostic workup and treatment initiated may often aggravate this condition. Therefore the importance of recognizing the atheromatous embolization syndrome cannot be overemphasized.

HISTORICAL BACKGROUND

Panum[3] is credited with the first description of atheromatous embolization in 1862. He described a case involving the famous Danish sculptor Thorwaldsen in which atheromatous material was found at autopsy. The first American report, noted by Doch in 1896,[4] involved coronary occlusion and death from multiple, cholesterol-rich emboli. By 1915 there was enough awareness of this syndrome that it was included in a textbook on diseases of the arteries,[5] although atheromatous embolization was still believed to be little more than an incidental finding at autopsy.

Flory[6] drew attention to atheromatous emboli in 1945 after reviewing 267 autopsies. He suggested that emboli containing cholesterol crystals produced infarction in multiple organs such as the kidney, spleen, or pancreas. He also speculated that atheroemboli may cause gangrenous changes in the lower extremities. Experimentally, he injected human atheromatous material into rabbit ears and found cholesterol crystals in the animals' arteries similar to those lesions he had earlier described in his autopsy studies. This work rekindled interest in atheromatous embolization.

Other investigators have played an important role in the better understanding and recognition of this condition. Snyder and Shapiro injected 16 rabbits and 9 dogs with cholesterol crystal suspensions.[7] All animals were later sacrificed and examined for the presence of cholesterol crystals. These studies demonstrated the persistence of arterial occlusions for extended periods (up to 160 days) and noted that these occlusions caused ischemia. Gore and Collins[8] reviewed the literature and reported 16 additional cases. They suggested that spontaneous atheromatous embolization was not an unusual complication of advanced atherosclerosis. Hoye et al[9] are credited with the first histologically proven case of peripheral atheromatous embolism. This patient developed gangrene that resulted in amputation. The source of the gangrene was either the abdominal aorta or the ileofemoral arteries. Handler[10] stressed the importance of atheromatous embolization that involved the kidney as a potential factor in the pathogenesis of hypertension. Thurlbeck and Castleman[11] found atheromatous material in the kidneys in 77% of patients who died after abdominal aneurysm surgery.

INCIDENCE

The exact incidence of atheroemboli is unknown. The presence of atheromatous emboli in an autopsy series or in a biopsy specimen merely indicates how often this entity is demonstrated pathologically but does not indicate how important it is clinically. In the late 1960s, 1970s, and early 1980s, numerous clinical pathologic conferences in the *New England Journal of Medicine*[12-19] illustrated different aspects of atheromatous embolization, suggesting that this disease was considered a curious or uncommon entity. Recently, however, there have been more studies that have been published with larger numbers of patients,[2,20-25] showing that clinical cholesterol embolization is not as rare as previously believed.

Atheromatous embolization is reported to be a common occurrence in individuals with advanced atherosclerosis.[6] The incidence clearly differs if patients with spontaneous embolization are compared with patients in autopsy series or with patients following surgery or other invasive procedures. In addition, the incidence increases in those patients with advanced atherosclerosis who receive anticoagulants. Spontaneous embolization is usually seen in the elderly patient with advanced atherosclerosis, diabetes, or hypertension.

In Flory's series,[6] the incidence of atheromatous embolization was 3.4% of 267 patients with advanced atherosclerosis at autopsy. The degree of aortic atherosclerosis predicted the likelihood of atheromatous emboli, and in those with the most severe degree of atherosclerosis, the incidence was 12.3%. In 100 consecutive autopsy cases, Maurizi, Barker, and Trueheart[26] examined the microscopic sections of muscles of the lower extremities and demonstrated atheromatous emboli in four patients (4%). In 25 patients with documented atheromatous emboli at autopsy, all patients had clinical features suggestive of atheromatous emboli (in retrospect), yet the diagnosis was not made until autopsy in 21 patients (84%)[26] When Wagner and Martin[27] reviewed 4635 cases of peripheral arterial emboli, they found only 1.4% attributed to atheroemboli. In a review of 2126 autopsies involving patients over 60 years of age, Kealy[28] found the incidence of atheroemboli to be 0.79%, although he suspected that this was probably an underestimation. Handler[10] reviewed 70 consecutive autopsies for evidence of cholesterol crystal embolization and found an incidence of 8.6%. In a review of 1352 autopsies, Sieniewicz et al[29] found atheromatous emboli in the kidneys of 3.47% of patients. The incidence clearly increased with age since the incidence was 11.76% in patients 80 to 89 years old. More recent studies[25,30,31] suggest that atheromatous embolization of the kidneys is a common histologic finding and may approach 15% to 30% in patients with severe aortic atherosclerosis or aneurysms of the abdominal aorta.[25,30,31] Clinical manifestations are clearly less common.

Over 30 years ago Thurlbeck and Castleman[11] demonstrated that 77% of patients who died after abdominal aortic aneurysm resection had atheromatous emboli in the kidney. In addition, 13 of 42 (31%) patients who were not operated on for abdominal aortic aneurysm and 6 of 38 patients (15.8%) with severe aortoiliac occlusive disease had atheromatous emboli at autopsy.

PRECIPITATING FACTORS

Although atheroembolization may be spontaneous, it occurs more often after surgery, arteriography, or anticoagulation (see the box below).

Arteriography is invaluable in the diagnosis and evaluation of the patient with vascular disease. Unfortunately, it is not without complications, including the potential to cause atheromatous embolization. This condition usually develops during or moments after the angiographic procedure. It may be heralded by an increase in blood pressure, pain, livedo reticularis pattern on the abdomen and lower extremities, or renal failure. Harrington et al[32] reported two cases in which progressive renal failure developed following retrograde renal arteriography. Others have reported similar findings with different techniques, including translumbar aortography and transaxillary angiography.[33-38] In a retrospective study of 71 autopsies, Ramirez et al[30] reported a 27% incidence of cholesterol embolization in patients who had arteriography performed before death, compared to a 4.3% incidence of spontaneous cholesterol emboli in an age- and disease-matched control group who did not undergo angiography.[30] When atheroemboli occur after arteriography, the risk of death increases considerably.[36,37,39,40] Whether the rigidity of the catheter or the force of contrast injection plays a role is unclear, but some have suggested that a softer, more flexible catheter may result in a lower incidence.[34,39] Probably the most important factor that determines who will or will not develop emboli is the severity of the atherosclerotic disease in the aorta[41] (Fig. 11-1).

Other invasive procedures that may lead to the atheromatous embolization syndrome include cardiac catheterization, percutaneous transluminal coronary angioplasty (PTCA), and peripheral angioplasty.[35,36,42,43] In a review of 4587 cardiac catheterizations, Drost et al[35] found seven cases of clinical cholesterol embolization (0.002%). Colt et al[36] found eight cases after heart catheterization, PTCA, and

Precipitating factors in atheroembolic disease*

1. Arteriography
2. Surgery
3. Anticoagulants
4. Thrombolytic agents

*Atheromatous embolization may also occur spontaneously

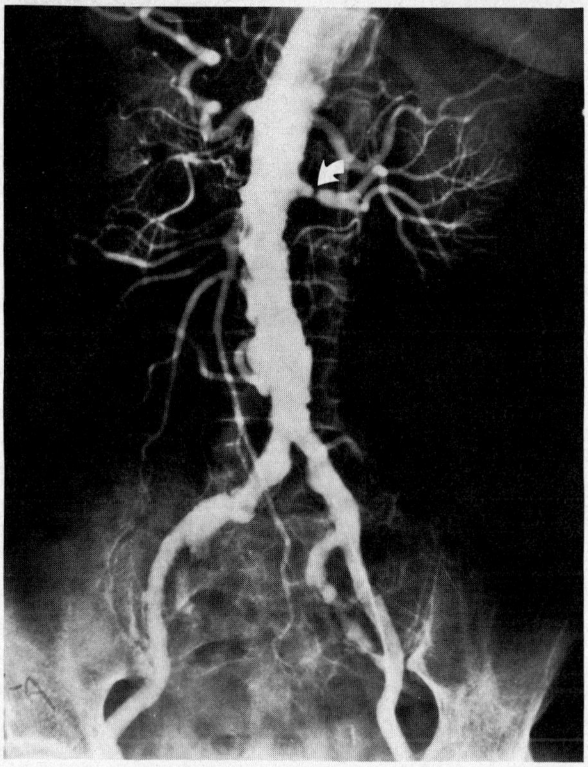

Fig. 11-1. Aortogram demonstrating severe erosive atherosclerosis of the aorta in a patient with atheromatous emboli. Note occlusion of the right renal artery and subtotal occlusion of the left renal artery (*arrow*).

Table 11-1. Clinical manifestations of atheromatous embolization

Skin	Purple or blue toes Gangrenous digits Livedo reticularis Nodules
Kidney	Uncontrolled hypertension Renal failure
Neurologic	Transient ischemic attack Amaurosis fugax Stroke Hollenhorst plaque
Cardiac	Myocardial infarction or ischemia
Gastrointestinal	Abdominal pain GI bleeding Ischemic bowel Acute pancreatitis
Constitutional symptoms	Fever Weight loss Malaise Anorexia

intraaortic balloon pumping involving 3733 procedures (0.002%). They also noted that there was no case reported of cholesterol embolization after cardiac catheterization when the brachial artery was used. These figures probably underestimate the true incidence in patients who undergo cardiac catheterization. Most likely only the severe cases were diagnosed, while many milder ones were not.

Atheroembolism has been associated with the use of anticoagulant and thrombolytic therapy.[44-51] "Purple toes" may occur at any time during anticoagulant therapy but typically occur within 4 to 12 weeks after therapy has been initiated. For years the relationship between purple toes and warfarin was believed to be the result of a direct toxic effect on the capillaries or a drug-induced vasculitis.[51] Moldveen-Geronimus and Merriam[1] postulated that the purple toe syndrome was caused by cholesterol embolization as a result of the anticoagulant. They believed that anticoagulants prevented clot formation over ulcerated plaques, thus allowing embolization to occur. Bruns, Segel, and Adler[46] noted clinical improvement in a patient when anticoagulants were discontinued. Most investigators recommend that warfarin be discontinued in patients who have an episode of cholesterol embolization.[44] Atheromatous emboli have also been associated with thrombolytic agents.[47-49] Other precipitating factors include surgery[11,52,53] and blunt trauma. Emboli may also occur spontaneously or after lifting or coughing.[54]

CLINICAL FINDINGS (Table 11-1)

Patients with atheromatous embolization usually have a history of atherosclerosis manifested clinically by angina, myocardial infarction, transient ischemic attacks, stroke, intermittent claudication, or gangrene. The patient is usually a man, over 60 years of age, and a smoker; however, atheromatous emboli may occur at any age and in either sex. Clinical signs and symptoms may be nonspecific and varied, depending on the number, size, and site of origin of the atheromatous material as well as on the end organ(s) affected. Patients with macroemboli may present with a catastrophic event such as an acutely ischemic leg, while those with microemboli may have milder localized signs or a clinical picture that suggests a systemic illness. Signs and symptoms suggestive of a multisystemic illness include fever, weight loss, anorexia, fatigue, myalgias, headache, nausea, vomiting, or diarrhea. Occasionally, the signs and symptoms may suggest necrotizing vasculitis, infective endocarditis, or malignancy.[51,54-58]

Skin manifestations

One of the most common clinical manifestations of atheromatous embolization is changes in the skin. These changes, generally found on the lower abdomen and legs, include livedo reticularis, gangrene, cyanosis, purple toes, ulcerations, nodules, and petechiae (Figs. 11-2 and 11-3). In a review of 221 histologically proven cases of cholesterol crystal embolization, cutaneous manifestations were noted

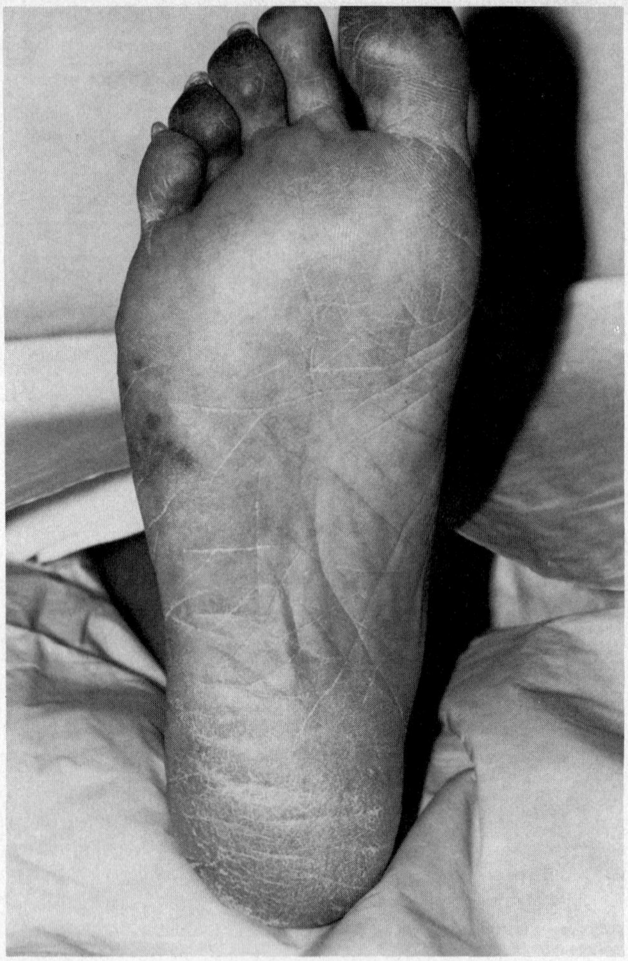

Fig. 11-2. The first, third, and fourth toes are cyanotic ("purple toes"), and the lateral aspect of the foot shows a patchy distribution of erythema and cyanosis in a patient with atheromatous emboli.

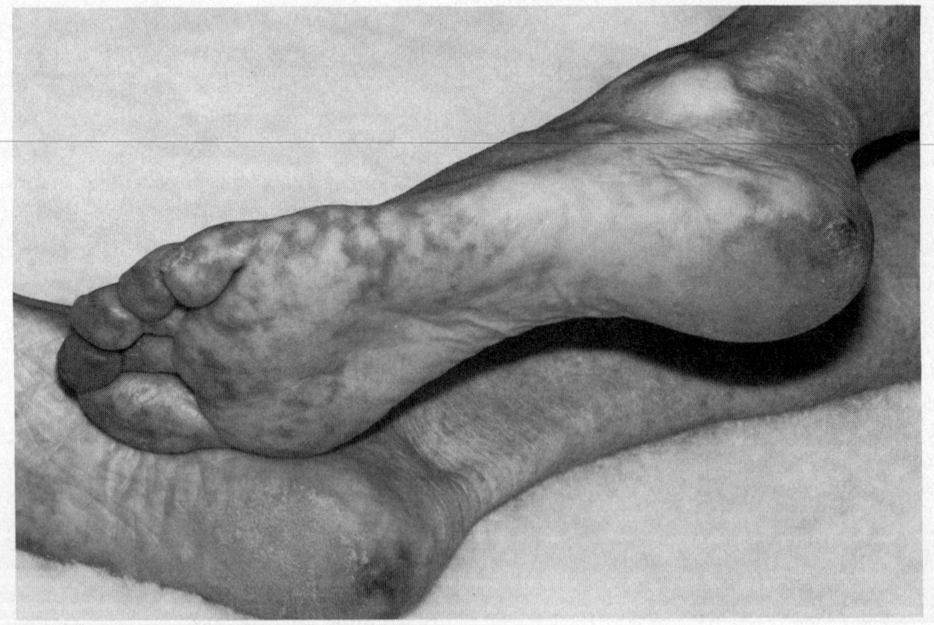

Fig. 11-3. Classic appearance of atheromatous emboli, with livedo reticularis on the lateral aspect of the foot and heel. The second toe is blue.

in over one third of patients.[20] This high incidence was confirmed in a recent review by Falanga, Fine, and Kapoor[59] in which cutaneous manifestations were the most common physical findings.

Livedo reticularis, a red-blue mottling or discoloration of the skin that occurs in a netlike fashion, is a common manifestation of atheromatous emboli.[60,61] Generally seen on the buttocks, thighs, or legs, it represents embolization to the dermal blood vessels (Fig. 11-3). Livedo reticularis is not pathognomonic of atheroemboli, since it may occur spontaneously or in other conditions, including vasculitis, particularly leukocytoclastic vasculitis. Livedo reticularis secondary to atheroemboli is rarely seen in the upper extremity.

Blue, cyanotic, or purple toes are frequently seen, and are usually painful (Fig. 11-2). Purple blotches or violaceous discoloration may also be seen on the sole of the foot (Figs. 11-2 and 11-3). These findings in the presence of palpable foot pulses are highly suggestive of atheromatous embolization. Ischemic or necrotic changes and frank gangrene of the lower extremities and toes are also common.

Necrosis of the penis and scrotum has been reported.[58] Nodules may occur on the calves and thighs.[60,62] They are painful, violaceous in appearance with a necrotic center, and they may mimic a necrotizing vasculitis such as polyarteritis nodosa. Other manifestations include muscle tenderness and burning, throbbing, or numbness of the feet or toes. Muscle cramps, nocturnal aching, and rare cases of restless leg syndrome secondary to atheromatous emboli have been reported.[63]

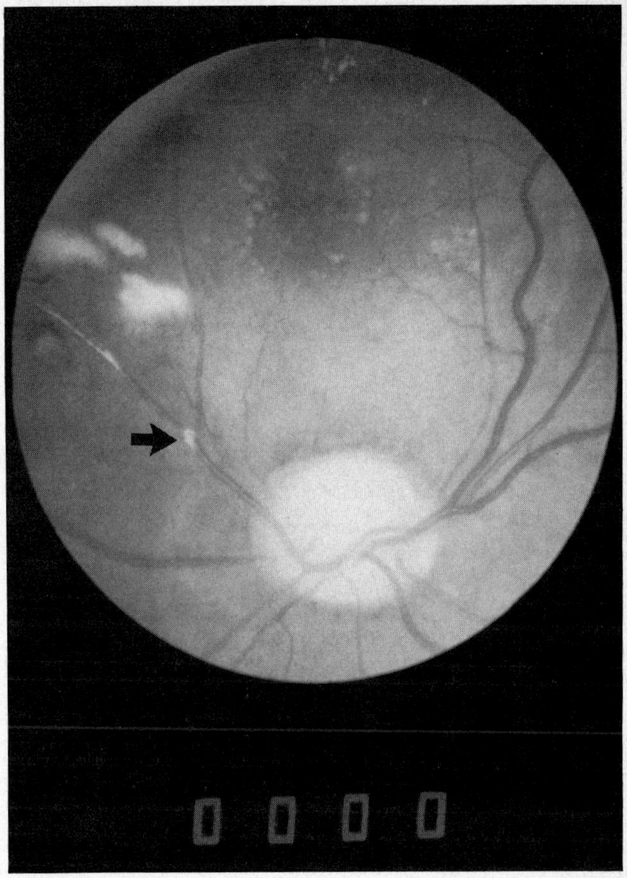

Fig. 11-4. Fundus showing a bright yellow refractile Hollenhorst plaque (*arrow*) representing atheromatous embolization to the retina.

Gastrointestinal tract

Atheroemboli may also involve the gastrointestinal tract. Frequently, this site is overlooked since clinical manifestations may be varied. Gore and Collins[8] have estimated that approximately 20% of patients with widespread atheromatous emboli have gastrointestinal involvement. Even more often the pancreas may be involved.[8,64] Patients may complain of generalized abdominal or periumbilical pain, nausea, vomiting, melena, or hematochezia. A guaiac positive stool may be noted. In severe cases frank bowel infarction may occur.[65] Cholesterol emboli to the gallbladder may cause acute gangrenous cholecystitis.[66]

Central nervous system and eye

The central nervous system and the retina may be involved with atheromatous emboli. Patients may develop visual disturbances such as amaurosis fugax or blindness caused by retinal artery occlusion. A Hollenhorst plaque may be seen on ophthalmoscopic examination as yellow, highly refractile atheromatous material that classically lodges in areas where vessels bifurcate (Fig. 11-4). Transient ischemic attack, stroke, headache, confusion, organic brain syndrome, and spinal cord infarction are other manifestations of central nervous system atheroemboli. The central nervous system is discussed further in Chapter 13.

Cardiac manifestations

Cardiac manifestations of atheroemboli, including angina pectoris and myocardial infarction, should be suspected in any high-risk patient, especially if other clinical findings suggest atheroemboli. Spontaneous atheroemboli to the coronary arteries have been reported. Intraoperative atheromatous embolization following coronary artery bypass surgery may also occur.[67,68]

Other areas

Atheromatous emboli have also been demonstrated in the spleen, bone marrow, muscle, and prostate.

Atheroembolic renal disease

When atheroembolic disease involves the kidneys, occlusion of multiple small arteries is seen leading to ischemic atrophy of segments of the kidney. This small vessel occlusive disease eventually may lead to uncontrolled hyper-

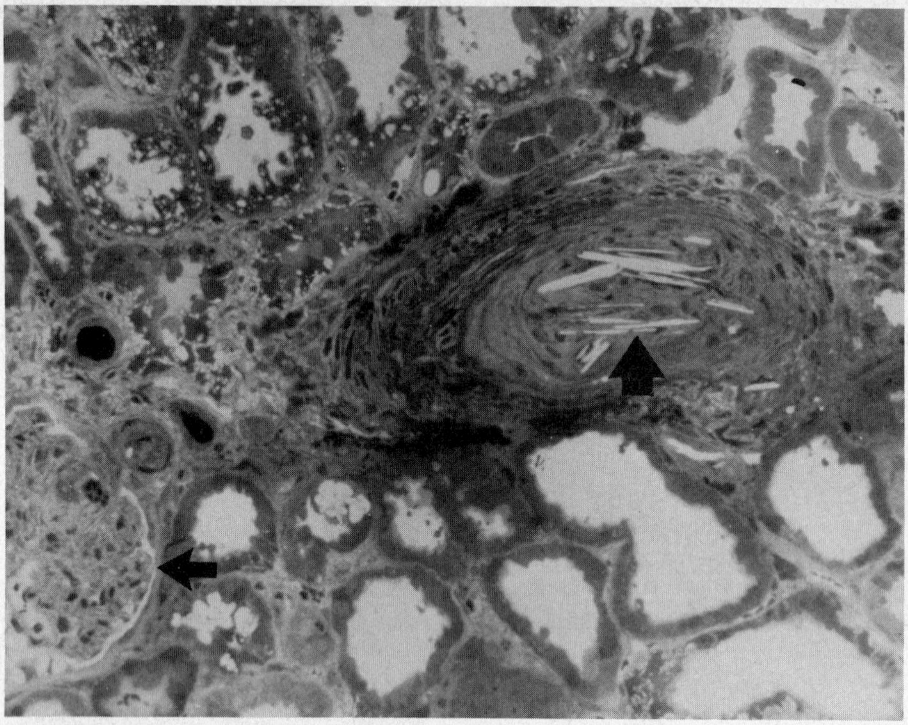

Fig. 11-5. Light microscopy showing multiple biconvex, needle-shaped cholesterol crystals in an arteriole in the kidney (*large arrow*). A glomerulus is seen in the left lower portion (*small arrow*). (Courtesy Gordon Gephardt, MD.)

tension, advanced renal failure, or end-stage renal disease. This disease differs from renal infarction from large *thromboemboli* originating from the heart or from emboli from a thrombus lining an aneurysm.

Renal atheroemboli originate from disease of the suprarenal aorta. The lining of the aorta may be covered with friable, shaggy cholesterol-rich atherosclerotic material (see Fig. 11-1). This material may be dislodged mechanically or spontaneously and lodge in the small arteries and arterioles of the kidney.

Pathologically, the interlobular and afferent arterioles (150 to 200 μm size) are usually involved. The material demonstrated in these arterioles is a biconvex cholesterol crystal. During histologic preparation, crystals dissolve and leave a space where the cholesterol crystals used to be (Fig. 11-5). Cholesterol embolization produces a foreign body reaction within the kidney, but the full-blown syndrome of renal failure and accelerated hypertension may take weeks or months to develop. Initially, polymorphonuclear leukocytes, macrophages, and multinucleated giant cells appear several days to several weeks after the inciting event. Eventually, this cellular infiltrate leads to thickening and fibrosis of the arterioles. Total occlusion of the blood vessel results from accumulation of fibrous material and connective tissue material. When large segments of small arterioles are occluded, ischemic atrophy of large portions of the kidney occurs. As glomerular filtration declines, the renin-angiotensin-aldosterone system is activated, and hypertension accelerates.[69-72]

The precipitating events associated in atheroembolic renal disease are identical to the precipitating events of atheromatous emboli, elsewhere in the body (see the box on p. 216).

Clinically, this disease occurs in the elderly who have evidence of atherosclerosis elsewhere in the body. Other evidence of atheroemboli may include livedo reticularis, stroke, amaurosis fugax, a Hollenhorst plaque, gastrointestinal bleeding, pancreatitis, or myocardial infarction. Some patients may exhibit multisystem failure, which suggests a necrotizing vasculitis.

Since patients with atheroembolic renal disease have many of the same precipitating factors as patients who develop acute tubular necrosis, other features may help to differentiate atheroembolic renal disease (Table 11-2). As a general rule, the urine sediment in patients with atheroembolic renal disease is benign or shows microhematuria with or without leukocyturia. By contrast, the urine sediment in patients with acute tubular necrosis often demonstrates pigmented granular casts (dirty brown casts) and renal tubular cells.

Patients who develop acute tubular necrosis may have no hypertension or mild hypertension only, whereas patients

Table 11-2. Differentiating acute tubular necrosis from atheroembolic renal disease

	Acute tubular necrosis	Atheroembolic renal disease
Precipitating factors	Hypotension Surgery Arteriography Drugs	Arteriography Surgery Anticoagulants Spontaneous
Urine sediment	Renal tubular cells Pigmented granular casts (dirty brown casts)	Benign or hematuria ± leukocyturia
Other associated laboratory findings	None	Eosinophilia and/or hypocomplementemia in some patients
Hypertension	None or mild	Often present, severe, and quite difficult to control; may be an early clue to atheroemboli renal disease
Rise in serum creatinine	1-2 days after insult, peak in 4-14 days	Usually begins 7-10 days after insult and slowly rises over weeks to months (Fig. 11-6)
Renal outcome	Full recovery is the rule if underlying precipitating factor is corrected	Progression to end-stage renal disease or advanced renal failure; stabilization or recovery of renal failure may sometimes occur

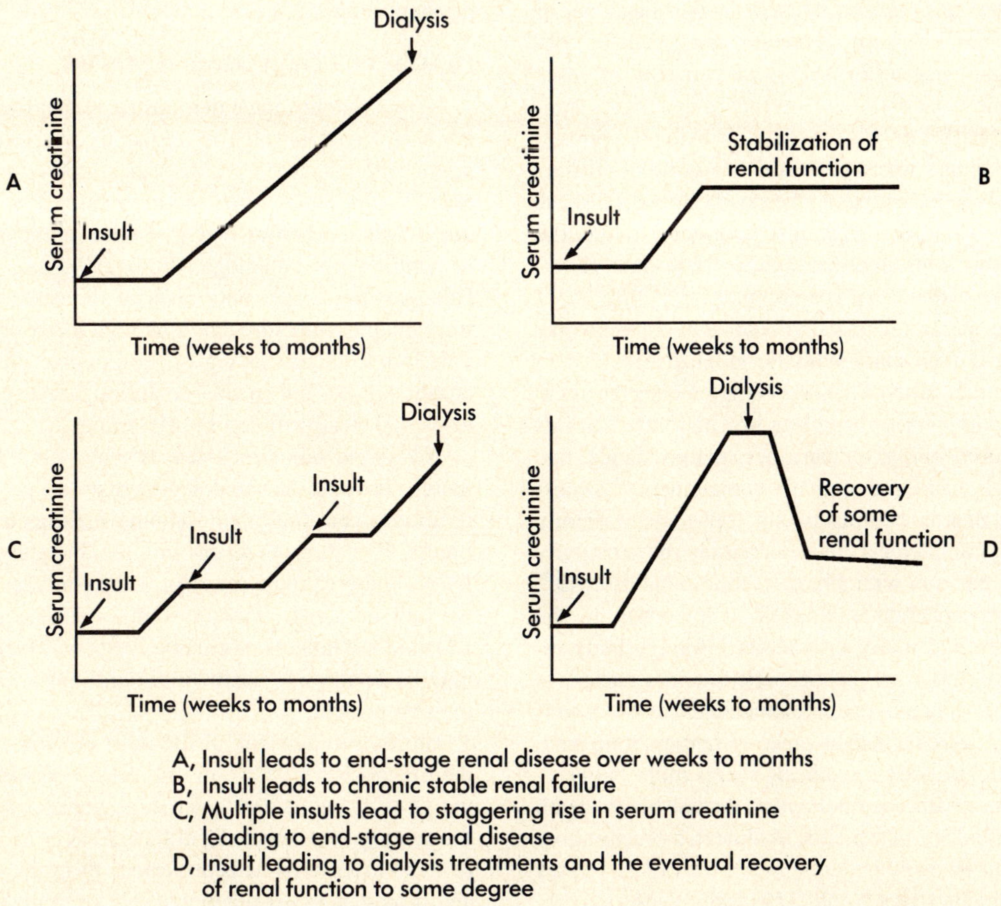

Fig. 11-6. Several patterns of renal failure in patients with atheroembolic renal disease.

with atheroembolic renal disease often experience an acceleration of their hypertension, which is often difficult to control. The hypertension is thought to be mediated through the renin-angiotensin-aldosterone system. In patients with acute tubular necrosis, the serum creatinine usually begins to rise soon after the insult peaks in 4 to 14 days, and often returns to normal if the precipitating event is corrected. On the other hand, in patients with atheroembolic renal disease the rise in serum creatinine is often delayed for 7 to 10 days. It is not uncommon for a patient to have an angiographic procedure performed, and to be discharged from the hospital only to return several weeks later with a markedly elevated serum creatinine. The serum creatinine may rise slowly and end-stage renal disease is not unusual.

Various patterns of renal insufficiency may occur in atheroembolic renal disease (Fig. 11-6). In the past it was thought that patients always progressed to end-stage renal disease that required dialytic support. However, in 1981 Smith, Ghose, and Henry[25] reported several cases in which renal function stabilized or even improved to the point where the patient no longer required dialysis. Since this report, others have also demonstrated that renal function may not always progress to end-stage renal disease.[2,42,73,74]

No laboratory tests uniformly help in the diagnosis of atheroembolic renal disease. Kasinath and Lewis[75,76] described eosinophilia as a clue that occurs in 80% of cases of atheroembolic renal disease. However, this effect is transient and may last for only a few days. It is thus important to check the patient's white blood cell count with a differential count early in the course if atheroembolic renal disease is suspected. In contrast to patients with acute interstitial nephritis, patients with atheroembolic renal disease generally do not have evidence of eosinophil*uria*.

Others have suggested that hypocomplementemia may occur in patients with atheroembolic renal disease.[77,78] In one series of nine patients whose complement was measured, the C3 complement level was low in seven.[77] In rats injected with homogenized human atheromatous plaque, five of eight animals had decreased C3 complement.[77] Others have suggested that the contrast media itself may transiently decrease serum complement, thus decreasing the sensitivity of this test for patients with atheroembolic renal disease.[79] Whether hypocomplementemia itself is important in the pathogenesis of renal injury or whether a foreign body reaction is a more important pathogenetic factor is unclear at the present time. Since hypocomplementemia is not a universal finding in patients with advanced atheroembolic renal disease, the foreign body hypothesis seems more likely.

The diagnosis of atheroembolic renal disease before death requires a high index of suspicion. Although a precipitating event may occur in many patients, in a review of 221 cases from the English literature[20] only 31% had at least one precipitating event. Evidence of atheroembolic disease elsewhere is helpful in making the diagnosis. Other disease entities such as atherosclerotic renal artery stenosis, renal artery thrombosis, infective endocarditis, vasculitis (such as polyarteritis nodosa), and other forms of acute renal failure need to be considered in the differential diagnosis. A definitive diagnosis of atheroembolic renal disease requires a renal biopsy specimen in which cholesterol clefts are demonstrated. Since the atheromatous emboli are patchy in distribution, they may be missed on a needle biopsy. Therefore when a biopsy is indicated, an open renal biopsy should be performed.

Once an episode of atheromatous emboli to the kidney has occurred, no direct treatment is able to reverse the damage already done. The best treatment is prevention. If a patient has evidence of atheromatous emboli, that segment of aorta thought to be the source of the emboli should be replaced if feasible. The patient should be dialyzed as necessary, and blood pressure should be meticulously controlled. Anticoagulants should be avoided since they may precipitate more atheroembolic events.

Atheroembolic renal disease carries a particularly poor prognosis since it is indicative of generalized atherosclerosis. In one series[20] 179 of 221 (81%) patients died. The most common causes of death were cardiac, renal, or multisystem illness.

DIAGNOSIS OF ATHEROEMBOLI

Several studies have demonstrated that the atheromatous embolization syndrome is frequently overlooked and diagnosed only at autopsy. Maurizi, Barker, and Trueheart[26] noted that in 84% of their autopsy cases atheroemboli were not diagnosed before death, despite clinical features corresponding to pathologic findings. Fine, Kapoor, and Falanga[20] noted that only 30% of the cases they reviewed were diagnosed before death. A high index of suspicion and a thorough understanding of the possible clinical manifestations are needed in this condition because prompt diagnosis and treatment can be lifesaving.

No single laboratory test is diagnostic. Some patients merely have an elevated sedimentation rate, leukocytosis, or anemia, but these are common findings in any systemic illness. Elevations in serum amylase, hepatic transaminases, BUN, and creatinine are seen if the pancreas, liver, or kidney are involved. Elevations in creatinine phosphokinase and aldolase reflect muscle involvement. The urine sediment may be abnormal. Eosinophilia and hypocomplementemia may be present.[75-78]

Biopsy remains one of the most effective ways to make the diagnosis.[62,69,73,80,81] In one series[80] random biopsies of the gastrocnemius and quadriceps muscles were helpful in diagnosing atheroemboli, although, skin or muscle biopsy from an involved area is preferred. Biopsies should be deep and should be examined in multiple sections. Other involved areas that may be biopsied include the kidney, bone marrow, amputated extremities, or gangrenous toes. The pathognomonic finding is the needle-shaped cholesterol cleft within the small vessels.

In the appropriate clinical setting, biplanar angiography can assist in confirming the suspected diagnosis. Generally a markedly irregular and shaggy aorta is demonstrated (see Fig. 11-1). If lesions involving the lower extremity are bilateral, an attempt should be made to obtain thoracic and abdominal aortography with runoffs to each leg. Noninvasive tests such as magnetic resonance imaging, computerized tomography, and ultrasound may also be helpful. These are especially valuable in confirming the presence of aneurysms or in demonstrating calcified plaques.

The differential diagnosis may be quite extensive and depends on the end organs involved. Atheromatous emboli may mimic a vasculitis such as polyarteritis nodosa, leukocytoclastic vasculitis, or cryoglobulinemia. The clinical manifestation may also suggest an underlying malignancy, nonbacterial thrombotic endocarditis, subacute bacterial endocarditis, multiple myeloma, or atrial myxoma. A cardiac source of emboli should always be excluded.

TREATMENT

Treatment should be directed toward three goals:

1. Removal of the source of atheromatous material, usually by surgery
2. Symptomatic care of the end organ where the emboli are located
3. Risk factor modification to prevent progression of the disease.

If embolization to the lower extremities has occurred, local care of ischemic ulcers is quite important. If significant gangrene is present, amputation may be required. However, if the amount of tissue loss is equivocal, local care with soaking in tepid soapy water and good skin care may expedite healing. Heel protectors should be used and lamb's wool placed between the toes. At times a chemical or surgical sympathectomy may be helpful. After the acute episode has stabilized, surgical replacement of the aorta or section of the artery that was the source of embolization should be strongly considered.

Medical therapy

The most accepted form of therapy for atheromatous embolization is surgical removal of the source where the emboli originated. However, under certain circumstances, medical therapy is indicated. Medical therapy should be considered if the source of embolization cannot be identified with certainty or if the patient is at a markedly increased surgical risk.

Anticoagulants, including heparin and sodium warfarin, should be avoided in patients who have suspected atheromatous embolization. Antiplatelet agents such as aspirin and dipyridamole have been advocated as the best available medical therapy. Unfortunately, there are no controlled studies demonstrating their efficacy. Morris-Jones et al[82] described reversal of pregangrenous changes in the toes in 19 of 35 patients who were treated with aspirin and dipyridamole. When antiplatelet therapy was discontinued, five patients had a recurrence of their symptoms. Waldin, Adar, and Mozes[83] noted improvement in the pregangrenous changes of the toes of 10 patients treated with aspirin and/or dipyridamole. While it is probably unreasonable to expect antiplatelet therapy itself to improve ischemia, it may prevent further episodes of embolization.

Other forms of therapy have been advocated such as corticosteroids, low molecular weight dextran, intraarterial papavarine, other vasodilatory agents, anticoagulants, and thrombolytic therapy. However, no controlled trials have shown that any of these forms of therapy are of benefit, and we do not recommend them. In fact, either anticoagulants or thrombolytic therapy can precipitate atheromatous embolization.

Surgical therapy

Surgical therapy is the preferred method of removing the source of proximal atheromatous embolic material. When the source is in the aortoiliac region, replacement of that segment of aorta or iliac arteries is warranted. When the atheromatous material is infrarenal, as is most common, an aortobiiliac or aortobifemoral bypass is indicated. However, if the suprarenal aorta is the source of atheromatous emboli, aortic replacement significantly increases the risk of surgical morbidity and mortality. In this situation, the potential benefits of surgery must be weighed against the known risks.

Patients who are poor surgical risks for aortic replacement may be candidates for ligation of the common femoral arteries followed by an extraanatomic bypass, such as an axillobifemoral bypass.[53] The ligation prevents further embolization from reaching the legs, although embolization to the intestines may still occur. The prognosis for patients undergoing axillobifemoral bypass is poor. In a recent study[53] of 4 patients, all were dead within 6 months of this surgical procedure.

No well-designed trials have compared medical and surgical therapy for treatment of atheromatous embolization. The most common types of surgery are resection and graft replacement or thromboendarterectomy. Several reports have suggested that these surgical procedures will prevent recurrences of atheromatous embolization.[84-86] However, not all reports show a correlation between therapeutic intervention (surgical, medical, or none) and results. Wingo et al[87] showed that surgical therapy did not predict whether the patient would suffer further atheroembolic episodes. They studied 67 extremities in 48 patients and observed these patients from 1 to 84 months (mean 26 months). Only 28 patients (44%) manifested an uncomplicated outcome, while 38% had evidence of tissue loss, and 14% had recurrent digital ischemia. Amputation was required for 14 limbs (22%), and 20% of the patients died. The outcomes did not correlate at all with the type of treatment, medical or surgical. A well-controlled trial is needed to compare the various treatment modalities for this condition.

Another complicating feature is that it is often difficult to determine the exact source of the atheromatous emboli. Many patients have involvement of the aortoiliac segments of the arterial tree as well as more distal disease, such as in the superficial femoral artery. When there is evidence of atheromatous embolization in both lower extremities, the lesion is generally in the aorta. However, when only one extremity is involved, it is often difficult to determine whether the emboli originate at the more proximal or the more distal site. Fisher et al[88] studied this question in six patients who developed unilateral blue toe syndrome. In each case the peripheral lesion was corrected first by either localized thromboendarterectomy or short reverse saphenous vein grafting. Two patients had concomitant moderately severe aortoiliac atherosclerosis and four patients had mild aortoiliac disease. Only one patient had recurrent embolization during a follow-up period of 8 to 24 months. These results suggest that if there is combined peripheral and aortoiliac atherosclerosis and the embolization is confined to one extremity, the more distal lesion should be corrected first. Only if the patient continues to embolize, should the aortic lesion be corrected.[57,88]

If areas of significant digital gangrene or ischemia occur, sympathectomy may be combined with the surgical procedure to remove the source of the emboli.[53,57,84-88] A lumbar sympathectomy may relieve pain and minimize loss of lower extremity tissue by improving blood flow and therefore tissue perfusion. Lee et al[86] demonstrated that the group who underwent concomitant sympathectomy had better healing of distal digital ischemic ulcers compared to a group of patients who did not undergo sympathectomy.

Amputation may also be required for patients who have atheromatous emboli to the toes or feet. While thromboendarterectomy or bypass surgery may prevent future embolization, these procedures do nothing to correct the ischemia from a previous embolic event. Therefore when the ischemia is extensive and the chance of healing is minimal with a sympathectomy, an amputation should be performed to relieve pain and remove gangrenous tissue. In a series by Wingo et al[87] 22% of patients underwent amputations.

Other interventional procedures

Recently, several investigators[89-92] have recommended percutaneous transluminal angioplasty, laser angioplasty, or percutaneous atherectomy for patients with atheromatous embolization. However, most of these reports are anecdotal. Brewer et al[89] advocated pretreatment with anticoagulants followed by percutaneous transluminal angioplasty for short segment stenosis or occlusions distal to the aortic bifurcation. In the six patients who underwent this procedure, rest pain was relieved, and peripheral pulses were reestablished. Most of the patients did not develop further evidence of atheromatous embolization. Kumpe, Zwerdlinger, and Griffin have similarly treated 10 patients with "classical blue digit syndrome" by percutaneous transluminal angioplasty.[90] Nine patients demonstrated clinical improvement and showed no evidence of recurrent embolization during a follow-up period of 7 to 86 months (mean, 28 months).

Several recent reports have suggested the removal of peripheral atheromatous plaques by means of an atherectomy device.[91,92] The short-term results in these studies are at least as good as those in patients who undergo percutaneous transluminal angioplasty or surgery. Percutaneous atherectomy makes more physiologic sense than percutaneous transluminal angioplasty for treating atheromatous embolization. In percutaneous transluminal angioplasty, the intima is cracked and remolded, and thus, theoretically, the chance of distal embolization should be increased. However, with percutaneous atherectomy, the plaque is actually shaved off the wall of the vessel and removed through a collection device.

It seems reasonable to try nonsurgical intervention for atheromatous embolization that arises from the vessels distal to the aortic bifurcation. If this intervention fails, surgery can then be considered. However, for most patients with atheromatous embolization the aortoiliac segments are the source of emboli, and surgery is the procedure of choice in this situation.

REFERENCES

1. Moldveen-Geronimus M and Merriam JC: Cholesterol embolization: from pathological curiosity to clinical entity, Circulation 35:946, 1967.
2. Dahlberg PJ, Frecentese DF, and Cogbill TH: Cholesterol embolism: experience with 22 histologically proven cases, Surgery 105:737, 1989.
3. Panum PL: Experimentelle Beitrage Zur Lehre Von der Embolie, Arch Pathol Anat Physiol Klin Med 25:308, 1862.
4. Doch G: Some notes on coronary arteries, M and S Reporter 75:1, 1896.
5. Albutt TC: Diseases of the arteries, including angina pectoris, London, 1915, MacMillan and Company.
6. Flory CM: Arterial occlusions produced by emboli from eroded aortic atheromatous plaques, Am J Pathol 21:549, 1945.
7. Snyder HE and Shapiro JL: A correlative study of atheromatous embolism in human beings and experimental animals, Surgery 49:195, 1961.
8. Gore I and Collins DP: Spontaneous atheromatous embolization: review of the literature and a report of 16 additional cases, Am J Clin Pathol 33:416, 1960.
9. Hoye SJ et al: Atheromatous embolization: a factor in peripheral gangrene, N Engl J Med 261:128, 1959.
10. Handler FP: Clinical and pathologic significance of atheromatous embolization, with emphasis on an etiology of renal hypertension, Am J Med 20:366, 1956.
11. Thurlbeck WM and Castleman B: Atheromatous emboli to the kidneys after aortic surgery, N Engl J Med 257:442, 1957.

12. Case Records of the Massachusetts General Hospital (Case 23-1974), N Engl J Med 290:1365, 1974.
13. Case Records of the Massachusetts General Hospital (Case 49-1975), N Engl J Med 293:1308, 1975.
14. Case Records of the Massachusetts General Hospital (Case 25-1967), N Engl J Med 276:1368, 1967.
15. Case Records of the Massachusetts General Hospital (Case 50-1977), N Engl J Med 297:1337, 1977.
16. Case Records of the Massachusetts General Hospital (Case 33-1974), N Engl J Med 291:406, 1974.
17. Case Records of the Massachusetts General Hospital (Case 4-1984), N Engl J Med 310:244, 1984.
18. Case Records of the Massachusetts General Hospital (Case 21-1972), N Engl J Med 286:1146, 1972.
19. Case Records of the Massachusetts General Hospital (Case 8-1972), N Engl J Med 286:422, 1972.
20. Fine MJ, Kapoor W, and Falanga V: Cholesterol crystal embolization: a review of 221 cases in the English literature, Angiology 38:769, 1987.
21. Rosman HS et al: Cholesterol emobilization: clinical findings and implications, J Am Coll Cardiol 15:1296, 1990.
22. Vidt DG et al: Atheroembolic renal disease: association with renal artery stenosis, Cleve Clin J Med 56:407, 1989.
23. Kassirer JP: Atheroembolic renal disease, N Engl J Med 280:812, 1969.
24. Meyrier A et al: Atheromatous renal disease, Am J Med 85:139, 1988.
25. Smith MC, Ghose MK, and Henry AR: The clinical spectrum of renal cholesterol embolization, Am J Med 71:174, 1981.
26. Maurizi CP, Barker AE, and Trueheart RE: Atheromatous emboli: a postmortem study with special reference to the lower extremities, Arch Pathol 86:528, 1968.
27. Wagner RB and Martin AS: Peripheral atheroembolism: confirmation of a clinical concept, with a case report and review of the literature, Surgery 73:353, 1973.
28. Kealy WF: Atheroembolism, J Clin Pathol 31:984, 1978.
29. Sieniewicz DJ et al: Atheromatous emboli to the kidneys, Radiology 92:1231, 1969.
30. Ramirez G et al: Cholesterol embolization: a complication of angiography, Arch Intern Med 138:1430, 1978.
31. Retan JW and Miller RE: Microembolic complications of atherosclerosis, Arch Intern Med 118:534, 1966.
32. Harrington JT, Sommers SC, and Kassirer JP: Atheromatous emboli with progressive renal failure: renal arteriography as the probable inciting factor, Ann Intern Med 68:152, 1968.
33. Pollitt J and Lee BM: Renal failure from atheroembolism after translumbar aortography, J Am Geriatr Soc 19:989, 1971.
34. Gaines PA et al: Cholesterol embolization: a lethal complication of vascular catheterisation, Lancet 1:168, 1988.
35. Drost H et al: Cholesterol embolization as a complication of left heart catheterization: report of 7 cases, Br Heart J 52:339, 1984.
36. Colt HG et al: Cholesterol emboli after cardiac catheterization: eight cases and a review of the literature, Medicine 67:389, 1988.
37. Nawar T et al: Widespread atheromatous emboli following abdominal aortography, Can Med Assoc J 100:1005, 1969.
38. Kennedy A, Cumberland D, and Gaines P: The pathology of cholesterol embolism arising as a complication of intra-aortic catheterization, Histopathology 15:515, 1989.
39. Rosansky SJ and Deschamps EG: Multiple cholesterol emboli syndrome after angiography, Am J Med Sci 288:45, 1984.
40. Gjesdal K, Orning OM, and Smith E: Fatal atheromatous emboli to the kidneys after left heart catheterization, Lancet 2:405, 1977.
41. Fisher ER, Hellstrom R, and Myers JD: Disseminated atheromatous emboli, Am J Med 29:176, 1960.
42. Tilley W et al: Renal failure due to cholesterol emboli following PTCA, Am Heart J 110:1301, 1985.
43. Labs JD, Merillat JC, and Williams GM: Analysis of solid phase debris from laser angioplasty: potential risks of atheroembolism, J Vasc Surg 7:326, 1988.
44. Hyman BT et al: Warfarin-related purple toes syndrome and cholesterol microembolization, Am J Med 82:1233, 1987.
45. Brenowitz JB and Edwards WS: The management of atheromatous emboli to the lower extremities, Surg Gynecol Obstet 143:941, 1976.
46. Bruns FJ, Segel DP, and Adler S: Control of cholesterol embolization by discontinuation of anticoagulant therapy, Am J Med Sci 275:105, 1978.
47. Ridker PM and Michel T: Streptokinase therapy and cholesterol embolization, Am J Med 87:357, 1989.
48. Shapiro LS: Cholesterol embolization after treatment with tissue plasminogen activator, N Engl J Med 321:1270, 1989 (letter).
49. Schwartz MW and McDonald GB: Cholesterol embolization syndrome: occurrence after intravenous streptokinase therapy for myocardial infarction, JAMA 258:1934, 1987.
50. Perdue GD and Smith RB: Atheromatous microemboli, Ann Surg 169:954, 1969.
51. Feder W and Auerbach R: "Purple toes": An uncommon sequelae of oral coumarin drug therapy, Ann Intern Med 55:911, 1961.
52. Mashiah A et al: Massive atheromatous emboli to both kidneys: a fatal complication following aortic surgery, J Cardiovasc Surg 29:60, 1988.
53. Kaufman JL, Stark K, and Brolin RE: Disseminated atheroembolism from extensive degenerative atherosclerosis of the aorta, Surgery 102:63, 1987.
54. Elliot RS, Kanjuh VI, and Edwards JE: Atheromatous embolism, Circulation 30:611, 1964.
55. Cappiello RA et al: Cholesterol embolism: a pseudovasculitic syndrome, Semin Arthritis Rheum 18:240, 1989.
56. Fischer DA and Kistner RL: Atherothrombotic emboli in the lower extremities, Arch Dermatol 104:533, 1971.
57. Karmody AM et al: "Blue toe" syndrome: an indication for limb salvage surgery, Arch Surg 111:1263, 1976.
58. Rosansky SJ: Multiple cholesterol emboli syndrome, South Med J 75:677, 1982.
59. Falanga V, Fine MJ, and Kapoor WN: The cutaneous manifestations of cholesterol crystal embolization, Arch Dermatol 122:1194, 1986.
60. Deschamps P et al: Livedo reticularis and nodules due to cholesterol embolism in the lower extremities, Br J Dermatol 97:93, 1977.
61. Kalter DC, Rudolph A, and McGavran M: Livedo reticularis due to multiple cholesterol emboli, J Am Acad Dermatol 13:235, 1985.
62. Richards AM et al: Cholesterol embolism: a multiple-system disease masquerading as polyarteritis nodosa, Am J Cardiol 15:696, 1965.
63. Harvey JC: Cholesterol crystal microembolization: a cause of the restless leg syndrome, South Med J 69:269, 1976.
64. Probstein JG, Jostic RA, and Blumenthal HT: Atheromatous embolization: etiology in acute pancreatitis, Arch Surg 75:566, 1957.
65. Hendel RC et al: Multiple cholesterol emboli syndrome: bowel infarction after retrograde angiography, Arch Intern Med 149:2371, 1989.
66. Thomas W and Zaret P: Cholesterol emboli causing acute gangrenous cholecystitis, Mt Sinai J Med 51:716, 1984.
67. Keon WJ, Heggtveit HA, and Leduc J: Perioperative myocardial infarction caused by atheroembolism, J Thorac Cardiovasc Surg 84:849, 1982.
68. FitzGibbon GM and Keon WJ: Atheroembolic perioperative infarction during repeat coronary bypass surgery: angiographic documentation in a survivor, Ann Thorac Surg 43:218, 1987.
69. Humphreys MH: Thromboembolic disorders of the major renal vessels. In Brener BM and Rector FC, eds: The kidney, Philadelphia, 1981, WB Saunders.
70. Otken IB: Experimental production of atheromatous embolization, Arch Pathol 68:685, 1959.
71. Warren BA and Vales O: The ultrastructure of the stages of atheroem-

bolic occlusion of renal arteries, Br J Exp Pathol 54:469, 1973.
72. Jones DB and Iannaccone PM: Atheromatous emboli in renal biopsies: an ultrastructural study, Am J Pathol 78:261, 1975.
73. McGowan JA and Greenberg A: Cholesterol atheroembolic renal disease: report of 3 cases with emphasis on diagnosis by skin biopsy and extended survival, Am J Nephrol 6:135, 1986.
74. Ho Sw-C, Thatcher GN, and Matz LR: Reversible renal failure due to renal cholesterol embolism, Aust N Z J Med 12:531, 1982.
75. Kasinath BS et al: Eosinophilia in the diagnosis of atheroembolic renal disease, Am J Nephrol 7:173, 1987.
76. Kasinath BS and Lewis EJ: Eosinophilia as a clue to the diagnosis of atheroembolic renal disease, Arch Intern Med 147:1384, 1987.
77. Cosio FG, Zager RA, and Sharma HM: Atheroembolic renal disease causes hypocomplementaemia, Lancet 2:118, 1985.
78. Firth JD and North JP: Does atheroembolic renal disease cause hypocomplementemia? Lancet 2:1133, 1985.
79. Gonsette R and Delnotte P: In vitro activation of serum complement by contrast media: a clinical study, Intervent Radiol 15(suppl):26, 1980.
80. Anderson WR and Richards AM: Evaluation of lower extremity muscle biopsies in the diagnosis of atheroembolism, Arch Pathol 86:535, 1968.
81. Carvajal JA et al: Atheroembolism: an etiologic factor in renal insufficiency, gastrointestinal hemorrhages, and peripheral vascular diseases, Arch Intern Med 119:593, 1967.
82. Morris-Jones W et al: Gangrene of the toes with palpable peripheral pulses: response to platelet suppressive therapy, Ann Surg 193:462, 1981.
83. Walden R, Adar R, and Mozes M: Gangrene of toes with normal peripheral pulses, Ann Surg 185:269, 1977.
84. Kempczinski RF: Lower-extremity arterial emboli from ulcerating atherosclerotic plaques, JAMA 241:807, 1979.
85. Mehigan JT and Stoney RJ: Lower extremity atheromatous embolization, Am J Surg 132:163, 1976.
86. Lee BY et al: Blue digit syndrome: urgent indication for digital salvage, Am J Surg 147:418, 1984.
87. Wingo JP et al: The blue toe syndrome: hemodynamics and therapeutic correlates of outcome, J Vasc Surg 3:475, 1986.
88. Fisher DF et al: Dilemmas in dealing with blue toe syndrome: aortic versus peripheral source, Am J Surg 148:836, 1984.
89. Brewer ML et al: Blue toe syndrome: treatment with anticoagulants and delayed percutaneous transluminal angioplasty, Radiology 166:31, 1988.
90. Kumpe DA, Zwerdlinger S, and Griffin DJ: Blue digit syndrome: treatment with percutaneous transluminal angioplasty, Radiology 166:37, 1988.
91. Hofling B et al: Percutaneous removal of atheromatous plaques in peripheral arteries, Lancet 1:384, 1988.
92. Dolmatch BL et al: Blue toe syndrome: treatment with percutaneous atherectomy, Radiology 172:799, 1989.

Chapter 12

ACUTE ARTERIAL OCCLUSION

Anthony J. Comerota
Eric Leefmans

An acute arterial occlusion is the abrupt interruption of blood flow within an artery. Manifestations of acute arterial occlusion reflect the pathophysiologic consequences of the end-organ supplied by the involved artery. Acute occlusion of a coronary artery can result in myocardial infarction; occlusion of a carotid or intracranial artery can result in stroke; occlusion of a renal artery results in severe hypertension associated with renal dysfunction; and, mesenteric arterial occlusion is associated with severe abdominal pain and intestinal ischemia and/or infarction. This chapter addresses only acute arterial occlusion of the extremities. Although the lower extremity is specifically addressed, upper extremity ischemia follows precisely the same principles.

The consequences of acute arterial occlusion depend on the degree of occlusion and the patient's underlying collateral circulation. Since acute arterial occlusion is usually indicative of significant underlying pathology (either of the blood vessel or the heart), it is important for the physician to diagnose the event properly and to identify its etiology since appropriate therapy can have a profound effect on long-term outcome.

ETIOLOGY

Acute arterial occlusions can be categorized as either extrinsic or intrinsic. The former is usually traumatic and the latter embolic or thrombotic. Either blunt or penetrating injuries can result in extrinsic occlusions. Both are generally apparent as wounds, and evidence of trauma accompanies acute arterial insufficiency. Acute venous obstruction on rare occasion can manifest as acute arterial insufficiency when massive venous occlusion causes venous pressures to rise to exceptionally high levels, thereby compromising arterial perfusion. This begins as a "physiologic occlusion." Limb swelling that precedes the signs of acute arterial insufficiency is a clue that acute venous obstruction may be responsible.

The dissecting hematoma of an acute aortic dissection can initially be seen as an acute arterial occlusion that obstructs flow through any branch of the aorta. The diagnosis is generally made through the associated extreme hypertension and by the tearing back and abdominal pain that usually begins in the interscapular area. It is beyond the scope of this chapter to deal but briefly with extrinsic occlusions; however, the ischemic consequences of acute arterial occlusion of both categories can be similar, but the treatment of the underlying lesion varies considerably.

The overwhelming majority of acute occlusions are either thrombotic or embolic. Acute thrombosis that occurs in a severely diseased artery because of atherosclerotic disease can be minimally symptomatic or asymptomatic; thus the actual acute occlusion may not be recognized.[1] Emboli, on the other hand, are much more likely to be acutely symptomatic since they can suddenly occlude minimally diseased or normal arteries (Table 12-1). Seventy-five percent to 90% of emboli originate in the heart.[1-5] The most common underlying cardiac pathology is atrial fibrillation, which occurs in up to 75% of patients with peripheral emboli.[1,6] Myocardial infarction with mural thrombi ranks second. Less common cardiac sources include prosthetic valves, dyskinetic cardiomyopathic ventricles, and ventricular aneurysms. Rarer causes of cardiac-derived emboli include atrial myxoma, cardioversion, marantic endocarditis, diseased cardiac valves, and paradoxic emboli.[7]

Arterial emboli may also originate from proximal ulcerated arterial plaque or thrombus, the so-called arterio-arterial emboli.[8,9] Small embolic occlusion of the digital vessels and other small end arteries is also known as the *blue toe syndrome* or *atheromatous emboli syndrome*. These terms indicate end-arterial occlusion and frequently are as-

Table 12-1. Acute arterial occlusion: embolism vs thrombosis

Characteristics of occlusion	Embolus	Thrombosis
Onset of symptoms	Rapid/immediate	Slower/insidious
Prior symptoms	Infrequent	Frequent
Duration of symptoms before presentation	Shorter	Longer
Opposite leg	Frequently normal examination	Frequently abnormal examination
Recent heart disease (artrial fibrillation, myocardial infarction)	Frequent	±
Goal of immediate therapy	Eliminate embolus	Correct underlying disease
Long-term pharmacologic prescription	Anticoagulation (if cardiac source)	Platelet inhibition (± anticoagulation)
Results of thromboembolectomy	Good	Poor
Amputation risk	Lower	Higher
Cause of subsequent mortality	Cardiac disease	Related to persistent limb ischemia

sociated with digital ischemia or necrosis. Patients may have associated areas of painful but punctate necrosis of the skin, with a surrounding area of cyanosis. The frequent confusion involved with the diagnosis and treatment of atheromatous emboli results from poor understanding of its pathophysiology. In general, patients with an atherothrombotic microembolism should not be considered in the same category as those with an acute large vessel occlusion. These patients most frequently have transient focal ischemia associated with minor tissue loss but no major foot or limb ischemia and should not be considered with those in the threatened limb categories.

Acute arterial thrombosis is the other common form of acute arterial ischemia. It generally is superimposed on a "low-flow" state during which the thrombotic threshold of a vessel is surpassed. Underlying atherosclerotic disease is the most commonly associated pathology. It is generally believed that limbs suffering acute ischemia after a thrombotic occlusion are associated with higher amputation rates than those with an embolic cause.[10,11] This observation is based on the results of surgical thromboembolectomy in which removal of an acute occluding embolus opens the majority of the occluded arterial tree and, in the absence of additional emboli, restores perfusion through a relatively nondiseased artery; removal of a thrombus from a diseased artery without definitive reconstruction leaves the pathology in place, resulting in reocclusion and progression of the ischemic process.[12] The clinical distinction between arterial embolism and arterial thrombosis is often difficult to make; however, a concerted effort must be made because of the short- and long-term therapeutic implications.

PATHOPHYSIOLOGIC CONSEQUENCES OF ACUTE ARTERIAL OCCLUSION

The consequences of an acute arterial occlusion hinge on several factors. Foremost is the degree of collateral circulation supplied to the tissue by the involved vessel.[13] If sufficient collateral flow is present, no clinical sequelae are discernable. This situation may occur when an acute thrombosis is superimposed on a chronic stenosis. A slowly progressing atherosclerotic stenosis allows time for the development of collaterals. An example is the patient without symptoms who is incidentally noted to have a superficial femoral artery thrombosis superimposed on chronic atherosclerotic disease. At the other extreme is the patient without peripheral vascular disease in whom an embolus suddenly moves from his heart to his femoral artery without his having had the opportunity to develop collaterals. This scenario will almost certainly lead to acute symptoms and a threatened limb. Between these extremes is a wide range of collateralization that permits the clinical spectrum of signs and symptoms that occur with acute occlusions.

If insufficient collaterals exist, tissue susceptibility to ischemia over time assumes paramount significance. It is well established that different tissues vary in their ability to tolerate ischemia. Nerve and skeletal muscle can suffer ischemia for only 4 to 6 hours before histologically demonstrable changes occur.[14] Skin will tolerate ischemia for 10 hours or more before irreversible changes become evident microscopically. Subcutaneous tissue resists ischemia even longer since it can be nourished by interstitial fluid. These susceptibilities are presumably a measure of the oxygen demand of the various tissues.

Recently Blebea et al[15] demonstrated the duration of ischemia required to induce irreversible injury in the gracilis muscle of a dog. They isolated the dog's gracilis muscle, leaving it attached only to its nutrient artery and vein. After arterial occlusion for 4, 6, or 8 hours, the accumulation of technetium-99m (^{99m}Tc) pyrophosphate in the injured muscle was measured. Only 8% more ^{99m}Tc pyrophosphate accumulated after 4 hours of occlusion than in controls, with 215% at 6 hours, and 400% to 500% at 8 hours. Histologic examination confirmed that irreversible cellular damage occurred after 6 hours of occlusion and reperfusion; however, the injury was reversible after 4 hours. Most of the observed injury centered around the gracilis arteries, suggesting that reperfusion may play a role in inducing injury after acute occlusion. An increase in free radical release near the source of the arterial flow may explain the distribution of injury.

Ricci et al,[16] pursuing the possibility that free radicals released on reperfusion may compound the injury, studied the effect of these free radical scavengers (superoxide dismutase and mannitol) on the isolated anterior compartment of the dog hind limb after 8 hours of acute ischemia. Thirty minutes before reperfusion they administered free radical scavengers intravenously. One hour after reperfusion, ^{99m}Tc pyrophosphate accumulation was assessed. There was significantly less muscle injury in the dogs receiving free radical scavengers than in the control animals. Muscle function studied 16 hours after reperfusion, however, demonstrated abnormal contractions even in the scavenger group. Thus free radical scavengers may decrease the muscle injury after acute arterial occlusion and reperfusion, but they did not appear to preserve normal muscle function.

Anoxia impairs cellular metabolism as anaerobic glycolysis assumes the burden of ATP formation. The lack of energy results in the loss of biocellular functions, including the active extrusion of sodium from cells. The increased intracellular sodium leads to cellular edema. If the ischemia is reversed before irreversible injury occurs, a reactivated sodium pump will re-extrude the sodium from the cell, thereby restoring normal cell volume. It has been suggested that the cellular edema may obstruct capillaries, thereby perpetuating cellular ischemia despite the restoration of blood flow.[17] This has been referred to as the *no-reflow* phenomenon. Experimentally, use of intravenous hypertonic mannitol has been effective in decreasing the cellular edema following ischemia by reducing the degree of tissue injury that follows transient compression of the renal artery.

The depletion of erythrocyte ATP by ischemia leads to loss of red cell deformibility, which may also impair the restoration of flow in ischemic tissues with edematous cells.[18]

In addition to cellular edema, distal propagation of thrombus, particularly within arterioles and capillaries, can prevent perfusion of tissue despite restoration of blood flow through major arteries.[19] Belkin, Valeri, and Hobson[20] studied the effect of urokinase on the acute occlusion of an isolated gracilis muscle preparation. After 5 hours of acute clamp occlusion of the gracilis artery, urokinase was injected into the artery for 5 minutes and was allowed to incubate in the gracilis muscle preparation for 15 minutes before reperfusion. The initial 30 ml of venous effluent were collected and discarded to avoid systemic effects of urokinase. The contralateral canine gracilis muscle exposed to the same degree of ischemia was used as a control. Triphenyltetrazolium chloride staining of the muscle preparation demonstrated 20.2% (±8.1%) infarction in the control muscle vs 8.6% (±6.2%) in the urokinase-infused preparations. There was a 33.6 (±5.9) g gain in weight in the control muscle vs 18.2 (±4.1) g in the urokinase-treated preparation. Both findings were statistically significant. Although gracilis muscle blood flow was better in the experimental group compared to the control group, the difference was not statistically significant. Overall blood flow per se may not be a good indicator of the success of reperfusion since overall flow does not reflect the distribution of flow through the ischemic tissue.

In 1960 Haimovici[21] initially described the systemic effect of reperfusion after an acute arterial occlusion. Restoration of flow to a profoundly ischemic limb results in the sudden overloading of the systemic circulation with lactate, potassium, myoglobin, and sometimes bacterial toxins. The consequence is a metabolic derangement, resulting in cardiovascular depression and renal impairment.[21-23] Besides the systemic effects, reperfusion also results in local injury, which is mediated in part by oxygen-free radicals as mentioned previously. Much of the reperfusion injury may simply be due to edema both intracellularly and in connective tissue as ischemic capillary walls lose their integrity, allowing leakage after reperfusion. Subfascial pressure may rise precipitously after reperfusion, resulting in a compartment syndrome limiting capillary perfusion and eventually resulting in muscle necrosis. As mentioned previously, Ricci et al[16] were unable to preserve muscle function using free radical scavengers despite their decreasing the extent of necrosis. Using fasciotomy after controlled arterial occlusion, however, they decreased muscle necrosis as measured by ^{99m}Tc pyrophosphate scanning and preserved normal muscle contraction. They concluded that early fasciotomy is the treatment of choice for the reperfusion compartment syndrome. These experimental observations fit well with the clinical findings of Lim et al[24] who treated vascular trauma of the popliteal artery by performing routine fasciotomy before vascular repair. In this traditionally morbid injury associated with a 20% to 30% limb loss, they found that prereperfusion fasciotomy offered significantly better limb salvage than previously reported.

Recently Breyersdorf et al[25] focused attention on the effects of reperfusion vs the direct effects of ischemia caused by acute arterial occlusion. Using the amputated hind legs of rats, they looked at the effects of standard uncontrolled reperfusion through the rat femoral arteries vs the effects of controlled reperfusion. Standard reperfusion was performed using Krebs-Hanseleit buffer at 37° C at a pressure of 100 mm Hg for 60 minutes. Controlled reperfusion was performed with a substrate-enriched modified perfusate at 37° C and a pressure of 50 mm Hg for 30 minutes. Thereafter this group was further perfused with standard Krebs-Hanseleit buffer at 100 mm Hg for 30 minutes. Uncontrolled reperfusion resulted in severe injury involving massive edema and the loss of contractile function, whereas controlled reperfusion preserved near-normal leg volume and contractile function. The authors emphasize maintaining the following three conditions for performing controlled reperfusion: (1) gentle perfusion pressures (50 mm Hg), (2) normothermia, and (3) prolonged duration of controlled reperfusion. Additionally, they emphasize that injury results directly from uncontrolled reperfusion and, perhaps more importantly, injury can be diminished significantly by decreasing reperfusion pressure. Their argument would be more convincing if they had used the same solution to reperfuse both limbs instead of adding a substrate-enriched solution to the controlled reperfused limb.

In addition to the local consequences of acute arterial occlusion, toxic metabolites distal to the occlusion may enter the systemic circulation, particularly during reperfusion, leading to systemic consequences. In 1960 Haimovici[21] reported two cases of acute massive muscle ischemia associated with myoglobinuria. Since then myoglobinuria with renal failure caused by muscle necrosis after acute arterial occlusion has been well described. Myoglobin released from necrotic muscle precipitates in renal tubules and may result in renal failure. Alkalinization of urine with a bicarbonate infusion and adequate hydration accompanied by administration of a loop diuretic help keep myoglobin soluble, thereby decreasing its likelihood of precipitation in the renal tubules.

In 1970 Fisher, Fogarty, and Morrow[26] reported the biochemical effects of prolonged transient acute femoral occlusion in four patients. Each artery was occluded by an embolus for at least 12 hours. The venous efflux of the ipsilateral femoral vein was assayed for partial pressure of oxygen (PO_2), creatine phosphokinase (CPK), pH, partial pressure of carbon dioxide (PCO_2), and potassium. These values were compared with those of systemic venous blood. The average venous PO_2 in the ischemic leg was significantly lower (18, ± 8 mm Hg) than the systemic venous value (40, ± 3 mm Hg). Five minutes after restoration of flow the venous PO_2 returned to normal in all four ischemic limbs. The average venous PCO_2 in the ischemic legs was 40 (± 5 mm Hg), and the systemic value was 32 (± 3 mm Hg) before restoration of flow. Although the venous pH was lower in all four ischemic legs compared to systemic values, 5 minutes after reperfusion the pH fell further to an average value of 7.07 (± 0.13). Potassium levels were normal and similar in both the ischemic leg and the systemic circulation before reperfusion. However, 5 minutes after reperfusion there was a marked increase in the venous potassium of the ischemic leg (6.2 and 6.6 mEq in two patients whose duration of occlusion exceeded 100 hours). Systemic venous CPK concentrations were elevated in all four patients before reperfusion (average, 26 U). The venous CPK in the ischemic legs was more remarkable (average 190 U). Five minutes after restoration of flow the CPK of the ischemic leg rose to an average of 456 U.

We have measured the degree and duration of hyperkalemia and acidosis following reperfusion of profoundly ischemic limbs. The magnitude of metabolic abnormalities was similar to that previously reported; however, the hyperkalemia and acidosis persisted well beyond the 15-minute period of monitoring. Clearly the biochemical effects of an acute arterial occlusion can be profound, and the release of these products into the systemic circulation with reperfusion can itself be life-threatening to a patient. A sudden drop in the pH or an elevation of potassium may lead to myocardial arrhythmias, and these metabolic abnormalities can persist for a prolonged period after revascularization.

CLINICAL MANIFESTATION

The classic presentation of acute arterial occlusion is described by the six "*p*'s": pain, pallor, paresthesias, pulselessness, paralysis, and polar (cold) sensation.

History

The patient frequently complains of a sudden onset of pain, coldness, and paresthesias distal to the site of occlusion. Occasionally he will be able to remember the precise instant the pain occurred. In such cases embolic arterial occlusion at a major bifurcation has occurred. As the peripheral nerves become affected by the ischemic process, paresthesias and then numbness develop. Finally, with severe late occlusion paralysis occurs.

Physical examination

Signs of ischemia generally are seen one joint distal to the level of arterial occlusion. A superficial femoral artery occlusion, for example, will generally cause ischemia distal to the knee joint. If examined within the first 8 hours of acute occlusion, the involved extremity will often be pale (pallor), which is due to the acute spastic reaction of the distal arterial tree following acute occlusion. After 12 to 24 hours the extremity may become cyanotic and mottled with intermittent patches of pallor. Spasm resolves with dilation of the involved arteries. Because of the profound stasis, prograde thrombosis is likely to continue, further jeopardizing the limb.

The acutely ischemic limb may appear withered and "doughy" to the touch. Palpable pulses are absent distal to the occlusion. A Doppler device is useful in verifying any pulsatile velocity signals within the distal arterial tree. The extremity is generally cold, and as one examines the more proximal limb, an area of temperature demarcation can be appreciated.

As the peripheral nerves suffer the consequences of ischemia, loss of light-touch sensation and/or position sense occurs. With more prolonged and severe ischemia the position sense becomes abolished, with loss of sensation to pinpricks and ultimately weakness and paralysis. Once paralysis occurs, the prognosis is poor, and irreversible ischemia is imminent if reperfusion is delayed. If ischemia progresses, the muscles become painful and firm and subsequently rigid. If all of these signs are present, the likelihood that revascularization and limb salvage are possible is exceedingly small; if they are attempted, the patient's life may be placed in jeopardy because of the severe metabolic derangement following revascularization.

The Ad Hoc Committee on Reporting Standards of the Society for Vascular Surgery and the North American Chapter of the International Society for Cardiovascular Surgery have suggested guidelines for identifying and reporting patients with acute ischemia.[27] The following categories of acute diffuse limb ischemia have been recommended (Table 12-2).

1. *Viable: extremity not immediately threatened.* The patient does not complain of ischemic rest pain, there is no neurologic deficit, and the skin capillary circulation appears adequate. On examination there are clearly audible Doppler pulsatile flow signals in the pedal arteries, with ankle pressures above 30 mm Hg.

Table 12-2. Clinical categories of acute limb ischemia

Category	Description	Capillary return	Muscle weakness	Sensory loss	Doppler signals: Arterial	Doppler signals: Venous
Viable	Not immediately threatened	Intact	None	None	Audible (AP >30 mm Hg)	Audible
Threatened	Salvageable if promptly treated	Intact	Mild, partial	Mild, incomplete	Inaudible	Audible
Irreversible	Major tissue amputation regardless of treatment	Absent (marbling)	Profound, paralysis (rigor)	Profound anesthetic	Inaudible	Inaudible

(From Ad Hoc Committee on Reporting Standards; J Vasc Surg 4:80, 1986.)

2. *Threatened viability: implies reversible ischemia and a foot that is salvageable without major amputation if the arterial obstruction is promptly relieved.* These patients complain of ischemic rest pain and have mild or incomplete neurologic defects (sensory loss involving vibration, light touch, position, or weakness of toes or foot on dorsiflexion). Audible arterial Doppler signals are not present in pedal arteries; however venous signals, especially with augmentation maneuvers, are demonstrable.
3. *Major, irreversible ischemic change: frequently requires major amputation of limb.* Findings include profound sensory loss and muscle paralysis, absent capillary skin blood flow, or evidence of more advanced ischemia such as muscle rigor or skin marbling. Neither arterial nor venous Doppler flow signals are audible.

DIAGNOSTIC STUDIES

In general, patients presenting with acute arterial ischemia undergo the routine blood studies evaluating renal and electrolyte status, blood cell count, cardiac enzymes, and blood gas determinations. An electrocardiogram and chest x-ray examination are also part of the routine evaluation. A rapid Doppler survey of the involved extremity and contralateral extremity is performed, and segmental pressures and pulse waveforms, if rapidly performed, lend additional objective evidence about the severity of ischemia and may be of some predictive value as well as serving as the patient's baseline.

Angiography

The use of angiography is not always advocated. When the site of an acute occlusion is clinically apparent and is surgically accessible and the cause is obviously embolic with the limb severely ischemic, no further diagnostic studies other than those that can be done at the bedside are indicated, and a surgical embolectomy is warranted. It might be judged that no additional information of therapeutic importance will likely be obtained from an angiogram. Additionally, the fear of delaying a needed embolectomy becomes real if angiography facilities or personnel are not readily available. Most patients, however, do not have a clear-cut presentation, and we generally recommend complete angiography (Fig. 12-1).

Our preference for preoperative angiography is based on its track record of safety, its ready availability, and its usefulness in helping to establish the diagnosis and in planning the surgical procedure. In recent years angiography has become important in evaluating and preparing the patient for percutaneous intraarterial thrombolytic therapy, which has evolved as an important therapeutic adjunct in many of these patients.[28]

In addition to helping differentiate embolic occlusion from thrombotic occlusion, the angiogram can identify instances of multiple-vessel occlusions, which often indicate an underlying embolic process. Angiography localizes the occlusive process, which in some cases can be atypical, especially in patients with extensive atherosclerosis, and offers important information about patent distal vessels should a bypass be required. Additionally, unusual causes of acute ischemia such as giant cell arteritis, dissecting aneurysms, and low-flow states can be appropriately identified.

MANAGEMENT

The most appropriate management of patients with acute arterial occlusion can be offered if the underlying cause (thrombosis vs embolus) is delineated.[4,12,29-33]

On presentation the patient is given a bolus of heparin, followed by a heparin infusion to maintain therapeutic anticoagulation. Data suggest that higher doses of heparin (2000 to 4000 U/hr) are more effective than standard doses without increasing the risk of bleeding complications.[34]

Providing rapid anticoagulation therapy is important to interrupt prograde and retrograde thrombosis, and it is also important to minimize the risk of additional embolic episodes; therefore our suggested bolus dose is 5000 to 20,000 U, depending on the degree of ischemia, the timing of arteriography, along with other patient care considerations.

The introduction of the Fogarty catheter[35] ushered in the modern era of vascular surgery and gave surgeons an im-

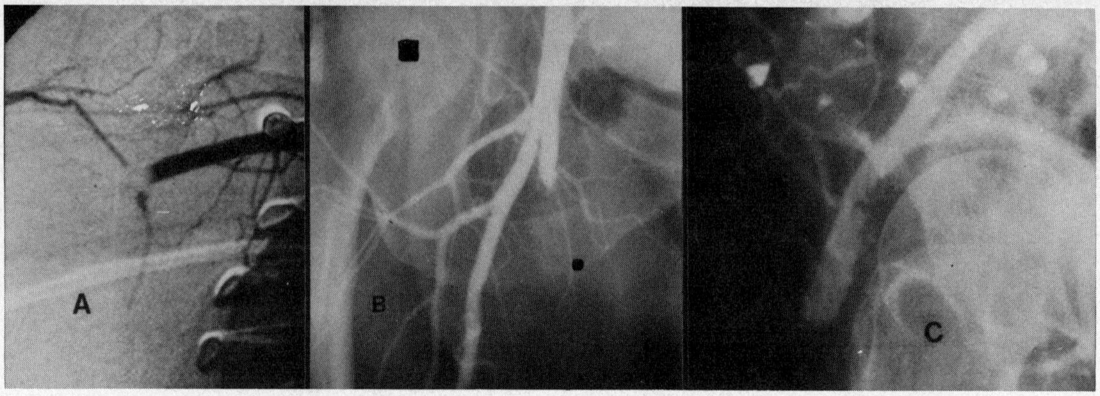

Fig. 12-1. Angiographic demonstration of three different types of acute arterial occlusion. **A,** Acute embolic occlusion of the axillary artery (note classical meniscus sign). **B,** Acute thrombotic occlusion of the superficial femoral artery. **C,** Acute iatrogenic occlusion of right common femoral artery caused by production of an atherosclerotic intimal flap during cardiac catheterization.

portant new technique for arterial thromboembolectomy. Seldom has a technical advance improved the surgical results of a procedure as has the Fogarty catheter. Good to excellent results increased by 75%, fair results decreased by 66%, and the death and amputation rates fell by 35% to 50%.[29,35-38]

EMBOLIC OCCLUSION

Compared to the experience with a single-extremity embolus, surgical treatment of carotid and visceral emboli continues to be poor.[29] The results in patients with simultaneous multiple emboli continue to carry an unfavorable prognosis, resulting in a 60% to 100% mortality rate.

As stated previously, although the differentiation between embolic occlusion and thrombotic occlusion may be difficult, it remains important because of the short- and long-term therapeutic implications. Early opinions stated that it was easy to differentiate embolic vs thrombotic occlusion since years ago acute embolic occlusion mainly occurred in patients with rheumatic heart disease. These patients were generally younger with much less associated vascular disease; therefore the acute occlusion of peripheral vessels was dramatic and instantly recognized, and treatment was instituted with frequent confirmation of the diagnosis. During the last two decades atherosclerotic heart disease occurring in an older population has become a more common source of embolism than rheumatic heart disease. Therefore the current principle source of emboli, atherosclerotic heart disease, occurs in patients likely to have existing peripheral vascular disease. Likewise, because of the increasing age of the U.S. population, patients requiring intervention for thrombotic arterial occlusion frequently have associated heart disease, contributing further to the dilemma of accurately differentiating between embolic and thrombotic occlusion.

In general terms, patients with an acute embolic occlusion have a higher mortality rate, reflecting the severity of their underlying cardiac condition. On the other hand, patients with an acute thrombotic occlusion have a higher limb-loss rate, indicative of the more severe underlying vascular disease and the inability to restore perfusion adequately with simple thrombectomy techniques. The mortality rate associated with acute arterial thrombosis apparently correlates with ongoing peripheral arterial ischemia and progression to gangrene.[1,4,10,11]

Jivegard, Holm, and Schersten[12] clearly demonstrated that surgical thrombectomy without definitive reconstruction for acute arterial thrombosis was associated with unacceptably high morbidity and mortality rates. These observations are supported by Field, Littoy, and Baker[30] who significantly improved limb salvage by performing a definitive reconstructive procedure at the time of initial exploration for acute limb ischemia after a thrombotic occlusion became evident. On the other hand, those patients having appropriate thromboembolectomy for acute embolic occlusion have significantly lower limb loss and their mortality rate, as mentioned, is directly related to their underlying cardiac disease.

Thus attention to the underlying cardiac disease is critical. There is stratification of cardiac mortality, however, within the group of patients suffering embolic occlusion. Patients with emboli resulting from acute myocardial infarction have a 40% mortality rate compared to a 9% mortality rate in those suffering emboli from atrial fibrillation not associated with acute myocardial infarction.[11]

After the expedient patient evaluation previously mentioned has been performed, the patient is prepared for angiography. Unless there is clear-cut evidence of a large-vessel acute embolic occlusion that is surgically accessible, angiography is routinely performed before intervention. The urgency of intervention is based on the severity and extent

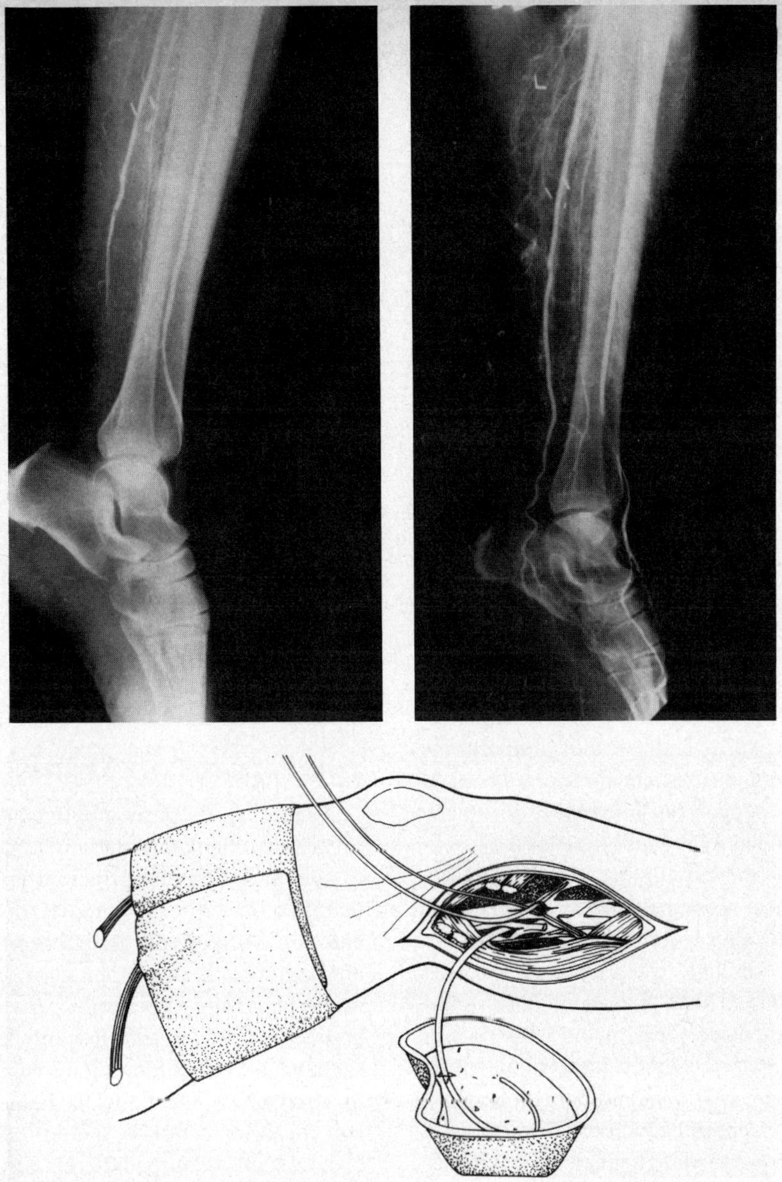

A

C

B

Fig. 12-2. Description of the intraoperative high-dose, isolated limb perfusion of urokinase for the treatment of multivessel distal acute arterial occlusion. This patient underwent an emergency coronary artery bypass and required the use of an intraaortic balloon for hemodynamic stabilization. Three days postoperatively the intraaortic balloon was percutaneously removed. Shortly thereafter the patient lost her previously palpable posterior tibial pulse, then lost her dorsalis pedis pulse, and finally lost her popliteal pulse. Her leg was profoundly ischemic. The patient was taken to the operating room where exposure of the distal popliteal artery and trifurcation was performed. Inflow to the popliteal artery was easily achieved. Direct thrombectomy of the anterior tibial, posterior tibial, and peroneal arteries was performed. After complete balloon catheter thrombectomy was performed, an intraoperative completion arteriogram was obtained. **A,** No contrast reached the foot despite direct injection into the anterior and posterior tibial arteries. Thinking that this condition would necessitate a major amputation, an isolated limb perfusion of high-dose urokinase was performed. The limb was raised, venous blood was exsanguinated with the use of an Esmarch bandage, and a thigh blood pressure cuff was applied and inflated to 300 mm Hg pressure. The popliteal vein was isolated and a venotomy performed, with a red rubber catheter placed distally to allow drainage of the venous effluent. Through the small Silastic catheters in the anterior tibial and posterior tibial arteries, 1,000,000 U of urokinase dissolved in 1000 L of saline solution were infused (500,000 U each through the anterior tibial and posterior tibial arteries). **B,** After the urokinase was infused, the limb was flushed with heparinized saline solution. The venotomy was closed primarily and the arteriotomy closed with a small PTFE patch. **C,** An intraoperative completion arteriogram was again obtained, demonstrating flow into the foot through both the anterior and posterior tibial arteries. The patient had a palpable dorsalis pedis pulse, and the foot was pink and warm at the completion of the procedure.

of ischemia. Most femoral emboli can be approached through an inguinal incision, exposing the common femoral, profunda, and superficial femoral arteries. Fogarty catheter embolectomy of these vessels remains the procedure of choice in most patients. A completion arteriogram is routinely performed to evaluate the distal vessels for occlusion and residual thrombus. If the popliteal artery and its terminal branches are involved, performing a complete embolectomy is difficult if not impossible through a femoral approach.[39] In such instances exposure of the popliteal artery and embolectomy of the popliteal trifurcation is suggested. This approach has resulted in improved limb salvage rates compared to the inadequate results obtained with a femoral exposure.

When failure of revascularization occurs after occurrence of an acute arterial embolus, it is usually due to distal small-vessel occlusion that defies removal by the Fogarty catheter. Additionally, Spencer and Eisman[40] noted extensive side-branch propagation of the clot occurring in patients having embolectomy more than 10 hours after the acute occlusion. Additionally, the presence of a residual clot after thromboembolectomy is common.[41] In such instances we have found the intraoperative, intraarterial infusion of thrombolytic agents highly beneficial in regaining patency of side branches and in clearing the distal circulation following performance of mechanical thrombectomy.[42] Our current recommendation is to infuse up to 250,000 U of urokinase over 30 minutes either through a continuous infusion through a distal arteriotomy or with a repeated bolus technique over the same time period. This method has proven safe in that we have not noted significant systemic fibrinolysis nor have we noted major bleeding complications.

In some instances the extent of distal thrombosis may be so extensive that it is not amenable to a single- or multiple-bolus technique, or the patient may have multivessel involvement and an absolute contraindication to any risk from systemic fibrinolysis. In these instances we have found performing isolated limb perfusion with high-dose urokinase (1,000,000 U) is effective (Fig. 12-2). Since regional drainage of the venous effluent is part of this technique, there is no danger of any degree of systemic fibrinolysis. This technique is particularly effective in patients suffering distal arterial occlusion with propagation of thrombus, which requires higher doses and more prolonged exposure to the lytic agent than can be obtained with a single or double bolus.

Numerous factors are used to differentiate between embolic and thrombotic occlusions (see Table 12-1). Cambria and Abbott[10] stated that atrial fibrillation was the only sign of discriminating value to differentiate acute embolic from thrombotic occlusion. Limb salvage clearly depends on the severity of ischemia. In Cambria's series 11% of patients with moderate ischemia lost their limb compared to 40% with severe ischemia.

Judgment must be shown when the profoundly ischemic limb is revascularized. Gregg and colleagues[11] reported that patients with embolic occlusion who had "recoverable" ischemia had a 90% limb-salvage rate and a mortality rate of 16% after embolectomy. On the other hand, those patients with rigidity of their involved muscles, indicating irreversible ischemia, uniformly lost their limbs and had an exceptionally high (73%) mortality rate. Therefore there are instances when primary amputation is justified. These instances occur in patients with profound ischemia in whom revascularization carries an exceptionally high risk to life and in those who are bedridden and unlikely to walk again.

Following restoration of perfusion to the ischemic limb after embolic occlusion, long-term anticoagulation therapy is critical unless the source of the embolus (e.g., proximal aneurysm) has been removed. The benefits of long-term anticoagulation therapy have been shown by Elliott et al[29] and Silvers, Royster, and Mulcare.[43] Permanent anticoagulation therapy has been associated with substantially lower mortality and recurrence rates (Fig. 12-3).

THROMBOTIC OCCLUSION

Patients initially seen with acute arterial thrombosis are given anticoagulation therapy as previously described. The important underlying principle in treating these patients is that they must have a definitive revascularization procedure and not just a simple thrombectomy. Therefore the use of arteriography is important in all these patients to identify properly the site of occlusion, the involved vessels, and the proper outflow vessels. Revascularization with autogenous saphenous vein is our preferred surgical approach in the majority of these patients. In some, however, if a localized lesion can be identified and corrected, a less extensive procedure such as an endarterectomy can be performed with excellent long-term results (Fig. 12-4).

During the past decade intraarterial infusion of thrombolytic agents has offered an important alternative therapeutic approach that has obvious advantages for many patients.[28] The concept is that segmental atherosclerotic disease, when severe enough, will precipitate thrombosis involving substantially longer segments of the arterial tree. Lysis of the thrombus with subsequent identification of the underlying atherosclerotic disease allows a more directed correction, either with percutaneous balloon dilation, atherectomy techniques, endarterectomy, or a much more limited bypass. Guidewire passage is attempted through the occluded arteries at the time of the initial arteriogram in all patients judged candidates for lytic therapy. If the guidewire passes, the likelihood of lysis is high (approximately 90% in our experience), and the patient is then prepared for the direct intrathrombus infusion of urokinase. We generally follow the technique established by McNamara and Fischer[44]; however, we have more recently been infusing higher doses (6000 U/min) and lacing the thrombus with

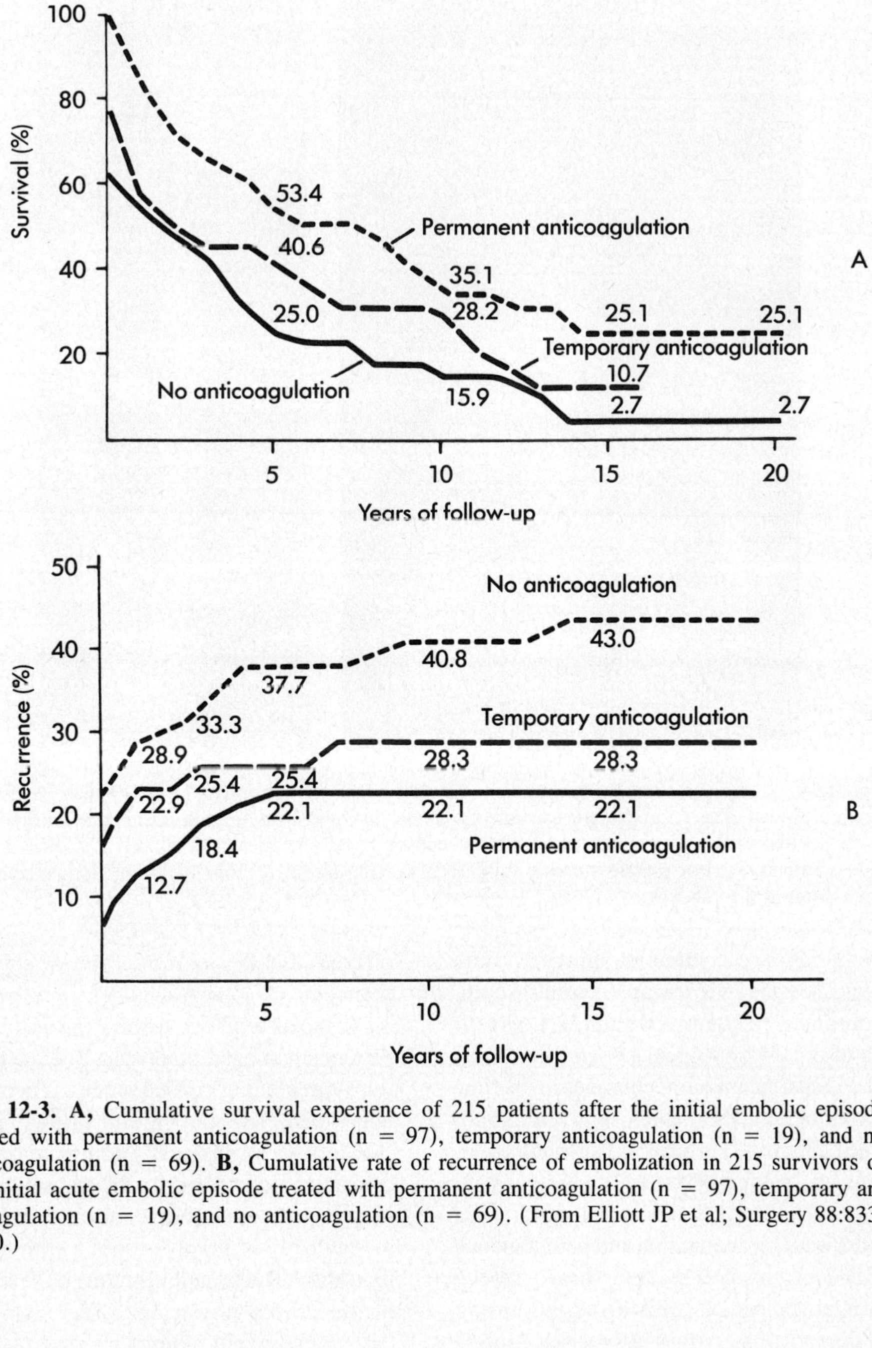

Fig. 12-3. A, Cumulative survival experience of 215 patients after the initial embolic episode treated with permanent anticoagulation (n = 97), temporary anticoagulation (n = 19), and no anticoagulation (n = 69). **B,** Cumulative rate of recurrence of embolization in 215 survivors of an initial acute embolic episode treated with permanent anticoagulation (n = 97), temporary anticoagulation (n = 19), and no anticoagulation (n = 69). (From Elliott JP et al; Surgery 88:833, 1980.)

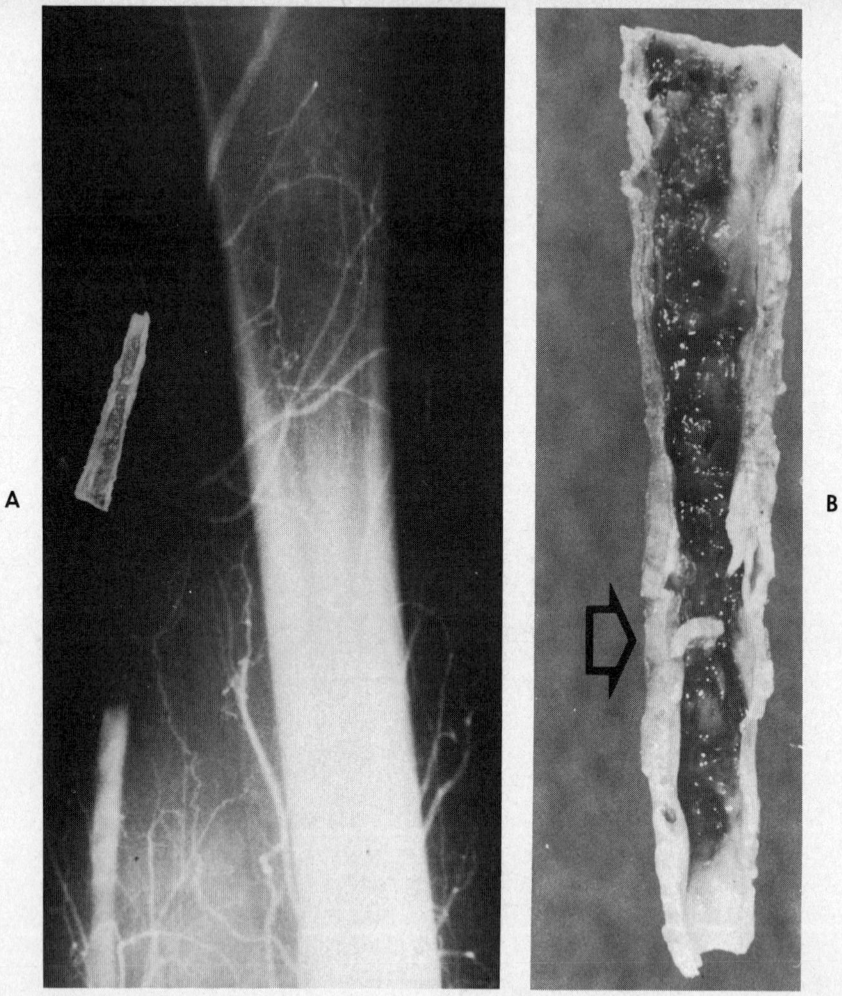

Fig. 12-4. A, Lower-extremity angiogram showing occlusion (thrombosis) of patient's superficial femoral artery. The focal plaque causing the acute thrombosis is juxtaposed to the arteriogram, showing that long-segment occlusion can be caused by short, focal lesions. **B,** Close-up of the excised atherosclerotic plaque showing small focal defect *(arrow)* responsible for the longer segment acute arterial thrombosis.

urokinase before beginning the continuous infusion. With this method of patient selection lytic therapy is usually completed within 24 hours and frequently within 12 hours. If definitive correction of the underlying atherosclerotic lesion is not accomplished with percutaneous techniques at the time of the completion arteriogram, the patient is given anticoagulation therapy until definitive surgical repair is achieved.

Fig. 12-5 provides an example of treating a patient with a 5-day thrombotic occlusion of his superficial femoral artery. This patient underwent recanalization and percutaneous balloon dilation in 1982. At his most recent follow-up office visit nearly 9 years later, he has palpable distal pulses and an ankle-brachial index of 0.95. Proper patient selection is critical for successful lytic therapy, and the guidewire test has been most helpful in this regard. If the guidewire cannot be passed through the occluded vessel, lytic therapy is not offered, and the most appropriate surgical reconstruction is planned.

Acute arterial occlusion is a vascular emergency in many patients; however, others can tolerate such occlusion without limb-threatening consequences. The physician who can obtain a complete and careful history, is aware of the subtle (and obvious) physical findings as well as their evolution, can accurately identify the cause, and can put into perspective the spectrum of therapeutic options will salvage the majority of involved limbs with the least morbidity and mortality. These patients require the interdisciplinary efforts of a team of physicians. The cooperative efforts of the vascular surgeon, radiologist, and cardiologist are important in the successful therapy of these patients. As new technology is developed, such interdisciplinary approaches will become even more important.

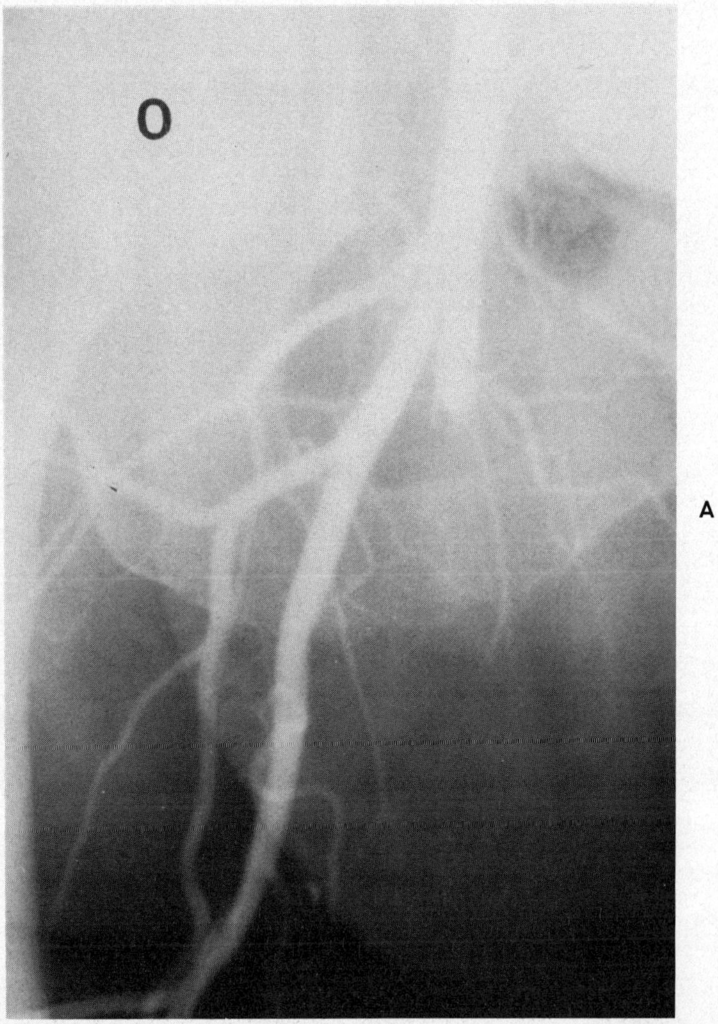

Fig. 12-5. Demonstration of the use of intraarterial delivery of thrombolytic therapy to dissolve the occluding thrombus and to identify and correct an underlying lesion. **A,** Arteriogram demonstrating acutely thrombosed superficial femoral artery in a letter carrier who complained of intolerable intermittent claudication.

Continued.

B

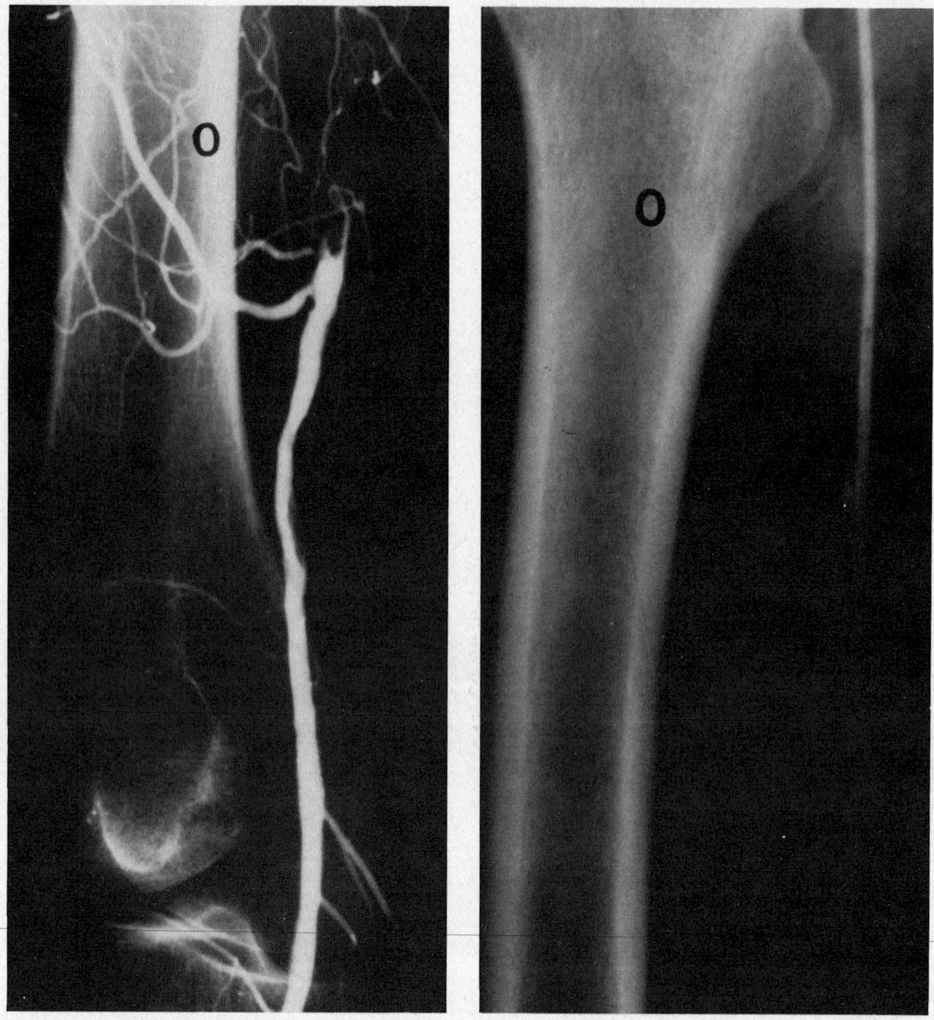

C

Fig. 12-5, cont'd. B, A patent popliteal artery; distal runoff was provided by all three intrapopliteal vessels. **C,** Infusion catheter threaded from the contralateral femoral artery and imbedded 6 to 8 inches into the occluding thrombus. Following infusion of the fibrinolytic agent, the thrombus was lysed and a stenosis demonstrated at the proximal superficial femoral artery. **D,** The stenosis *(arrow)* was dilated with good results. **E,** Two additional stenotic lesions *(arrows)* in the distal superficial femoral artery were likewise dilated with good results. **F,** Patient's initial pulse waveforms and ankle indexes on presentation and after therapy. Eight years after treatment the patient continues to have palpable distal pulses, nearly normal pulsewave forms, and an ankle index of 0.95.

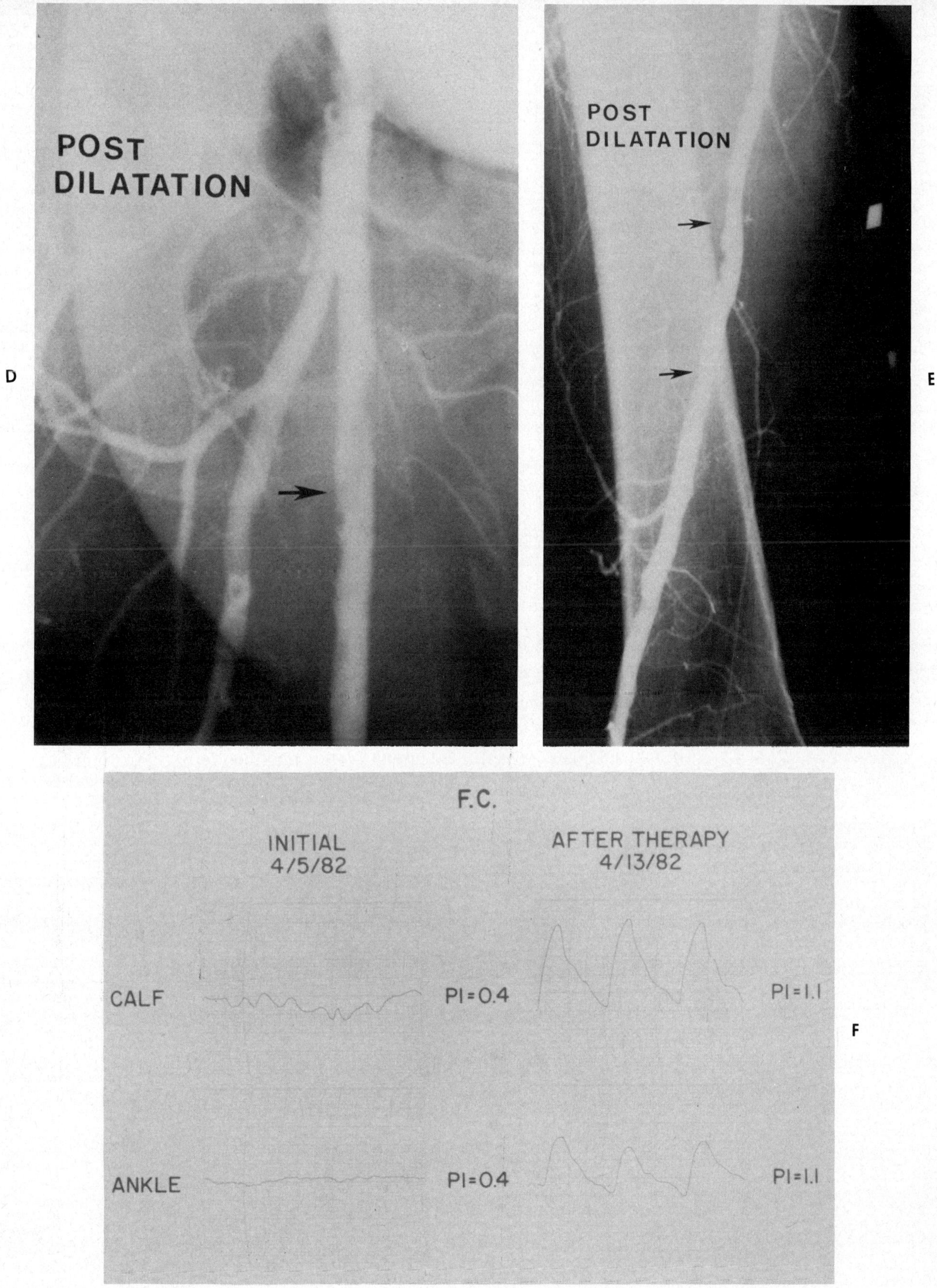

Fig. 12-5, cont'd. For legend see opposite page.

REFERENCES

1. Abbott WM et al: Arterial embolism: a 44 year perspective, Am J Surg 143:460-164, 1982.
2. Conett MC, Murray DA, and Wenneker WW: Peripheral arterial emboli, Am J Surg 148:14, 1984.
3. Cranley JJ et al: Peripheral arterial embolism: changing concepts, Surgery 55:57, 1964.
4. Dale WA: Differential management of the acutely ischemic leg, Trans South Surg 84:259, 1972.
5. Darling RC, Austen WG, and Linton RR: Arterial embolis, Surg Gynecol Obstet 124:106, 1967.
6. Balas P et al: Occlusion of the extremities, J Cardiovasc Surg 26:262, 1985.
7. Meister SG et al: Paradoxical embolism. Diagnosis during life, Am J Med 53:292, 1972.
8. Williams GM et al: Mural thrombus of the aorta, Ann Surg 194:737, 1981.
9. Wychulis AR, Spittell JA, and Wallace RB: Popliteal aneurysms, Surgery 68:942, 1970.
10. Cambria RP and Abbott WM: Acute arterial thrombosis of the lower extremity, Arch Surg 119:784, 1984.
11. Gregg RO et al: Embolectomy or heparin therapy for arterial emboli? Surgery 93:377, 1983.
12. Jivegard L, Holm J, and Schersten T: The outcome in arterial thrombosis misdiagnosed as arterial embolism, Acta Chir Scand 152:251, 1986.
13. Stallone RJ et al: Analysis of morbidity and mortality from arterial embolectomy, Surgery 65:207, 1969.
14. Malan E and Tattori Q: Physio and anatomo-pathology of acute ischemia of the extremities, J Cardiovasc Surg 4:212, 1963.
15. Blebea J et al: Technetium 99m pyrophosphate quantitation of skeletal muscle ischemia and reperfusion injury, J Vasc Surg 8:117, 1988.
16. Ricci MA et al: Are free radical scavengers beneficial in the treatment of compartment syndrome after acute arterial ischemia? J Vasc Surg 9:244, 1989.
17. Leaf A: Cell swelling: a factor in ischemic tissue injury, Circulation 47:455, 1973.
18. Summers WK and Jamison RL: The no reflow phenomenon in renal ischemia, Lab Invest 25:635, 1971.
19. Dunant JH and Edwards WS: Small vessel occlusion in the extremity after various periods of arterial obstruction: an experimental study, Surgery 73:240, 1973.
20. Belkin M, Valeri CR, and Hobson RW: Intra-arterial urokinase increases skeletal muscle viability after acute ischemia, J Vasc Surg 9:161, 1989.
21. Haimovici H: Arterial embolism with acute massive ischemic myopathy and myoglobinuria, Surgery 47:739, 1960.
22. Haimovici H: Muscular, renal and metabolic complications of acute arterial occlusions. Myonephropathic-metabolic syndrome, Surgery 85:461, 1979.
23. Haimovici H: Myopathic-nephrotic-metabolic syndrome associated with massive arterial occlusion, J Cardiovasc Surg 14:589, 1973.
24. Lim LT et al: Popliteal artery trauma, Arch Surg 115:1307, 1980.
25. Beyersdorf F et al: Avoiding reperfusion injury after limb revascularization: experimental observations and recommendations for clinical application, J Vasc Surg 9:757, 1989.
26. Fisher RD, Fogarty TJ, and Morrow AG: Clinical and biochemical observation of the effect of transient femoral artery occlusion in man, Surgery 68:323, 1970.
27. Ad Hoc Committee on Reporting Standards, SVS/NAISCVS: Suggested standards for reports dealing with lower extremity ischemia, J Vasc Surg 4:80, 1986.
28. Comerota AJ: Intra-arterial thrombolytic therapy. In Comerota AJ, ed: Thrombolytic therapy, Orlando, Fla, 1988, Grune & Stratton, Inc.
29. Elliott JP et al: Arterial embolization: problems of source, multiplicity, recurrence and delayed treatment, Surgery 88:833, 1980.
30. Field T, Littoy FN, and Baker WH: Immediate and long-term outcome of acute arterial occlusion of the extremities. The effect of added vascular reconstruction, Arch Surg 117:1156, 1982.
31. Hight DW, Tilney NL, and Couch NP: Changing clinical trends in patients with peripheral arterial emboli, Surgery 79:172, 1976.
32. McPhail NV et al: The management of acute thromboembolic limb ischemia, Surgery 93:381, 1983.
33. Murray DWG: Embolism in peripheral arteries, Can Med Assoc J 35:61, 1936.
34. Blaisdell FW, Steele M, and Allen RE: Management of acute lower extremity ischemia due to embolism and thrombosis, Surgery 84:822, 1978.
35. Fogarty TJ et al: A method for extraction of arterial emboli and thrombi, Surg Gynecol Obstet 116:241, 1963.
36. Cranley JJ et al: Catheter technique for arterial embolectomy: a seven-year experience, J Cardiovasc Surg 5:44, 1969.
37. Green RM, DeWeese JA, and Rob CG: Arterial embolectomy before and after the fogarty catheter, Surgery 77:24, 1975.
38. Thompson JE et al: Arterial embolectomy. A 20 year experience, Surgery 67:212, 1970.
39. Short D et al: The anatomic basis for the occasional failure of transfemoral balloon catheter thromboembolectomy, Ann Surg 190:555, 1979.
40. Spencer RC and Eisman B: Delayed arterial embolectomy. A new concept, Surgery 55:64, 1964.
41. Greep JM et al: A combined technique of peripheral arterial embolectomy, Arch Surg 105:869, 1972.
42. Comerota AJ, White JV, and Grosh JD: Intraoperative, intra-arterial thrombolytic therapy for salvage of limbs in patients with distal arterial thrombosis, Surg Gynecol Obstet 169:283, 1989.
43. Silvers LW, Royster TS, and Mulcare JR: Peripheral arterial emboli and factors in their recurrence rate, Ann Surg 192:232, 1980.
44. McNamara TO and Fischer JR: Thrombolysis of peripheral arterial and graft occlusions: improved results using high dose urokinase, AJR 144:769, 1985.

Chapter 13

EXTRACRANIAL CEREBROVASCULAR ARTERIAL DISEASE

D. Eugene Strandness, Jr.

The recognition that disease of the extracranial arterial system could be a cause of cerebral symptoms such as transient ischemic attacks (TIAs) and strokes is a relatively recent event. Although Hunt[1] discussed the relationship between carotid disease and stroke in 1914, it was not until 1951 that Fisher[2] clearly and unequivocally demonstrated that disease of the carotid artery was responsible for many of the ischemic syndromes involving the anterior circulation. These early studies were complemented by the delineation of the vertebrobasilar circulation and its problems by Millikan and Siekert[3] in 1955. Knowledge about this area of the circulation has been greatly enhanced by the availability of noninvasive tests, not only to detect the presence of disease but to follow its progress over time.

When reviewing the problems that can involve the extracranial arteries and secondarily the cerebral tissue they supply, several difficulties are encountered: (1) the diseases may involve multiple sites that include the vessels within the skull as well[4]; (2) stenoses and even occlusions are known to occur without producing symptoms or signs[5]; (3) data collected during life are often incomplete in defining the extent of involvement[6]; (4) occlusion of an intracranial artery may produce a clinical picture identical to that which occurs secondary to involvement of an extracranial artery; (5) the circle of Willis is very difficult to assess, and this difficulty may be a key factor in determining the effects of an occlusive event on outcome[6]; (6) ischemia of a particular area of the brain does not necessarily signify which vessel is responsible for the event; and (7) there are few data on the natural history of the diseases affecting the extracranial arterial circulation.

Before considering the diseases that affect the extracranial arteries, it is important to review briefly the pertinent anatomy because it can have a significant impact on the clinical presentation.

ANATOMY OF THE EXTRACRANIAL CIRCULATION

The arteries that arise from the aortic arch to supply the brain have a relatively constant configuration. In 80% of the population the three major trunks—the innominate, left common carotid, and left subclavian—have a constant configuration.[7] The more common anomalies are as follows: (1) in 16% of the population there will be a very close association between the innominate and left common carotid arteries; (2) in 8% the left common carotid artery will directly arise from the innominate artery; (3) in 6% the left vertebral artery will originate directly from the aortic arch; and (4) in approximately 1% the right subclavian artery will originate directly from the aortic arch.

The major vessels to the brain follow a relatively straight course. The carotid artery will bifurcate at approximately the level of the thyroid cartilage, providing branches for the face through the external carotid artery and for the brain through the internal carotid artery. At the level of this bifurcation the carotid bulb, or sinus, is found. This dilation is found there and nowhere else in the circulation. As will be noted, the disease atherosclerosis is largely confined to this arterial segment, with the internal carotid artery beyond the bulb being spared. The internal carotid artery has no branches in the neck in contrast to the external carotid artery, which has many.

The vertebral arteries also generally follow a straight course in the neck as they course through the transverse foramina of the cervical vertebrae up to the point where they join together to form the basilar artery.

The two carotid arteries and the two vertebral arteries join at the base of the brain to form the circle of Willis, which is, in theory, the ideal anastomotic network of any organ in the body. Since it joins all four vessels together, one vessel alone could theoretically supply the entire brain. Although the circle exists to some degree in all brains, there is frequent variability in the size and potential of various components. Riggs and Rupp[8] in a study of 700 autopsy specimens found that segments were frequently incomplete. Although accurate figures are difficult to obtain, it is thought that up to 50% of the population may have one or more segments of the circle that are functionally and perhaps anatomically incomplete. It appears that the most frequent anomaly affects the posterior communicating arteries.

Potential collateral sources are available for providing normal or near-normal blood flow to an area of brain that may be deprived of its supply through the normal route. The circle not only provides protection anteriorly to posteriorly but also from side to side through the anterior communicating arteries. In addition, a common source of collateral input is through the external carotid artery, which can feed directly into the ophthalmic artery through its connections with the medial frontal and supraorbital arteries.

CEREBROVASCULAR INSUFFICIENCY

Symptoms occur whenever the blood flow is reduced below that level required to maintain neuronal function. One of the major difficulties in sorting out the causes of cerebrovascular insufficiency is that the site of flow reduction may be anywhere from the level of the aortic arch to the arterioles at the cortical level. The symptoms that occur do not come with a label as to the cause but can be helpful in suggesting a possible etiology. One of the best examples of this is amaurosis fugax, which, as is discussed later, occurs most frequently secondary to emboli that originate in the carotid bifurcation. It is important to distinguish between ischemia and infarction. Ischemia can be and often is transient, whereas infarction represents loss of actual cortex and, many times, the functions that are subserved by the involved segments.

In practical terms it is useful to attempt to classify the initial events as hemispheric or nonhemispheric. In present usage hemispheric symptoms most often are ascribed to problems that occur in the distribution of the carotid artery's territory. They include contralateral hemiparesis or monoparesis, contralateral hemimonoparesthesias or monoparesthesias, dysphasia, and ipsilateral monocular blindness. The differential diagnosis often includes hemiplegic or ophthalmoplegic migraine headache, focal convulsive events, position-related arm numbness or paresis, and a variety of central and peripheral neuropathies. The nonhemispheric symptoms often labeled as vertebrobasilar include dysarthria, dysphasia, global aphasia, diplopia, visual blurring, and brainstem ischemia, which includes drop attacks, vertigo, visual blurring, syncope, dizziness, and transient confusion. The nonhemispheric symptoms are the most difficult to sort and to relate to specific involvement of the extracranial arterial system.

The event must be classified in temporal terms to indicate the potential severity of the attack and to aid in planning the diagnostic workup and the therapeutic approaches. This classification includes describing the duration and symptom complex of the event and its degree of permanence. The term *transient ischemic attack* (TIA) is used to describe a neurologic deficit that is transient and reversible. Although the time interval that is used to describe such an event varies, it is usually in terms of minutes to hours at best. To fit this description properly, the patient must be neurologically normal after the event has subsided. It is also known that TIA when repetitive may be identical in character, suggesting that there is a repeatable mechanism that is resulting in the flow deficit. This is most evident with recurrent retinal ischemia (amaurosis fugax), which is typically described as a window shade being drawn down over the eye, causing transient monocular blindness.

Another term for ischemic involvement that is frequently used is *reversible ischemic neurologic deficit* (RIND). This event will last in excess of 24 hours, but like the TIA it does not result in any permanent deficits. If on the other hand the deficit does not resolve, a completed stroke has occurred, which signifies permanent damage to the involved area of cortex. In some cases only the passage of time will tell how much recovery, if any, occurs.

When an area of the brain is infarcted, several distinct changes can occur that may be relevant to the initial event and outcome as well. Those areas of infarction with hemorrhage are referred to as *hemorrhagic infarcts,* whereas those that do not have this as a component are referred to as *ischemic infarcts*. In recent years more attention has been paid to infarcts that occur in the deep penetrating arteries—so-called lacunar infarcts—and appear related to hypertension and not secondary to diseases of the extracranial arteries. It is very important to recognize these infarcts since the treatment of hypertension often prevents their recurrence.

MECHANISMS OF CEREBROVASCULAR ISCHEMIA

The major factors that may lead to ischemia include emboli, thrombosis, intracerebral hemorrhage, and subarachnoid hemorrhage. In addition, other events may lead to transient and permanent changes in the cortex, including a systemic drop in blood pressure and diversion of blood away from the cortex such as occurs in some of the steal syndromes. Some of the processes that may lead to acute and chronic ischemia are shown in the box on p. 243.

For all of the entities shown in the accompanying box, it is clear that, at least in the Western world, atherosclerosis is the most common cause of cerebral ischemia, accounting for more than 90% of the patients seen with this problem. How does atherosclerosis affect these vessels and what are the mechanisms responsible for the ischemic events?

Causes of acute and chronic cerebral ischemia

Atherosclerosis
Fibromuscular hyperplasia
Aneurysms (developmental, infectious, posttraumatic)
Arteriovenous malformations
Segmental lipohyalinosis
Arteritis (temporal arteritis, Takayasu's disease, collagen vascular disorders)
Vasospasm after subarachnoid hemorrhage
Moyamoya disease
Spontaneous dissection
Trauma
Anomalies (loops, kinks)
Cystic medial necrosis
Radiation arteritis

Atherosclerotic plaque

Atherosclerosis is a disease of branch points and bifurcations, and its distribution in the extracranial arteries is consistent with this premise. One of the more extensive arteriographic studies done to confirm the location of such lesions was that done by Hass et al[9] who reviewed the distribution of lesions in 3788 symptomatic patients who underwent four-vessel arteriography. As noted in Fig. 13-1, most lesions were located at branch points, areas in which the vessel was fixed, and curvatures. In 75% of the cases the lesions were accessible to some form of surgical intervention. However, intracranial lesions were noted in 40% of patients. The most common sites were the carotid siphon, the terminal portions of the vertebral artery, and the basilar artery (Fig. 13-2).

Disease involving an extracranial artery indicates that other areas of the arterial circulation are also often involved. In the Framingham study 70% of the patients who had an atherothrombotic stroke also had hypertension, 70% had coexisting cardiac disease, 30% had peripheral vascular disease, and approximately 15% had diabetes mellitus.[10] These results highlight the importance of considering atherosclerosis a systemic disease whose manifestations in other beds may be more important than that involving the extracranial arterial segments.

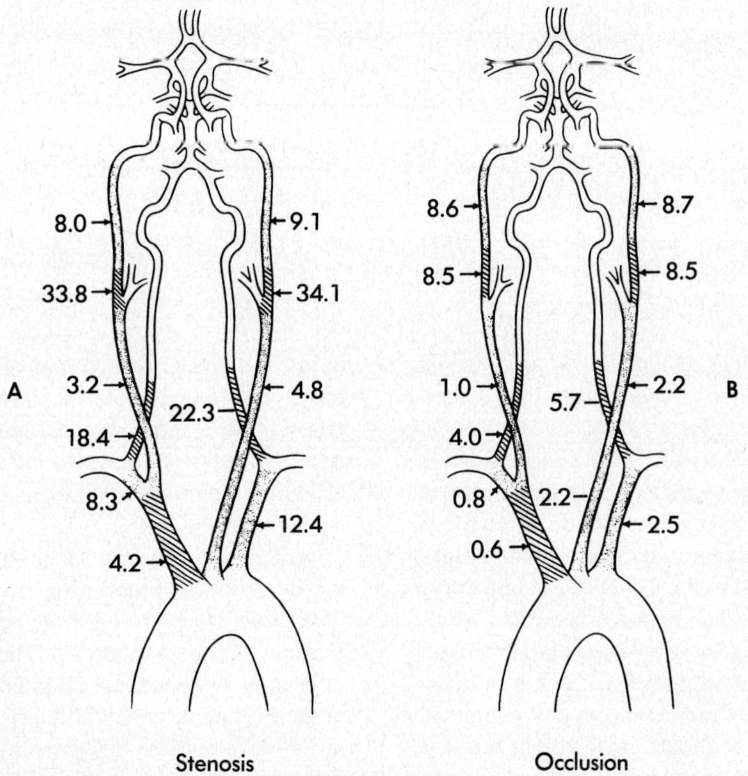

Fig. 13-1. Frequency of disease in stenoses, **A,** and occlusion, **B,** in the surgically accessible extracranial arteries. (From Hass WK et al: JAMA 203:961, 1968.)

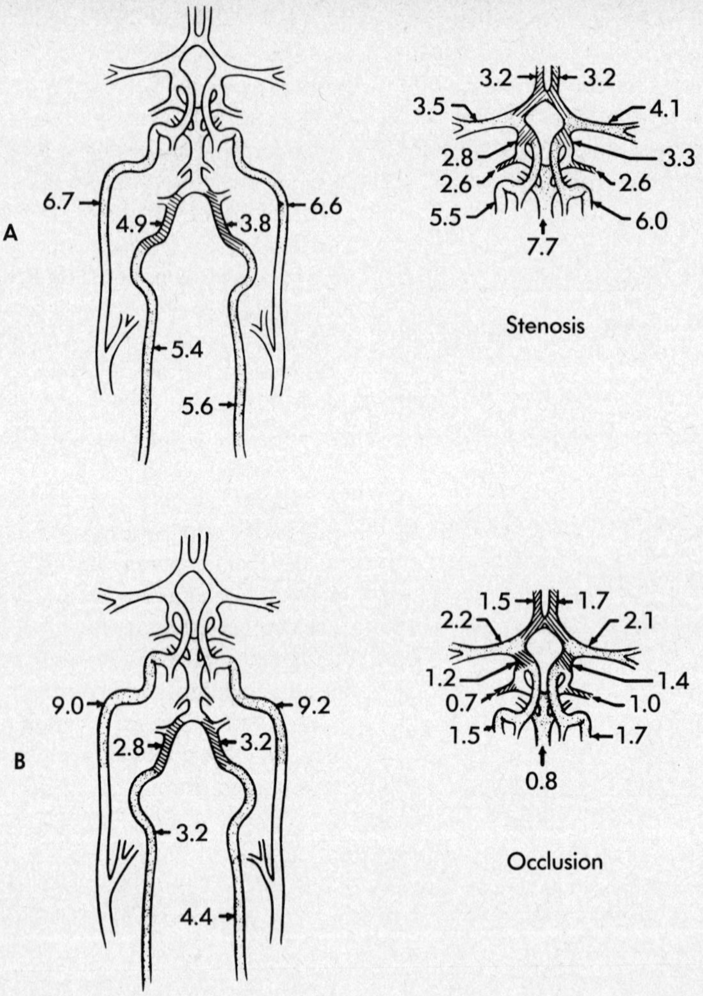

Fig. 13-2. Frequency of lesions by percentage in the intracranial arteries. **A,** Stenosis; **B,** occlusion. (From Hass WK et al: JAMA 203:961, 1968.)

How do atherosclerotic lesions cause problems? Two major mechanisms appear operative and provide the source of the problems seen clinically. The first and the most widely accepted theory is the embolic one, which suggests that the ulcerating lesion, by virtue of its exposure of the flowing blood to subendothelial collagen, is a frequent site for the accumulation of platelet thrombi that can at some point in time become embolic to the brain.[11-13] The second theory is that when a lesion narrows the artery by more than 50% in terms of diameter, the change may produce a fall in pressure and flow to the ipsilateral hemisphere and lead to symptoms. This theory has been nearly impossible to prove clinically because so many patients with very tight lesions and even in some cases total occlusions never become symptomatic. However, in recent years evidence has accumulated that some lesions—particularly the high-grade ones (>80% in terms of diameter reduction)—are prone to develop thrombosis, resulting in total occlusion of the internal carotid artery.[14] This sudden reduction in flow may lead to the development of an ischemic event, particularly if the circle of Willis is not adequate to maintain flow to the involved hemisphere.

Another mechanism for the production of symptoms is the diversion of blood away from the brain because of a high-grade stenosis and in some cases a total occlusion at the level of the aortic arch.[15] The most common example is of lesions of the subclavian artery in which reversal of flow in the ipsilateral vertebral artery may in some patients lead to the development of symptoms of vertebrobasilar insufficiency. As noted in Fig. 13-3, this occurrence is also possible if there are lesions of the innominate artery depriving blood not only to the basilar artery territory but to

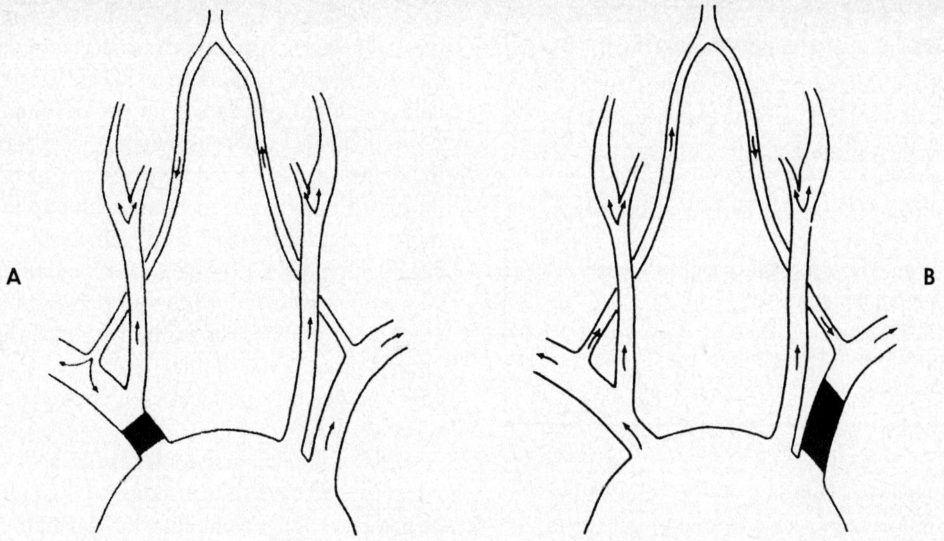

Fig. 13-3. A, Proximal occlusion of the innominate artery causes retrograde flow down the right vertebral artery to feed both the right subclavian and carotid arteries. **B,** Occlusion of the proximal subclavian artery on the left tends to reverse flow in the vertebral artery. (From Roederer GO et al: Cerebral arterial flow and cerebral vascular insufficiency. In Condon RE and DeCosse JJ, eds: Surgical care II, Philadelphia, 1985, Lea & Febiger.)

the anterior circulation as well. In addition, it is possible to have a situation in which the reverse flow component can involve the common carotid artery as well.

Fibromuscular dysplasia

Fibromuscular dysplasia was first described by Paulbinskas and Ripley[16] in 1964, with increasing numbers being reported in the literature. Osborne and Anderson[17] classified the lesions into three categories, according to their appearance on angiography.

The most common site of involvement is the mid- and distal cervical carotid artery, which rarely extends beyond the point of entry into the skull. When found, the disease is usually bilateral and may also involve the vertebral arteries. Interestingly, when this disease occurs, intracranial aneurysms are also noted in up to 50% of the patients. This disorder is confined to whites, with two thirds of those affected female. The disease is most commonly discovered at approximately age 50, but it has been recorded for every decade of life. Houser and Baker[18] in a review of 7500 arteriograms at the Mayo Clinic found 52 patients with this disorder. Only 10 of these patients had ischemic symptoms.

Embolic events

Although there is no doubt that the carotid arteries can be the source of emboli, several other entities may give rise to emboli to the brain. Some are listed in the box. As noted, in many instances it is necessary to consider causes for emboli other than ulceration of a carotid bifurcation plaque.

Cardiac causes of cerebral embolism

- Mural thrombi (cardiomyopathy, congestive heart failure, postmyocardial infarction)
- Rheumatic heart disease
- Chronic or paroxysmal atrial fibrillation
- Mitral valve prolapse
- Acute and subacute bacterial endocarditis
- Cardiac valve prostheses
- Others (atrial myxoma, congenital heart disease, marantic endocarditis)
- Pulmonary vein thrombi
- Fat
- Air
- Tumor metastases

This additional list of causes may greatly complicate and extend the workup in patients whose underlying cause for an ischemic event may not be at all clear.

Although this chapter focuses primarily on the role of extracranial arterial disease, two other phenomena that produce ischemia must always be kept in mind: intracranial hemorrhage and subarachnoid bleeding.

Intracranial hemorrhage. This most commonly occurs with uncontrolled hypertension.[19] When intracranial hemorrhage occurs, the actual disruption of the intracerebral arteries that occurs produces displacement, compression, and finally destruction of brain tissue, leading to the de-

Common causes of intracranial hemorrhage

Hypertension
Ruptured aneurysm
Ruptured arteriovenous malformation
Trauma
Hematologic disorders (leukemia, thrombocytopenia purpura)
Hemophilia, collagen disorders, anticoagulant therapy
Hemorrhage into a brain tumor
Hemorrhagic infarction
Septic embolism and mycotic aneurysm
Cerebral venous thrombosis

velopment of a space-occupying lesion that may, by compression of vital centers, lead to coma and death. In 90% of the cases there will be some communication with the ventricular system, giving rise to blood in the cerebrospinal fluid. When this occurs, the prognosis is not good, with 60% to 90% of the patients dying within 30 days. A summary of the various causes of intracranial hemorrhage is shown in the accompanying box.

Subarachnoid hemorrhage. In most cases the cause of subarachnoid bleeding is a ruptured berry aneurysm or, less frequently, rupture of an arteriovenous malformation.[20] These are developmental lesions that usually manifest themselves between the ages of 35 and 65 years. The clinical picture when they do become symptomatic is often dramatic and difficult to confuse with other entities. The diagnosis is made through the combination of a CT scan and arteriography.

STROKE RISK

Stroke-related deaths have declined in this country.[21] Although this decline apparently is a real phenomenon, it is not clear what factors are responsible. Some relate it to the aggressive treatment of hypertension, but although this is undoubtedly a factor, the decline preceded the active treatment of hypertension. The role of hypertension is clear from the Framingham data.[10] It is present in 70% of the patients who have a stroke. Men and women over the age of 50 show a fourfold to eightfold increase in the incidence of atherothrombotic stroke if they have had hypertension (defined as 160/95 mm Hg or greater). In addition, patients with high-grade lesions of their carotid bifurcation apparently have a higher systolic and diastolic blood pressure than do age- and sex-matched controls.[22] There is convincing evidence from the Veterans Administration Study that control of hypertension will reduce the incidence of stroke.[23] Other important factors are diabetes mellitus and cigarette smoking. In the type II diabetic the incidence of stroke is two times greater than that of age- and sex-matched controls. In addition, diabetics have eight times the incidence of high-grade lesions of the carotid bifurcation. Only recently has the connection between cigarette smoking and stroke became apparent. Cigarette smoking is now recognized as being a potent risk factor for the development of stroke.

Another fact that must never be forgotten is the very high incidence of associated involvement in other arterial beds. At least three of four patients with stroke will have one or more of the following findings of cardiac disease—electrocardiographic (ECG) changes, myocardial hypertrophy, or congestive heart failure[24]—further highlighting the importance of heart disease as the major cause of death in this patient group. Myocardial infarction is the most common cause of death in patients with stroke secondary to atherosclerosis.[25]

From a clinical standpoint the risk of subsequent stroke when carotid disease is discovered is of ultimate importance in patient management. For the asymptomatic patient who has carotid disease discovered and verified by duplex scanning, the risk of an ischemic event is very low (2% to 4%/yr). This is when all patients are considered without regard for the degree of involvement and the degree of stenosis. When patients are stratified by the degree of narrowing, the risk of an ischemic event increases dramatically when the very tight stenoses (>80% diameter reduction) are considered. In this group up to 48% will have an event, usually within the first 6 months after discovery of the lesion (mean interval, 4.9 months).[14] The events are TIAs, strokes, or total occlusion of the internal carotid artery. Although statements have been made that nearly all strokes are preceded by a warning TIA, this has not been our experience. In the two prospective series this author has conducted, the strokes that occurred were not preceded by a warning TIA.[14,26]

If one considers only the greater than 80% diameter-reducing stenoses that are not treated surgically, 19% of the patients had a TIA and 12% a completed stroke. The events occurred early, with 62% developing in the first 6 months and 85% within the first year after discovery of the lesion.

When a patient has as the first event a TIA, the historical controls would suggest that the risk of a subsequent stroke is not insignificant. The Committee on Health Care Issues of the American Neurological Association[27] addressed this issue and concluded that the stroke rate could be expected to be 5% per year in the first 3 years and 3% per year thereafter.

What of the patient who occludes his internal carotid artery but at the time of the event does not sustain a stroke? Data from Cote, Barnett, and Taylor[28] and Nicholls et al[29] suggest that the annual stroke rate is similar to that which occurs when a TIA is the presenting complaint. In the former study the annual incidence of strokes on the side of the occlusion was 5%. In our own study of 212 patients with total occlusions, the annual stroke rate was 3%.[29] Thus it appears clear that, although it is possible to occlude the internal carotid artery without the development of symptoms, this event should not be considered a benign occurrence.

What is the risk of having an ischemic event with development of a total occlusion of the internal carotid artery? Roederer et al,[14] in studying the natural history of asymptomatic patients with carotid disease, found a total of 11 occlusions out of 267 patients with documented carotid artery disease. Three were in the less than 80% diameter-reducing lesions, with the remaining eight occurring in the greater than 80% stenosis group. Four strokes (36%) developed in response to the occlusion. Moneta et al[26] reviewed the outcome in 73 patients who had not undergone surgery but had greater than 80% stenoses. There were 9 strokes (12%) in patients followed up to 3 years. Of these nine strokes, five were associated with the development of a total occlusion, giving a stroke rate of 56%.

In a more recent review of the outcome associated with total occlusion of the internal carotid artery, Nicholls, Bergelin, and Strandness[30] were able to collect a total of 24 patients who progressed to a total occlusion of the carotid artery. In this group were 6 immediate strokes (25%), 4 TIAs (16%), and 1 nonhemispheric attack (5%). During follow-up, which extended to 31 months (mean, 12 months), there were 2 additional strokes, 4 TIAs, and the onset of nonhemispheric symptoms in an additional 6 patients. By life-table analysis, the adjusted stroke rate for the first 2 years was 13% for both stroke and TIAs. The combined rate for both stroke and TIA was 23% per year.

Although bilateral occlusion of the internal carotid artery can occur, data on the outcome are sparse since it is possible that many lead to stroke-related death. Fields, Edwards, and Crawford[31] reported that, although the initial occlusion may be well tolerated, events can often occur with obstruction of the contralateral side. Six of the 16 cases reported had minimal permanent neurologic defects with excellent collateral circulation. We have been able to document bilateral occlusions in five patients, with two having permanent deficits as the result.

EVALUATION OF THE PATIENT

At the time the patient suspected of having extracranial arterial disease is first seen, several aspects of the clinical presentation must be clearly defined. Some of the salient features are as follows:

1. If the patient is asymptomatic, what is the extent of the disease as documented by noninvasive testing?
2. For the symptomatic patients it is important to note the following:
   a. Time of day the event occurred
   b. Temporal profile for the event
   c. Detailed description of the event
   d. Duration of the event
   e. Extent of any residual deficit
   f. History of similar episodes in the past

In addition to the above, every workup must evaluate the patient's coexisting disorders that may be relevant such as hypertension, diabetes mellitus, and cardiac disease and risk factors such as cigarette smoking and hyperlipidemia.

The physical examination includes a close examination of the neck to detect the telltale bruits of carotid disease and measurement of blood pressures in both arms. However, the character of the detected bruits is of little value in predicting the status of the arteries from which the noises arise. As Ziegler et al[32] have shown, carotid stenosis can be present without a bruit. Conversely, in another study by David et al[33] 14% of asymptomatic patients with bruits had arteries that were normal as determined by arteriography.

The physical examination should also include a careful neurologic examination, particularly in the early phases of an ischemic event to document the extent of the impairment. This examination will serve as the baseline from which to estimate the degree of recovery that occurs. As noted previously, this provides good evidence about the location and extent of the damage that may have occurred.

A funduscopic examination must be done since it provides the only accessible window to the cerebral circulation. Although one must look for the telltale signs of hypertensive and diabetic retinopathy, signs of retinal emboli and ischemia should be looked for. The orange color of the cholesterol emboli can be distinguished from the whitish appearance of platelet-fibrin aggregates and the white, angular calcium fragments that may on occasion be seen.[13]

Testing procedures

The workup that is done depends on the clinical presentation and the need for additional information. If the extracranial arterial circulation is suspect as the cause of the event, a duplex scan of the neck must be obtained. It provides with a high degree of accuracy information on the status of all of the major vessels in the neck.[34] For details of this examination and its accuracy see Chapter 3.

Lumbar puncture. Lumbar puncture is most commonly performed when there is a question about the presence of subarachnoid hemorrhage or intracerebral hemorrhage. When blood is found in the cerebrospinal fluid, it is good evidence that one or the other has occurred. A major application of this method in the acute situation is when there is some concern about using anticoagulants during the acute phase of the illness. Obviously, finding blood in the cerebrospinal fluid is solid evidence that heparin should not be given.

Electroencephalography. Although there is no doubt that acute ischemic events can produce changes in the electrical activity of the cortex, the findings of electroencephalography are not specific and are of little value. On occasion, the testing will be helpful if a seizure disorder is suspected. Many centers use this test routinely in the monitoring of patients at the time of endarterectomy.

Computed tomography. Computed tomography (CT) has become one of the most commonly performed tests since it can provide information about both ischemic and nonischemic lesions of the brain.[35] It can provide not only topographic information but, with the administration of contrast material, information about the status of the blood-brain barrier. Infarcts are seen as lesions of low absorption, whereas fresh hematomas stand out as areas of higher density. A negative CT scan does not, however, rule out ischemic damage to the cortex. More recently magnetic resonance imaging has arrived on the scene. What its role will be requires further study. Another interesting method that is still in evolution is positron emission tomography, which has the potential not only for identifying lesions in the brain but also for providing information about the brain's blood flow and the metabolic activity of the cortex.

Noninvasive testing. The noninvasive tests that have been used include the indirect methods that infer changes in the carotid bulb from physiologic changes detected at the level of the eye. The most frequently performed tests include supraorbital Doppler examination[36] and the use of oculopneumoplethysmography.[37,38] Although these tests can be used to detect the presence of high-grade lesions in the carotid distribution, they are not sensitive to all categories of involvement. In addition, they cannot be used to distinguish stenoses from occlusions—a serious problem. Also, once the test becomes positive, further changes in the status of the disease cannot be detected. All of these tests have been largely replaced by the use of ultrasonic duplex scanning. These tests are discussed in more detail in Chapter 3.

Cerebral arteriography. Opacification of the vessels of the neck and those inside the skull remains in many cases the definitive test to document the exact location and extent of disease. At the present time cerebral arteriography should be done only if there is some question about the cause of an event or if some form of surgical intervention is being contemplated. Several innovative changes in the method have modified the approach used. The most important is the introduction of digital methods to process images.[39,40] When this method was first introduced, there was interest in using intravenous administration of the contrast agent to allow performance of the procedure on an outpatient basis and with very little risk. This did not turn out to be a very satisfactory approach because of the large volumes of contrast material required and the large number of studies ($\approx$20%) that did not provide the necessary morphologic data needed. However, many radiologists currently use the intraarterial method of injection, which can in most cases provide satisfactory images of all sites of interest.

Although in most centers arteriography is currently considered an outpatient procedure, it does have serious limitations that restrict its use. It does carry a small risk secondary to the arterial puncture and the use of contrast material, which can in a small percentage of cases lead to problems. One of its major drawbacks is the difficulty in using this test to document changes in the status of the patient over time. This is one area in which the noninvasive tests have become very important.

THERAPY

There are few areas in cardiovascular medicine in which there is more dispute than in the area of therapy for atherosclerotic lesions, particularly of the carotid bifurcation.[41-43] Because of the uncertainty about the role of carotid endarterectomy, three national trials have been mounted to study the role of this operation. Two involve the randomization of asymptomatic patients, and one is examining use of the procedure in patients with either TIAs or strokes. The results of these trials are years away, so we are forced at the present time to design our therapy based on data that do not satisfy the requirements of a randomized trial. Before considering the indication for surgical therapy, it is important to review the evidence that is available concerning the use of antiplatelet therapy, particularly aspirin.

The most recent and complete evaluation of aspirin therapy was reported in 1988.[44] This collaboration reviewed the results of 31 randomized trials of patients with a history of TIAs, occlusive stroke, unstable angina, and myocardial infarction. The technique of meta-analysis was used to evaluate the data and draw conclusions about the efficacy of this approach to the treatment of extracranial arterial disease. The studies evaluated included a total of 29,000 patients. Antiplatelet therapy had no apparent effect on nonvascular mortality rates but did reduce the vascular mortality rate by approximately 15% and the nonfatal vascular events by 30%. It was concluded that if good compliance to therapy was achieved, the vascular mortality rate might be reduced by one sixth and other vascular events by approximately one third. No difference was noted between the different types of antiplatelet treatment tested, which included 300 to 325 mg aspirin daily, higher doses of aspirin, sulfinpyrazone, or high doses of aspirin with dipyridamole. The balance of risk vs benefit was for only secondary prevention.

In practical terms the most important factor is the absolute reduction in risk through the use of antiplatelet therapy. As the trial collaborators noted, for 100 patients with a cardiovascular event to enter a trial with antiplatelet therapy, one could expect to avert one vascular death and two nonfatal vascular events. This is not a dramatic form of therapy, with the results somewhat less than expected. On the other hand, the weakly effective therapy provided is clearly evident in the sample size required to reach any conclusions at all about the effect of therapy.

Other points to consider when examining this form of therapy are rarely mentioned by those conducting the trials but are becoming of greater importance. Aspirin is at best a weakly effective antithrombotic agent if at all. Why is this fact relevant to the treatment of carotid artery disease? It is becoming recognized that high-grade carotid lesions, as is the case of similar plaques in the coronary arteries, have as a very common end point, thrombosis with total occlusion of the artery with a sudden reduction in blood flow to the tissue supplied by the artery. There is no evidence that antiplatelet therapy will prevent this end point from occurring. Another critical factor that is never mentioned is that no evidence exists that any of the antiplatelet agents affect the progression of the atherosclerotic lesions themselves. Any form of therapy, be it for primary or secondary prevention, will only succeed if it interferes with the progression of the lesion and all the consequences that follow.

The initial results for the use of ticlopidine in the treatment of thromboembolic stroke appeared in 1989.[45] The study of this drug was a double-blind randomized, placebo-controlled trial involving 25 centers. A total of 1072 patients entered into the trial 1 week to 4 months after suffering a stroke. The patients were followed for a mean period of 24 months. The event rate per year for stroke, myocardial infarction, or vascular death when considered together was 15.3% for the placebo-treated patients and 10.8% in the Ticlopidine group, representing a risk reduction of 30.2% ($P = 0.006$). The reduction in events apparently is the same for both men and women. The complications encountered with the drug were severe neutropenia in 1% and skin rash and diarrhea in 2% of cases. The neutropenia reversed itself when the drug was stopped.

CAROTID ENDARTERECTOMY

The issues surrounding the use of endarterectomy can be considered in two categories: (1) safety of the procedure and (2) long-term results when compared to nonoperative therapy. With regard to the risks of the procedure, the reported results have been a source of great concern, particularly when city-wide experiences have been reported. Two reports—one from Springfield, Illinois,[46] the other from Cincinnati[47]—reported perioperative stroke and death rates of 21.1% and 11.4%, respectively. Knowing the natural history of carotid artery disease makes these rates unacceptable. On the other hand, a review of institutional results is much better, and the stroke and death rate ranges from 1.5% to 4.7%, clearly placing these institutions in a competitive position for stroke prevention.[48]

In such a controversial area on which statistics can one rely when considering the use of carotid endarterectomy? In our own series of 200 consecutive patients the perioperative stroke rates were 2.3% in the patients with TIAs, 2.8% in those who had a stroke, and 1.3% in the asymptomatic patients.[49] There was one perioperative death, giving a rate of 0.5%. Till et al[50] reviewed their experiences spanning a period of 10 years and showed a dramatic reduction in risks associated with the operation. In 1978 they reported a 16% morbidity rate and a 6% mortality rate. In their latter series the 30-day morbidity/mortality rate had dropped to 3%.

In 1989 Beebe et al[51] issued a report for health care professionals to serve as guidelines for assessing the risk associated with carotid endarterectomy. The limits they considered acceptable are as follows for combined morbidity/mortality rates according to indication for surgery:

1. Absence of symptoms, less than 3%
2. TIA, less than 5%
3. Ischemic stroke, less than 7%
4. Recurrent carotid disease in the same artery after endarterectomy, less than 10%

In recommending these limits it is clear the authors attempted to stratify the risk by indications and, presumably, the potential for problems that each group of patients presented. Whether these guidelines are too liberal or not will await further studies. In our case as well as others, it appears that better results are achievable.

The operation itself is designed to remove the lesion at the carotid bifurcation and restore the internal carotid artery to as near normal status as is possible. The lesion will extend down into the media of the vessel, but the plaque itself rarely extends beyond the distal limits of the bulb. For reasons that are unknown the internal carotid artery is not frequently involved, permitting the surgeon to achieve a suitable end point that is very smooth and free of atheroma. It may be necessary to tack down the intima at the distal end of the endarterectomy, but this can usually be accomplished without difficulty. The operation is one that must be done with great care since any technical problem is likely to lead to an adverse outcome.

Asymptomatic patient

A great deal of opinion suggests that carotid endarterectomy should never be performed for asymptomatic patients. This opinion is based primarily on the low level of risk patients with disease have when followed expectantly. For example, the annual stroke risk for the entire group of patients with disease is approximately 2% to 4%/yr. If this truly represents the stroke risk for those patients to whom the operation is being applied, it would be difficult to support an aggressive approach since the combined morbidity and mortality rates in even the best surgical series are generally in this range. However, a different picture emerges when one stratifies the disease by the degree of narrowing that is present and how it changes over time.

It was not until 1984 that the first opportunity arose to examine the relationship between the degree of narrowing and the outcome when asymptomatic patients were followed serially to examine outcome. In our initial study patients with an 80% to 99% stenosis were followed; 47% sustained either a TIA, stroke, or total occlusion of the internal carotid artery, usually within 6 months of discovery of the lesion.[14] Studies by Chambers and Norris[52] and Bogousslavsky,

Despland, and Regli[53] have also confirmed that the high-grade lesions are the most dangerous and predictive of subsequent outcome.

Although many do not consider the development of a total occlusion of the internal carotid artery as an adverse outcome unless it is associated with the development of an ischemic event, this author does not agree with this view. Studies by Cote, Barnett, and Taylor[28] and Nicholls, Bergelin, and Strandness[29] have clearly shown that the annual stroke rate on the side of the occlusion is approximately 5% per year, which is equivalent to the risk one is facing when a TIA is the presenting complaint.

For the subset of patients with high-grade stenoses (>80%) surgery apparently is a satisfactory form of therapy if the surgical complications are low. Although no exact figure for what an acceptable stroke rate should be is available, a combined morbidity/mortality rate of 3% of less would be acceptable.[53] This rate has been achieved in many centers that have surgeons with a special interest in this area.[48]

Are there any exceptions to the above guidelines as they relate to indications for carotid endarterectomy? For one category of patient there are no data, but one may be justified to proceed with the operation. This is the patient who has an occlusion of one carotid artery and a 50% to 79% stenosis of the other carotid artery. If one chooses a nonoperative approach, frequent follow-up with repeat duplex scanning would appear to be in order because some lesions progress rapidly and can be detected only by serial studies, preferably every 3 months. On the other hand, this author believes it is justified to offer an operation to ensure that the remaining carotid artery stays patent. This represents a very conservative course. In our studies of asymptomatic patients with carotid artery disease as documented by duplex scanning, only 7% of such patients will have such a high-grade lesion at the time they are initially screened.[26] In addition, once lesions are found, they may not be as stable as once thought. In our experience the annual rate of progression from less than to greater than 50% diameter-reducing stenosis is 8% per year.[14]

Symptomatic patient

It would appear that the guidelines for treating the symptomatic patient are more clear-cut in that patients with focal TIAs and strokes (with considerable recovery) should be considered candidates for this operation if there is an appropriate lesion found in the carotid artery supplying the affected area of the brain. Although there is no doubt that lesions of all stenotic severity can lead to embolic and thrombotic events, the majority of patients in this category will have advanced lesions. When we examined this issue, we noted the following distribution of lesions in 200 consecutive patients who underwent the operation: 1% to 15% stenosis, 5 sides (2.5%); 16% to 49% stenosis, 19 sides (9.5%); 50% to 79% stenosis, 83 sides (41.5%); and 80% to 99% stenosis, 93 sides (46.5%).[49]

Special situations

One area of great interest and concern is the patient with carotid artery disease who is about to undergo major vascular or cardiac surgery.[54] Should carotid endarterectomy be done before or at the time of the procedure? Surgery has been recommended on the basis that a drop in systemic blood pressure at the time of the operation in combination with a high-grade carotid artery stenosis may be responsible for precipitating an ischemic event. In the case of aortocoronary bypass grafting, the incidence of perioperative stroke has remained in the 2% to 5% range, with the supposition being that the stroke may be secondary to the presence of carotid artery lesions that may have been undetected or untreated by surgical means.[55] This has remained a controversial subject, but it appears that many surgeons would now recommend leaving the carotid lesion alone unless the patient is having symptoms of cerebral ischemia.[56-59] In this circumstance it would not appear unreasonable either to treat the carotid lesion first or to repair it in conjunction with the other procedure. The studies done to date could not relate the occurrence of perioperative stroke with the status of the carotid artery.

VERTEBROBASILAR INSUFFICIENCY

In 1961 Reivich et al[15] described a new clinical syndrome associated with reversal of flow in the vertebral artery when there was significant stenosis or occlusion of the subclavian artery. This entity, referred to as the *subclavian steal syndrome,* was thought responsible for intermittent brainstem ischemia because of the diversion of blood down the vertebral artery, which was then serving as a major collateral source of blood to the arm. In some cases arm exercise that increased the amount of flow down the vertebral artery was often associated with the development of symptoms. From a hemodynamic standpoint the explanation would appear quite simple and straightforward, but subsequent experience has proved that this is not the case.

With the accumulation of more data, it is clear that subclavian stenosis and occlusion are not uncommon findings and when they occur, flow will be reversed in the vertebral artery. In the study by Bornstein and Norris[60] reversal of flow was found in 6.4% of 500 patients who were asymptomatic but had neck bruits. The association of the steal with vertebrobasilar symptoms is rare. It is thought that patients become symptomatic only when there may be associated vascular lesions that may contribute to the production of symptoms.

In our laboratory we were able to identify 43 patients over a 5-year period who had reverse flow in one vertebral artery at the time of a duplex scan. They were subdivided into the following groups—those with the subclavian steal syndrome, those with nonhemispheric symptoms, those with hemispheric symptoms, and those who were asymptomatic. One third of the patients were asymptomatic, with only 7% having the classical syndrome of developing symptoms with arm exercise. Those patients with hemispheric symptoms usually had an associated disease of the carotid artery. We concluded that reversal of flow in the vertebral artery in and of itself was probably an innocuous finding.

When a patient is initially seen with brainstem ischemia, Brain[61] has suggested that at least four possible causes should be considered: cervical spine injury, cervical spondylosis, lesions of the vertebral and/or basilar artery, and brain tumor of the posterior fossa. Clearly surgery must be withheld until all other causes of the events are ruled out. One other factor of importance is that vertebrobasilar symptoms are often short lived and may disappear without any therapy at all.

REFERENCES

1. Hunt JR: Role of carotid arteries in causation of vascular lesions of the brain: with remarks on special features of symptomatology, Am J Med Sci 147:704, 1914.
2. Fisher CM: Occlusion of the internal carotid artery, Arch Neurol Psychiatr 65:346, 1951.
3. Milliken CH and Siekert RG: Studies in cerebrovascular disease. I. The syndrome of intermittent insufficiency of the basilar arterial system, Proc Staff Meet Mayo Clin 30:61, 1955.
4. Hutchinson EC and Yates PO: Carotid-vertebral stenoses, Lancet 1:2, 1957.
5. Mitchell JRA and Schwartz CJ: Arterial disease in different sites. In Mitchell JRA and Schwartz CJ, eds: Arterial disease, Philadelphia, 1965, FA Davis Co.
6. Wiener LM, Berry RG, Kundin J: Intracranial circulation in carotid occlusion, Arch Neurol 11:554, 1964.
7. Bosniak MA: An analysis of some anatomo-roentgenologic aspects of the brachio-cephalic vessels, Am J Roentgen 91:1222, 1964.
8. Riggs HE and Rupp C: Variation in the form of Circle of Willis: the relation of variations to collateral circulation: anatomic analysis, Arch Neurol 8:8, 1963.
9. Hass WK et al: Joint Study of Extracranial Arterial Occlusion. II. Arteriography, techniques, sites and complications, JAMA 203:961, 1968.
10. Wolf PA, Kannel WB and Dawber TR: Prospective investigation: the Framingham Study and the epidemiology of stroke, Adv Neurol 19:107, 1978.
11. Fisher CM: Transient monocular blindness associated with hemiplegia, Arch Ophthalmol 47:167, 1952.
12. Russell RWR: Observation on the retinal blood vessels in monocular blindness, Lancet 2:1422, 1981.
13. Hollenhorst RW: Significance of bright plaques in the retinal arterioles, JAMA 178:123, 1961.
14. Roederer GO et al: The natural history of carotid arterial disease in asymptomatic patients with cervical bruits, Stroke 15:605, 1984.
15. Reivich M et al: Reversal of blood flow through the vertebral artery and its effect on cerebral circulation, N Engl J Med 265:878, 1961.
16. Palubinskas JA and Ripley HR: Fibromuscular hyperplasia in extrarenal arteries, Radiology 82:451, 1964.
17. Osborne AG and Anderson RE: Angiographic spectrum of cervical and intracranial fibromuscular dysplasia, Stroke 8:617, 1977.
18. Houser WO and Baker HL Jr: Fibromuscular dysplasia and other uncommon diseases of the cervical carotid artery. Angiographic aspects, Am J Roentgenol 104:201, 1968.
19. Kase CS and Mohr JP: General features of intracerebral hemorrhage. In Barnett HJM et al, eds: Stroke, New York, 1986, Churchill Livingstone, Inc.
20. Mohr JP et al: Intracranial aneurysm. In Barnett HJM et al, eds: Stroke, New York, 1986, Churchill Livingstone, Inc.
21. Levy RJ: Stroke decline: implications and prospects, N Engl J Med 300:490, 1979.
22. Duncan GW et al: Concomitants of atherosclerotic carotid artery stenosis, Stroke 8:665, 1977.
23. Veterans Administration Cooperative Study Group on Antihypertensive Agents: Effects of treatment on morbidity in hypertension, JAMA 202:1028, 1970.
24. Shurtleff D: Some characteristics related to the incidence of cardiovascular disease and death. The Framingham study: 18-year follow-up, Washington DC, 1974, Department of Health Education and Welfare.
25. Hertzer NR and Lees CO: Fatal myocardial infarction following carotid endarterectomy: three-hundred thirty-five patients followed 6-11 years after operation, Am Surg 194:212, 1981.
26. Moneta GL et al: Operative versus nonoperative management of asymptomatic high-grade internal carotid artery stenosis: improved results with endarterectomy, Stroke 18:1005, 1987.
27. Committee on Health Care Issues ANA: Does carotid endarterectomy decrease stroke and death in patients with transient ischemic attacks? Ann Neurol 22:72, 1987.
28. Cote R, Barnett HJM, and Taylor DM: Internal carotid artery occlusion. A prospective study, Stroke 14:898, 1983.
29. Nicholls SC et al: Carotid artery occlusion: natural history, J Vasc Surg 4:479, 1986.
30. Nicholls SC, Bergelin RO, and Strandness DE Jr: Neurological sequelae of unilateral carotid artery occlusion. Immediate and late, J Vasc Surg 10:542, 1989.
31. Fields WS, Edwards WH, and Crawford ES. Bilateral carotid artery thrombosis, Arch Neurol 4:369, 1961.
32. Ziegler DK et al: Correlation of bruits over the carotid artery with angiographically demonstrated lesions, Neurology 21:860, 1971.
33. David TE et al: A correlation of neck bruits and arteriosclerotic carotid arteries, Arch Surg 107:729, 1973.
34. Langlois YE et al: Evaluating carotid artery disease. The concordance between pulsed Doppler/spectrum analysis and angiography, Ultrasound Med Biol 9:51, 1983.
35. New PFJ and Scott W: Computed tomography of the brain and orbit (EMI scanning), Baltimore, 1975, The Williams & Wilkins Co.
36. Barnes RW et al: The Doppler cerebrovascular examination: improved results with refinements in techniques, Stroke 8:468, 1977.
37. Gee W: Carotid physiology with ocular pneumoplethysmography, Stroke 13:666, 1982.
38. Gee W: Ocular pneumoplethysmography, Surv Ophthalmol 29:276, 1985.
39. Mistretta CA and Crummy AS: Diagnosis of cardiovascular disease by digital subtraction angiography, Science 214:761, 1981.
40. Little JR et al: Progress in cerebrovascular disease: digital subtraction angiography in cerebrovascular disease, Stroke 13:557, 1982.
41. Barnett HJM, Plum F, and Walton JM: Carotid endarterectomy: an expression of concern, Stroke 15:941, 1984.
42. Chambers BR and Norris JW: The case against surgery for asymptomatic carotid stenosis, Stroke 15:964, 1984.
43. Dyken ML and Pokras R: The performance of endarterectomy for disease of the extracranial arteries of the head, Stroke 15:948, 1984.
44. Secondary prevention of vascular disease by prolonged antiplatelet treatment: antiplatelet trialists collaborators, Br Med J 296:320, 1988.
45. Gent M et al: The Canadian American Ticlopidine Study (CATS) in thromboembolic stroke, Lancet 1:1215, 1989.

46. Easton JD and Sherman DG: Stroke and mortality rate in carotid endarterectomy: 228 consecutive operations, Stroke 8:565, 1977.
47. Brott T and Thalinger K: Carotid endarterectomy in Cincinnati, 1980. Indications and morbidity in 431 cases, Neurology 33(suppl):93, 1983.
48. Roederer GO, Langlois YE, and Strandness DE Jr: Cerebral arterial flow and cerebral vascular insufficiency. In Condon RE and De Cosse H, eds: Surgical care II, Philadelphia, 1984, Lea & Febiger.
49. Healy DA et al: Immediate and long-term results of carotid endarterectomy, Stroke 20:1138, 1989.
50. Till JS et al: Declining morbidity and mortality of carotid endarterectomy: The Wake Forest University Medical Center Experience, Stroke 18:823, 1987.
51. Beebe HG et al: Assessing risk associated with carotid endarterectomy (special report), Stroke 20:314-315, 1989.
52. Chambers BR and Norris JW: Outcome in patients with asymptomatic neck bruits, N Engl J Med 315:860, 1986.
53. Bogousslavsky J, Despland PA, and Regli F: Asymptomatic tight stenosis of the internal carotid artery: long-term prognosis, Neurology 36:861, 1986.
54. Hertzer NR et al: Staged and combined surgical approach to simultaneous and coronary vascular disease, Surgery 84:803, 1978.
55. Reul GJ et al: Current concepts in coronary artery surgery. A critical analysis of 1287 patients, Ann Thorac Surg 14:243, 1972.
56. Barnes RW, Marzalek PB, and Rittgers SF: Asymptomatic carotid disease in preoperative patients, Stroke 2:136, 1980 (abstract).
57. Breslau PJ et al: Carotid arterial disease in patients undergoing coronary artery bypass operations, J Thorac Cardiovasc Surg 82:765, 1981.
58. Ivey TD et al: Management of patients with carotid bruit undergoing cardiopulmonary bypass, J Thorac Cardiovasc Surg 87:183, 1984.
59. Turnipseed WD, Berkoff HA, and Belzer FO: Postoperative stroke in cardiac and peripheral vascular disease, Am Surg 192:365, 1980.
60. Bornstein NM and Norris JW: Subclavian steal: a harmless hemodynamic phenomenon, Lancet 2:303, 1986.
61. Brain WR: Vertebral artery syndromes, J Neurol Neurosurg Psychiatry 26:558, 1963.

Chapter 14

VISCERAL ISCHEMIC SYNDROMES

Robert A. Graor
Patrick J. Ginley III

In 1936 Dunphy identified a syndrome of abdominal pain followed by ischemia and gangrene of the gut secondary to mesenteric arterial occlusion.[1] In 1957 Mikkelsen suggested the term intestinal angina to identify this syndrome, which "may for a period of months to years precede complete mesenteric arterial occlusion."[2] In this publication Mikkelsen suggested that chronic atherosclerotic occlusive disease of the superior messenteric artery might be treated by a bypass graft or repair and reimplantation of this artery. In 1957 Shaw reported the first thromboendarterectomy of the superior mesenteric artery, and in 1959 Mikkelsen et al successfully opened an occluded superior mesenteric artery with the use of a Cannon loop dissector.[3,4]

Despite the enormous advances in noninvasive technology, perioperative care, and surgical technique, acute and chronic intestinal ischemia and infarction continue to be associated with an exceedingly high mortality. Recent large series have indicated that mortality rates from 60% to 85% can be expected.[5,6,7] There are three reasons why relatively little improvement has been made in the outcome of this disease. First, the early symptoms of vascular insufficiency to the bowel are mild and can be dismissed by the physician who rarely sees this unusual disease. Only 1% to 2% of patients treated for an acute abdomen have intestinal gangrene. Most patients who are treated for ischemia are in the early phase without evidence of an acute abdomen, thus the correct diagnosis is frequently delayed and only made at laparotomy. Second, intestinal ischemia frequently occurs in the very elderly patient with severe associated cardiopulmonary disease and other comorbid conditions, which predispose the patient to a high mortality. Third, the results of mesenteric circulation interruption adversely affect the outcome of surgical revascularization because of frequent and serious infections, superoxide radicals, and severe acidosis, which accompany this entity. A more successful outcome will only be effected if management of these secondary problems improves. The complexity of this disease reflects in part the fact that although obstruction of the mesenteric arterial or venous flow has a primary role in the ischemia, inadequate collateral flow, arterial spasm, and a decrease in perfusion pressure, at times initiate or accentuate the extent of the ischemic injury.

ANATOMY

The visceral arteries consist of the celiac, superior mesenteric, and inferior mesenteric arteries. The celiac axis arises at the first lumbar vertebra and divides into the splenic, hepatic, and left gastric artery branches (Fig. 14-1). The right gastric and the gastroduodenal arteries arise from the hepatic artery. The gastroduodenal artery later divides into the right gastroepiploic and the superior pancreaticoduodenal arteries. The superior pancreaticoduodenal artery often forms an important anastomosis with the inferior pancreaticoduodenal artery (the first branch of the SMA), and thereby provides a collateral flow for occlusion of either the celiac or the superior mesenteric artery.

The superior mesenteric artery arises from the aorta anteriorly between the lumbar 1 and 2 vertebral bodies and supplies the critical blood flow for the greatest portion of the gastrointestinal tract. This gives off vessels to the duodenum, jejunum, and ileum as well as branching to the middle, right, and ileocolic vessels (Fig. 14-2). The anastomotic arcades in the small intestine are extensive, as they are fewer in number and are located further apart than those of the large intestine.

The inferior mesenteric artery arises proximal to the aortic bifurcation and supplies the left colic artery and other

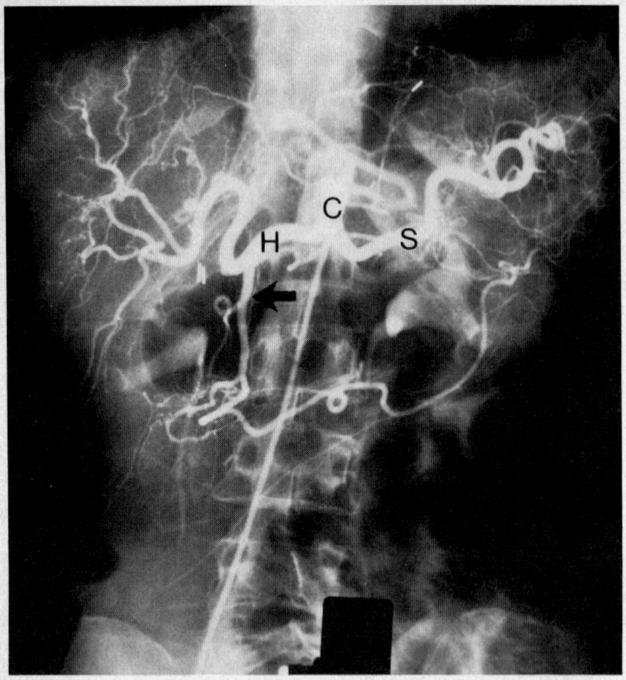

Fig. 14-1. A selective injection of the celiac axis demonstrates the main body of the axis *(C)*. The celiac bifurcates to form the splenic artery *(S)* and the common hepatic artery *(H)*. The gastroduodenal *(arrow)* further subdivides into the pancreaticoduodenal arteries.

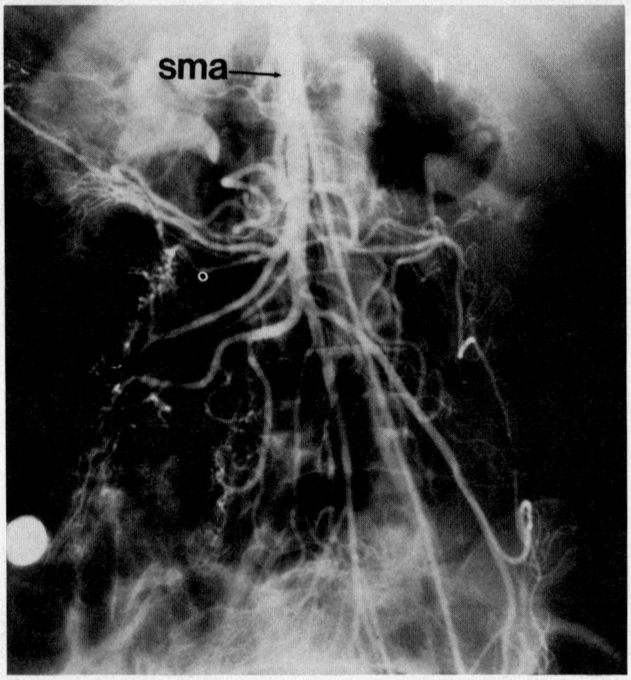

Fig. 14-2. This selective anterior to posterior view of the superior mesenteric artery demonstrates its normal divisions to the small and large intestine. The main body of the superior mesenteric artery is marked *SMA*. The SMA projects anteriorly off the aorta, and in this view, the origin of the superior mesenteric artery is not well visualized.

branches to the left colon including the sigmoid and superior hemorrhoidal arteries (Fig. 14-3). The left colic artery anastomosis with the middle colic artery provides collateral distribution to the superior mesenteric artery. This left colic artery becomes enlarged when the superior mesenteric artery is occluded and has been referred to as "the meandering mesenteric artery," "the arc of Riolan," "the artery of Gonzales," or "the artery of Moskowitz." It should be noted that the left colic artery is not the marginal or wandering artery of Drummond, which is an artery that runs independently and immediately adjacent to the colon. In the presence of severe occlusive disease, the superior mesenteric artery fills retrograde through the wandering artery of Drummon (Fig. 14-4). The superior hemorrhoidal vessels anastomose freely with the middle and inferior hemorrhoidal vessels derived from the internal iliac arteries.

PATHOPHYSIOLOGY

Despite the different clinical manifestations or anatomic causes of acute intestinal ischemia, the final pathway leading to irreversible intestinal infarction is the same. The gross lesions in humans are nearly identical to those induced experimentally in animals. In 1875 Litten performed the classical demonstration of acute intestinal ischemia.[8] A ligature was applied to the superior mesenteric artery and Dr. Litten noted "the moment the ligature was tightened, the circulation in the region immediately stopped and every trace of pulsation ceased. The loops of the bowel became bluish white, rippled, and strongly contracted."

When blood flow ceases or perfusion pressure falls below a critical level to the bowel, compensatory mechanisms attempt to restore flow and prevent ischemia. On the macroscopic level, collateral flow between adjacent mesenteric vessels and the mesenteric arcades may supply substantial blood flow. Although there is rich interconnecting submucosal blood flow, this collateral network is insufficient to maintain long segments of bowel viable. Intestinal blood flow is maintained by autoregulation, and as perfusion drops, vasodilatation occurs and blood flow remains constant over a broad range of perfusion pressures.[9] Redistribution of flow begins as perfusion pressure is decreased and flow is then redistributed from the muscularis to the mucosal layers.

At the microscopic level cell tissue oxygen extraction increases with reduced blood flow.[10,11] When blood flow decreases below a critical level, ischemic changes ensue and rapidly become irreversible. As the ischemic period pro-

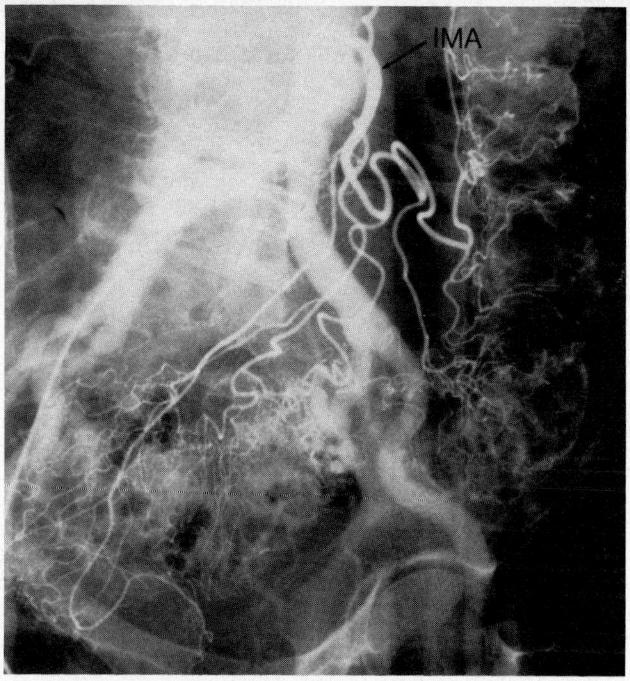

Fig. 14-3. This demonstrates the inferior mesenteric artery *(IMA)* and its branches from a selective injection. The inferior mesenteric artery supplies the distal third of the colon and rectosigmoid section.

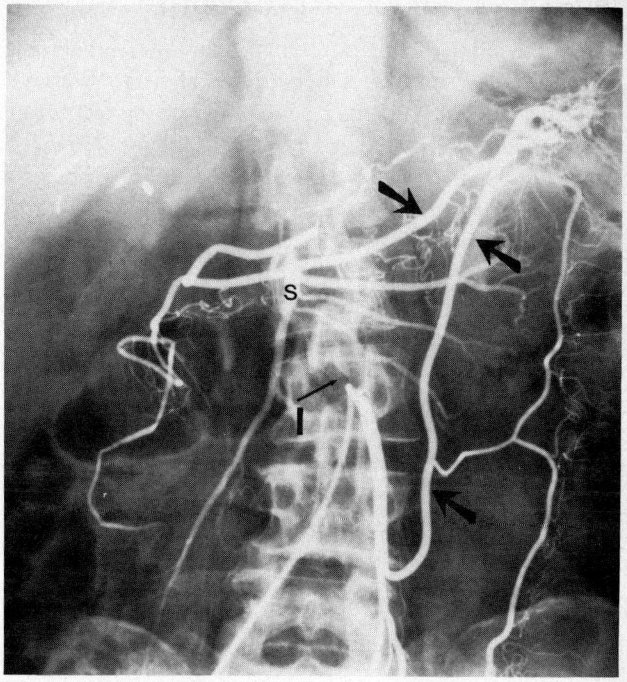

Fig. 14-4. This selective injection in the anterior-posterior view of the inferior mesenteric artery demonstrates the collateral filling of the wandering artery of Drummond. The inferior mesenteric artery origin is labeled *I,* and the wandering artery of Drummond is outlined by the large arrows. At the superior most portion of the wandering artery the superior mesenteric artery *(S)* is filling through the middle colic branches of the superior mesenteric artery.

gresses, adenosine triphosphate (ATP) is depleted and converted to adenosine monophosphate (AMP). The AMP undergoes catabolization to adenosine, inosine, and hypoxanthine. Xanthine dehydrogenase is then converted to xanthine oxidase in the ischemic tissue. When reperfusion occurs and reoxygenation results, the superoxide radical O_2^- is produced. These superoxide radicals then may be mediators for further tissue damage during reperfusion. With prolonged complete arterial occlusion, cell death occurs irrespective of oxygen radical blockade, and microvascular patency is lost. Once this occurs, restoration of macrovascular blood flow is of no value.

Early histologic changes occur within 10 minutes of the onset of ischemia.[12] Damage to the endoplasmic reticulum and mitochondrial alterations are the early cellular changes; however, it is not until the lysosomal membranes rupture that the hydrolytic enzymes contained within the cell are released into the circulation.[13] The lysosomal rupture releases autolytic enzymes as a result of anoxia and acidosis that injure adjacent cells, setting up a vicious cycle of continual intestinal death.[11,14]

The later stages include hemorrhagic infarction with bowel edema that is infiltrated with blood and lead to further mucosal necrotic changes. Ultimately bacterial peritonitis occurs when perforation ensues. Histologically, hemorrhagic necrosis is present with extensive submucosal edema, which worsens as mucosal cells lose their ability to produce mucus and protect themselves. The bowel wall then becomes highly permeable, and bidirectional fluid flow occurs, resulting in massive loss of plasma-like high-protein content fluid.[15]

The systemic effects of acute intestinal infarction are characterized by early detection of neutrophilic leukocytosis (>20,000 white blood cells per cubic mm).[16] An increase in hemoglobin and hematocrit concentration is usually present, reflecting the hemoconcentration produced by volume loss into the extravascular space. This latter change reverses itself as hemorrhage occurs into the gastrointestinal tract. A metabolic acidosis ensues once lactic acid from bacterial digestion is released into the system. Hypoamylasemia is noted early after the onset of acute mesenteric insufficiency and is thought to be caused by plasma loss into the intestine. Later, amylase levels return to normal and subsequently begin to rise. Other late findings in the course of mesenteric infarction include the release of lactic dehydrogenase, serum glutamic oxaloacetic transaminase, serum glutamic pyruvic transaminase, and a marked elevation in creatine phosphokinase.[13,17]

CLASSIFICATION OF VISCERAL DISEASE

Although it may be preceded by a long history of chronic symptoms, visceral infarction occurs as an acute event. Of the cases of acute mesenteric infarction diagnosed before death, about 50% have been the result of superior mesenteric artery occlusion, 25% have been the result of nonocclusive infarction, and an additional 25% have been the result of inferior mesenteric artery occlusion, mesenteric venous thrombosis, or arteritis.[18,19]

In the 50% of cases resulting from occlusion of the SMA, atherosclerotic disease leading to thrombosis and cardiac embolization to the SMA occur with about equal frequency. When thrombotic occlusion occurs, it most commonly occupies the first 1 to 3 cm of the vessel and is generally a result of thrombosis in situ in the presence of an atherosclerotic plaque. Emboli lodge at bifurcations of this vessel or in a finely tapering branch (Fig. 14-5).

In the presence or absence of atherosclerotic changes involving the mesenteric vessels, nonocclusive bowel infarction results from diminished cardiac output and low arterial perfusion of the mesenteric bed. Management of such cases either requires reperfusion by increasing the cardiac output, or a reduction of factors producing regional blood flow abnormalities. In this setting bowel infarction is generally spotty, can often be of partial thickness, and may recover without treatment if reperfusion can occur.

Occlusion of the inferior mesenteric artery is common and rarely results in colonic ischemia. Most reported cases of ischemia have resulted from surgical ligation of the artery during aortic surgery.[20] Management involves close observation following ligation of the artery and revascularization if necessary.

Superior mesenteric vein thrombosis leading to infarction may reflect extension of a thrombus from the portal vein or may result from thrombosis of the superior mesenteric vein itself. The condition has been associated with many other pathologic processes, including the use of oral contraceptives, impairment of the fibrinolytic system, hypercoagulable states, and rapidly advancing tumors or tumor with associated hypercoagulable states (see the accompanying box).[21-28] Thrombosis of the superior mesenteric vein is characterized by the thrombus extending in a fanlike fashion to the mesenteric border. This unusual characteristic distinguishes this diagnosis. Usually the middle portion of the small bowel is involved and colon infarction is rare. Because of the extension of the thrombus to the bowel wall, throm-

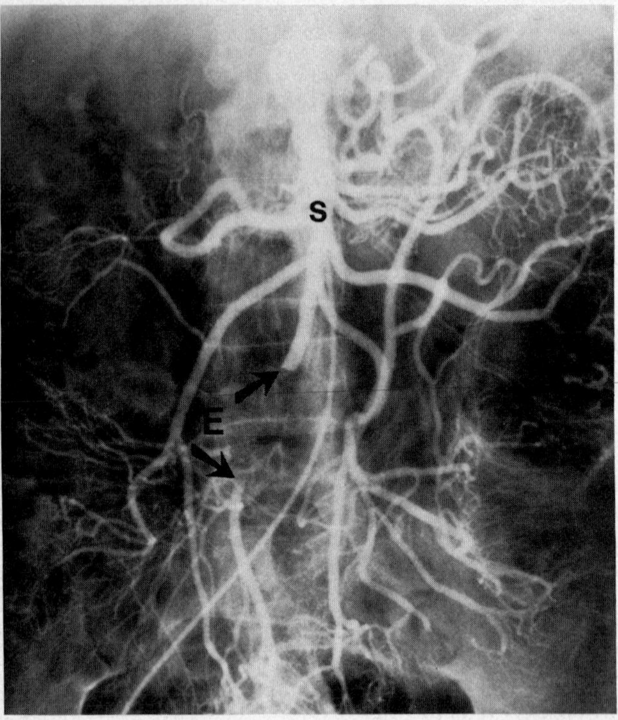

Fig. 14-5. This is a selective injection of the superior mesenteric artery *(S)* and demonstrates an embolus *(E)* in the main superior mesenteric artery after several branches. The abrupt cutoff at the level of the arrows is the meniscus commonly seen following embolization. Collaterals fill the distal portion of the SMA.

Conditions associated with mesenteric venous thrombosis

Portal hypertension

Cirrhosis
Congestive splenomegaly

Inflammation

Peritonitis (e.g., appendicitis, perforated viscus)
Inflammatory bowel disease
Pelvic or intraabdominal abscess
Diverticular disease

Postoperative state and trauma

Splenectomy and other postoperative states
Blunt abdominal trauma*

"Hypercoagulable" states

Neoplasms (especially intraabdominal, e.g., colonic or pancreatic)
Oral contraceptive use
Pregnancy*
Migratory thrombophlebitis
Antithrombin III deficiency
Peripheral deep vein thrombosis
Polycythemia vera
Thrombocytosis

Other conditions

Renal disease (including kidney transplantation*)
Cardiac disease

*Rare, isolated reports.

bectomy is of little value. Resection of a generous portion of the bowel is mandatory and subsequent infarction at suture lines is common. Second look operations are often indicated.

Vasculitis may also produce mesenteric infarcts.[29] These infarcts tend to be small and superficial, but they can result in perforation. Bowel infarct lesions from vasculitis are distinct in the sense that they are of varying age and depth. Some appear as fresh infarctions, while others will show exudation and scarring as part of the healing process. In addition to acute mesenteric ischemic syndromes, other signs of vasculitis are frequently present.

The celiac axis compression syndrome is characterized by abdominal pain and narrowing of the celiac axis at its origin.[30-32] The anatomic finding may be demonstrated by arteriography. The compression is caused by the inferior margin of the median arcuate ligament (Fig. 14-6). Since collateral flow into the celiac axis should support the needs of the organs supplied by this artery, there is serious doubt that this lesion can produce symptomatic ischemia despite documented case reports. Nonetheless, it has been our view that a subgroup of patients appear to exist for whom celiac compression is a clinicopathologic variant and not an anatomic one. The ability to preoperatively identify the patient who will benefit from operative treatment of this condition is a major concern. Ischemia in this syndrome is either caused by obstructed blood flow or emboli or mesenteric steal; however, there is no documentation of the exact process.

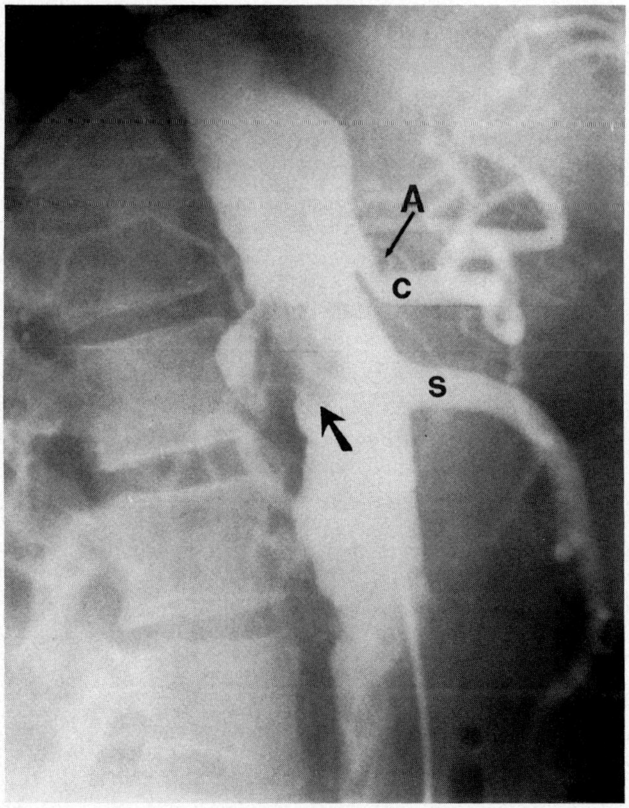

Fig. 14-6. A lateral view of the aorta demonstrates the origin of the celiac axis *(C)* and the superior mesenteric artery *(S)*. The arrow with the letter *A* denotes the arcuate ligament compressing the origin of the celiac axis. A large posterior plaque in the aorta is identified and appears to be ulcerated *(arrow)*.

CLINICAL PRESENTATION

The signs and symptoms associated with mesenteric ischemia are not specific, although 100% of patients with mesenteric infarction will be found to have abdominal pain if they are alert and can experience the sensation of abdominal pain. The clinical mimicry of bowel ischemia and infarction by other critical illnesses causing abdominal pain, tenderness, diarrhea, obtundation, and hypotension leads to considerable difficulty in establishing the diagnosis without direct examination and on clinical grounds alone. The misdiagnosis of bowel infarction cannot be attributed to the rarity of the problem alone. Four specific problems result in the misdiagnosis of bowel infarction: (1) Failure to recognize patients at risk, (2) insufficient appreciation of the typical nonspecific presentation, (3) misplaced confidence in the sensitivity and specificity of certain laboratory tests, and (4) preferential selection of more familiar medical and surgical diagnoses.

In a study done at the Mayo Clinic by Hallet et al[33] the clinical presentation included postprandial abdominal pain in 100% of patients, epigastric bruit in 75% of patients, and the fear of eating with associated weight loss in 98% of patients. The average duration of symptoms in their study before the diagnosis was 12 months. Rheudasil et al[34] reported similar findings in patients with chronic mesenteric ischemia (Table 14-1), whereas the findings of mesenteric

Table 14-1. Signs and symptoms of chronic mesenteric ischemia and associated common conditions

Signs and symptoms at presentation	No. of patients	%
Pain	31	100
Weight loss	28	90
Nausea, vomiting	26	84
Abdominal bruit	21	68
Previous abdominal surgery	21	68
Diarrhea	10	32
Constipation	8	26
Associated conditions	**No. of patients**	**%**
Tobacco abuse	36	88
Atherosclerotic/valvular heart disease	23	56
COPD	20	49
Cerebrovascular disease	19	50
Peripheral atherosclerotic disease	18	45
Renal hypertension	14	34
Chronic renal insufficiency	9	22
Diabetes mellitus	5	12

Table 14-2. Clinical presentation of mesenteric ischemia caused by venous thrombosis

Symptom	No. of patients (%)
Abdominal pain	12 (75)
Gastrointestinal bleeding	3 (19)
Malaise	1 (6)
Associated complaints	
Anorexia	7 (44)
Nausea with vomiting	3 (19)
Nausea without vomiting	3 (19)
Diarrhea	2 (13)

venous thrombosis resulting in bowel ischemia are slightly different and are best described by Harward et al[35] in Table 14-2.

Abdominal pain, intestinal angina, will be present, often with significant weight loss, and will classically begin 30 to 90 minutes after eating. It may persist for a variable period of time, usually not exceeding 2 to 3 hours. The associated weight loss is not caused by anorexia but by food avoidance, which the patient cognitively undertakes to avoid the painful postprandial syndrome. The pain typcially is located near the midabdomen or epigastrium and frequently may radiate to the back. It usually is a dull ache and the severity correlates with the amount of food ingested. As the severity of the ischemia progresses, smaller amounts of food will induce pain.

Acute infarction classically occurs with sudden pain, with or without vomiting, and a crampy bowel evacuation type of bloody diarrhea. Abdominal tenderness is frequently found but is a later manifestation. Findings other than pain are inconsistent. Rarely do patients actually feel constipated, nausea and vomiting are uncommon, and malabsorption is rare.

On physical examination a patient with chronic intestinal ischemia generally appears chronically ill and often looks emaciated, as if he has cancer. Systolic or diastolic bruits may be heard over the abdomen, but these are nonspecific diagnostic signs. The presence of mesenteric symptoms following acute myocardial infarction and superior mesenteric artery embolization from a left ventricular thrombus is also common. Nonocclusive, low-flow bowel ischemia and mesenteric venous thrombosis symptoms are more insidious until actual bowel infarction occurs. At that time there is generally an associated acute abdominal pain that is periumbilical, and the abdomen may be soft or only slightly tender. In the early phase as the ischemic syndrome progresses and infarction occurs, the abdomen becomes more tender and progresses to rigidity as perforation occurs.

Less typical symptoms of chronic visceral arterial insufficiency can occur, including a long history of uncomfortable postprandial abdominal bloating before classic intestinal angina begins. Consequently, chronic intestinal ischemia must remain high on the differential diagnosis list of any clinician evaluating patients with intermittent chronic abdominal pain and weight loss, especially if there are symptoms of atherosclerosis elsewhere, including angina pectoris and claudication.

Predisposing factors

Advanced age, hypertension, smoking, elevated cholesterol, and diabetes all may be predisposing factors in mesenteric arterial occlusive disease. In the case of superior mesenteric embolization, cardiac disease is most commonly suspected, and evaluation for chamber thrombi, arrhythmias, and valvular defects should be undertaken. Other sources of large vessel emboli include the aorta and occasionally embolization originating from arteriosclerosis at the origin of the superior mesenteric or other mesenteric arteries. As a result of vasculitis such as lupus erythematosus, rheumatoid arthritis, or other types of vasculitis, patients may develop occlusive disease. Fibrous dysplasia of the mesenteric arteries has been described but rarely results in infarction. Patients with hypercoagulable states can develop arterial or venous thrombotic mesenteric disorders. These patients are described in Chapter 4. Low-flow bowel ischemia (hypoperfusion) and nonocclusive bowel ischemia commonly result from low cardiac output, which can be induced in many clinical situations. Profound sepsis and heart failure are the two most common hypotensive states that lead to bowel infarction.

DIAGNOSIS

Noninvasive diagnosis

Only recently have reliable noninvasive methods for diagnosing chronic visceral arterial occlusive disease become available. While angiography has been considered the definitive diagnostic test, it has not provided quantitative, physiologic, or hemodynamic data regarding splanchnic blood flow. Now, however, it is possible to assess noninvasively blood flow dynamics in the human superior mesenteric artery using a duplex system, the B-mode ultrasound and Doppler.[36,37] Hemodynamic studies of patients at rest and after a test meal indicate a sharp increase in blood flow across the superior mesenteric within 15 minutes after the test meal.[33] The increase continues and is maximal at 45 minutes after food intake and then begins a slow decline. Most remarkable is the acceleration of diastolic forward flow that occurs during the augmented phase of superior mesenteric artery flow.

In a study by Nicholls et al four patients with symptoms of intestinal angina underwent duplex scanning and subsequent angiography of the mesenteric circulation.[37] All four exhibited loss of reverse flow in the superior mesenteric artery. The change in diastolic foward flow in the superior mesenteric artery was statistically significant when compared to normal subjects. Changes were also noted in peak systolic velocity in the celiac artery. Angiography confirmed severe superior mesenteric artery stenosis in these patients.

Nicholls et al also observed that the celiac artery blood flow was normal in the subjects with severe superior mesenteric artery stenosis, suggesting that this vessel's contribution to splanchnic flow is limited, and that its flow characteristics are determined by the hepatic and splenic runoff vessels. In addition, no significant change in flow in the celiac artery was noted during digestion. These authors also demonstrated that failure to identify the inferior mesenteric artery with the ultrasound equipment did not imply occlusion of this vessel.

In a report from the Mayo Clinic selected patients were imaged and Doppler determinations were obtained prior to and following a high-calorie liquid diet.[33] They demonstrated that within 30 to 45 minutes following the diet, blood flow in the superior mesenteric artery increased normally. They also demonstrated that if superior mesenteric artery flow fails to increase or shows a more turbulent pattern, a significant visceral artery stenosis should be suspected and confirmed by visceral arteriography.

Larson et al described two other noninvasive studies that may soon be used to assist in the diagnosis of chronic intestinal ischemia by assessing mucosal perfusion with reflectance spectrophotometry and tonometric measurements of mucosal pH.[38] Reflectance spectrophotometry allows rapid and repeated measurement of an index of mucosal hemoglobin concentration and an index of oxygen saturation based on spectral analysis of light reflected from the musosal surface. They have confirmed the correlation that changes in reflectance correlate linearly with changes in superior mesenteric artery blood flow. Technical difficulties make this test inappropriate at present to use in the human clinical setting.

Tonometry uses a semipermeable balloon in the gut lumen to measure indirectly intraluminal pH as a metabolic marker of the adequacy of oxygenation, and therefore a reflection of blood supply to the intestine. Tonometry has a nonlinear response to superior mesenteric blood flow reduction. The mucosal pH is constant at 75% of superior mesenteric artery flow but decreases thereafter, suggesting that a critical threshold for blood flow–dependent oxygen delivery is less than 75% of normal flow.

Since radiologic studies are paramount in establishing the correct diagnosis, the plain abdominal x-ray examination is usually the first radiologic study to be performed. In several small series, this study has been abnormal in 50% to 75% of patients.[39-41] Although a nonspecific ileus or evidence of ascites may be the only finding, marked bowel wall thickening, mucosal irregularity, separation of bowel loops and thickening of the valvulae conniventes are strongly suggestive, but not diagnostic, of intestinal ischemia. Infrequently, gas may be seen in the bowel wall or the portal system, but this is usually a late finding signifying extensive bowel infarction. Clemett and Chang reported eight patients for whom they felt the diagnosis was strongly suggested on the basis of barium studies of the small intestine.[42] These patients all had marked thickening of the bowel wall and valvulae conniventes resulting from congestion and edema, with mesenteric thickening contributing to separation of the bowel loops. Thumb printing caused by bowel wall edema and focal hemorrhage were found occasionally in their patients.

Scott et al evaluated plain abdominal x-ray films and small bowel studies in 74 patients with intestinal ischemia due to mesenteric arterial or venous occlusive disease.[41] Their data have shown that the extent of ischemic mucosal patterns seen on x-ray films did not correspond to the anatomic extent of infarction seen at the time of surgery or autopsy.

Invasive diagnostic studies

Arteriography is the diagnostic study of choice for all patients with all types of mesenteric ischemia. A lateral view of a flush aortogram is invaluable in obtaining adequate visualization of the origin of the celiac and superior mesenteric arteries (Fig. 14-7). If necessary, this is followed by selective injections of the superior mesenteric artery and celiac artery. The contrast volume should be kept to a minimum since patients with this diagnosis may already have reduced renal blood flow and compromised multisystem disease.

Nonocclusive bowel ischemia. Nonocclusive bowel ischemia may be diagnosed angiographically when nonspecific signs of mesenteric vasoconstriction are seen in the patient with a clinical picture of mesenteric ischemia.[42] Angiographic findings may vary from localized spasm to a diffuse pruned appearance of the entire mesenteric tree and may be consistent with nonocclusive ischemia also.[43] Papaverine or some other vasodilator agent should be infused in all patients once the diagnosis of nonocclusive bowel ischemia has been established. Commonly, papaverine is infused with a pump through the angiographic catheter, which is left within the SMA origin. Based on the angiographic appearance and the clinical course of the patient, decisions on the need for continued infusions can then be made.

SMA embolic bowel ischemia. The diagnosis of superior mesenteric artery embolization is generally made easily with a flush lateral aortogram or a selective injection of the superior mesenteric artery (see Fig. 14-5). Emboli will usually lodge in areas of branching or where the size of the embolus becomes disproportionate to the size of the artery. Emboli often result in a characteristic meniscus sign within the mesenteric artery.

Chronic visceral ischemia. Atherosclerotic disease leading to bowel ischemia is a multivessel occlusive disease involving the proximal segment of the mesenteric arteries. In chronic visceral ischemia, at least two of the three mesenteric vessels are usually occluded or severely stenotic. A large central anastomotic, or wandering mesenteric artery, is often present and indicates the presence of severe occlu-

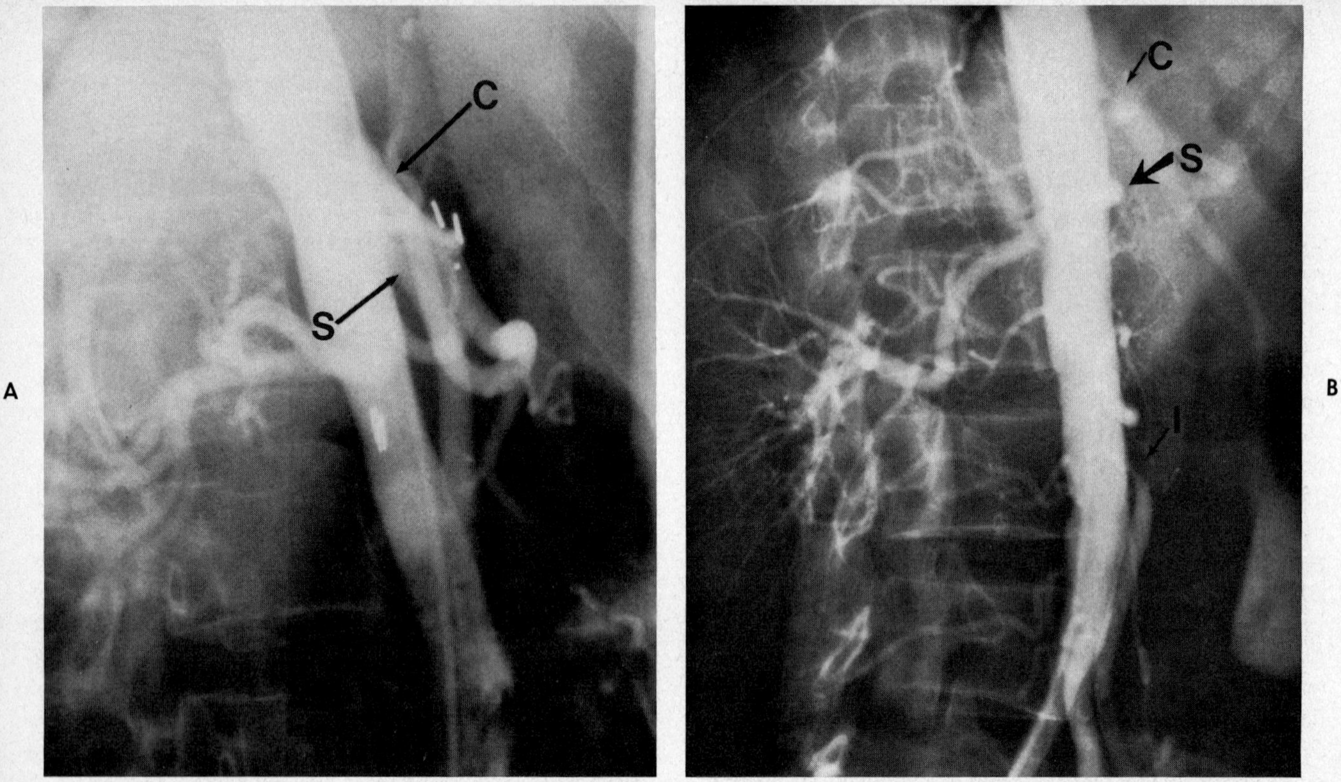

Fig. 14-7. A, This lateral view of the aorta demonstrates a normal origin of the celiac axis *(C)* and the superior mesenteric artery (S). **B,** This view shows the aorta in the lateral projection with the celiac axis *(C),* tightly stenotic at the origin. The large arrow denotes the superior mesenteric artery *(S)* and is occluded with a stump only at its origin. The inferior mesenteric artery *(I)* with the small arrow demonstrates the origin to be tightly stenotic. This arteriogram represents the typical angiographic manifestation for a patient who may be symptomatic with chronic mesenteric ischemia.

sive or stenotic disease of either the superior mesenteric or inferior mesenteric artery (see Fig. 14-4). If this collateral, or anastomotic, artery, is able to dilate appreciably in size, it may provide adequate blood flow to the intestines and the patient may be without symptoms. In general, if stenosis of 50% or more is seen in at least two or more of the three mesenteric vessels, the diagnosis can be established and early revascularization of the stenotic or occluded vessels should be considered.

Venous thrombotic ischemia. The diagnosis of mesenteric venous thrombosis is difficult. The use of the venous phase of selective mesenteric arteriograms may be helpful, but often it is difficult to detect the actual filling defects within the venous system. Therefore the diagnosis has depended on indirect findings such as incomplete venous filling. More recently, contrast-enhanced abdominal computerized tomography (CT) scanning has been shown to accurately detect portal vein, ovarian vein, and mesenteric vein thrombosis.[35,44-46] In the Harward et al series, a contrast-enhanced CT scan was done to search for abdominal disease after other evaluations were nondiagnostic.[35] This technique correctly established the diagnosis in 10 of 11 patients (91%). In one patient the CT scan initially was interpreted as normal, but later subtle findings were seen that changed the interpretation to mesenteric venous thrombosis. Harward et al speculate that magnetic resonance imaging (MRI) may be of even better diagnostic quality than CT scanning.

Colonoscopy or proctosigmoidoscopy can be of diagnostic benefit if the ischemic segment of bowel is situated within viewing reach of the scopes. This diagnostic test does not aid in determining the cause of the bowel ischemia, but can establish that infarcted or ischemic bowel does exist. Barium studies of the colon and small bowel are of limited or no value in diagnosing this disease.

TREATMENT

Treatment of visceral ischemia, whether embolic occlusive, nonocclusive, or venous thrombotic in origin, first requires a prompt, precise diagnosis angiographically. Exclusion of other common diseases that mimic bowel ischemia is essential since the treatment is radically different. Once the cause of the bowel ischemia has been established, a treatment decision can be implemented. This treatment may vary according to the cause of the ischemia, but when

Table 14-3. Operative mortality rates for various types of mesenteric ischemia and infarction

Causes of ischemia	Mortality rates (%)
Acute ischemia-thrombotic acute abdomen	60-90
Chronic ischemia-elective operation	5-24
Mesenteric venous occlusion	10-25

infarcted bowel is present, surgery will be required or death will occur.

The clinical manifestations of bowel infarction are nonspecific, and therefore the signal to initiate the chain of events that lead to surgery can be misleading. Although abdominal tenderness is usually present, only approximately 75% of patients will present with this symptom. Therefore nearly 25% of patients may have minimal signs of bowel infarction. This characteristic absence of signs early in the process makes the usual terms "nonsurgical abdomen" and "surgical abdomen" unfortunate, as the benefit of surgical intervention in bowel infarction is greatest when performed early. The best benefit from surgery, then, will be obtained when the abdomen is a nonsurgical abdomen. Once the development of peritonitis occurs, this indicates that infarction is advanced and the prognosis is poor. Therefore, the association of severe abdominal pain and minimal physical findings should always prompt a high suspicion for bowel infarction.

Improvements in surgical technique and perioperative management has greatly decreased the mortality associated with this surgery in the past. Hallett et al[33] have reviewed the surgical management of bowel ischemia and have noted three trends: (1) the patients are getting older, (2) surgical treatment has included more antegrade mesenteric bypass grafts or transaortic endarterectomies, and (3) late recurrence of symptoms has been minimized by attention to a more complete revascularization.[33] The fact that patients tolerate the initial surgery and subsequent second-look surgery is attributed to improved technology and skill. Most current studies show operative mortalities of <15% for patients with chronic ischemia symptoms and >75% for acute syndromes (Table 14-3).[5,33] As increasing experience is acquired with noninvasive studies, earlier recognition of this disease process should be possible, resulting in a further reduction of mortality.

Shaw and Rutledge initially described the concept of a second-look procedure and its importance was further emphasized by Zuidema.[47,48] However, the data supporting the second-look operation are not clear. Zuidema et al reported 49 successful cases of bowel revascularization and resection; however, only seven patients were subjected to a second look and only two of these needed further intestinal resection at the second operation.[49] Although second operations are strongly recommended based upon information derived during the first operation, a patient's postoperative course will not provide useful information to determine the need for a second-look procedure. In general, this procedure is performed 18 to 24 hours after the first operation. This interval should be used for vigorous resuscitation of the patient, including correction of any cardiovascular, hemodynamic, or renal problems.

General treatment measures

Treatment for all types of mesenteric ischemia should begin with rapid fluid replacement, correction of electrolyte imbalances, correction of hypotension and acidosis, and optimizing the cardiac and renal status. Optimizing cardiac performance is critical since cardiac disease predisposes to both nonocclusive and occlusive embolic bowel ischemia. Low cardiac output and increased venous pressure associated with congestive heart failure can produce splanchnic vasoconstriction with blood shunting away from the bowel and can further worsen the ischemia. Cautious use of digoxin, α-adrenergic agonists, and vasopressors is necessary since these agents can also decrease mesenteric blood supply. Cardiac diseases that are known to cause mesenteric emboli include ventricular thrombi following myocardial infarction, dilated cardiomyopathy, valvular disease, and atrial fibrillation. Broad-spectrum antibiotics are appropriate if perforation and peritonitis are suspected. Paramount in the nonoperative treatment is the rapid replacement of lost plasma volume and the correction of hemoconcentration. A Swan-Ganz catheter is recommended to optimize fluid replacement decisions, since large quantities of fluid will be extravasating out of the bowel wall.

Anticoagulation is indicated in patients who have embolic and venous thrombotic causes for their bowel ischemia.[50] Anticoagulation has not been shown to be helpful for chronic bowel ischemia. The cautious addition of dextran may help improve collateral blood flow, although some studies do not support this treatment.[51-53]

Intraarterial papaverine has proven to be helpful in many patients with nonocclusive bowel ischemia where vasodilation improves regional bowel flow in the distribution of the superior mesenteric artery.[54] Pharmacologic therapy with papaverine should be considered in patients who have angiographically demonstrated good perfusion of the vascular bed supplying the bowel but who have had an episode of hypotension or low flow that resulted in the bowel ischemia. The infusion should be at a constant rate of 30 to 60 mg/hr. Continuous monitoring of systemic arterial pressure and cardiac rate and rhythm is indicated since this amount of papaverine could have systemic effects. Other agents such as verapamil hydrochloride, nitroglycerine, and various other vasodilators have been tried but have not been shown to be superior to papaverine infusions. Papaverine infusions should continue for approximately 24 hours, and a repeat arteriogram should then be performed.

Dietary manipulations including frequent small feedings

and liquid meals may reduce symptoms and improve nutrition prior to surgical intervention in the patients with chronic mesenteric ischemia. Hyperalimentation is recommended when the patient has a long history of food avoidance and is in a malnourished state. Several days of such treatment may improve the ability of the patient to heal and tolerate the surgical intervention required.

Other medical treatment options for patients suffering from visceral ischemic symptoms are limited. A rare patient will experience symptomatic improvement using long-acting nitrates with meals or similar benefit from calcium channel blockers. While it is unclear why these medications may help selected patients, it is likely that these agents work by altering resistance in the mesenteric vascular bed.[55] There are no data demonstrating that patients derive long-term improvement from medical treatment. Hyperalimentation and other medical measures may improve the preoperative and postoperative courses but will not directly affect the course of the disease.

Specific therapy for chronic visceral ischemia

Surgery for mesenteric vascular disease in the asymptomatic patient is not indicated. For the symptomatic patient, numerous surgical approaches have been described. Some surgeons[56-58] prefer the transaortic endarterectomy of the visceral orifice, while other surgeons prefer bypass grafting. Considerable discussion has centered around the use of the supraceliac aorta for the bypass graft origination with antegrade flow vs a bypass originating from the infrarenal aorta with retrograde flow to the superior mesenteric artery.[33,56]

While both saphenous vein and synthetic grafts have been used as bypass material, initial reports of Dacron bypass grafts have found them to be at least as good as saphenous vein without any greater tendency for thrombosis.[57] Recent studies, however, have found prosthetic grafts to be better than vein bypasses because they have demonstrated less tendency to kink, less fibrotic constriction, easier surgical attachment, and they are readily available.[56,58]

The optimal number of vessels to be revascularized is still controversial. Some authors have advised revascularization of only one vessel because of the large collateral flow in the mesenteric vessels.[56-58] Others[59] believe that multivessel revascularization may be superior.

As an alternative to surgical management, several successful percutaneous transluminal angioplasties of the mesenteric vessels have been reported.[60-62] While long-term follow up data are not yet available, early results are promising. Instituting thrombolytic infusion prior to balloon dilation has also been reported with varied results.[61] Thrombolysis alone is generally not recommended for chronic mesenteric ischemia.

Since patients with chronic mesenteric ischemia are often chronically ill, malnourished, and anergic, preoperative hyperalimentation can be a valuable addition to therapy. If preoperative hyperalimentation cannot be done because of time constraints, postoperative hyperalimentation should be instituted.

Specific therapy for acute embolic mesenteric ischemia

Embolization to the superior mesenteric artery is the most common cause of intestinal infarction and the easiest to treat. An embolectomy can usually be done to restore blood flow.[63] If fragmentation of the embolus has occurred and emboli exist in branches, attempts should be made to remove as many of the emboli as possible. Bowel resection should be done if the emboli have resulted in infarction. If the superior mesenteric artery has thrombosed distally, formal revascularization, if possible, may need to be undertaken.

Tests of intestinal viability include clinical judgment, fluorescein dye, trypan blue, patent blue 5, Doppler probe, electromyography, pH readings, bowel temperature, oxygen electrodes, radionuclides, and tetrazolium analysis of mucosa.[64-67] Fortunately, clinical judgment has an overall accuracy of greater than 90%, which compares favorably with fluorescein-induced fluorescence.

The Doppler examination is sensitive and accurate.[66,67] The Doppler probe is placed on the mesenteric surface while the surgeon listens for arterial signals. Although the presence of arterial signals does not guarantee survival of the intestine, it strongly suggests that the bowel can be left in place rather than resected. The absence of arterial signals is certain evidence that irreversible ischemic damage has occurred.

The decision to perform a second-look operation will be derived from the surgeon's impression of the blood supply to the bowel and bowel viability obtained during the first operation. This procedure is usually performed 18 to 24 hours after the first. It is unusual for the postoperative course to predict the need for a second-look procedure unless the patient has decompensated significantly.

Specific therapy for mesenteric vein thrombosis treatment

Mesenteric vein thrombosis is a dangerous and somewhat uncommon abdominal catastrophe that has received little attention or study because of the small numbers of patients. Treatment is often hampered by the fact that approximately 50% of patients experience symptoms for 5 to 30 days prior to seeking medical attention.[68] Approximately 25% of patients report abdominal pain for more than 1 month.[68] It is difficult to project what percentage of patients with mesenteric vein thrombosis proceed to mesenteric infarction. In one study 5 of 16 patients (31%) developed severe peritonitis secondary to intestinal necrosis.[38]

Treatment is dictated by the extent of bowel involvement. The most common area of involvement is the superior mesenteric vein, and thrombosis here can produce ischemia in the middle portion of the small intestine. The colon is usually not affected by mesenteric venous thrombosis.

The initial steps of treatment include volume expansion. Broad-spectrum antibiotics with coverage for anaerobic organisms are recommended to diminish the septic complications that result from the bowel infarction. Anticoagulation is essential to prevent extension of the thrombotic process and worsening of the syndrome.[35,68,69] When possible, anticoagulation should begin preoperatively and the addition of low molecular weight dextran may also be helpful in establishing a rheologic effect. A second-look operation is mandatory.[71] Approximately 60% of cases will have additional areas of infarction at the time of the second-look operation.[69,72,73]

Although anecdotal reports suggest that venous thrombectomy may be useful, it should be considered only in those rare cases in which acute occlusion of the major splanchnic venous trunks is associated with extensive bowel ischemia and the thrombotic process does not extend into the smaller veins.[68,74,75]

A theoretically ideal method of treatment would be thrombolytic agents; however, many patients do not seek treatment until long after the initial appearance of symptoms, by which time the thrombus is organized and less amenable to thrombolysis. If the symptoms are relatively acute and the bowel is viable, systemic thrombolysis or thrombolysis using a catheter placed in the superior mesenteric artery can be attempted. We have achieved encouraging results infusing urokinase in three of five patients using this technique.

Specific therapy for nonocclusive mesenteric ischemia

Management of nonocclusive ischemia requires correcting the cause of the decreased perfusion, and intestinal resection if full-thickness infarction is present. Papaverine infusions have been of benefit in some patients with vasospasm. The addition of low molecular weight dextran serves a dual purpose because of its effect as a plasma expander and its potential value in decreasing sludging in the microcirculation. Anticoagulants may be of value in nonocclusive bowel ischemia, but this has never been proven. Intestinal decompression by nasogastric suction and optimization of the cardiac output are both essential. Laparotomy is indicated in patients who are felt to have bowel infarction. Short segments of bowel should be resected if they are nonviable or questionably viable. If extensive segments of bowel are involved, resection of the frankly necrotic bowel should be done at the initial operation followed by a second-look operation to reexplore the areas of marginally ischemic bowel.

CELIAC ARTERY COMPRESSION SYNDROME

In 1963 Harjola described a clinical picture characterized by postprandial abdominal pain of varying duration and invariably associated with the finding of a systolic epigastric bruit.[76] Dunbar et al described this as the median arcuate ligament syndrome with the most common anatomic pattern showing involvement of the celiac axis and superior mesenteric artery.[77] Many authors have reported experiences with symptomatic patients who were found to have compression of only the celiac axis by either the left crus of the diaphragm or the celiac ganglion.[32,78,79]

Symptoms

The selection of patients suitable for surgical repair is difficult because of the vague symptoms and sparsity of clinical signs. Most patients complain of abdominal pain commonly situated in the epigastrium. A distinguishing characteristic of these patients is that some feel that the pain is related to activity and posture as well as to the amount of food ingested. In a proportion of patients there is no relationship to food at all, and other nonspecific complaints and findings occur. This condition usually occurs in younger patients and more commonly in females. A bruit in the epigastrium is frequently audible, and all laboratory investigations with the exception of arteriography are normal.

In most patients lateral arteriography demonstrates indentation of the anterior wall of the celiac artery at its origin (see Fig. 14-6). Collateral channels may develop, particularly in the pancreaticoduodenal and the gastroduodenal arteries, and may produce retrograde filling of the hepatic artery.

Operative management

The literature describing operative management of patients with arcuate ligament syndrome is somewhat confusing. The selection of patients is often complicated by vague symptoms, paucity of physical signs, and the unreliability of the epigastric bruit. Edwards et al[80] reported asymptomatic bruits in 6.5% of 200 adults between 17 and 30 years of age. Arteriography performed in patients with unrelated symptoms has shown narrowing of the celiac artery in 24% of cases. Drapanas and Bron have reported a high incidence of psychologic disturbance in patients with typical symptoms of celiac artery compression. Other investigators have postulated that division of nerve fibers of the celiac ganglia for purposes of access could possibly explain the relief of pain from the operation.[81] This explanation seems somewhat unlikely since the dissection described in some of the surgical papers is not extensive enough to result in damage to the ganglia. It is likely that this disease entity truly exists without firm diagnostic criteria.

In reviewing 238 surgically treated patients Lord and Tracy found 83% remained asymptomatic.[82] Evans reviewed 59 cases over a period of 8 years and identified no correlation between initial symptoms and results. As the period of follow-up became longer, the success rate fell to 41%.[83]

It is clear that selection of patients for surgery with this diagnosis is made difficult by the vague symptoms and sparsity of clinical findings. Arteriographic findings are also unfortunately nonpredictive of a good outcome. There is little question that this is a true clinical entity, but at this time data are not adequate to predict outcomes.

CHRONIC MESENTERIC ISCHEMIA IN CHILDHOOD AND ADOLESCENCE

Chronic mesenteric ischemia is uncommon in adults and extremely rare in childhood. Meacham and Dean reported four children treated for chronic mesenteric ischemia.[84] Their ages ranged from 30 months to 17 years, and the initial symptoms varied from a clinically silent ischemia in the 30-month-old child to gastrointestinal infarction in the 17-year-old adolescent. Abdominal coarctation was present in three of the four cases. The fourth case had the appearance of fibromuscular dysplasia. Operative treatment was undertaken in all patients, resulting in substantial improvement.

CONCLUSION

As the U.S. population ages, chronic mesenteric ischemia will likely become an increasing problem. Fortunately, duplex scanning has provided a noninvasive method to demonstrate the hemodynamic compromise that occurs during obstruction of mesenteric flow. These noninvasive tests will allow earlier recognition in treatment of patients with chronic mesenteric ischemia. A more aggressive approach to the early recognition and surgical intervention of chronic and acute mesenteric symptoms must occur before mortality will be lessened. The concept of an acute abdomen needs to be relaxed when one considers the possibility of acute embolic, venous thrombotic, or arterial thrombotic ischemia leading to bowel infarction. The earlier the operation, the better the outcome.

REFERENCES

1. Dunphy JE: Abdominal pain of vascular origin, Am J Med 192:109, 1936.
2. Mikkelsen WP: Intestinal angina: its surgical significance, Am J Surg 94:262, 1957.
3. Shaw RS and Rutledge RH: Superior mesenteric artery embolectomy in the treatment of massive mesenteric infarction, N Engl J Med 252:595, 1957.
4. Mikkelsen WP and Zaro JA Jr: Intestinal angina: report of a case with preoperative diagnosis and surgical relief, N Engl J Med 260:912, 1959.
5. Bergan JJ et al: Nontraumatic mesenteric vascular emergencies, J Vasc Surg 5:903, 1987.
6. Rogers DM et al: Mesenteric vascular problems: a 26-year experience, Ann Surg 195:554, 1982.
7. Rosenman LD and Gropper AN: Small intestine stenosis caused by infarction: an unusual sequel of mesenteric artery embolism, Ann Surg 14:254, 1955.
8. Litten M: Uber die Folgen des Verschlusses der Arteria Mesaraica Superior, Arch pathol Anat 63:289, 1875.
9. Bailey RW et al: Pathogenesis of nonocclusive mesenteric ischemia: studies in a porcine pig model induced by periocardial tamponade, Surg Forum 33:14, 1982.
10. Bulkley GB, Kvietz PR, and Granger DN: Relation between intestinal blood flow and oxygen uptake, Am J Physiol 244:6605, 1983.
11. Chiu C-H, Scott HJ, and Gurd FN: Circulatory collapse following the restoration of blood flow to the occluded superior mesenteric artery, Surg Forum 21:47, 1970.
12. Brown RA et al: Ultrastructural changes in the canine mucosal cell after mesenteric arterial occlusion, Arch Surg 101:290, 1970.
13. Calman C et al: Serum lactic dehydrogenase in diagnosis of the acute surgical abdomen, Surgery 44:43, 1958.
14. Glenn TM and Lefer AM: Role of lysosomes in the pathogenesis of splanchnic ischemia shock in cats. Circ Res 27:783, 1970.
15. Schennach W and Dorfmann A: Problem of acute obstruction of the mesenteric arteries, Thoraxchirurgie 20:457, 1972.
16. Marston A: Causes of death in mesenteric arterial occlusion. II. Observations on revascularization of the ischemic bowel, Ann Surg, 158:960, 1963.
17. Vyden JK: The systemic effects of acute superior mesenteric vascular insufficiency. In Boley SJ, ed: Vascular Disorders of the Intestines, New York, 1971, Appleton-Century-Crofts.
18. Ottinger LW and Austen WG: A study of 136 patients with mesenteric infarction, Surg Gynecol Obstet 124:251, 1967.
19. Boley SJ, Brandt LJ, and Veith FJ: Ischemic disorders of the intestine, Curr Probl Surg 15:1, 1978.
20. Ottinger LW et al: Left colon ischemia complicating aorto-iliac reconstruction, Arch Surg 105:841, 1972.
21. Mathews JE and White RR: Primary mesenteric venous occlusive disease, Am J Surg 122:579, 1971.
22. Johnson CC and Baggenstoss AH: Mesenteric vascular occlusion. I. Study of 99 cases of occlusion of veins, Mayo Clin Proc 24:628, 1949.
23. van Way CW III, Brockman SK, and Rosenfeld L: Spontaneous thrombosis of the mesenteric veins, Ann Surg 173:561, 1971.
24. Gruenberg JC, Smallridge RC, and Rosenberg RD: Inherited anti-new clinical entity, Ann Surg 181:791, 1975.
25. Collins GJ et al: Hypercoagulability in mesenteric venous occlusion: report of two cases, Am J Surg 132:390, 1976.
26. Peters TG et al: Antithrombin III deficiency causing postsplenectomy mesenteric venous thrombosis coincident with thrombocytopenia, Ann Surg 185:229, 1976.
27. Green D, Granger DR, and Blei AT: Protein C deficiency in splanchnic venous thrombosis, Am J Med 82:1171, 1987.
28. Hoyle M et al: Small bowel ischaemia and infarction in young women taking oral contraceptives and progestational agents, Br J Surg 64:533, 1977.
29. Williams LF Jr: Vascular insufficiency of the intestines, Gastroenterology 61:757, 1971.
30. Brandt LJ and Boley SJ: Celiac axis compression syndrome: a critical review, Am J Dig Dis 23:633, 1978.
31. Evans WE: Long-term evaluation of the celiac band syndrome, Surgery 76:867, 1974.
32. Szilagyi DE et al: The celiac artery compression syndrome: does it exist? Surgery 72:849, 1972.
33. Hallett JW et al: Recent trends in the diagnosis and management of chronic intestinal ischemia, Ann Vasc Surg 4:126, 1990.
34. Rheudasil JM et al: Surgical treatment of chronic mesenteric arterial insufficiency, J Vasc Surg 8:495, 1988.
35. Harward TRS et al: Mesenteric venous thrombosis, J Vasc Surg 9:328, 1989.
36. Jager K et al: Measurement of mesenteric blood flow by duplex scanning, J Vasc Surg 3:462, 1986.
37. Nicholls SC et al: Use of hemodynamic parameters in the diagnosis of mesenteric insufficiency, J Vasc Surg 3:507, 1986.
38. Larson MV et al: Assessment of intestinal ischemia by endoscopic measurement of mucosal perfusion: a pilot study in dogs, Gastroenterology 1990 (in press).
39. Thomas ML: Radiology-plain films and barium studies of the ischemic bowel, Clin Gastroenterol 1:581, 1972.
40. Tomchik FS, Wittenberg J, and Ottinger LW: The roentgenographic spectrum of bowel infarction, Radiology 96:249, 1970.
41. Scott JR et al: Acute mesenteric infarction, Am J Roentgenol 113:269, 1971.

42. Clemett AR and Chang J: The radiologic diagnosis of spontaneous mesenteric venous thrombosis, Am J Gastroenterol 63:209, 1975.
43. Bookstein JJ et al: Angiographic aspects of experimental nonocclusive intestinal ischemic injury, Am J Roentgenol 128:923, 1977.
44. Rosen A et al: Mesenteric vein thrombosis: CT identification, Am J Roentgenol 143:83, 1984.
45. Vogelzang RL et al: Thrombosis of the splanchnic veins: CT diagnosis, Am J Roentgenol 150:93, 1988.
46. Miller VE and Berland LL: Pulsed Doppler duplex sonography and CT of portal vein thrombosis, Am J Roentgenol 145:73, 1985.
47. Shaw RS and Rutledge RH: Superior mesenteric artery embolectomy in the treatment of massive mesenteric infarction, N Engl J Med 252:595, 1957.
48. Zuidema GD: Surgical management of superior mesenteric arterial emboli, Arch Surg 82:267, 1961.
49. Zuidema GD et al: Superior mesenteric artery embolectomy, Ann Surg 159:548, 1964.
50. Vellar ID et al: Superior mesenteric artery embolism, Med J Aust 1:801, 1973.
51. D'Angelo CJ, Ameriso LM, and Tredway JB: Survival after mesenteric arterial occlusion by treatment with low molecular weight dextran, Circulation 27:662, 1963.
52. Frajndlich D, Taylor RL: Infarction of the small bowel, JAMA 189:327, 1965.
53. Serjeant JCB: Mesenteric embolus treated with low molecular weight dextran, Lancet 1:139, 1965.
54. Renton CJC. Non-occlusive intestinal infarction, Clin Gastroenterol 1:655, 1972.
55. Granger DN et al: Intestinal blood flow, Gastroenterology 78:837, 1980.
56. Ricotta JJ and Williams GM: Endarterectomy of the upper abdominal aorta and visceral arteries through an extraperitoneal approach, Ann Surg 192:633, 1980.
57. Pokrovsky AV and Kasantchjan PO: Surgical treatment of chronic occlusive disease of the enteric visceral branches of the abdominal aorta: experience with 119 operations, Am Surg 191:51, 1980.
58. Rapp JH et al: Durability of endarterectomy and antegrade grafts in the treatment of chronic visceral ischemia, J Vasc Surg 3:799, 1986.
59. Stanton PE et al: Chronic intestinal ischemia: diagnosis and therapy, J Vasc Surg 4:338, 1986.
60. Levy PJ, Haskell L, and Gordon RL: Percutaneous transluminal angioplasty of splanchnic arteries: an alternative method to elective revascularization in chronic visceral ischemia, Eur J Radiol 7:239, 1987.
61. Kohler M et al: (Successful treatment of superior mesenteric artery thrombosis with local high-dose urokinase therapy) Erfolgreiche Behandlung einer Thrombose der Arteria Urokinasetherapie, Klin Wochenschr 63:722, 1985.
62. Roberts L Jr et al: Transluminal angioplasty of the superior mesenteric artery: an alternative to surgical revascularization, Am J Roentgenol 141:1039, 1983.
63. Bergan JJ and Hoehn J: Superior mesenteric artery embolectomy, JAMA 188:935, 1964.
64. Cooperman M, Martin EW Jr, and Carey LC: Evaluation of ischemic intestine by Doppler ultrasound, Am J Surg 139:73, 1980.
65. Locke R, Hauser CJ, and Shoemaker WC: The use of surface oximetry to assess bowel viability, Arch Surg 119:1252, 1984.
66. Marfuggi RA and Greenspan M: Reliable intraoperative prediction of intestinal viability using a fluorescent indicator, Surg Gynecol Obstet 152:33, 1980.
67. Wright CB and Hobson RW: Prediction of intestinal viability using Doppler ultrasound technique, Am J Surg 129:642, 1975.
68. Matthews JE and White RR: primary mesenteric venous occlusive disease, Am J Surg 122:579, 1971.
69. Abdu RA, Zakhour BJ, and Dallis DJ: Mesenteric venous thrombosis-1911 to 1984, Surgery 101:383, 1987.
70. Grendell JH and Ockner RK: Mesenteric venous thrombosis, Gastroenterology 82:358, 1982.
71. Trinkle JK et al: The operative management of idiopathic mesenteric venous thrombosis with intestinal infarction, Ann Surg 35:338, 1969.
72. Jona J et al: Recurrent primary mesenteric venous thrombosis, JAMA 227:1033, 1974.
73. Carr N and Jamieson MH: Superior mesenteric venous thrombosis, Br J Surg 68:343, 1981.
74. Inahara T: Acute superior mesenteric venous thrombosis: treatment by thrombectomy, Ann Surg 174:956, 1971.
75. Polk HC: Experimental mesenteric venous occlusion. III. Diagnosis and treatment of induced mesenteric venous thrombosis, Ann Surg 163:432, 1966.
76. Harjola PT: A rare obstruction of the celiac artery, Ann Chir Gynaecol 52:547, 1963.
77. Dunbar JD et al: Compression of the celiac trunk and abdominal angina: preliminary report of 15 cases, Am J Roentgenol Radium Ther Nucl Med 95:731, 1965.
78. Brandt LJ and Boley SJ: Celiac axis compression syndrome: a critical review, Dig Dis Sci 23:633, 1978.
79. Reilly LM et al: Late results following operative repair for celiac artery compression syndrome, J Vasc Surg 2:79, 1985.
80. Edwards AJ et al: Experience with coeliac axis compression syndrome, Br Med J 1:342, 1970.
81. Drapanas T and Bron KM: Stenosis of the celiac artery, Ann Surg 164:1085, 1966 (editorial).
82. Lord RS and Tracy GD: Coeliac artery compression, Br J Surg 67:590, 1980.
83. Evans WE: Long-term evaluation of the celiac band syndrome, Surgery 76:867, 1974.
84. Meacham PW and Dean RH: Chronic mesenteric ischemia in childhood and adolescence, J Vasc Surg 2:878-885, 1985.

Chapter 15

RENOVASCULAR DISEASE

Jeffrey W. Olin
Andrew C. Novick

HISTORICAL PERSPECTIVE

Richard Bright first demonstrated an association between hypertension and the kidney. This association was taken several steps forward in 1934 when Harry Goldblatt elucidated the pathogenesis of renovascular hypertension based upon experimental renal artery constriction in animals.[1] Shortly thereafter, Page and Helmer and Braun-Menendez et al published reports describing a renal pressor system, which led to an early understanding of the renin angiotensin system.[2,3] Since these early times, much has been learned about the pathogenesis, diagnosis, and treatment of renovascular disease, and several excellent accounts of the history are described in more detail elsewhere.[4-6]

Exactly how common renovascular disease and renovascular hypertension are is a matter of dispute. The prevalence of renovascular *hypertension* varies between 0.2% and 32%.[7,8] The higher percentages occur among tertiary referral centers and highly selected populations. Renovascular hypertension is much less common in blacks than in whites.[9] It has been suggested that less than 0.5% of an entire hypertensive population has renovascular hypertension.[10]

These data on prevalence of renovascular hypertension are difficult to interpret for several reasons. The only true way to diagnose renovascular hypertension is to correct the renal artery stenosis (surgery or percutaneous transluminal angioplasty) and demonstrate cure of the hypertension. The prevalence of renovascular *disease* is much higher than renovascular *hypertension*. We have just completed a study to determine the prevalence of atherosclerotic renal artery stenosis in 395 consecutive patients who have atherosclerosis elsewhere.[11] There was greater than 50% renal artery stenosis in 38% of patients with abdominal aortic aneurysms, 33% in patients with aortoocclusive disease, and 39% in patients with lower extremity occlusive disease. These patients did not have the usual clinical clues to suggest renal artery stenosis. High-grade bilateral disease was present in approximately 13% of patients. Similar associations have been documented in patients with coronary disease.[12]

The average age of patients with generalized atherosclerosis is approximately 65 to 70 years. The prevalence of hypertension among this age group is approximately 65%. Thus there is a high prevalence of renovascular disease and a high prevalence of hypertension in the elderly population. However, renovascular hypertension per se is much less common. Some patients have renal artery stenosis and essential hypertension. Also, not all patients who have anatomic evidence of renal artery stenosis have hypertension. Dustan et al[13] demonstrated that only 50% of the people with significant renal artery stenosis in fact had hypertension.

With the advent of newer and more potent antihypertensive agents, control of blood pressure is not as much of a problem as it was in the past. However, with the higher prevalence of unilateral and bilateral significant renovascular disease, patients now undergo intervention more often for preservation of renal function than they do for control of blood pressure.[14]

CLASSIFICATION OF RENOVASCULAR DISORDERS

Atherosclerosis

Approximately 65% to 70% of all renovascular lesions are caused by atherosclerosis. This disease may be limited to the renal artery but more commonly is a manifestation of generalized atherosclerosis involving the abdominal aorta and coronary, cerebral, and lower extremity vessels. Atherosclerotic stenosis usually occurs in the proximal 2 cm of the renal artery, and distal arterial or branch involvement is distinctly uncommon (Fig. 15-1).

Because of the proximal location of these lesions, oblique aortic views are often needed to adequately visualize the

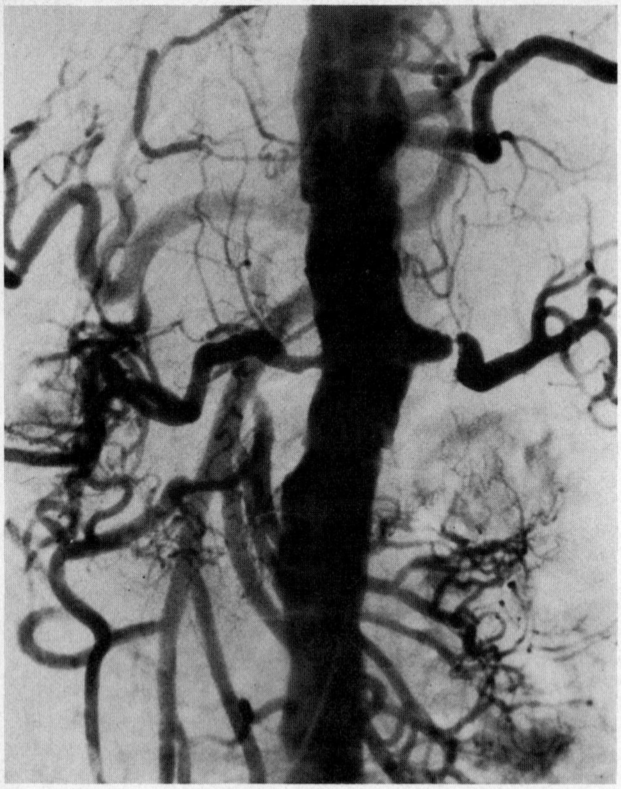

Fig. 15-1. This aortogram demonstrates a severely atherosclerotic aorta. The right renal artery demonstrates an osteal lesion that reduces the lumen by 50% to 60%. The left renal artery shows an atherosclerotic lesion several centimeters distal to the takeoff in which the lumen is reduced by >95%. This is a typical nonostial lesion.

area of stenosis. The lesion involves the intima of the artery and in two thirds of the cases appears as an eccentric plaque. In the remainder the vessel is circumferentially involved with narrowing of the lumen and destruction of the intima. Dissecting hematomas may complicate this disease, sometimes resulting in thrombosis of the entire vessel.

There have been relatively few published reports on the natural history of atherosclerotic lesions in patients managed nonoperatively. The available data suggest that progressive arterial stenosis, occasionally resulting in total occlusion, is a relatively common sequela of this disease. In 1968 Wollenweber, Sheps, and Davis[15] reviewed 30 patients with atherosclerotic renovascular disease who had been followed up with serial renal arteriograms from 3 to 88 months apart; progressive renal artery stenosis was observed unilaterally in 13 patients (43%) and bilaterally in 6 patients (20%). Also in 1968, Meaney, Dustan, and McCormack reported progression of atherosclerotic renal artery stenosis in 14 of 39 patients (36%) followed with serial arteriography during intervals ranging from 6 months to 7 years.[16]

More recently, Schreiber and co-workers reviewed the outcome of atherosclerotic renovascular disease in 85 patients treated medically and followed with sequential renal arteriography during intervals of 3 to 172 months.[17] The mean angiographic follow-up interval was 52 months, and the mean clinical follow-up period in these patients was 87 months. Progressive renal artery obstruction from atherosclerosis was observed in 37 patients (44%), including 14 patients (16%) who developed complete arterial occlusion. Clinical follow-up checks revealed that serial decreases in both overall renal function ($P < .02$) and the size of the involved kidney ($P < .001$) occurred more commonly in patients who developed progressive renovascular disease than in those who did not. However, serial blood pressure control was no different in these two groups, and therefore it was not a useful marker for progressive disease. This study indicates not only that atherosclerotic renal artery disease progresses in a large number of patients, but also that such progression is commonly associated with clinically detectable loss of functioning renal parenchyma.

Fibrous dysplasia

Fibrous dysplasias comprise approximately 40% of all renovascular disorders. These lesions are considered to be congenital dysplasias with maldevelopment of the fibrous, muscular, and elastic tissues of the renal artery. They are subcategorized according to the layer of the arterial wall involved.[18] This classification is important since each type of fibrous dysplasia has distinct histologic and angiographic features, and each type occurs in a different clinical setting.

Primary intimal fibroplasia occurs in children and young adults, and accounts for approximately 10% of the total number of fibrous lesions. This lesion is characterized by a circumferential accumulation of collagen inside the internal elastica lamina. Disruption and duplication of the elastica interna occur more often in younger patients, with dissecting hematomas as a complication in some patients. Intimal fibroplasia with complicating medial dissection is characterized pathologically by large dissecting channels in the outer one half of the media. These lesions are thought to develop because of defects in the internal elastica with resultant medial dissection and aneurysmal dilation.

Arteriography in primary initial fibroplasia reveals a smooth, fairly focal stenosis, usually involving the midportion of the vessel or its branches (Fig. 15-2). Dissecting hematomas may distort the area of the stenosis. With nonoperative management, progressive renal artery obstruction and ischemic atrophy of the involved kidney invariably occur. Severe intimal fibroplasia may subsequently develop de novo in the contralateral renal artery. Although primary intimal fibroplasia most commonly affects the renal arteries, this may also occur as a generalized disorder with concomitant involvement of the carotid, upper and lower extremities, and mesenteric vessels.

Medial fibroplasia is the most common of the fibrous lesions, making up 75% to 80% of the total number. It tends to occur in 25- to 50-year-old women and often involves

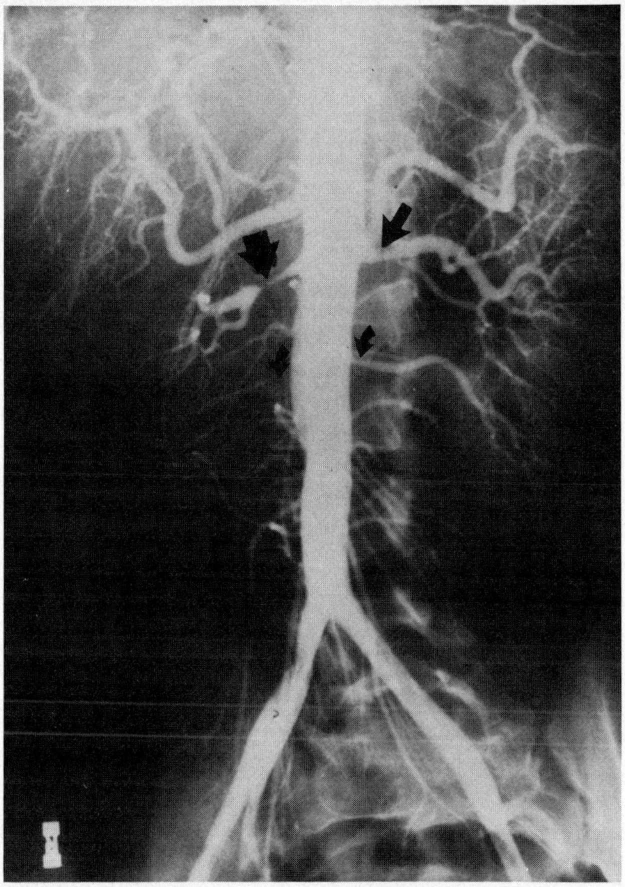

Fig. 15-2. This aortogram demonstrates the classic arteriographic appearance of intimal fibroplasia. The left renal artery stenosis demonstrates a focal area of narrowing simulating a band around the renal artery (*arrow*). The right renal artery demonstrates a long smooth area of narrowing (*large arrow*). The lower pole renal arteries bilaterally also demonstrate smooth long areas of narrowing (*small arrows*).

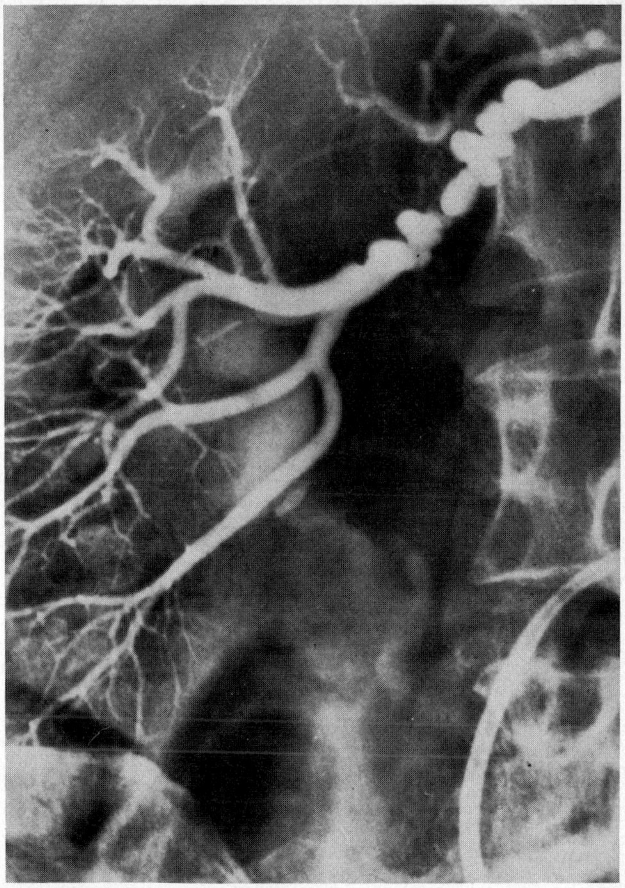

Fig. 15-3. This renal arteriogram demonstrates typical medial fibroplasia of the renal artery. The "string of beads" appearance of the renal artery involves the distal portion of the main renal artery and the "beads" are larger than the normal diameter of the artery.

both renal arteries. It may involve other vessels in the body, most notably the carotid, mesenteric, and iliac arteries. Microscopically, the internal elastic membrane is focally variably thinned and lost. Within the alternating thickened areas much of the muscle is replaced by collagen, hence the term *medial fibroplasia*. In other areas, thinning of the media occurs to the point of complete loss, and microaneurysms can be seen as saccules lined by only the external elastica. In extreme cases, giant aneurysms may be found in association with medial fibroplasia.

Arteriographically, medial fibroplasia demonstrates a typical "string of beads" appearance involving the distal two thirds of the main renal artery and branches (Fig. 15-3). The areas of stenosis are often overshadowed by contrast medium in the microaneurysms, making the degree of actual stenosis difficult to assess. The aneurysms themselves are greater in diameter than the normal renal artery proximal to the disease, and extreme collateral circulation is absent. These are important features in differentiating the lesion from perimedial fibroplasia.

Schreiber, Novick, and Pohl[17] studied the natural history of renal artery disease caused by medial fibroplasia in 66 patients who had follow-up serial angiograms. Progressive renal artery stenosis occurred in 22 patients (33%) and contrary to an earlier report, this occurrence was no different in patients 40 years of age or older. Significantly, there were no cases of progression to total arterial occlusions in this group. Also, clinical follow-up studies revealed that serial decreases in either overall renal function or the size of the involved kidney seldom occurred in patients with progressive medial fibroplasia, suggesting that the risk of losing renal function is relatively small in patients with this disease who are managed medically.

Perimedial fibroplasia occurs predominantly in 15- to 30-year-olds and therefore has been referred to as "girlie disease." Of all fibrous lesions 10% to 15% are perimedial fibroplasias. These tightly stenotic lesions only occur in the renal artery and consist pathologically of a collar of dense collagen enveloping the renal artery for variable lengths and thicknesses. The collagen is deposited in the outer border of the media and usually replaces a considerable portion of the media; in some areas it may completely replace the media. Islands of smooth muscle are occasionally seen trapped within the collagenous ring. Special stains show that the lesion is confined within the external elastic lamina and contained in all cases by intact adventitial connective tissue. The arterial lumen may be further compromised by a process of secondary intimal fibroplasia. It has been suggested that this secondary thickening of the intima is related to slowing of blood flow through a narrowed arterial segment, with resultant platelet and fibrin deposition and subsequent fibrous organization.

The arteriogram of perimedial fibroplasia may give the appearance of arterial beading, but careful observation shows that the caliber of the normal segment of the vessel is not exceeded by the "bead." This fact, along with the frequent occurrence of external collateral circulation, differentiates this lesion angiographically from that of medial fibroplasia (Fig. 15-4). Perimedial fibroplasia produces severe stenosis and, although complicating thrombosis or dissection is relatively uncommon, progressive obstruction with ischemic renal atrophy occurs in almost all patients managed nonoperatively.

Fibromuscular hyperplasia is an extremely rare disease, comprising only 1% to 2% of fibrous lesions, and tends to occur in children and young adults. This is the only renal arterial disease in which true hyperplasia of the smooth muscle cells is present. The renal artery shows a concentric thickening of its wall with a mixture of proliferating smooth muscle and fibrous tissue in variable quantity. Arteriographically, fibromuscular hyperplasia appears as a smooth stenosis of the renal artery or its branches and, from a radiographic standpoint, may be indistinguishable from intimal fibroplasia. Follow-up serial angiographic studies have shown that most patients with this disease have developed progressive vascular obstruction.

Renal artery aneurysms

Renal artery aneurysms may require surgical treatment when they are the cause of significant hypertension or to obviate the risk of rupture. The latter is of greatest concern with aneurysms that are larger than 2 cm in diameter and

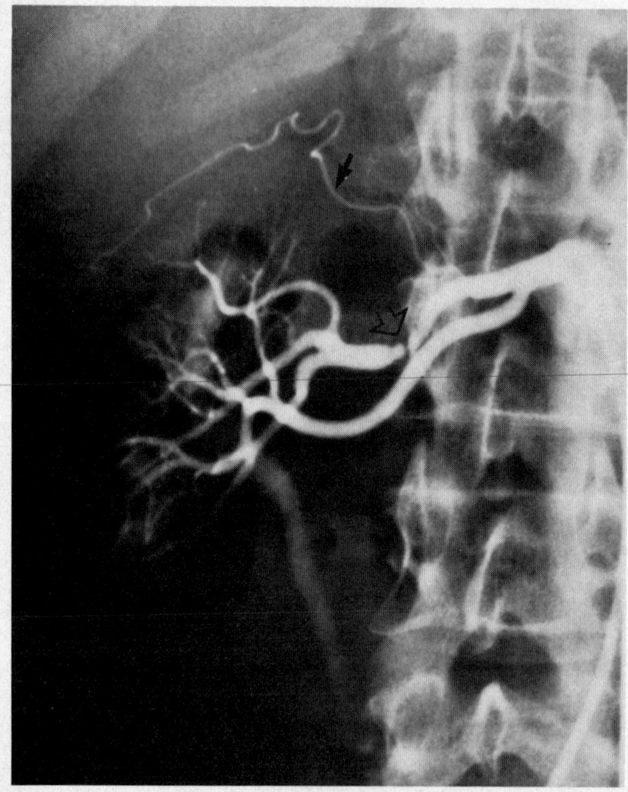

Fig. 15-4. Perimedial fibroplasia. Note the tightly stenotic lesion in the distal right renal artery. One may appreciate the appearance of arterial beading but the "bead" is smaller than the normal vessel. (*open arrow*). A collateral vessel is noted (*closed arrow*).

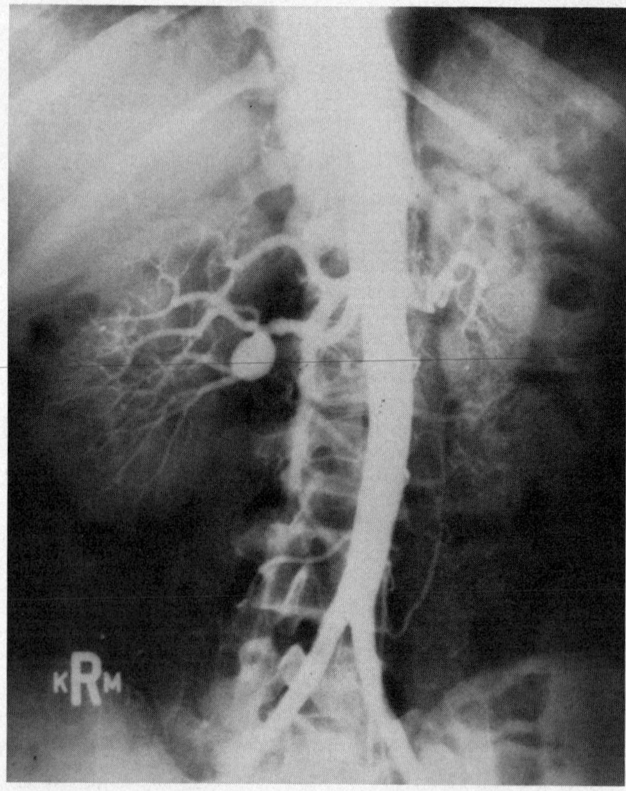

Fig. 15-5. Saccular right renal artery aneurysm.

noncalcified, particularly when they occur in premenopausal women because of the predisposition for aneurysmal rupture during pregnancy.[19] According to the classification of Poutasse, there are four basic types of renal artery aneurysms: saccular, fusiform, dissecting, and intrarenal.[20]

Saccular aneurysms, which account for about 75% of renal artery aneurysms, are the most common. They generally occur at the bifurcation of the renal artery, perhaps due to an inherent weakness in the wall of the artery at this point (Fig. 15-5). Because of this location, branch arterial involvement is common. These aneurysms may become involved with secondary atherosclerotic degeneration and/or intramural calcification. There are several mechanisms by which saccular aneurysms may be causally related to hypertension. These include compression or displacement of renal artery branches with resulting ischemia, aneurysmal erosion into a renal vein with formation of an arterial venous fistula, mural thrombus formation within the aneurysm with peripheral renal embolization, and the association of some aneurysms with stenosing fibrous renal artery disease. It is also well appreciated that saccular aneurysms can cause hypertension in the absence of these sequelae, most likely because of relative renal ischemia caused by the turbulent flow of blood as it passes through the aneurysmally dilated arterial segment. Saccular aneurysms may be quite variable in their location and extent. The incidence of bilateral and multiple renal aneurysms is approximately 25%.

Fusiform renal artery aneurysms are almost always associated with stenosing fibrous renal artery disease. The latter is the cause for the severe hypertension generally seen in these patients. Fusiform aneurysms actually represent a severe post stenotic dilation of the renal artery. Dissecting renal artery aneurysms are most often a complication of primary intimal fibroplasia or atherosclerosis. These are often manifested clinically by the sudden onset of pain that stimulates renal colic. In some patients, the dissection in the wall of the vessel may reenter the lumen more distally. In other patients, total arterial occlusion with renal infarction may ensue. Intrarenal arterial aneurysms are of mixed origin and may be congenital, post traumatic, iatrogenic, neoplastic, or associated with polyarteritis nodosa. Intrarenal aneurysms that occur following blunt trauma or closed renal biopsy will occasionally resolve spontaneously with expectant management. Intrarenal aneurysms do have the propensity for rupture, and surgical treatment may be indicated if their diameter is greater than 2 cm.

Renal arteriovenous fistulas

Renal arteriovenous fistulas are relatively uncommon lesions that are generally discovered during the course of angiographic evaluation for suspected renal or renovascular disease.[19] The most common clinical symptoms are hematuria, high output cardiac failure, and diastolic hypertension. Congenital or cirsoid fistulas comprise approximately 25% of these lesions and are the result of a developmental anomaly of the involved renal vessels. The angiographic appearance is one of multiple small interconnecting arterial and venous channels with impaired distal renal parenchymal vascularity and early filling of the renal vein. Idiopathic fistulas make up only 3% to 5% of these lesions and have no apparent cause. They are considered to develop as a result of venous erosion by a preexisting arterial aneurysm. Acquired fistulas are the most common type, accounting for 70% to 75% of all renal arteriovenous fistulas. By far the most common cause is iatrogenic trauma resulting from needle biopsy of the kidney. The majority of the latter will close spontaneously. Fistulas may also be acquired through blunt or penetrating trauma, tumor, inflammation, or prior renal surgery.

Renal artery thrombosis or embolism

Acute occlusion of the renal artery or its branches may result from thrombosis or embolism. Embolic occlusions may occur as a complication of rheumatic heart disease, infective endocarditis, cardiac operations, saccular aneurysm of the renal artery, or renal artery catheterization. Thrombosis of the renal artery is somewhat less common and is associated with a variety of diseases such as intimal fibroplasia, segmental arteritis, polycythemia vera, tumors, trauma, or umbilical arterial catheterization. Blunt trauma to the renal artery may result in disruption of the intima with subsequent dissection and thrombotic occlusion.

Miscellaneous

Middle aortic syndrome, Takayasu's arteritis, and neurofibromatosis are all associated with renal artery stenosis. External compression or obstruction of the renal arteries by neural tissue, musculocutaneous fibers, or diaphragmatic crura rarely occur.

PATHOGENESIS OF RENOVASCULAR HYPERTENSION

In 1934 Goldblatt et al first demonstrated that constriction of the main artery in dogs produced elevation in blood pressure, which was sustained.[1] The mechanism of the hypertension was not known at the time of these experiments. Since then a number of humoral factors have been shown to play an important role in the generation and maintenance of hypertension.

Animal models for renovascular hypertension include the two kidney-one clip (2K-1C) model, which is a model for unilateral renal artery stenosis and the one kidney-one clip (1K-1C) model of renovascular hypertension, which is the model for renal artery stenosis to a solitary functioning kidney or bilateral renal artery stenosis. Although the acute phases of both of these models are similar, different events occur in the chronic phase.

In the 2K-1C model (unilateral renal artery stenosis) de-

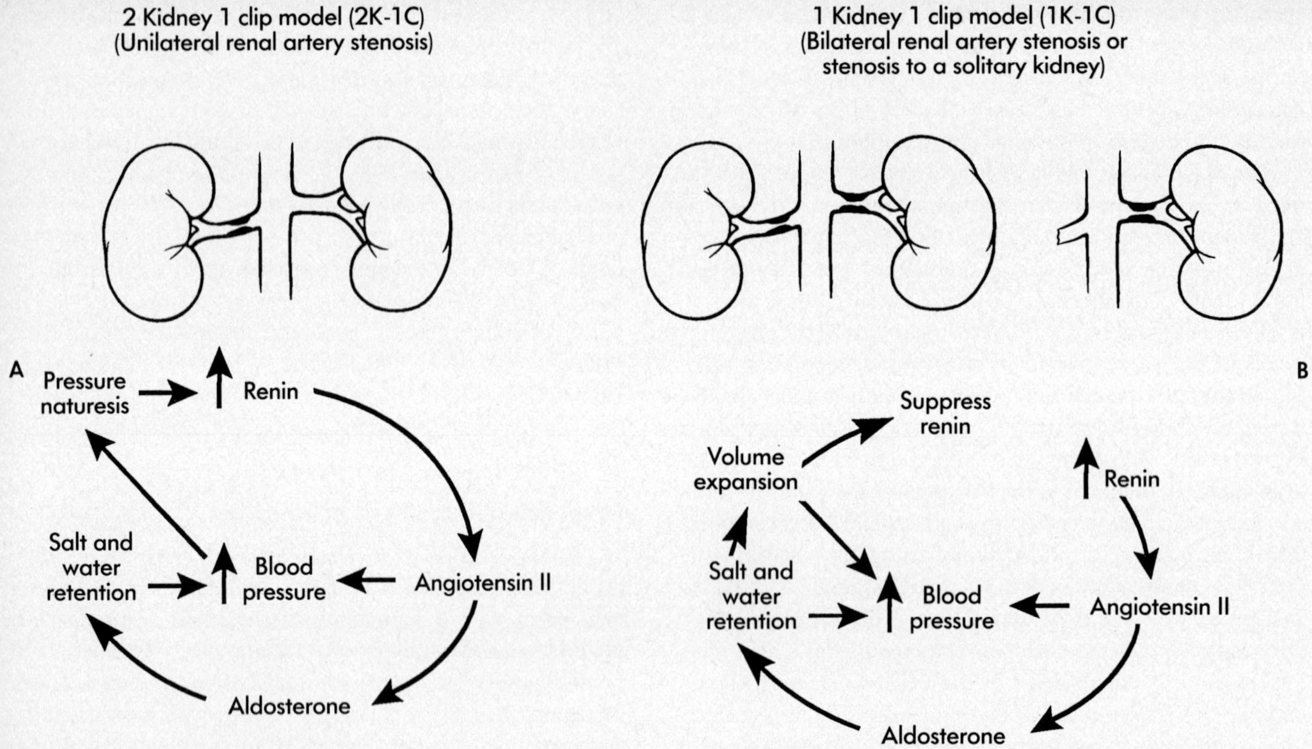

Fig. 15-6. Pathogenesis of renovascular hypertension in unilateral and bilateral renal artery stenosis.

creased renal blood flow stimulates the production of renin (Fig. 15-6, *A*). Renin cleaves the proenzyme angiotensinogen to form angiotensin I and in the presence of angiotensin converting enzyme is converted to angiotensin II. Angiotensin II has several important functions: (1) It elevates blood pressure directly by causing systemic vasoconstriction. (2) It stimulates aldosterone secretion, causing sodium reabsorption and potassium and hydrogen ion secretion in the cortical collecting duct. (3) It changes the intrarenal hemodynamics, such as diminishing glomerular filtration, by decreasing glomerular capillary surface area and redistributing intrarenal blood flow. The salt and water retention caused by excess aldosterone production is rapidly excreted by the contralateral (normal) kidney by pressure naturesis. This produces a cycle of renin-dependent hypertension.[21-24] Administration of an angiotensin converting enzyme inhibitor blocks the vicious cycle and early in the course of renovascular hypertension returns the blood pressure to normal. There is decreased blood flow to the kidney with the clipped (stenotic) artery, increased renin secretion from the ischemic kidney, and suppressed renin secretion from the contralateral kidney in the 2K-1C model.

In the 1K-1C model of renovascular hypertension, there is a similar decrease in blood flow to the affected kidney(s), acutely causing the secretion of renin and synthesis of angiotensin II and aldosterone (Fig. 15-6, *B*). Angiotensin II directly elevates blood pressure and aldosterone causes salt and water retention. Now there is not a normal kidney that can *sense* the elevated blood pressure, therefore, no pressure naturesis occurs. The increased aldosterone causes sodium and water retention and volume expansion. The expanded plasma volume suppresses plasma renin activity, thus converting the animal from renin-mediated hypertension to volume-mediated hypertension.[23-25] During this stage, administration of an angiotensin converting enzyme inhibitor or angiotensin II antagonist does not decrease blood pressure or change renal blood flow.[25] Dietary restriction of sodium or administration of diuretics will convert the animal to a renin-mediated form of hypertension, and the animal will then become sensitive to a converting enzyme inhibitor or angiotensin II antagonist. As will be discussed later in this chapter, functional renal insufficiency may occur in humans when converting enzyme inhibitors are administered to patients with bilateral renal artery stenosis or renal artery stenosis to a solitary kidney.

The time course for the chronic phase to occur may be weeks in the 1K-1C rat model whereas it may take up to 4 months in the 2K-1C rat model.[26] In the 2K-1C model loss of renin sensitivity in the chronic state may also occur and is caused by an inability of the contralateral (normal) kidney to excrete an increased sodium load when the blood pressure is increased (pressure naturesis). This attenuation is thought to be produced by changes in intrarenal hemodynamics and structural changes in the microvasculature of the kidney.[27] A whole host of other mechanisms have been implicated such as impairment of sodium transport by an ouabain-like naturetic factor, elevated levels of vasopressin, which acts as a potent vasoconstrictor and antidiuretic hormone as well as increased sensitivity of the vascular smooth muscle to the effects of angiotensin II.[28]

CLINICAL MANIFESTATIONS OF RENOVASCULAR DISEASE

There are a number of clinical features that may be present in patients with renovascular disease (see the accompanying box). None of these features alone can be used with certainty to make the diagnosis. However, the presence of one or more of these features will increase the likelihood of finding renal artery stenosis. In a series of 76 patients with one or more of the following clinical clues, renal arteriography demonstrated significant renal artery stenosis to be present in 70% of patients.[11]

Clinical clues to suggest renovascular disease

1. Onset of hypertension before the age of 30 or after the age of 55
2. Hypertension that was well controlled and has become difficult to control
3. Malignant or accelerated hypertension
4. Resistant hypertension
5. Epigastric bruit (systolic/diastolic)
6. Atrophic kidney or discrepancy in size between the two kidneys
7. Azotemia while receiving angiotensin converting enzyme (ACE) inhibitors
8. Azotemia in the elderly patient with atherosclerosis elsewhere
9. Patients with generalized atherosclerosis

Onset of hypertension before the age of 30 or after the age of 55 years

The onset of primary (essential) hypertension is usually between the ages of 30 and 55. When hypertension begins below the age of 30, secondary causes should be sought, and fibromuscular dysplasia would be one of the more common secondary causes in this age group. When hypertension appears for the first time in a patient over the age of 55, a likely diagnosis is atherosclerotic renovascular disease.

Hypertension that was well controlled and has become more difficult to control

When the blood pressure has been reasonably well controlled on a particular blood pressure regimen and the blood pressure suddenly becomes more difficult to control, one should suspect a secondary cause. Often the secondary cause, such as renovascular disease, is superimposed upon previously diagnosed essential hypertension.

Malignant or accelerated hypertension

Patients with Grade III or Grade IV hypertensive retinopathy have an extremely high prevalence of renovascular disease.[29] Davis et al[8] demonstrated that renovascular hypertension was present in 32% of 76 white patients and 11% of 29 black patients studied with arteriography.

Resistant hypertension

Renovascular disease and renovascular hypertension occur in patients with mild, moderate, or severe hypertension. As discussed earlier, patients with renal artery stenosis may also have normal blood pressure. The likelihood of having renal artery stenosis is increased in patients with truly resistant hypertension. In one study 72% of patients with atherosclerotic renovascular disease and 65% of patients with fibromuscular dysplasia had increased blood pressure despite a good medical regimen.[30] This report was published before many of the newer antihypertensive agents were available, leading some investigators to believe that normalization of blood pressure may occur as frequently in patients with renovascular disease as it does in patients with essential hypertension.[31]

Resistant hypertension is defined as failure to normalize blood pressure (<140/90 mm Hg) following a good medical regimen consisting of at least three drugs with different mechanisms of action such as a diuretic, sympathetic inhibiting agent, and a vasodilator. Under this circumstance, the presence of renovascular hypertension should be strongly considered.

Epigastric bruit

In the cooperative study of renovascular hypertension, abdominal bruits were detected in only 9% of patients with essential hypertension compared with 46% of patients with renovascular hypertension.[29] Patients with fibromuscular dysplasia were more likely to have bruits than patients with atherosclerotic renovascular disease (57% vs 41%).

The presence of a short systolic bruit in the epigastrium is frequently not significant. However, a holosystolic epigastric bruit, or more importantly a systolic/diastolic epigastric bruit, increases the likelihood of renovascular disease. A systolic/diastolic bruit more often occurs in patients with fibromuscular disease (53%) than in patients who have atherosclerotic disease (12.5%).[32] Hunt et al found a systolic/diastolic bruit in one third of patients with atherosclerotic renovascular disease and in 75% of patients with fibromuscular disease.[30] The presence of a bruit is helpful, but the absence does not exclude the diagnosis of either atherosclerotic renovascular disease or fibromuscular dysplasia.

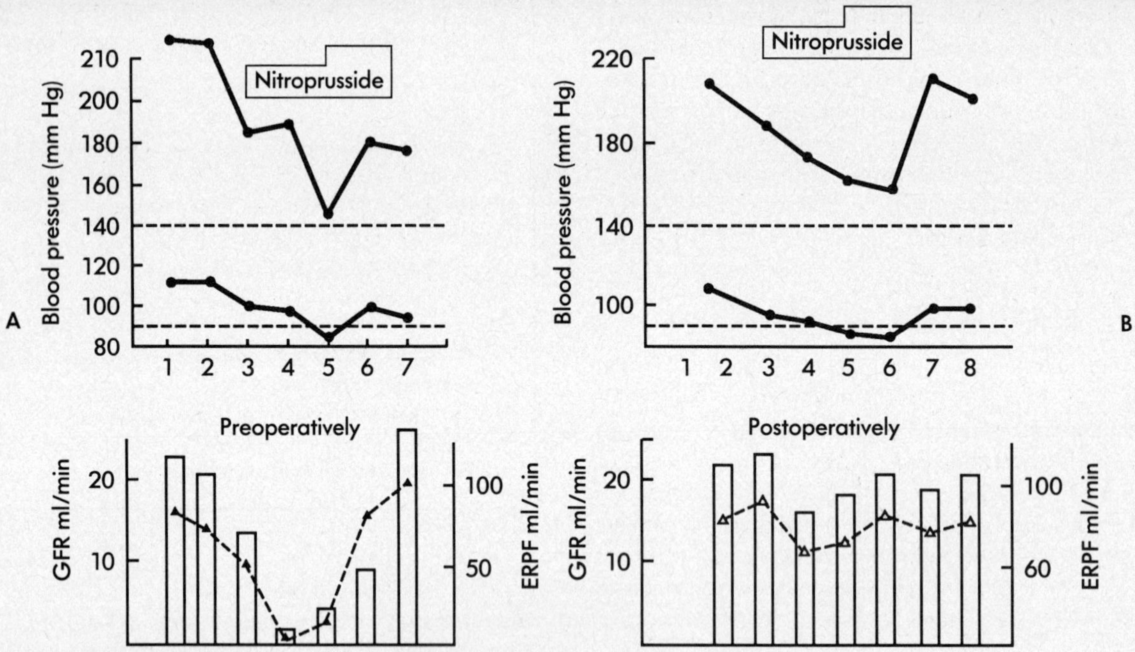

Fig. 15-7. A, Glomerular filtration rate (*GFR*) and renal blood flow (*ERPF*) decreases markedly as blood pressure is lowered with sodium nitroprusside in a patient with bilateral renal artery stenosis. **B,** This is reversible following unilateral renal revascularization. (From Textor SC et al: AM J Med 76(5B):29, 1984.)

Atrophic kidney or discrepancy in size between the two kidneys

In the past, an atrophic kidney was thought to be due to chronic pyelonephritis. While this may be true in the pediatric population, several studies have demonstrated that a small kidney in adults is most often associated with renovascular disease. Gifford et al[33] demonstrated total occlusion or severe stenosis of the renal artery supplying the atrophic kidney in 53/75 patients (71%). More importantly, 22 patients (42%) had significant stenosis of the contralateral (normal sized kidney) renal artery. Similarly, in a group of 40 patients with a totally occluded renal artery, there was associated contralateral renal artery stenosis in 31 patients (78%).[34] If an atrophic kidney or a discrepancy in size between the kidneys is discovered in an adult, a thorough investigation for the presence of renovascular disease should be undertaken.

Azotemia while receiving angiotensin converting enzyme (ACE) inhibitors

There are numerous reports suggesting that patients who develop azotemia while receiving angiotensin converting enzyme (ACE) inhibitors have either bilateral renal artery stenosis, renal artery stenosis to a solitary kidney, or decompensated congestive heart failure in the sodium depleted state.[35-38]

There are two mechanisms by which renal functional impairment may occur with the use of antihypertensive agents. The first may occur with any antihypertensive agent and occurs when a critical perfusion pressure is reached below which the kidney is no longer able to be perfused (Fig. 15-7). This has been shown by the infusion of sodium nitroprusside in patients with high-grade bilateral renal artery stenosis. When the critical perfusion pressure was reached, urine output, renal blood flow, and glomerular filtration rate declined and later returned to normal when the blood pressure increased above this critical perfusion pressure.[35] The exact pressure necessary to perfuse a kidney with renal artery stenosis varies with the degree of stenosis and is different among different patients.

The second mechanism is confined to patients receiving angiotensin converting enzyme inhibitors and may occur despite no significant change in blood pressure (Fig. 15-8). Patients with high-grade bilateral renal artery stenosis or renal artery stenosis to a solitary kidney may be highly dependent on angiotensin II for glomerular filtration. This is particularly common in patients who receive a combination of ACE inhibitor and diuretic[39] or in patients who are placed on a sodium restricted diet.[40] Under these circumstances, the constrictive effect of angiotensin II on the efferent arteriole allows for the maintenance of normal transglomerular capillary hydraulic pressure, thus allowing glomerular filtration to remain normal in the presence of markedly diminished blood flow (Fig. 15-9). In this instance glomerular filtration is highly dependent on angiotensin II, and when an angiotensin converting enzyme inhibitor is administered, the efferent arteriolar tone is no longer maintained and glomerular filtration is therefore decreased. A

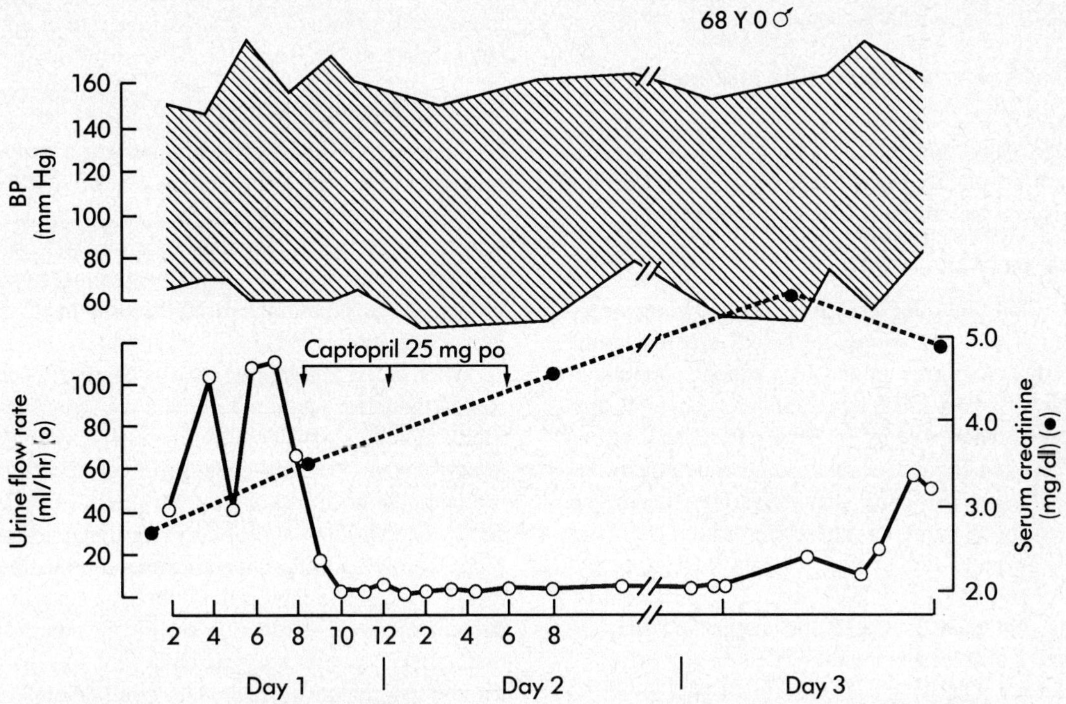

Fig. 15-8. This patient had renal artery stenosis to a solitary kidney. After the administration of captopril, the urine ouput decreased, and serum creatinine increased despite no change in the systemic blood pressure. (From Textor SC et al: AM J Med 76(5B):29, 1984.)

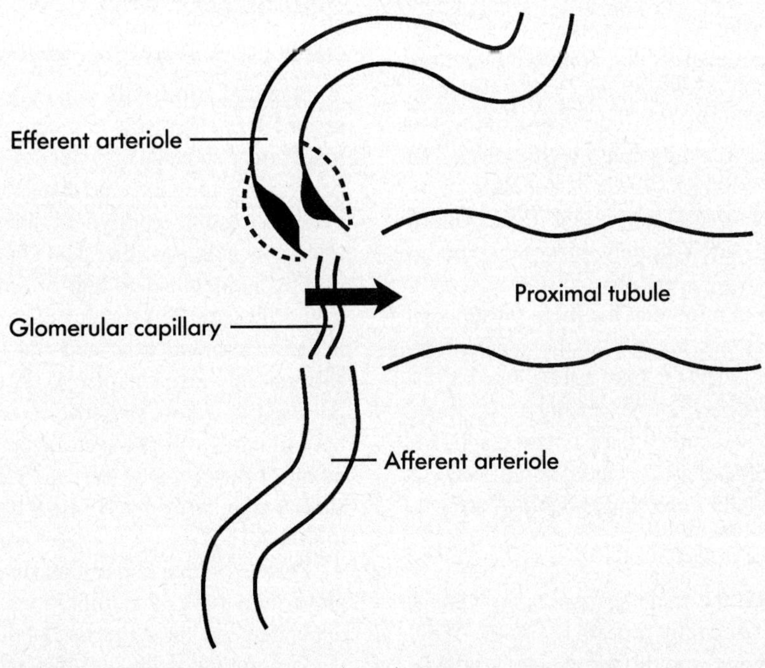

Fig. 15-9. Patients with high-grade bilateral renal artery stenosis or renal artery stenosis to a solitary kidney may be highly dependent on the efferent arteriolar constriction caused by angiotensin II in preserving transglomerular capillary hydraulic pressure (*arrow*) and glomerular filtration rate. When an ACE inhibitor is given, the efferent arteriole dilates (*dotted line*), and blood is shunted past the glomerulus.

similar situation is seen in patients with decompensated congestive heart failure who are sodium depleted.[38]

Azotemia in the elderly patients with atherosclerosis elsewhere

It has been suggested that an elderly patient who has azotemia with no readily explainable cause should have a careful search for the presence of renovascular disease.[10,37]

EPIDEMIOLOGY

Generally, fibromuscular disease occurs in a younger patient population (usually women) whereas atherosclerotic renal artery disease occurs in an older patient population. Renovascular disease is much more common in whites than it is in blacks.[9] There seems to be a particularly strong correlation between cigarette smoking and renovascular disease.[41,42] This is not surprising since cigarette smoking is quite prevalent in all forms of atherosclerosis.

There are no good studies that evaluate the role of hypercholesterolemia in patients with atherosclerotic renal artery stenosis, but there is one report suggesting that aggressive control of hyperlipidemia may cause regression of an atherosclerotic renal artery lesion.[43] In all likelihood hypercholesterolemia is as strong a risk factor for atherosclerotic renal artery stenosis as it is for all other forms of atherosclerosis.

DIAGNOSTIC STUDIES FOR RENOVASCULAR DISEASE

There are a number of screening tests for renovascular disease. These have differing sensitivities and specificities and will be discussed in detail in the following section. These include newer noninvasive techniques that either directly visualize the renal arteries (i.e., duplex scanning) or use pharmacologic agents to exaggerate the stimulation of the renin-angiotensin-aldosterone system or decrease in renal blood flow and glomerular filtration rate in the kidney with renal artery stenosis. Arteriography, however, remains the gold standard.

It is important to keep in mind that the mere presence of renal artery stenosis does not mean that the renal artery lesion is functionally significant. It may not be causing the high blood pressure, and it may not be causing a decrement in renal function. Hopefully, some of these newer diagnostic tests will not only define the anatomy but also will sort out which lesions are functionally important and which are not.

Intravenous urography

Maxwell et al described the rapid sequence intravenous pyelogram as a useful screening procedure in the early 1960s.[44] Since that time many studies have demonstrated an extremely high false positive and false negative rate. In the cooperative study of renovascular hypertension[45] 11.4% of patients with essential hypertension had an abnormal intravenous urogram and 17% of patients with documented significant renal artery stenosis by arteriography had a normal intravenous urogram. A false positive rate of up to 41% has been reported.[46,47]

Nuclear imaging modalities

Radionuclide imaging techniques are a noninvasive and relatively safe way of evaluating renal blood flow and excretory function. However, they have similar degrees of sensitivity as the intravenous urogram and are much less specific in that many patients with essential hypertension or glomerular or tubulointerstitial diseases have abnormal radionuclide studies.[14,46]

When an ACE inhibitor such as captopril is added to the standard nuclear medicine studies, the sensitivity and specificity increases considerably especially for unilateral renal artery stenosis.[48-50] This technique involves using glomerular radionuclide tracers such as ^{99m} tc-diethylenetriaminepentaacetic acid (DTPA) and performing dynamic renal scintigraphy before and one hour after the administration of captopril, 25 mg. The captopril produces an acute and reversible decrement in renal function on the ipsilateral side to the renal artery stenosis whereas renal function (glomerular filtration) will remain normal on the contralateral (nonstenotic) side. Prime activity curves will show a delayed uptake of technetium^{-99m} labeled DTPA as well as delayed excretion. These early reports show excellent sensitivity and specificity of this test for unilateral renal artery stenosis. However, this may not be demonstrated in patients with bilateral renal artery stenosis or with renal artery stenosis to a solitary functioning kidney.[51]

Duplex scanning of the renal arteries

Standard ultrasonic imaging provides an accurate assessment of renal size and contour. However, patients with renal artery stenosis may not demonstrate an atrophic kidney or a discrepancy in renal size. Recently, with the advent of better ultrasonic equipment, duplex scanning of the renal arteries is now possible. The Doppler spectra from the renal arteries is identical to that of a normal carotid artery flow. When the arterial segment is stenotic, there are alterations in laminar blood flow and the Doppler signature changes substantially (see Chapter 3). A number of Doppler criteria are used to assess the severity of the stenosis such as the ratio of renal to aortic systolic peak velocities and the broadening of the Doppler spectra. These techniques give a sensitivity ranging from 83% to 91% with a specificity of 95% to 100%.[52,53]

This technique is particularly attractive because it is safe and noninvasive. The limitations are that its quality is highly dependent on the expertise of the physician or technician performing the study and the study is time-consuming. Excessive weight and bowel gas may limit the quality of the study. As ultrasonic equipment improves, this technique, no doubt, will play a more prominent role in screening for renovascular disease.

Arteriography

Several angiographic techniques have been used to visualize the renal arteries. These include intravenous digital subtraction, intraarterial digital subtraction, or standard cut film arteriography.

The intravenous digital subtraction arteriogram has been used by many as an initial screening test for renovascular disease.[54] This technique is noninvasive in that the contrast medium is injected directly into a peripheral vein or into a catheter advanced into a more central vein such as the superior vena cava. Often the proximal renal arteries are well visualized. However, there may be difficulty visualizing the distal main renal artery or its branches, thus making it a poor screening test when searching for fibrous disease of the renal arteries. The amount of contrast medium needed is much more than that for an intraarterial digital subtraction arteriogram (DSA) and often approaches that necessary for standard cut film arteriography. Havey et al[54] has reviewed the literature of 406 hypertensive patients who had intravenous digital subtraction arteriograms and standard arteriograms. They found a sensitivity and specificity of the intravenous DSA to be 87.6% and 89.5%, respectively. In this same report 7.4% of 965 intravenous digital subtraction arteriograms were considered uninterpretable because of technical problems. Therefore the intravenous DSA seems to be a reasonable screening test for patients suspected of having atherosclerotic renovascular disease. In our institution we are using this method to follow the natural history of atherosclerotic renal lesions. The intravenous DSA, however, is poor for patients with fibromuscular dysplasia and should not be used under these circumstances.

The intraarterial DSA is performed by inserting a catheter into the femoral artery by the Seldinger technique and injecting contrast medium. A digital computer allows subtraction of the bone and soft tissues. This technique provides excellent resolution of the aorta, main renal arteries, and its branches. There are several advantages of this technique. An aortogram with visualization of the main renal arteries can be accomplished with much smaller amounts of contrast medium than standard cut film arteriography. The resolution is much better than with intravenous digital subtraction arteriography and is at least as good as cut film arteriography for the aorta and main renal arteries. The disadvantage of this technique is that the smaller renal arteries cannot be visualized as well as with cut film arteriography.[14] When diseases of the smaller vessels are searched for such as emboli, aneurysms, vasculitis, and certain forms of fibromuscular disease, standard arteriography with selective renal artery injections should be performed.

Standard cut film arteriography is the gold standard for the diagnosis of renal artery stenosis. It is no more invasive than the intraarterial DSA. However, the resolution may be slightly better.

When patients undergo arteriography, a lateral view of the aorta should be obtained to assess the origin of the celiac and superior mesenteric arteries if surgical revascularization is contemplated and a hepatorenal or splenorenal bypass is considered. It is important to know the status of inflow (proximal celiac artery) before either of these operations is performed.

DETERMINING THE FUNCTIONAL SIGNIFICANCE OF A STENOTIC RENAL ARTERY

Once renal artery stenosis is demonstrated on arteriography, it becomes important to determine whether or not it is functionally significant. In other words, is the lesion causing the patient's hypertension or leading to a decrement in renal function? The captopril stimulated renogram, which was discussed earlier in this chapter, may prove to be useful in separating out those lesions that have a propensity to decrease renal function from those that do not.

Plasma renin activity (PRA)

Maxwell et al[55] reviewed 540 patients reported in the literature to assess the value of plasma renin activity in the diagnosis of renovascular hypertension. There is a sensitivity of 57% and a specificity of 66%. The false negative and false positive rates were extremely high at 43% and 34%, respectively. The PRA did not predict which patients benefited from renal revascularization. Elevated plasma renin activity may be present in approximately 15% of patients with essential hypertension.

In an attempt to increase the utility of measuring plasma renin activity, Muller and colleagues administered captopril, 50 mg orally, and obtained PRA 60 minutes later.[56] In patients with normal renal function, the test correctly identified all 56 patients with proven renovascular disease. False positive results occurred in only 2 of 112 patients (1.8%) with essential hypertension.

Renal vein renin ratios

Measurement of renin produced from the renal vein of the kidney with renal artery stenosis compared to the renal vein of the "normal" kidney has been used as a method for predicting which patients may benefit from intervention such as surgery or percutaneous transluminal angioplasty. A number of factors can interfere with renin measurements, which will limit the utility of this particular test. If patients are not receiving any medications that suppress renin production, and if furosemide or converting enzyme inhibitors are administered before blood is taken from the renal vein, the test may be accurate in predicting in whom a cure of renovascular hypertension may occur.[50,57]

A renal vein renin ratio of 1.5:1 or greater with suppression of renin production by the contralateral (nonstenotic) kidney is considered a positive renal vein renin response. Hughes et al demonstrated that when a renal vein renin ratio greater than 1.4:1 was combined with a duration of hypertension of less than 5 years, 19 out of 20 patients

(95%) had a cure of their renovascular hypertension.[58] A number of reports have now been published that show that renal vein renin lateralization does not predict which patient will have an *improvement* in blood pressure after surgical revascularization or percutaneous transluminal angioplasty.[59-62] The renal vein renin ratio may be helpful in selecting a patient in whom one can expect a cure in hypertension, but it does not predict which patient will show an improvement after interventional therapy. Therefore this test is somewhat limited in its overall usefulness.

TREATMENT OF RENOVASCULAR DISEASE

The three modalities available for the treatment of renovascular disease include medical therapy, surgical therapy, and percutaneous transluminal angioplasty (PTA). In the near future atherectomy or laser therapy of the renal arteries may be useful, but these techniques are not currently available in most centers and their effectiveness is unknown.

The best treatment for renovascular disease is not known because there have been no controlled prospective randomized trials comparing medical therapy with either surgical therapy or PTA. Currently a study is under way at our institution in which patients with high-grade bilateral atherosclerotic renal artery stenosis are randomly assigned either medical therapy or surgical therapy. It is hoped that this study will provide an answer to this very important question.

The usual reasons for intervention in renal artery disease include failure to adequately control blood pressure, despite a good antihypertensive regimen, or renal artery lesions, which have the potential to jeopardize or already have jeopardized renal function. Failure to control blood pressure may appear as truly drug-resistant hypertension (elevated blood pressure despite maximal doses of a good triple drug regimen), intolerable side effects to antihypertensive medications, noncompliance, or the opinion that it may not be desirable to keep a young person on antihypertensive medications for the next 30 or 40 years.

The therapeutic options available will be discussed in the following sections for both of the most common underlying types of renovascular disease, atherosclerosis, and fibromuscular disease.

Medical therapy

The same principles apply to treating patients medically with renovascular disease as they do to treating patients with essential (primary) hypertension. With a few minor modifications, the principles of drug therapy are the same as those discussed in the previous chapter. One should begin with one antihypertensive agent. If the blood pressure is not controlled, a second agent of a different pharmacologic class should be added and a third agent with a different mechanism of action added if necessary.

If the patient has a known unilateral renal artery stenosis, an ACE inhibitor either alone or with a diuretic is the preferred initial therapy. If, however, the patient has high-grade bilateral renal artery stenosis or significant renal artery stenosis to a solitary functioning kidney, an ACE inhibitor should either not be used or should be used with great caution because of the possibility of causing renal insufficiency. Case et al demonstrated the long-term efficacy of captopril in renovascular hypertension in approximately 90% of patients.[63] Havelka et al[64] have demonstrated that captopril plus a diuretic and β-blocker was more effective at one month and 30 months in patients with atherosclerotic renovascular disease than was standard triple therapy of a diuretic, a sympathetic inhibiting agent, and a direct vasodilator.

In addition to simply treating the blood pressure, all cardiovascular risk factors need to be modified. Almost all patients with atherosclerotic renal artery disease die from complications of atherosclerosis such as myocardial infarction and stroke. The same approach should be taken with these patients as with patients who have atherosclerosis elsewhere. The incidence of coronary artery disease is very high in this patient population, therefore the presence of coronary artery disease should be carefully searched for. Patients should be encouraged to stop smoking and their diabetes and lipid disturbances should be aggressively treated.

Surgical revascularization

Operative techniques and mortality. The operative mortality for surgical revascularization has varied greatly in the past from 0% to 9.3%.[14,61,65-70] In an initial series from our institution, Novick et al demonstrated a 2% operative mortality in 100 consecutive patients with atherosclerotic renal artery stenosis undergoing renal revascularization.[61] This extremely low operative mortality is caused by meticulous perioperative screening for other cardiovascular risk factors such as coronary artery disease and carotid artery disease. These extrarenal manifestations of atherosclerosis are corrected before considering the patient for surgical revascularization of the renal arteries. An additional reason for the low operative morbidity and mortality is advances in surgical techniques. In a more recent series of 241 patients with atherosclerotic renal artery disease, the operative mortality was 2.1%.[14] This acceptably low operative mortality has occurred despite changes in the type of renal artery disease that is currently being encountered. In the earlier years, more patients developed focal renal artery stenosis, but as the age of our population increases, more patients are developing diffuse atherosclerosis in conjunction with their atherosclerotic renal artery disease. From 1981 to 1984 at the Cleveland Clinic, 87% of the patients had diffuse atherosclerosis.

Whenever possible, autogenous tissue such as saphenous vein or native artery should be used. In patients with renal artery stenosis and a relatively normal aorta, an aortorenal saphenous vein bypass can be performed. In patients who have significant disease of the aorta, in which there are no indications for aortic replacement, a hepatic artery to renal artery saphenous vein bypass can be performed on the right, splenorenal bypass can be performed on the left, and iliorenal bypass can be performed on either side. In the past superior mesenteric artery to renal artery bypasses have been performed, but this procedure has been largely abandoned. If a splenorenal bypass or hepatorenal bypass is to be considered, a lateral view of the aorta should be obtained to assess the patency of the proximal celiac artery. If a stenosis to the celiac artery is present, neither of these procedures would be acceptable because of poor inflow. In the period from 1975 to 1980 at the Cleveland Clinic, 72% of all renal artery bypasses were aortorenal bypasses or endarterectomies.[14] Since 1981, a larger number of hepatorenal or splenorenal bypasses were performed in order to avoid manipulating a severely diseased aorta.

Whereas the operative mortality is quite low for renal revascularization alone or aortic replacement alone, a combined procedure carries a higher mortality. This mortality for aortic replacement and renal revascularization is between 3% and 30%.[71-74] In a series of 89 patients undergoing concomitant renal revascularization and aortic replacement, there was an operative mortality of 7% when unilateral renal artery revascularization was undertaken and 15% when bilateral renal artery revascularization was performed.[72] The overall operative mortality was 10% with the principal cause of death being oliguric renal failure in five patients, myocardial infarction in two patients, and cardiac arrhythmia and respiratory failure in one patient each. Most of these patients were elderly and had generalized atherosclerosis. All patients underwent either coronary arteriography or stress thallium testing, and in all patients extracranial carotid artery disease was searched for. The incidence of acute tubular necrosis postoperatively was 25% in the unilateral renal artery stenosis group and 48% in the patients with bilateral disease.

In another series of 21 elderly patients undergoing surgical renal revascularization, the mortality was 4%.[62] However, the one patient who died postoperatively underwent aortic replacement and renal revascularization, so, in fact, the mortality for patients undergoing renal revascularization alone in this series was 0%.

Recently, O'Mara et al[74] studied 32 patients undergoing simultaneous aortic reconstruction and bilateral renal revascularization and demonstrated an operative mortality of 3%. The reason for the higher operative mortality in most series of patients undergoing simultaneous procedures is not clear. Possible causes include an extended time of operation, the need to clamp above the renal arteries for longer periods of time, larger fluid shifts when aortic reconstruction is performed, and the extremely high incidence of acute tubular necrosis, which carries at least 50% to 60% mortality in its own right. Since all the patients are carefully screened for coexisting cardiovascular disease, this cannot be implicated as a cause for the increasing mortality. Why there was a significantly lower mortality in O'Mara's series[74] is also not clear.

Because of this unacceptably high mortality among patients undergoing combined procedures in most series, one should use alternate surgical techniques such as the splenorenal, hepatorenal, or iliorenal bypass if the aorta is significantly diseased. Only if there is a true indication for aortic replacement (i.e., abdominal aortic aneurysm, symptomatic aortoocclusive disease, or atheromatous emboli) (see Chapter 9) should concomitant aortic replacement and renal revascularization be considered. Whether or not staged procedures will lower the operative mortality and morbidity is not known.

There was a 0% operative mortality in 104 patients with fibromuscular dysplasia and in 16 patients with renal artery aneurysms who underwent surgical revascularization.[14] In this group of patients recent technical advances now allow exvivo reconstruction of branch renal arteries with autotransplantation.

Revascularization for blood pressure control. At the Cleveland Clinic between 1975 and 1980, 41% of patients underwent surgical renal revascularization for control of blood pressure alone, whereas only 26% underwent revascularization for control of blood pressure between 1981 and 1984.[14] We suspect that this number is decreasing because more effective antihypertensive agents are available that successfully control blood pressure in many patients.

The results of surgical treatment for atherosclerotic renovascular hypertension are summarized in Table 15-1.

Table 15-1. Surgical treatment of atherosclerotic renovascular hypertension

Series	Year	No. of patients		No. cured (%)	No. improved (%)	No. failed (%)
Ernst et al[66]	1973	68				
		32	focal	10 (31)	18 (56)	4 (13)
		36	gen ASO	9 (25)	10 (28)	17 (47)
Foster et al[70]	1973	78		41 (53)	28 (36)	9 (11)
Dean et al[75]	1977	23		7 (30)	11 (48)	5 (22)
Askari et al[76]	1982	35		18 (51)	14 (40)	3 (9)
Starr, Lawrie, and Morris[68]	1980	137		109 (80)	?	?
Fry and Fry[67]	1982	22		12 (55)	9 (41)	1 (4)
Novick et al[14]	1987	180		55 (30.6)	110 (61.1)	15 (8.3)
Libertino et al[77]	1988	88		38 (44.2)	44 (51.2)	4 (4.7)

Many series demonstrated cure or improvement rates of approximately 90%.[14,62,66,67] In 180 patients revascularized for atherosclerotic renovascular hypertension at our institution, 55 patients (30.6%) were cured, 110 patients (61.1%) were improved, and 15 patients (8.3%) were not improved.[14] In a subgroup of 20 patients over 64 years old, 25% were cured and 65% had improvement in blood pressure control.[62] Dean et al[75] demonstrated a cure or improvement in blood pressure control in 78% of patients with bilateral renal artery stenosis and Askari[76] similarly showed that 32 of 35 patients (91%) undergoing revascularization to a solitary functioning kidney had improvement in blood pressure control. Despite extremely high rates of generalized atherosclerosis, exceptionally good results in blood pressure control are often obtained.

At the Cleveland Clinic surgical revascularization was performed in 104 patients with fibrous dysplasia and in 16 patients with renal artery aneurysms.[14] Of these patients 59 had branch renal artery disease. The indication for surgical revascularization in all patients with fibrous dysplasia was renovascular hypertension. Eighty-two patients underwent aortorenal bypass, while 37 patients underwent extracorporeal branch arterial reconstruction and autotransplantation. Four patients underwent splenorenal bypass, two patients underwent renal artery aneurysectomy and patch angioplasty, and one patient underwent autotransplantation alone. Branch renal artery revascularization was performed in 61 of these patients (24 in situ and 37 extracorporeal revascularization).

Hypertension was cured postoperatively in 66 of 104 patients with fibromuscular dysplasia (63%), improved in 31 patients (30%), and not changed in 7 patients (7%). In the 16 patients with renal artery disease caused by aneurysm, all were normotensive postoperatively. Early bypass thrombosis occurred in four patients, and stenosis of the bypass graft occurred late in two patients (1 month and 5 years).

Occasionally, a nephrectomy will be needed either alone or combined with contralateral renal artery revascularization for control of blood pressure. However, with the advent of newer and more effective antihypertensive agents, nephrectomy is less commonly performed.

Surgical revascularization for preservation of renal function. There is sufficient indirect evidence to suggest that renal function can, in fact, be salvaged. Case reports have been published demonstrating that renal function can be salvaged by surgical revascularization after total occlusion of a renal artery to a solitary functioning kidney even after periods of anuria ranging from 48 to 75 hours.[78-80] The most dramatic case of restoration of renal function was recently described by Perona et al.[81] A 23-year-old woman had total occlusion of a renal artery to a solitary kidney secondary to fibromuscular dysplasia. The patient was anuric for 31 days and required dialytic support. She was revascularized and within a period of 2 months, renal function returned to normal with a serum creatinine of 1.0 mg/dl.

Other examples of restoration of renal function include patients who have renal artery thromboembolism and then undergo successful thrombolysis with direct renal artery infusions of streptokinase.[82] We have recently reported on a group of three patients who underwent intraarterial administration of urokinase for thrombosis of renal artery bypass grafts (two patients) and occlusion of a native renal artery (one patient).[83] Restoration of renal function after a 6 to 12-hour period of intraarterial urokinase occurred in one patient.

There are several clues that may predict which patients can expect improvement in renal function after renal revascularization or percutaneous transluminal angioplasty. These include a renal artery length greater than 8 to 9 cm on laminograms, late filling of the distal renal artery via collaterals and/or the presence of a late nephrogram, a renal biopsy demonstrating intact viable glomeruli independent of what the tubulointerstitial and vascular structures show, and significant back bleeding at the time of operation.[84,85] When stenosis develops slowly (i.e., atherosclerosis), a good collateral circulation is more likely to develop, even after the renal artery is totally occluded. On the other hand, if there is sudden occlusion of the renal artery (i.e., occlusion of a bypass graft or embolism to a main renal artery), the likelihood for an adequate collateral circulation is much less.

Revascularization to preserve renal function is often ineffective in patients with severe azotemia (serum creatinine greater than 4 to 5 mg/dl). In these situations, advanced renal parenchymal disease is often present. However, this general rule is not invariable, and individual patients may demonstrate a significant improvement in renal function even with markedly elevated levels of serum creatinine.[62,83]

Patients with malignant or accelerated hypertension have a much higher incidence of renovascular disease.[8] Ying et al showed that when patients with severe elevations in blood pressure are treated medically, renal function often worsens.[86] In their series of eight patients, surgical revascularization or percutaneous transluminal angioplasty improved renal function in every patient. In a series of 161 patients in whom surgical revascularization was performed for the purpose of preservation of renal function, 93 patients (57.7%) were improved, 50 patients (31.1%) had stable renal function, and 10 patients (11.2%) grew worse.[14] Age was not an important predictor in patients in whom renal function was either improved or unchanged. In a series from Mayo Clinic in 98 patients with chronic renal insufficiency undergoing renal revascularization, 69% of patients had improvement or stabilization in renal function and 90% of the patients avoided dialysis.[87] Other reports have similarly demonstrated a favorable response to renal revascularization and preservation of renal function.[86,88-90]

Renal function has been successfully restored in patients with totally occluded renal arteries.[91,92] Improvement can be expected when the parameters outlined earlier regarding renal salvageability in totally occluded renal arteries are followed.

Whether or not intervention for high-grade bilateral renal artery stenosis or high-grade stenosis to a solitary kidney will prevent the need for future dialysis is unclear. Novick et al published a series on 25 patients with end-stage renal disease secondary to atherosclerotic renal artery stenosis. Of these patients, 17 underwent chronic dialytic therapy and 13 (77%) were dead in a mean period of 8.7 months, whereas in the eight patients who underwent surgical revascularization, only two patients (25%) were dead after a mean period of 96 months.[93] This was not a controlled series and there is no way to determine why some patients were maintained on chronic dialysis and others underwent surgical revascularization. However, these data suggest that patients who have end-stage renal disease secondary to renal artery stenosis do more poorly on dialysis than the general dialysis population.

Percutaneous transluminal angioplasty (PTA)

Percutaneous transluminal angioplasty for renal artery stenosis was first reported by Andreas Grüntzig in 1978 when he successfully dilated a 61-year-old patient with hypertension.[94] PTA is quite effective in treating patients with fibromuscular disease. However, we and others have been uniformly disappointed with its use in treating atherosclerotic renal artery stenosis.[95,96] Hayes et al[95] reported on 55 patients with atherosclerotic renal artery stenosis who underwent PTA. A successful clinical outcome was achieved in only 12 patients (26.1%) with atherosclerotic disease. The nonostial lesions fared better than ostial lesions (50% improvement vs 15.4%).

Cicuto et al have demonstrated that patients with ostial lesions fare much worse than those who have lesions distal to the takeoff of the renal artery.[97] Sos and colleagues[96] report that when angioplasty was technically successful, 84% of patients with atheromatous disease demonstrated a cure or improvement in blood pressure control. Unfortunately, these data are misleading in that only 57% of patients with unilateral atheromatous disease had technically successful angioplasty, and only 10% of patients with bilateral disease had a technically successful angioplasty. Therefore when all patients are considered, of the 51 patients with atherosclerotic renal artery stenosis, only 33.3% had either a cure or improvement in blood pressure control. Those with bilateral disease fared worse than those with unilateral disease, and those with ostial lesions did worse than those with nonostial lesions.

In one recent report[98] there were technical success rates of 76.2%, 74.1%, and 67.7% for unilateral renal artery disease (n = 42), bilateral disease (n = 27), and disease in a solitary kidney (n = 31). Of those patients who had technical successes, 43 of 73 patients (59%) demonstrated significant improvement in blood pressure control. These patients were observed for a mean period of 29 months. As in most other series, ostial lesions fared worse than those that were nonostial. Another recent report has suggested that if patients demonstrate sustained reduction in blood pressure on ACE inhibitors and have a renal vein renin ratio greater than 1.5 : 1, the chance of successful blood pressure lowering with percutaneous transluminal angioplasty is much greater than if neither of these features are present.[99]

Percutaneous transluminal angioplasty has also been shown to be effective in the preservation of renal function.[100,101] Canzanello et al[98] reported that in 69 patients who had a technically successful first percutaneous transluminal renal angioplasty, the renal function was improved or stable in 17 out of 32 patients (53%) with unilateral disease, 11 out of 18 patients (61%) with bilateral disease, and 8 out of 19 patients (42%) with a solitary functioning kidney. There are reports of restoration of renal function after dilation of an occluded renal artery.[102,103] We[95] as well as others[104] have had dismal results when trying to improve renal function using percutaneous transluminal angioplasty for atherosclerotic renovascular disease.

A note of caution should be interjected here. Reports appear in the literature that describe technical successes but fail to report on the clinical outcome. For example, one series demonstrated excellent technical success in both angiographic appearance and reduction in pressure gradient across an area of stenosis but failed to mention the effect on blood pressure lowering or renal function.[105]

Complications can occur with percutaneous transluminal angioplasty. In Sos' series[96] of 51 patients (70 arteries) undergoing angioplasty, 3 patients required surgery for puncture site trauma, 4 patients had nonocclusive renal artery dissection, of which 3 underwent a successful renal revascularization. Two patients had transient acute renal failure and one patient had transient myocardial ischemia. Acute rupture of the renal artery at the time of renal artery angioplasty[106] and delayed rupture of the renal artery up to 9 days after percutaneous transluminal angioplasty[107] have been reported.

We use percutaneous transluminal angioplasty for atherosclerotic renovascular disease in focal nonostial renal artery lesions and only dilate patients with diffuse disease or ostial lesions if no other options are available. However, the focal lesions are clearly less common than ostial lesions or more diffuse atherosclerosis. Therefore the utility of PTA in atherosclerotic renovascular disease is limited.

PTA is the preferred modality in many patients with fibromuscular disease. The results are superior to, and the complication rate less than, the results in patients with atherosclerosis.[96] In Sos' series of 31 patients, 27 (87.1%) had a technically successful dilation. Of those who were successfully dilated, 16% of the patients had a cure in their blood pressure (59.3%), nine patients had improvement (33.3%) and two patients had failed to improve (7.4%). When there was a successful response in lowering blood pressure, it was usually sustained. Although recurrence of stenosis is common in atherosclerotic disease, it is particularly uncommon in patients with fibromuscular disease. In a series of 31 patients in whom 34 arteries were dilated, there was no mortality, one nonocclusive renal artery dissection, and one occlusive renal artery dissection. Similar good results have been reported in other series in which patients underwent percutaneous transluminal angioplasty for fibromuscular disease.[108,109]

The main limitation of percutaneous transluminal renal angioplasty for patients with fibromuscular disease is that it is usually effective only for patients who have disease in the main renal arteries. Medial fibroplasia and perimedial fibroplasia often involve the branches of the renal artery and these may be technically difficult or impossible lesions to dilate. Therefore patients with branch disease often must undergo extracorporeal reconstruction and autotransplantation.

In summary, percutaneous transluminal angioplasty is the procedure of choice for patients who have main renal artery disease secondary to fibromuscular dysplasia. However, if branch disease is involved, surgical revascularization is often necessary.

REFERENCES

1. Goldblatt H et al: Studies in experimental hypertension. I. The production of persistent elevation of systolic blood pressure by means of renal ischemia, J Exp Med 59:347, 1934.
2. Page IH and Helmer M: A crystalline pressor substance (angiotonin) resulting from the reaction between renin and renin activator, J Exp Med 71:29, 1940.
3. Braun-Menendez E et al: The substance causing renal hypertension, J Physiol 98:283, 1940.
4. Dustan HP: History of clinical renovascular hypertension. In Stanley JC et al, eds: Renovascular hypertension, Philadelphia, 1984, WB Saunders Co.
5. Hoobler SW: History of experimental renovascular hypertension. In Stanley JC et al, eds: Renovascular hypertension, Philadelphia, 1984, WB Saunders Co.
6. Page IH: Hypertension research: a memoir 1920, New York, 1988, Pergamon Press.
7. Gifford RW Jr: Evaluation of the hypertension patient with emphasis on detecting curable causes, Milbank Memorial Fund Quart 47:170, 1969.
8. Davis BA et al: Prevalence of renovascular hypertension in patients with Grade III or IV hypertensive retinopathy, N Engl J Med 301:1273, 1979.
9. Keith TA: Renovascular hypertension in black patients, Hypertension. 4:438, 1982.
10. Working Group on Renovascular Hypertension: Detection, evaluation and treatment of renovascular hypertension, Arch Intern Med 147:820, 1987.
11. Olin JW et al: Prevalence of atherosclerotic renal artery stenosis in patients with atherosclerosis elsewhere, Am J Med, 88:46 N, 1990.
12. Landwehr DM et al: Association of renal artery stenosis with coronary artery disease in patients with hypertension and/or chronic renal insufficiency, Kidney Int 25:171 1984 (abstract).
13. Dustan HP et al: Normal arterial pressure in patients with renal arterial stenosis, JAMA 187:1028, 1964.
14. Novick AC et al: Trends in surgical revascularization for renal artery disease: ten years experience, JAMA 257:498, 1987.
15. Wollenweber J, Sheps SG, and Davis GD: Clinical course of atherosclerotic renovascular disease, Am J Cardiol 21:60, 1968.
16. Meaney TF, Dustan HP, and McCormack LJ: Natural history of renal arterial disease, Radiology 91:881, 1968.
17. Schreiber MJ, Novick AC, and Pohl MA: The natural history of atherosclerotic and fibrous renal artery disease, Urol Clin North Am 116:1408, 1981.
18. Harrison HG and McCormack LJ: Pathologic classification of renal artery disease in renovascular hypertension, Mayo Clin Proc 46:161, 1971.
19. Novick AC: Renal artery aneurysm and arteriovenous malformation. In Novick AC and Straffon RA, eds: Vascular problems in urologic surgery, Philadelphia, 1982, WB Saunders Co.
20. Poutasse EF: Renal artery aneurysms, J Urol 113:443, 1975.
21. Gross F: The renin-angiotensin system in hypertension, Ann Intern Med 75:777, 1971.
22. Mohring J et al: Salt and water balance and renin activity in renal hypertension of rats, Am J Physiol 228:1847, 1975.
23. Dzau VJ, Gibbons GH, and Leven DC: Renovascular hypertension: an update on pathophysiology, diagnosis and treatment, Am J Nephrol 3:172, 1983.
24. Vaughan ED: Renovascular hypertension, Kidney Int 27:811, 1985.
25. Vaughan ED Jr et al: Renovascular hypertension; renin measurements to indicate hypersecretion and contralateral suppression, estimate renal plasma flow and score for surgical curability, Am J Med 55:402, 1973.
26. Dzau VJ et al: Sequential renal hemodynamics in experimental, benign and malignant hypertension, Hypertension 3:(suppl I):63, 1981.
27. Rostand SG et al: Attenuated pressure naturesis in hypertensive rats. Kidney Int 21:330, 1982.
28. Gavras H et al: Angiotensin-sodium interaction and blood pressure maintenance of renal hypertensive and normotensive rats, Science 180:1369, 1973.
29. Simon N et al: Clinical characteristics of renovascular hypertension: cooperative study of renovascular hypertension, JAMA 220:1209, 1972.
30. Hunt JC et al: Renal and renovascular hypertension, Arch Intern Med 133:988, 1974.
31. Gifford RW Jr: Epidemiology and clinical manifestations of renovascular hypertension. In Stanley JC, Ernst CB, and Fry WJ, eds: Renovascular hypertension, Philadelphia, 1984, WB Saunders Co.
32. Eipper DF et al: Abdominal bruits in renovascular hypertension, Am J Cardiol 37:48, 1976.
33. Gifford RW Jr, McCormack LJ, and Poutasse EF: The atrophic kidney: its role in hypertension, Mayo Clin Proc 40:834, 1965.
34. Lawrie GM, Morris GC, and Debakey ME: Long-term results of treatment of the totally occluded renal artery in 40 patients with renovascular hypertension, Surgery 88:753, 1980.
35. Textor SC et al: Regulation of renal hemodynamics and glomerular filtration rate in patients with renovascular hypertension during converting enzyme inhibition with captopril, Am J Med 76(5B):29, 1984.
36. Silas JH et al: Captopril induced reversible renal failure: a marker for renal artery stenosis affecting a solitary kidney, Br Med J 286:1702, 1983.
37. Jacobson HR: Ischemic renal disease: an overlooked clinical entity? Kidney Int 34:729, 1988.
38. Packer M et al: Functional renal insufficiency during long-term therapy with captopril and enalapril and severe congestive heart failure, Ann Intern Med 106:346, 1987.
39. Watson ML et al: Captopril/diuretic combinations in severe renovascular disease: a cautionary note, Lancet 2:404, 1983.
40. Hricik D et al: Captopril-induced functional renal insufficiency in

patients with bilateral renal-artery stenosis or renal-artery stenosis to a solitary kidney, N Engl J Med 308:373, 1983.
41. Nicholson JP et al: Cigarette smoking and renovascular hypertension, Lancet 2:765-766, 1983.
42. Black HR and Cooper KA: Cigarette smoking and atherosclerotic renal artery stenosis, J Clin Hyper 4:322, 1986.
43. Basta LL et al: Regression of atherosclerotic stenosing lesions of the renal arteries and spontaneous cure of systemic hypertension through controlled hyperlipidemia, Am J Med 61:420, 1976.
44. Maxwell MH et al: Use of the rapid sequence intravenous pyelogram: the diagnosis of renovascular hypertension, N Engl J Med 270:213, 1964.
45. Bookstein JJ et al: Radiologic aspects of renovascular hypertension. II. The role of urography and unilateral renovascular disease: co-operative study of renovascular hypertension, JAMA 220:1225, 1972.
46. Kaufman JJ: Renovascular hypertension: the UCLA experience, J Urol 121:139, 1979.
47. Thornbury JR, Stanley JC, and Fryback DG: Hypertensive urogram: A nondiscriminatory test for renovascular hypertension, AJR 138:43, 1982.
48. Fommei E et al: Renal scintigraphic captopril test in the diagnosis of renovascular hypertension, Hypertension 10:212, 1987.
49. Nally JV et al: Captopril renography for the detection of renovascular hypertension, Cleve Clin J Med 55:311, 1988.
50. Wilcox CS et al: Diagnostic uses of angiotensin-converting enzyme inhibitors in renovascular hypertension, Am J Hypertens 1:344S, 1988.
51. Nally JV: Renal scinitography in the evaluation of renovascular hypertension: a note of optimism yet caution, J Nucl Med 28:1501, 1987.
52. Robertson R, Murphy A, and Dubbins PA: Renal artery stenosis: the use of duplex ultrasound as a screening technique, Br J Radiol 61:196, 1988.
53. Taylor DC et al: Duplex ultrasound scanning in the diagnosis of renal artery stenosis: a prospective evaluation, J Vasc Surg 7:363, 1988.
54. Havey RJ et al: Screening for renovascular hypertension: is renal digital-subtraction angiography the preferred non-invasive test? JAMA 254:388, 1985.
55. Maxwell MH, Rudnick M, and Waks AU: New approaches to the diagnosis of renovascular hypertension. In Bach JF et al, eds: Advances in nephrology 14:285, 1985.
56. Muller FB et al: The captopril test in identifying renovascular disease in hypertensive patients, Am J Med 80:633, 1986.
57. Re R et al: Inhibition of angiotensin-converting enzyme for diagnosis of renal artery stenosis, N Engl J Med 298:582, 1978.
58. Hughes JS et al: Duration of blood pressure elevation in acutely predicting surgical cure of renovascular hypertension, Am Heart J 101:408, 1981.
59. Maxwell MH et al: Predictive value of renin determinations in renal artery stenosis, JAMA 238:2617, 1977.
60. Marks LS et al: Renovascular hypertension: does the renal vein renin ratio predict operative results? J Urol 115:365, 1976.
61. Novick AC et al: Diminished operative morbidity and mortality in renal revascularization, JAMA 246:749, 1981.
62. Olin JW et al: Renovascular disease in the elderly: an analysis of 50 patients, J Am Coll Cardiol 5:1232, 1985.
63. Case DB et al: Long-term efficacy of captopril in renovascular and essential hypertension, Am J Cardiol 49:1440, 1982.
64. Havelka et al: Long-term experience with captopril in severe hypertension, Br J Pharmacol 14(suppl 2):71S, 1982.
65. Lawrie GM et al: Late results of reconstructive surgery for renovascular disease, Ann Surg 191:528, 1980.
66. Ernst CB et al: Renal revascularization for arteriosclerotic renovascular hypertension: prognostic implications for focal renal arterial vs. overt generalized arteriosclerosis, Surgery 73:859, 1973.
67. Fry RE and Fry WJ: Renovascular hypertension in the patient with severe atherosclerosis, Arch Surg 117:938, 1982.
68. Starr DS, Lawrie GM, and Morris GC: Surgical treatment of renovascular hypertension: long-term follow-up of 216 patients up to 20 years. Arch Surg 115:494, 1980.
69. Franklin SS et al: Operative morbidity and mortality in renovascular disease, JAMA 231:1148, 1975.
70. Foster JH et al: Ten years experience with surgical management of renovascular hypertension, Ann Surg 117:755, 1973.
71. Brewster DC et al: Combined aortic and renal revascularization, Am J Med 131:457, 1976.
72. Tarazi RY et al: Simultaneous aortic reconstruction and renal revascularization: risk factors and late results in 89 patients, J Vasc Surg 5:707, 1987.
73. Dean RH et al: Aortic and renovascular disease: factors affecting the value of combined procedures, Ann Surg 200:336, 1984.
74. O'Mara CS et al: Simultaneous aortic reconstruction and bilateral renal revascularization: is this a safe and effective procedure? J Vasc Surg 8:356, 1988.
75. Dean RH et al: Bilateral renal artery stenosis and renovascular hypertension, Surgery 81:53, 1977.
76. Askari A et al: Surgical treatment of renovascular disease in the solitary kidney: results in 43 cases, J Urol 127:20, 1982.
77. Libertino JA et al: Changing concepts in surgical management of renovascular hypertension, Arch Intern Med 1988;148:357, 1988.
78. Smith SP et al: Occlusion of the artery to a solitary kidney: restoration of renal function after prolonged anuria, JAMA 231:1306, 1974.
79. Williams B et al: Recovery of renal function after delayed revascularization of acute occlusion of the renal artery, Br Med J 296:1591, 1988.
80. Sheil AGR et al: Reversal of renal failure by revascularization of kidneys with thrombosed renal arteries, Lancet 2:865, 1973.
81. Perona PG et al: Successful revascularization of an occluded renal artery after prolonged anuria, J Vasc Surg 9:817, 1989.
82. Skinner RE et al: Recovery of function in a solitary kidney after intra-arterial thrombolytic therapy, J Urol 141:108, 1989.
83. Olin JW, Young JR, and Graor RA: Thrombolytic therapy for the treatment of renal artery occlusions, Cleve Clin J Med 56:432, 1989.
84. Scheft P et al: Renal revascularization in patients with total occlusion of the renal artery, J Urol 124:185, 1980.
85. Libertino JA et al: Renal artery revascularization: restoration of renal function, JAMA 244:1340, 1980.
86. Ying CY et al: Renal revascularization in the azotemic hypertensive patient resistant to therapy, N Engl J Med 311:1070, 1984.
87. Hallett JW et al: Renovascular operations in patients with chronic renal insufficiency: do the benefits justify the risk? J Vasc Surg 5:622, 1987.
88. Dean RH et al: Retrieval of renal function by revascularization: study of preoperative outcome predictors, Ann Surg 202:367, 1985.
89. Mestres CA et al: Improvement of renal function in azotaemic hypertensive patients after surgical revascularization, Br J Surg 75:578, 1988.
90. Lawrie GM, Morris GC, and DeBakey ME: Long-term results of treatment of the totally occluded renal artery in 40 patients with renovascular hypertension, Surgery 88:753, 1980.
91. Alexander RH and Brient BW: Revascularization of kidneys with totally occluded renal arteries, South Med J 75:1087, 1982.
92. Zinman L and Libertino JA: Revascularization of chronic totally occluded renal artery with restoration of renal function, J Urol 118:517, 1977.

93. Novick AC et al: Revascularization to preserve renal function in patients with atherosclerotic renovascular disease, Urol Clin North Am 11:477, 1984.
94. Grüntzig A et al: Treatment of renovascular hypertension with percutaneous transluminal dilatation of renal/artery stenosis, Lancet 1: 801, 1978.
95. Hayes JM et al: Experience with percutaneous transluminal angioplasty for renal artery stenosis at the Cleveland Clinic, J Urol 139:488, 1988.
96. Sos TA et al: Percutaneous transluminal renal angioplasty in renovascular hypertension due to atheroma or fibromuscular dysplasia, N Engl J Med 309:274, 1983.
97. Cicuto KP et al: Renal artery stenosis: anatomic classification for percutaneous transluminal angioplasty, AJR 137:599, 1981.
98. Canzanello VJ et al: Percutaneous transluminal renal angioplasty in management of atherosclerotic renovascular hypertension: result in 100 patients, Hypertension 13:163, 1989.
99. Staessen J et al: Blood pressure during long-term converting enzyme inhibition predicts the curability of renovascular hypertension by angioplasty, Am J Hypertens 1:208, 1988.
100. Madias NE, Kwon OJ, and Millan VG: Percutaneous transluminal renal angioplasty: a potentially effective treatment for preservation of renal function, Arch Intern Med 142:693, 1982.
101. Martin LG, Casarela WJ, and Gaylord GM: Azotemia caused by renal artery stenosis: treatment by percutaneous transluminal angioplasty, AJR 150:839, 1988.
102. Gutierrez OH, Izzo JL, and Burgener FA: Transluminal recanalization of an occluded renal artery: reversal of anuria in a patient with a solitary kidney, AJR 137:1254, 1981.
103. Mann JFE et al: Dilatation to avoid dialysis: angioplasty of an occluded renal artery with a coronary guiding catheter, Lancet 1:579, 1985.
104. Beebe HG et al: Results of renal artery angioplasty and its indications, J Vasc Surg 8:300, 1988.
105. Martin LG et al: Renal artery angioplasty: increased technical success and decreased complications in the second 100 patients, Radiology 159:631, 1986.
106. Dixon GD, Anderson S, and Crouch TT: Renal arterial rupture secondary to percutaneous transluminal angioplasty treated without surgical intervention, Cardiovasc Intervent Radiol 9:83, 1986.
107. Olin JW and Wholey M: Rupture of the renal artery 9 days after percutaneous transluminal angioplasty, JAMA 257:518, 1987.
108. Tegtmeyer CJ et al: Percutaneous transluminal angioplasty: treatment of choice for renovascular hypertension due to fibromuscular dysplasia, Radiology 143:631, 1982.
109. Archibald GR, Beckmann CF, and Libertino JA: Focal renal artery stenosis caused by fibromuscular dysplasia: treatment by percutaneous transluminal angioplasty, AJR 151:593, 1988.

Chapter 16

HYPERTENSION

Donald G. Vidt

Approximately 60 million individuals in the United States have arterial hypertension, which is defined as systolic blood pressure (SBP) greater than or equal to 140 mm Hg and/or diastolic blood pressure (DBP) greater than or equal to 90 mm Hg, and/or the taking of antihypertensive medication. Prevalence of hypertension increases with advancing age, and blacks are affected more than whites.[1,2] Hypertension is the most common public health problem in the United States today. It has been clearly demonstrated that cardiovascular risk increases progressively as systolic and diastolic blood pressure levels rise.[3] While incremental risk is apparent in both men and women, the overall mortality experienced at any given range of blood pressure is lower among women than it is among men. The absolute cardiovascular risk of any given blood pressure level depends on the presence or absence of other associated cardiovascular risk factors.

HISTORICAL PERSPECTIVE

Risks of morbidity and mortality related to blood pressure levels are generally recognized as a continuum, without clear demarcation between segments of the population at different degrees of risk.[4,5] Definitions of hypertension have evolved over the last 30 years, in part, from knowledge derived from epidemiologic studies in defined populations. From these studies, baseline blood pressure levels were analyzed to derive predictions of morbidity and mortality over varied intervals of follow-up. A second major development relates to the availability of effective and well-tolerated antihypertensive therapy. The development of effective treatment in the 1950s stimulated several prospective intervention trials, which demonstrated the beneficial effects of treatment on hypertension-related cardiovascular events. Diastolic pressures have assumed primacy over systolic pressures as the result of the design of most clinical trials. Yet, systolic pressure is a more accurate predictor of cardiovascular risk than diastolic pressure.

PATHOGENESIS

In 1949 Page proposed his mosaic theory of multifactorial causation for essential hypertension.[6] At the time the theory was proposed, hypertension was assumed to result from a single cause. A major difficulty was that each investigator selected his or her own cause, tending to rule out all others. Applied to the circulation, most of the known and many of the unknown control factors could be accommodated as long as they were in equilibrium, maintaining blood pressure and tissue perfusion, while adapting to tissue needs. Essential hypertension was thus designated a disease of control or regulation, without necessarily having a single constant dominant cause. Today it is recognized that 90% to 95% of all patients with hypertension have what is termed *essential or primary hypertension,* that is, the pathogenesis of the disease remains unclear. There has been an extraordinary development in the knowledge of regulatory mechanisms of blood pressure control, as well as numerous other factors that may contribute to our understanding of essential hypertension. The role of heredity in the etiology of essential hypertension cannot be discounted. Population studies have clearly demonstrated the tendency for hypertension to aggregate within family groups; however, the manner in which heredity affects the numerous mechanisms involved in the control of blood pressure remains uncertain. More recently, intensive investigation has focused on mechanisms of sodium and other cation transport, as well as the role of the central nervous system and the renin-angiotensin-aldosterone system in blood pressure control. In addition, distinct racial influences on the prevalence of blood pressure have been well recognized, as well as the role of socioeconomic environment, obesity, physical inactivity, cigarette smoking, and alcohol consumption.

New drug development over the last several decades has certainly reflected the multiple mechanisms that influence blood pressure. The selection of drugs and regimens for controlling blood pressure continues to evolve. As new information becomes available, we can expect that future drug development will reflect evolving knowledge regarding mechanisms and other factors inherent in the onset and natural history of essential hypertension.

There are also many secondary forms of hypertension, such as renal artery stenosis,[7] adrenal cortical adenomas,[8] coarctation of the aorta, and pheochromocytoma.[9] With these causes, correcting the initiating factor often leads to reversal of the hypertension. In addition, hypertension associated with numerous causes of progressive renal parenchymal disease is now well recognized as a treatable, but not necessarily a correctable, form of secondary hypertension. In contrast, an increasing incidence of hypertensive end-stage renal disease is apparent, in opposition to the declining mortality from hypertensive heart disease and stroke. Progressive renal failure as a consequence of untreated or inadequately treated malignant hypertension is well recognized. While the incidence of malignant hypertension has decreased dramatically with new drug development and more aggressive treatment of hypertension, the incidence of progressive renal failure in young, predominantly black individuals with hypertension has certainly not declined.[10] There is a growing body of experimental and clinical data suggesting a cause-and-effect relationship for progressive renal failure in association with mild to moderate arterial hypertension.[11,12] These data suggest that more aggressive treatment and blood pressure control is indicated in patients with mild to moderate hypertension. Yet there are no data from carefully controlled clinical trials to show that renal protection will result from more aggressive blood pressure control. Again, current and future studies with newer classes of antihypertensive agents to assess the potential for "renal protection" through effects on intrarenal hemodynamics may affect future treatment considerations.

DIAGNOSIS

The recommendations of the Joint National Committee on Detection, Evaluation, and Treatment of High Blood Pressure (JNC IV) are useful for the practicing physician.[13] The diagnosis of hypertension in adults is confirmed when the average of two or more diastolic measurements on at least two office visits is greater than or equal to 90 mm Hg or when the average of multiple systolic measurements on two or more visits is greater than or equal to 140 mm Hg. A recommended classification for categorizing arterial pressure in individuals 18 years or over is listed in Table 16-1. Blood pressure confirmation on subsequent visits will help determine whether initial elevations remain high and therefore require further evaluation and therapy, or whether they have returned to normal and may therefore require only periodic remeasurement. The diagnosis of hypertension and treatment decisions must never be made on the basis of a single blood pressure reading. Blood pressure measurement techniques as outlined by the American Heart Association are recommended.[14]

Table 16-1. Classification of blood pressure* in adults age 18 years or older

Range (mm Hg)	Category†
Diastolic	
<85	Normal blood pressure
85-89	High normal blood pressure
90-104	Mild hypertension
105-114	Moderate hypertension
≥115	Severe hypertension
Systolic (when diastolic blood pressure is <90)	
<140	Normal blood pressure
140-159	Borderline isolated systolic hypertension
≥160	Isolated systolic hypertension

(From the 1988 report of the Joint National Committee on Detection, Evaluation, and Treatment of High Blood Pressure, Arch Intern Med 148:1023-1038, 1988.)

*Classification based on the average of two or more readings on two or more occasions.

†Classification of borderline isolated systolic hypertension (SBP 140 to 159 mm Hg) or isolated systolic hypertension (SBP ≥160 mm Hg) takes precedence over high normal blood pressure (diastolic blood pressure 85 to 89 mm Hg) when both occur in the same person. High normal blood pressure (DBP 85 to 89 mm Hg) takes precedence over a classification of normal blood pressure (SBP <140 mm Hg) when both occur in the same person.

EVALUATION OF THE HYPERTENSIVE PATIENT

With approximately one quarter of the population at risk from hypertension and its complications, initial evaluation of the new hypertensive patient should be thorough but must also be cost-effective. The initial evaluation of patients with sustained hypertension should be designed to answer several questions:

1. Is target organ involvement present?
2. Are cardiovascular risk factors other than hypertension present?
3. Does the patient have primary or secondary hypertension?

Historically, physicians have been overly reliant on increasingly sophisticated laboratory measurements in an effort to identify secondary and potentially curable causes of hypertension, when, in fact, a careful and thorough history and physical examination will enable the exclusion of most causes of secondary hypertension. A few carefully selected and easily performed laboratory studies will help establish the severity of the hypertension, enable exclusion of most secondary causes, and provide an estimation of the patient's overall cardiovascular risk status.[13]

The medical history should include any family history of hypertension, premature cardiovascular disease or mortality, diabetes, renal disease, or pheochromocytoma. If the patient has been previously diagnosed as hypertensive, the duration of disease should be established as well as prior antihypertensive therapy prescribed, response to therapy, and adverse effects of treatment. A careful history of both prescription and over-the-counter medications should be obtained for all patients since numerous agents may interact with antihypertensive drugs to raise blood pressure or block the effectiveness of antihypertensive medications. The presence or absence of other cardiovascular risk factors such as obesity, smoking, hyperlipidemia, and carbohydrate intolerance must be established. Psychosocial and environmental factors such as emotional stress, socioeconomic status, or specific cultural food practices that may have a bearing on blood pressure control and on subsequent compliance with medication regimens should be noted. In particular, an estimate of daily sodium intake and alcohol use should be established. The use of oral contraceptives in younger women and excessive alcohol intake in both men and women represent the two most common causes of reversible hypertension.

Symptoms of target organ involvement may be revealed by obtaining a history of transient ischemic attack, stroke, myocardial infarction, angina pectoris, atherosclerotic heart disease, or lower extremity arteriosclerosis obliterans. A change in the diurnal pattern of urine flow may be an early clue to concentrating defects secondary to hypertension-induced renal disease or other forms of renal parenchymal disease.

The physical examination should help verify the degree of target organ involvement and may also provide additional clues to secondary causes of hypertension. Careful measurement of blood pressure, height, and weight, and a thorough funduscopic evaluation for evidence of arteriolar narrowing, arteriovenous compression, hemorrhages, exudates, or papilledema should be made. Auscultation and palpation of the neck should be performed for evidence of carotid bruits, distended neck veins, or an enlarged thyroid gland. Examination of the heart should establish size, rate, and rhythm, as well as the presence or absence of murmurs or gallop sounds. Careful auscultation of the lungs for rhonchi, rales, or wheezes will help establish the presence or absence of congestive heart failure or possibly chronic pulmonary disease. Examination of the abdomen should include both auscultation and palpation for evidence of bruits, enlarged kidneys, other abdominal masses, or dilation of the abdominal aorta. Examination of the extremities may reveal diminished or absent peripheral arterial pulses, bruits, or edema, and careful neurologic assessment will establish the presence of fixed neurologic deficits.

The history and physical examination should be complemented by a few carefully selected laboratory studies, preferably performed before initiating therapy. The determination of a hemoglobin, hematocrit, urinalysis, serum potassium, serum creatinine, and an electrocardiogram will help determine the severity of vascular disease or the presence of target organ involvement and may provide clues to secondary hypertension. The addition of a lipid profile, se-

Clinical clues for secondary causes of hypertension

Renovascular hypertension

- Systolic-diastolic epigastric bruit
- Accelerated or malignant hypertension
- Unilateral small kidney discovered by an investigative study
- Onset of hypertension before the age of 30 or after the age of 50
- Resistant hypertension
- Hypertension and unexplained impairment in renal function
- Impairment in renal function in response to angiotensin converting enzyme inhibitor
- Evidence of extensive arteriosclerosis obliterans: carotid, coronary, peripheral

Coarctation of the aorta

- Absent or reduced pulses in the lower extremities
- Palpable pulsations over intercostal arteries in the posterior thorax
- Bruits over the intercostal arteries
- Rib notching on chest x-ray
- Absent aortic knob

Cushing's syndrome

- Recent change in physical appearance and weight gain
- Extreme weakness with muscle wasting
- Typical body habitus with moon facies, skin changes, and hirsutism
- Glucose intolerance
- Neutrophilia with relative lymphocytopenia

Pheochromocytoma

- Symptomatic paroxysms of hypertension with headache, tachycardia, palpitations, tremor, and sweating
- History of labile blood pressure
- Substandard weight or recent weight loss
- A pressor response to antihypertensive drugs or during induction of anesthesia
- Refractory hypertension
- Occasional occurrence with neurocutaneous syndromes
- Unusual lability of blood pressure or orthostatic hypotension
- Abnormal glucose tolerance

Primary aldosteronism

- Weakness, periodic paralysis, paresthesia, and tetany (rare)
- Hypokalemia with inappropriate kaliuresis
- Resistant hypertension

rum calcium, fasting blood sugar, and serum uric acid will help identify other cardiovascular risk factors. Many of these studies are easily obtainable today as part of an automated blood chemistry profile. The decision to perform additional diagnostic studies should be determined by the presence or absence of clinical clues to secondary hypertension uncovered in the course of the history, physical examination, and screening studies. Clinical clues that may be helpful in identifying secondary and potentially reversible causes of hypertension are outlined in the box on p. 287.

When the diagnosis of hypertension has been established, the process of patient education should be initiated. For subsequent therapy to be successful, patients must recognize that hypertension is a lifelong disease, that it is usually asymptomatic since the symptoms do not correlate with blood pressure levels, and that therapy will, in most instances, have to be maintained for life. Patients must recognize that effective therapy will control hypertension and that optimal control is usually compatible with an excellent long-term prognosis and quality of life. Adherence with a prescribed regimen is the key to successful therapy and will relate directly to the patient's willingness to comply with recommended medications and, when appropriate, to undertake selected behavioral modification.

NONPHARMACOLOGIC THERAPY

The benefits of therapy have been demonstrated in numerous clinical trials during the last 20 years. The decision to initiate therapy in the individual patient requires that both the severity of the hypertension and the presence or absence of other cardiovascular risk factors or disease conditions be considered. Nonpharmacologic approaches have received increasing attention in recent years as evidence has continued to mount regarding the effectiveness of selected nonpharmacologic measures in the control of blood pressure, particularly in patients with mild hypertension. Selected nonpharmacologic interventions can also be of adjunctive value in patients with more severe hypertension receiving pharmacologic therapy.

The use of nondrug therapies as initial treatment for most patients, at least for the first 3 to 6 months after recognition of their hypertension, has been widely advocated.[15,16] Nonpharmacologic measures include appropriate reduction of calories, salt, alcohol, and fat consumption. In addition to these measures, avoidance of tobacco, participation in regular exercise, and the role of behavioral modification need to be considered.

Sodium restriction

Moderate dietary sodium restriction carries no risk for the hypertensive individual and may benefit selected patients by modest reductions in blood pressure. Almost half the patients who reduce their daily sodium intake into the range of 2 g of sodium or 5 to 6 g of salt will lower their blood pressure by about 5 mm Hg. In some mild hypertensive patients this may be sufficient to normalize blood pressure without medication, while in others sodium restriction will enhance the antihypertensive efficacy of most antihypertensive medications.[17] Since a high proportion of daily sodium intake comes from prepared foods, merely undertaking a no-added-salt diet at the table or in food preparation may not be sufficient in many individuals. Thus appropriate counseling should include educational information regarding the labeling of processed foods and an increased awareness of the sodium content of frequently purchased foods.

The role of other cations such as potassium, calcium, and magnesium in the genesis of hypertension remains controversial. A modest beneficial effect on blood pressure has been noted after potassium supplementation in hypertensive patients who have been rendered hypokalemic from using diuretics; thus potassium supplements and prevention of hypokalemia in diuretic-treated patients may be beneficial.[18] Preliminary nutritional data have suggested that calcium intake is lower among hypertensive individuals than normotensive individuals, and that calcium supplementation may lower blood pressure in hypertensive patients.[19,20] Calcium supplements may be considered for patients in whom rigid restriction of dairy products has been undertaken for control of hyperlipidemia. Similarly, lower magnesium levels have been noted in hypertensive individuals.[21] Diuretic therapy may induce hypomagnesemia along with hypokalemia, and, if documented, supplementation may be considered in the diuretic-treated hypertensive patient.

Weight reduction

The relationship between obesity and blood pressure has now been clearly established from numerous epidemiologic and intervention studies.[22,23] It is appropriate to recommend weight reduction for all obese hypertensive patients, with the goal of reducing body weight to within 15% of ideal weight. There is now evidence to suggest that upper body obesity correlates to hypertension, impaired glucose tolerance, and hypertriglyceridemia.[24] An increased coronary risk has also been associated with upper body obesity, thus suggesting that the risks related to obesity may not be a matter of weight alone, but also may be related to the distribution of that increased weight.[25] While blood pressure reduction represents the primary benefit of weight reduction, favorable effects on plasma lipid abnormalities should also be considered. The rate of recidivism following successful weight reduction is well recognized, stressing the importance of ongoing, long-term counseling and reassurance.

Restriction of alcohol

Heavy alcohol consumption (more than 1 oz daily of ethanol alcohol) may elevate arterial pressure.[26] One oz of ethanol is contained in 2 oz of 100-proof whiskey, 8 oz of wine, or 24 oz of most beers. Hypertensive patients who drink should be encouraged to moderate their ethanol alcohol intake to comply with these limits.

Cessation of smoking

Although there is little evidence to suggest that smoking is a risk factor for the development of hypertension, avoidance of tobacco products can considerably improve the overall cardiovascular health of the hypertensive patient. Smokers clearly increase their risks for cancer and chronic pulmonary disease, more than double their risk for coronary artery disease and sudden death, and increase their risk of stroke from twofold to tenfold.[27] Smokers may require higher dosages of a β-blocker to control blood pressure than nonsmokers might. Avoidance of smoking should be strongly encouraged in hypertensive patients regardless of their age.

Exercise

A regular program of aerobic (isotonic) exercise facilitates cardiovascular conditioning, can aid the obese hypertensive individual in weight reduction, and may provide some benefit in reducing blood pressure.[28] Physical fitness is associated with lower all-cause mortality as well as cardiovascular and cancer mortality.[29] Additional benefits may be reflected in favorable changes in the lipid profile. A regular isotonic exercise program is strongly encouraged, while isometric exercise, such as that associated with weight lifting, should be discouraged because of exaggerated rises in systolic and diastolic blood pressure observed with this form of exercise.

Relaxation

Considerable data have accumulated demonstrating modest reductions in blood pressure in association with relaxation and behavioral modification techniques. Modest long-term reductions in blood pressure have been demonstrated in selected patients.[30,31] Behavioral methods may be of particular relevance for the treatment of mild hypertension, but most have not yet been subjected to comparative clinical trials with other forms of hypertension therapy and should not be considered as definitive therapy for all patients with hypertension.

Fat and fish oils

Studies have demonstrated that diets low in saturated fats and high in polyunsaturated fats are associated with a modest reduction in systolic and diastolic blood pressure. Eating fish that are rich in the polyunsaturated omega-3 fatty acids may lower blood levels of triglycerides and therefore may have a beneficial effect on the coronary risk profile. Unfortunately, the use of omega-3 fatty acid supplements has failed to document an antihypertensive effect and may be associated with deficient blood clotting and excessive bleeding. There is insufficient evidence to recommend the routine use of fish oil supplements at this time.

Caffeine

Although acute ingestion of caffeine may raise blood pressure, chronic, moderate caffeine ingestion appears to have no significant effects upon blood pressure.[32] In higher doses caffeine may induce tachycardia and even cardiac arrhythmias. A brief increase in cardiac output and a transient vasodilatory effect may be noted. In effect, there is no evidence to support a long-term pressor effect from the chronic ingestion of caffeine.

CURRENTLY AVAILABLE ANTIHYPERTENSIVE AGENTS

Drug treatment of hypertension has changed significantly in the past decade. Many new classes of antihypertensive agents have been introduced for clinical use such as the α- and β-adrenergic blockers, the angiotensin converting enzyme inhibitors and calcium channel blocking drugs. The effectiveness of these agents, their favorable adverse effect profiles, and the high degree of patient acceptance have led to their rapidly increasing popularity and significant changes in physician prescribing patterns. The primary attention of clinicians is no longer focused on the safety and efficacy issues of available drugs, since all approved agents share these characteristics. Rather, attention is now focused on selection of agents for initial and subsequent therapy that control blood pressure and provide an optimal quality of life for the treated hypertensive patient, thus ensuring better patient adherence with long-term therapy. Another important trend in therapy has been the use of lower doses of individual agents, which is probably best demonstrated by the change in prescribing of thiazide diuretics.

The next section will address all of the currently available classes of antihypertensive agents, but I have allowed current prescribing habits to dictate the attention directed to each class. The accompanying box lists characteristics that would seem desirable for the optimal antihypertensive agent. The following section focuses on special character-

Characteristics of the optimal antihypertensive agent

- Once-a-day dosage
- Few side effects (quality of life): subjective, electrolyte, biochemical
- Compatibility with other antihypertensives and other drugs
- Beneficial effect on concomitant diseases
- Freedom from serious adverse effects
- Long-term blood pressure lowering effects regardless of age or race
- Improvement of the hemodynamic abnormality

Table 16-2. Currently available antihypertensive drugs

Agent	Trade name	Usual daily dose[a] (mg)	Precautions and special considerations
Thiazides and related sulfonamide diuretics			
Bendroflumethiazide	Naturetin	2.5-5	May be ineffective in renal failure. Hypokalemia increases digitalis toxicity. May cause an increase in blood levels of lithium.
Benzthiazide	Exna Aquatag	12.5-50	
Chlorothiazide	Diuril	125-500	
Chlorthalidone	Hygroton	12.5-50	
Hydrochlorothiazide	HydroDIURIL Esidrix	12.5-50	
Hydroflumethiazide	Saluron	12.5-50	
Inadapamide	Lozol	2.5-5	
Methyclothiazide	Enduron	2.5-5	
Metolazone	Zaroxolyn Diulo	1.25-10	
	Mykrox	0.5-1	
Polythiazide	Renese	2-4	
Quinethazone	Hydromox	25-100	
Trichlormethiazide	Naqua	1-4	
Loop diuretics[b]			
Bumetanide[c]	Bumex	0.5-5	Effective in chronic renal failure.
Ethacrynic acid[c]	Edecrin	25-100	
Furosemide[c]	Lasix	20-320	
Potassium-sparing agents			
Amiloride	Midamor	5-10	Danger of hyperkalemia or renal failure in patients treated with an ACE inhibitor or a nonsteroidal antiinflammatory drug. May increase blood levels of lithium.
Spironolactone	Aldactone	25-100	
Triamterene	Dyrenium	50-150	
β-blockers[d]			
Acebutolol	Sectral	200-1200	Should not be used in patients with asthma, chronic obstructive pulmonary disease (COPD), congestive heart failure, heart block (greater than first-degree), or sick sinus syndrome. Use with caution in insulin-treated diabetics and patients with peripheral vascular disease. Should not be discontinued abruptly in patients with ischemic heart disease.
Atenolol	Tenormin	25-150	
Carteolol	Cartrol	2.5-10	
Labetalol[c,e]	Normodyne Trandate	200-1800	
Metoprolol	Lopressor	50-200	
Nadolol	Corgard	40-320	
Penbutolol	Levatol	20-80	
Pindolol[c]	Visken	10-60	
Propranolol[c]	Inderal	40-320	
Propranolol, long-acting (LA)	Inderal LA	60-320	
Timolol maleate[c]	Blocadren	20-80	

(Modified from the 1988 report of the Joint National Committee on Detection, Evaluation, and Treatment of High Blood Pressure.)

[a]The dosage range may differ slightly from recommended dosage in *Physicians' Desk Reference* or package insert. Given once daily unless otherwise indicated.

[b]Larger doses of loop diuretics may be required in patients with renal failure.

[c]This drug is usually given in divided doses twice daily.

[d]Atenolol, metoprolol, and acebutolol are cardioselective; pindolol, carteolol, penbutolol, and acebutolol have partial agonist activity (ISA).

[e]Combined α- and β-blocker.

[f]This drug is usually given in divided doses three or four times daily.

[g]This drug is administered as a skin patch once weekly.

[h]Given IV 100 mg injected rapidly; repeat every 5-10 minutes.

[i]Given 5 μg/min-100 μg or more.

[j]Given IV 0.5-10 μg/kg/min continuous infusion in continuous monitoring.

Table 16-2. Currently available antihypertensive drugs—cont'd

Agent	Trade name	Usual daily dose[a] (mg)	Precautions and special considerations
ACE inhibitors			
Captopril[c]	Capoten	25-300	Can cause reversible, acute renal failure in patients with bilateral renal arterial stenosis or unilateral stenosis in a solitary kidney. Proteinuria may occur (rare at recommended doses). Hyperkalemia can develop, particularly in patients with renal insufficiency. Rarely can induce neutropenia. Hypotension has been observed with initiation of ACE inhibitors, especially in patients with high plasma renin activity or in those receiving diuretic therapy.
Enalapril	Vasotec	2.5-40	
Lisinopril	Zestril	5-40	
	Prinivil		
Calcium antagonists			
Benzothiazepine derivative			
Diltiazem[f]	Cardizem	60-360	Relatively contraindicated for congestive heart failure, sick sinus syndrome, or greater than first-degree heart block. May cause liver dysfunction.
Diltiazem SR[c]	Cardizem SR	90-360	
Diphenylalkylamine derivative			
Verapamil[f]	Calan	120-480	As above.
Verapamil SR	Isoptin		
	Calan SR	120-480	
	Isoptin SR		
Dihydropyridines			
Nifedipine[f]	Procardia	30-180	As above.
	Adalat		
Nifedipine XL	Procardia XL	90-120	
Nicardipine[f]	Cardene	60-120	
Isradipine[c]	DynaCirc	5-120	
Nitrendipine	Baypress	5-40	
Adrenergic inhibitors			
Centrally acting α agonists			
Clonidine[c]	Catapres	0.1-1.2	Rebound hypertension may occur with abrupt discontinuance, particularly with prior administration of high doses or with discontinuation of concomitant β-blocker therapy
Clonidine TTS (patch)[g]	Catapres-TTS	0.1-0.3	
	Wytensin		
Guanabenz[c]	Tenex	4-64	
Guanfacine		1-3	
Methyldopa[c]	Aldomet	250-2000	May cause liver damage and Coombs'-positive hemolytic anemia. Use cautiously in elderly patients because of orthostatic hypotension. Interferes wtih measurements of urinary catecholamine levels by fluorimetric methods.
α-$_1$ adrenergic blockers			
Prazosin[c]	Minipress	1-20	Use cautiously in elderly patients because of orthostatic hypotension
Terazosin	Hytrin	1-20	
Peripheral-acting adrenergic antagonists			
Guanadrel sulfate[c]	Hylorel	10-100	Use cautiously because of orthostatic hypotension.
Guanethidine	Ismelin	10-150	
Rauwolfia alkaloids			
Rauwolfia serpentina (whole root)	Raudixin	50-100	Contraindicated in patients with history of mental depression. Use with caution in patients with history of peptic ulcer.
Reserpine	Serpasil	0.1-0.25	
	Sandril		

Continued.

Table 16-2. Currently available antihypertensive drugs—cont'd

Agent	Trade name	Usual daily dose[a] (mg)	Precautions and special considerations
Vasodilators			May precipitate angina pectoris in patients with coronary artery disease.
Hydralazine[c]	Apresoline	50-300	Lupus syndrome may occur (rare at recommended doses)
Minoxidil[c]	Loniten	2.5-80	May cause or aggravate pleural and pericardial effusions
Diazoxide[h]	Hyperstat IV		Effects persist for 12 hours or longer.
Nitroglycerin[i]	Tridil Nitrostat IV Nitro-Bid IV Nitroglycerin injection Nitrol IV		Close observation necessary because of rapid onset of action. Special infusion set necessary because of absorption with plastic.
Sodium nitroprusside[j]	Nipride Nitropress		Close observation necessary because of rapid onset of action. Rapidly degraded by exposure to light. Monitor thiocyanate levels, especially with renal or liver disease.

istics, as well as potential advantages or disadvantages of different classes and selected agents. A review of the pharmacologic and metabolic properties of antihypertensive drugs is beyond the scope of this chapter but is available from other sources.[2,33-35] A complete listing of currently available drugs and recommended dosages is provided in Table 16-2.

Thiazide and related sulfonamide diuretics

Diuretics have been the cornerstone of antihypertensive therapy since the introduction of the prototype agent chlorothiazide in 1958. These agents have been an integral part of every major clinical trial on hypertension during the past 25 years. Two important observations have significantly affected the use of diuretics in recent years and have led to a trend toward the use of lower doses of these agents. The first has been the clarification that therapeutic efficacy is obtained with once-a-day administration of doses ranging from 12.5 to 50 mg of hydrochlorothiazide or chlorthalidone in many patients (compared to doses of 50 to 100 mg, which were used previously). The second has been the accompanying observation that adverse effects such as hypokalemia and the risk of cardiac arrhythmias are less commonly observed with lower doses.

Clinical trials, which included diuretics, demonstrated that optimal blood pressure control can drastically reduce cardiovascular morbidity and mortality, particularly the risk of stroke. The failure to achieve reductions in coronary mortality comparable to those observed in stroke mortality has focused concern on selected metabolic abnormalities induced by the thiazide and thiazide-like diuretics. This concern, which has focused primarily on the abnormalities in electrolytes and in glucose and lipid metabolism, is the focus of continued debate and has clearly led to significant changes in prescribing habits in hypertension management.

Approximately 50% of mild to moderate hypertensive individuals will have a suitable blood pressure response to 12.5 to 50 mg of hydrochlorothiazide per day or its equivalent.[34] Thiazide diuretics are particularly effective in managing black individuals with hypertension, possibly because more blacks have a salt-sensitive, low-renin hypertension with a normal to modestly expanded plasma volume. Despite the fact that elderly individuals with hypertension tend to have a decreased plasma volume and a high peripheral resistance, diuretics are nevertheless effective as initial or subsequent therapy. In particular, preliminary data from the Systolic Hypertension in the Elderly Program (SHEP) revealed that 88% of elderly persons with isolated systolic hypertension achieved a goal blood pressure after approximately 1 year of chlorthalidone therapy.[34] Not only was diuretic therapy well tolerated, but 56% of the group required no more than 25 mg of hydrochlorothiazide daily to achieve a goal blood pressure.

The most common adverse effects associated with the thiazide or thiazide-like diuretics are volume depletion and electrolyte imbalance. Chronic administration predisposes patients to hypokalemia. It is apparent that the general trend toward lower doses of these agents has resulted in fewer problems with symptomatic hypokalemia. Hypomagnesemia, associated with weakness, tremors, and anorexia, can also be observed as a dose-related complication of thiazide therapy. Hyperuricemia is commonly associated with administration of these agents, but symptomatic gout seldom occurs unless the patient has a family or personal history of acute podagra. In the patient with a history of gout in whom thiazides are deemed necessary for control of hypertension, hyperuricemia can usually be controlled by the concomitant administration of allopurinol.

The major concern for the hypokalemic individual with hypertension relates to a possible increased risk for ventricular arrhythmias and sudden death in the setting of intrinsic cardiac disease or in the patient receiving a digitalis preparation.[36,37] Severe hypokalemia (less than 3 mEq/L) is less common with the use of low doses of diuretics. Probably the most effective way to prevent significant hypokalemia during thiazide therapy is to ensure that a patient adheres to a modest sodium-restricted diet. The use of potassium supplements, potassium-sparing diuretics, or ACE inhibitors also minimizes the risk of hypokalemia (less than 3.5 mEq/L).

Undoubtedly, the major current debate regarding the use of thiazide diuretics relates to their potential adverse effects upon carbohydrate and lipid metabolism. Thiazide therapy has been associated with increases in plasma glucose and with the development of overt diabetes mellitus in selected patients. The mechanism of thiazide-induced impaired glucose tolerance probably relates to impaired insulin release and/or peripheral insulin resistance.[38] These changes may occur within weeks of initiation of diuretic therapy and are reversible upon discontinuation of these agents. The risk of impaired glucose tolerance appears to be enhanced by diuretic-induced hypokalemia.

In the management of the hypertensive diabetic with established nephropathy and edema, the use of a diuretic is often mandatory for adequate control of edema. Risk of deterioration in glycemic control associated with diuretic therapy is probably small if obesity and caloric intake can be carefully controlled. Prevention of hypokalemia and prudent use of recommended lower doses of diuretics can further reduce the risk of thiazide-induced hyperglycemia. Concurrent use of an ACE inhibitor will further blunt diuretic-induced hypokalemia.

Multiple observations have demonstrated elevations of total cholesterol, LDL cholesterol, and triglycerides in association with thiazide diuretic therapy.[39,40] Careful adherence with a low-cholesterol diet during therapy has been shown to blunt the hyperlipidemic effects. Although there is no direct evidence to confirm that thiazide-induced lipid changes increase coronary heart disease risk in the hypertensive patient, this has done little to quiet the concern of many clinicians that these lipid changes may serve to blunt the expected reductions in coronary heart disease mortality despite improved control of high blood pressure. These concerns will continue to influence the choice of initial therapy for many patients with mild to moderate hypertension.[41] It would seem prudent to avoid diuretics, at least as initial therapy, in patients with hypertension and hyperlipidemia, particularly those with LDL cholesterol levels greater than 160 mg/dl. In these high-risk patients, suitable initial alternative therapies are available that do not adversely affect the lipid profile. When diuretic therapy is indicated in the hypertensive, hyperlipidemic patient, concurrent treatment with a low-cholesterol, controlled caloric intake, liberal use of increased soluble dietary fiber, and the lowest effective diuretic dosage is recommended.

Loop diuretics

The antihypertensive effects of loop diuretics are similar to those of the thiazide and thiazide-like agents. Unlike thiazides, the potency of loop diuretics can be increased by increasing the dose of furosemide or bumetanide in stepwise fashion, and it is often possible to establish diuresis in patients who are otherwise refractory to thiazide diuretics. Loop diuretics may be preferable to thiazide diuretics in patients with refractory hypertension or congestive heart failure and in patients with impaired renal function (serum creatinine greater than 2.5 mg/dl and GFR less than 25 ml/min). Ethacrynic acid has never attained the popularity enjoyed by furosemide or bumetanide but may be a useful alternative for patients with known hypersensitivity to these agents.

Intravenous administration may be preferred in patients with refractory edema and as concurrent therapy with other parenteral agents in the management of hypertensive urgencies or emergencies. Transient deafness has been reported with furosemide and ethacrynic acid and is most common with administration of high parenteral doses in patients with renal insufficiency. The ototoxic potential from bumetanide is significantly less than that observed with other loop diuretics.

Indapamide

Indapamide is an indoline derivative that differs chemically from the thiazide diuretics in that it contains only one sulfonamide group and no thiazide ring system. Although the mechanism of action is primarily a result of its diuretic activity as with the thiazides, it also reduces peripheral vascular resistance, possibly by exerting a calcium channel blocking effect.

A major potential advantage of indapamide in the treatment of hypertension is an apparent absence of observed effects on blood lipids.[42,43] In fact, HDL cholesterol levels may increase modestly during indapamide therapy. Impaired glucose tolerance is infrequently observed, while adverse effects, such as hypokalemia and hyperuricemia, are similar to those observed with thiazides.

Potassium-sparing diuretics

The potassium-sparing agents include spironolactone, triamterene, and amiloride. Unfortunately, spironolactone and amiloride are less potent diuretic and antihypertensive agents than are the thiazides, and triamterene has no significant antihypertensive effects when used alone, making them inappropriate agents for initial therapy of patients with mild to moderate essential hypertension.

Potassium-sparing agents reduce potassium losses secondary to other diuretics and in states of increased circulating aldosterone. They may potentiate the effectiveness of a thiazide or loop diuretic when used concurrently.

Hyperkalemia is the most common adverse effect of potassium-sparing agents, and severe renal insufficiency represents an absolute contraindication to their administration because of the danger of inducing hyperkalemia. Concurrent therapy with potassium-sparing agents, ACE inhibitors, and oral potassium supplements should be avoided because of the risk of hyperkalemia.

Adrenergic blocking agents

The maintenance of an elevated blood pressure is not caused by any single pressor mechanism but rather by complex interactions between numerous pressor mechanisms. As such, increased activity of the sympathetic nervous system alone is not responsible for maintaining elevated blood pressure in patients with essential hypertension, rather, there are complex interrelationships of the adrenergic nervous system with other pressor mechanisms. The antihypertensive effects of adrenergic blocking agents may be caused by prevention of sympathetic responses to changes in posture, exertion, and plasma volume deficits, or to suppression of renin secretion by selected sympathetic depressant drugs. Prevention of vasoconstriction in the arterial vascular bed results in a modest reduction in blood pressure. The normal baroreceptor influences mediated by sympathetic nerves are blunted under the influence of sympathetic depressant drugs. Cardiac contractility, heart rate, and cardiac output may be reduced, while decreased sympathetic activity in the veins results in increased venous capacitance, decreased cardiac output, and possibly postural hypotension. Subtle changes in renal plasma flow and glomerular filtration rate following reduction of blood pressure may lead to salt retention and increase in plasma volume, a consequence of therapy with most of the sympathetic depressant drugs.

β-Adrenergic blocking agents

Currently, nine β-adrenergic blockers have been approved for hypertension, and when used in appropriate doses, there is little evidence to suggest that any one has major advantages over the others in hypertension control. There are, however, differences in the clinical pharmacology of these agents that affect their use in associated diseases and may contribute to specific differences in the adverse effect profiles of these drugs.

All β-blockers, including those with cardioselectivity and partial agonist activity, can induce bronchoconstriction in patients with poorly controlled asthma. These agents may aggravate heart failure in patients with preexistent cardiac disease. β-blockers can aggravate claudication symptoms in hypertensives with peripheral vascular insufficiency.

In insulin-dependent diabetics, who are prone to hypoglycemia, premonitory symptoms may be masked by β-blockade, and there is some evidence to suggest that prolonged therapy with propranolol may impair carbohydrate tolerance.[38] An area of current concern relates to the effects of some β-blockers on lipid metabolism.[44] Nonselective agents appear to increase plasma triglycerides as well as VLDL cholesterol, and may decrease the HDL cholesterol. The propensity for these adverse lipid changes is lessened in the presence of cardioselectivity or partial agonist activity.[45]

All β-blockers cross the blood-brain barrier to some degree, although higher central nervous system concentrations have been evidenced with the more lipophilic agents. As a result, symptoms of fatigue, depression, sleep disturbances, and occasional nightmares have been commonly observed with this class of agents. Clinical experience suggests that the hydrophilic β-blockers have less propensity for these central nervous system adverse effects. β-blockers should be used with caution in patients receiving digitalis glycosides, since excessive bradycardia has been reported in patients receiving both agents.

Some β-adrenergic blockers are less effective in lowering blood pressure in black individuals with hypertension, and, as should be apparent from previous discussion, side effect profiles may vary from agent to agent. The β-blockers are the only antihypertensive drugs shown to reduce the risk of ischemic heart disease, particularly as it relates to morbidity and mortality following an initial myocardial infarction. In general, immediate reductions in blood pressure are not expected with administration of a β-blocker. Continued therapy for several days to a week or longer is needed to appreciate the full pharmacologic effects of these agents.

A recently released parenteral β_1 cardioselective β-blocker, esmolol, has demonstrated immediate antihypertensive effects. It is ultrashort acting and is used primarily for the control of supraventricular tachycardia, but it has been tested successfully for the control of perioperative hypertension, including postcoronary artery bypass surgery. After a loading dose of 500 μg/kg is administered over 1 minute, a maintenance infusion of 25 to 200 μg/kg/min is titrated by increments of 50 μg/kg/min at 5- to 10-minute intervals. Increments in dosage may be preceded by reboluses of 500 μg/kg.

Combined α- and β-blocker

Labetalol differs from currently available β-adrenergic blocking agents in its ability to block both α- and β-adrenergic receptors. Systemic vascular resistance and arterial blood pressure are reduced, while heart rate is unchanged or slightly suppressed and cardiac output is generally unaffected. This hemodynamic profile is observed within minutes of an intravenous injection of labetalol, and changes persist during long-term oral administration. Labetalol also demonstrates mild intrinsic agonist activity for β_2-adrenergic receptors, an effect that may help explain its improved tolerance in patients with asthma or COPD. Clinical studies have demonstrated labetalol to be more effective in black and elderly individuals than other β-blockers.

As with other β-adrenergic blockers, labetalol should be avoided or used with caution in patients with asthma, heart block greater than first-degree, severe sinus bradycardia, or decompensated congestive heart failure. The most common adverse effect observed with oral administration of labetalol is postural hypotension, a manifestation of the α-blocking properties of this agent.

The immediate effectiveness of labetalol by intravenous infusion or intermittent pulse administration has made labetalol the drug of choice for many clinicians in the initial management of hypertensive urgencies or emergencies, including pheochromocytoma.[46,47] The observation of peak antihypertensive effects within 90 to 120 minutes after oral administration has led to increasing usage in the initial management of severe hypertension or hypertensive urgencies.

Central adrenergic inhibitors

The four agents in this family of drugs, methyldopa, clonidine, guanabenz, and guanfacine, appear to exert their major effects upon central nervous system vasomotor centers. These agents function primarily by decreasing sympathetic outflow from the central nervous system.

Dryness of the mouth and drowsiness occur frequently with these agents and are the most common adverse effects. No significant adverse effects have been reported on either carbohydrate metabolism or blood lipid concentrations. In fact, clinical trials have suggested that guanabenz may reduce total cholesterol and triglycerides. The decrease in cholesterol appears primarily because of a reduction in the low-density lipoprotein fraction. A pronounced withdrawal reaction may develop within 12 to 48 hours after sudden discontinuation of clonidine or guanabenz therapy. The withdrawal syndrome occurs most commonly in patients receiving larger doses of either agent and is associated with restlessness, irritability, tremors, tachycardia, abdominal pain, and marked rebound hypertension. The hypertension is associated with increased plasma and urinary catecholamines. Patients must be warned of the risk of this withdrawal syndrome, should they abruptly discontinue medication. A longer duration of action of guanfacine enables once-daily administration, while other agents in this class are administered twice daily.

Clonidine may be administered transdermally in an adherent skin patch that provides sufficient drug treatment for 7 days at a time. The transdermal preparation is available in sizes delivering the equivalent of 0.1 mg, 0.2 mg, or 0.3 mg of clonidine per day. While the incidence of drowsiness and dry mouth appear less with the transdermal preparation, a major limitation in its usage has been the development of localized skin reactions with pruritus.[48]

The central α-agonists are useful in treating a broad range of patients with hypertension, including those with renal insufficiency, asthma, or chronic obstructive pulmonary disease, and diabetes mellitus. The absence of adverse metabolic effects, particularly on plasma lipid profiles, provides a potential advantage in treating hypertensives at high risk for progression of atherosclerosis. Adverse effects can be minimized by concomitant administration of a small dose of a diuretic to enable smaller daily dosages of the agent of choice.

α-Adrenergic blocking agents

Two early α-adrenergic blockers, phentolamine and phenoxybenzamine, are currently reserved for the diagnosis and treatment of hypertensive states associated with high circulating levels of catecholamines. Intravenous administration of phentolamine is followed by a transient α-adrenergic blockade. Significant cardiac stimulation with tachycardia and occasional cardiac arrhythmias may be associated with its use. A transient and sometimes marked reduction in blood pressure will be observed in patients with high circulating levels of catecholamines from an actively secreting tumor, or from rebound hypertension following abrupt discontinuation of clonidine or guanabenz.

Similarly, oral phenoxybenzamine is still used in the preoperative management of patients with pheochromocytoma. It is a short-acting agent, and its administration is also associated with profound postural hypotension and reflex tachycardia.

Prazosin induces functional blockade of postsynaptic α_1-adrenergic receptors to reduce peripheral vascular resistance. It dilates both arterioles and veins, and, unlike phentolamine or phenoxybenzamine, does not induce reflex tachycardia. The most common side effect of prazosin is postural hypotension, which can often be minimized by initiating therapy with a low dosage and increasing it gradually. Terazosin is also a selective postsynaptic α_1-blocker, differing from prazosin in having more predictable absorption and better bioavailability following oral administration and a longer duration of action that enables once-daily administration.

Both prazosin and terazosin can be administered to hypertensives with renal insufficiency without changing the dosage. Use of these agents in hypertensive patients with congestive heart failure has not been associated with any significant reduction in mortality. These agents have no detrimental effects on pulmonary function and can be useful in hypertensive patients with asthma. No adverse effects have been demonstrated in carbohydrate metabolism or in lipid levels. In fact, clinical studies have suggested a slight decrease in total cholesterol and a rise in the HDL cholesterol with long-term therapy, making prazosin and terazosin suitable treatment choices for high-risk hypertensive patients with hyperlipidemia. Because of the propensity for postural hypotension following α_1-blockade, these agents must be used with caution in patients with autonomic impairment, including elderly individuals, in whom baroreceptor responses are often impaired.

Rauwolfia alkaloids

The rauwolfia alkaloid compounds, including reserpine, were among the earliest available sympathetic inhibiting agents for treating hypertension. The use of reserpine has declined progressively over the last two decades with the emergence of many new classes of effective and better-tolerated agents.

The major limitations in the use of reserpine have been its modest efficacy and significant adverse effect profile. The sedative and depressive effects of reserpine are subtle, and have been mostly observed with dosages exceeding 0.25 mg daily. It is expected that the use of reserpine will continue to progressively decline.

Postganglionic sympathetic compounds

Guanethidine and guanadrel inhibit the function of postganglionic sympathetic neurons by accumulation and displacement of norepinephrine from neuronal storage granules. Blood pressure reduction is associated with a decrease in cardiac output, caused primarily by pooling of blood in capacitance vessels and decreased venous return to the heart. The use of these agents today is reserved for patients with severe or refractory hypertension in whom combinations of other, better-tolerated agents have been ineffective.

The clinical pharmacology and problems experienced with guanethidine are similar to guanadrel, with one caveat. The major advantage of guanadrel over guanethidine is its shorter duration of action, an advantage that is most notable in the patient who develops incapacitating postural symptoms on guanethidine. The potential for drug interactions is the same as that observed with guanethidine. These compounds are infrequently required in the therapy of hypertension today since the vast majority of patients can be controlled with one or a combination of other agents that are far better tolerated.

Direct vasodilating agents

Since direct vasodilators reduce peripheral vascular resistance, the primary hemodynamic abnormality in essential hypertension, they should be preferred therapeutic agents. Unfortunately, their effectiveness is limited by the responsiveness of homeostatic mechanisms, which tend to blunt the pharmacologic response to vasodilators (increased cardiac output, increased plasma renin activity, and increased plasma volume). Vasodilators have largely been relegated to use in combination with adrenergic blocking agents and diuretics.

Hydralazine. Hydralazine lowers peripheral vascular resistance by a direct effect on arteriolar smooth muscle.[49] Reflex increases in heart rate and cardiac output accompany its use as monotherapy because it has little effect on venous capacitance; in patients with coronary artery disease, the increased cardiac work may precipitate anginal symptoms. Stimulation of the renin-angiotensin-aldosterone system contributes to sodium and water retention and expansion of plasma volume, which may lead to rapid pseudotolerance.

The major metabolism of hydralazine occurs in the liver by ring hydroxylation and subsequent conjugation. Most reported cases of hydralazine toxicity, including the development of antinuclear antibodies and rheumatoid arthritis-like symptoms, have probably occurred in slow acetylators.[50] Patients with renal failure acetylate hydralazine more slowly, and adjustment in dosage may be required because of slow acetylation and decreased renal clearance of the unchanged drug.

Hydralazine has been used parenterally to manage selected hypertensive emergencies. Although affording the convenience of either intramuscular or intravenous administration, it is not as consistently effective as newer vasodilating agents such as diazoxide or sodium nitroprusside. Hydralazine remains a favorite with some clinicians to manage eclampsia of pregnancy.

Minoxidil. Minoxidil is an extremely potent vasodilating agent with hemodynamic actions similar to those of hydralazine. Vasodilation is accompanied by reflex tachycardia, increased cardiac output, and a propensity for sodium and water retention. Minoxidil added to a β-blocker to control reflex cardiac stimulation and a loop diuretic to control fluid retention is a potent combination in the management of severe or refractory hypertension.

While the drug has a relatively short plasma half-life of approximately 4 hours, once-daily administration is effective in most patients. The most common adverse effects are those common to direct vasodilating agents, such as headache, tachycardia, palpitations, and aggravation of anginal symptoms. A common adverse effect of prolonged use, hirsutism, can be of considerable cosmetic concern to some patients. The use of topical minoxidil in the treatment of pattern baldness has not been associated with any adverse effects upon blood pressure in hypertensive patients.

Diazoxide. When administered intravenously, diazoxide is a potent arteriolar vasodilator with rapid onset of action. The maximum hypotensive effect is usually observed within 3 to 5 minutes following injection and may persist for variable periods of 1 to 12 hours or longer.[51] The rapid, dose-related reduction in blood pressure has been associated with impaired regional blood flow in patients with significant coronary or cerebrovascular disease. It is recommended that diazoxide be administered in repeated, small pulse doses of 50 to 75 mg, given at intervals of 5 to 15 minutes. With repeated pulse administration, a more gradual and controllable reduction in blood pressure can be obtained, thus minimizing the risk of cerebral or myocardial ischemia.[52] Concomitant administration of a β-adrenergic blocker is useful in patients with coronary artery disease to prevent reflex tachycardia, and concomitant administration of a loop diuretic is recommended to prevent sodium and water retention with repeated dosages.

Diazoxide induces hyperglycemia; occasionally, adjustments in insulin dosage may be required in diabetic patients. The hypotensive effects of diazoxide may be exaggerated by concomitant administration of other antihypertensive agents, particularly other vasodilators, and by intravascular volume depletion. Since diazoxide displaces coumarin anticoagulants from their binding sites on serum albumin, reduction of the anticoagulant dose may be necessary in patients receiving both diazoxide and a coumarin derivative. Diazoxide should only be considered in the initial management of patients with severe hypertension or in hypertensive emergencies.

Sodium nitroprusside. This agent differs from other direct vasodilators in that both resistance and capacitance vessels are affected; thus decreases in both arterial pressure and central venous pressure accompany its use.[53] Because of its ability to improve left ventricular function without inducing reflex tachycardia, it has been a particularly useful agent in managing the hypertensive crisis associated with congestive heart failure or following acute myocardial infarction. The rate of reduction in blood pressure during intravenous administration of sodium nitroprusside depends on the rate of infusion. Its rapid onset of effect, and rapid disappearance following discontinuation, necessitate administration of a controlled infusion in an intensive care environment with constant nursing supervision. Nitroprusside is almost universally effective and will lower blood pressure when other potent antipressor agents have failed.

Sodium nitroprusside is rapidly metabolized to cyanogen and subsequently converted to thiocyanate, which is excreted by the kidneys. Acute toxicity is primarily related to excessive vasodilation and hypotension, and symptoms disappear promptly when the infusion is stopped or slowed. In patients with renal failure, excessive accumulation of thiocyanate may occur after several days of administration and may produce manifestations of toxicity ranging from weakness, nausea and tinnitus, to overt psychosis. There is a small but significant risk of cyanide toxicity, which has been observed with prolonged use of nitroprusside in patients with refractory heart failure and poor tissue perfusion.[54] Rapid decomposition of nitroprusside on exposure to light necessitates the use of opaque wrappings during administration and periodic replacement with fresh solutions.

Nitroglycerin. Intravenous nitroglycerin shares several of the advantages of sodium nitroprusside, including its rapid onset and offset of action and the ability to titrate the drug to a desired goal blood pressure under close supervision. Unlike nitroprusside, nitroglycerin predominantly dilates venous capacitance vessels, but when large doses are administered, arteriolar dilation may also be observed. By reducing both left ventricular filling pressure and mean arterial pressure, end-diastolic volume and pressure and myocardial oxygen demand are reduced. Collateral coronary blood vessels are also dilated and improved perfusion to ischemic areas and myocardium can be observed, as opposed to sodium nitroprusside, which decreases flow to ischemic myocardium. Thus nitroglycerin is efficacious in hypertensive patients with significant coronary artery disease and has proved particularly effective in the management of hypertensives following coronary artery bypass surgery.[55,56] It is also a treatment of choice in congestive heart failure when blood pressure before treatment is normal or only modestly elevated.

Nitroglycerin's ultrashort half-life, measured in minutes, requires close and constant supervision of continuous infusions. Headache, flushing, and dizziness may be observed during infusion, but can usually be minimized by starting with small initial infusion rates. Because of variable absorption by plastic containers and tubing, glass containers must be employed for dilution and storage, combined with nonabsorbing administration tubing. Nitroglycerin may be useful in managing hypertension with renal failure, since it lacks the risk of cyanide and/or thiocyanate toxicity.

Angiotensin converting enzyme (ACE) inhibitors

Experience with these agents has clearly demonstrated that blood pressure can be substantially reduced in a majority of patients by blockade of the renin-angiotensin-aldosterone system.[57,58] The major action of the ACE inhibitors resides in their ability to inhibit the conversion of angiotensin I to the potent vasoactive peptide, angiotensin II, thus inducing vasodilation and reduced peripheral vascular resistance. A secondary decrease in aldosterone secretion prevents sodium and water retention and adds to the utility of this class of agents as monotherapy in managing mild and moderate hypertension. Their combined vasodilator and natriuretic effects have led to their wide acceptance as primary agents in managing congestive heart failure with or without complicating hypertension. Vasodilation and reduced blood pressure are accomplished without reflex cardiac stimulation, possibly caused in part by the parasympathomimetic action of these agents. Other potential mechanisms of action may include accumulation, via ACE inhibition, of vasodilator bradykinins and prostaglandins, or possibly by interactions within the central nervous system, as well as the peripheral sympathetic nervous system to blunt baroceptor responsiveness. Emerging evidence suggests the existence of tissue-specific renin-angiotensin systems, including vascular endothelium. It is intriguing to consider the possibility that future developments may provide ACE inhibitors with different tissue-specific responses.[57]

ACE inhibitors are excreted wholly or in part by the kidney, and adjustments in dosage may be required in patients with renal insufficiency. These agents have no adverse effects on lipid metabolism, pulmonary function, or carbohydrate metabolism, and recent studies suggest that ACE inhibitors reduce proteinuria and may have the potential for preservation of renal function in hypertensive diabetics with diabetic nephropathy. Clinical experience suggests that ACE inhibitors, when used as monotherapy, are more effective in whites and younger individuals than they are in blacks or older individuals. When combined with a diuretic, additive effects are noted on blood pressure, and the age and racial differences are no longer apparent.

Several adverse effects occur with ACE inhibitors as a class that deserve attention. Potentially hazardous hypotension may follow the initial dose of an ACE inhibitor if administered to a patient who is volume-depleted. It is appropriate to discontinue diuretics for several days before initiating ACE inhibitor therapy. If this is not practical, the first dose should be administered under close clinical surveillance. Sudden, severe hypotension and oliguric renal failure has been observed with ACE inhibitors administered to patients with bilateral high-grade renal artery stenosis or high-grade stenosis to a solitary functioning kidney.[59] The increasing prevalence of generalized arteriosclerotic occlusive disease, including renovascular disease or cholesterol emboli and azotemia, in older patients makes this a noteworthy caution when considering ACE inhibitors in this population.[60]

Hyperkalemia is routinely observed with ACE inhibitors, and, while these agents may blunt the tendency toward hypokalemia when used with diuretics, the clinician must be aware of a significant risk of hyperkalemia if potassium-sparing agents or potassium supplements are used concurrently. A dry, nonproductive cough is now clearly the most common adverse effect observed with ACE inhibitors, and, when searched for, may be observed in as many as 10% of patients.[61,62] While the mechanism for cough is unclear, a possible pulmonary effect of accumulated bradykinin is suspected. While rarely observed, angioedema is a potentially life-threatening adverse effect. Adverse effects such as leukopenia, nephrotic-range proteinuria, dysgeusia, and skin rashes are rarely observed with current, therapeutic doses of captopril and have rarely been observed with subsequent generations of ACE inhibitors.

Much recent attention has been focused on the quality of life of patients undergoing long-term antihypertensive therapy.[63] The ACE inhibitors clearly possess many of the features considered desirable in the optimal antihypertensive agent, and this recognition has contributed to the rapid growth in physician prescribing and patient acceptance of this class of agents.

Calcium channel blockers

Calcium channel blockers have had a major impact on the treatment of patients with ischemic heart disease and a variety of cardiovascular and noncardiovascular disorders.[64] The antihypertensive effects of calcium channel blockers have been known for many years, but only recently have they received approval as antihypertensive agents in the United States. Although representing a chemically diverse group of compounds, calcium channel blockers all act by selective inhibition of calcium influx through cell membranes. Despite sharing the same pharmacologic mechanism of action at the cell level, clinical effects of subgroups of calcium channel blockers are quite different, particularly as they relate to the contractile process of the heart, vascular smooth muscle and skeletal muscle, and cardiac nodal conduction tissue.[65] These differences apparently relate to differences in relative specificity of different calcium channel blockers for effector tissues.

Extensive first-pass metabolism and short plasma half-lives once necessitated frequent doses to maintain an adequate clinical response. The recent availability of long-acting preparations of currently available agents, verapamil, diltiazem, and nifedipine, now enables once-daily or twice-daily administration in most patients.

Calcium channel blockers have no adverse effects on lipid metabolism or carbohydrate metabolism with prolonged use and can be safely administered to the asthmatic hypertensive patient. A natriuretic and diuretic effect observed with most calcium channel blockers may explain the lack of sodium and volume retention, which enables administration of these agents as monotherapy.

Clinical observations suggest that calcium channel blockers are particularly efficacious in older and black hypertensive patients, who share a tendency toward normal to low plasma renin activity. Use of calcium channel blockers need not be restricted to these groups since their efficacy in younger, white hypertensive patients has also been observed.

Nifedipine deserves special mention, since it has emerged as an agent of choice in the initial treatment of patients with hypertensive urgencies or emergencies.[66] The ease of administration sublingually or orally and a rapid dose response within 30 to 60 minutes have undoubtedly contributed to its popularity. However, a word of caution must be offered. In older patients with significant occlusive cerebral or coronary vascular disease, the uncontrolled, initial response to nifedipine may be accompanied by symptomatic cerebral or coronary ischemia.

The predominant vasodilator effects of dihydropyridine derivatives such as nifedipine and nicardipine may cause headache, reflex tachycardia, dizziness, and edema. The latter is caused by fluid redistribution, not retention. Constipation is the most prominent side effect of negative inotropic agents such as verapamil and diltiazem. Diltiazem and verapamil should be used with caution in combination with β-blockers in patients with atrial ventricular conduction disturbances.

The efficacy of the calcium channel blockers, together with their high degree of patient acceptance, has contributed to their rapid increase in clinical use.[67] Experimental observations suggesting a potential antiatherogenic effect and an ability to mitigate renal ischemia, together with a host of other noncardiovascular effects, tend to enhance the future promise of this class of agents.

USEFULNESS OF PHARMACOLOGIC THERAPY

Combined clinical trials over the last 30 years have demonstrated reduced cardiovascular mortality and morbidity with reduction of blood pressure, particularly in patients with diastolic blood pressures greater than 104 mm Hg.[68,69] In patients with mild hypertension (DBP 90 to 104 mm Hg), clinical trials have shown protection against stroke, congestive heart failure, progression to more severe levels of hypertension, and all-cause mortality.[70,71] In addition, a 30% to 50% reduction in both fatal and nonfatal strokes has been demonstrated with therapy. Protection against the complications of coronary artery disease as a result of antihypertensive therapy has not been convincingly demonstrated.[68] Analysis of the major clinical trials shows a trend of reduced mortality from coronary artery disease in intervention groups, but the differences do not reach statistical significance. While numerous explanations have been offered for the lack of demonstrated benefit for coronary artery disease, it is not known whether these explanations account for the failure of studies to demonstrate significant effects of therapy on the incidence of coronary artery disease.

For the initial treatment of patients with diastolic pressures between 90 and 94 mm Hg who are otherwise at low risk for developing cardiovascular disease, JNC IV recommends initial therapy with nonpharmacologic measures, which have been reviewed in an earlier section of this chapter.[13] As a consensus document, JNC IV suggests that some clinicians may wish to initiate pharmacologic therapy in those patients whose diastolic pressures remain above 90 mm Hg despite a period of 3 to 6 months of vigorous nonpharmacologic therapy. Physicians who elect not to initiate drug therapy for patients in this range must accept the responsibility for monitoring patients closely, since some will progress to higher levels of blood pressure, with attendant higher risks, that clearly warrant drug treatment.

Individualized stepped-care therapy (JNC IV recommendations)

The 1984 report of the Joint National Committee on Detection, Evaluation, and Treatment of High Blood Pressure (JNC III) recommended that a thiazide diuretic or a β-adrenergic blocker be used as initial therapy in most patients, unless contraindications to their use exist.[72] Clinical experience with ACE inhibitors and calcium antagonists, demonstrating comparable efficacy, encouraged JNC IV (1988) to include these two classes of agents along with diuretics and β-blockers as recommended classes of drugs for initial therapy.

A scheme for individualizing stepped-care therapy was outlined by JNC IV (Fig. 16-1). It was noted that the large number of effective antihypertensive agents currently available provide many excellent options for effective therapy with minimal side effects. If after several months of initial therapy, blood pressure has not been controlled, several options for subsequent therapy are offered: (1) Increase the dose of the initial drug. (2) Add an agent from another class. (3) Discontinue the initial choice and substitute a drug from another class as monotherapy. If a diuretic is not chosen as

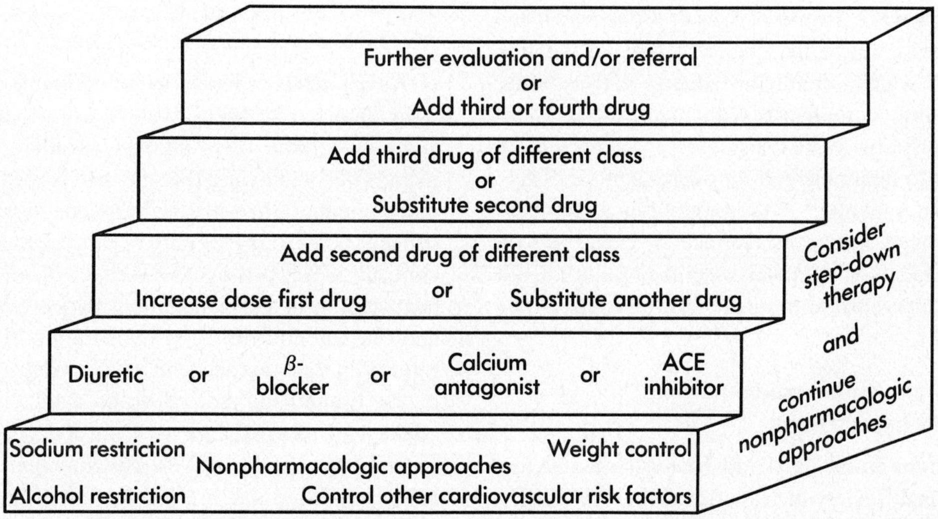

Fig. 16-1. Individualized stepped-care therapy for hypertension. For some patients, nonpharmacologic therapy should be tried first. If blood pressure goal is not achieved, add pharmacologic therapy. Other patients may require pharmacologic therapy initially. In these instances, nonpharmacologic therapy may be a helpful adjunct. ACE indicates angiotensin converting enzyme.
(From The 1988 report of the Joint National Committee on Detection, Evaluation, and Treatment of High Blood Pressure, Arch Intern Med 148:1023, 1988.)

the initial drug, it will often be advisable as a second agent since fluid retention may be responsible in part for the suboptimal response to some nondiuretic agents. Before proceeding to each subsequent treatment step, physicians should look for possible reasons for nonresponsiveness to initial therapy. JNC IV also emphasized the importance of step-down therapy for patients with mild hypertension whose blood pressure has been adequately controlled for periods of 1 year or longer. Obviously, if discontinuation of antihypertensive agents is possible, regular follow-up examinations must be maintained since blood pressure can rise again to hypertensive levels even after years without therapy.

JNC IV also emphasizes the usefulness of other clinical factors that may be helpful in the selection or tailoring of initial therapy, particularly in patients with mild or uncomplicated hypertension who are likely to require only one drug for adequate control. Studies have indicated that blacks and older patients tend to respond better to diuretics or calcium antagonists than to β-blockers or ACE inhibitors. Gender has not been found to be a factor in control of blood pressure with currently available agents. Clinicians must be aware of the fact that antihypertensive drugs may worsen some diseases while improving other conditions. For example, β-blockers may worsen asthma and arteriosclerosis obliterans of the lower extremities but may improve symptoms of angina pectoris and certain migraine or vascular headaches. Awareness of the more common adverse effects of the different classes of antihypertensive agents is critical to optimal tailoring of initial and subsequent antihypertensive therapy.[73] Patients will not tolerate undesirable symptoms, a particular problem of some centrally acting agents, while other drugs with β-adrenergic blocking properties may reduce exercise tolerance. Newer classes of drugs may offer the opportunity to optimize the quality of life of the hypertensive patient while minimizing adverse effects, thus optimizing long-term compliance with medication.[63] The cost of therapy must always be considered and represents a significant barrier to treatment and long-term control of hypertension in some patients.[74] A thorough clinical appreciation of the beneficial and adverse effects of each class of antihypertensive agents is extremely useful in tailoring the selection of antihypertensive drugs for the individual patient.

World Health Organization guidelines for treatment of mild hypertension

Recommendations from the World Health Organization and the International Society of Hypertension (WHO/ISH) relative to the therapy of mild hypertension differs somewhat from attitudes in the United States as proposed by JNC IV. The WHO/ISH recommend concentrating on nonpharmacologic treatment in patients whose diastolic blood pressure averages less than 100 mm Hg, while initiating drug therapy if diastolic pressure averages greater than 100 mm Hg over a 3-month period.[75] After a more prolonged period of observation and nonpharmacologic therapy (3 to 6 months), drug therapy may be considered for diastolic pressures greater than or equal to 95 mm Hg. WHO/ISH notes that individuals whose diastolic pressures remain greater than 95 mm Hg also have an increased risk of cardiovascular disease, which is more marked in smokers, diabetics, and those with hypercholesterolemia. Drug therapy is recommended for those with diastolic blood pressures of 90 to 95 mm Hg who are at higher risk because of associated cardiovascular risk factors. Any of the available classes of antihypertensive agents are suggested as appropriate initial therapy. The value of both diuretic and nondiuretic-containing drug combinations of agents is also noted.

Criticisms of JNC IV

Some clinicians feel that JNC IV did not go far enough in its recommendations. In particular, criticism has been directed toward a failure to break away from the stepladder or stepped-care approach to drug additions.[76] It is also noted that the JNC IV report failed to emphasize the importance of the J-curve for coronary mortality, despite the fact that multiple reports have now documented that reduction of diastolic pressures below 85 to 90 mm Hg is associated with increased coronary mortality.[77,78] The report has also been criticized because only four classes of antihypertensive agents were suggested as being most appropriate for initiation of treatment in patients with mild hypertension, as well as the report's recommendation that most patients with diastolic pressures of 90 to 94 mm Hg will benefit from drug therapy. As noted, this remains a point of disagreement between most clinicians in the United States and those outside the United States.

A reasoned approach to treatment

As one reads or listens to the continuing debate regarding individualized stepped-care versus tailored care or discussions in defense of traditional vs alternative therapy, clinicians become aware that the differences expressed appear more semantic than real.[79,80] Opponents of the stepped-care concept point to the rigidity of this approach today. Yet, the concept of stepped care was never meant to be a rigid sequence of drug additions, but always provided for flexibility and the potential for drug substitution. The appearance of rigidity in this approach, in its early days, was more related to the limited number of drugs available at the time the concept of stepped-care was introduced. Subsequent JNC reports have recognized the development of new drugs and have broadened the "menu" for initial therapy.

There is sufficient evidence from comparative clinical trials to suggest that all of the currently available classes of antihypertensive agents are efficacious and will in fact control blood pressure in about one half of those mild hypertensives treated with initial therapy. It is interesting that two drugs in combination, as long as they are not two drugs in the same class, will control blood pressure in more than 85% to 90% of patients with mild to moderate hypertension. Recognizing that we can control the vast number of patients with hypertension with available therapy, the issues come down to those of understanding the clinical pharmacology of the available antihypertensive agents to take advantage of selected clinical parameters, which enables skillful individualization or tailoring of treatment to the hypertensive patient.[73]

There have been no carefully controlled clinical trials providing convincing evidence that traditional agents, diuretics and β-blockers, can be incriminated in the failure of hypertension control to show greater reductions in coronary mortality. On the other hand, these agents have been part of the majority of major clinical trials during the last several decades, all of which have demonstrated reduced cardiovascular morbidity and mortality associated with improved blood pressure control. These agents are cost-effective and have proved to be efficacious and safe during prolonged use. As we view the newer classes of agents, they clearly are not associated with the degree of adverse metabolic and electrolyte adverse effects seen with older agents, and their vasodilator effects do address the primary abnormality in most hypertensive patients, an elevated peripheral vascular resistance. On the down side, there are as yet no long-term data (over 5 years) regarding adherence, safety or efficacy, and outcome with these newer classes of drugs. At this time, we do not know whether a change to newer agents will in fact be associated with a greater reduction in cardiovascular mortality than has been observed with older, traditional therapies.

As we view cost effectiveness, it is true that older agents are inexpensive by today's standards, which can be a major factor in long-term patient adherence to therapy. On the other hand, newer classes of agents clearly have very favorable adverse effect profiles, and may in fact provide a better quality of life than that observed on some older therapies. The quality of life issue also represents an important factor from the standpoint of long-term adherence to therapy. The bottom line regarding cost-effectiveness is clearly the ability to maintain optimal adherence and ensure long-term control of blood pressure, to minimize morbid events and the extraordinary costs associated with these events.

For patients with mild hypertension not controlled with a single agent, or patients with moderate to severe hypertension requiring two or three drugs in combination, it is not necessary to proceed to the maximum recommended dosage of each agent used in the regimen before considering the addition of another drug. It is appropriate to ascertain that a patient tolerates a given dosage of a medication with few if any adverse effects, when considering the addition of a second or third drug to the regimen. The adverse effects of most agents are dose-related, and utilization of smaller doses of two or more agents in combination may ensure fewer side effects, better long-term compliance, and therefore a better quality of life for the patient being treated. Nowhere is this better demonstrated than in the trend toward reduced doses of oral diuretics. A dosage of 50 mg of hydrochlorothiazide, or its equivalent, is now considered maximal, with many patients responding to doses of 12.5 to 25 mg daily. Doses as low as 6.25 mg of hydrochlorothiazide may, in fact, provide additive effects when combined with other classes of antihypertensive drugs. It is likely that use of smaller doses of other classes of agents will also be pursued, particularly in combination, in an effort to minimize well-recognized adverse effects of individual drugs. Fortunately, there are few adverse drug-drug interactions between currently available classes of antihypertensive agents that would discourage combination use.

MANAGEMENT OF RESISTANT HYPERTENSION

Resistant hypertension may be defined as the persistence of blood pressure greater than 150/100 mm Hg in a patient receiving at least three different pharmacologic agents, including an oral diuretic. Hypertension truly resistant to currently available drugs is uncommon in clinical practice.[81,82] Thus difficulties experienced in the control of blood pressure today must be placed in appropriate perspective. The most common reason for inadequate control of blood pressure is poor patient adherence (patient resistance) with nonpharmacologic treatment, prescribed drugs, or recommended follow-up. Conversely, it may be the physician who is resistant if treatment is unsuccessful in a patient who has received inadequate education regarding his or her disease process, an inadequate or inappropriate drug regimen, or who has not been dissuaded from use of other interfering drugs. Keep in mind that aspirin, nonsteroidal antiinflammatory drugs, oral contraceptive agents, tricyclic antidepressant compounds, and other drugs may antagonize the effectiveness of certain antihypertensive agents. Thorough knowledge of a patient's concomitant disease conditions and related symptoms is critical in drug selection if undesirable adverse effects are to be minimized.

In evaluating resistant hypertension, the clinician must not be misled by the patient whose blood pressure is elevated only in the office (office hypertension) or by the patient with generalized atherosclerosis who may demonstrate pseudohypertension with auscultatory measurements of blood pressure.

Sodium and volume play a major role in patients with resistant hypertension.[83] Failure to appropriately control salt intake may lead to blood pressure that is refractory to many antihypertensive agents, even when a diuretic is a part of the treatment regimen. In the patient with progressive renal parenchymal disease, retention of salt and water occurs early to contribute to the establishment of hypertension, and as the disease progresses other hemodynamic and humoral factors contribute to its persistence. Associated obesity and excessive alcohol consumption can contribute to sustained hypertension despite apparently adequate drug treatment.

Finally a presumptive diagnosis of essential hypertension in the patient with unsuspected secondary hypertension (pheochromocytoma, aldosteronism, and renovascular hypertension) may result in hypertension resistant to therapy. Having considered these factors and before considering the patient truly resistant, a further search for a secondary cause of hypertension is often indicated. Only after consideration of these factors in a patient who is apparently unresponsive to appropriate medication should a diagnosis of resistant hypertension be entertained.

HYPERTENSION IN THE ELDERLY

Evidence supporting benefits from the treatment of hypertension in elderly patients is much less than the extensive clinical trial evidence reported in younger hypertensive populations. Several clinical trials have included hypertensive patients between 60 and 69 years of age and have demonstrated lower rates of cardiovascular events.[84-86] All patients entered in these trials had diastolic pressures greater than 90 to 95 mm Hg. A more recent study, the European Working Party on Hypertension in the Elderly (EWPHE), included elderly subjects between 60 and 97 years of age at entry.[87] Treatment appeared beneficial for individuals with entry systolic pressures greater than 160 mm Hg and those with entry diastolic pressures greater than 95 mm Hg. The sample size in this study of individuals above age 80 years was small, negating firm recommendations for individuals in this older age group. A significant 38% decrease in overall cardiovascular mortality was observed; a 32% reduction in cerebrovascular mortality did not quite reach statistical significance. Concern has been expressed about aggressive overtreatment of elderly patients because of observations that those with the lowest treated levels of diastolic pressure actually may have a higher risk of myocardial infarction.[77,78] Contrary to this, another study has confirmed the J-shaped relation in treated blood pressures and subsequent rates of fatal and nonfatal myocardial infarction, but noted that this relationship is observed in both treated and placebo groups.[88] When all cardiovascular risk factors are considered in the elderly patient, an increased systolic blood pressure is the single greatest risk factor, other than age, for increased cardiovascular morbidity and mortality.[89] The Systolic Hypertension in the Elderly Program (SHEP) is currently ongoing, but it is too early yet to determine if aggressive treatment of systolic hypertension will indeed be indicated. A pilot study of the SHEP program reported excellent control of systolic hypertension in elderly patients with very small doses (12.5 to 25 mg) of chlorthalidone.[90]

For treatment in the elderly, it is suggested that diastolic blood pressures be controlled to less than 90 mm Hg, as with younger hypertensive individuals. An acceptable goal for systolic blood pressure reduction would appear to be a range of 140 to 160 mm Hg.[91] Treatment decisions should be based on careful assessment, as with younger patients, in an effort to address problems with concomitant diseases and medications and the quality of life for the elderly patient on therapy.[92] Despite declining renal function with age, there is little evidence to suggest that currently available antihypertensive medications carry any risk of precipitating marked deterioration of renal function or renal failure. An exception with ACE inhibitors in patients with renal artery stenosis has been previously noted. Adverse effects of diuretics on either carbohydrate metabolism or blood lipids in the elderly appear minimal and transient, possibly because of metabolic differences with age or possibly because of the lower doses of diuretics currently in use. Evidence suggesting that β-blockers and ACE inhibitors are less effective in older patients does not mean they cannot be used, particularly when combined with a small dose of a diuretic. While adrenergic inhibitors such as β-blockers, methyldopa, clonidine, and guanabenz may be useful in the elderly, care must be taken to evaluate mentation and cognitive function before and during treatment in view of the central adverse effects associated with these agents. The effect of β-blockers to decrease cardiac output must also be considered in the elderly hypertensive patient who may have marginal left ventricular function. While older patients appear to tolerate medications well and demonstrate compliance comparable to that in younger hypertensives, care should be taken to simplify the regimen, ensure regular and frequent review of medications and dosing schedules, and assess patients carefully for adverse effects and potential drug interactions. Several studies have suggested that calcium channel blockers may be particularly effective in the elderly, but may be associated with peripheral edema and constipation that can be troublesome for many elderly individuals. Drugs that induce or exacerbate postural hypotension should be avoided in the elderly patient whenever possible.

Whatever the choice of initial and subsequent therapy in the elderly hypertensive patient, it is wise to initiate therapy with very small doses (one half the usual adult dose) and proceed slowly with drug titration. Blood pressures higher than suggested goal pressures are acceptable in the face of continued, disabling adverse effects.

HYPERTENSIVE URGENCIES AND EMERGENCIES

Most hypertensive urgencies and emergencies arise as a result of poorly controlled chronic hypertension from primary or secondary causes. Increased awareness, widespread detection efforts, and more aggressive therapy of mild and moderate hypertension have contributed to a progressive decline in the incidence of hypertensive urgencies and emergencies. A distinction between a hypertensive urgency and a true emergency can be helpful in determining the required expediency for therapy as well as the selection and route of administration of appropriate drugs.[93,94] A true hypertensive emergency represents a life-threatening condition in which blood pressure should be lowered to a safer level within minutes to 1 hour. Hypertensive urgencies are those situa-

Table 16-3. Drugs for the management of hypertensive emergencies

Preparation	Method of administration IM	Intermittent IV	Continuous IV
Vasodilating drugs*			
Sodium nitroprusside			0.5-10 μg/kg/min
Nitroglycerin			5-200 μg/min
Diazoxide		50-100 mg bolus injection	15-30 mg/min until the desired effect is achieved
Hydralazine hydrochloride	10-50 mg†	10-20 mg/20 ml‡	100-200 mg/L
Nifedipine	10-20 mg	Perforated capsule sublingually or orally	
Verapamil		5-10 mg	3-25 mg/hr
Enalaprilat		1.25 mg every 6 hours	
Sympathetic inhibiting drugs*			
Labetalol		20-80 mg by intermittent injection every 10-15 min	0.5-2.0 mg/kg/min
Trimethaphan camsylate			0.8-6 mg/min
Phentolamine	5-10 mg†	5-10 mg bolus injection	0.1-100 μg/kg/min
Reserpine	1-5 mg†	1-5 mg from syringe over 3-5 min	
Methyldopa		250-500 mg in 100 ml over 30-60 min	
Esmolol		500 μg/kg bolus injection	25-200 μg/kg/min§

*In most cases, a rapidly acting diuretic should be given intravenously at the beginning and at appropriate intervals throughout the treatment.
†Start with smallest dose listed.
‡Inject from syringe at rate of 1 mg/min until the desired effect is obtained.
§Titration every 5 min with reboluses each time.

tions in which the immediate risk to the integrity of the cardiovascular system is less, but prompt institution of drug therapy (usually oral) and reduction of blood pressure over several hours to 24 hours will be appropriate. Several agents have been successfully used by repeated administration or "loading dosages" to induce progressive but controlled reduction of blood pressure in hypertensive urgencies. These agents include clonidine, minoxidil, nifedipine, captopril, and more recently, labetalol. The rapid onset of effect, within 15 to 30 minutes, following administration of nifedipine has led to its becoming the most popular agent in this group.

Those parenteral agents currently available for treatment of the hypertensive emergency are listed in Table 16-3. These agents generally fall into two classes, direct vasodilating drugs and those agents that act through inhibition at various sites in the sympathetic nervous system. Nifedipine, while not administered intravenously, has also become a very popular drug for the initial treatment of hypertensive emergencies because of its ready availability and rapid onset of action, within 15 to 30 minutes.

In managing the hypertensive emergency or urgency, prompt initiation of therapy should take precedence over time-consuming diagnostic procedures. The agent selected, and the method of administration, should enable a controlled reduction of blood pressure to a safer level, usually a diastolic pressure in the range of 100 to 110 mm Hg. Additional diagnostic studies, if considered necessary, can be undertaken after blood pressure has been safely controlled. A thorough knowledge of the pharmacologic properties and proper indications of the currently available agents is essential for optimal management.

REFERENCES

1. Cornoni-Huntley J, LaCroix AZ, and Havlik RJ: Race and sex differentials in the impact of hypertension in the United States: the National Health and Nutrition Examination Survey I epidemiologic follow-up study, Arch Intern Med 149:780, 1989.
2. Ibrahim M et al: Hypertension prevalence and the status of awareness, treatment, and control in the United States: final report of the Subcommittee on Definition and Prevalence of the 1984 Joint National Committee, Hypertension 7:457, 1985.
3. Kannel WB: Role of blood pressure in cardiovascular morbidity and mortality, Prog Cardiovasc Dis 17:5, 1974.
4. Pooling Project Research Group: Relationship of blood pressure, serum cholesterol, smoking habit, relative weight, and ECG abnormalities to incidence of major coronary events: final report of the Pooling Project, J Chron Dis 31:201, 1978.
5. Society of Actuaries and Association of Life Insurance Medical Directors of America: blood pressure study, Chicago, 1979 and 1980.
6. Page IH: The mosaic theory. In Page IH: Hypertension mechanisms, New York,1987, Grune & Stratton, Inc.
7. Working Group on Renovascular Hypertension: Detection, evaluation, and treatment of renovascular hypertension, Arch Intern Med 147:820, 1987.
8. Bravo EL et al: The changing clinical spectrum of primary aldosteronism, Am J Med 74:641, 1983.
9. Bravo EL and Gifford RW Jr: Pheochromocytoma: diagnosis, localization and management, N Engl J Med 311:1298, 1984.

10. Eggers PW, Connerton R, and McMullan M: The Medicare experience with end-stage renal disease trends in incidence, prevalence, and survival, Health Care Financing Review 5:69, 1984.
11. Hostetter TH, Rennke HG, and Brenner BM: The case of intrarenal hypertension in the initiation and progression of diabetic and other glomerulopathies, Am J Med 72:375, 1982.
12. Lindeman RD, Tobin JD, and Shock NW: Association between blood pressure and the rate of decline in renal function, Kidney Int 26:861, 1984.
13. Joint National Committee on Detection, Evaluation, and Treatment of High Blood Pressure: The 1988 report of the Joint National Committee on Detection, Evaluation, and Treatment of High Blood Pressure, Arch Intern Med 148:1023, 1988.
14. Frohlich ED et al: Recommendations for human blood pressure determination by sphygmomanometers: report of a special task force appointed by the Steering Committee, American Heart Association, Hypertension 11:209A, 1988.
15. Kaplan NM: Treatment of hypertension: nondrug therapy and the rationale for drug therapy. In Kaplan NM: Clinical hypertension, ed 4, Baltimore, 1986, Williams & Wilkins.
16. Nonpharmacologic approaches to the control of high blood pressure: final report of the Subcommittee on Non-Pharmacologic Therapy of the Joint National Committee on Detection, Evaluation, and Treatment of High Blood Pressure, Hypertension 8:444, 1986.
17. Erwteman TM et al: B blockade, diuretics, and salt restriction for the management of mild hypertension: a randomised double blind trial, Br Med J 289:406, 1984.
18. Kaplan NM et al: Potassium supplementation in hypertensive patients with diuretic-induced hypokalemia, N Engl J Med 312:746, 1985.
19. McCarron DA: Calcium, magnesium, and phosphorus balance in human and experimental hypertension, Hypertension 4 (suppl III):III-27, 1982.
20. Resnick LM, Nicholson JP, and Laragh JH: Outpatient therapy of essential hypertension with dietary calcium supplementation, J Am Coll Cardiol 3:616, 1984 (abstract).
21. Resnick LM, Gupta RK, and Laragh JH: Intracellular free magnesium in erythrocytes of essential hypertension: relation to blood pressure and serum divalent cations, Proc Natl Acad Sci USA 81:6511, 1984.
22. Aristimuno GG et al: Influence of persistent obesity in children on cardiovascular risk factors: the Bogalusa heart study, Circulation 69:895, 1984.
23. Barrett-Connor E and Khaw KT: Is hypertension more benign when associated with obesity? Circulation 72:53, 1985.
24. Haffner SM et al: Do upper body and centralized adiposity measure different aspects of regional body fat distribution? Relationship to non-insulin-dependent diabetes mellitus, lipids, and lipoproteins, Diabetes 36:43, 1987.
25. Donahue RP et al: Central obesity, and coronary heart disease in men, Lancet 1:821, 1987.
26. MacMahon SW and Norton RN: Alcohol and hypertension: implications for prevention and treatment, Ann Intern Med 105:124, 1986.
27. Dawber TR: The Framingham Study: the epidemiology of atherosclerotic disease, Cambridge, Mass, 1980, Harvard University Press.
28. Kaplan NM: Therapy for mild hypertension: toward a more balanced view, JAMA 249:365, 1983.
29. Blair SN et al: Physical fitness and all-cause mortality: a prospective study of healthy men and women, JAMA 262:2395, 1989.
30. Health and Public Policy Committee, American College of Physicians: Biofeedback for hypertension, Ann Intern Med 102:709, 1985.
31. Engel BT, Glasgow MS, and Gaarder KR: Behavioral treatment of high blood pressure. III. Follow-up results and treatment recommendations, Psychosom Med 45:23, 1983.
32. Robertson D et al: Caffeine and hypertension, Am J Med 77:54, 1984.
33. AMA Drug Evaluations, ed 5, Chicago, 1983, American Medical Association.
34. McMahon FG: In management of essential hypertension: the new low dose therapy ed 2, Mount Kisco, NY, 1984, Futura Publishing Co.
35. Vidt DG: Antihypertensive agents. In Wang RIH, ed: Practical drug therapy, Milwaukee, 1987, Medstream Press.
36. Holland OB, Nixon JV, and Kuhnert L: Diuretic-induced ventricular ectopic activity, Am J Med 70:762, 1981.
37. Hollifield JW and Slaton PE: Thiazide diuretics, hypokalemia, and cardiac arrhythmias, Acta Med Scand Suppl 647:67, 1981.
38. Houston MC: The effects of antihypertensive drugs on glucose intolerance in hypertensive nondiabetics and diabetics, Am Heart J 115:640, 1988.
39. Ames R: Effects of diuretic drugs on the lipid profile, Drugs 36 (suppl 2):33, 1988.
40. Weidmann P and Gerber A: Effects of treatment with diuretics on serum lipoproteins, J Cardiovasc Pharmacol 6:S260, 1984.
41. Kaplan NM: Importance of coronary heart disease risk factors in the management of hypertension: an overview, Am J Med 86 (suppl 1B):1, 1989.
42. Beling S et al: Long-term experience with indapamide, Am Heart J 106:258, 1983.
43. Meyer-Sabellek W et al: Serum lipoprotein levels during long-term treatment of hypertension with indapamide, Hypertension 7 (suppl II):II-170, 1985.
44. Pollare T et al: Sensitivity to insulin during treatment with atenolol and metoprolol: a randomised, double blind study of effects on carbohydrate and lipoprotein metabolism in hypertensive patients, Br Med J 298:1152, 1989.
45. Chait A: Effects of antihypertensive agents on serum lipids and lipoproteins, Am J Med 86 (suppl 1B):5, 1989.
46. Dal Palu C et al: Intravenous labetalol in severe hypertension, Br J Clin Pharmacol 13 (suppl 1):978, 1982.
47. Vidt DG: Intravenous labetalol in the emergency treatment of hypertension, J Clin Hypertens 2:179, 1985.
48. Chen S and Vidt DG: Patient acceptance of transdermal clonidine: a retrospective review of 25 patients, Cleve Clin J Med 56:21, 1989.
49. Koch-Weser J: Hydralazine, N Engl J Med 295:320, 1976.
50. Perry HM Jr: Late toxicity to hydralazine resembling systemic lupus erythematosus or rheumatoid arthritis, Am J Med 54:58, 1973.
51. Miller WE et al: Management of severe hypertension with intravenous injections of diazoxide, Am J Cardiol 24:870, 1969.
52. Wilson DJ, Lewis RC, and Vidt DG: Control of severe hypertension with pulse diazoxide. In Vidt DG, ed: Cardiovascular Clinics, Philadelphia, 1982, FA Davis Co.
53. Cohn JN and Burke LP: Nitroprusside, Ann Intern Med 91:752, 1979.
54. Vesey CJ, Cole PV, and Simpson PJ: Cyanide and thiocyanate concentrations following sodium nitroprusside infusion in man, Br J Anaesth 48:651, 1976.
55. Cottrell JE and Turndorf H: Intravenous nitroglycerin, Am Heart J 96:550, 1978.
56. Flaherty JT et al: Comparison of intravenous nitroglycerin and sodium nitroprusside for treatment of acute hypertension after coronary artery bypass surgery, Circulation 65:1072, 1982.
57. Frohlich ED: Angiotensin converting enzyme inhibitors, Hypertension 13 (suppl I):I-125, 1989.
58. Williams GH: Converting-enzyme inhibitors in the treatment of hypertension, N Engl J Med 319:1517, 1988.
59. Hricik DE et al: Captopril-induced functional renal insufficiency in patients with bilateral renal artery stenosis or renal artery stenosis in a solitary kidney, N Engl J Med 303:373, 1983.
60. Vidt DG et al: Atherembolic renal disease: association with renal arterial stenosis, Cleve Clin J Med 56:407-413, 1988.
61. Coulter DM and Edwards IR: Cough associated with captopril and enalapril, Br Med J 294:1521, 1987.
62. Hood S, Nichollas MG, and Gilchrist NL: Cough with angiotensin converting enzyme inhibitors, N Z Med J 100:6, 1987.

63. Croog SH et al: The effects of antihypertensive therapy on the quality of life, N Engl J Med 314:1657, 1986.
64. Braunwald E: Mechanism of action of calcium-channel-blocking agents, N Engl J Med 307:1618, 1982.
65. Kates RE: Calcium antagonists: pharmacokinetic properties, Drugs 25:113, 1983.
66. Bertel O et al: Nifedipine in hypertensive emergencies, Br Med J 286:19, 1983.
67. Kaplan NM: Calcium entry blockers in the treatment of hypertension: current status and future prospects, JAMA 262:817, 1989.
68. MacMahon SW et al: The effects of drug treatment for hypertension on morbidity and mortality from cardiovascular disease: a review of randomized controlled trials, Prog Cardiovasc Dis 24 (suppl 1):99, 1986.
69. Strasser T and Genten D, eds: Mild hypertension: from Drug Trials to Practice, New York, 1987, Raven Press.
70. Alderman MH: Mild hypertension: new light on an old clinical controversy, Am J Med 69:653, 1980.
71. Swales JD et al: Treating mild hypertension: agreement from the large trials. Report of the British Hypertension Society working party, Br Med J 298:694, 1989.
72. Joint National Committee on Detection, Evaluation, and Treatment of High Blood Pressure: The 1984 report of the Joint National Committee on Detection, Evaluation, and Treatment of High Blood Pressure, Arch Intern Med 144:1045, 1984.
73. Reid JL: First-line and combination treatment for hypertension, Am J Med 86(suppl 4A):2, 1989.
74. Shulman NB et al: Financial cost as an obstacle to hypertension therapy, Am J Public Health 76:1105, 1986.
75. Amery A et al: 1986 Guidelines for the treatment of mild hypertension: memorandum from the WHO/ISH, Hypertension 8:957, 1986.
76. Kaplan NM: Critical comments on recent literature: the 1988 report of the Joint National Committee, Am J Hypertens 2:72, 1989.
77. Beevers DG: Overtreating hypertension: mortality from coronary artery disease may be increased if pressures are dropped too low, Br Med J 297:121, 1988.
78. Cruickshank JM: Coronary flow reserve and the J curve relation between diastolic blood pressure and myocardial infarction, Br Med J 297:1227, 1988.
79. Moser M: In defense of traditional antihypertensive therapy, Hypertension 12:324, 1988.
80. Zusman RM: In defense of alternative antihypertensive therapy, Hypertension 12:327, 1988.
81. Gifford RW Jr and Tarazi RC: Resistant hypertension: diagnosis and management, Ann Intern Med 88:661, 1978.
82. Vidt DG: Accelerated hypertension, malignant hypertension, and hypertensive emergencies. In Bayless TM, Brain MC, and Cherniak RM, eds: Current therapy in internal medicine 1984-1985, Philadelphia, 1984, BC Decker, Inc.
83. Vidt DG: The patient with resistant hypertension: cations, volume and renal factors, Hypertension 11 (suppl II):II-76, 1988.
84. Hypertension Detection and Follow-up Cooperative Group: Five-year findings of the Hypertension Detection Follow-up Program, JAMA 242:2562, 1979.
85. Management Committee of the Australian Therapeutic Trials in Mild Hypertension: the Australian therapeutic trial, Lancet 2:1261, 1980.
86. Veterans Administration Cooperative Group: Effects of treatment in hypertension. II. Results in patients with diastolic blood pressure averaging 90 through 114 mm Hg, JAMA 213:1143, 1970.
87. Amery A et al: Mortality and morbidity results from the European Working Party on High Blood Pressure in the Elderly trial, Lancet 2:1349, 1985.
88. Coope J and Warrender TS: Randomized trial of treatment of hypertension in elderly patients in primary care, Br Med J 293:1145, 1986.
89. Kannel WB and Gordon T: Evaluation of cardiovascular risk in the elderly: the Framingham study, Bull NY Acad Med 54:573, 1978.
90. Hulley SB et al: The Systolic Hypertension in the Elderly Program (SHEP): antihypertensive efficacy of chlorthalidone, Am J Cardiol 56:913, 1985.
91. Working Group on Hypertension in the Elderly: Statement on hypertension in the elderly, JAMA 256:70, 1986.
92. Applegate WB: Hypertension in elderly patients, Ann Intern Med 110:901, 1989.
93. Garcia JY and Vidt DG: Current management of hypertensive emergencies, Drugs 34:263, 1987.
94. Vidt DG and Gifford RW Jr: A compendium of the treatment of hypertensive emergencies, Cleve Clin Q 51:421, 1984.

Chapter 17

ANEURYSMS

John A. Spittell, Jr.
Peter C. Spittell

An aneurysm may be defined as a permanent localized dilation of an artery. Unless aneurysms are the result of penetrating trauma, they tend to develop at a point where the artery is subject to frequent bending or is not supported by skeletal muscle. Once initiated, an aneurysm tends to enlarge gradually, and this, along with the usual laminated thrombus that develops within the aneurysm, leads to the usual complications of aneurysms—pressure on surrounding structures, rupture, thrombosis, and distal embolization. For reasons unknown, however, aneurysms in certain locations are prone to develop one type of complication more often than others, and awareness of this aspect is important in clinical management. With the exception of some in visceral arteries, aneurysms are about 10 times as frequent in men as in women, and, for the most part, occur after the age of 50.

Since arteriosclerosis is the most common cause of arterial aneurysms today, aneurysmal disease and its complications are frequent clinical problems. Because arteriosclerosis is a multifocal process, coronary artery disease, cerebral vascular disease, and aneurysms at multiple locations are common in persons with atherosclerotic aneurysms[1,2] and are conditions to constantly keep in mind in the management of the person with aneurysmal disease.

While advances in imaging and surgical techniques have greatly enhanced our recognition and successful treatment of aneurysms, their protean manifestations can challenge the best of clinicians at times, making the aphorism of Sir William Osler, "There is no disease more conducive to clinical humility than aneurysm of the aorta,"[3] appropriate even today.

ETIOLOGY

The most common cause of arterial aneurysms today is arteriosclerosis. Less common causes include congenital defects of the arterial wall, trauma (both blunt and penetrating types), sudden deceleration and entrapment, infection including syphilis, polyarteritis, and other types of necrotizing arteritis and hereditary abnormalities of connective tissue (see the accompanying box). Of note, hypertension seems to enhance aneurysm formation.[4]

Arteriosclerosis

A combination of factors, such as "wear and tear" and impaired nutrition, over time, results in weakening of the

Etiology of arterial aneurysms

I. Arteriosclerosis
II. Congenital defects
    A. Localized defects of the arterial wall
    B. Fibromuscular dysplasia
    C. Hereditary connective tissue abnormalities
        1. Marfan syndrome
        2. Ehlers-Danlos syndrome
III. Trauma
    A. Penetrating arterial trauma
    B. Blunt arterial trauma
    C. Sudden deceleration
    D. Entrapment (poststenotic dilation)
IV. Infection
    A. Syphilitic
    B. Mycotic
V. Arteritis
    A. Polyarteritis nodosa
    B. Giant cell arteritis
    C. Associated with ankylosing spondylitis
    D. Associated with atrial myxoma
    E. Associated with relapsing polychondritis
    F. Associated with Behçet's syndrome

medial coat of the arterial wall leading to tortuosity, dilation, and aneurysm formation in atherosclerotic arteries. Serum collagenolytic activity, abnormalities of trace metal metabolism (particularly copper) and of ascorbic acid metabolism (particularly in smokers), in addition to genetic factors, may also condition the atherosclerotic aneurysmal response.[5] Busuttill, Abou-Zamzam, and Machleder have reported that increased degradative collagenase and elastase activity correlates with aneurysm size and is much higher in ruptured aneurysms.[6]

Atherosclerotic aneurysms tend to develop where the artery is not supported by skeletal muscle or is subject to frequent bending with physical activity. Thus the most common locations for arteriosclerotic aneurysms are the thoracic and abdominal aorta, the iliac arteries, and the femoral and popliteal arteries. The frequent association with and enhancement of arteriosclerotic aneurysmal disease by hypertension, whether direct, indirect, or both, is notable from the standpoint of management as well as etiology.[4]

Congenital defects

Absence or poor development of the media in segments of some arteries results in aneurysms that are usually saccular. These aneurysms frequently occur in the intracerebral arteries (often in association with coarctation of the aorta or polycystic disease of the kidneys) and are less frequently seen in some visceral arteries and arteries in the extremities.

Fibromuscular dysplasia, which may represent a developmental abnormality of vascular smooth muscles, most often affects the renal arteries and less often other visceral arteries and the carotids, and usually produces multiple medial ridges in the affected artery with interspersed mural aneurysms, which produces the characteristic "string of beads" seen on arteriograms of affected arteries.

Among the heritable disorders of connective tissue, the two best known to result in aneurysm formation are Marfan syndrome and Ehlers-Danlos syndrome.[7] In Marfan syndrome the connective tissue disorder usually results in aortic root dilation and ascending thoracic aortic aneurysm, while in Ehlers-Danlos syndrome multiple aortic aneurysms may occur.

Trauma

Penetrating trauma of any type may result in an aneurysm anywhere in the body. More often it is a false aneurysm than a true aneurysm. Blunt trauma, particularly repetitive, to superficial arteries can result in a true aneurysm. Deceleration stress may result in partial rupture of the aortic isthmus with subsequent false aneurysm formation; this type of injury occurs most often with automobile accidents but may also occur in falls. The aortic rupture at the isthmus is no doubt caused by the relative fixation of the proximal descending thoracic aorta at this point.[8]

While the exact mechanism of dilation of an artery beyond a constriction—poststenotic dilation—is not known, this phenomenon is likely the basis for aneurysm formation in thoracic outlet compression of the subclavian artery, in popliteal artery entrapment syndrome, and some cases of femoropopliteal artery aneurysm in the lower medial thigh just beyond the exit of the artery through the adductor tendon.

Infection

Syphilitic aneurysms, a late manifestation of syphilis, most commonly involve the ascending thoracic aorta and aortic arch. An inflammatory process involving the vasa vasorum leads to slow degeneration of muscle fibers and weakening of the arterial wall and then formation of an aneurysm of either the fusiform or saccular type.

Infections other than syphilis may involve existing aneurysms or cause aneurysms via infection of the arterial wall by septic emboli of the vasa vasorum (as in the case of infective endocarditis or other types of bacteremia) or by involvement of the arterial wall by contiguous suppuration. Aneurysms caused by nonluetic infections—so-called mycotic aneurysms—most often occur in the ascending aorta, less often in arteries to the viscera, and least often in the extremity arteries.[9,10] In recent years staphylococcal and salmonella infections are the most frequent types of infected aneurysms encountered,[11] but virtually any organism can infect an existing aneurysm given the chance, even *Campylobacter* fetus.[12] Among those infections that may involve the aorta and its branches, usually by direct spread from infected contiguous structures is tuberculosis, an important infection to keep in mind.[13]

Arteritis

Polyarteritis nodosa and other types of arteritis can cause localized medial necrosis and result in aneurysm formation. In polyarteritis small arteries, especially in the kidney, are involved with multiple aneurysms in more than half the patients.[14] Other types of arteritis that may lead to aneurysm formation include giant cell (temporal, cranial) arteritis, and the aortitis associated with relapsing polychondritis[15] or with ankylosing spondylitis.[16] Another rare type of aneurysm, whose cause is unclear, can occur in persons with atrial myxoma.[17]

PATHOLOGY

From the pathologic standpoint, aneurysms are of several types. Fusiform aneurysms, are localized rather uniform dilations of an artery, while the term *saccular* is used to describe an outpouching of an artery at a point where the medial cost is thinned. A false aneurysm results from the development of a sac around a hematoma that maintains a communication with the lumen of an artery whose wall has ruptured or been penetrated. At times a dissecting hematoma is referred to as a dissecting aneurysm because the hematoma in the arterial wall can form a localized enlargement of the involved artery.

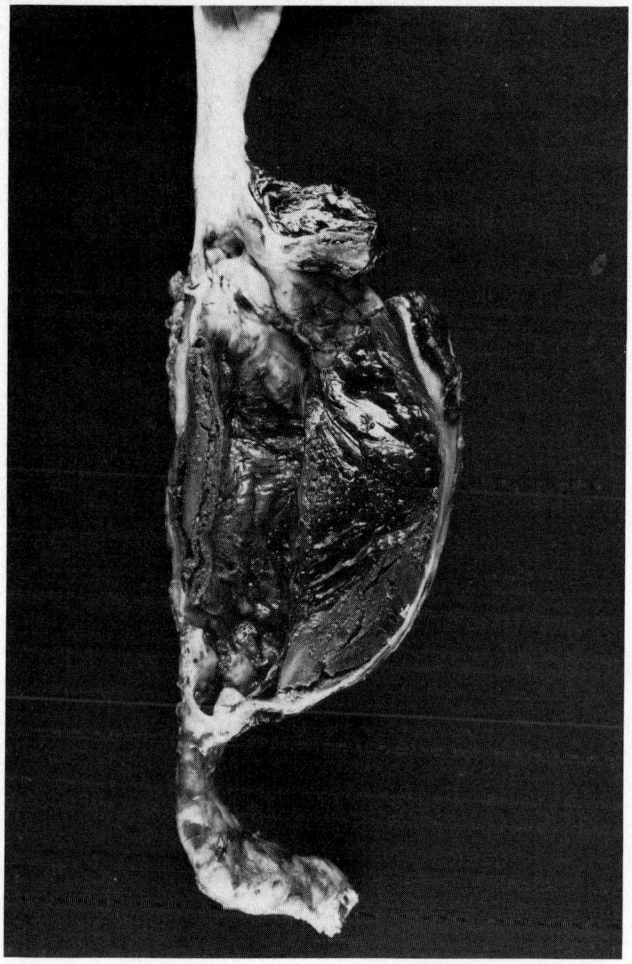

Fig. 17-1. Aneurysm of the abdominal aorta contains laminated thrombus. (From Spittell JA Jr: Cardiovasc Clin 3[1]:114, 1971.)

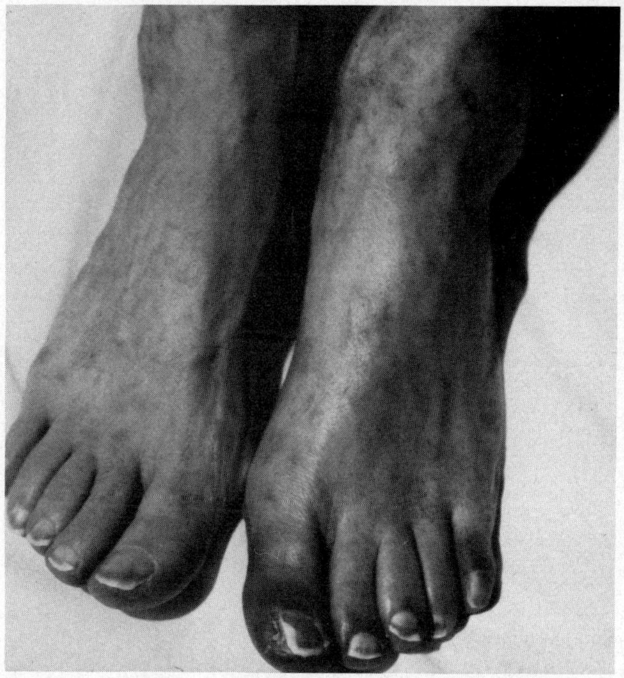

Fig. 17-2. Thromboembolism and atheroembolism from abdominal aortic aneurysm; livedo reticularis and multiple blue toes. (From Spittell JA Jr: Curr Prob Cardiol 5[5]:6, 1980.)

The most common cause of aneurysms, as has been noted, is arteriosclerosis, which weakens the arterial wall allowing the development of either a fusiform or saccular type of aneurysm. Why some persons develop occlusive arterial disease and others develop an aneurysm is not known, but several factors, including heredity,[18] coexisting hypertension,[4] and smoking[19] appear important. Once formed atherosclerotic aneurysms tend to enlarge progressively,[20] but specific factors that influence the rate of enlargement, other than the hydraulic stresses, remain unclear.[18] The laminated thrombus (Fig. 17-1) that so often develops, producing a lumen of near-normal caliber through the aneurysm, may represent an attempt to slow the progressive enlargement. The complication of thromboembolism (Fig. 17-2) results from the embolization to distal dermal arterioles and other arteries by portions of the mural thrombus dislodging from the aneurysm. Atheroembolism may also occur (see Chapter 11). At times the thrombotic process within an aneurysm results in complete occlusion, a complication that occurs most often in popliteal artery

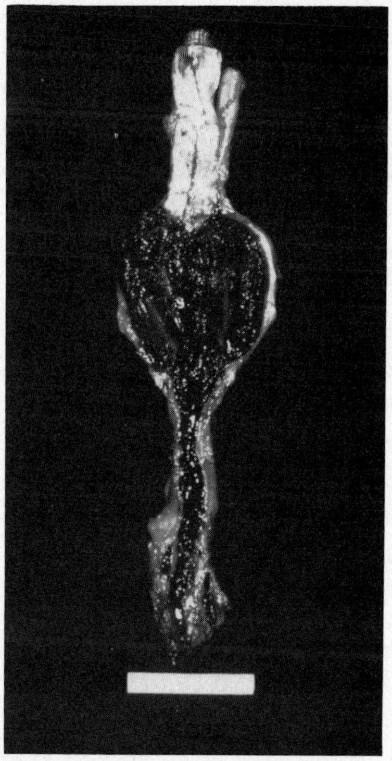

Fig. 17-3. Arteriosclerotic aneurysm of popliteal artery completely filled with thrombus. (From Juergens JL et al, eds: Peripheral vascular diseases, ed 5, Philadelphia, 1980, WB Saunders Co.)

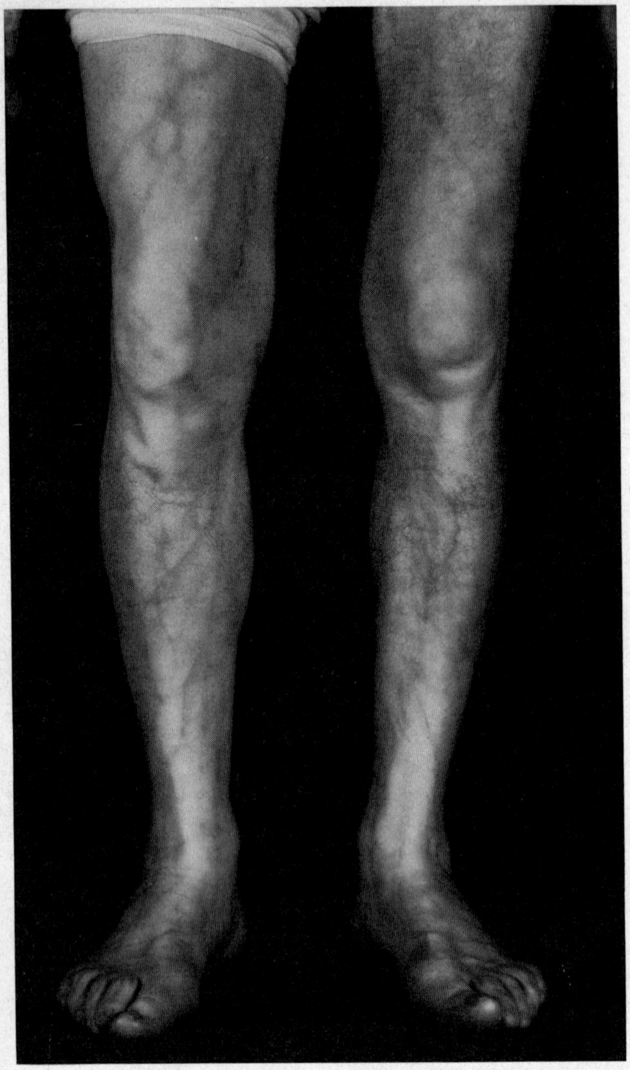

Fig. 17-4. Edema and increased venous pattern of the right leg and thigh of a 70-year-old man with a common femoral artery aneurysm compressing the femoral vein. The venous compression was relieved by resection of the aneurysm. Arterial continuity was restored with a prosthetic graft (infrared photograph). (From Spittell JA Jr: Curr Prob Cardiol 5[5]:6, 1980.)

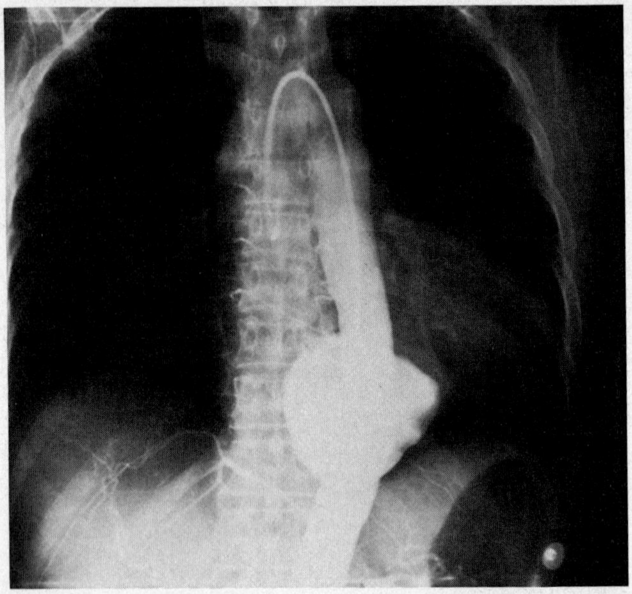

Fig. 17-5. Aortagram demonstrating a mycotic aneurysm of the descending thoracic aorta of a 64-year-old woman.

aneurysm (Fig. 17-3). With progressive enlargement, an aneurysm may compress surrounding structures (Fig. 17-4), a phenomenon most often seen with aneurysm of the thoracic aorta, the femoral artery and the popliteal artery whose locations in rather confined anatomic spaces favor this complication. The frequency of rupture in aneurysms of the aorta seems related to size[21] and associated hypertension,[4,22] but data on size in relation to rupture is incomplete for aneurysms of other arteries.

Syphilitic aneurysms of the aorta may be fusiform or saccular, with the latter type often becoming quite large and compressing contiguous structures or eroding bone.

Mycotic aneurysms (Fig. 17-5) occur most often in the aorta with the visceral arteries, intracranial arteries, and arteries of the extremities, in decreasing frequency, as other sites.[9] Septicemia of any variety may produce mycotic aneurysms, but infective endocarditis probably still remains the leading cause. Various stages of the inflammatory process may be found in different parts of a mycotic aneurysm and in mycotic aneurysms at different locations according to Stengel and Wolferth.[9] The chief complication of mycotic aneurysm is rupture, caused, no doubt, by the destructive effect of the infection on the arterial wall.

The phenomenon of poststenotic dilation applies to the pathogenesis of aneurysms at only a few locations (principally the subclavian artery [Fig. 17-6] and the popliteal artery [Fig. 17-7]) but deserves comment because studies of this phenomenon contribute to our knowledge of factors involved in progressive enlargement of an aneurysm. The physical phenomena distal to a stenotic segment of artery were described in 1954 by Holman[23] as the simple mechanical effect of hydraulics governing the flow of liquid through a conduit. He concluded further that once the dilation is initiated, the process is enhanced according to the Bernoulli theorem—that is, a widened lumen slows the stream, thereby increasing the lateral pressure and further dilating the lumen. Other theories have been proposed but the exact pathophysiology of poststenotic dilation remains to be defined.

THORACIC AORTIC ANEURYSM

Effective antiluetic therapy has changed the etiologic spectrum of thoracic aortic aneurysm so that luetic aneurysms are rare while arteriosclerotic aneurysms have become

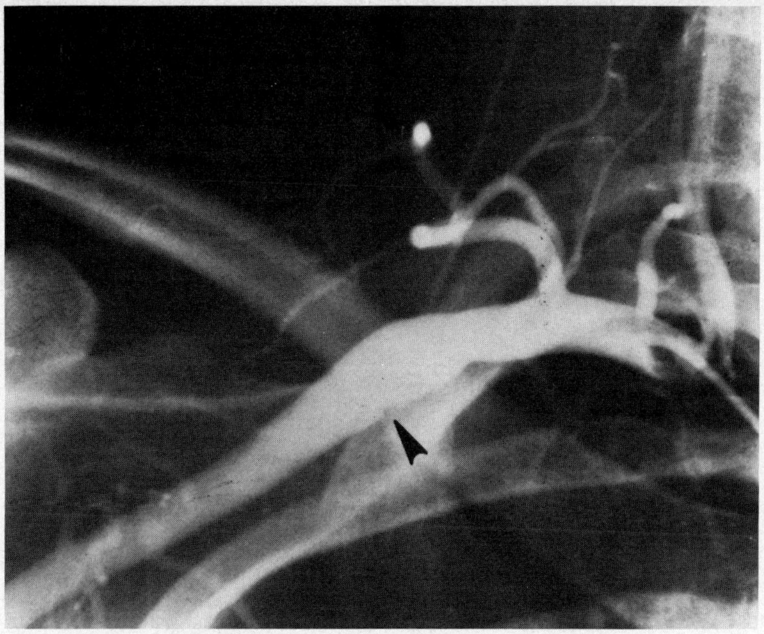

Fig. 17-6. Selective arteriogram of the right subclavian artery demonstrating aneurysmal (post-stenotic) *(arrowhead)* dilation of the artery just distal to its compression by the uppermost rib in a 20-year-old woman with the thoracic outlet compression syndrome.

the most common type because of the aging U.S. population. Thus the most common location of thoracic aneurysms is in the descending thoracic aorta; they are more common in men than in women and occur most frequently after the age of 60. Less frequent types of aneurysms of the thoracic aorta are those caused by incomplete aortic rupture,[8] arteritis of various types,[15,16] mycotic aneurysms,[9,10] and Marfan syndrome.

Most aneurysms of the thoracic aorta are asymptomatic and can be identified on chest roentgenograms.[24,25] When thoracic aortic aneurysms enlarge to the point of encroaching on surrounding structures, they may cause back pain, hoarseness, cough, dyspnea, stridor, or dysphagia. As a result of pressure on surrounding structures physical signs such as distended neck veins (Fig. 17-8, *A*) or a fixed vocal cord appear. In cases of ascending aortic aneurysm there is dilation of the aortic root, and aortic valve regurgitation results.

On plain chest roentgenograms a thoracic aortic aneurysm appears as an abnormal smooth density in the central portion of the chest (Fig. 17-8, *B*), and unless there is calcification in the wall of the aneurysm it may simulate an intrathoracic neoplasm.[26] Aortography has been the classic method to diagnose thoracic aortic aneurysm, but computed tomography (Fig. 17-8, *C*), particularly with intravenous contrast media enhancement, has now become the standard imaging procedure.

Contrary to earlier studies[24,25] a more recent study[22] has demonstrated that patients with untreated thoracic aortic aneurysms have a poorer prognosis than those with untreated abdominal aortic aneurysms. The one- and three-year survival rates of untreated thoracic aortic aneurysm patients in the latter study were 58.2% and 25.7% respectively. Of the 24 nondissecting aneurysms in the latter study 51% ruptured, and incidentally, all of these patients had hypertension.[22]

Because of the poor prognosis of untreated thoracic aortic aneurysm, surgical treatment is warranted unless associated conditions contraindicate operation. From the natural history studies cited, indications for surgical resection of atherosclerotic thoracic aortic aneurysm include:

1. a symptomatic aneurysm.
2. an aneurysm 6 cm in diameter or larger.
3. an aneurysm enlarging on serial observation.
4. an aneurysm in a person with significant and/or poorly controlled hypertension.

Unless there are contraindications elective surgical resection of thoracic aortic aneurysms resulting from trauma, even when asymptomatic, is indicated because of the unpredictability of these aneurysms.[8,27] Prophylactic surgical

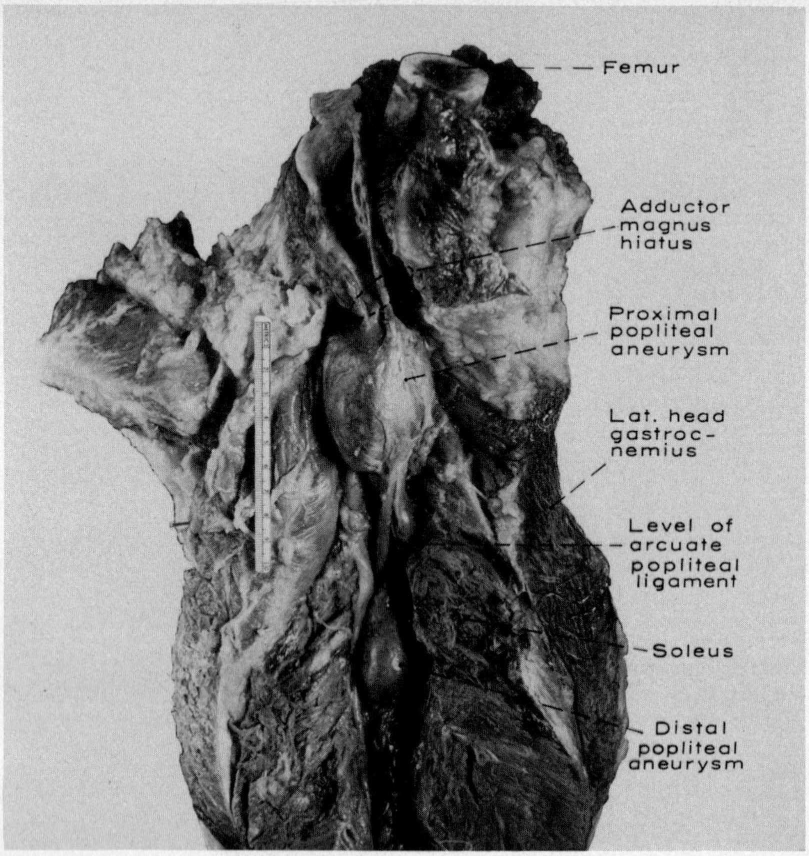

Fig. 17-7. Photograph of popliteal fossa in dissected amputated limb of patient having proximal and distal popliteal aneurysms. (From Gedge SW et al: Circulation 24:270, 1961.)

treatment of aortic root dilation greater than 5.5 cm in diameter in the person with Marfan syndrome is advisable to prevent the complications of aortic dissection and rupture.[28]

ABDOMINAL AORTIC ANEURYSM

Like most other aneurysms, those in the abdominal aorta are usually caused by arteriosclerosis. As noted earlier in this chapter, in addition to the usual risk factors for arteriosclerosis, smoking, heredity, and hypertension appear to be important etiologically in aneurysm of the abdominal aorta. In the aging U.S. population abdominal aortic aneurysm occurs in about 2% of persons over 60 years of age, and they occur more often in men than in women. Trauma, syphilis, mycotic aortitis, and nonbacterial arteritis are rare causes of abdominal aortic aneurysm.

Most abdominal aortic aneurysms are asymptomatic,[29] their discovery being incidental on careful physical examination or on roentgenograms of the abdomen or lumbar spine for other reasons (Fig. 17-9). The most common symptom in a series of 191 cases was awareness of a pulsating mass in the abdomen with or without pain (21.4%) followed by abdominal pain (10.5%), abdominal and back pain (7.3%), back pain (4.7%), groin pain (2.1%), and flank pain (2.1%).[30] The larger the aneurysm the greater the frequency of symptoms.

An abdominal pulsating mass is the most frequent physical finding in a patient with an abdominal aortic aneurysm, but care must be taken to differentiate tumors exhibiting transmitted pulsation and the prominent pulsation of a tortuous sclerotic nonaneurysmal aorta. Thus the admonition of Osler,[31] "A mistake is not likely to occur if it is remembered that no pulsation, however forcible, no thrill, however intense, no bruit, however loud—singly or together—justify the diagnosis of an aneurysm of the abdominal aorta, *only* the presence of a palpable, expansile tumor" remains pertinent today. While 90% of large abdominal aortic aneurysms can be diagnosed on physical examination,[32] smaller aneurysms and aneurysms in obese persons are not so readily diagnosed.

While roentgenograms of the abdomen or lumbar spine will often demonstrate an abdominal aortic aneurysm (see Fig. 17-9), ultrasound (Fig. 17-10) and computed tomography are more accurate methods to confirm the diagnosis of an abdominal aortic aneurysm.[33] Ultrasound has the ad-

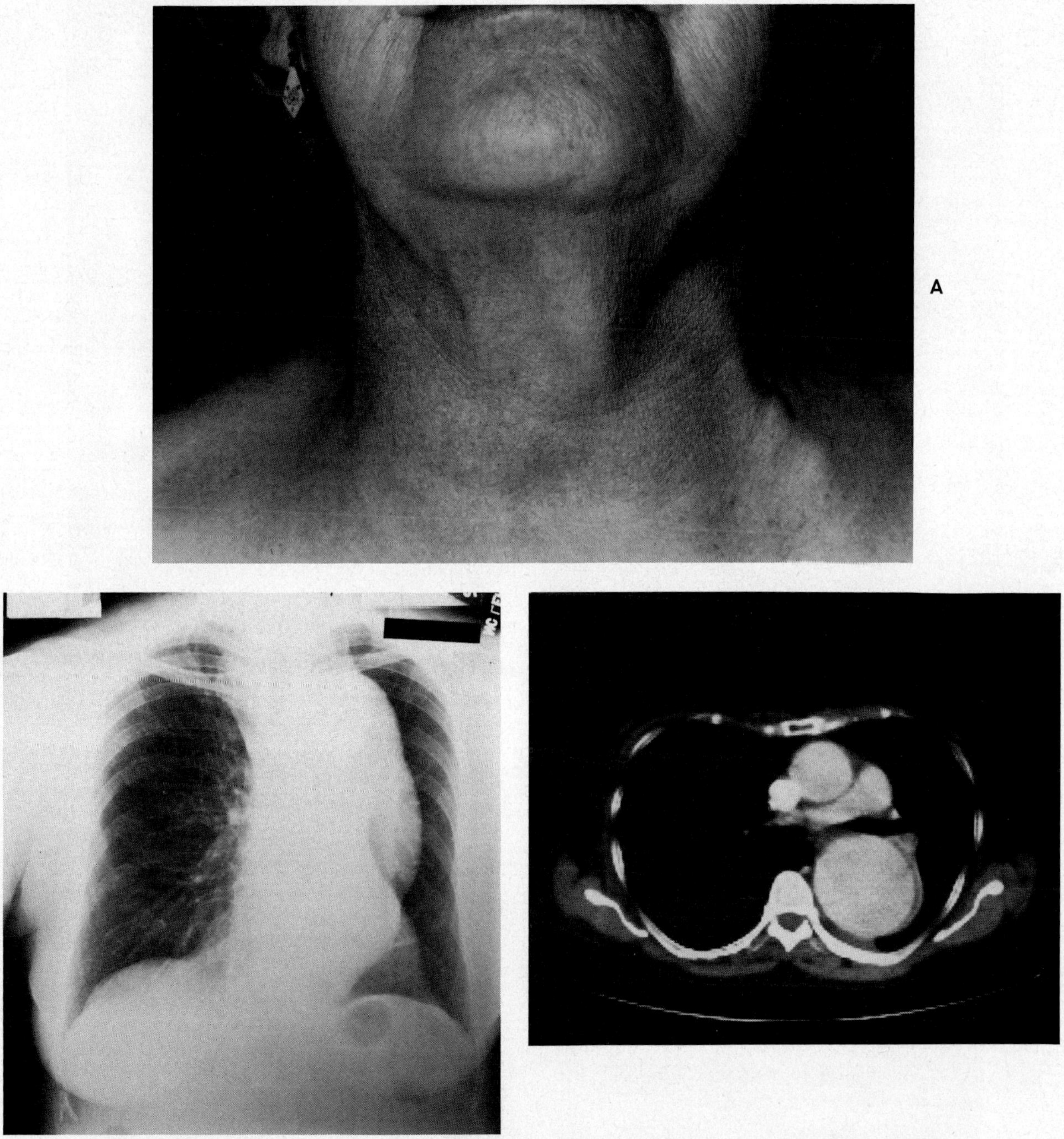

A

B

C

Fig. 17-8. Aneurysm of thoracic aorta in a 65-year-old woman. **A,** Unilateral *(left)* jugular vein distention caused by compression of the left innominate vein by the aneurysm. **B,** Chest roentgenogram showing the large aneurysm of the descending thoracic aorta. **C,** Computed tomography with contrast enhancement demonstrating the aneurysm of the descending thoracic aorta.

A

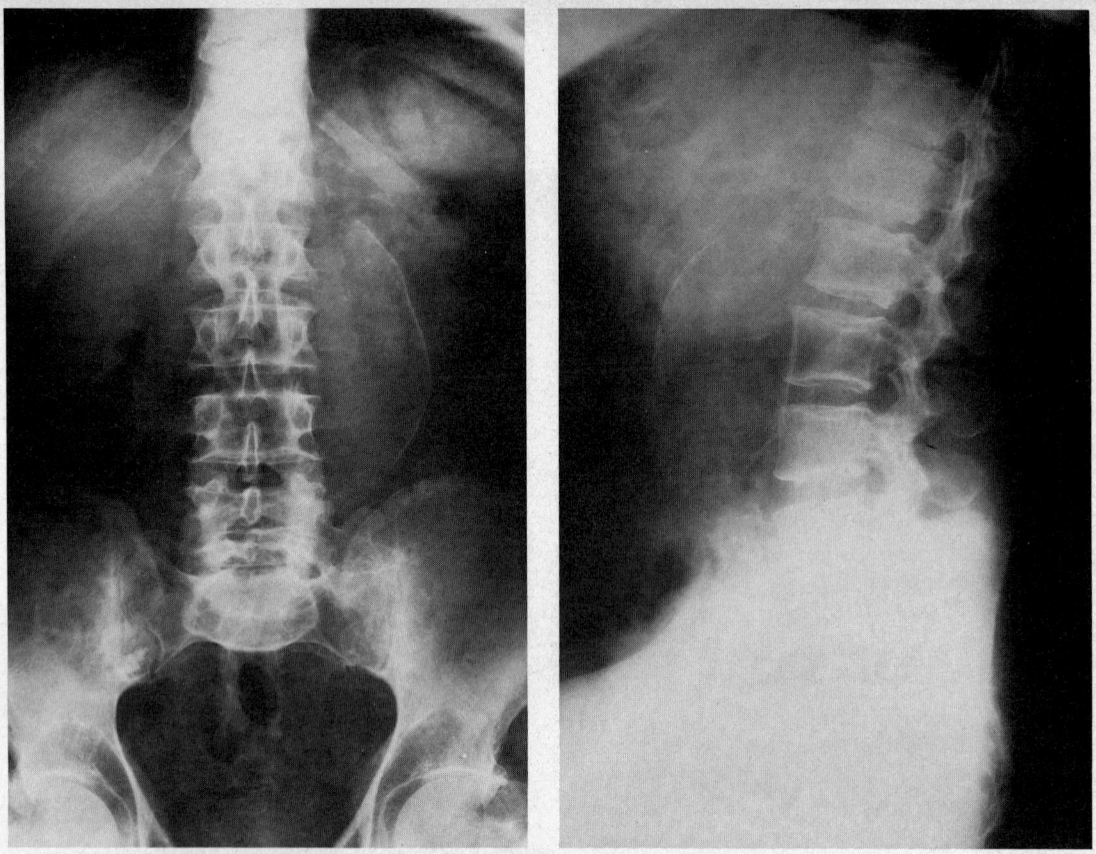

B

Fig. 17-9. Large aneurysm of abdominal aorta with calcification of aneurysmal wall. **A,** Anteroposterior view. **B,** Lateral view. (From Spittell JA et al, eds: Peripheral vascular diseases, ed 5, Philadelphia, 1980, WB Saunders Co.)

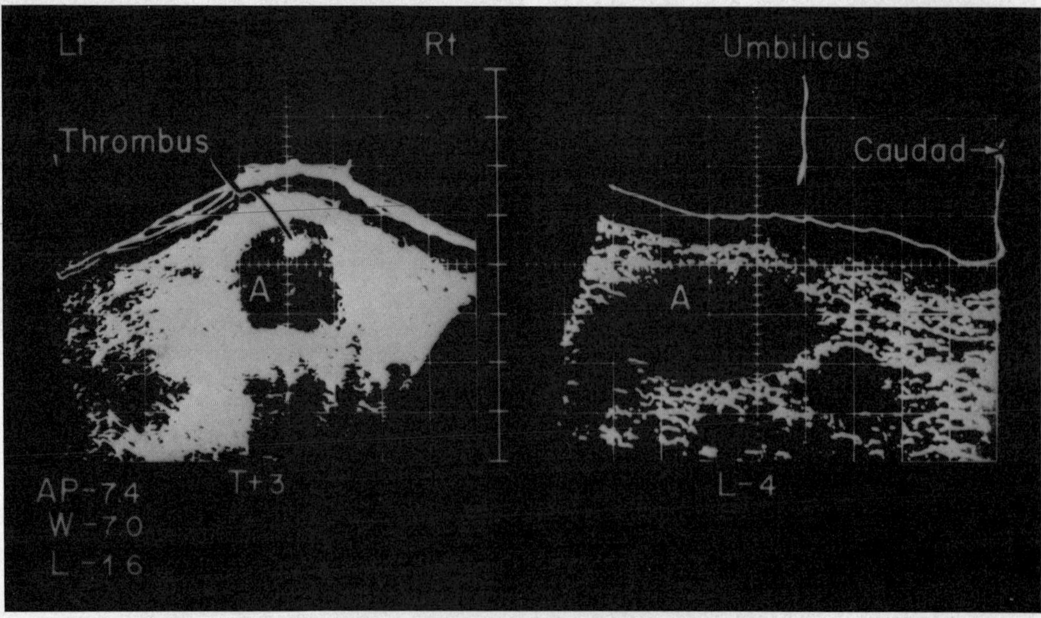

Fig. 17-10. Ultrasound scans of an abdominal aortic aneurysm as well as mural thrombus. Transverse scan (*left*) indicates aneurysm with an internal diameter of 6 cm, an anteroposterior diameter of 7.1 cm, and an anterior wall thrombus. Longitudinal scan (*right*) indicates anteroposterior diameter is actually 7.4 cm and shows aneurysm of left common iliac artery, which is the echo-free space caudad to the large defect (grid scale 3 cm) (From Spittell JA Jr: Abdominal aortic aneurysms, Hosp Pract 21:105, 1986.)

vantage of being less costly and devoid of radiation exposure, but computed tomography is more useful, in the obese patient, to identify rupture with either contained or retroperitoneal bleeding and to demonstrate suprarenal extension of the aneurysm. Computed tomography scan with contrast is also quite useful when associated renovascular disease or renal anomalies that may complicate surgical treatment are suspected. Aortography is utilized to varying degrees by different centers in the evaluation of an abdominal aortic aneurysm; it is clearly indicated when the patient has significant associated occlusive aortoiliac disease or renovascular disease that may be repaired at the time of aneurysm surgery.[34]

The most frequent complication of abdominal aortic aneurysm is rupture, which occurs most often in those 5 cm in diameter or greater.[21] Rupture causes pain, typically in one or both flanks with radiation to the lower abdomen, groin, or genitalia. If the aneurysm ruptures into the adjacent vena cava, rather than retroperitoneally or intraabdominally, producing an aortocaval fistula, the patient develops a sudden increased venous pressure in the lower extremities, acute right heart failure, or both. Rarely, an abdominal aortic aneurysm can rupture into the gastrointestinal tract and causes gastrointestinal bleeding.

Less common than rupture, other complications of abdominal aortic aneurysm are thromboembolism or atheroembolism (see Fig. 17-2), pressure on surrounding structures (see Figs. 17-4 and 17-8, *A*) and infection, all of which produce interesting syndromes. With cholesterol embolization the patient develops blue toes, livedo reticularis, hypertension, and renal insufficiency. The blue toes and livedo reticularis result from embolization to digital arteries and cutaneous arterioles, while microembolism of renal arterioles accounts for the renal insufficiency and hypertension.[35]

When an abdominal aortic aneurysm becomes infected, the most common organism causing the infection is salmonella.[11]

Because abdominal aortic aneurysms are atherosclerotic, coronary artery disease, and cerebral vascular disease must always be kept in mind because of their frequency.[1,2] In some centers coronary angiography is performed in all persons with an abdominal aortic aneurysm to identify those in whom coronary artery surgery is deemed advisable before aneurysm surgery to lessen the risk of the latter. Other groups perform coronary arteriography before aneurysm surgery only in those patients with symptomatic coronary disease or with an abnormal exercise study or dipyridamole-thallium scan.[36]

For different reasons the kidneys also deserve special attention in the patient with an abdominal aortic aneurysm.[37] In addition to their involvement in atheroembolism, the kidneys may be affected when the aneurysm encroaches on one or both ureters producing hydronephrosis or oliguria. Associated renal anomalies, particularly horseshoe kidney, may require preoperative selective renal angiography to identify any anomalous renal arteries and special care to avoid symphysiotomy at the time of resection of the aneurysm.[38] As mentioned earlier, associated renal artery stenosis is common in patients with abdominal aortic aneurysms and may warrant repair at the time of surgery for the aneurysm.[34]

The multiple studies of the natural history of abdominal aortic aneurysms show clearly that if the patient with an aneurysm 5 cm in diameter or larger does not have significant cardiovascular or other life-threatening disease, death is more likely to result from rupture of the aneurysm than from anything else.[21,32] Elective resection and graft replacement has a surgical mortality of less than 5%, but emergent surgical treatment after the aneurysm has ruptured has a much higher mortality.[1] The identification and surgical treatment of significant correctable coronary artery disease prior to elective resection of abdominal aortic aneurysm has been shown to reduce the incidence of postoperative myocardial infarction and mortality.[1]

In the poor-risk patient with an aneurysm smaller than 5.0 cm in diameter, observation of the aneurysm with ultrasonographic examination every 3 or 4 months is appropriate. There is some evidence that long-term β-blockade may be associated with a decreased rate of expansion of abdominal aortic aneurysm.[39] In the patient with a large or symptomatic abdominal aortic aneurysm and serious noncorrectable coronary artery disease causing poor left ventricular function, support with intraaortic balloon assist in the early postoperative period has been useful.[40]

Another special circumstance is the patient with a thoracoabdominal aortic aneurysm whose surgical repair has been associated with a broad spectrum of complications and a formidable surgical mortality. Nonetheless, elective resection is desirable, and with careful preoperative evaluation and preparation, intraoperative reduction in visceral ischemia time, and intensive postoperative support can produce acceptable postoperative morbidity and mortality rates.[41]

ILIAC ARTERY ANEURYSM

Aneurysms of the common iliac artery are similar in etiology to but distinctly less common than those of the abdominal aorta.[42] They are noteworthy because of the unusual symptoms they may produce as a result of encroachment on pelvic structures—the ureters and urinary bladder, the sacral plexus, and the iliac veins. Less than 40% of iliac artery aneurysms are palpable as a pulsating lower abdominal or rectal mass. Thus, as noted by Lipoff et al,[43] iliac artery aneurysm should be suspected when a patient develops unexplained obstructive urologic symptoms, unexplained pain in the groin or perineum, or signs of proximal venous obstruction of a lower extremity. Currently, computed tomography with contrast enhancement is the diagnostic procedure of choice, though aortography has been the standard and is still a definitive procedure. As with other aneurysms the treatment is surgical resection with graft replacement because of the frequency of rupture.

VISCERAL ARTERY ANEURYSMS
(other than renal artery aneurysm)

Aneurysms of the visceral arteries—splenic, celiac, hepatic, mesenteric and gastric—are unusual but not rare. Etiologic factors are the same as for other aneurysms but vary in frequency with specific aneurysms. If calcified they may be noted as curvilinear or round shadows of calcification, but again the frequency of calcification varies with aneurysms of different arteries. Computed tomography with contrast media enhancement or aortography are the best methods to confirm the diagnosis. For all but renal artery aneurysms (which are covered in Chapter 15), rupture is the most common complication, and its frequency justifies surgical treatment once diagnosed.[44-46]

Splenic artery aneurysm is the most common visceral artery aneurysm and is distinctive from aneurysms of other arteries in being more frequent in women than in men. Medial degeneration appears to be the most common cause of splenic artery aneurysms, which are usually saccular.[46] These aneurysms are often suspected from the observation of a curvilinear shadow of calcification in the left upper abdomen on roentgenograms performed for an unrelated problem (Fig. 17-11, *A*), but differentiation from other causes of left upper abdominal calcification requires aortography (Fig. 17-11, *B*). Most often splenic artery aneurysm is asymptomatic prior to rupture but at times patients will have abdominal pain or splenomegaly.[44] With rupture, which for an unexplained reason often occurs in the third trimester of pregnancy, the patient may exhibit signs of acute intraabdominal bleeding or if the aneurysm ruptures into the stomach, gastrointestinal bleeding. Rupture into the adjacent splenic vein may produce symptomatic portal vein hypertension.[47] The incidence of rupture appears to be somewhere between 6.6% and 8.2% so that for a patient who is otherwise well, and particularly a woman of childbearing age, elective resection of splenic artery aneurysm seems appropriate.[44,46]

Aneurysms of other visceral arteries are much less common than splenic artery aneurysm. They are rarely calcified so their diagnosis depends on arteriography or direct observation at surgery. Unless the clinical problems associated with visceral artery aneurysm are kept in mind, they are easily overlooked. Hepatic artery aneurysms may mimic cholecystitis or present as unexplained gastrointestinal bleeding when they rupture into the biliary tract, producing hematobilia and gastrointestinal bleeding or biliary obstruction and jaundice. Except for those of the superior mesenteric artery, other visceral artery aneurysms, if symptomatic, produce gastrointestinal bleeding. In the superior mesenteric artery, however, the most common cause of aneurysm is mycotic; thus the development of epigastric pain and a tender abdominal mass in a patient with infective endocarditis should raise the question of mycotic aneurysm of the superior mesenteric artery. On the basis of available evidence, aneurysms of the visceral arteries warrant surgical treatment if the patient is an acceptable surgical candidate.[46]

A

B

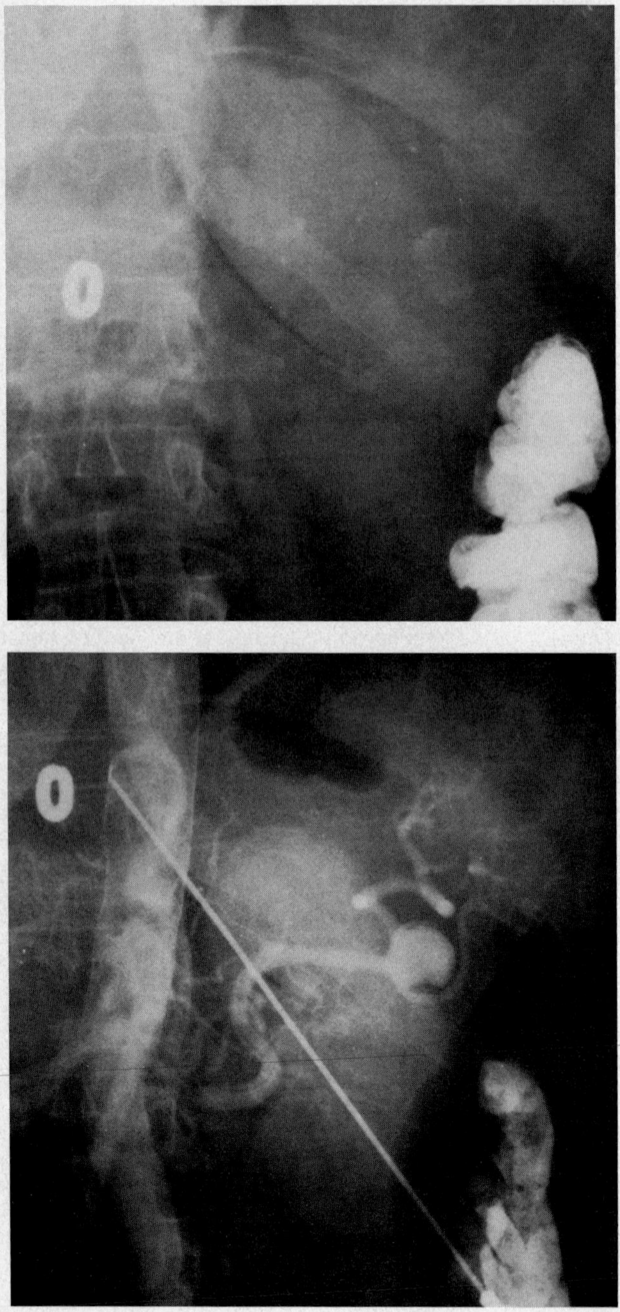

Fig. 17-11. A, Curvilinear shadow of calcification in left upper portion of abdomen seen in colon roentgenogram. Shadow suggests aneurysm of splenic artery. **B,** Translumbar aortogram of same patient demonstrates aneurysm at bifurcation of splenic artery. (From Spittell JA Jr et al: Aneurysm of splenic artery, JAMA 175:452, 1961.)

ANEURYSMS OF EXTREMITY ARTERIES

Typical of arteriosclerosis, which is the cause of most aneurysms of extremity arteries, aneurysms are much more common in the lower than in the upper extremities. In fact, in the upper extremity, aneurysm of the subclavian artery (see Fig. 17-6), often the result of thoracic outlet compression, is commonly encountered clinically.

Since arteriosclerosis is the most common cause of femoral and popliteal artery aneurysms, they occur mostly in men over the age of 60. Aneurysms of the femoral artery occur in Scarpa's triangle, a point of frequent bending of the artery, and in the distal medial thigh, just beyond the tendinous hiatus of the adductor magnus muscle. It is unclear whether poststenotic dilation plays a role in aneurysm formation in the popliteal artery. An increasingly frequent type of femoral aneurysm in the groin is femoral anastamotic aneurysm after aortofemoral grafting.[48]

The common location for popliteal artery aneurysm is just below the level of the knee joint where the artery bends frequently and also may be constricted by muscles, tendons, or ligaments.[49,50] Aneurysms of the popliteal artery are distinctive in that they are bilateral in more than half the patients with a popliteal artery aneurism and are associated with aneurysms of other arteries, usually the abdominal aorta or femoral artery, in more than 40% of cases.[51]

Aneurysms of arteries of the lower extremity are readily diagnosed if the groin, thigh, and popliteal space are carefully examined. B-mode ultrasound is the most reliable diagnostic procedure for aneurysms of the femoral and popliteal arteries and reliably differentiates aneurysm from cysts and tumors that can be problematic in the popliteal space in particular,[52] but before surgical treatment arteriography should be performed to evaluate the distal circulation.

The most frequent complications of femoral and popliteal artery aneurysms are thrombosis (see Fig. 17-3) and distal embolization (Fig. 17-12, *A*).[51,53] The ischemia they produce can vary from intermittent claudication to cutaneous infarction of the foot to digital artery occlusion to gangrene of the leg and foot (Fig. 17-12, *B*). Because of the proximity of the companion vein and the confined space in the extremity, femoral and popliteal aneurysm can cause venous obstruction and mimic thrombophlebitis (see Fig. 17-4). Because of the severity of their complications, elective resection and grafting of femoral and popliteal artery aneurysms is desirable when the distal arterial circulation is adequate and the surgical risk is reasonable. The results of

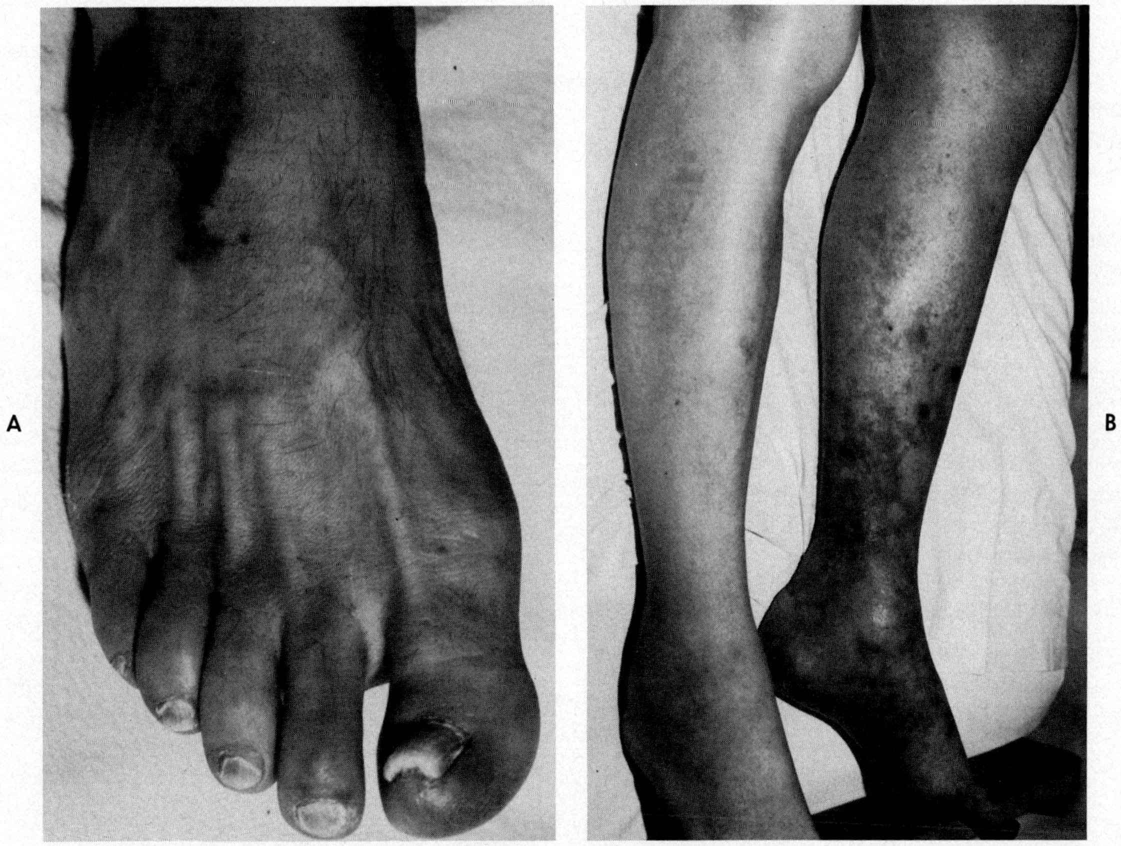

Fig. 17-12. A, Skin infarction of the dorsum of the foot in a patient with emboli from popliteal aneurysm. **B,** Gangrene of the left foot and leg as a result of thrombosis of a popliteal aneurysm. (From Spittell JA Jr: Curr Prob Cardiol 5[5]:6-35, 1980.)

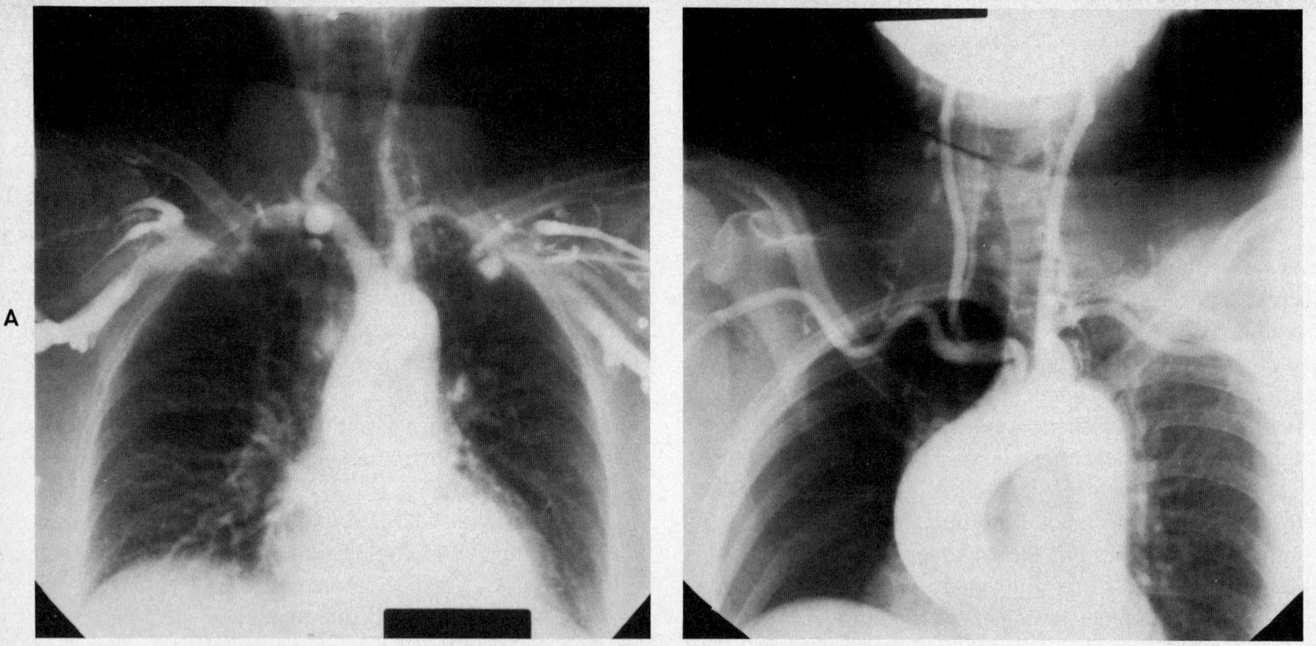

Fig. 17-13. Thoracic aortograms demonstrating buckling of carotid artery (A) and innominate artery (B). (From Spittell JA et al, eds: Peripheral vascular diseases, ed 5, Philadelphia 1980, WB Saunders Co.)

surgical treatment, after complications occur, are far less acceptable, and the risk of limb loss is substantial after thromboembolic complications.

Aneurysms of the subclavian and axillary arteries are uncommon. Most are caused by atherosclerosis, but trauma and poststenotic dilation are also important causes.[54] These aneurysms are more common in men than in women and often are asymptomatic appearing as a pulsatile mass. When symptomatic, the usual complaint is pain in the upper extremity, varying from "intermittent claudication of the arm" to ischemic rest pain caused by more severe ischemia of the hand or fingers if distal embolization from mural thrombus in the aneurysm has occurred. If the subclavian aneurysm is related to thoracic outlet compression, resection of the uppermost rib and resection of the aneurysm with arterial reconstruction is advisable.

CAROTID ARTERY ANEURYSM

Aneurysms of the common carotid artery and its two major branches in the neck are uncommon.[55] Most carotid aneurysms involve the common carotid artery, usually at its bifurcation and are atherosclerotic in origin, though in years past, syphilis was the usual cause. Aneurysms of the extracranial portion of the internal carotid artery are rare. They may be asymptomatic or appear as a mass in the neck or internally in the lateral pharyngeal wall.[56] More common than carotid aneurysm, though often confused with it, are the syndromes of "buckled carotid artery" and "buckled innominate artery" (Fig. 17-13), which may include prominent pulsation, suggestive of aneurysm, in the right side of the neck. "Buckling" of the carotid and innominate arteries occurs almost exclusively in elderly women with significant hypertension. The buckling results from elongation and tortuosity of the aortic arch and its branches caused by advanced arteriosclerosis. Chemodectoma of the carotid body may exhibit pulsation that is difficult to distinguish from an aneurysm. Both buckled arteries and chemodectoma can be readily differentiated from carotid artery aneurysm by ultrasound scanning or carotid angiography. The natural history of carotid artery aneurysm is not defined because of the paucity of cases, but assuming their behavior to be similar to other aneurysms, aneurysmectomy with restoration of arterial continuity is recommended for suitable surgical candidates.

REFERENCES

1. Hertzer NR et al: Coronary artery disease in peripheral vascular patients: a classification of 1000 coronary angiograms and results of surgical management, Ann Surg 199:223, 1984.
2. Spittell JA Jr: Clinical aspects of aneurysmal disease, Curr Probl Cardiol 5:6, 1980.
3. Osler W: Quoted by Bean WB, ed. "Sir William Osler Aphorisms," Springfield, Ill, 1961, Charles C. Thomas.
4. Spittell JA Jr: Hypertension and arterial aneurysm, J Am Coll Cardiol 1:533, 1983.
5. De Palma RG: Biochemical abnormalities and atherosclerotic aneurysms. In Bergan JJ and Yao JST, eds: Aneurysm: diagnosis and treatment, New York, 1982, Grune & Stratton.
6. Busuttel RW, Abou-Zamzam AM, and Machleder HI: Collagenase activity of the human aorta, Arch Surg 115:1373, 1980.
7. Glesby MJ and Pyeritz RE: Association of mitral valve prolapse and systemic abnormalities of connective tissue, JAMA 262:523, 1989.
8. Fleming AW and Green DC: Traumatic aneurysms of the thoracic aorta: report of 43 patients, Ann Thorac Surg 18:91, 1974.
9. Stengel A and Wolferth CC: Mycotic (bacterial) aneurysms of intravascular origin, Arch Intern Med 31:527, 1923.
10. Mundth ED et al: Surgical management of mycotic aneurysms and the complications of infection in vascular reconstructive surgery, Am J Surg 117:460, 1969.
11. Davies OD Jr, Thorburn JD, and Powell P: Cryptic mycotic abdominal aortic aneurysms, Am J Surg 136:96, 1978.
12. Marty AT et al: Inflammatory abdominal aortic aneurysm infected by *Campylobacter* fetus, JAMA 249:1190, 1983.
13. Mulmed LN et al: Femoral tuberculous arteritis, Minn Med 62:271, 1980.
14. Dornfield L, Lecky JW, and Peter JB: Polyarteritis and intrarenal renal artery aneurysms, JAMA 215:1950, 1971.
15. Cipriano PR et al: Multiple aortic aneurysms in relapsing polychondritis, Am J Cardiol 37:1097, 1976.
16. Tucker CR et al: Aortitis in ankylosing spondylitis: early detection of aortic root abnormalities with two dimensional echocardiography, Am J Cardiol 49:680, 1982.
17. Leonhardt ETC and Kullenberg KPG: Bilateral atrial myxomas with multiple arterial aneurysms—a syndrome mimicking polyarteritis nodosa, Am J Med 62:792, 1977.
18. Johansen K: Aneurysms, Sci Am 247:110, 1982.
19. Auerbach O and Garfinkel L: Atherosclerosis and aneurysm of the aorta in relation to smoking habits and age, Chest 78:805, 1980.
20. Bernstein EF et al: Growth rates of small abdominal aortic aneurysms, Surgery 80:765, 1976.
21. Nevitt MP, Ballard DJ, and Hallet JW: Prosnosis of abdominal aortic aneurysms: a population based study, N Engl J Med 321:1009, 1989.
22. Bickerstaff LK et al: Thoracic aortic aneurysms: a population based study, Surgery 92:1103, 1982.
23. Holman E: The obscure physiology of poststenotic dilatation: its relation to the development of aneurysms, J Thorac Surg 28:109, 1954.
24. Joyce JW et al: Aneurysms of the thoracic aorta: a clinical study with reference to prognosis, Circulation 29:176, 1964.
25. Pressler V and McNamara JJ: Thoracic aortic aneurysm: natural history and treatment, J Thorac Cardiovasc Surg 79:489, 1980.
26. Shabian DM et al: Lesions of the thoracic aorta and its arch simulating neoplasm, J Thorac Cardiovasc Surg 81:251, 1981.
27. Quaini E et al: Chronic traumatic aneurysms of the descending thoracic aorta, Texas Heart Inst J 12:143, 1985.
28. McDonald GR et al: Surgical management of patients with the Marfan syndrome and dilatation of the ascending aorta, J Thorac Cardiovasc Surg 81:180, 1981.
29. Bickerstaff LK et al: Abdominal aortic aneurysms: the changing natural history, J Vasc Surg 1:6, 1984.
30. Ryan EA, Spittell JA, Jr, and Kincaid OW: Roentgenographic manifestations of abdominal aortic aneurysm, Postgrad Med 36:77, 1964.
31. Osler W: Aneurysm of the abdominal aorta, Lancet 2:1089, 1905.
32. Estes JE, Jr: Abdominal aortic aneurysm: a study of one hundred and two cases, Circulation 2:258, 1950.
33. Maloney JD et al: Ultrasound evaluation of abdominal aortic aneurysms, Circulation 56:80, 1977.
34. Olin JW et al: Prevalence of atherosclerotic renal artery stenosis in patients with atherosclerosis elsewhere, Am J Med 88:46N-51N, 1990.
35. Kazmier FJ et al: Livedo reticularis and digital infarcts: a syndrome arising from atheromatous abdominal aortic aneurysms, Vasc Dis 3:12, 1966.
36. Eagle KA et al: Dipyridamole-thallium scanning in patients undergoing vascular surgery, JAMA 257:2185, 1987.
37. Spittell JA Jr and Hunt JC: Abdominal aortic aneurysm and the kidney, Med Clin North Am 50:1021, 1966.
38. Sidell PM et al: Horseshoe kidney associated with surgery of the abdominal aorta, Mayo Clin Proc 54:97, 1979.
39. Leach SD et al: Effect of β-adrenergic blockade on the growth rate of abdominal aortic aneurysms, Arch Surg 123:606, 1988.
40. Hollier LH, Spittell JA Jr and Puga FJ: Intra-aortic balloon counterpulsation as adjunct to aneurysmectomy in high risk patients, Mayo Clin Proc 56:565, 1981.
41. Hollier LH et al: Thoracoabdominal aortic aneurysm repair: analysis of postoperative morbidity, Arch Surg 123:871, 1988.
42. Lowry SF and Kraft RO: Isolated aneurysms of the iliac artery, Arch Surg 113:1289, 1978.
43. Lippoff O et al: Initial report of a mycotic aneurysm of the common iliac artery with compression of the ipsilateral ureter and femoral vein: literature review and case report, Texas Heart Inst J 13:321, 1986.
44. Spittell JA Jr et al: Aneurysm of the splenic artery, JAMA 175:452, 1961.
45. Sweetman WR and Weinstein MJ: Hepatic and celiac artery aneurysms, JAMA 197:221, 1966.
46. Stanley JC, Thompson NW, and Fry WJ: Splanchnic artery aneurysms, Arch Surg 101:689, 1970.
47. Cassel WG et al: Arteriovenous fistula of splenic vessels producing ascites, Circulation 16:1077, 1957.
48. Hollier LH, Batson RC, and Cohn I Jr: Femoral anastomotic aneurysms, Ann Surg 191:715, 1980.
49. Gedge SW, Spittell JA Jr, and Ivins JC: Aneurysm of the distal popliteal artery and its relationship to the arcuate popliteal ligament, Circulation 24:270, 1961.
50. Rich NW and Hughes CW: Popliteal artery and vein entrapment, Am J Surg 113:696, 1967.
51. Wychulis AR, Spittell JA Jr, and Wallace RB: Popliteal aneurysms, Surgery 68:942, 1970.
52. Carpenter JR et al: Ultrasound evaluation of the popliteal space: comparison with arthrography and physical examination, Mayo Clin Proc 51:498-503, 1976.
53. Pappas G et al: Femoral aneurysms, JAMA 190:489-493, 1964.
54. Pairolero PC et al: Subclavian-axillary artery aneurysms, Surgery 90:757-763, 1981.
55. Raphael HA et al: Cervical carotid aneurysms: treatment by excision and restoration of arterial continuity, Am J Surg 105:771-778, 1963.
56. Mokri B et al: Extracranial internal carotid artery aneurysms, Mayo Clin Proc 57:310-321, 1982.

Chapter 18

DISSECTION OF THE AORTA AND OTHER ARTERIES

John A. Spittell, Jr.
Peter C. Spittell

Acute dissection of the thoracic aorta is the most common acute aortic lesion encountered clinically, and because of its protean manifestations, it has challenged clinicians for decades. The development of noninvasive imaging techniques, which have remarkable diagnostic accuracy, should significantly improve the previous high degree of misdiagnosis and nondiagnosis. The most important ingredient in accurate diagnosis, however, is clinical suspicion, which depends not only on knowledge of the varied historical features and physical findings but also on awareness of the usual settings in which acute aortic dissection can occur. Increased awareness of acute aortic dissection, better diagnosis, and aggressive pharmacologic and surgical therapy have all contributed to the improved survival rate in acute aortic dissection.

Spontaneous dissection in branches of the aorta is less common than in aortic dissection. The unusual clinical syndromes produced by these lesions are being recognized more frequently now than in the past because of wider application of angiography and other imaging techniques. Although the pathology of a hematoma dissecting the media is similar in peripheral arteries and the aorta, the etiology and natural history of spontaneous dissection in peripheral arteries appears to differ from that of aortic dissection in other respects, so that the correct approach to management must be individualized.

AORTIC DISSECTION

Etiology

The etiologic basis of the medial degeneration, a prerequisite for aortic dissection, has held the interest of investigators since the time of Erdheim who described "medionecrosis aorta idiopathic cystica."[1] More recent studies suggest that the basic lesion involves the muscle and elastic tissue of the media and is neither necrotic nor cystic.[2] It has been proposed that the medial degeneration is the principal lesion in persons more than 40 years of age,[3] while the less common elastic tissue degeneration occurs mainly in younger persons, particularly in persons with Marfan syndrome.[4] The basis of the medial degeneration is not definitely known. It is not clear whether disturbed nutrition of the media caused by changes in the vasa vasorum, aggravated by hypertension, or injury and repair of the media consequent to hydrodynamic forces are responsible.[5]

The frequency with which aortic dissection occurs in certain conditions suggests that multiple risk factors are involved. The frequency of aortic dissection in persons with Marfan syndrome certainly implies a genetic predisposition. Medial changes secondary to abnormal hemodynamic forces distal to aortic stenosis[6-8] and congenital abnormalities of the aortic valve[9] give support to the concept of a hemodynamic factor. The frequency of hypertension—essential or secondary (e.g., coarctation of the aorta or pregnancy)—also implicates it as a major risk factor for aortic dissection. Arteriosclerosis has only recently been shown to be a risk factor in some patients with the "penetrating atherosclerotic ulcer" syndrome of the descending thoracic aorta.[10] These patients are usually elderly and hypertensive. An ulcerating atherosclerotic placque disrupts the internal elastic lamina exposing the media to the intraluminal pressures leading to intramural hematoma formation.

Pathology

An intramural hematoma has been considered the initial event in acute aortic dissection, with rupture of the vasa vasorum being considered the underlying cause of the intramural hematoma. Some investigators suggest that the intimal tear, exposing the aortic media to the intraluminal pulsatile pressure, is a secondary event, while others continue to believe that the intimal tear is primary. While this sequence appears to be the most frequent pathogenesis of classic aortic dissection, medial dissection may occur with a penetrating aortic ulcer causing intramedial hemorrhage.[10] An important difference between classic aortic dissection and that secondary to penetrating aortic ulcer is the location of the proximal intimal tear, which is most often in the ascending aorta in the former[11] and always in the descending thoracic aorta in the latter.[10] Larson and Edwards observed that the intimal tears in cases of dissection beginning in the descending thoracic aorta were associated with extensive atherosclerosis in the majority of patients. They proposed that rupture of an atherosclerotic plaque might have initiated the intimal tear,[12] a point supported by the observations of others.[13,14] Another distinction between proximal and distal aortic dissections is the greater frequency of hypertension in cases of distal dissection compared to proximal aortic dissection,[15] an observation that may bear on pathogenesis.

Whatever its origin, the intimal tear exposes the aortic media to pulsatile flow, which, as Prokop, Palmer, and Wheat have shown,[16] effects rapid cleavage of the aortic media in its outer portion. The outer layer of the false channel thus created in the wall of the aorta is consideraly thinner than the inner layer, likely accounting for the higher frequency of external rupture of the dissecting hematoma than internal rupture into the true aortic lumen (reentry). As noted by Roberts, "The thinner the outer wall of the false channel, the greater the likelihood of fatal rupture."[11] External rupture, the most frequent cause of death in untreated cases, most often occurs into the pericardium and, in decreasing frequency, into the left pleural cavity, the right pleural cavity, the mediastinum, and the abdomen.

The usual course of the dissecting column of blood is along the greater curvature of the thoracic aorta, involving a variable portion of the circumference of the aorta but usually no more than one-half.[11] When the origin of branches of the aorta are encountered by the dissecting column of blood, they may be sheared off or occluded by extension of the dissection into the wall of the branch or spared by a division of the dissection around the origin of the branch artery. Accordingly, occlusion of a major branch of the aorta may be the dominant feature[17] or become the focus of treatment.[18]

When attachment of one or more of the aortic valve cusps to the aortic ring is disrupted by the dissecting column of blood, aortic insufficiency results and may be severe enough to cause left ventricular failure and sometimes death.

Clinical manifestations

The protean manifestations and variety of clinical manifestations of acute aortic dissection likely account for the high rate of misdiagnosis or nondiagnosis in the past. It is important to consider the diagnosis of aortic dissection whenever one encounters a patient who has a catastrophic illness and signs or symptoms of ischemia to various organ systems.[19] The condition can occur at any age but is most common between the ages of 40 to 70 years. Aortic dissection occurs two or three times as often in men as in women. Of note, in younger women it most often occurs in the third trimester of pregnancy.

As noted, dissection usually manifests itself as a catastrophe with the sudden onset of severe pain often described as "tearing" or "ripping" in the chest. The pain tends to move distally to the back, abdomen, and lower extremities as the aortic dissection progresses distally. The location of the initial pain is usually located in the anterior chest, raising the question of acute myocardial infarction, but occasionally the pain occurs in the interscapular area or high in the epigastrium, raising the question of an acute intraabdominal process. Much less often the pain begins in the neck or shoulder. Pain may be absent in some patients. Syncope or collapse may occur at the onset of the dissection, usually caused by rupture into the pericardium causing tamponade. The pain may be persistent or may subside with treatment. In the latter instance, any recurrence of pain suggests extension of the dissection or external rupture.

Of some interest is the activity of the patient at the time of onset of the dissection. In a series of 39 patients in whom we could determine this, only 7 were working or lifting, while 5 were asleep, and another 4 were lying down.[20]

The patient with an acute aortic dissection commonly exhibits a shock-like appearance—pallid and sweating—but with a moderately or severely elevated blood pressure. Elevated blood pressure is present in 70% of cases. Hypertension is more common and often more severe in patients whose initial tear is in the proximal descending thoracic aorta than when the initial tear is in the ascending aorta. Cardiac examination may reveal only a moderate tachycardia. When the dissection involves the aortic valve, the decrescendo diastolic murmur of aortic insufficiency may be heard. However, if there is acute severe aortic insufficiency and significant left ventricular failure, one may not hear a murmur. If the dissection has extended to the root of the aorta, it may extend into the pericardium causing a pericardial friction rub or tamponade.[21] Since the dissection may involve the branches of the aorta, diminution of one or more arterial pulsations in the extremities[17,18] or neck may be noted. Neurologic findings include syncope, seizure, stroke, or paraplegia caused by involvement of the arterial supply to the spinal cord or an ischemic peripheral neuropathy resulting from the dissection extending to a peripheral artery.

Should the dissection compromise the renal arterial circulation, severe hypertension, hypertensive crisis, or acute anuric or oliguric renal failure can complicate acute aortic dissection. The enlargement of the thoracic aorta caused by the intramural hematoma can cause symptoms resulting from pressure on mediastinal structures—hoarseness, dysphagia, or the superior vena cava syndrome.[22] Extension of the dissection into the abdominal aorta can raise the question of an abdominal aortic aneurysm because of the tenderness and increased aortic diameter produced by the intramural hematoma. Aortic dissection may occasionally be accompanied by fever of uncertain origin.[23] These unusual features should not exclude aortic dissection from consideration, if other features such as sudden catastrophic illness, chest or back pain, and hypertension are present.

Diagnosis

Laboratory tests are of limited value in the diagnosis of acute aortic dissection but are useful in the exclusion of other possible diagnoses. The electrocardiogram is of greatest value in differentiating acute myocardial infarction from acute aortic dissection. Rarely the dissection occludes the ostium of one of the coronary arteries and produces myocardial ischemia. As mentioned earlier pericarditis and/or acute tamponade with acute aortic dissection occasionally occurs. The most common electrocardiographic abnormality in acute aortic dissection is that of left ventricular hypertrophy.[24]

Multiple abnormalities may be seen on plain roentgenographic films of the chest (Table 18-1).[25] The most common is an increase in the diameter of the supracardiac aorta; this

Table 18-1. Plain film radiographic findings in 74 cases of thoracic aortic dissection

Finding	Patients No.	Patients %
Abnormalities in region of aortic knob	49	66
Change from previous films	9*	47*
Irregular aortic contour	28	38
Discrepancy in diameters of ascending and descending aorta	25	34
Pleural effusion	20	27
Left	15	
Bilateral	4	
Right	1	
Indistinct aortic margin	13	18
Mediastinal widening	8	11
Displacement of calcified intima	5	7
Negative chest or nonspecific findings	13	18

(From Earnest F et al: Roentgenographic findings in thoracic aortic dissection, Mayo Clin Proc 54:43-50, 1979. Used with permission.)

*Previous films were available in 19 cases.

A

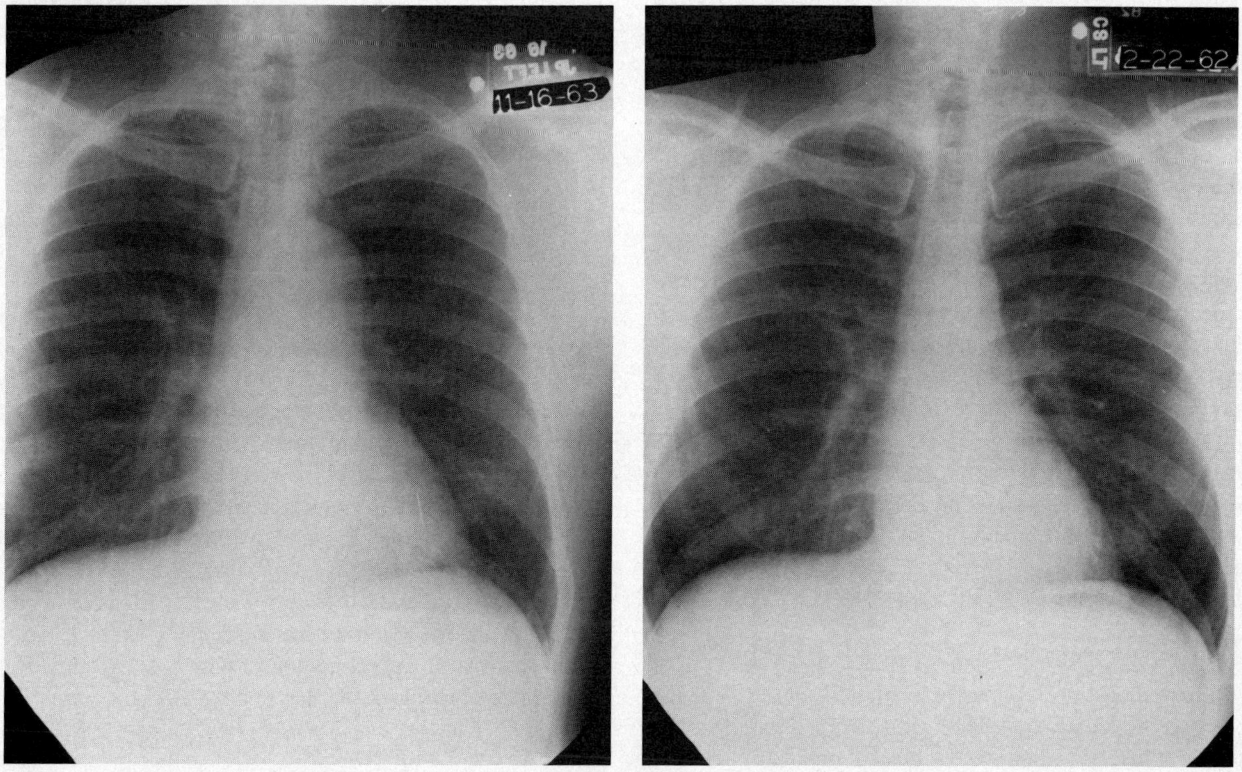

B

Fig. 18-1. A, Widening of supracardiac aortic shadow in patient with aortic dissection. **B,** Same patient 1½ years earlier. (From Spittell JA Jr and Wallace RB: Aortic dissection, Am Fam Physician 1:89-98, 1970.)

finding is particularly significant if a change can be confirmed by comparing a prior chest roentgenogram with the current films (Fig. 18-1). It should be emphasized that a negative chest roentgenogram does not exclude acute aortic dissection.

Echocardiography is emerging as a useful (perhaps preferred) noninvasive method to diagnose aortic dissection. Prior to the development of transesophageal echocardiography, conventional transthoracic echocardiography was of value in diagnosis only when the dissection involved the ascending aorta. Now, with a combination of transthoracic and transesophageal echocardiography, the accurate diagnosis of aortic dissection is possible. Erbel et al recently reported a sensitivity of 99% and a specificity of 98% with transesophageal echocardiography.[26] Diagnostic difficulty is encountered only in dissections limited to the arch of the aorta whose scanning is limited by the trachea. Employing color-coded Doppler imaging further enhances the diagnosis of aortic dissection, allowing identification of intimal tears and the true and false lumens.[27]

Computed tomography (CT) scanning with intravenous contrast infusion is another accurate and readily available screening technique that can be used when acute aortic dissection is suspected,[28] but it is not available for bedside use as is echocardiography, and there is a slight risk associated with the administration of contrast media not associated with the echocardiography. Magnetic resonance imaging (MRI) certainly has potential for demonstrating aortic dissection at any location, and without ionizing radiation, but its expense and limited availability will limit its use to the most difficult or unusual cases.[29]

Angiography is still the definitive method for the diagnosis and localization of aortic dissection. The angiographic findings in aortic dissection include opacification of the false lumen, deformity of the true lumen, and visualization of an intimal flap.[25] Aortograms are not diagnostic in all cases, however. Falsely negative aortograms can occur when there is only very faint opacification of the false channel or when there is simultaneous and equal opacification of the true and false lumens.[30] In one series an incidence of about 2% false negative aortograms has been reported.[31]

In the patient with suspected penetrating aortic ulcer, CT scan without contrast is the recommended imaging procedure since the use of contrast media may make appreciation of an intramural hematoma difficult.[32] The penetrating ulcer, usually in the descending thoracic aorta, may be demonstrated by aortography as well (Fig. 18-2).

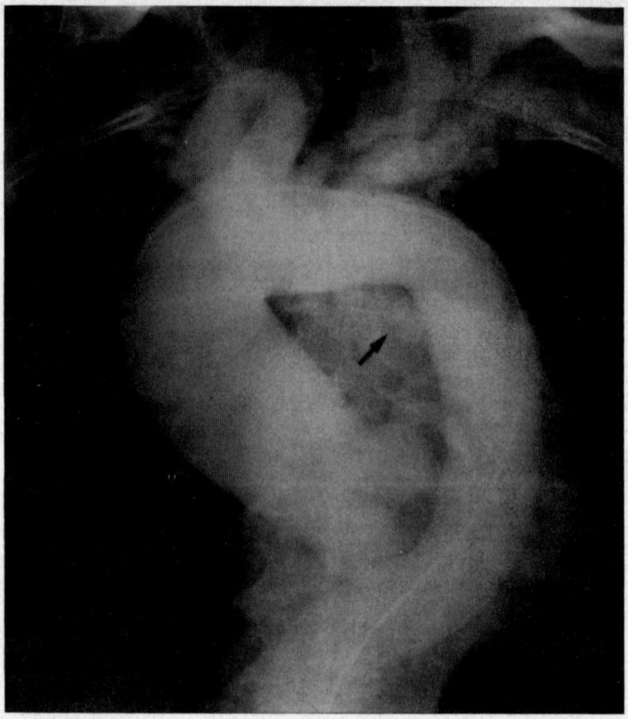

Fig. 18-2. Thoracic aortogram of a 71-year-old man, demonstrating a penetrating aortic ulcer (*arrow*) of the upper descending thoracic aorta at the level of the ligamentum arteriosum.

Localizing the dissection

Since management of acute aortic dissection depends mainly on the location of the primary tear and on any compromise of arterial blood supply to vital organs by the dissection, determination of the location and extent of the dissection is essential.

Several systems of classification of aortic dissection have been proposed. The most widely used is that proposed by DeBakey et al[33]—namely Types I, II, and III (Fig. 18-3). Other systems use the terms "Type A," "proximal," or "ascending" for Type I of DeBakey and "Type B," "distal," or "descending" for Type III of DeBakey.[33] As noted by Miller,[34] the "cardinal feature of all classification systems today is whether or not the ascending aorta is involved by the dissecting process."

While either angiography, CT scan, or echocardiography will provide the definitive information on the location of the dissection, clinical features can often suggest the type of dissection. Involvement of the ascending aorta is suggested by substernal pain, aortic diastolic murmur, pericardial friction rub, electrocardiographic evidence of pericarditis or myocardial ischemia, and significant diminution in the pulse and blood pressure in the right arm. Also, dissection involving the ascending aorta is the usual type seen in persons with Marfan syndrome. Hypertension is more common in dissection of the descending thoracic aorta.[15] Also, an interscapular location of pain is suggestive of dissection originating in the descending thoracic aorta.[35]

Differential diagnosis

In our experience, acute aortic dissection has been misdiagnosed as acute myocardial infarction, acute stroke,

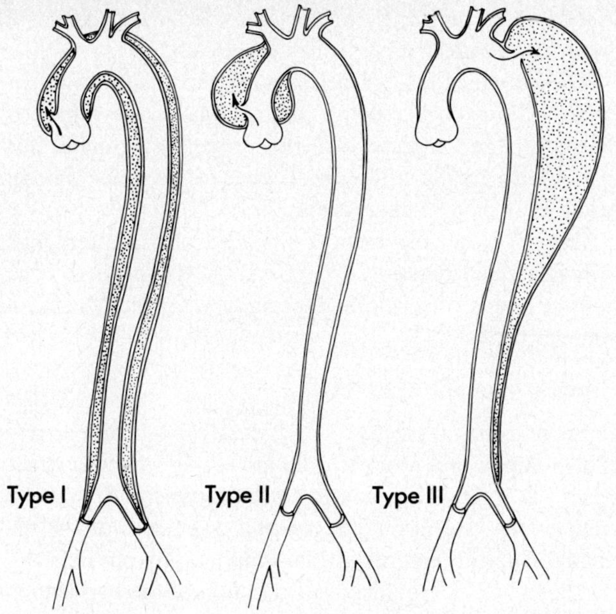

Fig. 18-3. Classification of aortic dissection. *Type I*, primary tear in ascending aorta and dissection involving aortic arch and distal aorta for a variable distance. *Type II*, dissection involving only ascending aorta. *Type III*, primary tear just distal to the origin of the left subclavian artery and extending distally for a variable distance. (Modified from DeBakey ME et al: Surgical management of dissecting aneurysms of the aorta, J Thorac Cardiovasc Surg 49:130-148, 1965.)

acute intraabdominal process, acute peripheral arterial occlusion, or acute renal failure.[17,18,31,36] Less often acute dissection has been confused with pulmonary embolism (particularly if there is a pleural effusion present), other causes of acute aortic insufficiency, and acute pericarditis.[21]

Prognosis

The poor prognosis for untreated acute aortic dissection is well established by several studies.[20,24,37] Seventy percent or more of patients die within the first 2 weeks without treatment, and half or more of the persons who survive the first 2 weeks die within 1 year if untreated. In general involvement of the ascending aorta carries a worse prognosis than when the descending thoracic aorta is involved. The presence of other cardiovascular disease—coronary artery disease, cerebrovascular disease, and abdominal aortic aneurysm—also worsen the prognosis in acute aortic dissection.[37] Younger patients seem to have a slightly more favorable prognosis.[20]

Treatment

Fortunately, good emergent treatment and definitive surgical management of aortic dissection have evolved through the efforts of many, but specifically through the pioneering efforts of DeBakey,[33] Wheat,[38] and their associates. Today in most centers the approach to acute aortic dissection is individualized, using both pharmacologic therapy and surgical treatment according to the type of dissection and any associated complications.

When the diagnosis of acute aortic dissection is suspected, intensive pharmacologic therapy to control hypertension and decrease the force of ventricular contraction is started and continued while the diagnostic procedures are being performed. The treatment of choice for acute aortic dissection is sodium nitroprusside combined with intravenous β-blockade to decrease the force of left ventricular ejection.[39] One should start with an initial dose of nitroprusside of 0.05 μg/kg/min and titrate the dose to the lowest systolic blood pressure, which allows adequate perfusion to the vital organs (usually 90-110 mm Hg). β-blockers are administered to keep the heart rate at about 60 beats per minute. If the blood pressure is normal, β-blockade alone may be used to slow the heart rate. Recently, the use of intravenous labetalol has been proposed for the emergent treatment of acute aortic dissection. This agent has both α- and β-adrenoreceptor blocking action.[40] In some centers this has replaced sodium nitroprusside as the drug of choice in acute aortic dissection. If β-blockers or labetolol cannot be used, trimethaphan camsylate (Arfonad) can be used. It is initially effective but has undesirable side effects (e.g., bowel and bladder atony and pupillary dilation) and tachyphylaxis develops rapidly.

Unless some associated condition limiting the patient's life expectancy coexists, dissections of the ascending aorta are best treated by urgent surgical repair to prevent intrapericardial hemorrhage, aortic valve insufficiency, and coronary artery occlusion. Resection of the ascending aorta and replacement with a Dacron graft is the usual surgical procedure.[34,41] If there is associated aortic valvular insufficiency, resuspension of the valve, if possible, is preferred, but if there is associated annuloaortic ectasia, a valved conduit may be used.[41]

In dissections of the descending thoracic aorta, management following the initial emergent period is controversial. Our approach has been to continue pharmacologic therapy, if the patient is stable and without evidence of progressing dissection, for 2 to 3 weeks before advising surgical repair, given a patient without other life-threatening conditions. If evidence of progressing dissection or expansion of the intramural hematoma develops then prompt surgical treatment is undertaken. Others have recommended long-term pharmacologic therapy for dissections of the descending thoracic aorta, closely monitoring the patient for evidence of increasing aortic size, development of an enlarging saccular aneurysm or the development of pain or other symptoms related to the chronic dissection, all of which warrant surgical intervention. One feared complication of replacement of the descending aorta is paralysis from interruption of

Causes of primary dissection of the peripheral arteries

Spontaneous
Trauma
Hypertension
Fibromuscular dysplasia
Degenerative arterial disease
Cystic medial necrosis

blood supply to the spinal cord.

The objectives of surgical treatment are the prevention of further or recurrent dissection, elimination of the risk of external rupture, correction of any aortic valve incompetence, and restoration of patency of any occluded branches of the aorta. These objectives are met by resecting the segment of aorta in which the primary tear is located, closing the false channel proximally and distally and repairing or, if necessary, replacing an incompetent aortic valve. Any significant branch of the aorta whose compromise is not relieved by closing the false channel can be repaired or replaced surgically if the blood supply to a vital organ remains extremely compromised.

DISSECTING ANEURYSM OF OTHER ARTERIES

Primary dissecting aneurysms of the arteries of the extremities without involvement of the aorta are rare. Wychulis, Kincaid, and Walbee[42] reported 110 cases of primary dissecting aneurysms of the peripheral arteries with only 9 of these cases involving arteries leading into or entirely within an extremity.

Primary dissecting aneurysms of the peripheral arteries are most common in the renal arteries, followed by the intracranial, pulmonary, and mesenteric arteries in decreasing order of frequency. Usually only one artery is involved but primary dissecting aneurysms of 2 or more peripheral arteries have been reported.[43-46]

The causes of dissecting aneurysms of the peripheral arteries are listed in the accompanying box. Primary dissecting aneurysms of the peripheral arteries are more common in males (male/female ratio is 2:1) less than 50 years old, and in persons with hypertension or a history of trauma. Dissections are rarely found in association with arteriosclerosis.[47]

Primary dissecting aneurysms of the peripheral arteries occur most frequently either within the media proper or between the media and external elastica layers of the arterial wall. The dissection occurs most frequently in medium- to small-sized muscular arteries, close to their origins from the aorta, the regions of marked rheologic change. The dissection generally involves more than 50% of the circumference of the artery and the occurrence of symptoms depends largely on the degree of ischemia produced by compression of the arterial lumen. Significant atherosclerotic changes in the invovled artery are unusual, as already noted.[48]

The complications of peripheral arterial dissections include arterial occlusion by obliteration of the lumen or thrombosis and rupture with hemorrhage. Thrombus formation can greatly affect the degree of ischemia and can result in an acute ischemic episode.

Primary dissecting aneurysm of a peripherial artery must always be considered in the differential diagnosis of acute limb or visceral ischemia, especially when this occurs in younger patients.

Cervical cephalic arteries

Spontaneous dissection of the cervical cephalic arteries is uncommon, but not rare. The increasing frequency of its diagnosis is probably related to the more frequent use of angiography and also to a growing awareness of the distinctive clinical features of this syndrome by physicians.

The cause of spontaneous dissection of the cervical cephalic arteries is not known. Trauma, often trivial, has been implicated in some cases. The angiographic features of fibromuscular dysplasia have been noted in the internal carotid artery, vertebral artery, or renal artery of 14% of patients with spontaneous dissection of the cervical cephalic arteries.[45]

Clinically, most patients exhibit one of two clinical syndromes, either hemicrania with oculosympathetic paresis or hemicrania associated with delayed focal cerebral ischemic symptoms. Onset of pain is usually abrupt, and headache often precedes the onset of cerebral ischemic symptoms by several hours or days. Other associated symptoms include syncope, light-headedness, subjective bruits, pulsatile tinnitus, amaurosis fugax, impairment of tongue motion, neck swelling, and dysgeusia. Occasionally, symptoms and signs of subarachnoid hemorrhage can occur.

Like dissecting aneurysms of other peripheral arteries, dissection involving the cervical cephalic arteries are more common in persons under 50 years of age and in patients with hypertension. Other associated factors include smoking, history of migraine headache, and current or prior use of oral contraceptives.[45] Spontaneous dissection of the cervical cephalic arteries has a slightly greater predilection for women.

The diagnosis of dissecting aneurysm of the cervical cephalic arteries is often suggested by the presenting symptoms and signs alone. Angiographic findings in spontaneous dissection are distinctive and diagnostic. Typically, a long tapering stenosis is seen with irregular narrowing of the internal carotid artery from the carotid sinus to the base of the skull, termed the "string sign" (Fig. 18-4).

Various modalities have been used in the treatment of spontaneous dissection of the cervical cephalic arteries. Observation, antiplatelet therapy, anticoagulation, and surgery have all been tried. A survey of patients with regard to outcome shows that the prognosis in all the aforementioned

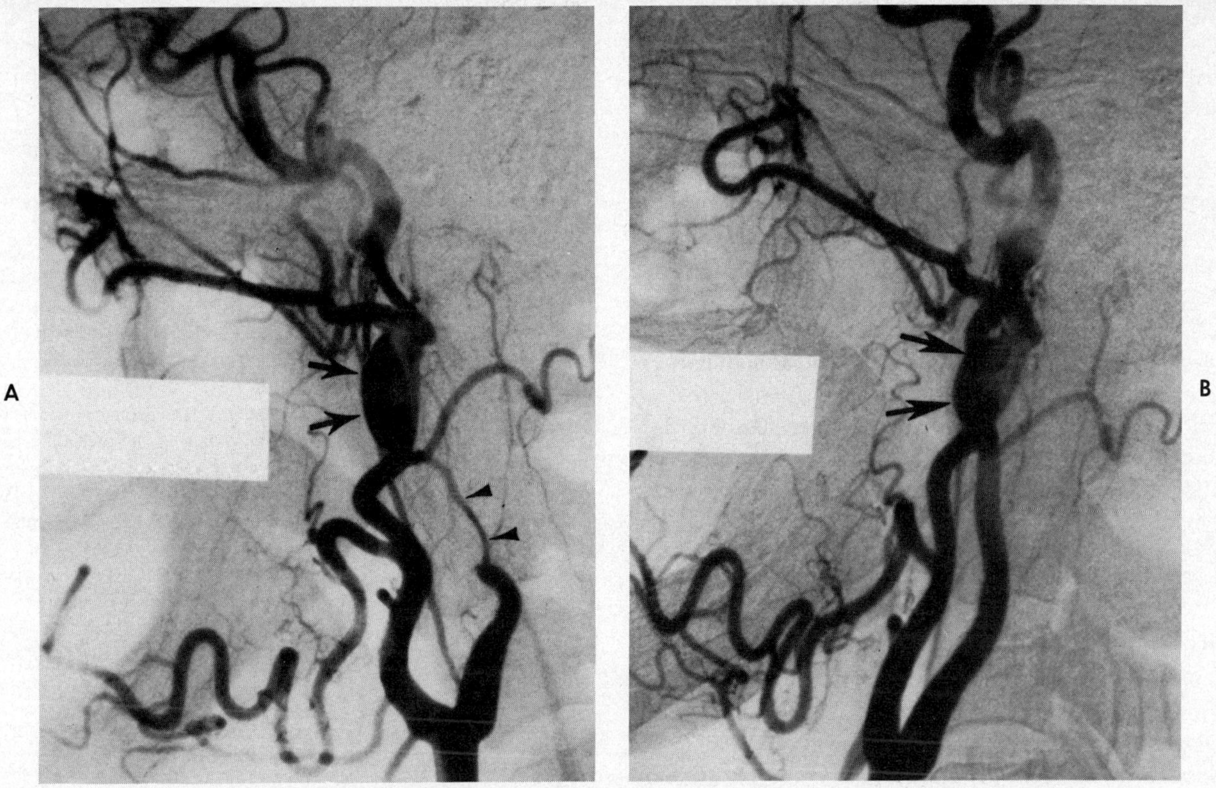

Fig. 18-4. Left carotid angiograms. **A,** Long-segment narrowing of internal carotid artery as a result of dissection (*arrowheads*) and more distal dissecting aneurysm (*arrows*). **B,** Arterial stenosis has resolved, but dissecting aneurysm *(arrows)* has remained essentially unchanged almost 4 months later. (From Mokri B et al: Spontaneous dissection of the cervical internal carotid artery, Ann Neurol 19:126-138, 1986.)

treatments was good,[45] with most patients experiencing an excellent or complete recovery. Follow-up angiography has shown that the stenosis has either completely resolved or improved by angiography in 85% of patients.[45] Recurrences are rare, but spontaneous dissection of the cervical cephalic arteries has been associated with dissection of other peripheral arteries, even much later.[43]

Subclavian artery

Primary dissecting aneurysms of the subclavian artery are extremely rare, first being reported in 1969 by Wychulis, Kincaid, and Walbee.[42] The patients with dissection will commonly have a history of trauma, and usually complain of pain in the ipsilateral shoulder region with radiation to the neck and arm. Paresthesia and coolness of the ipsilateral extremity have been noted.

On examination a bruit over a pulsatile mass in the supraclavicular fossa may be heard. A difference in blood pressure or peripheral pulses may be present in the upper extremities. Findings compatible with syphilis, cervical rib, and arteriosclerosis should be sought, since all may cause aneurysm of the subclavian artery.

Diagnosis is accomplished by arteriography and treatment is surgical resection with autogenous vein or prosthetic graft interposition to prevent peripheral thromboembolism.

Visceral arteries

The superior mesenteric artery is the visceral artery most frequently affected by spontaneous dissection.[47,49] Reports of spontaneous dissection of the gastroduodenal,[50] hepatic,[51] and splenic[47] arteries have also been reported. Spontaneous dissection of a visceral artery may accompany profound shock caused by abdominal apoplexy, or symptoms and signs of bowel ischemia. Hypertension is commonly associated with spontaneous dissection of a visceral artery, and some cases closely follow abdominal surgical procedures.[51]

In most patients with bleeding caused by rupture of a visceral artery, rupture of an atherosclerotic aneurysm is the cause, but occasionally rupture occurs secondary to spontaneous dissection.[52,53] Spontaneous dissection of a visceral artery should be included in the differential diagnosis of an acute abdomen with hemoperitoneum, especially if there is a history of hypertension, recent abdominal surgery, or preexisting arterial disease.

The key to the diagnosis of spontaneous dissection of a visceral artery is a high index of suspicion about patients at risk; prompt definitive diagnosis by arteriography is indicated.

Treatment of visceral artery dissections, if recognized, includes initial stabilization of the patient, followed by excision of the dissecting aneurysm with autogenous vein or prosthetic graft placement or endoaneurysmorrhaphy. The majority of the patients with spontaneous dissection of a visceral artery with subsequent rupture will also require bowel resection and splenectomy—survival is uncommon.

Femoropopliteal artery

Primary dissecting aneurysm of the femoral and/or popliteal arteries is extremely rare, with less than 5 cases reported in the literature.[42] Femoral and popliteal artery dissecting aneurysms are usually of atherosclerotic origin but may also occur secondary to blunt or penetrating trauma, degenerative arterial disease, or inflammatory arterial disease.

The degree of symptoms depends on the severity of limb ischemia secondary to compression of the true lumen by the arterial dissection. Patients may experience pain following trauma, with a picture of acute arterial occlusion, or with intermittent claudication of new onset.

Diagnosis is by angiography, and treatment is surgical resection with autogenous vein or prosthetic graft interposition.

Renal artery

Spontaneous dissection of one or both renal arteries is rare, and its cause remains unclear. It was first described by Bumpus in 1944,[54] and subsequently over 90 cases have been reported in the English literature.[43,44]

Spontaneous dissection of the renal arteries is observed with higher frequency in patients with fibromuscular dysplasia[43,44,55] and involvement is commonly bilateral.[44] Unlike the more prevalent finding of fibromuscular dysplasia in women, renal artery dissection coincident with renal artery fibromuscular dysplasia is most common in middle-aged men.

Patients may be asymptomatic,[56] but most patients develop severe, new onset, or transient hypertension and signs of renal infarction.

The diagnosis is made by angiography. Surgery should be delayed if possible since the prognosis of spontaneous renal artery dissection is good. Rupture is uncommon, as is progression of the dissection. The more typical course is one of arterial recanalization over a period of time with conservative treatment. Most importantly, associated hypertension should be treated aggressively and follow-up angiography should be performed. Surgery is indicated if hypertension is refractory to medical therapy or if both renal arteries are involved, and renal function is jeopardized.

REFERENCES

1. Erdheim J: Medionecrosis aortac idiopathica cystica, Virchows Arch (A) 276:187, 1930.
2. Hirst AE and Gore I: Is cystic medionecrosis the cause of dissecting aortic aneurysm? Circulation 53:915, 1976 (editorial).
3. Hurley JV: Dissecting aneurysm of the aorta: histological appearances and an hypothesis of pathogenesis, Australas Ann Med 8:297, 1959.
4. Gore I: Dissecting aneurysm of the aorta in persons under forty years of age, Arch Path 55:1, 1953.
5. Schlatmann TJM and Becker AE: Pathogenesis of dissecting aneurysm of the aorta: comparative histopathologic study of significance of medial changes Am J Cardiol 39:21, 1977.
6. McKusick VA, Logue RB, and Bahnson HT: Association of aortic valvular disease and cystic medial necrosis of the ascending aorta: report of four instances, Circulation 16:188, 1957.
7. Heath D, Edwards JE, and Smith LA: The rheologic significance of medial necrosis and dissecting aneurysm of the ascending aorta in association with calcific aortic stenosis, Proc Staff Meet Mayo Clin 33:228, 1958.
8. Flanders JF, Ashley PF, and Durham JR: Rupture of the aorta associated with aortic stenosis, JAMA 193:614, 1965.
9. Edwards WO, Leaf DS, and Edwards JE: Dissecting aortic aneurysm associated with congenital bicuspid aortic valve, Circulation 57:1022, 1978.
10. Stanson AW et al: Penetrating atherosclerotic ulcers of the thoracic aorta: natural history and clinicopathologic correlations, Ann Vasc Surg 1:15, 1986.
11. Roberts WC: Aortic dissection: anatomy, consequences, and causes, Am Heart J 101:195, 1981.
12. Larson EW and Edwards WD: Risk factors for aortic dissection: a necropsy study of 161 cases, Am J Cardiol 53:849, 1984.
13. Willius FA and Cragg RW: A talk on dissecting aneurysm of the aorta, Proc Staff Meet Mayo Clin 16:41, 1941.
14. Slater EE and DeJanatis RW: The clinical recognition or dissecting aortic aneurysm Am J Med 60:625, 1976.
15. Spittell JA Jr: Hypertension and arterial aneurysm, J Am Coll Cardiol 1:533, 1983.
16. Prokop EK, Palmer RF, and Wheat MW: Hydrodynamic forces in dissecting aneurysms: in-vitro studies in a tygon model and in dog aortas, Circ Res 27:121, 1970.
17. Amer NC et al: Aortic dissection presenting as iliac artery occlusion: an aid to early diagnosis, N Engl J Med 266:1040, 1962.
18. Cambria RO et al: Vascular complications associated with spontaneous aortic dissection, J Vasc Surg 7:199, 1988.
19. Spittell JA Jr: Dissecting aneurysm (dissecting hematoma) of the aorta, Mod Concepts Cardiovasc Dis 33:837, 1964.
20. McCloy RM, Spittell JA Jr, and McGoon DC: The prognosis in aortic dissection, Circulation 31:665, 1965.
21. Greenberg DI et al: Dissecting aortic aneurysm manifesting as acute pericarditis, Arch Intern Med 139:108, 1979.
22. Spitzer S et al: Superior vena cava obstruction and dissecting aortic aneurysm, JAMA 233:164, 1975.
23. Mackowiak PA et al: Dissecting aortic aneurysm manifested as fever of unknown origin, JAMA 236:1725, 1976.
24. Hirst AE Jr, Johns VJ Jr, and Kime SW Jr: Dissecting aneurysm of the aorta: a review of 505 cases, Medicine (Baltimore) 37:217, 1958.
25. Earnest F IV, Muhm JR, and Sheedy PF II: Roentgenographic findings in thoracic aortic dissection, Mayo Clin Proc 54:43, 1979.
26. Erbel R et al: Echocardiography in diagnosis of aortic dissection, Lancet 1:457, 1989.
27. Hashimoto S et al: Assessment of transesophageal Doppler echocardiography in dissecting aortic aneurysm, J Am Coll Cardiol 14:1253, 1989.

28. Moncada R et al: Diagnosis of dissecting aortic aneurysm by computed tomography, Lancet 1:238, 1981.
29. Fruehwald FXV et al: Cine-MR in dissection of the thoracic aorta, Eur J Radiol 9:37, 1989.
30. Shuford WH, Sybers RG, and Weens HS: Problems in the aortographic diagnosis of dissecting aneurysm of the aorta, N Engl J Med 280:225, 1969.
31. Eagle KA et al: Spectrum of conditions initially suggesting acute aortic dissection but with negative aortagrams, Am J Cardiol 57:322, 1986.
32. Hussain S et al: Penetrating atherosclerotic ulcers of the thoracic aorta J Vasc Surg 9:710, 1989.
33. DeBakey ME et al: Surgical management of dissecting aneurysms of the aorta, J Thorac Cardiovasc Surg 49:130, 1965.
34. Miller DC: Acute dissection of the aorta—continuing need for earlier diagnosis and treatment, Mod Concepts Cardiovasc Dis 54:51, 1985.
35. Burchell HB: Aortic dissection (dissecting hematoma; dissecting aneurysm of aorta), Circulation 12:1068, 1955.
36. Spittell JA Jr: Differential diagnosis of dissecting aneurysm, Prog Cardiovasc Dis 14:225, 1971.
37. Grondin C et al: Dissecting aneurysms of the thoracic aorta: a review of 52 cases with consideration of factors influencing prognosis, Ann Thorac Surg 4:29, 1967.
38. Wheat MW et al: Treatment of dissecting aneurysms of the aorta without surgery, J Thorac Cardiovasc Surg 50:364, 1965.
39. Cooke JP and Safford RE: Progress in the diagnosis and management of aortic dissection, Mayo Clin Proc 61:147, 1986.
40. Grubb BP, Sirio C, and Zelis R: Intravenous Labetalol in acute aortic dissection, JAMA 258.78, 1987.
41. Jex RK et al: Repair of ascending aorta dissection, J Thorac Cardiovasc Surg 93:375, 1987.
42. Wychulis AR, Kincaid OW, and Walbee RB: Primary dissecting aneurysm of peripheral arteries, Mayo Clin Proc 44:804, 1969.
43. Mokri B, Stanson AW, and Houser OW: Spontaneous dissections of the renal arteries in a patient with previous spontaneous dissections of the internal carotid arteries, Stroke 16:959, 1985.
44. Edwards BS et al: Isolated renal artery dissection: presentation, evaluation, management, and pathology, Mayo Clin Proc 57:564, 1982.
45. Mokri B, Houser OW, and Sundt TM Jr: Idiopathic regressing arteriopathy, Ann Neurol 2:466, 1977.
46. Fisher CM, Ojemann RG, and Roberson GH: Spontaneous dissection of cervicocerebral arteries, Can J Neurol Sci 5:9, 1978.
47. Foord AG and Leurs RD: Primary dissecting aneurysms of peripheral and pulmonary arteries, Arch Path 68:553, 1959.
48. Page MH, Leslie GJ, and Thorburn C: Dissecting aneurysm of the femoral and popliteal arteries, Med J Aust 140:24, 1984.
49. Krupski WC, Effeney DJ, and Ehrenfeld WK: Spontaneous dissection of the superior mesenteric artery, J Vasc Surg 2:731, 1985.
50. Dvorak A and Gassaniger A: Dissecting aneurysm of the gastroduodenal artery: anatomic basis for the clinical syndrome of abdominal apoplexy, Ann Surg 169:425, 1969.
51. Larson CJ, Geier GR, and Edwards WD: Fatal acute dissection of the right hepatic artery after appendectomy, Arch Pathol Lab Med 111:300, 1987.
52. Kleinsasser LJ: Abdominal apoplexy: report of 2 cases and review of the literature, Am J Surg 120:623, 1970.
53. McNamara MF and Griska LB: Superior mesenteric artery branch aneurysms, Surgery 88:625, 1980.
54. Bumpus HC Jr: A case of renal hypertension, J Urol 52:295, 1944.
55. Kinearol OW et al: Fibromuscular dysplasia of the renal arteries: arteriographic features, classification, and observations on the natural history of the disease, AJR 104:271, 1968.
56. Hasday JD, Sterns RH, and Karch FB: Renal infarction due to renal artery dysplasia with dissection, Am J Med 76:943, 1984.

Chapter 19

THROMBOANGIITIS OBLITERANS (BUERGER'S DISEASE)

John W. Joyce

After decades of controversy thromboangiitis obliterans (Buerger's disease) has emerged as a well-defined, distinctive clinicopathologic entity. It is a vasculitis of small- and medium-size veins and arteries. Thromboangiitis obliterans (TAO) is unique and contrasts with atherosclerosis obliterans in that the process starts distally and progresses cephalad, and also because both lower and upper extremities are usually involved. It is a disease of the second through fourth decades seen predominantly in men, although the incidence in women is increasing. Tobacco use is the sole known etiologic factor and probably triggers TAO through autoimmune mechanisms.

The evolution of our current knowledge of TAO has been slow. Felix von Winiwarter, an Austrian surgeon working with Billroth, described an initial case in 1879.[1] The eponym "von Winiwarter-Buerger's Disease" is commonly used in Europe. It was in 1908 that Leo Buerger of New York published his first observations on a small group of patients, defining the disease and naming it "thromboangiitis obliterans."[2] His description of the clinical feature is superb and remains valid to this day. Buerger also provided histopathologic observations that were quite sound, particularly a description of superficial veins in the acute phase, the focal and segmental distribution of lesions, and an early appreciation of different tissue responses as the disease progressed. However, Buerger's differentiation of the acute arterial lesion from bland thrombus and some of his wording about atherosclerosis obliterans left confusion, resulting in overdiagnosis of the disease for many years.[3,4]

Wessler et al challenged these original observations in 1960. They noted a dramatic drop in the diagnosis of Buerger's disease at their hospital, when tobacco use was increasing. After careful retrospective reviews of both clinical and pathology material, they correctly concluded that premature atherosclerosis was greatly underappreciated and found that histopathologic criterion were not specific as being applied. They asked if idiopathic thrombosis and systemic embolization might not explain most of the cases studied and, indeed, questioned if TAO as a distinct entity existed.[5,6]

The original and subsequent reports of Wessler et al gave impetus to several valuable studies in response. McPherson, Juergens, and Gifford noted that the survival of patients with TAO approximated that of an age/sex matched population without the disease, in contrast to a third group with premature atherosclerosis, whose survival was significantly shorter because of atherosclerotic cardiac and cerebral events.[7] McKusick et al reconfirmed both the clinical profile and the histopathology of TAO. They carefully pointed out that interpretation of tissue specimens was dependent on the site of the biopsy and the stage of the disease at that time and site.[8,9] Then, of prime importance, angiography was established as the third modality for diagnosing TAO. The work of McKusick et al, particularly of Szilagyi, and of several subsequent European authors correlated clinical and histologic features with radiographic images and established clear, diagnostic criteria for angiographic confirmation of the diagnosis.[9,10]

It remains an observation of referral practice that the diagnosis of TAO may yet be ignored or invoked too readily. Vascular disease in general is not fully taught clinically in most medical schools, and the incidence of TAO is small, perhaps 2 to 4 cases each year in active vascular practices.[11,12] These observations help explain underdiagnosis.

In turn, the diagnosis is often assigned when other conditions causing digital, microcirculatory, or distal arterial disease occur in the young. These are delineated in the discussion of differential diagnosis. TAO can be diagnosed on clinical grounds by attention to its common patterns and by exclusion of these other processes. The diagnosis is then strongly supported by angiography, and when available, confirmed by histopathology.

PATHOGENESIS

Early studies supported that TAO occurred exclusively in males, most of Jewish heritage, and Buerger strongly suspected it was of infectious origin. Each of these concepts has been altered by subsequent observations.

Buerger's reports indicated that TAO was primarily a disease of Jews, but clearly this reflected the population he attended. The disease has a broad ethnic base and occurs worldwide, with a greater incidence apparent in the Orient, Southeast Asia, India, and Israel.[13-17] Blacks have a low rate of reported occurrence, but a contemporary study is desirable.[18]

Women constitute only 1% to 2% of the patients in early reports. This has increased to 11% to 19% in the period 1971 to 1986.[12,13] This may indicate that women now have better access to health care, or that the accuracy of diagnosis has improved in the face of the long-standing belief that TAO is a male disease. It should also represent, however, the increased use of tobacco by women in America in recent decades. TAO is equally as severe in women as in men.[12]

The prevalence of TAO diagnosed has dropped most significantly in recent decades. At the Mayo Clinic, the diagnosis per 100,000 patients per year was 114.3 in 1947, 61.1 in 1956, 18.8 in 1966, 9.9 in 1976, and 12.6 in 1986.[19] Although this may represent a change in referral patterns, I suspect that an appreciation of premature atherosclerosis and other causes of distal ischemia since the challenge of Wessler, and the common use of angiography is responsible for this manyfold drop and recent stabilization in diagnosis. In Japan where care is more centralized and less subject to referral bias, a similar dramatic reduction has taken place, and the current incidence is 5 cases per 100,000 patients each year.[20]

The definitive etiology of TAO is unknown, but it is universally observed that the disease and its exacerbations occur in active smokers, and that cessation of smoking brings remission. Most reports document use of 20 to 40 cigarettes daily. The author has noted exacerbation of TAO in patients acknowledging only 4 to 8 cigarettes daily for 2 or 3 weeks and has also observed florid TAO in a man who never smoked more than 3 to 6 cigarettes a few days each week for 3 years. McKusick, Harris, and Ottesen have made a similar observation.[9] The disease has been reported in pipe smokers and in a patient using only chewing tobacco.[21,22] In the face of continued smoking, progression is usual, but not inevitable.[3,23] The effect of passive exposure to smoke is unknown but should probably be minimized for the patient with TAO.

The fact that only a miniscule percentage of heavy smokers develop TAO in contrast to the almost inevitable multiple manifestations of atherosclerosis obliterans in heavy smokers, and in the face of the observation that the disease can occasionally occur unrelated to a large volume or long duration of smoking, again true of atherosclerosis, strongly suggests that an additional factor specific to these patients is present. Both genetic and immunologic mechanisms have been implicated to explain the pathogenesis of TAO.

An increased incidence of various HLA antigens has been noted in some patient populations with Buerger's disease, but the findings were not universal, and other studies could not make this observation.[13,24] Autoimmune mechanisms remain the most plausible cause of TAO, based on our current understanding of cellular mechanisms. Evidence for this is based on the findings of increased complement, sensitivity to types I and III human collagen, and the presence of anticollagen antibodies in some patients with TAO.[25,26] Further details and confirmation are awaited. No evidence for a hypercoagulable state was found in a small group of patients, using contemporary hematologic tests.[13] At this time, the specific cause of TAO has not been found, but tobacco use is clearly a contributing factor.

PATHOLOGY

General characteristics of specimens taken from legs amputated for TAO include focal, segmental thrombotic occlusion of arteries and adjacent veins with normal proximal vessels, the absence of atherosclerosis, involvement of digital vessels, and various stages of evolution on histologic examination of different sites.

The acute lesion is now considered diagnostic.[2,4,9,12] The artery or vein is modestly swollen, and there is a moderate infiltrate of the adventitia and media. The lumen is occluded by a highly cellular thrombus, with characteristic microabscesses in the thrombus. Lymphocytes exceed neutrophils, and occasional giant cells, and some eosinophils may be seen. The elastic laminae of arteries are intact. In the subacute phase cellularity of the vessel wall and thrombus is less, microabscesses have disappeared, and recanalization has begun (Fig. 19-1). Late lesions consist of organized and recanalized thrombus in fibrotic, small vessels. These lesions are compatible with several forms of vascular injury.

Specimens from an acutely inflamed superficial vein are an excellent source of diagnostic biopsy. TAO has also been diagnosed in acutely inflamed temporal and epididymal arteries.[9,27,28] Acute occlusion of an ectatic or frankly aneurysmal politeal artery, with additional distal manifestations, is an occasional manifestation of TAO. When a youthful smoker has such an event, both the thrombus and a portion of the arterial wall warrant histologic study.[21,22,29] It is also

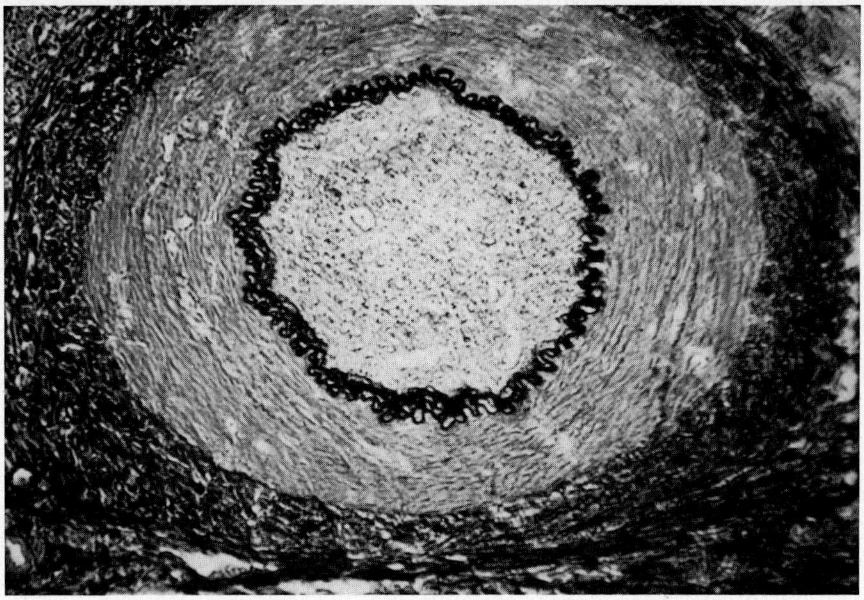

Fig. 19-1. Artery, dorsum of foot. Organizing, highly cellular thrombus, early recanalization; subacute stage; mild infiltrate media. Note intact elastic membrane. (Elastin stain; ×40.)

important to examine multiple specimens of mesenteric vessels when bowel ischemia occurs in TAO of the limbs.[30]

CLINICAL ASPECTS

TAO can usually be distinguished from premature atherosclerosis and other processes causing distal ischemia by its clinical features. It is almost always seen in young smokers. The initial manifestations are bilateral leg ischemia or claudication that begins quite distally and progresses proximally. The tempo of progression may be just 2 to 3 years or 5 to 7 years from onset to tissue loss. The incidence of associated upper extremity involvement, superficial phlebitis, and Raynaud's phenomenon increase as the disease progresses. Several well-documented experiences are recommended.[3,19,23,29,31]

The disease is seen in persons between ages 16 and 45, rarely beyond, and the average age at diagnosis is in the mid-30s. At the time of initial diagnosis, two or more limbs are always involved. In one of the excellent reports of Shionoya, two limbs were affected in 16%, three limbs in 41%, and all limbs in 43%.[29] The patient may develop superficial migratory phlebitis; cool, dysesthetic feet; claudication or rest pain; and gangrene. Raynaud's phenomenon of the fingers and sometimes the toes occurs in up to a third of patients.[13]

A significant number of patients, up to a fifth, will experience migratory, recurrent crops of superficial phlebitis as the initial symptom for a year or two prior to arterial symptoms.[13,23] Biopsy confirming the diagnosis at this time is an opportunity to abort the disease, if the patient can stop tobacco use. The phlebitis occurs in episodes lasting 2 to 3 weeks any time during the course of active disease. Most lesions are linear or branched, but some may be small nodules of 0.5 to 1 cm in diameter.

As the disease often starts in digital and pedal vessels, about a third of patients will first note dysesthesias, cold sensitivity, and rubor or cyanosis.[29] Claudication of the foot or low calf first brings the patient to medical attention in another third of patients. Pedal claudication is a characteristic of TAO, in contrast to atherosclerosis, and patients often seek orthopedic or podiatric help before the disease is fully appreciated. Claudication extends proximal as the disease progresses, and may involve the thigh in 6% to 10% of cases later because of profunda femoris or external iliac involvement. Aortoiliac involvement is rare, and usually from clot propagating from below.[32] Rest pain and gangrene or ulceration are the initial symptoms in 10% to 20% of patients and eventually afflicts two thirds or more.[14,29] While these ischemic manifestations may occur spontaneously, more often they follow trauma such as nail trimming or pressure from foot wear (Fig. 19-2). Secondary infection and further destruction of poorly nourished adjacent tissue is common.

Reports of upper extremity involvement in TAO give an incidence ranging from 15% to 100%, most citing a 50% to 60% figure. Hirai studied 34 consecutive patients with upper extremity TAO. Six had ischemic symptoms but 22 had pulse deficits. Arteriography was performed on all, and 91% had involvement of the digital, radial, and ulnar arteries. Higher lesions were not seen.[33] Digital disease was

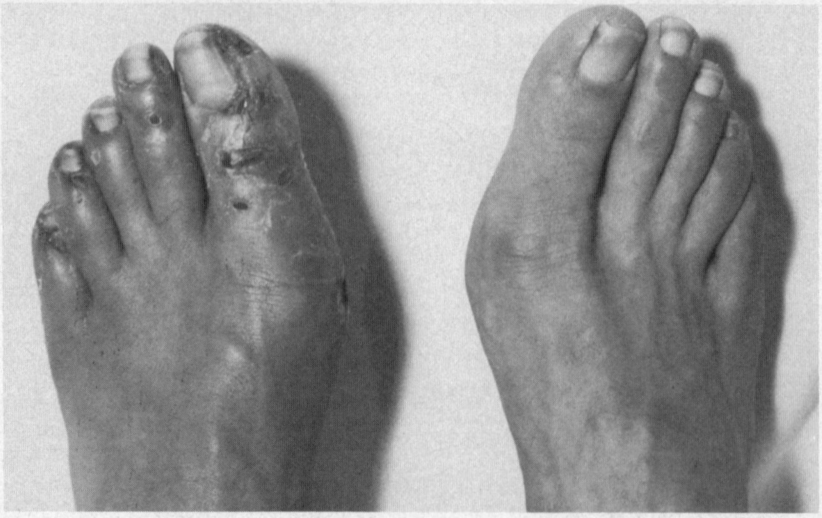

Fig. 19-2. Man, 36. Recurrent crops of nodular phlebitis of calves, 4 years. Claudication pedal arches 2 years. Hand claudication while water skiing 6 months. Rest pain has occurred in left foot since new boots induced skin lesions. Absent wrist and pedal pulses. Note multiple ischemic traumatic ulcers.

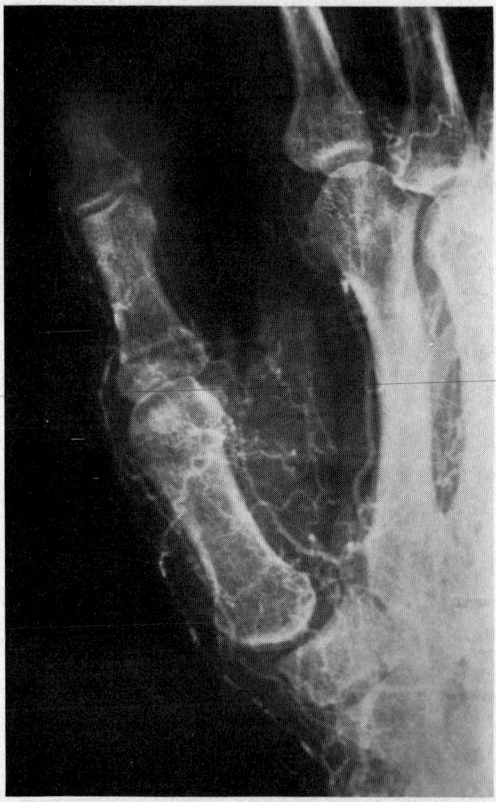

Fig. 19-3. Woman, 41. Bilateral arch claudication 6 years. Presented with cyanosis and rest pain left second, third, and fourth fingers. Note multiple smooth stenosis, many occluded vessels.

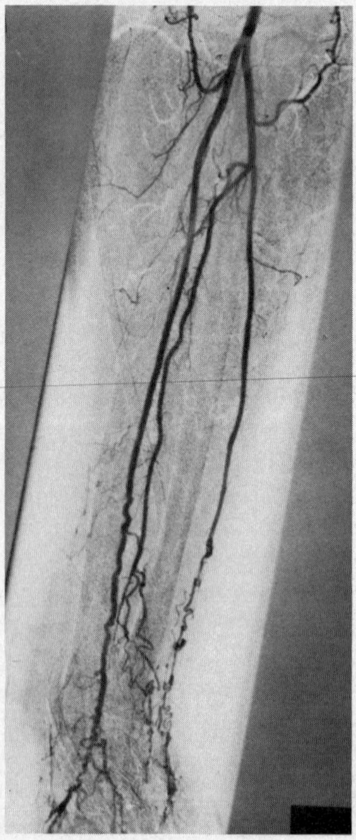

Fig. 19-4. Same patient as in Fig. 19-3. Normal proximal arteries. Multiple focal stenosis of ulnar artery. Corkscrewing of radial artery. Occluded interosseous with "tree root" distal collaterals.

the most frequent finding, followed by focal lesions of the radial and ulnar vessels just above the wrist (Figs. 19-3 and 19-4). I have experience with one case having brachial lesions that resulted in bilateral upper arm amputation.

TAO is not a lethal disease. Most recorded deaths are from complications of surgery or, on occasion, from mesenteric vascular insufficiency.[30] Random cases of cerebral TAO have been documented.[34,35]

Angiographic correlations

Arteriography has played an essential role in the contemporary understanding and definition of TAO. It is utilized routinely to confirm the clinical diagnosis of Buerger's disease at our institution, and on occasion confirms the feasibility of proximal or distal bypass grafting for relief of ischemia. The essential findings are multiple, bilateral focal segments of stenosis or occlusion with normal proximal vessel. The lesions may be a few millimeters or several centimeters long. An intraluminal filling defect is often apparent in stenosis, and occlusions tend to taper in some distal vessels. Collaterals are usually generous and can be "tree-root," spider-like, or corkscrew. The latter term is used to describe what are clearly nearby collaterals but also named, involved vessels that are apparently recanalizing. It is debated if the corkscrew appearance of some vessels represents vasa vasorum. Involved digital arteries are attenuated, may be tortuous, and have abrupt cutoffs (see Fig. 19-3).[9,10,17,36,37]

The patterns of occlusive disease seen by angiography parallel both the distribution and severity of the clinical picture. Digital, pedal, and low-calf vessel involvement is almost universal.[17,37] Bilateral infrapopliteal occlusive disease was seen in all of 210 limbs studied by Shionoya: 90% of anterior tibial, 80% of posterior tibial, and 50% of peroneal arteries were diseased. The peroneal often serves as an important collateral. He observed that toe ulceration occurred in 57% of patients with three obstructed infrapopliteal vessels, but that ulcers occurred in only 7% when at least one vessel reached the foot. An additional "skip area" of the disease at the femoropopliteal segment was noted at the time of diagnosis in 41% of patients, and that an additional 40% of patients later showed progression at this level.[17] Ectasia of the popliteal segment is an occasional finding. Involvement of the common and profunda femoris arteries is seen in about 10%, and of the external iliac in 6%. (Fig. 19-5).[29,32]

Differential diagnosis

Premature atherosclerosis is the most common cause of leg claudication and ischemia in young men and women. Pairolero et al studied 50 consecutive patients under age 35 whose symptoms warranted arteriography. Twenty-four had premature atherosclerosis, 14 had TAO, and 12 had a diversity of other illness. It was striking that all but one of those with premature atherosclerosis were heavy smokers. Diabetes was also present in 10 patients, and increased lipids, or hypertension, was present in 8 patients.[38]

Such patients are usually identified by their more proximal symptoms and have characteristic arteriographic findings. Patients with embolic occlusive disease almost always have an acute onset, and an obvious cardiac source for the embolus. Rare sources of either progressive claudication and/or distal emboli are the popliteal entrapment syndrome and cystic disease of the popliteal or common femoral artery, both of which occur in the age range of TAO. The unusual heritable disorders of connective tissue, Ehlers-Danlos syndrome and pseudoxanthoma elasticum, can manifest themselves in the young. The former can occlude arteries both by rupture with thrombosis or aneurysm with embolization, and pseudoxanthoma elasticum can cause chronic occlusion of the forearm, thigh, and calf arteries. Pseudoxanthoma elasticum is diagnosed by its specific cutaneous manifestations, and the Ehlers-Danlos syndrome by its cutaneous, ocular, and musculoskeletal defects.

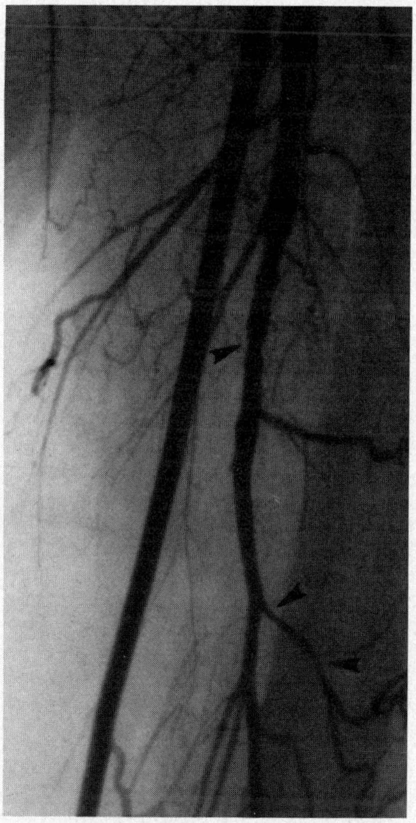

Fig. 19-5. Man, 29. Veins of both calves stripped 6 years earlier for recurrent phlebitis. Bilateral foot, calf claudication 4 years. Left thigh claudication 1 year. Acrocyanotic left foot with rest pain. Absent pedal pulses bilaterally. Note focal stenosis in left profunda femoris artery *(upper arrow)* and focal smooth zones of narrowing in branch *(lower arrows)*.

Digital occlusive disease is often a major manifestation of collagen-vascular and hematologic disorders. Scleroderma, polyarteritis nodosa, and systemic lupus erythematosus are each accompanied by other manifestations and yield to clinical diagnosis, supported by laboratory testing or biopsy. However, lupus may be initiated by a specific clotting problem, a circulating inhibitor, that causes clots in veins, and large or digital arteries. Anticardiolipin antibodies or plasma clot time support the diagnosis. It should be noted that serologic and immunologic tests are normal in TAO.[13] Thrombocytosis, polycythemia, intravascular coagulopathy, and dysproteinemia can also be associated with major and microcirculatory occlusion. These are uncommon in the young, and each can be tested for. In essence, the clinical picture of TAO, knowledge of the natural history of the other lesions listed (with selective testing when indicated), and angiography will establish the diagnosis of TAO in most instances.

THERAPY

Only total abstinence from tobacco will halt the progression and prevent recrudescence of TAO. This must be conveyed clearly and unequivocally to the patient and supporting family or friends, but firmness must be matched with concern, kindness, and patience in seeking to establish patient motivation. Smoking clinics, even inpatient psychiatric support, can be most useful. Photos, anecdotes, and visiting with another patient with TAO may assist selected patients. Some patients stop only after several ischemic episodes, some never. Many patients with TAO have well-developed denial patterns of behavior and skip from one source of care to another, seeking pain medication. Continuity of care in a supportive setting, a well-informed and interested family, and economic security are highly desirable for the difficult problem of tobacco withdrawal.

Patients with rest pain and ischemic lesions warrant hospitalization. Adequate pain control is an essential first step. Assessment of the degree of ischemia by clinical examination and noninvasive testing allows judging whether local digital amputation or debridement will succeed. Infection should be treated by drainage and culture-directed antibiotics.

When ischemia is intermediate, and smoking cessation is accomplished, vasodilation by calcium channel blockers or prazosin may be effective, but they are disappointing in most patients. Surgical sympathectomy has long been a standard of treatment. It too has its best success in the absence of tobacco and with intermediate ischemia. Few reports give information that defines the degree of ischemia, correlation of the anatomic pattern, and whether smoking was controlled when reporting results of lumbar sympathectomy. One report does state a 71.4% improvement following lumbar sympathectomy in 57 patients. While more encouraging than earlier anecdotal information, the criterion for measuring improvement and its duration, and the relationship to smoking are not cited.[39]

Direct arterial repair is feasible in TAO. Shionoya found that distal disease precluded direct repair in the majority of 148 patients studied. However, 22 bypass grafts using autologous saphenous vein were accomplished and only six remained patent for the first 1 to 5 years of follow-up. The successful grafts terminated above the popliteal bifurcation. It is not clear from this report[40] or a subsequent review[29] however, what long-term benefits were accomplished.

The past 15 years have seen the careful evaluation of prostaglandin E1 (PGE1) because of its vasodilator effect and its capacity to inhibit platelet aggregation. Preliminary studies demonstrated improved healing of superficial wounds and clearing of rest pain but required repetitive intraarterial infusions over several weeks. Iloprost, a prostacyclin analogue, has undergone a clinical trial by the European group for the study of TAO. The drug was administered in intravenous infusions on a daily basis for 4 weeks and compared with a similar group of patients treated with aspirin. Approximately 85% of those being treated responded, and 63% had total relief of rest pain. This compares with 17% responders and 28% relief of rest pain in those treated with aspirin. Follow-up studies at 6 months showed that much of the gain had been maintained, but additional follow-up studies have not yet been accomplished. All patients had rest pain and angiographic proof of the diagnosis.[41] It is noteworthy that there were responders in both groups who continued to use tobacco. A specific agent has not yet been identified because the cause of TAO is not clear; this indirect approach on known pathogenetic mechanisms is encouraging.

When ischemic pain, ulceration, and gangrene cannot be controlled by the measures discussed within the first 2 to 3 weeks of hospitalization, early amputation should be considered as a positive tool for rehabilitation.

REFERENCES

1. von Winiwarter F: Ueber eine eigenthumliche Dorm von Endarteritis und Endophlebitis mit Gangran des Fusses, Arch Klin Chirur 23:202, 1879.
2. Buerger L: Thrombo-angiitis obliterans: a study of the vascular lesions leading to presenile spontaneous gangrene, Am J Med Sci 136:567, 1908.
3. Eastcott HHG: Buerger's disease. In Bergan JJ and Yao JST, eds: Evaluation and treatment of upper and lower extremity circulatory disorders, New York, 1984, Grune & Stratton.
4. Lie JT: II. Thromboangiitis obliterans (Buerger's disease) revisited. Pathol Annu 23:257, 1988.
5. Wessler S et al: A critical evaluation of thromboangiitis obliterans: the case against Buerger's disease. N Engl J Med 262:1149, 1960.
6. Wessler S: Buerger's disease revisited, Surg Clin North Am 49:703, 1969.
7. McPherson JR, Juergens JL, and Gifford RW: Thromboangiitis obliterans and arteriosclerosis obliterans: clinical and prognostic differences, Ann Intern Med 59:288, 1963.

8. McKusick VA and Harris WS: The Buerger syndrome in the Orient, Bull Johns Hopkins Hosp 109:241, 1961.
9. McKusick VA et al: Buerger's disease: a distinct clinical and pathologic entity, JAMA 181:5, 1962.
10. Szilagyi ED, DeRusseo FJ, and Elliot JP Jr: Thromboangiitis obliterans: clinico-angiographic correlations, Arch Surg 88:824, 1964.
11. Goodman RM et al: Buerger's disease in Israel, Am J Med 39:601, 1965.
12. Lie JT: Thromboangiitis obliterans (Buerger's disease) in women. Medicine (Baltimore) 66:65, 1987.
13. Mills JL, Taylor LM Jr, and Porter JM: Buerger's disease in the modern era, Am J Surg 154:123, 1987.
14. Hill GL and Smith AH: Buerger's disease in Indonesia: clinical course and prognostic factors, J Chronic Dis 27:205, 1974.
15. Kjeldsen K and Mozes M: Buerger's disease in Israel, Acta Chir Scand 135:495, 1969.
16. Rao AS, Rao GN, and Vasantha VC: Thromboangiitis obliterans: a clinicopathologic study, J Indian Med Assoc 66:98, 1976.
17. Shionoya S, Hiari M, and Kawai S: Pattern of arterial occlusion in Buerger's disease, Angiology 33:375, 1982.
18. Davis HA and King LD: A comparative study of thromboangiitis in white and negro patients, Surg Gynecol Obstet 85:597, 1947.
19. Lie JT: The rise and fall and resurgence of thromboangiitis obliterans (Buerger's disease), Acta Pathol Jpn 39:153, 1989.
20. Kimoto S: The history and present status of aortic surgery in Japan particularly for aortitis syndrome, J Cardiovasc Surg 20:101, 1979.
21. Case Records of the Massachusetts General Hospital (Case 16-1989), N Engl J Med 320:1068, 1989.
22. Lie JT: Thromboangiitis obliterans (Buerger's disease) and smokeless tobacco, Arthritis Rheum 31:812, 1988.
23. Schatz IJ, Fine G, and Eyler WR: Thromboangiitis obliterans, Br Heart J 28:84, 1966.
24. Numano F et al: HLA in Buerger's disease, Clin Immunogenet 3:195, 1986.
25. Adar R et al: Cellular sensitivity to collagen in thromboangiitis obliterans, N Engl J Med 308:1113, 1983.
26. Gulati SM et al: Immunologic studies in thromboangiitis obliterans (Buerger's disease), J Surg Res 27:287, 1979.
27. Ferguson GT and Starkebaum G: Thromboangiitis obliterans associated with idiopathic hypereosinophilia, Arch Intern Med 145:1726, 1985.
28. Lie JT and Michet CJ Jr: Thromboangiitis obliterans with eosinophilia (Buerger's disease) of the temporal arteries, Hum Pathol 19:598, 1928.
29. Shionoya S: Buerger's disease (thromboangiitis obliterans). In Rutherford RB, ed: Vascular Surgery, Philadelphia, 1989, WB Saunders Co.
30. Wolf EA, Sumner DS, and Strandness DE Jr: Disease of the mesenteric circulation in patients with thromboangiitis obliterans, Vasc Surg 6:218, 1973.
31. Ohta T and Shionoya S: Fate of the ischemic limb in Buerger's disease, Br J Surg 75:259, 1988.
32. Shionoya S et al: Involvement of the iliac artery in Buerger's disease: a pathogenesis and arterial reconstruction, J Cardiovasc Surg 19:69, 1978.
33. Hirai M and Shionoya S: Arterial obstruction of the upper limb in Buerger's disease: its incidence and primary lesion, Br J Surg 66:124, 1979.
34. Biller J et al: A case for cerebral thromboangiitis obliterans, Stroke 12:686, 1981.
35. Drake ME: Winiwarter-Buerger disease (thromboangiitis obliterans) with cerebral involvement, JAMA 246:1170, 1982.
36. Hagen B and Lohse S: Clinical and radiologic aspects of Buerger's disease, Cardiovasc Intervent Radiol 7:283, 1984.
37. Suzuki S et al: Buerger's disease (thromboangiitis obliterans): an analysis of the arteriograms of 119 cases, Clin Radiol 33:235, 1982.
38. Pairolero PC et al: Lower limb ischemia in young adults: prognostic implications, J Vasc Surg 1:459, 1984.
39. Shionoya S et al: Diagnosis, pathology, and treatment of Buerger's disease, Surgery 75:695, 1974.
40. Shionoya S et al: Vascular reconstruction in Buerger's disease, Br J Surg 63:841, 1976.
41. Fiessinger JN and Schafter M: Trial of iloprost versus aspirin for critical limb ischemia of thromboangiitis obliterans, Lancet 335:555, 1990.

Chapter 20

SYSTEMIC VASCULITIS

Leonard H. Calabrese
John D. Clough

While the vast majority of patients with ischemic vascular disease have conditions that are noninflammatory in nature, no textbook of peripheral vascular disease would be complete without a thorough consideration of inflammatory vascular disease as well. The term *vasculitis* is generally used interchangably with the term *necrotizing vasculitis*, which refers to a heterogeneous group of disorders all sharing in varying degrees the pathologic features of vascular inflammation and vascular necrosis. Generally speaking, while inflammation may accompany a wide variety of vascular syndromes, the term necrotizing vasculitis is not used to refer to the incidental inflammatory reactions that may occur in other vascular diseases or to vascular inflammation resulting from simple mechanical or chemical trauma. The vasculitides encompass those syndromes that are either suspected or proven to be immune mediated and frequently with distinctive clinical pictures.

The clinical approach to vascular inflammatory disease has been evolving since the first detailed description of polyarteritis nodosa over 100 years ago. This approach has been influenced by our improved understanding of these disorders, particularly in the following areas:

1. Immune mechanisms responsible for these diseases
2. Pathologic spectrum of the disorders
3. Identification of certain etiologic agents
4. Promising therapies for what used to be considered frequently fatal disorders

This chapter will review our current understanding of the pathogenesis, classification, and clinical spectrum of these disorders and will also provide a practical diagnostic and therapeutic approach.

PATHOGENESIS

Immunologic factors are believed to be central in the pathogenesis of most vasculitic syndromes, though no uniform mechanism is likely to be operative in all cases. Recent advances in our understanding of humoral and cellular immunology have provided a clearer view of the underlying immunologic events causing vascular inflammation.

The greatest body of experimental and clinical data support convincingly an important role for circulating immune complexes in the pathogenesis of necrotizing vasculitis. Supportive evidence for such a role includes:

1. Animal models of immune complex disease and vasculitis
2. Identification of immune complexes in tissues
3. Identification of immune complexes in the sera of patients with necrotizing vasculitis
4. Identification of discrete antigens responsible for certain immune complex disorders

The most important animal model supporting the role of circulating immune complexes in necrotizing vasculitis is that of serum sickness, elucidated by Dixon over 20 years ago.[1] In this model certain animals immunized with nontoxic protein antigens develop an immune complex disease characterized by widespread vascular inflammation. Furthermore, the appearance of these vascular lesions in the experimental animals coincides with detection of immune complexes in their serum and the onset of hypocomplementemia. A variety of factors appears critical in this and other models of immune complex disease including the genetic ability of the host to respond to the inciting antigen, the avidity of the humoral response, the size and charge of the resulting immune complexes, as well as the ability of the host to clear these immune complexes by the reticuloendothelial system. These factors are also likely to be important in human forms of immune complex disease.

In humans evidence of immune complexes in vasculitis include their identification in tissues and blood. Immunopathologic analysis of vascular lesions in a wide variety of disorders (but not all) have revealed varying degrees of immunoglobulin and complement deposition. Identification of these products appears highly dependent on the timing and the site of biopsy tissue.[2] Additionally, numerous studies over the past decade have identified soluble immune complexes in the sera of patients with a variety of forms of vasculitis, and some have correlated their presence and concentration to disease activity.[3] It should be noted that these circulating immune complexes have not been identified in all vasculitic syndromes and not even uniformly within a single syndrome. Furthermore, circulating immune complexes have been detected in a variety of other conditions not characterized by vascular inflammation. The reason for these variations is unclear but may relate to the technical limitations of detection methods or the fact that immune complexes may only represent a secondary phenomena in many of these conditions.

Lastly, in support of an immune complex theory of pathogenesis, there has been the identification of certain etiologic agents such as hepatitis B, which has been found in association with a number of vasculitic syndromes including polyarteritis nodosa, urticarial vasculitis, and small vessel vasculitis associated with cryoglobulinemia. The hepatitis B antigen has been identified in both circulating immune complexes and vascular tissues.[4] Unfortunately, the discovery of additional etiologic agents has been slow and difficult.

While it has generally been presumed that immune complexes mediate vascular damage as a result of their deposition in vascular tissues or their in situ formation within the vasculature, more recent studies suggest that alternative forms of immunologically mediated vascular injury, such as that found in systemic lupus erythematosus, may occur. In this condition, even in the absence of vascular immune complex deposition, complement activation with release of C3a and C5a can lead to mast cell degranulation and the chemotaxis of polymorphonuclear leukocytes, which then become adherent to vascular endothelium and thus lead to vascular injury. This mechanism is analogous to a localized Shwartzman reaction.[5]

Other vascular syndromes, such as giant cell arteritis, Takayasu's arteritis, Wegener's granulomatosis, and lymphomatoid granulomatosis, bear little resemblance to immune complex disease. In these conditions cell-mediated responses are much more likely to be important. Recent studies have revealed that vascular endothelium is an immunologically competent tissue and is capable of the dynamic expression of cell surface class II histocompatibility antigens. These Dr-like or Ia-like antigens are similar to those present on antigen-presenting cells, such as macrophages, and can be induced by cytokines, such as interferon gamma, and probably directly by agents such as viruses. These transformed endothelial cells may then be capable of serving as a focus for cell-mediated or granulomatous reactions.

CLASSIFICATION

Since the earliest descriptions of necrotizing vasculitis in the nineteenth century, numerous attempts have been made to classify these disorders and thus provide clinicians a useful basis for approaching them. The desire to separate these disorders on some rational basis has been limited by the simple fact that the vascular system has a limited range of responses to noxious stimuli and that the resultant end-organ damage caused by vasculitis is not unique but simply that of vascular ischemia, regardless of the underlying vascular pathology. As a result, attempts to separate these disorders by various criteria or variables has been problematic.

Early classification schemes were based on a variety of factors such as the pathologic picture including the presence or absence of fibrinoid necrosis, giant cells, granulomas, eosinophils or other morphologic features. Unfortunately, many diseases such as Henoch-Schönlein purpura, systemic lupus erythematosus, hepatitis B associated vasculitis, and vasculitis associated with malignancies frequently yielded the identical histopathologic picture. Other more specific morphologic findings such as those found in allergic granulomatous angiitis and Wegener's granulomatosis may at times be distinct but do not assist in the separation of the remainder of the vasculitic syndromes.

Classification schemes have also been proposed based on characteristic distribution of target organ damage, but these, too, have not been uniformly successful. For example, most cases of polyarteritis nodosa appear to spare the lungs, but the now recognized overlap syndrome or polyangiitis may demonstrate lung involvement as well as the other clinical and pathologic features identical to classic

Spectrum of vasculitides

Polyarteritis nodosa group of systemic necrotizing vasculitis

Classic polyarteritis nodosa
Allergic granulomatosis (Churg-Strauss syndrome)

Hypersensitivity vasculitis group

True hypersensitivity vasculitis
Henoch-Schönlein purpura
Mixed cryoglobulinemia with vasculitis
Vasculitis with connective tissue disease
Vasculitis associated with malignancies
Urticarial vasculitis (hypocomplementemic vasculitis)
Vasculitis associated with other primary disorders

Wegener's granulomatosis group

Classic Wegener's granulomatosis
Limited Wegener's granulomatosis
Lymphomatoid granulomatosis
Benign lymphocytic angiitis

Giant cell arteritis group

Temporal arteritis
Takayasu's arteritis

Miscellaneous vasculitides

polyarteritis nodosa.[6] Classification schemes based purely on laboratory findings such as the presence or absence of immune complexes or based on identification of etiologic agents have been less rewarding.

In 1978 Fauci, Haynes, and Katz at the National Institutes of Health proposed a classification scheme that has now been widely accepted[7] with several minor modifications (see box on p. 340). This classification scheme is based on an admixture of clinical, pathologic, immunologic and therapeutic variables that yield a scheme that is not only approachable in its clarity but clinically useful. Diseases are grouped into headings that frequently serve as points of differential diagnosis and thus assist diagnostic and therapeutic decision-making by clinicians. For example, the hypersensitivity group all share the features of near-universal involvement of the skin and the fact that these diseases tend to involve the smallest branches of the vascular system though etiologically they are diverse. When confronted with such a patient with a small-vessel cutaneous vasculitis, this group of disorders forms a logical starting place in the differential diagnostic process. The remainder of this chapter will discuss the clinical and pathologic features of the main forms of necrotizing vasculitis as well as provide a diagnostic and therapeutic approach to their management.

POLYARTERITIS NODOSA

Polyarteritis nodosa (PAN) was first described by the term periarteritis nodosa by Kussmaul and Maier over 100 years ago. The prefix "peri" referred to the fact that the disease could be identified grossly by the presence of visible nodules found along the course of muscular arteries. Over the ensuing years many similar cases were described by the same gross appearance. These cases all shared the clinical features of a general sparing of the tissues of the lungs and the microscopic features of tendencies of involving the bifurcations of the muscular arteries as well as sparing the smallest branches of the intrinsic vascular system. Unfortunately, because of a lack of appreciation of the broader spectrum of necrotizing vasculitis, the term polyarteritis, or periarteritis, was also applied to other vasculitic syndromes, both primary and secondary, not recognized to be nosologically distinct. Rheumatic fever, syphilis, Wegener's granulomatosis, hypersensitivity vasculitis, and others were all included under the same heading, thus leaving considerable confusion and controversy in subsequent attempts to classify these disorders. In the 1970s the recognition that the hepatitis B virus was etiologically responsible for some cases of PAN gave new insight into the pathogenesis of the disorder and new controversy about whether it represented a single entity or was multifactorial in its origin.

Clinical features

Though the incidence of PAN is not precisely known, it is generally considered to be clinically rare. There is a sex predilection for males over females of approximately 2-3:1. The disease has been recognized in virtually all age groups but appears to peak in the fourth and fifth decades.[8,9]

The most common signs of PAN relate to its devastating multisystem inflammatory nature. Constitutional symptoms including malaise and weakness accompanied by varying degrees of fever and weight loss are common. Other clinical findings depend on the distribution of target organ involvement, which may be highly variable. Musculoskeletal symptoms including inflammatory polyarthritis mimicking rheumatoid disease is not uncommon. Muscle involvement characterized by either muscle pain and/or proximal weakness mimicking polymyositis can also be observed. Symptoms relating to the presence of a sensory and/or motor neuropathy are also quite common. Abdominal pain, which may be mild to severe, may represent gastrointestinal involvement.[8,9]

Kidneys. The kidneys are involved in the vast majority of patients estimated to be between 75% and 85%. The renal manifestations of PAN are varied and may consist of glomerulonephritis, renal vasculitis or aneurysms of the renal vascular system. The clinical sequellae of this pathologic involvement can be asymptomatic or life-threatening. The glomerular disease of PAN is that of focal segmental necrotizing glomerulonephritis.[9] Immunoglobulin or complement deposition is variably present. Necrotizing vasculitis of the renal vessels is found in over half of autopsied cases but is rarely encountered in percutaneous renal biopsies. This finding is frequently misinterpreted by clinicians as a strong negative indicator of disease presence. Microaneurysms identified by arteriography when present in medium or small caliber vessels are considered almost pathognomonic of polyarteritis nodosa, but they may be observed in other types of vasculitis and rarely in nonvasculitic conditions such as atrial myxoma.[10]

The clinical sequellae of renal involvement include hypertension, which is seen in the majority of patients and, at times, can be clinically severe. The mechanism of this hypertension appears to be renin mediated from diffuse intrarenal vascular disease and may persist after the disease is adequately treated. Renal failure is seen in a varying number of patients and may be responsible for death in up to 50% of patients with PAN.[9]

Neurologic system. The central nervous system is involved in as many as 25% of patients with PAN when it is assessed by clinical findings or autopsy results. This may be manifested by strokes, altered mental status, cognitive impairment, seizures, or hemorrhage.[9]

Peripheral neurologic lesions are seen in nearly half the patients with PAN. Several patterns of clinical involvement of the peripheral nerves have been reported including mononeuritis multiplex (the most characteristic), symmetric sensory involvement (glove and stocking neuropathy) and a lesion known as dense mononeuritis multiplex resulting from the infarction of multiple peripheral nerves in one extremity leading to profound weakness of the affected limb.[11] Isolated mononeuropathies may be observed as well. The new appearance of mononeuritis multiplex in the absence of diabetes or trauma should be considered presumptive evidence of necrotizing vasculitis until proven otherwise.

Musculoskeletal system. PAN may appear as a symmetric polyarthritis mimicking rheumatoid arthritis. The differential diagnosis is further complicated by the fact that many patients with PAN may have elevated sedimentation rates and rheumatoid factors. There is generally a discordance between the amount of systemic disease and the amount of arthritis in PAN as opposed to rheumatoid. In PAN there is often prominent constitutional symptoms from the outset in the presence of arthritis that is nonerosive. In rheumatoid arthritis, on the other hand, the arthritis is usually the earliest manifestation of the disease and significant constitutional symptoms usually arise further along in the clinical course.

Muscle involvement may be manifested by simple myalgias or a proximal myopathy mimicking polymyositis. Muscle enzymes may be slightly elevated and electromyographic examination may be consistent with a patchy inflammatory myopathy. Rarely does PAN cause dramatic proximal muscle weakness, but because of clinical similarities, it is important to differentiate these conditions because of differences in therapy and prognosis.

Gastrointestinal system. Gastrointestinal involvement is present in nearly half the patients with PAN. The clinical manifestations relate to underlying ischemia, which may involve the mucosa, submucosa, or the entire thickness of the bowel. Other organs within the gastrointestinal system may be involved including the liver and pancreas. Occasionally, in patients with PAN with gastrointestinal involvement there will be the typical symptoms of "intestinal angina." This symptom complex consists of postprandial abdominal pain and cramping. The most severe complication of gastrointestinal involvement by PAN is visceral perforation. This is a catastrophic complication because it generally occurs when the underlying disease is uncontrolled and in need of immunosuppressive therapy, and the resultant complication is a septic process in need of strengthened host defenses.

Virtually every part of the gastrointestinal tract can be involved by PAN and the diagnosis has occasionally been made by biopsy of gastric polyps, cholecystectomy, and appendectomy. Of important clinical note is the syndrome of isolated gallbladder or appendiceal involvement by PAN. In this clinical situation the histopathology of the resected gallbladder or appendix is typical of PAN with fibrinoid necrosis of medium-sized muscular arteries, but there is no evidence of systemic disease, and long-term follow-up care of several of these patients has revealed a benign prognosis.

Cardiac involvement. Cardiac involvement occurs in up to 80% of patients with PAN and is second only to renal disease as a cause of death.[9] Cardiac involvement is generally difficult to detect and the most common expression of its presence is congestive heart failure. All anatomic areas of the heart including the endocardium, myocardium, and pericardium may be involved by the vasculitic process. Conduction abnormalities have been observed and are clinically rare.

Miscellaneous findings. Skin involvement in PAN is relatively infrequent when compared to other categories of systemic vasculitis (e.g., hypersensitivity vasculitis). The most common cutaneous manifestations are nonspecific vascular rashes, such as palpable purpura, nonblanching maculopapular lesions or urticaria. This may cause some confusion with diseases within the hypersensitivity vasculitis group, but the presence of extensive involvement of larger caliber vessels should help clarify the situation. The most characteristic cutaneous finding is the subcutaneous inflammatory nodule, which may occur in as many as 10% or 15% of patients. The syndrome of subcutaneous PAN is characterised by skin lesions that are highly inflammatory and painful and pathologically display necrotizing vasculitis of muscular vessels within the subcutaneous tissue but are unassociated with systemic disease.[12]

Ocular involvement can be seen in 10% to 15% of cases. This may be manifested by hemorrhages, conjunctivitis, iritis, or also by involvement of the corroid leading to retinal detachment.

Testicular involvement has been mentioned as a common clinical finding and a source of diagnostic material. Orchitis occurs in approximately 10% to 15% of male patients and, when present, may be useful as a source for pathologic documentation.

Involvement of the lungs is distinctly uncommon in classic PAN and usually suggests another form of angiitis such as Wegener's granulomatosis. The involvement of the lungs in the overlap syndrome or polyangiitis representing an admixture of the clinical findings of several different vasculitic syndromes should be kept in mind.[6] While the pulmonary circulation is generally spared, the bronchial circulation may be affected in classic PAN and secondary pulmonary disease such as infection complicating immunosuppressive therapy may be seen.

Laboratory

There is no specific laboratory test for PAN and the most sensitive laboratory findings in this disease are elevation of the erythrocyte sedimentation rate, white blood cell count, and the presence of anemia.[9] The absence of all of these findings in an individual suspected of having PAN would be strong evidence of its absence. The presence of elevated circulating immune complexes and hypocomplementemia are helpful when present but are absent in the majority of patients. Rheumatoid factor may be found in a sizable number of patients with PAN. The remainder of the laboratory studies reflect the presence or absence of various target organ damage including kidneys, central nervous system, gastrointestinal, etc.

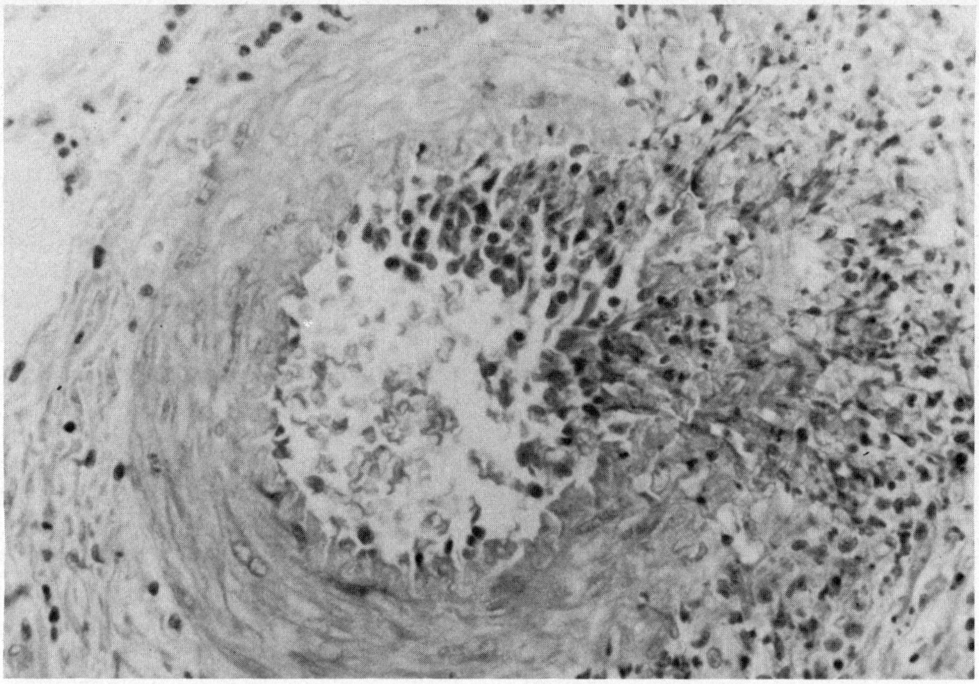

Fig. 20-1. Vessel biopsy from a patient with PAN demonstrating vascular wall necrosis and acute inflammation.

Pathophysiology

In the 1970s it was reported that hepatitis B surface antigen could be found in the majority of patients with PAN. This finding prompted an aggressive search for other etiologic agents that could explain this disease. Unfortunately, current estimates suggest that only about 15% of patients with PAN have evidence of hepatitis B infection with the remaining patients representing an admixture of idiopathic disease and those associated with a variety of other findings. Other underlying diseases and problems that have been associated with the presence of a PAN-like syndrome include hairy cell leukemia, endocarditis, connective tissue disease, and drug abuse.[9]

Diagnosis

The diagnosis of PAN can be highly problematic but must first start with a high suspicion of its presence. Fever of unknown origin, unexplained multisystem disease, mononeuritis multiplex, unexplained inflammatory disease of muscle or joints may all be the initial manifestations of PAN. There are no laboratory tests that can diagnose the presence of this condition, though, as stated previously, a normal hemoglobin, white count, and sedimentation rate strongly suggest its absence. The presence of numerous symptoms or signs consistent with PAN in conjunction with elevated circulating immune complexes and hypocomplementemia would strongly support its presence.

The diagnosis of the condition must be based on either tissue evidence of necrotizing vasculitis or angiographic evidence of multiple microaneurysms. The pathologic lesion is characterized by a predilection for medium-sized muscular arteries with a tendency to involve the bifurcations (Fig. 20-1). There is significant debate as to which is the first test to choose when trying to diagnose this condition, but several generalizations can be made. First in the absence of any obvious target organ involvement, such as renal, gastrointestinal, or neurologic, panabdominal arteriography is the diagnostic mode of choice. Approximately 70% to 80% of patients with PAN will have abnormal abdominal arteriograms with three fourths of these patients demonstrating classic multiple microaneurysms (Fig. 20-2).[10] In the presence of documented peripheral neurologic disease by either clinical exam or EMG, a sural nerve biopsy has extremely high yield.[13] Blind biopsies of the muscle, kidney, and testicle in the absence of clinical signs or symptoms of their involvement is rarely productive. Skin biospy alone is inadequate evidence of the presence of PAN. Percutaneous renal biopsies may be employed with the recognition that they will rarely demonstrate extraglomerular vasculitis, but rather a segmental necrotizing glomerulonephritis.

Treatment

Untreated, the 5-year survival rate for PAN is 10% to 15%. With the use of corticosteroids the 5-year survival rate was noted to improve to nearly 50%. In recent years, the use of combination therapy with cyclophosphamide and high-dose steroids has been reported to increase the 5-year

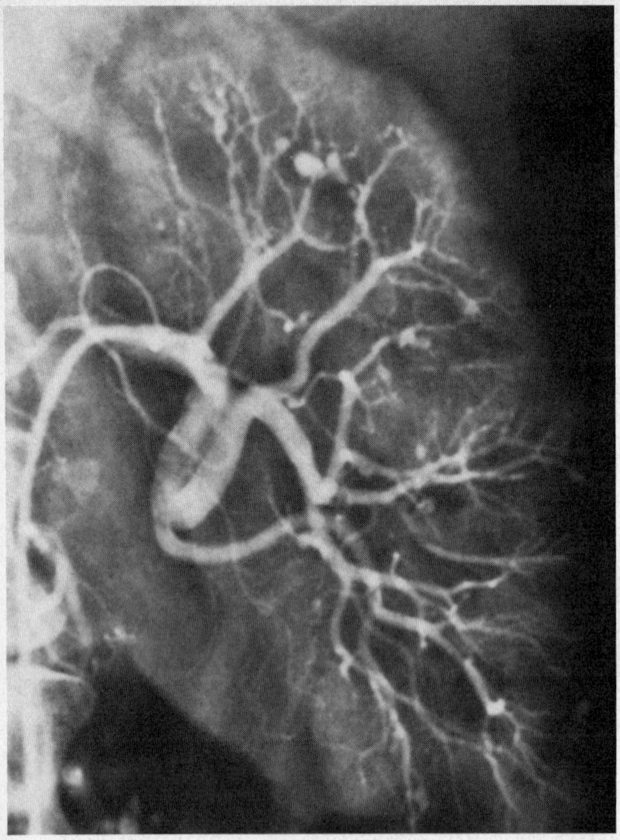

Fig. 20-2. Renal arteriogram demonstrating multiple microaneurysms.

survival rate to 80% or more.[14] Treatment of this condition is generally instituted with doses of cyclophosphamide in a range of 1 to 2 mg/kg/day and prednisone 1 mg/kg/day. Treatment is prolonged, and it may require several years to allow for total control of the disease.

ALLERGIC GRANULOMATOUS ANGIITIS AND ALLERGIC GRANULOMATOSIS (CHURG-STRAUSS SYNDROME)

In 1951 Churg and Strauss described 13 cases of systemic necrotizing vasculitis that had a variety of distinguishing features from classic PAN.[15] These patients had a predominance of involvement of the pulmonary circulation, a frequent history of adult onset asthma, and striking peripheral eosinophilia. It also bore a variety of similarities to classic PAN, including the predominance of medium-sized vessel involvement and, with the exception of the lungs, a similar array of target organ involvement.[16]

The syndrome is clinically rare and in the largest series of patients reported from the Mayo Clinic there was a predominance of males over females by a 2:1 ratio. The mean age is approximately 47 years but has been reported in both children and the elderly.[17]

The lungs are nearly always involved with x-ray changes being noted in over 90% of patients. Skin involvement is also present in approximately two thirds of patients manifested by palpable purpura or inflammatory nodules. Peripheral neurologic involvement as seen in classic PAN is also frequently observed with mononeuritis multiplex being the most common complication. Involvement of the gastrointestinal, cardiac, and renal systems are also not infrequent.[16,17]

There is a striking history of asthma in the vast majority of patients with the symptoms often antedating the vasculitis by approximately 2 years. We have noticed that in several patients with the disorder, the asthma may actually become less severe or go into a clinical remission at the time of the onset of the vasculitis.

The laboratory hallmark of this disorder is a striking degree of peripheral eosinophilia, generally in excess of 1500 cells/mm^3. Elevation of IgE has also been described. The pathology of the disorder is a necrotizing vasculitis involving medium- and small-sized muscular arteries. In distinction to PAN, eosinophils and granulomata are seen in and around the vascular infiltrates.

The prognosis of this disorder is not as well documented as that of classic PAN, though some observers have considered it similar. The initial treatment of the disorder is generally with high-dose corticosteroids. For those failing to respond to corticosteroids alone or those with unacceptable toxicities from these agents, the use of additional immunosuppressive drugs such as cyclophosphamide has been reported to be successful.[14]

Polyangiitis overlap syndrome

In addition to classic PAN and allergic granulomatosis, the polyangiitis, or overlap syndrome, has been included under the heading of systemic necrotizing vasculitis. The legitimization of this disorder as a distinct nosologic entity within the necrotizing vasculitides is supported by the recognition that there are patients with both classic PAN and Churg-Strauss syndrome bearing features of each condition but not precisely fitting the clinical descriptions of either.[6,7]

In addition to bearing features of each of these conditions, patients with polyangiitis may demonstrate clinical features of other vasculitic syndromes such as hypersensitivity vasculitis or giant cell arteritis.[6,7]

Examples of patients with polyangiitis may be individuals with classic PAN without lung involvement but with a high degree of peripheral eosinophilia. Alternatively, patients with a classic picture of Churg-Strauss syndrome with multiple microaneurysms on abdominal angiography may also fit this description. In a series of 10 patients with this disorder reported from the National Institutes of Health, cutaneous disease was the most common feature frequently and mistakenly diagnosed as a disorder from the hypersensitivity vasculitis group.[6] While many of these patients displayed features of either PAN or Churg-Strauss syndrome, others had features of disorders such as temporal arteritis, Takayasu's arteritis, Henoch-Schönlein purpura or Wegener's granulomatosis.

The prognosis of this disorder is unclear at the present time. Patients fitting this description should be approached diagnostically and therapeutically in a similar fashion to PAN or Churg-Strauss. Overall, in the National Institutes of Health experience, the mean duration of remission was 45.9 months with a mean follow-up period of 58.4 months. All patients were treated with a combination of cyclophosphamide and corticosteroids.[6]

THE HYPERSENSITIVITY VASCULITIS GROUP

The concept of vasculitis secondary to allergic or hypersensitivity mechanisms was first proposed by Zeek, Smith, and Weeter in 1948.[18] Support for this rationale included a series of experimental and clinical observations distinguishing this disorder from other recognized vasculitic conditions. These distinguishing features included the frequent precipitation by a drug or serum, prominent involvement of the skin and pathologically the tendency to involve the small vessels and display leukocytoclasis (nuclear fragmentation).

Despite the distinguishing features of hypersensitivity vasculitis, it has subsequently been recognized that many patients with these clinical and pathologic findings have no history of exposure to drugs or toxins. Additionally, a wide variety of disorders with mechanisms other than hypersensitivity have also been noted to have the same clinical and pathologic picture. These conditions include certain cases of vasculitis secondary to connective tissue disease (e.g., rheumatoid arthritis, Sjögren's syndrome, and systemic lupus erythematosus), Henoch-Schönlein purpura, certain malignancies, the presence of mixed cryoglobulins in the serum and even occasional patients with systemic necrotizing vasculitis. At present the term hypersensitivity vasculitis group (HVG) refers to a heterogeneous group of disorders all displaying the clinical and pathologic features previously referred to. The presence of these findings (i.e., vasculitic rash, which upon biopsy displays a small vessel vasculitis with leukocytoclasia) should serve as a clinical starting point for a differential diagnosis of those disorders referred to in the classification scheme under this heading (see the box on the right).

Pathogenesis

The causes of the disorders within the hypersensitivity vasculitis group are diverse, but there is strong evidence that they all share a similar mechanism of vascular inflammatory disease; namely, that mediated by immune complexes. Evidence supporting an immune complex pathogenesis includes the experimental model of serum sickness elucidated by Dixon over 20 years ago.[1] In this model rabbits immunized with a nontoxic protein antigen develop specific antibodies to the antigen resulting in soluble circulating immune complexes. At the point in time where the concentration of these soluble circulating immune complexes is maximal, evidence of complement activation and the coincidental production of a variety of target organ manifestations including carditis, glomerulonephritis, arthritis, and vasculitis is observed. In humans with small vessel vasculitis caused by hypersensitivity to proteins or drugs, there has been identification of soluble circulating immune complexes both in the peripheral blood and in the tissues. While these findings are not universal, this is understandable since detection of circulating immune complexes is greatly influenced by detection techniques as well as the timing and nature of the biopsy sample.[19]

Specific diseases

Diseases that frequently share the cardinal features of the hypersensitivity vasculitis group (cutaneous involvement, small vessel vasculitis, and leukocytoclasis) are listed below:

1. True hypersensitivity vasculitis. This term should be limited to those conditions strongly linked to exposure to an exogenous antigen (e.g., drug, serum, toxin, infection).
2. Henoch-Schönlein purpura.
3. Cryoglobulinemia of essential origin.
4. Vasculitis associated with certain connective tissue disease (e.g., rheumatoid arthritis, systemic lupus erythematosus, Sjögren's syndrome).
5. Vasculitis associated with malignancies.
6. Urticarial vasculitis (hypocomplementemic vasculitis).
7. Vasculitis associated with systemic diseases. These diseases include, but are not limited to, inflammatory bowel disease, primary biliary cirrhosis, Behçet's syndrome, Goodpasture's syndrome, and retroperitoneal fibrosis.

True hypersensitivity vasculitis. True hypersensitivity vasculitis, which is caused by exposure to an exogenous antigen, is the most common syndrome within the hypersensitivity vasculitis group. Incriminate antigens that have been associated with this syndrome are listed in the accompanying box. The typical case of hypersensitivity vasculitis

Antigenic exposures causing hypersensitivity vasculitis

I. Drugs	*II. Infections*	*III. Chemicals*
Penicillin	Streptococcus	Insecticides
Sulfa	Staphylococcus	Herbacides
Iodides	Subacute bacterial endocarditis	
Griseofulvin	Meningococcus	*IV. Immunizations*
Quinidine	Leprosy	Influenza
Tetracycline	Malaria	Allergy
Dilantin	Tuberculosis	
	HIV	
Phenylbutazone	Hepatitis B	*V. Miscellaneous*
Allopurinol	Cytomegalovirus	Foreign protein
ASA phenacetin	Epstein-Barr virus	Insect bites
Phenothiazine	Others	Others

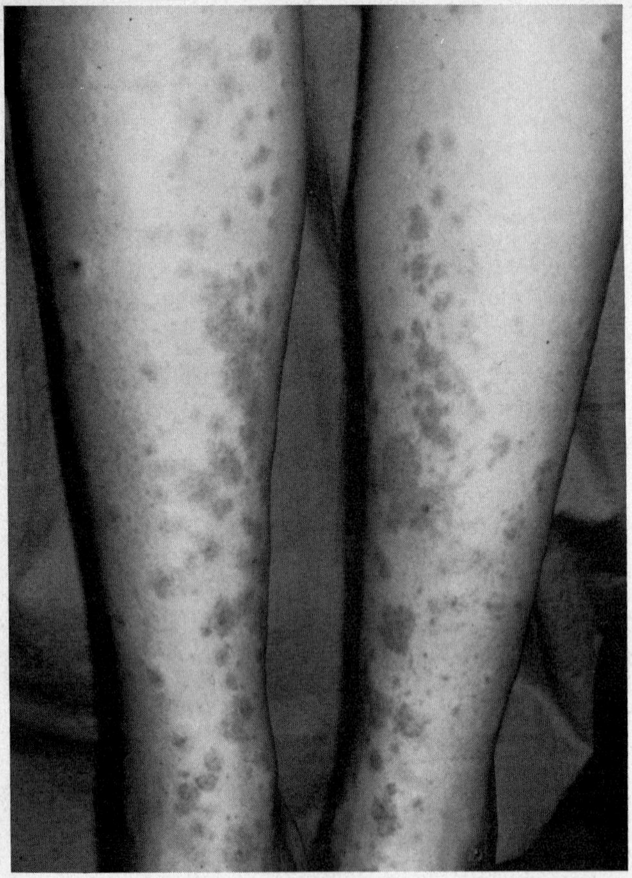

Fig. 20-3. Typical lesions of palpable purpura and maculopapular rash in a patient with hypersensitivity vasculitis.

occurs 7 to 10 days following the initial exposure to incriminate antigen. The disease is frequently heralded by the development of the characteristic rash. The most common rash is palpable purpura (Fig. 20-3), though a variety of other cutaneous findings such as ulcers, nodules, bullae or urticaria may be seen. All the lesions tend to be at one anatomic stage and, when biopsied, display typical histopathologic features. These include the presence of polymorphonuclear leukocytes and associated leukocytoclasis, but at times the infiltrates may be predominantly mononuclear in nature (Fig. 20-4). Immunofluorescent studies often demonstrate the deposition of complement and immunoglobulins in vessel walls. The laboratory may reveal evidence of soluble immune complexes detected by a variety of techniques as well as evidence of complement activation.[20] These laboratory findings, however, are neither universal nor necessary for the diagnosis.

The clinical course of patients with hypersensitivity vasculitis is variable, but is is usually self-limited. Varying degrees of constitutional symptoms including fever, malaise, and weight loss may be observed. Occasionally, more significant target organ involvement may be present including the muscle, joint, renal, pulmonary, and central nervous systems. At times the disorder may become chronic or recurrent. The treatment of true hypersensitivity vasculitis should focus primarily on removal of the inciting antigen. If the antigen is a drug, it should be discontinued, and if there is an incriminate infection, it should be treated. Mild cases may require no treatment at all while more advanced cases may require the use of a variety of modalities including

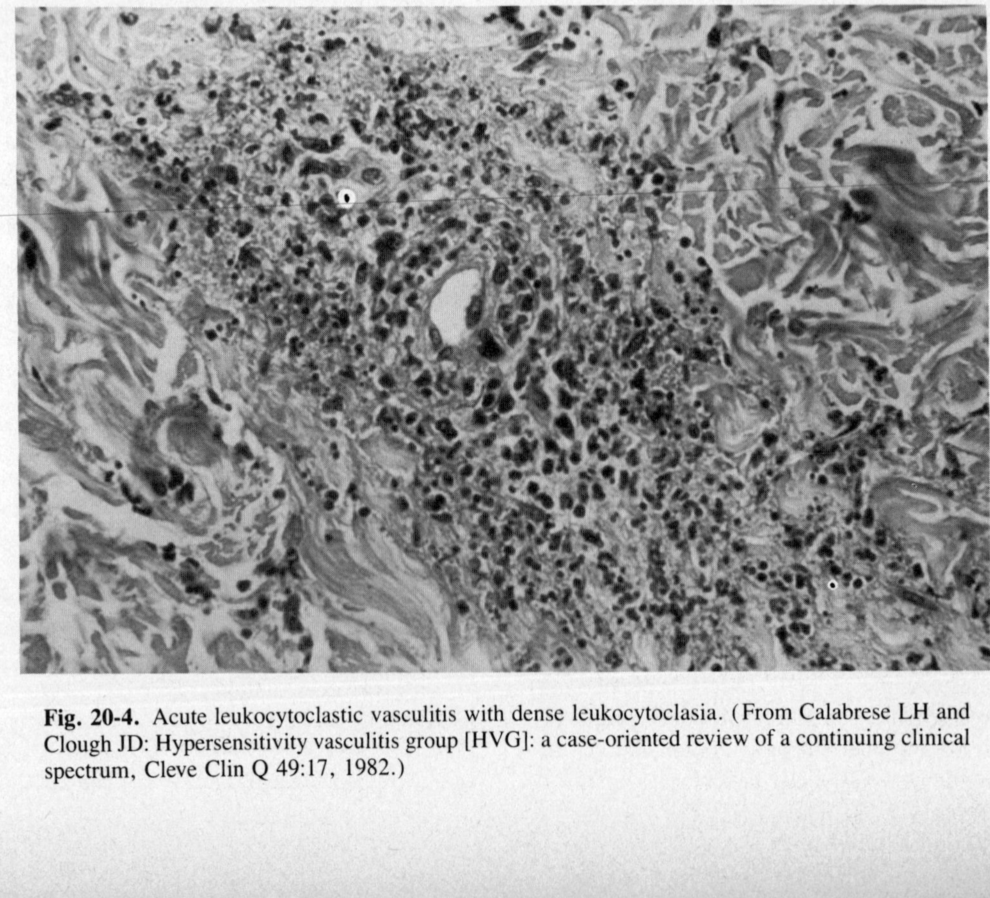

Fig. 20-4. Acute leukocytoclastic vasculitis with dense leukocytoclasia. (From Calabrese LH and Clough JD: Hypersensitivity vasculitis group [HVG]: a case-oriented review of a continuing clinical spectrum, Cleve Clin Q 49:17, 1982.)

antihistamines, colchicine, corticosteroids, and for severe cases, cytotoxic drugs.[20] In fulminant hypersensitivity vasculitis caused by an exogenous antigen, plasmapheresis has been occasionally reported to be of dramatic benefit, though there are no controlled studies of this or any other modality in this disorder.[21]

Henoch-Schönlein purpura. Henoch-Schönlein purpura is a syndrome characterized by the presence of palpable purpura and varying degrees of gastrointestinal ischemia and glomerulonephritis. Other symptoms such as arthritis, fever, and constitutional symptoms are not uncommon. Topically, the lesions of Henoch-Schönlein purpura may be identical to true hypersensitivity vasculitis and the conditions may be confused since Henoch-Schönlein purpura is frequently reported following an upper respiratory infection, and children are often given an antibiotic incriminated in hypersensitivity vasculitis for their condition.[19] Useful points of differentiation include the facts that Henoch-Schönlein purpura occurs most often in the spring, displays a high frequency of gastrointestinal involvement including colicky abdominal pain and gastrointestinal bleeding, and occurs in individuals under 18 years of age, though adults may occasionally be affected.[22] Immunopathologically, Henoch-Schönlein purpura is distinguished by the presence of IgA containing circulating immune complexes and the deposition of IgA containing immune complexes within the vasculitic tissues.[23] An IgA associated glomerulonephritis is identified in about half the patients, and while generally mild and self-limiting, may infrequently be severe and persistent. The treatment of Henoch-Schönlein purpura depends upon the severity of the syndrome with mild disease requiring essentially no therapy while life-threatening visceral disease may require high-dose corticosteroids and possibly the addition of cytotoxic drugs.

Cryoglobulinemia of essential origin. Occasionally, patients with the clinical and pathologic features of the hypersensitivity vasculitis group may have high concentrations of cryoprecipitable proteins in their blood without an identifiable reason for their presence such as chronic infection or connective tissue disease. Such patients are said to have essential cryoglobulinemia. Recent studies have identified that many patients with circulating immune complexes caused by identifiable factors such as subacute bacterial endocarditis, hepatitis B, or connective tissue disease have cryoglobulins in their blood that merely represent soluble immune complexes. Thus the term essential should be reserved for those patients without identifiable causes for the presence of immune complexes.[24] While topically the cutaneous involvement of cryoglobulinemia of essential origin does not differ from other members of the hypersensitivity vasculitis group, the clinical course is generally chronic with 50% of the patients developing significant renal disease, which is a major cause of morbidity and mortality in this disorder.[19,20,24] Varying degrees of other target organ involvement including the muscle, joint, and peripheral nervous system may be present.

While the overall prognosis for patients with this disorder is good, it depends upon the degree of visceral target organ involvement, in particular the kidneys. In our experience, in patients with mild disease little treatment is needed other than nonsteroidal antiinflammatory agents, antihistamines, and low-dose corticosteroids. Colchicine has been reported to be effective, though in our experience it is of little value. Plasmapheresis may be beneficial for patients with serious disease, but this procedure is costly and must be continued on a long-term basis. Patients with significant renal disease may require combinations of high doses of corticosteroids and immunosuppressive therapy for control of their disease.

Vasculitis associated with connective tissue disease. Small vessel vasculitis may be observed in association with a variety of connective tissue diseases.[19] Though this presentation is not the only manifestation of vasculitis in this disorder, it is probably the most frequent. Patients with rheumatoid arthritis, systemic lupus erythematosus and Sjögren's syndrome may occasionally display cutaneous vasculitic involvement, including palpable purpura. These disorders, however, may also be associated with larger vessel disease reminiscent of systemic necrotizing vasculitis. The identification of these disorders as a cause for hypersensitivity vasculitis is generally readily apparent on clinical and serologic grounds. The treatment for hypersensitivity vasculitis in patients with connective tissue disease is based on control of the underlying connective tissue disease.

Hypersensitivity vasculitis associated with malignancy. Occasionally vasculitis may be a manifestation of an underlying malignancy. Those conditions most frequently associated with vasculitis include lymphoproliferative or myeloproliferative disorders.[19,25] In the majority of cases the vasculitis antedates the malignancy by many months, but occasionally the vasculitis may appear after the malignancy. The most common manifestations include palpable purpura, petechial lesions, maculopapular rashes, and ulcers. Though systematic investigations for the deposition of immunoglobulin and complement have been largely unrevealing, we have identified the presence of a paraprotein within the vascular lesions in a patient with chronic lymphocytic leukemia. The symptoms of vasculitis associated with malignancy are generally poorly responsive to therapy but may remit with the underlying therapy of the condition.

Urticarial vasculitis. While the most classic cutaneous manifestation of small vessel vasculitis is palpable purpura, a variety of other cutaneous findings may occasionally be encountered. A syndrome predominantly associated with urticaria, which upon biopsy reveals leukocytoclastic vasculitis, has been named urticarial vasculitis or hypocomplementemic vasculitis.[26,27] While hypocomplementemia is a prominent part of this disorder, it should be noted that complement levels may be normal in some cases of urticarial vasculitis and that hypocomplementemia may readily be observed in cutaneous vasculitis without urticaria. Patients with this syndrome clinically have attacks of urticaria that frequently last for greater than 24 hours at a time. Consti-

Miscellaneous conditions associated with cutaneous vasculitis mimicking hypersensitivity vasculitis

Celiac disease
Inflammatory bowel disease
Primary biliary cirrhosis
Behçet's syndrome
Goodpasture's syndrome
Retroperitoneal fibrosis
Transplant vasculitis

tutional symptoms including arthralgias and low-grade fever are prominent features. Angioneurotic edema of the face and bowel may occasionally be encountered. Renal disease is not generally observed though occasionally cases of glomerulonephritis are reported. A unique syndrome of urticarial vasculitis, membranoproliferative glomerulonephritis and pseudotumor cerebri has been reported in six patients and is not completely understood.[28] Many patients with urticarial vasculitis have many features of systemic lupus erythematosus but do not satisfy the American College of Rheumatology criteria for the diagnosis.[29]

Laboratory studies in patients with this disease frequently reveal evidence of hypocomplementemia with marked depressions of C1 through C3. It should be noted that urticaria may also be observed in a variety of other immune complex conditions including serum sickness, Henoch-Schönlein purpura, connective tissue disease, and hepatitis B. Therefore the presence of urticaria and immune complexes is not specific for this disease but depends on a careful exclusion of a variety of other conditions and appropriate documentation by biopsy. The treatment of this disorder is generally accomplished by a combination of medications including antihistamines, colchicine and corticosteroids.

Hypersensitivity vasculitis associated with systemic diseases. As previously mentioned the presence of a cutaneous vasculitic condition associated with leukocytoclasis should aid the clinician in formulating a differential diagnosis that centers around the classification scheme (see the box on p. 345). While the vast majority of these cases may be caused by conditions such as hypersensitivity to drugs, infections, toxins, Henoch-Schönlein purpura, or connective tissue disease, it must be noted that there are a variety of systemic diseases that have been reported in association with small vessel vasculitis similar to that reported in these conditions.[19,30,31] The box above contains a partial list of those disorders that must be searched for when confronted with a patient with a small vessel vasculitic condition with prominent skin involvement.

WEGENER'S GRANULOMATOSIS

Wegener's granulomatosis (WG) is a granulomatous inflammatory disease of unknown cause. It affects small- and medium-sized blood vessels throughout the body with major manifestations in the upper and lower respiratory tract and the kidneys. It was definitively described in 1939[32] and was more recently subdivided into "classical" and "limited" forms, the difference being absence of renal manifestations in the latter form.[33] Until recognition that alkylating agents, especially cyclophosphamide, could be used to control the disease in most patients, WG was always fatal. Although the cause remains unknown, recent developments in both diagnosis and therapy of WG offer the clinician powerful tools for early recognition and management of this disease.

Clinical aspects

Although WG can begin at any age, onset most commonly occurs in the 40s. Males are affected slightly more frequently than females (3:2). No racial or geographic predilections have been reported, and, although there is a single report of two sisters with WG,[34] no other evidence of a genetic pattern has emerged. The leading candidates for cause are infection and autoimmunity, but there is little hard evidence for any specific agent or pathogenic mechanism.

In classic WG all three target areas (upper airways, lungs, kidneys) are typically involved at onset or soon thereafter; however, cases have been reported in which delays of up to several years elapsed between the onset of disease and involvement of all three areas. On the other hand, WG may affect other organ systems, making diagnosis more difficult. There have been reports of patients with breast mass, prostatic nodule, gastrointestinal hemorrhage or diarrhea, palpable purpura, cranial nerve palsies, scleritis, unilateral parotid enlargement, or erosive arthritis. Since an infectious process is often suspected initially, the correct diagnosis is often delayed, especially when the symptoms are unusual.

Upper airway involvement is often destructive; the nasal mucosa is obscured by purulent crusts, and perforation of the nasal septum may soon follow, with collapse of the nose resulting in the typical "saddle-nose" deformity (Fig. 20-5). Nasal drainage is often bloody or tarry in appearance. Chronic sinusitis is frequent and often painful. Even when the sinuses are asymptomatic, x-ray studies often reveal opacification of the sinuses. The middle ear may be involved, presenting as otitis media. Damage to the inner ear may result in sensorineural hearing loss and/or vertigo; in a recent study this was found to be caused by vasculitis of the vessels of the endolymphatic sac, with no abnormalities of the other vessels of the inner ear.[35] Oral involvement is uncommon, most frequently manifested by hypertrophic gingivitis with loosening of the teeth. Tracheal and laryngeal stenosis have also been reported. Upper airway involvement must be differentiated from malignancy or idiopathic midline destructive disease (IMDD). Biopsy is the usual method for this, although less invasive procedures, such as MRI, may be helpful.

Pulmonary involvement usually produces symptoms suggestive of pneumonia, including fever, cough, and often chest pain. The cough may be productive, but sputum cul-

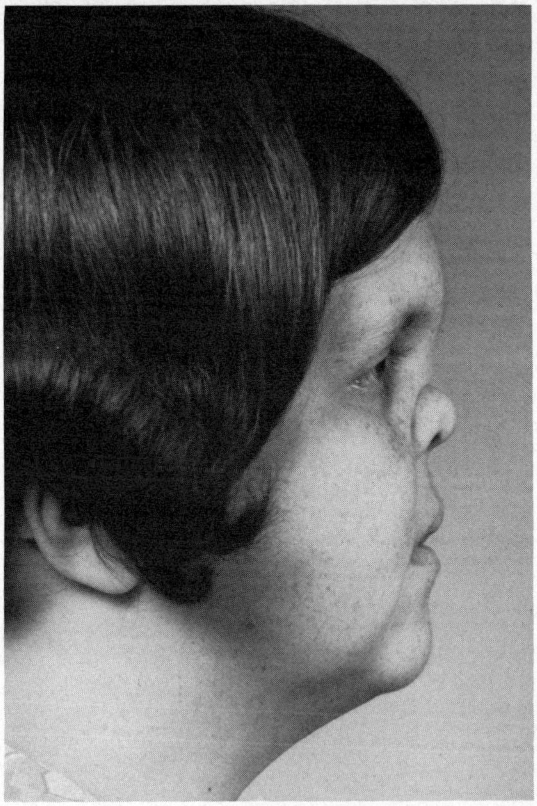

Fig. 20-5. Young woman with Wegener's granulomatosis, showing the typical "saddle-nose" deformity, seen in patients with extensive destruction of nasal cartilage and loss of the nasal septum. (From Orlowski JP, Clough JD, and Dyment PG: Wegener's granulomatosis in the pediatric age group, Pediatrics 61:83, 1978.)

tures grow normal flora. Chest x-ray studies typically show nodules or infiltrates, which are often bilateral, with a tendency to cavitate. Occasionally WG appears as diffuse alveolar hemorrhage with massive hemoptysis.[36] In the presence of renal involvement, this clinical picture resembles Goodpasture's syndrome, and antibodies against glomerular basement membrane have been rarely reported in this setting. A less dramatic presentation is that of a pleural mass. Confirmation of the diagnosis of WG requires biopsy, and the lung is the site most likely to yield definitive histopathology in WG. Tissue may be obtained either by thoracotomy or bronchoscopy, although the former method is more likely to be successful.

Renal disease is the third component of the classic triad.[33] If it is absent, the condition is referred to as limited WG. Symptoms and signs of renal involvement may be those of rapidly progressive glomerulonephritis. They include malaise, edema, proteinuria, active urinary sediment, and rising serum creatinine. Even in the face of severe renal disease, biopsy of the kidney may not produce diagnostically specific findings, and the kidney is not the ideal biopsy site if WG is suspected.

Arthritis is common, but it is usually mild. Patients often complain of arthralgias when the disease is active. Occasionally, erosive arthritis has been described. Joint pain, especially in the hips, may also result from avascular necrosis of bone in patients treated with corticosteroids; it is important to distinguish this from arthritis because of therapeutic implications.

Skin lesions are occasionally present and are sometimes the initial manifestation. Several types of lesions have been described, ranging from palpable purpura, typical of leukocytoclastic angiitis, to pyoderma-like skin ulcerations resembling Weber-Christian panniculitis. Skin biopsy is unlikely to yield a definitive diagnosis.

Ocular manifestations are common.[37] Most ominous is the appearance of an orbital mass with the potential to displace and destroy the eyeball. This usually presents as painful unilateral or asymmetrically bilateral proptosis with impaired vision on the involved side. Computed tomography of the orbits is helpful in detecting and monitoring this condition. Most frequently seen are episcleritis and scleritis. Uveitis can also occur. Lacrimal gland involvement has been described as well.

The nervous system may be affected either centrally or peripherally.[38] Both cerebral infarction and diffuse cerebritis have been described. Multiple cranial nerve palsies have also been observed.

Gastrointestinal manifestations are less common in WG than in other forms of necrotizing arteritis, but they may be severe and life-threatening when they occur. Abdominal pain is the most frequent symptom of intestinal vasculitis, followed by diarrhea and hemorrhage. Abnormal liver function tests have also been described.[39] Colonic lesions may be identified and biopsied endoscopically.

Cardiac involvement may occur in the form of myocardial infarction, cardiomyopathy, conduction system abnormalities, or valvulitis. Although significant cardiac symptoms are uncommon, like gastrointestinal WG, they may be quite severe.[38]

Finally, WG may appear as a mass almost anywhere. There have been several reports of breast masses, identified either at examination or mammography, found to be WG by biopsy. WG also appears occasionally as a prostatic lesion, sometimes causing gross hematuria. Splenic involvement has also been described.

The histopathologic hallmarks of WG are granuloma formation and necrotizing vasculitis of small- and medium-sized arteries. This picture is seen in its most complete and diagnostically useful form in the lung (Fig. 20-6), which is the preferred biopsy site for this reason.[40] Recent studies of involved lung tissue suggest that although vasculitis is an important component of WG, the disease has a significant extravascular component, and vasculitic lesions are not always found. Both vascular and extravascular collagen and reticulum are affected. The granulomas, which often contain giant cells, differ from the compact granulomata typically seen in infectious processes (such as tuberculosis) and sarcoidosis in that the cells are lined up in palisades. The lesions pass through stages of micronecrosis with neutrophilic microabscesses, then macronecrosis (which is more widespread), and finally fibrosis.[41] Not all patients show these findings to the same degree, and the findings can be classified into four histologic types that have prognostic significance:

1. The fulminant type (most severe, poorest prognosis)
2. The granulomatous type (little evidence of vasculitis in some cases)
3. The fibrous scar type (most protracted course)
4. The mixed type[42]

Renal biopsies often show evidence of crescentic glomerulonephritis. Granuloma formation may not be evident, and specimens often have little diagnostic specificity for WG. The characteristic lesion is focal in distribution, often involving less than half the glomeruli; it is a segmental necrotizing glomerulonephritis (SNGN). Most studies show little or no evidence of immune complex deposition using immunohistochemical methods and/or electron microscopy, although fibrin deposition is usually present. Findings have been interpreted as suggesting that glomerulothrombosis, rather than immune complex deposition, is the primary event.[43]

Diagnosis

WG is suspected in patients who have fever, malaise, and multisystem disease with prominent lung and upper airway symptoms. Physical examination will often disclose crusts on the nasal mucosa and sometimes perforation of the nasal septum.

A

B

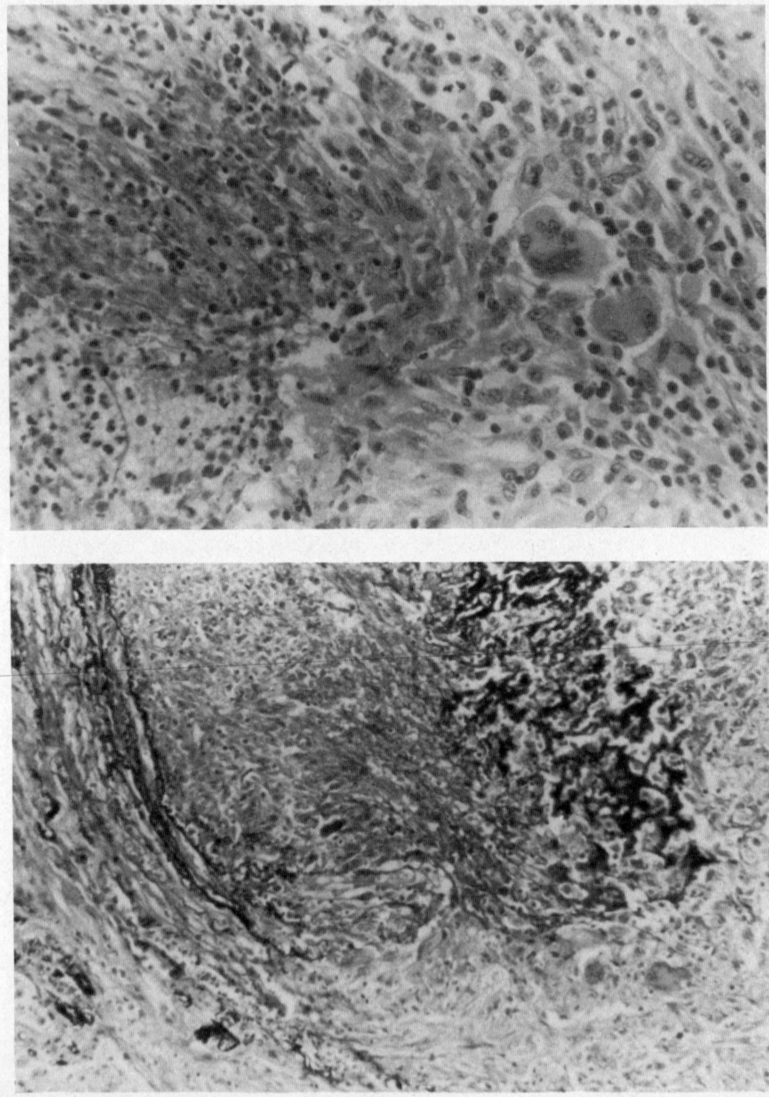

Fig. 20-6. Lung biopsy from a patient with Wegener's granulomatosis showing (**A**) a lymphocytic/histiocytic infiltrate with multinucleated giant cells adjacent to a necrotic area at the lower left (hematoxylin-eosin stain; × 340) and (**B**) destruction of elastin in an arterial wall (Van Gieson stain; × 140). (Courtesy GN Gephardt, MD, Cleveland Clinic Foundation.)

Routine laboratory studies suggest acute and chronic inflammation. Anemia, leukocytosis, thrombocytosis, polyclonal hypergammaglobulinemia, and elevated acute phase reactants are usually found. C-reactive protein has been reported to be a more sensitive indicator of active inflammation in WG than the erythrocyte sedimentation rate. In the majority of cases circulating immune complexes are not detected by the Raji cell assay, cryoglobulin assay, or the C1q-binding assay. Complement levels are usually normal.

Antibodies against neutrophilic cytoplasm (ANCA) have recently been described in WG.[44] These antibodies, which are detected by indirect immunofluorescence using ethanol-fixed human neutrophils as substrate (Fig. 20-7), appear to have a high degree of specificity (greater than 90%) for WG. Sensitivities vary in different studies from 58% to 96%. Studies to determine the exact antigenic specificity of the antibodies have yielded conflicting results, but they bind 1.8, 6.2, and 100 kD cytoplasmic components on Western blot studies.[45] Of great interest also is the finding that ANCA titers correlate with disease activity better than other parameters commonly used for this in WG. The exact role of ANCA in the diagnosis and management of WG remains to be defined, and it is premature to consider a positive ANCA result as a satisfactory substitute for histologic confirmation of the diagnosis, but the studies available to date appear quite promising.

The diagnosis of WG is confirmed by ruling out infection and by obtaining appropriate histologic confirmation through biopsy of the involved areas. As noted above if there is clinical evidence of lung involvement, the lung is the most appropriate biopsy site. However, biopsies may be obtained from upper airways or other locations if the lung is not considered practical. The kidney is usually not a suitable site.

Three major categories of disease constitute the bulk of the differential diagnosis of WG: infection, malignancy, and connective tissue disease, including other forms of vasculitis. Chronic infections have many features in common with WG, and there is, in fact, some evidence that WG itself is an infection with an as yet unidentified agent. Mycobacterial and fungal infections must be differentiated by appropriate cultures and immunologic methods. Malignant diseases, such as lymphomatoid granulomatosis, Hodgkin's disease, and idiopathic midline destructive disease are typically distinguished by biopsy. Other forms of vasculitis and connective tissue disease, such as polyarteritis nodosa, allergic granulomatous vasculitis, giant cell arteritis with pulmonary nodules, Goodpasture's syndrome, and bronchocentric granulomatosis, can be differentiated by a combination of histologic, serologic, and clinical criteria. ANCA may turn out to be useful as a differentiating factor.

Treatment

Two important developments in the treatment of WG have occurred during the past decade. The first was the recognition that cyclophosphamide has a potent suppressive effect on WG.[38] The second was the most recent recognition that trimethoprim-sulfamethoxazole appears to be able to induce remission in at least some patients with WG.[46]

Based on the widely held concept that WG is an autoimmune disease (for which there is, however, little evidence), as well as the recognition that corticosteroids are ineffective in the long-term management of WG, several immunosuppressive agents have been tried, and anecdotal reports of response to a variety of drugs including azathioprine, chlorambucil, methotrexate, and cyclophosphamide have appeared. Fauci, Haynes, and Katz assembled a convincing, though uncontrolled, body of data on the favorable response

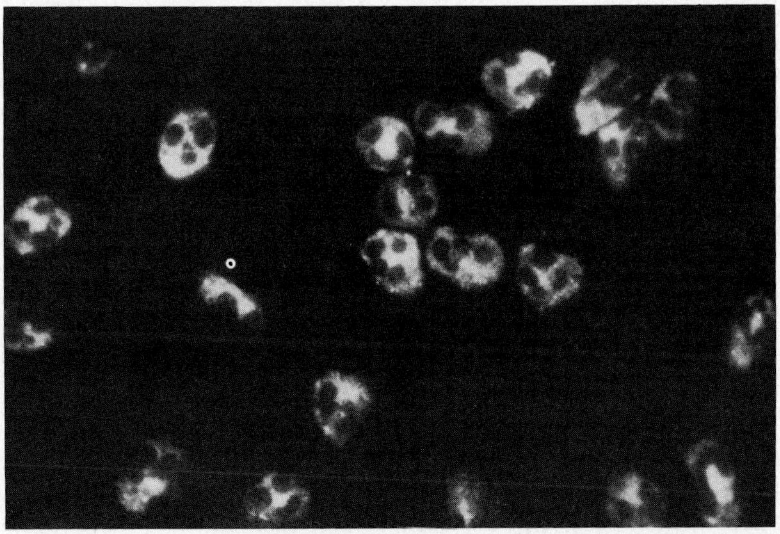

Fig. 20-7. Detection of anti-neutrophil cytoplasm antibody (ANCA) by indirect immunofluorescence. This antibody is a marker for diagnosis and disease activity in Wegener's granulomatosis.

to cyclophosphamide from the National Institutes of Health series, which led to the widespread acceptance of this modality.[38] The preferred regimen is daily oral cyclophosphamide 100 to 150 mg/day for 1 year, with or without low-dose prednisone, followed by taper and discontinuance. We have found that rapid control of the disease may be achieved by preceding the initiation of cyclophosphamide therapy with a course of intravenous nitrogen mustard (0.3 mg/kg).[47] Unlike cyclophosphamide, which is also sometimes administered intravenously to achieve more rapid results, this drug is not affected by impaired renal function, a considerable advantage in classic WG. Although the early results suggested that remissions induced in this way might be permanent, it has since become clear that many patients relapse after periods of a few months to a few years. There are, moreover, significant short- and long-term adverse effects associated with the use of cyclophosphamide, including marrow suppression, increased susceptibility to infection, hemorrhagic cystitis, sterility, alopecia, and malignancy.

The initial report of efficacy of trimethoprim-sulfamethoxazole in WG was greeted with some skepticism, but recent confirmatory studies from a number of different centers have supported the original findings of DeRemee, McDonald, and Wieland.[46] Most, but not all, reported cases of successful use of this drug combination have been in patients who had already had one or more courses of cytotoxic drug treatment. The success rate in such patients is impressive and warrants consideration of this preparation in patients with WG. The usual course of treatment is trimethoprim 160 mg/day and sulfamethoxazole 800 mg/day.

High-dose corticosteroid therapy is the treatment of choice for serious ocular problems,[37] although the process may recur when the steroid dose is lowered. A granulomatous mass behind the eyeball can cause excrutiating pain, which can be temporarily relieved by corticosteroids. Surgical decompression may be necessary, but this is technically difficult and may result in further loss of vision.

Other treatments include intensive plasmapheresis for patients with severe active glomerulonephritis, other cytotoxic agents, and cyclosporin, although none of these is in widespread use at present. No controlled trials are available.

LYMPHOMATOID GRANULOMATOSIS AND BENIGN LYMPHOCYTIC ANGIITIS

Lymphomatoid granulomatosis (LG) is a vasculocentric granulomatous disease, first described in 1972,[48] with many clinical similarities to Wegener's granulomatosis. It affects primarily the lungs, skin, central nervous system, and kidneys. As understanding of and experience with this condition have progressed, the preponderance of evidence increasingly supports the concept of LG as a premalignant or malignant disease of T lymphocytes.[49] Moreover, there is a close relationship of LG to idiopathic midline destructive disease (polymorphic reticulosis), and some investigators regard these conditions to be different clinical presentations of the same nosologic entity.[50]

There is considerable variability in clinical course and severity of illness among patients with LG; Fauci et al have suggested that LG should be viewed as a spectrum from benign to malignant.[51] Saldana and colleagues have classified pulmonary angiitis with granulomatosis into three categories: (1) lymphocyte-depleted angiitis and granulomatosis (Wegener's granulomatosis), (2) benign lymphocytic angiitis and granulomatosis, and (3) malignant lymphoproliferative angiitis and granulomatosis (LG).[52] We consider benign lymphocytic angiitis and granulomatosis (BLAG) to be at the mild end of the spectrum of LG, a nonvasculitic malignant process, while WG is an inflammatory, vasculitic process that lies outside this spectrum.

LG is a rare disease with a 3:1 male predominance. The cause is unknown. It responds poorly to treatment, and the mortality rate varies in different series from 38% to 85%[38,53] with some patients recovering spontaneously. BLAG responds well to treatment with alkylating agents but not corticosteroids and generally has a good prognosis. These differences may result from difficulties in the classification of some patients.

Clinical aspects

The most common target organ for LG is the lung.[48] Although some cases have been discovered in asymptomatic individuals at the time of routine chest x-ray, patients most commonly develop cough, fever, night sweats, chest pain, and dyspnea. Hemoptysis is uncommon. The typical chest x-ray shows multiple bilateral nodules with a tendency to cavitate; hilar adenopathy is unusual. BLAG is usually limited to the lung[52]; cough and dyspnea are the usual initial symptoms, and the chest x-ray shows multiple bilateral nodules.

The second most frequently involved site for LG is the skin.[48] Nodules may be present on the face or the trunk. Annular infiltrated or ulcerating lesions, often resembling those of Weber-Christian disease, may be present.

Slightly less frequently patients will have central or peripheral nervous system involvement. Presentation may suggest brain tumor, cranial or peripheral motor neuropathy. Central nervous system LG has been seen with some frequency in acquired immunodeficiency syndrome (AIDS).

Although renal involvement occurs in about a third of the patients, it is not as severe as that seen in WG.[48] While glomerulonephritis has been reported in one case, the usual lesion is an interstitial infiltration that does not severely affect renal function.

The lower urinary tract and prostate may also be affected. Other tissues that may be involved include bone marrow, lymph nodes, spleen, and liver.

Several authors have raised the possibility that IMDD may be the upper airway manifestation of LG, and this is supported by recent reports of co-occurrence of classic LG and IMDD.[50] This combination appears to be quite unusual, however, and would present a clinical picture highly reminiscent of WG, from which it must be differentiated.

The disease follows a progressive course in most instances. Although the malignant nature of the process may not be apparent at the outset, development of frank lymphoma is the usual outcome. Occasional spontaneous remissions have been described.

The characteristic lesion of LG has been classically described as "angiocentric and angiodestructive lymphoreticular proliferative and granulomatous".[48] The lungs are involved in 57% to 90% of patients, the skin in 20% to 46%, and the nervous system in 21% to 33%. The granulomata are pleomorphic and necrotic. The histologic appearance resembles IMDD. Infiltrating lymphocytes have been characterized as T cells bearing either the CD4 or CD8 phenotype. In most, but not all, cases that have been examined, rearrangement of genes for the T cell receptor has been found, indicating restricted clonality and a malignant process.[50]

In BLAG the characteristic lesion is a vasculocentric, nonnecrotizing infiltration with mature-appearing lymphocytes. Gene rearrangement studies have not been reported for BLAG, although a recent study has documented malignant transformation in three of nine patients with this lesion.[54]

Diagnosis

LG and BLAG are diagnosed by histopathologic examination of involved tissue. Depending on the organ system(s) affected, the differential diagnosis includes infections (especially mycobacterial and fungal), other malignancies, and "collagen-vascular" diseases (especially WG). Southern blotting studies to detect the characteristic T cell receptor gene rearrangement may be diagnostically helpful.[50] Several investigators have commented on findings suggesting impaired cellular immunity (skin test anergy and depressed lymphocyte transformation)[55] in contrast with WG, where these findings tend to be normal.

Treatment

Although one study has indicated optimistic results of treatment with cyclophosphamide and prednisone in a protocol similar to that used in WG,[51] LG is clearly less responsive to this than WG. Most authors recommend combination chemotherapy and/or irradiation regimens similar to those employed in the treatment of more classic lymphoproliferative malignancies. Irradiation is clearly the treatment of choice for IMDD. Surgical removal of mass lesions may be helpful at times, but it is generally not curative. Treatment for LG remains unsatisfactory.

BLAG generally has a good prognosis, responding to corticosteroids sometimes combined with a cytotoxic agent.[52] The most critical factor in the natural history of BLAG is whether or not lymphoma develops.

GIANT CELL ARTERITIS

The term giant cell arteritis (GCA) is commonly used to refer to granulomatous arteritis of unknown cause, predominantly affecting large arteries with prominent destruction of the internal elastic lamina. Giant cells are often but not invariably present in positive biopsies. Moreover, giant cells are also frequently found in other forms of granulomatous vaculitis, such as Wegener's granulomatosis. Thus the term GCA is a something of a misnomer.

Two syndromes have been recognized under the general heading of GCA, temporal arteritis[56] and Takayasu's arteritis.[57] The major differences between these syndromes are the age at which they occur (temporal arteritis generally occurs in individuals over 50), the distribution and severity of vascular involvement (more widespread and severe for Takayasu's arteritis), and the racial distribution (predominantly white for temporal arteritis and oriental for Takayasu's arteritis). During the past few years increasing numbers of cases have been recognized in which these distinctions are blurred,[58] and it is not at all clear that these are two separate entities.

It may be more sensible to view GCA as a spectrum of disease severity with temporal arteritis (with or without polymyalgia rheumatica) at the mild end and Takayasu's arteritis at the more severe end. Other presentations of GCA, not easily classified under either syndrome, would occupy positions along the spectrum determined by the systems or organs affected and the patient's responsiveness to treatment.

Temporal arteritis

The most common syndrome of GCA is temporal arteritis. Its major importance stems from its threat to vision. It is frequently seen in association with the clinical syndrome of polymyalgia rheumatica (PMR), but the basis for this association is unknown.

Clinical aspects. Temporal arteritis affects the elderly and increases in frequency with age. It is seldom seen before the age of 50. It has a predilection for whites of northern European descent; the largest demographic studies have been done in Scandinavia and Minnesota, where large numbers of Americans of Scandinavian descent reside.[58] The disease is uncommon in blacks, but it has been reported.

Classic symptoms are persistent headache, often in the temporal areas, which may be locally tender over the superficial temporal arteries; transient visual disturbances (amaurosis fugax), usually manifested by dimming or "graying" of vision but sometimes by blurring or diplopia; and jaw claudication. This picture is even more characteristic when it occurs in a patient with PMR, a clinical syndrome characterized by acute onset of proximal muscular stiffness and pain on active motion.[59] The relationship between these two conditions has never been satisfactorily explained, but it is close enough that asymptomatic temporal arteritis is often sought and sometimes found in patients with PMR.

Temporal arteritis may also be identified without typical symptoms in up to one sixth of elderly patients with fever of unknown origin.

On physical examination tenderness and swelling are often found in the temporal arteries, which may be pulseless, but these findings are not invariable, and the physical examination is frequently normal. If the patient has PMR, active motion of limb and pelvic girdle muscles is usually more painful than passive motion; muscle strength is not affected but may be difficult to test because of pain.

Complications are more common in males than females. These include permanent partial or complete visual loss (the most frequent complication), necrosis of the tongue, paresthesias of the face, multiple cranial nerve palsies, hearing loss, diabetes insipidus, stroke, and other ischemic phenomena in the head and neck region. Blindness can result from occlusion of the central retinal artery.

Involvement outside the area of the head and neck may occur in patients with or without temporal arteritis. Unless the temporal arteries are involved, this is more properly referred to as GCA or, in the proper clinical setting, as Takayasu's arteritis (see next section).

In temporal arteritis, the characteristic lesion is granulomatous inflammation of the arterial wall with destruction of the internal elastic lamina and giant cell formation (Fig. 20-8). Immunoglobulin deposits in the region of the internal elastic lamina have been detected in some patients by direct immunofluorescence. The cellular infiltrate contains many lymphocytes, which have been characterized as CD4-positive T cells, an elevated percentage of which bear class II histocompatibility antigens and interleukin-2 receptors, indicating activation. Activated macrophages are also present. Smooth muscle cells have been shown not to express class II antigens; this suggests that these cells are not functioning as antigen-presenting cells.[60]

Although there is some controversy over the distribution of the granulomatous lesion, most authorities agree that it is a skip lesion and that small biopsy specimens may not show evidence of disease in affected individuals. Another area of controversy is the ability to diagnose "healed" temporal arteritis from biopsy material; most authorities now believe that the findings on which such conclusions are based are too nonspecific to warrant this.

Diagnosis. Biopsy of the temporal artery is the "gold standard" for the diagnosis of temporal arteritis. However, in clinical situations where the degree of certainty about the diagnosis before biopsy is high, it is reasonable to make the diagnosis tentatively and begin treatment without the biopsy result. Prednisone therapy changes the biopsy findings relatively slowly, and there is evidence of active arteritis in specimens obtained up to 7 weeks after initiation of treatment.[61] The improvement of symptoms after initiation of treatment, however, is rapid in most cases, and the observation of rapid disappearance of headache and PMR (generally within 24 hours) provides additional support for the diagnosis. Patients failing to respond rapidly to prednisone and ultimately having negative biopsies have turned out most frequently to have either malignancy or diabetes mellitus.

The only helpful laboratory test is the erythrocyte sedimentation rate (ESR), which is usually markedly elevated. Although cases of otherwise typical temporal arteritis with normal ESR have been described, this test has such a high sensitivity for temporal arteritis that other diagnostic pos-

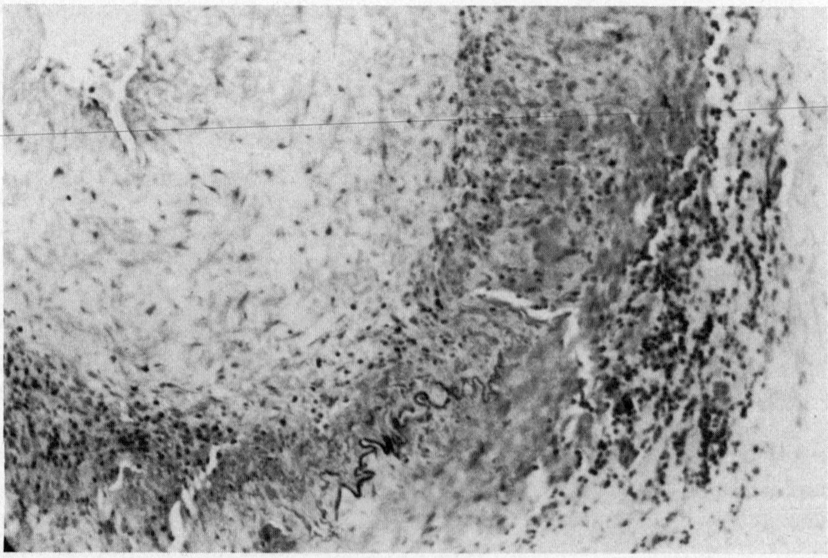

Fig. 20-8. Biopsy of the superficial temporal artery from a patient with temporal arteritis showing disruption of the internal elastic lamina, granulomatous infiltrate, and giant cells. (Silver stain; × 140.)

sibilities should be strongly considered when it is normal. The role of the ESR in monitoring patients for response to treatment and relapse is controversial. Although ESR is widely used for this, some authorities recommend monitoring clinical symptoms only, since it may rise again without clinical relapse.[61] Other acute phase reactants (fibrinogen, C-reactive protein, haptoglobin) have been found not to be as useful or dependable as ESR. The von Willebrand factor is often elevated in temporal arteritis, and levels have been reported higher in GCA than in "pure" PMR and certain other rheumatic conditions, but this has no recognized diagnostic utility at present.[62]

HLA-DR4, a class II histocompatibility antigen associated with several "autoimmune" diseases (most notably rheumatoid arthritis), has been found with increased frequency in patients with temporal arteritis (40%, compared to 20% of controls). This increased frequency is almost entirely segregated to the group with PMR, 59% of whom have HLA-DR4, compared to the group without PMR, 19% of whom are positive for this antigen.[63]

The differential diagnosis of temporal arteritis depends on the clinical presentation. Classically the presentation is so typical that other explanations are unlikely. Occasionally systemic lupus erythematosus presents a PMR-like picture that may be associated with headache and retinal vasculitis leading to visual symptoms. The presence of other features of lupus as well as the typical serologic findings can usually make this distinction. Malignancy and diabetes mellitus have already been referred to. Patients who have fever of unknown origin, infections, and other connective tissue diseases also become part of the differential diagnosis.

Treatment. Prednisone remains the treatment of choice. Classically the recommendation was low-dose prednisone (15 mg/day) for PMR without evidence of temporal arteritis but much higher doses (60 to 100 mg/day) for patients with temporal arteritis. High-dose prednisone would be continued for 6 weeks, then tapered to the lowest dose that would maintain freedom from symptoms (with or without maintenance of normal ESR). Low-dose prednisone would be continued for as long as necessary to prevent relapse upon discontinuing the drug.

Prednisone, however, has many side effects, not the least of which is osteoporosis in the elderly, predominantly female population. There has been considerable interest in minimizing exposure to prednisone to the least necessary amount, and some investigators have shown results equal to those obtained with high-dose prednisone using more moderate doses (20 to 40 mg/day) with considerable reduction of side effects.[64] However, temporal arteritis has developed in some patients with "clinically pure" PMR while on treatment with low-dose prednisone with good control of symptoms and normal ESR. Furthermore, development of ischemic optic neuropathy has been reported despite high-dose prednisone treatment. An alternative approach is to take advantage of the steroid-sparing potential of certain chemotherapeutic agents such as azathioprine[65] in clinical situations that warrant it (e.g., preexisting osteoporosis or severe diabetes mellitus).

The relapse rate on discontinuing prednisone is high; in several studies it approached 50% whether high- or low-dose prednisone was used. Approximately 40% of patients required prednisone for more than 4 years. Reported mean durations of therapy ranged from 2 to 6 years, but many patients required treatment for more than 10 years. Fortunately, once the disease is controlled, the required dose is generally low enough not to pose much of a problem for most patients (less than 10 mg/day).

GENERALIZED GIANT CELL ARTERITIS AND TAKAYASU'S ARTERITIS

Takayasu's arteritis is a special case of generalized GCA that occurs in young oriental females.[57] It has also been described in young females of other races, including blacks and whites. However, other than this demographic peculiarity, there is little to distinguish this as a nosologic entity from generalized GCA, which sometimes occurs in the elderly with or without temporal arteritis. Since the cause of GCA is unknown, regardless of the location of the lesion or the age, race, and sex of the patient, we will discuss the generalized forms of GCA, including Takayasu's arteritis, together.

Clinical aspects

The clinical manifestation of generalized GCA is entirely dependent on the location of major involvement. The most common manifestation is claudication of the upper extremities, but involvement of the aorta and its major branches other than the subclavian arteries has also been described, leading to wide variations in clinical manifestations in different patients.[66]

Claudication of the upper extremities occurs when the subclavian arteries are severely involved. This is accompanied by reduced or undetectable radial, ulnar, and brachial pulses and often by bruits over the subclavian arteries. Although it may be asymmetrical in severity, both sides are usually involved. Raynaud's phenomenon is not usually present.

Lower extremity involvement may also be seen. Ischemic manifestations are usually more severe in the lower extremities and often lead to skin breakdown and gangrene, sometimes requiring amputation. Although this is more common in older individuals, GCA should be included in the differential diagnosis of younger individuals with intermittent claudication or ischemic ulcerations of the lower extremities as well.

Involvement of the aorta may lead to aneurysm formation, either in the thoracic or abdominal aorta. The diagnosis of GCA in this setting is often made unexpectedly at the time of histopathologic examination of the surgical specimen. If the ascending aorta is affected, this may lead to dilation of the aortic valve ring with aortic insufficiency, which may necessitate valve replacement.[67]

Coronary artery involvement, gastrointestinal ischemia, and mononeuritis multiplex are all less common than in polyarteritis nodosa, but have been described in GCA. Other unusual manifestations include pulmonary artery involvement, cranial neuropathies, infarction of the spinal cord, erythema nodosum, and masses in the breast, ovary, or prostate. Kidney and lung involvement are uncommon.

There is no histologic difference between the lesion seen in generalized GCA and that seen in temporal arteritis; the only difference is in the distribution. Temporal arteries may or may not be involved when the disease is generalized.

Diagnosis. GCA is often diagnosed angiographically when it occurs in sites not readily amenable to biopsy. Long segments of narrowing are seen in affected arteries, often producing a "string sign" (Fig. 20-9). Collateral circulation may be well developed, especially if the process is longstanding. If surgery is needed, vascular tissue may be available for examination, and typical GCA is identified.

Laboratory studies are not particularly helpful, although, as in temporal arteritis, the ESR is usually markedly elevated. There is no association with any specific immunologic response, and evidence of infection with hepatitis viruses or other agents has not been demonstrated.

The differential diagnosis includes other vascular occlusive diseases, especially other forms of vasculitis (e.g., polyarteritis nodosa) and atherosclerosis.

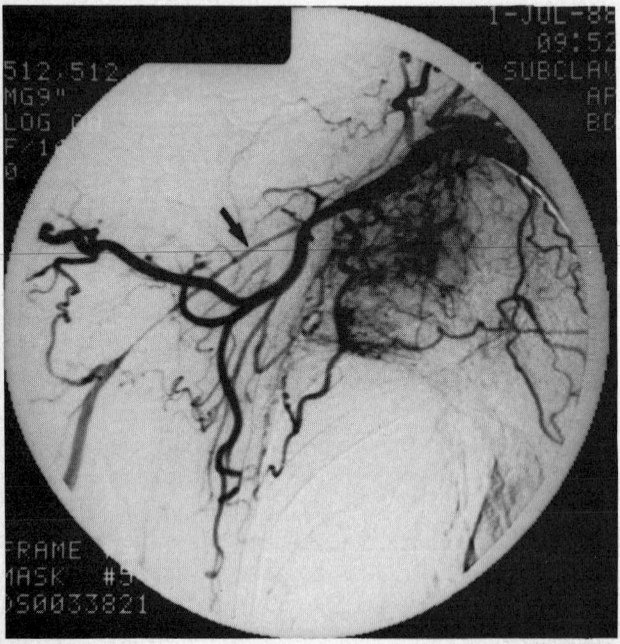

Fig. 20-9. Digital subtraction arteriogram showing involvement of the right subclavian artery producing a "string sign" (*arrow*) in a patient with giant cell arteritis (Takayasu's arteritis); notice the extensive collateral circulation.

Treatment. Although corticosteroid treatment may be effective in generalized GCA, many patients require more aggressive treatment, and our practice is to treat this condition much the same as Wegener's granulomatosis and polyarteritis nodosa, that is with cyclophosphamide and prednisone. We have had good results in individual cases with a starting regimen of prednisone (1 mg/kg/day orally) and mechlorethamine (nitrogen mustard) (0.3 mg/kg total dose given intravenously in 2 to 3 mg increments over a week). After completion of the mechlorethamine, cyclophosphamide is begun (2 mg/kg/day orally) and continued for a year. After the first few weeks, prednisone is tapered to an eventual maintenance dose (less than 10 mg/day). With this regimen there may be some initial evidence of improved circulation; pulses may return or become stronger, claudication may lessen or disappear, and skin ulcers may begin to heal. In addition the ESR usually returns to normal within a few days or weeks.

Surgical intervention is often required in severe generalized GCA. Acute disasters, such as aortic rupture or perforation of the bowel, require immediate surgical intervention to save the patient's life. Bypass surgery or aneurysm repair may be indicated if ischemia is severe and unresponsive to medical treatment. Skin grafting or amputation may be necessary, particularly with lower extremity involvement.

CLINICAL APPROACH

Diagnosis

The vasculitides as a group of disorders remain a formidable challenge to clinicians from both the diagnostic and therapeutic perspectives. Diagnostically, the signs and symptoms of vasculitis are generally nonspecific since they represent those of vascular ischemia regardless of the cause. Certain vasculitic syndromes represent greater diagnostic challenges than others because of the nature and distribution of their target organ involvement. For example, when the skin is involved, such as in the hypersensitivity vasculitides, it is generally apparent that vasculitis is the underlying process, but a greater challenge is to determine the precise cause and thus the prognosis and treatment. In the absence of topical signs of vasculitis such as a characteristic rash or signs of peripheral ischemia, systemic vasculitis may mimic a wide variety of nonvasculitic diseases.

The box on p. 357 enumerates a series of warning signs or symptoms of systemic vasculitis. These findings should alert clinicians to the possibility of systemic vasculitis when a careful workup for other causes is unrevealing. Clearly, certain of these signs or symptoms have greater degrees of sensitivity or specificity depending upon the clinical situation. The following is a brief description of the significance of these warning signs or symptoms:

1. Fever of unknown origin. Virtually all the vasculitic syndromes are capable of producing fever. The differential diagnosis of fever of unknown origin centers around infections, malignancies, and connective tissue diseases. Among the connective tissue diseases, systemic vasculitis remains among the most prominent possibilities.
2. Unexplained multisystem disease. Because of the potential widespread distribution of vascular inflammatory disease, multisystem organ dysfunction is not uncommon in systemic vasculitis. While there are many other diagnostic considerations including disseminated infection, disseminated cancer, and other infiltrating and inflammatory diseases (e.g., amyloidosis or sarcoidosis), systemic vasculitis should be kept in mind.
3. Mononeuritis multiplex. The clinical involvement of isolated peripheral nerves in differing anatomic sites is probably the most specific warning sign of underlying systemic vasculitis. Mononeuritis multiplex may be seen in a variety of vasculitic syndromes. While other patterns of peripheral neurologic involvement may be seen including symmetric polyneuropathy, pure sensory neuropathy, or the diffuse involvement of peripheral nerves in a single limb, mononeuritis multiplex is the most common problem. In the absence of diabetes or trauma, mononeuritis multiplex should be considered vasculitic until proven otherwise.
4. Unexplained inflammatory arthritis. Associated with a number of the vasculitic syndromes including polyarteritis nodosa, Wegener's granulomatosis, certain of the hypersensitivity vasculitides, and others, articular disease may be prominent. In general the arthritic picture associated with systemic vasculitis is one of a symmetric polyarthritis that is nonerosive and may be clinically severe. Because of the frequent presence of rheumatoid factor, it is not uncommon for inflammatory arthritis to be misdiagnosed as rheumatoid arthritis. The presence of severe constitutional signs and symptoms in the presence of unexplained inflammatory arthritis should always raise the diagnostic possibility of systemic vasculitis.
5. Unexplained inflammatory myositis. Muscle is a frequent target organ of systemic vasculitis and may produce an angiocentric myositis. The myositis of systemic vasculitis may be associated with elevated muscle enzymes and varying degrees of muscle pain or weakness. Electromyographic studies of these patients will usually reveal evidence of a patchy inflammatory myopathy, which may be confused with idiopathic polymyositis. In our experience the primary muscle weakness associated with vasculitic muscle involvement is generally not as severe as that seen in polymyositis, and the symptoms of muscular pain and tenderness are somewhat more prominent.
6. Unexplained glomerulonephritis. Glomerulonephritis can be caused by a variety of systemic and immunologic diseases. There is no specific finding in the urinary sediment or in the associated laboratory tests that has a high degree of predictive value for the presence of systemic vasculitis. Frequently, patients with renal involvement and systemic vasculitis develop severe hypertension or a syndrome of rapidly progressive glomerulonephritis.
7. Unexplained cardiac, gastrointestinal, or CNS ischemia. This is probably the least specific of all the warning signs or symptoms of vasculitis but still must be considered in appropriate clinical context. Obviously, a stroke in an octagenerian would not raise a high degree of suspicion regarding the possibility of CNS angiitis, but a TIA in a 15-year-old girl certainly would. Similarly, ischemic events involving the cardiovascular or gastrointestinal systems should be considered potentially vasculitic if no other causes are apparent after careful investigation.

Conditions mimicking vasculitis

It should be kept in mind that there are a variety of conditions that can closely mimic the presence of systemic vasculitis. These conditions can lead to vascular occlusion, and thus ischemic symptomatology, but are generally noninflammatory. A partial listing of these mimicking syndromes is listed in the box below.

Among these syndromes cholesterol embolization perhaps represents the greatest challenge at differentiation from systemic vasculitis. Cholesterol microembolization may produce a variety of signs or symptoms resembling a multisystem disorder by virtue of its involvement of the nervous system, skin, heart, muscle, kidney, and gastrointestinal

Warning signs and symptoms of vasculitis

1. Fever of unknown origin
2. Unexplained multisystem disease
3. Mononeuritis multiplex
4. Unexplained inflammatory arthritis
5. Unexplained inflammatory myositis
6. Unexplained glomerulonephritis
7. Unexplained cardiac, gastrointestinal, or CNS ischemia

Conditions mimicking systemic vasculitis

Cholesterol embolism
Atrial myxoma
Sarcoidosis
Fibromuscular dysplasia
Angioendotheliomatosis
Ergotism
Neuroectodermal dysplasia

systems. Laboratory abnormalities may include leukocytosis, eosinophilia, hypocomplementemia, and elevated erythrocyte sedimentation rates. A recent study by Cappiello[68] has revealed the occasional presence of antinuclear antibodies and rheumatoid factors. To diagnose cholesterol embolization, a high degree of suspicion must exist based upon the clinical findings. The definitive diagnosis depends on histologic demonstration of needle-shaped cholesterol clefts on biopsy of an affected target organ. The amputated tissue may be a prime source for this characteristic finding. The condition should be suspected when a patient develops signs or symptoms of multifocal vascular ischemia and occlusion following an arteriographic procedure or while on warfarin therapy.

DIAGNOSTIC APPROACH

The diagnosis of the systemic vasculitides represents a formidable challenge in both recognition that a syndrome exists, and also in its precise nosologic classification. The precise approach is highly dependent on which syndrome is primarily suspected. Certain vasculitic syndromes such as hypersensitivity vasculitis are not difficult to recognize because of their prominent cutaneous involvement, but further identification of the precise cause and therefore prognosis, and appropriate treatment may be quite challenging. Giant cell arteritis is generally diagnosed by a temporal artery biopsy and Takayasu's arteritis is generally diagnosed by angiography for obvious reasons.

The overlap of the systemic necrotizing vasculitides, polyarteritis nodosa, Churg-Strauss syndrome, and polyangiitis is most challenging to diagnose. Numerous algorithms have been proposed based on a series of laboratory tests, organ biopsies, and the use of visceral angiography. There are no laboratory tests that have an extremely high predictive value in diagnosing these conditions, but certain combinations of tests may be extremely helpful. For example, the presence of elevated circulating immune complexes and a depressed level of serum complement in the presence of mononeuritis multiplex would certainly strongly suggest an underlying vasculitic condition, whereas the same laboratory findings in a person with merely a fever of unknown origin may not be nearly as predictive. Generally speaking, biopsies in patients suspected of having systemic necrotizing vasculitis are best directed at obvious clinically involved organs. Blind biopsies of asymptomatic tissues such as muscle, nerve, kidney, or testicle are generally unrewarding.[69] Recent studies have suggested that a clinically or electrically documented involved sural nerve may yield an extremely high sensitivity for picking up systemic necrotizing vasculitis.[70]

Visceral abdominal angiography has been reported to be abnormal in up to 70% to 80% of patients with PAN though not all patients have equally characteristic findings. The presence of multiple saccular aneurysms in the distribution of the renal arteries or celiac axis is highly predictive of PAN while the presence of isolated vessel cutoff or mild luminal irregularities is far less specific.[10]

The diagnosis of Wegener's granulomatosis is basically a clinical pathologic one based on the characteristic distribution of target organ involvement. The diagnosis is secured when the characteristic histopathology is identified in the appropriate clinical setting. While any clinically involved organ may be the candidate source for biopsy material, the lung is generally the end organ with the highest yield. This overall approach may be drastically changed if the predictive value of antineutrophil cytoplasm antibody holds up to prospective evaluations of its diagnostic utility.

Pitfalls in the diagnosis of systemic necrotizing vasculitis

Since there is no single test or combination of tests that is totally sensitive for the presence of systemic vasculitis, the clinician must be both patient and persistent to secure the diagnosis. Since most vasculitic lesions may be patchy by their nature, false negative biopsies are not uncommon. Certain tissues such as muscle, nerve, temporal artery, kidney, and testicle are well known for this problem. Certain organs such as the kidney may reveal nonvascular pathology that must be appropriately interpreted. For example, a closed-needle biopsy of a kidney in a patient with PAN or Wegener's granulomatosis is more likely than not to *fail* to reveal frank vasculitis of the renal vasculature. Similarly, the same technique is likely to yield evidence of a focal segmental necrotizing glomerulitis in the presence of an active urinary sediment or azotemia. Thus recognizing the characteristic finding of glomerulonephritis as opposed to vasculitis of the renal vasculature may secure the diagnosis. Another situation that is frequently encountered is a false negative nasal biopsy in patients with Wegener's granulomatosis. Because of the highly destructive nature of the lesions, the pathology may reveal only inflammation and necrosis. This should not be cast off as evidence of a nonvasculitic cause but should stimulate the clinician to further pursue securing the diagnosis of Wegener's if clinical suspicion is high. Collectively, the diagnosis of vasculitis remains clinically and pathologically based on a combination of history and physical findings, laboratory data, organ biopsy, and the selected use of vascular imaging studies.

REFERENCES

1. Dixon FJ: The role of antigen-antibody complexes in diseases, Harvey Lect 58:21, 1963.
2. Winkelman RK: The spectrum of cutaneous vasculitis, Clin Rheum Dis 6:413, 1980.
3. Nydegger VE and Lambert PH: The role of immune complexes in the pathogenesis of necrotizing vasculitis, Clin Rheum Dis 6:255, 1980.
4. Levo Y et al: Association between hepatitis B virus and essential mixed cryoglobulinemia, N Engl J Med 296:1501, 1977.

5. Phillips MR, Abramson SB, and Weissmann G: Neutrophile adhesion and autoimmune vascular injury, Clin Aspects Autoimmune 3:6, 1989.
6. Leavitt RY and Fauci AS: Polyangiitis overlap syndrome, Am J Med 81:79, 1986.
7. Fauci AS, Haynes B, and Katz P: The spectrum of vasculitis: clinical pathologic, immunologic and therapeutic considerations, Ann Intern Med 89:660, 1978.
8. Guillevin L et al: Clinical findings and prognosis of polyarteritis nodosa and Churg-Strauss angiitis: a study of 165 patients, Br J Rheumatol 27:258, 1988.
9. Cupps TR and Fauci AS: The vasculitides. Chapter 4: Systemic necrotizing vasculitis of the polyarteritis nodosa group, Philadelphia, 1981, WB Saunders Co.
10. Travers RL et al: Polyarteritis nodosa: a clinical angiographic analysis of 17 cases, Semin Arthritis Rheum 8:184, 1979.
11. Moore PM and Fauci AS: Neurologic manifestations of systemic necrotizing vasculitis: a retrospective and prospective analysis of the clinical pathologic features and responses to therapy in 25 patients, Am J Med 71:517, 1981.
12. Diaz-Perez JL and Winkelman RK: Cutaneous periarteritis nodosa: a study of 33 patients. In Wolf K and Winkelman RK, eds: Vasculitis, Philadelphia, 1980, WB Saunders Co.
13. Wees SJ, Sunwoo IN, and Oh SJ: Sural nerve biopsy in systemic necrotizing vasculitis, Am J Med 71:525, 1981.
14. Cupps TR, and Fauci AS: Management and treatment. In Cupps R and Fauci AS, eds: The vasculitides, Philadelphia, 1981, WB Saunders Co.
15. Churg J and Strauss L: Allergic granulomatosis, allergic angiitis and periarteritis nodosa, Am J Pathol 27:277, 1951.
16. Lanham JG et al: Systemic vasculitis with asthma and eosinophilia: a clinical approach to the Churg-Strauss syndrome, Medicine (Baltimore) 63:65, 1984.
17. Chumbley LC, Harrison EG, and DeRemee RD: Allergic granulomatosis and angiitis (Churg-Strauss syndrome): report and analysis of 30 cases, Mayo Clin Proc 52:477, 1977.
18. Zeek PM, Smith CC, and Weeter JC: Studies on periarteritis nodosa. III. The differentiation between the vascular lesions of periarteritis nodosa and of hypersensitivity, Am J Pathol 24:889, 1948.
19. Calabrese LH and Clough JD: Hypersensitivity vasculitis group (HVG): a case-oriented review of a continuing clinical spectrum, Cleve Clin Q 49:17, 1982.
20. Cupps TR and Fauci AS: Hypersensitivity vasculitis. In: Cupps TR and Fauci AS, eds: The Vasculitides, Philadelphia, 1981, WB Saunders Co.
21. Wysenbeck AJ et al: Limited plasmapheresis in fulminant leukocytoclastic vasculitis, J Rheumatol 9:315, 1982.
22. Cream JJ, Gumpel JM, and Peachy AOG: Schönlein-Henoch purpura in the adult: a study of 77 adults, Q J Med 39:461, 1970.
23. Levy M et al: Anaphylactoid purpura nephritis in children: natural history and immunopathology, Adv Nephrol 6:183, 1976.
24. Gorevic PD et al: Mixed cryoglobulinemia: clinical aspects and long-term follow-up of 40 patients, Am J Med 69:287, 1980.
25. Greer JM et al: Vasculitis associated with malignancy, Medicine 67:220, 1988.
26. Zeiss CR et al: A hypocomplementemic vasculitic urticarial syndrome: report of four new cases and definition of the disease, Am J Med 68:867, 1980.
27. McDuffie FC et al: Hypocomplementemia with cutaneous vasculitis and arthritis: possible immune complex syndrome, Mayo Clin Proc 48:340, 1973.
28. Lieberman J, Gephardt G, and Calabrese LH: Chronic urticarial disease associated with pseudotumor cerebri membranoproliferative glomerulonephritis and hypocomplementemia: case report and review of the literature, Cleve Clin J Med, 1990, (in press).
29. Agnello V: Complement deficiency states, Medicine (Baltimore) 57:1, 1978.
30. Ekenstam EA and Callen JP: Cutaneous leukocytoclastic vasculitis: clinical and laboratory features of 82 patients seen in private practice, Arch Dermatol 120:484, 1984.
31. Gilliam JN and Smiley JD: Cutaneous necrotizing vasculitis and related disorders, Ann Allergy 37:328, 1976.
32. Wegener F: Ueber eine eigenartige rhinogene Granulomatose mit besonderer Beteiligung des arteriensystems und der Nieren, Beitr Pathol Anat Allgemein Pathol 102:36, 1939.
33. Carrington CB and Lieblow AA: Limited forms of angiitis and granulomatosis of the Wegener's type, Am J Med 41:497, 1966.
34. Muniain M, Moreno JC, and Gonzalez Campora R: Wegener's granulomatosis in two sisters, Ann Rheum Dis 45:417, 1986.
35. Leone CA, Feghali JG, and Linthicum FH Jr: Endolymphatic sac: possible role in autoimmune senorineural hearing loss, Ann Otol Rhinol Laryngol 93:208, 1984.
36. Haworth SJ et al: Pulmonary hemorrhage complicating Wegener's granulomatosis and microscopic polyarteritis, Br Med J 290:1775, 1985.
37. Haynes BF et al: The ocular manifestations of Wegener's granulomatosis: fifteen years experience and review of the literature, Am J Med 63:131, 1977.
38. Fauci AS: Wegener's granulomatosis: prospective clinical and therapeutic experience with 85 patients for 21 years, Ann Intern Med 98:76, 1983.
39. Camiller M et al: Gastrointestinal manifestations of systemic vasculitis, Q J Med 52:141, 1983.
40. Churg J and Churg A: Idiopathic and secondary vasculitis: a review, Med Pathol 2:144, 1989.
41. Mark EJ et al: The pulmonary biopsy in the early diagnosis of Wegener's (pathergic) granulomatosis: a study based on 35 open lung biopsies, Hum Pathol 19:1065, 1988.
42. Yoshikawa Y and Watanabe T: Pulmonary lesions in Wegener's granulomatosis: a clinicopathologic study fo 22 autopsy cases, Hum Pathol 18:401, 1986.
43. Weiss MA and Crissman JD: Renal biopsy findings in Wegener's granulomatosis: segmental necrotizing glomerulonephritis with glomerular thrombosis, Hum Pathol 15:943, 1984.
44. Van der Woude FJ et al: Antibodies against neutrophils and monocytes: Tool for diagnosis and marker of disease activity in Wegener's granulomatosis, Lancet 1:425, 1985.
45. Lockwood CM et al: Association of alkaline phosphatase with an autoantigen recognized by circulating anti-neutrophil antibodies in systemic vasculitis, Lancet 1:716, 1987.
46. DeRemee RA, McDonald TJ, and Wieland LH: Wegener's granulomatosis: observations on treatment with antimicrobial agents. Mayo Clin Proc 60:27, 1985.
47. Orlowski JP, Clough JD, and Dyment PG: Wegener's granulomatosis in the pediatric age group, Pediatrics 61:83, 1978.
48. Liebow AA, Carrington CRB, and Friedman PJ: Lymphomatoid granulomatosis, Hum Pathol 3:457, 1972.
49. Weis JW et al: Peripheral T-cell lymphomas: histologic, immunohistologic, and clinical characterization, Mayo Clin Proc 61:411, 1986.
50. Gaulard P et al: Lethal midline granuloma (polymorphic reticulosis) and lymphomatoid granulomatosis: evidence for a monoclonal T-cell lymphoproliferative disorder, Cancer 62:705, 1988.
51. Fauci AS et al: Lymphomatoid granulomatosis: prospective clinical and therapeutic experience over 10 years, N Engl J Med 306:68, 1982.
52. Saldana MJ et al: Pulmonary angiitis and granulomatosis: the relationship between histological features, organ involvement, and response to treatment, Hum Pathol 8:391, 1977.
53. Koss MN et al: Lymphomatoid granulomatosis: a clinico-pathologic study of 42 patients, Pathology 18:283, 1986.

54. Lipford EH et al: Angiocentric immunoproliferative lesions: a clinico-pathologic spectrum of post-thymic T-cell proliferations, Blood 72:1674, 1988.
55. Firstater E et al: Lymphomatoid granulomatosis with impaired cellular immunity: eight year survial without treatment, Chest 84:777, 1983.
56. Hamilton CR Jr, Shelley WM, and Tumulty PA: Giant cell arteritis: including temporal arteritis and polymyalgia rheumatica, Medicine (Baltimore) 50:1, 1971.
57. Ishikawa K: Natural history and classification of occlusive thromboarthropathy (Takayasu's disease), Circulation 57:27, 1978.
58. Klein RG: Large artery involvement in giant cell (temporal) arteritis, Ann Intern Med 83:808, 1975.
59. Harmin B: Polymyalgia arteritica, Acta Med Scand Suppl 533:1, 1972.
60. Andersson R et al: HLA-DR expression in the vascular lesion and circulating T lymphocytes of patients with giant cell arteritis, Clin Exp Immunol 73:82, 1988.
61. McDonnell PJ et al: Temporal arteritis: a clinico-pathologic study, Ophthalmology 83:518, 1986.
62. Healey LA and Wilske KR: Polymyalgia rheumatica and giant cell arteritis, West J Med 141:64, 1984.
63. Cid MC et al: Polymyalgia rheumatica: a syndrome associated with HLA-DR4 antigen, Arthritis Rheum 31:678, 1988.
64. Delecoeuillerie G et al: Polymyalgia rheumatica and temporal arteritis: a retrospective analysis of prognostic features and different corticosteroid regimens (11 year survey of 210 patients), Ann Rheum Dis 47:733, 1988.
65. DeSilva M and Hazleman BL: Azathioprine in giant cell arteritis/polymyalgia rheumatica: a double-blind study, Ann Rheum Dis 45:136, 1986.
66. Cupps TR and Fauci AS: Chapter 8: Giant cell arteritides. In The Vasculitides, Philadelphia, 1981, WB Saunders Co.
67. Marchioni N et al: Giant cell arteritis causing severe aortic regurgitation secondary to aneurysm of ascending aorta: a case report, Angiology J Vasc Dis 38:712, 1987.
68. Cappiello RA: Cholesterol emoblism: a pseudovasculitic syndrome, Semin Arthritis Rheum 18:240, 1989.
69. Dahlberg PJ, Lockhart JM, and Overholt EL: Diagnostic studies for systemic necrotizing vasculitis, Arch Intern Med 149:161, 1989.
70. Wees SH, Sunwoo IN, and OH SJ: Sural nerve in systemic necrotizing vasculitis, Am J Med 71:525, 1981.

Chapter 21

VASOSPASTIC DISEASES

Jay D. Coffman

Vasospastic diseases of the extremities include Raynaud's phenomenon, acrocyanosis, and livedo reticularis. Vasospasm implies reversible localized or diffuse vasoconstriction of arteries or smaller blood vessels. If the vasospasm is short-lived, the ischemia is reversible, and permanent damage does not result. Therefore patients may have vasospastic attacks for many years with no trophic changes of the digits. However, prolonged vasospasm with ischemia may lead to tissue damage with loss of subcutaneous tissue, ulcers, or gangrene. Raynaud's phenomenon, acrocyanosis, and livedo reticularis each occur in an idiopathic or primary form, that is, the underlying cause cannot be found. Usually the idiopathic varieties are benign and little permanent ischemic damage results. However, each of the entities may occur secondary to underlying conditions, and then the tissue damage can be extreme. Evidently, any disease, persistent vasoconstrictor stimulus, or constant trauma that causes damage to blood vessels or tissue may lead to one of the vasospastic syndromes, perhaps by the common mechanism of ischemia.

PRIMARY RAYNAUD'S DISEASE

Maurice Raynaud described Raynaud's phenomenon in 1888.[1] The clinical picture is characteristic with the occurrence of episodic attacks of well-demarcated discoloration of the digits brought on by cold. Between attacks, the digits appear normal, or they may be cool and moist.

Sex and age

Women are predominantly affected in a ratio of four females to one male.[2,3] The onset of the disease usually occurs in the second to fourth decade in both sexes.[2-4]

Prevalence

Studies of the prevalence of Raynaud's phenomenon in a general population have yielded estimates of 4.6% to 30% of randomly questioned people.[5-8] The largest survey[8] favors the smaller number but was performed in a warmer climate than other studies. These studies did not distinguish between primary and secondary Raynaud's phenomenon.

Pathology

There are few studies on the pathology of primary Raynaud's disease. Lewis found no abnormalities in the digital arteries in two patients with mild disease.[9] In patients with more severe disease intimal hyperplasia, narrowing or total occlusion of the digital arteries, or thrombi were present. Other studies[10,11] describe inflammatory destruction of the capillary bed or fibrinoid degeneration of the capillaries, and various abnormalities at the cellular level and in the basement membranes, but whether these were primary or secondary changes caused by the ischemic episodes is unknown. There are conflicting reports of abnormalities in the digital arteries by arteriography in patients with primary Raynaud's disease with some studies finding normal vasculature[12] and others reporting digital artery stenoses and occlusions.[13,14] It is probable that the digital arteries are normal in early primary Raynaud's disease.

Pathophysiology

In normal subjects digital blood flow is primarily controlled by the sympathetic nervous system. It is decreased by activation of the sympathetic nerves and increased by withdrawal of sympathetic activity. Reflex sympathetic digital vasoconstriction results from body cooling or application of cold to other parts of the body, which is absent in sympathectomized or nerve-blocked digits. In vitro experiments using pharmacologic agonists and antagonists on hand arteries and veins have shown that α_1-adrenoceptors and α_2-adrenoceptors are present.[15,16] In human subjects intra-arterial phenylephrine, an α_1-adrenoceptor agonist, and clonidine, an α_2-adrenoceptor agonist, produce dose-related decreases in total finger blood flow and increases in vascular resistance.[17] These responses are blocked by the appropriate antagonists. The α_2-adrenoceptors have been shown to be most important during reflex sympathetic vasoconstriction induced by body cooling.

In addition to the capillary circulation, human digits contain a large number of arteriovenous anastomoses, which directly connect the arterial with the venous circulation, bypassing the capillary bed. These shunts allow a very large blood flow to pass through the digits in a warm environment and to close during cold exposure, allowing the body to regulate its core temperature. They are mainly under the control of the sympathetic nervous system via the α_2-adrenoceptors.[17] During body cooling the arteriovenous shunts constrict, but capillary or nutritional blood flow is maintained in normal subjects.[18]

Serotonin may also be important in reflex sympathetic vasoconstriction induced by body cooling in normal subjects. In vitro pharmacologic studies have shown that 5-hydroxytryptamine$_2$ receptors (5-HT$_2$) are present in human hand arteries and veins.[16] In normal subjects intraarterial 5-HT produces a dose-dependent decrease in total finger blood flow and an increase in vascular resistance, which is blocked by a specific 5-HT$_2$ antagonist, ketanserin.[19] Ketanserin also causes a large increase in total finger blood flow during reflex sympathetic vasoconstriction, which is not related to α_1-adrenoceptor or α_2-adrenoceptor antagonism.

As is true of most vascular beds, digital blood flow is integrated and regulated by the central nervous system via the sympathetic nervous system. The arteriovenous anastomoses are controlled by the hypothalamus to regulate body temperature; emotional responses also occur through the hypothalamus. The latter receives messages from the cerebral cortex and passes them on to the pressor and depressor vasomotor centers in the medulla oblongata. Baroreceptors, chemoreceptors, and somatic afferent nerves also influence the vasomotor centers. Messages from the medulla travel in the intermediolateral cell columns to the sympathetic ganglia and then to the sympathetic nerves.

In a 28.3° C or 20° C room total finger blood flow is decreased in patients with primary Raynaud's disease compared with normal subjects.[20] The hand blood flow is also abnormally low in a 20° C room with the hand in 32° C water but hand blood flow rises to normal levels with body warming and with the hand in 42° C water.[21,22] Capillary blood flow in the finger is significantly less in both warm and cool environments in patients with primary and secondary Raynaud's phenomenon compared with that in normal subjects.[20] A decrease in capillary blood flow with body cooling in these patients contrasts with the lack of change in normal subjects. This decrease is very important since capillary flow provides the nutritional support for the tissues.

The cause of the decreased finger blood flow or vasospastic attacks of the digits in primary Raynaud's phenomenon is unknown. The two classic theories are a local fault, that is, an abnormality at the level of the digital artery and an overactivity of the sympathetic nervous system. Lewis[23] proposed the local fault theory after finding that local cooling produced ischemic attacks in a single finger and that attacks could be produced in sympathetically blocked fingers. He also showed that an ulnar nerve block, which blocks the sympathetic nerves, did not relieve vasospasm in the fifth finger. Jamieson, Ludbrook, and Wilson[24] found an enhancement of local cooling of the hand by reflex sympathetic vasoconstriction produced by ice application to the neck in patients with primary Raynaud's disease or scleroderma compared with normal subjects. They postulated that cold sensitized the α-adrenoceptor mediated vasoconstriction of vascular smooth muscle. In support of this hypothesis increased levels of α_2-adrenoceptors of platelets have been reported in patients with primary Raynaud's disease compared with normal subjects or patients with secondary Raynaud's phenomenon.[25] The local fault theory is logical but remains to be proved.

Lewis[23] also presented evidence that the vasospasm occurred in the digital arteries and not the arterioles. Cooling the proximal finger with the distal finger kept warm induced vasospastic attacks, and resolution of attacks occurred by proximal and not distal warming of the finger. Digital artery vasospasm is substantiated by a fall in digital systolic pressure to zero after fingers are cooled to temperatures below 15° C during occlusion of blood flow in most patients with primary Raynaud's disease, while normal subjects show a gradual reduction in systolic pressure.[26]

Raynaud[1] considered that an overactivity of the sympathetic nervous system was the cause of vasospastic attacks in Raynaud's phenomenon. In support of this theory is the fact that patients attain normal hand blood flow during body and hand warming[21,22] and have an exaggerated vasoconstrictor response of digital blood flow to changes in body posture, which is a sympathetic nervous system response.[27] In some patients, emotional stress induces attacks that could be explained by this theory but not by the local fault theory. Evidence against overactivity of the sympathetic nervous system is the recording by microelectrodes of normal sympathetic nerve activity with and without sympathetic stimulation,[28] a normal vasoconstriction of the ipsilateral hand to cooling of the opposite hand,[29] and normal blood and urine catecholamine levels in patients with primary Raynaud's disease.[30,31]

Associated factors are also important in either helping to induce or maintain digital vasospastic attacks but are probably not the definitive abnormality. Patients with primary Raynaud's disease have a lower brachial and finger systolic blood pressure and fingertip perfusion pressure than normal subjects.[32] This would result in a decreased arterial transmural distending force, and less external pressure would be required to stop blood flow.

However, not all subjects with low finger blood pressure have vasospastic attacks. Increased blood or plasma viscosity has been investigated as a causative factor in primary

Raynaud's disease but studies have been conflicting.[33-36] Viscosity is probably not of pathogenetic significance in the primary disease but may be important in secondary Raynaud's phenomenon because of cryoglobulinemia, polycythemia, and cold agglutinins. Serotonin has been implicated in vasospasm in some vascular beds in humans and animals and may be involved in the pathogenesis of Raynaud's phenomenon.[37] It may be important in persistence of vasospastic attacks but is probably not the instigating factor.[38]

A significant correlation of Raynaud's phenomenon and migraine headaches in patients with variant angina pectoris, which is considered to be caused by coronary artery vasospasm, has been reported.[39] Another example of possible vasospasm in more than one vascular bed is the rare condition of primary pulmonary hypertension and Raynaud's phenomenon with no underlying disease. A blood-borne or neurologic factor or a generalized functional abnormality of vascular smooth muscle has been postulated to explain generalized vasospasm.[40]

In secondary causes of Raynaud's phenomenon, decreased blood flow or blood pressure in the digits is usually present, which accounts for the vasospastic attacks. Low blood pressure occurs distal to digital or larger vessel obstructions or stenoses in connective tissue diseases, vinyl chloride disease, and obstructive arterial diseases. A decreased blood flow would occur from hyperviscosity in cryoglobulinemia and other blood abnormalities or from persistent vasoconstriction with drug therapy or sympathetic nerve irritation in the thoracic outlet syndrome. With a low digital blood flow or blood pressure, a normal sympathetic stimulus or external pressure on the digits could induce abrupt closure of blood vessels.

Clinical picture

Most patients have vasospastic attacks only in the fingers.[4] Less than half the patients also have attacks in the toes. Only a few patients have only the toes involved. The nose, ears, face, chest, and lips have been affected in some patients. When the disease first appears, only one or two fingers may be affected. Later, more fingers become involved and sometimes the toes; the thumbs are often spared.

Classically, the digits turn white or sometimes yellow and numb because of the cessation of blood flow. The hands are not involved. As slow blood flow returns, the digits turn blue because of the desaturation of the blood. When the digital arteries fully reopen, the digits become red from reactive hyperemia. During this last phase, a throbbing pain may occur. Pallor is often the only color change; the three-phase color change has been reported to occur in 4% to 65% of patients.[2,4,8] Exposure to cold is the precipitating factor of vasospastic attacks in all patients, but emotions may also cause attacks in some patients. In a large study reported in 1957, 13% of patients had ulcerations, chronic paronychia, necrosis, scarring, or fissuring of the fingers; sclerodactyly occurred in 12%.[4]

The patient's physical examination is normal except for cool digits and sometimes excess sweating of the hands. Radial, ulnar, dorsalis pedis, and posterior tibial pulses are present.

Diagnosis

The diagnosis of Raynaud's phenomenon can usually be made from the patient's description of the attacks. In primary Raynaud's disease, vasospastic attacks are usually difficult to induce in the physician's office. Well-demarcated, episodic white or blue discoloration of one or more digits or digital segments on exposure to cold is characteristic. The fingers may first turn white and numb, then blue, and finally bright red with throbbing pain as the circulation returns. This classic triad of colors is not always present; only one of the ischemic phases may occur or only two of the color changes.

After the physician is satisfied that a patient has Raynaud's phenomenon, then it must be determined if there is a secondary cause or if the syndrome is primary (idiopathic). In 1932 Allen and Brown[41] proposed the following criteria to distinguish primary from secondary Raynaud's phenomenon:

1. Vasospastic attacks precipitated by exposure to cold or emotional stimuli.
2. Bilateral involvement of the extremities.
3. Absence of gangrene or if present, limited to the skin of the fingertips.
4. No evidence of an underlying disease that could be responsible for vasospastic attacks.
5. A history of symptoms for at least 2 years.

These criteria may help in the diagnosis of primary Raynaud's disease, but connective tissue diseases, such as scleroderma, can develop several years after the onset of Raynaud's phenomenon. Involvement of the hands may occur in secondary cases of Raynaud's phenomenon but not in the primary disease. The criteria can be strengthened by measurement of antinuclear antibodies, sedimentation rate, and examination of nail fold capillaries. Secondary causes of Raynaud's phenomenon should be more actively sought in men, in women who develop vasospastic attacks after age 40, and in patients with sclerodactyly, ulcers, or gangrene.

Measurement of finger systolic blood pressure during ischemia combined with local cooling is a useful diagnostic test for Raynaud's phenomenon that has primary or secondary causes.[26] The digit is cooled by circulating water through a cuff around the proximal finger at 20° C, 15° C, 10° C, and 5° C for 5-minute intervals. To aid the finger to approximate the external temperature, blood flow is stopped by inflating another digital cuff to suprasystolic pressure during cooling. Patients with Raynaud's phenomenon have a greater reduction in finger systolic pressure or digital arterial closure at higher pressures than normal subjects following ischemic cooling. If the body is also cooled during the test, about 80% of patients show a positive response.[42] This test does not help differentiate primary from secondary Raynaud's phenomenon.

The capillaries of the skin of the nail fold can be visualized using a microscope or even an ophthalmoscope. They are spaced regularly with hairpin loops aligned along the axis of the digit. Patients with primary Raynaud's disease usually have a normal nail fold capillary pattern. In scleroderma, mixed connective tissue disease, and dermatomyositis there are a decreased number of capillaries that are enlarged and deformed, and avascular areas are present.[43] In systemic lupus erythematosus abnormal capillary loops are present and the subpapillary venous plexus is more prominent than in normal subjects. Other diseases may also have abnormal capillaries. The value of this test is that an abnormal capillary plattern indicates a secondary cause of Raynaud's phenomenon; a normal pattern is not diagnostic but favors the primary disease.

The sedimentation rate is normal in patients with primary Raynaud's disease and often elevated in the connective tissue diseases. However, it can be normal in the latter diseases. Therefore the value of measuring the sedimentation rate is to determine if it is elevated and then secondary causes of Raynaud's phenomenon should be sought.

The presence of antinuclear antibodies in patients with Raynaud's phenomenon usually indicates that a systemic disease is present or will manifest itself later. Elderly patients may have a titer as high as 1:64 without systemic disease, but younger patients rarely exceed 1:16. A speckled pattern is often present in scleroderma. Anticentromere antibodies are present in the majority of patients with CREST syndrome.[44] A homogeneous pattern of antinuclear antibodies with antibodies to desoxyribonucleic acid is often present in systemic lupus erythematosus. Antinuclear antibodies and rheumatoid factor may be present in other connective tissue diseases, and can also be induced by some drugs.

Since the majority of patients with Raynaud's phenomenon have the benign, primary disease, a young woman with no other symptoms and a normal physical exam should have a minimum laboratory workup.[45] If a complete blood count, sedimentation rate, urinalysis, and chest x-ray film show any abnormalities, a more extensive workup searching for a secondary cause should be instituted.

Prognosis

In a long-term study[4] of 307 patients with Raynaud's phenomenon, primary by the criteria of Allen and Brown,[41] 38% had stable disease, 36% improved, 16% became worse, and the syndrome disappeared in 10%. Sclerodactyly disappeared in 19 of 27 patients and was unchanged in 7 patients; it developed in 3.3%. Only 0.4%, or 2 patients, had digital amputations, but 13% had ulceration, chronic paronychia, necrosis of the skin, scarring, or fissuring. Tobacco smoking did not affect the prognosis. Symptoms were alleviated in just over half of the 44 patients who moved to a warmer climate. In another study[3] that included surgically treated patients, 40% remained the same, 48% had slight to severe progression, and 12% had regression or disappearance of vasospastic attacks. Medical or surgical treatment did not affect the prognosis.

The presence of sclerodactyly with Raynaud's phenomenon does not predict an adverse prognosis.[46] Of 71 patients with sclerodactyly and primary Raynaud's disease by the Allen and Brown criteria,[41] 28% improved, 22.5% deteriorated, and 40.8% were unchanged over an average 10-year follow-up study. Six patients died of unrelated causes. Scleroderma developed in only 4% (3 patients).

Evidently, connective tissue disease does not frequently develop over the ensuing years in patients diagnosed as having primary Raynaud's disease. Of 87 patients followed up for an average of 5.1 years after the onset of symptoms, 5% developed scleroderma of the CREST variety, although 17% of these patients had antinuclear antibodies.[47]

SECONDARY CAUSES OF RAYNAUD'S PHENOMENON

Raynaud's phenomenon may be caused by drugs; connective tissue diseases; constant trauma to the fingers; compression of nerves or blood vessels; obstruction of blood vessels; increased blood viscosity, or sludging of blood; vasculitis; or endocrine disorders. The most common causes are drugs and the connective tissue diseases.

Drugs

β-Adrenoceptor antagonists are the most common drugs inducing Raynaud's phenomenon. Both nonselective and cardioselective agents have been implicated[48] although β_2-adrenoceptors predominate in the peripheral circulation. Unlike primary Raynaud's disease, males and females are equally afflicted, and all ages may be affected.[49,50] There is no apparent relationship to dose. The incidence has been reported as 4.1% to 40% of patients taking these agents.[49-51] Almost every β-adrenoceptor blocking drug has been reported to cause vasospastic attacks. Substitution with β-blocking drugs with α-adrenoceptor antagonist[52] or intrinsic sympathetic activity does not always alleviate the syndrome. However, administration of β-adrenoceptor blocking agents to patients who already have Raynaud's phenomenon does not appear to aggravate the vasospastic attacks.[52,53] How these agents induce Raynaud's phenomenon is unknown, but the phenomenon may be caused by unopposed α-adrenoceptor vasoconstrictor activity, a decrease in cardiac output or blood volume with reflex vasoconstriction, or central cardiovascular depressant effects with increased reflex sympathetic vasoconstriction.

Ergot produces intense vasospasm of the digits and large blood vessels by stimulation of α-adrenoceptors. Ergot intoxication can occur from ingestion of rye contaminated with the fungus, *Claviceps purpurea*, but the most common cause is the use of ergotamine preparations for migraine headaches. Pathologic studies in humans have shown proliferation of the endothelium, thrombosis, hyaline degeneration, and fibrosis of the vascular wall in severe cases. Vasospasm occurs from excess doses of the drugs, usually greater than 10 mg per week.[54] Females are affected more frequently than males; the incidence of toxicity is 0.01% of patients using the drug. Digital, carotid, axillary, renal, coronary, ophthalmic, and splanchnic vessels may be involved.[55] Patients develop painful, cold, discolored extremities or intermittent claudication. Occasionally, an intense burning pain in the extremities called St. Anthony's fire occurs.[54] Only the large vessel pulses may be palpable. Gangrene may occur. The diagnosis is usually easily made by a careful history and physical exam. Arteriograms show uniform smooth tapering of large and medium size arteries, and the vessels often disappear at the forearm or calf level.[56] In patients who do not have limb-threatening vasospasm, conservative therapy with heparin and bed rest is the best course since the blood vessels usually relax within 3 days. Many drugs have been recommended for the more severe cases; intraarterial or intravenous nitroprusside with or without oral nifedipine is as successful as any regimen.[57,58]

Methysergide is a congener of lysergic acid diethylamide, which has both serotonin antagonist and agonist activity. About 3% of patients who take this drug for migraine headaches develop ischemia of the upper and lower extremities.[59] This complication may occur with as small a dose as 1 mg. The clinical manifestation and treatment are similar to ergot toxicity.

Vinblastine and bleomycin therapy for a variety of tumors may induce Raynaud's phenomenon in 2.6% to 37% of patients.[60,61] It is not known whether one or both agents is the cause. Vinblastine can cause neuropathy and bleomycin can cause cutaneous toxicity. Symptoms usually appear after 10 months of therapy. Arteriograms show diffuse digital arterial narrowing or multiple digital or palmar arterial occlusions. Symptoms may improve when chemotherapy is terminated, but many patients continue to have vasospastic attacks.[61]

Other drugs that have rarely been reported to induce Raynaud's phenomenon are bromocriptine, clonidine, imipramine, amphetamine, cyclosporine, and withdrawal from chronic nitroglycerin exposure. Oral contraceptives have also been incriminated, but the data are inconclusive.[62]

Connective tissue diseases

Scleroderma. Approximately 90% of patients with scleroderma (systemic sclerosis) have Raynaud's phenomenon or persistent digital vasospasm.[63] It is the initial complaint in almost 50% of patients. In the CREST syndrome Raynaud's phenomenon accompanies subcutaneous calcifications, esophageal motility abnormalities, skin thickening or tightness, and telangiectasias. More advanced cases of scleroderma may also have sclerodactyly, arthralgias or arthritis, and pulmonary or renal involvement. Digital ulcerations from ischemia of the fingertips is common in scleroderma but may also be caused by subcutaneous diffuse or localized calcifications. The claw finger deformity of the hands, caused by thickened skin and contracture of the phalangeal joints, is not diagnostic of scleroderma since only 3 of 71 patients with sclerodactyly observed for an average of 10 years developed the systemic disease.[46]

Laboratory studies in scleroderma can be normal. The sedimentation rate is increased in about two thirds of patients. Antinuclear antibodies are usually present in the advanced disease and are directed against a soluble nuclear antigen called SCL-70, nucleolar ribonucleic acid, or the centromere of chromosomes. The CREST syndrome usually has the anticentromere antibody,[64] while the other antibodies occur in the systemic disease. Barium swallow examination or esophageal manometry may reveal the motor abnormality, which is limited to the lower smooth muscle part of the esophagus. Chest x-ray films may show linear streaks of fibrosis in the basal areas of the lungs. Nailbed microscopic examination may reveal sparse, dilated, and convoluted capillaries and avascular areas. The preliminary criteria recommended by the American Rheumatism Association for the diagnosis of scleroderma are shown in the accompanying box. The cause of scleroderma is unknown. Pathologic studies show cutaneous edema and chronic inflammatory cells with homogeneous, acellular deposits of collagen in indistinct bundles. Capillaries may be sparse and arterioles may show hyaline. The cause of Raynaud's phenomenon is unknown, but the walls of small arteries and arterioles may be thickened, and also the blood vessels may be entrapped in nondistensible fibrous tissue.

Systemic lupus erythematosus. Raynaud's phenomenon has been reported in 10% to 44% of patients with systemic lupus erythematosus.[65,66] Systemic lupus erythematosus occurs mostly in women in their third to fourth

Preliminary criteria for classification of scleroderma*

Major criterion

Sclerodermа skin changes proximal to acral parts

Minor criteria

Sclerodactyly
Digital pitting scars
Bibasilar pulmonary fibrosis

*The presence of either the major criterion or two or more of the minor criteria determines the diagnosis.

From Masi AT and Rodnan GP: Preliminary criteria for the classification of systemic sclerosis (scleroderma), Arthritis Rheum 23:581, 1980.

American Rheumatism Association 1982 revised criteria for classification of systemic lupus erythematosus

For the purpose of identifying patients in clinical studies, a person shall be said to have the disease if any 4 or more of the following 11 criteria are present, serially or simultaneously, during any interval of observation.

- Malar rash (butterfly)
- Discoid rash
- Photosensitivity
- Oral ulcers
- Arthritis (nonerosive) in 2 or more peripheral joints
- Serositis (pleuritis or pericarditis)
- Persistent proteinuria (>0.5 g per day) or cellular casts
- Seizures or psychosis with no other cause
- Hemolytic anemia with reticulocytosis or leukopenia ($<4000/mm^3$ on two occasions) or lymphopenia ($<1500/mm^3$ on two occasions) or thrombocytopenia ($<100{,}000/mm^3$)
- Positive LE cell preparation or anti-DNA, anti-Sm, or false positive serologic test for syphilis for at least 6 months
- Abnormal titer of antinuclear antibody

Modified from Tan EM et al: The 1982 revised criteria for the classification of systemic lupus erythematosus, Arthritis Rheum 25:1271, 1982.

decade, and the disease is more common in blacks than whites. The vasospastic attacks may precede other disease manifestations but usually develop later in the course of the disease. This multisystem disease should be suspected in young women with Raynaud's phenomenon who have a photosensitive rash on the face in a butterfly pattern, arthralgias or arthritis, seizures, psychosis, alopecia, pericarditis, or nephritis. Criteria for the diagnosis of SLE recommended by the American Rheumatism Association are shown in the box above. Anemia, leukopenia, and thrombocytopenia are common. A circulating anticoagulant may cause a prolongation of the partial thromboplastin time. The sedimentation rate is usually elevated. Complement levels are often low. A large number of antibodies to nuclear and cytoplasmic constituents may be present and are usually homogeneous. Antibodies to double-stranded deoxyribonucleic acid (DNA) and Sm antigen are characteristic. The cause of systemic lupus erythematosus is unknown, but it is considered to be an autoimmune disease. Immune complexes are deposited in various organs and tissues, producing an inflammatory response. The pathologic picture is that of a vasculitis affecting arterioles and venules; fibrinoid necrosis of blood vessels is commonly present. In most cases it is believed the patient is reacting against his or her own tissues. Many popular drugs, including procainamide, isoniazid, and hydralazine, can induce a similar disease.

Rheumatoid arthritis. Raynaud's phenomenon may occur in rheumatoid arthritis. Focal ischemic lesions and microinfarctions also occur in the periungal areas and digital pulp. Pathologically, there may be an obliterative intimal proliferation of the digital arteries,[67] and arteriograms often show occlusions of one or more digital arteries.[68]

Sjögren's syndrome. Patients who develop Raynaud's phenomenon and who have dry eyes and mouth with enlargement of the salivary or lacrimal glands should be investigated for primary or secondary Sjögren's syndrome. The secondary syndrome occurs most frequently in rheumatoid arthritis and systemic lupus erythematosus. The majority of patients with primary Sjögren's syndrome have antibodies to SS-A antigen, and about 50% have antibodies to SS-B.[69] These antibodies are not frequent in rheumatoid arthritis but do occur in systemic lupus erythematosus. However, patients with primary Sjögren's syndrome rarely have antibodies to double-stranded DNA and lack sufficient clinical features for the diagnosis of systemic lupus erythematosus. Antibodies to salivary gland ducts occur in rheumatoid arthritis but not in primary Sjögren's syndrome.

Polymyositis and dermatomyositis. Polymyositis occurs more often in women in their fifth and sixth decades than it does in men, while dermatomyositis is more common in children. Patients develop symmetrical weakness of proximal muscles but may also have arthritis or arthralgias, an erythematous skin rash, dysphagia, dysarthria, and pulmonary fibrosis. Raynaud's phenomenon occurs in about one third of patients. A heliotrope or purplish discoloration of the upper eyelids is a characteristic finding. Elevated levels of creatine phosphokinase and aldolase are usually present. In polymyositis muscle fiber degeneration, necrosis, and fibrosis with a mononuclear cell infiltrate is seen by muscle biopsy, but sclerotic changes in small vessels and arterioles may be seen in dermatomyositis.[70]

Mixed connective tissue disease. Patients with mixed connective tissue disease have many features of other connective tissue diseases such as joint, muscle, pulmonary, and renal involvement.[71] Swelling of the dorsum of the hands and fingers with a sausage-shaped appearance of the digits is characteristic. Raynaud's phenomenon may precede other manifestations of the disease by many years; it may occur in up to 85% of patients. Antinuclear antibodies of a speckled pattern are often found, and a high titer of antibodies to extractable ribonuclease antigens is diagnostic. Rheumatoid factor and an increased sedimentation rate are also common. Raynaud's phenomenon may improve with steroid therapy.

Traumatic vasospastic disease

Raynaud's phenomenon may occur in people engaged in occupations in which their fingers are constantly exposed to trauma or vibratory tools. Traumatic vasospastic disease has also been called vibration-induced white fingers or Raynaud's phenomenon of occupational origin. Pneumatic hammers, chain saws, riveting machines, pounding and lasting machines, and brush saws are the most common offenders, but telephone operators, typists, pianists, meat cutters, and sewing machine operators have also been affected. Of workers who use vibratory tools 30% to 84% develop vasospastic symptoms,[72-74] usually after 6000 to 7000 hours of exposure.[75] The vasospastic attacks are manifested by blanching and numbness of the fingers, but pain and cyanosis are uncommon.[76] Both hands may be involved, but the feet are asymptomatic. Attacks are produced not only by exposure to the tools but also to cold. Gangrene or loss of fingers is rare.

Some investigators[77,78] consider that there is a syndrome of muscle and joint pain or weakness, hearing loss, headache, forgetfulness, fatigability, tinnitus, impotence, dizziness, and palmar hyperhidrosis with Raynaud's phenomenon. Pathologic studies of biopsies of fingers have shown a normal picture[76] or medial muscular hypertrophy and subintimal fibrosis of the digital vessels.[77] Angiography only showed tapered forearm arteries. The pathophysiology of traumatic vasospastic disease is unknown. Some improvement in symptoms may occur after cessation of tool exposure, but sensitivity to cold often remains.[79] Prognosis for recovery is better in brush saw than chain saw workers. Prevention of traumatic vasospastic disease includes training in the easiest way to use the tools, use of multiple layers of warm gloves inside an outer waterproof glove, and frequent changes of gloves if the hands become wet.[77] Using antivibratory saws and limiting the duration of tool use to 2 hours per day has decreased the incidence of the disease.[75] In an open study[80] diltiazem, 30 mg three times a day, decreased a variety of subjective symptoms and improved the rewarming time of hands immersed in 10° C water in patients with traumatic vasospastic disease.

Hypothenar hammer syndrome

About 2 cm distal to the wrist, the ulnar artery is protected only by skin, subcutaneous tissue, and the palmar brevis muscle. Trauma to the vessel by hammering with the palm of the hand, for instance, practicing karate and using bowling balls or walkers, may cause ulnar artery occlusion.[81-83] Patients with the hypothenar hammer syndrome can develop Raynaud's phenomenon involving one hand. Pallor or cyanosis with numbness occurs on exposure to cold, but a reactive hyperemia phase does not develop. The inciting trauma may not seem important to the patient, but calluses over the hypothenar eminences suggest the diagnosis. There may also be a tender mass in the area. Radial and ulnar pulses are normal at the wrist. Allen's test, which is done by compression of the radial artery while the patient exercises the hand above heart level, produces a pale hand that regains color on release of the radial artery. Normally, the ulnar artery would supply the hand, and the hand would retain normal color with radial artery occlusion. Doppler flow examination of the superficial palmar arch during compression of the radial artery will document that flow sounds disappear. About 1.7% of patients with Raynaud's phenomenon will have this entity[82]; men are mainly afflicted in their third to fifth decade. Pathologically, the ulnar artery is occluded and often aneurysmal. Angiography is diagnostic, showing thrombosis, irregularity, or aneurysm of the ulnar artery in the region of the hamate bone.[82,84] Multiple digital artery occlusions may also be present, which are probably the result of emboli. The treatment is initially conservative since symptoms often abate in a few months.[82] Resection of the diseased segment of artery,[83] sympathectomies or sympatholytic agents, and even fibrinolytic agents[85] have been used with some success.

Causes of the carpal tunnel syndrome

- Idiopathic
- Pregnancy
- Fractures or dislocations
- Bee stings
- Nonspecific tenosynovitis
- Median artery thrombosis
- Hemorrhage into the tunnel
- Anomalous or accessory muscles
- Systemic diseases
  - Arthritis (osteoarthritis, rheumatoid, and gout)
  - Sarcoidosis
  - Connective tissue diseases (scleroderma, lupus erythematosus, and polymyositis)
  - Amyloidosis (also in hemodialysis patients)
  - Diabetes mellitus
  - Hypothyroidism
  - Acromegaly
- Infections of forearm or hand
- Tumors (neuromas, fibromas, lipomas, and ganglions)

Carpal tunnel syndrome

Patients with the carpal tunnel syndrome complain of numbness, burning, or tingling in the first three fingers. Pain may radiate to the arm or shoulder. Symptoms are usually bilateral. Raynaud's phenomenon is commonly present and may precede other symptoms by 6 to 12 months.[86] Examination may reveal weakness and atrophy of muscles of the thenar eminence. Sensory changes only occur distal to the wrist, and usually only the first three fingers are involved. There are many causes of carpal tunnel syndrome (see the box above) but no underlying cause can be found in many patients. The carpal tunnel consists of the carpal bones covered by the transverse ligament running across the ventral surface of the wrist. Any increase in pressure in the tunnel by swelling, inflammation, or deposition or infiltration of tissue may compress the median nerve. The diagnosis is made by nerve conduction studies, which reveal prolonged sensory latencies of the median nerve and decrease sensory potentials in 85% to 95% of patients. Delayed motor latencies occur in few cases.[87] Reproduction of symptoms by tapping the median nerve at the wrist (Tinel's sign) or maximal wrist flexion (Phalen's sign) may be present but are not reliable tests.[88] Surgical decompression of the carpal tunnel by section of the transverse ligament is the preferred treatment with an 80% to 90% cure rate.[89] Injection of steroids into the tunnel,[90] splinting of the wrist, and vitamin B_6 have been advocated.[91] Diuretics may be of value in pregnancy.[92] The vasospastic attacks may or may not be helped by successful treatment of the entrapped nerve.

Thoracic outlet syndromes

As many as 38.6% of patients with the hyperabduction syndrome[93] and 5.3% of patients with different types of thoracic outlet syndromes[94] manifest Raynaud's phenomenon. The vasospastic attacks may be caused by compression of the sympathetic nerves in the thoracic outlet, but some patients have digital arterial emboli from thrombi in the subclavian artery.[95] There may be an aneurysmal dilation with thrombi distal to the point of subclavian artery compression. The thoracic outlet syndromes may be caused by compression of the neurovascular bundle by cervical ribs or the scalenus anticus muscle, between the first thoracic rib and clavicle (costoclavicular syndrome) or by the pectoralis minor tendon (hyperabduction syndrome). Cervical ribs occur in 0.5% to 1% of the population, but only 10% cause symptoms.[96]

When a cervical rib is present, the subclavian artery passes higher than usual as it leaves the thorax, making it susceptible to kinking or distortion. In the scalenus anticus syndrome, there may be a fibrous band at the border of the muscle, or the muscle may have an abnormal insertion. With cervical ribs or scalenus muscle syndrome, the subclavian vein is not affected because it lies anterior to the muscle. Adson's maneuver is used to detect these two entities.[97] The neck is fully extended with the chin turned toward the side being examined, and the patient holds a deep breath while the examiner palpates the radial pulse. Many patients without thoracic outlet syndromes diminish or lose the radial pulse, so only production of symptoms is diagnostic. Compression of the subclavian artery between the first rib and clavicle is detected by the production of symptoms or signs, while the patient pulls the shoulders backward and down into an exaggerated military position and takes a deep breath. In the hyperabduction syndrome, the arm is raised above head level and rotated away from the body to reproduce symptoms or signs. Production of a systolic bruit in the supraclavicular or infraclavicular areas with any of these maneuvers supports the diagnosis. Both the costoclavicular and hyperabduction syndromes may have arm swelling caused by subclavian vein compression.

When Raynaud's phenomenon is present, the manifestations are typical, with attacks induced by cold and emotions. It may involve one or both hands. Neurologic symptoms are much more frequent than vascular symptoms in these syndromes. Pain, numbness, and paresthesias of the neck, arm, or hand are usually present. The ulnar nerve distribution of symptoms and signs is most common because of the compression of nerves C8 and T1 in the brachial plexus. Symptoms usually develop in the fourth decade whether or not congenital or anatomic abnormalities are present; this may be caused by the drooping of the shoulder girdle with age. Certain positions such as reaching above the head, combing the hair, or sleeping on an arm may induce the symptoms. Physical findings are few, but supraclavicular or axillary area tenderness is common,[94] and systolic bruits may be present over the subclavian artery. Weakness of hand or arm muscles may be present.[98] Arterial pulses are usually normal.

The maneuvers just described are most useful in the diagnosis. A chest x-ray film can reveal the cervical ribs. Nerve conduction studies may or may not be abnormal.[99,100] Treatment of the thoracic outlet syndromes has alleviated or even cured some patients who had vasospastic attacks as a manifestation. Conservative therapy of exercises to strengthen the muscles of the shoulder girdle and improve posture should be prescribed first. Such exercises result in remarkable improvement in about 70% of patients.[101] Surgical treatment should be reserved for those for whom conservative measures fail since the results are variable. With careful selection, 80% to 95% of patients can have good to excellent results with various surgical procedures, and those with significant vascular symptoms or with cervical ribs may obtain the best relief.[94,98]

Cryoproteinemia, cold agglutinins, and polycythemia

Patients with cold agglutinins, polycythemia, or cryoproteinemia may develop Raynaud's phenomenon, probably because of the intravascular clumping of red blood cells or precipitated proteins decreasing or obstructing blood flow in small blood vessels. Of 100 patients with polycythemia vera, 3 had attacks of pallor of single digits, which were relieved by decreasing the blood volume,[102] but this is a rare cause of vasospastic attacks. Patients with Waldenström's macroglobulinemia have been reported to have Raynaud's phenomenon, but they may also have cryoglobulins.[103]

Patients with cryoglobulinemia develop purpura of the lower legs, joint pains, leg ulcers, renal failure, and occasionally Raynaud's phenomenon.[104] Ten percent of patients with essential cryoglobulinemia may have vasospastic attacks. The disease is twice as common in females as males, and symptoms usually occur in the patient's third or fourth decade. Secondary cryoglobulinemia may develop in a variety of disorders including infections, autoimmune or connective tissue diseases, lymphoproliferative disease, and liver disease. Occasionally, cryofibrinogens may also cause Raynaud's phenomenon.[105] The symptoms and signs of cryoglobulinemia are evidently caused by the precipitation of the proteins at low temperatures. The precipitates then act as immune complexes inciting an inflammatory reaction. However, the cryoglobulins may also increase blood and plasma viscosity, leading to a decrease in hand blood flow.[106] Cryoglobulinemia has been successfully treated with alkylating agents plus prednisone[107] or plasmapheresis[108] but not with prednisone alone.

Raynaud's phenomenon may occur in patients with cold agglutinins. Cold agglutinins may develop in viral infections or lymphomas. In elderly patients cold agglutinins may be found with no underlying disease and may cause cyanosis, hemolytic anemia, and hemoglobulinuria.[105] Males are affected twice as commonly as females, and patients are usually 30 to 90 years of age.[109] Cold agglutinins are antibodies of the γ-IgM type and are usually present in titers greater than 1:128 when symptoms and signs occur. Although Raynaud's phenomenon may occur, pallor or cyanosis may involve the whole hand. Necrosis and gangrene of the fingers may develop. The pathophysiology is caused by intravascular clumping of red blood cells with a blockage of blood flow in small vessels.[110] Treatment is nonspecific and depends on avoidance of cold. Chlorambucil will reduce the quantity of cold agglutinins, but it must be given for prolonged periods, and toxicity is a problem.

Vinyl chloride disease

Vinyl chloride exposure may cause a multisystem disease resembling scleroderma with thickening of the skin of the hands and forearms, nodule formation, thinning of bones, thrombocytopenia, hepatic and pulmonary dysfunction, and angiosarcoma of the liver.[111] Raynaud's phenomenon is common. The disease occurs mainly in workers who clean autoclaves. Circulating immune complexes occur in over 60% of symptomatic workers with a polyclonal increase in immunoglobulins, usually IgG.[112] Antinuclear antibodies may be present in low titers. Their fingernail beds show dilated capillary loops, disarray of capillary polarity, and avascular areas.[113] Angiography shows stenoses or occlusions of digital arteries.[114] Skin biopsies reveal thickened dermis, nonfibrillary homogenization of collagen, and swollen, thickened collagen. Treatment is removal from exposure to polyvinyl chloride.

Obstructive arterial diseases

Raynaud's phenomenon may occur in limbs affected by arteriosclerosis obliterans, thromboangiitis obliterans, or arterial emboli. In arteriosclerosis obliterans, usually only one or two toes of the affected extremity show attacks of pallor or cyanosis.[115] A reactive hyperemia phase does not occur. The diagnosis is made by the occurrence of vasospastic attacks only in the lower extremity of one limb, absence of pulses in the extremity, and usually a history of intermittent claudication. Raynaud's phenomenon may occur in as many as 57% of patients with thromboangiitis obliterans.[116] The cause of this disease is unknown, but it occurs most often in young male smokers, and episodes of superficial thrombophlebitis are frequent. Pathologically, there is inflammation of the walls of arteries and veins with secondary thromboses. The thrombi contain foci of leukocytes surrounded by giant cells. The lower extremities are affected most often, but the upper extremities may be involved in greater than 70% of patients. Digital ulcers and gangrene are common and the pain is often excruciating. Arteriography shows segmental involvement of medium to small arteries with intervening normal areas, absence of atheroma, and a tree-root pattern of collateral vessels springing from the thrombosed end of the arteries. Blood vessel biopsy during the acute stages is required for a definite diagnosis. Raynaud's phenomenon may occur in the fingers or toes in a limb or digit that has had a previous arterial embolus.

Reflex sympathetic dystrophy

Extreme, constant pain that persists after the healing phase of major or minor trauma, fractures, or surgery is termed reflex sympathetic dystrophy. Initially, the affected part is dry, swollen, and warm but then becomes persistently cold, swollen, and pale or cyanotic. Raynaud's phenomenon may occur in the latter stage. The cause is unknown, but it may be injured sensory nerve fibers transmitting constant signals to the spinal cord, which results in increased sympathetic outflow to the limb.[117] In support of this theory sympathectomy performed early in the course of reflex sympathetic dystrophy can result in a cure. Reflex sympathetic dystrophy can be a very disabling syndrome, preventing use of the extremity. Intensive physical therapy should be instituted. If this fails, pharmacologic sympathetic blocks may produce relief, although surgical sympathectomy may finally be necessary. Many other therapies have been recommended without consistent beneficial results.

Vasculitis

Any of the many diseases causing vasculitis may also cause Raynaud's phenomenon. They may manifest immune complexes, which can induce inflammatory reactions in small vessels. The connective tissue diseases, periarteritis nodosa and hepatitis B antigenemia, are examples.[118-120]

Arteriovenous fistula

Greater than 50% of patients with arteriovenous fistulas may manifest Raynaud's phenomenon.[121] Diminished blood flow and blood pressure distal to the fistula may result in peripheral coldness and trophic changes. Other factors than decreased blood flow may be involved, since an abnormal response of digital artery blood pressure to cooling occurs in the opposite hand.[122] Arteriovenous shunts are seen most frequently in patients who need hemodialysis. Renal transplantation has been reported to improve the cold sensitivity.

Renal disease

Patients with severe renal disease may have cool, cyanotic hands, and gangrene may develop. These patients often have calcification of their medium sized and digital arteries. Occlusions of radial and ulnar arteries have been shown by arteriography. The pathogenesis of the ischemia is unknown since medial calcification of blood vessels occurs in many patients with renal or other diseases without vasospastic manifestations. Parathormone, hypercalcemia, steroid or immunosuppressive therapy, and mechanical obstruction resulting from calcium deposition have been postulated as etiologically important.[123] Some patients have responded to parathyroidectomy.

Hypothyroidism

Raynaud's phenomenon is seen in some patients with hypothyroidism, and improvement has occurred with thyroid therapy.[124] The incidence may be as high as 24%.[125] The extremity blood flow is decreased in patients with myxedema. Their decreased heat production may induce peripheral vasoconstriction in an attempt to conserve body heat. It is also possible that thickening of the blood vessel walls by edema could lead to closure of blood vessels with normal sympathetic stimuli.

Neoplasms

Raynaud's phenomenon or digital ischemia and gangrene may occur in neoplastic diseases without the presence of cryoglobulinemia, cold agglutinins, carpal tunnel syndrome, or compression of the cervical sympathetic chain. These reports include cancers of the stomach, kidney, colon, ovary, cervix, and lung and leukemias. In one patient with a high level of γ-globulins, skin biopsy showed leukocytoclastic angiitis.[126] Fibrinoid necrosis, intimal proliferation, and inflammatory cell infiltration of the digital vessels, suggesting a vasculitis, were also described in another patient. Raynaud's phenomenon of 2 years' duration in a 59-year-old woman was resolved with resection of a small bowel adenocarcinoma and did not recur in the next 5 years.[127] In a review of 180 cases of malignancy associated with Raynaud's phenomenon over a 6-year period, 63 cases preceded tumor discovery by an average of 9.3 years.[127] Breast and lung cancer were the most common malignancies. Raynaud's phenomenon did not resolve in any patient after tumor resection. No information is given regarding abnormal proteins or metastases in these patients, so it is difficult to analyze the cause of the vasospastic attacks.

Heavy metals

Raynaud's phenomenon has been attributed to toxicity from lead, arsenic, thallium, and mercury. Substantial evidence has not been presented that they induce typical episodic vasospastic attacks.

Primary pulmonary hypertension

Several patients with primary pulmonary hypertension have been reported to have Raynaud's phenomenon but no other evidence of a systemic disease.[128,129] Marked intimal thickening or concentric proliferation has been described in pulmonary arterioles,[128] but skin or muscle biopsies have shown no vascular changes. An incidence of Raynaud's phenomenon of 10% to 30% has been reported in two series of patients with primary pulmonary hypertension.[130,131] Whether a separate disease entity of pulmonary hypertension and Raynaud's phenomenon exists is unknown, but it has been postulated that vasospasm may occur in both circulations because of a neurohumoral mechanism and that recurrent episodes of vasospasm could lead to pathologic changes in small blood vessels.[40]

Primary biliary cirrhosis

Patients with primary biliary cirrhosis who also have Raynaud's phenomenon, calcinosis cutis, telangiectasias, and thickened, tight skin resembling scleroderma have been described.[132,133] Skin biopsies have suggested scleroderma. Antinuclear antibodies are present in some, but not all, patients but can occur in primary biliary cirrhosis without scleroderma. Hepatitis B antigen is not present. A common immunologic mechanism has been suggested for both the liver and skin disease.

TREATMENT OF RAYNAUD'S PHENOMENON

Conservative therapy

Many patients who experience few vasospastic attacks never seek a physician's advice. Of those who do reassurance that the disease is benign and does not lead to loss of digits or limbs often suffices. It is always helpful to give patients a few suggestions on living with their problem. Mittens are better than gloves because the fingers can share their heat. Pressure plus cold is likely to induce attacks, for instance, holding cold steering wheels and iced drinks. Body plus hand chilling is also likely to cause attacks; shopping in the frozen food section of a supermarket is a good example. It should be explained to patients that they must keep the whole body warm, since chilling most parts of the body can lead to digital vasoconstriction. Although a connection with tobacco smoking has not been made for primary Raynaud's disease, smoking should be avoided, since nicotine causes cutaneous vasoconstriction via the sympathetic nervous system. There are various foot or hand warming devices, battery operated or chemical, that may be helpful to some patients.

Drug therapy

If, despite conservative therapy, vasospastic attacks interfere with the patient's daily activities or employment or if trophic digital lesions occur, drug treatment should be considered. However, drug therapy is nonspecific and often produces intolerable side effects. The most common agents used are calcium entry blockers or sympatholytic drugs.

Nifedipine is the calcium entry blocker with the most potent peripheral vasodilator action and has been shown to decrease the frequency, duration, and severity of vasospastic attacks in about two thirds of patients with Raynaud's phenomenon in several placebo-controlled studies.[134,135] Doses of 10 to 20 mg three times a day are used. Side effects include headache, dizziness, flushing, palpitations, edema, dyspepsia, and pruritus. Diltiazem in doses of 30 to 120 mg three times a day has also been reported to have favorable effects[136,137] although one study[138] failed to find a beneficial response. Side effects are fewer than with nifedipine and include headache, flushing, dizziness, nausea, and edema. Verapamil has not been shown to be of value.[139] Newer calcium entry blockers have not been adequately studied.

Reserpine and guanethidine are agents that interfere with sympathetic vasoconstriction and have been shown to increase digital capillary blood flow in Raynaud's phenomenon.[140-142] Adequate placebo-controlled studies have not been performed, but these agents have been used with benefit in patients with Raynaud's phenomenon.[142] Both drugs must be carefully titrated to the relief of symptoms or the production of side effects to be sure an adequate dose is being used. For reserpine, 0.125 to 0.5 mg daily is recommended. Intraarterial reserpine has also been used but probably is no more beneficial than oral administration.[143] Side effects of reserpine are bradycardia, postural hypotension, dyspepsia, edema, lethargy, and depression. It should never be given to a depressed patient or a patient with a history of depression. Recommended doses of guanethidine are 10 to 50 mg daily, and side effects are diarrhea, postural hypotension, and impotence. It can be used in patients with depression. One advantage of reserpine and guanethidine is once-daily administration.

Prazosin is an α_1-adrenoceptor antagonist that has been shown to decrease the frequency, duration, or severity of vasospastic attacks in patients with Raynaud's phenomenon in placebo-controlled studies.[144,145] The favorable effects are moderate and occur in about two thirds of patients. However, improvement may dissipate with time.[144] Recommended doses are 2 to 8 mg daily. Side effects of nausea, headache, palpitations, dizziness, fatigue, edema, dyspnea, rash, and diarrhea often prevent its use. Phenoxybenzamine is a potent α-adrenoceptor blocking agent, which has been recommended for the treatment of Raynaud's phenomenon.[146,147] Placebo-controlled studies have not been performed. Usual dosage has been 10 to 30 mg four times a day. Side effects often preclude its use and include postural hypotension, nasal congestion, palpitations, impotence, and gastrointestinal symptoms. Methyldopa, which decreases peripheral sympathetic vasoconstriction by stimulation of central inhibitory α-adrenoceptors, has been used in patients with Raynaud's phenomenon. In an uncontrolled study[148] 75% of patients improved with 1 to 2 g daily, while no benefit was apparent at an average dose of 704.3 mg daily in a study[149] comparing it with other drugs. Side effects are edema, drowsiness, headache, postural hypotension, diarrhea, nasal congestion, and rarely fever and hemolytic anemia.

Tolazoline is an α-adrenoceptor antagonist with a histamine-like effect, which increases skin blood flow. It has been recommended for the treatment of Raynaud's phenomenon in doses of 25 to 100 mg daily.[40] Placebo-controlled studies have not been performed. The oral preparation of tolazoline is no longer available in the United States.

Nitroglycerin is a direct acting vasodilator, which has been used as an ointment in the treatment of Raynaud's disease for many years. Nitroglycerin ointment, compared with lanolin placebo, improved patients in one study of patients with secondary Raynaud's phenomenon, who were on maximally tolerated doses of sympatholytic agents.[150] Reports of the use of transdermal nitropaste plasters in Raynaud's phenomenon have indicated variable results.[151,152] Headache often precludes the use of nitroglycerin preparations and postural hypotension and paresthesias may also occur.

Prostaglandins, which induce vasodilation and inhibit platelet aggregation are being used in severe Raynaud's phenomenon, but must be given intravenously. A multicenter study of PGE_1 found no benefit over placebo[153] in patients with primary or secondary Raynaud's. Studies of prostacyclin (PGI) are more promising with long-term beneficial effects after the infusions are stopped.[154,155] Hypotension, headache, facial flushing, abdominal colic, nausea, vomiting, and diarrhea may occur during the infusions.

Ketanserin is a selective 5-hydroxytryptamine$_2$ antagonist and has some α_1-adrenoceptor blocking activity. It inhibits the vasoconstriction and platelet aggregation caused by serotonin. In several placebo-controlled studies, ketanserin in a daily dose of 80 to 120 mg orally has been reported to improve or have no benefit in patients with Raynaud's phenomenon.[156-158] In the largest multicenter study performed in patients with Raynaud's phenomenon, ketanserin significantly decreased the frequency of, but not the duration or severity of, vasospastic attacks.[159] Patients and their physicians rated the drug better than placebo. Side effects of ketanserin are dizziness, sedation, edema, dry mouth, and anxiety. It also may prolong the QT interval.

Captopril inhibits the enzyme converting angiotensin I to angiotensin II and kinase II, allowing bradykinin to accumulate. It has been reported to improve patients with primary or secondary Raynaud's phenomenon in uncontrolled studies.[160-162] It is effective treatment for the hypertension occurring in some patients with scleroderma but needs to be studied with suitable controls in the treatment of Raynaud's phenomenon.

Other vasodilator drugs, including niacin derivatives, papaverine, cyclandelate, griseofulvin, and isoxsuprine, have not been shown to be of benefit in Raynaud's phenomenon.

Plasmapheresis

Plasma exchange has been reported as beneficial in patients with severe Raynaud's phenomenon.[163] In one study[164] it was superior to placebo tablets or intermittent intravenous heparin therapy. Plasma exchange has not been studied adequately by other groups.

Conditioning and biofeedback

Pavlovian conditioning has been used to treat patients with Raynaud's phenomenon.[165] Patients immerse their hands in 43° C water while their bodies are exposed to 0° C temperature for about 30 minutes a day. Patients with Raynaud's phenomenon, compared with normal subjects, showed a significant increase in finger temperature during cold exposure. Patients also reported subjective benefit, which sometimes lasted 9 to 12 months.

Many forms of biofeedback have been used to treat patients with Raynaud's phenomenon,[166-168] and patients generally show improvement. The type of behavioral therapy does not seem to make a difference although finger temperature feedback has been most successful in some studies.

Pavlovian conditioning or biofeedback may benefit some patients and have no side effects. They are therefore worth a trial if the patient is willing to spend the time involved.

Sympathectomy

Sympathectomy of the upper extremities may benefit 50% to 60% of patients with Raynaud's phenomenon.[169-172] However, vasospastic attacks often recur within 6 months to 2 years.[173,174] Lumbar sympathectomy for Raynaud's phenomenon in the toes is successful in over 80% of patients and the results persist longer.[169,175] In the upper extremities, sympathetic vasoconstrictor activity often returns after sympathectomy. This has been attributed to incomplete denervation, reinnervation, or denervation hypersensitivity. The evidence is strong that sympathetic activity returns, but the mechanism is unknown.

SUMMARY

Most patients with Raynaud's phenomenon, especially the primary disease, will respond to conservative measures and reassurance. Conditioning or biofeedback may be helpful for some patients but is time consuming. When drug therapy is necessary, nifedipine, guanethidine, or reserpine yield the most beneficial effects if the side effects can be tolerated. Prazosin, diltiazem, and dibenzyline may give some relief. Ketanserin and prostacyclin are promising therapeutic agents. The benefits of plasmapheresis need more documentation. Sympathectomy is not indicated in Raynaud's phenomenon.

ACROCYANOSIS

Patients whose hands and feet became blue on exposure to cold were described by Crocq[176] in 1896. Patients with acrocyanosis have persistent cyanosis and coldness of the digits in the hands and feet, and sometimes the distal arms, face, and ears are involved. The blueness intensifies with cold and is relieved by warming.[177,178] Trophic changes such as ulceration, severe pain, or contractures do not occur. In some patients, edema and excess sweating of the hands and feet may occur.[177] Idiopathic acrocyanosis is a benign condition that is mainly a cosmetic problem to patients. Secondary acrocyanosis may occur in association with connective tissue diseases or any disease complicated by central cyanosis.

The cause of idiopathic acrocyanosis is unknown. Only one study[177] reported pathologic findings of skin biopsies. Findings were nonspecific with thickening of the medial layers of the arterioles. Nail fold capillary studies have shown dilated capillary loops, a decreased number of capillaries, and an inhomogeneous capillary flow.[179,180] The pathophysiology evidently involves arteriolar spasm, but the reason is not known. Elevation of the cyanotic hand above heart level produces pallor, ruling against venous obstruction.[181] With body heating the temperature of the fingers becomes normal and reactive hyperemia of the fingers is normal, ruling against structural arterial disease. Also, ulnar nerve blockade relieves cyanosis in the fifth finger. Since the color of the digit did not change until the temperature of the digit rose 7° C, the digital arteries probably opened before the arterioles. Patients have normal hand blood flows during local warming to 42° C but low blood flow at 32° C.[178,182] In one child the cyanotic limbs became warm and red during sleep. This was considered evidence for an abnormal vascular response originating in the central nervous system and against a local hypersensitivity of digital blood vessels to cold.[183]

The incidence of acrocyanosis is unknown, and there is no sex predominance. The age range in one study was 20 to 45 years.[177] Physical examination and laboratory studies are normal.

The differential diagnosis of acrocyanosis is Raynaud's phenomenon, connective tissue diseases, and central cyanosis. In Raynaud's phenomenon, the vasospastic attacks are episodic, the color changes are only in the fingers and are well-demarcated, and females are predominantly affected. History, physical examination, and laboratory tests will rule out the connective tissue diseases. If central cyanosis is suspected, it can be confirmed by an arterial oxygen saturation measurement.

Treatment is usually unnecessary since this is a benign disease. For the few patients who request therapy, small doses of reserpine or guanethidine may relieve some of the manifestations.

LIVEDO RETICULARIS

There are at least three types of livedo reticularis. The benign form is a mottled discoloration of the extremities and sometimes the trunk of the body in a reticular or lacelike pattern. It is intensified by cold exposure and relieved by warming. Besides livedo reticularis, this form has also been called cutis marmorata, livedo racemosa, livedo annularis, sympathetic or idiopathic livedo reticularis, and aphyxia reticularis. Livedo reticularis with ulceration (livedo vasculitis, livedoid vasculitis, atrophie blanche en plaque) is either a vasculitis or vascular thrombosis causing the same skin pattern but is usually irreversible with warming. Secondary livedo reticularis occurs in connective tissue diseases and with the use of amandatine hydrochloride.

Pathologic findings in the benign form are nonspecific although increased numbers of dilated capillaries may be present.[184,185] In livedo reticularis with ulceration, a segmental hyalinizing vasculitis affects the middle dermal vessels.[184,186,187] Infarcts of the skin are caused by obstructed arterioles. Some investigators believe that thrombosis of arterioles resulting from blood or tissue abnormalities causes the disease rather than vasculitis, since a defect in the fibrinolytic system and abnormalities of platelet aggregation may be present.[188-191]

The reticular pattern on the skin is considered to be secondary to vasospasm or obstruction of small perpendicular arterioles in the dermis.[192] The red to blue periphery of each reticulum is caused by deoxygenated blood in the surrounding horizontally arranged venous plexuses.[193] Increased sympathetic nervous system activity is considered to cause the benign form because it is reversible by warming and use of sympathetic blocking agents. Arteriolar obstruction caused by vasculitis or thrombosis may cause livedo reticularis with ulceration. Amantadine releases norepinephrine from nerves and enhances the action of norepinephrine and dopamine on peripheral vessels, which could cause arteriolar vasoconstriction.[194]

Benign livedo reticularis is common in women during their second to fifth decades. Livedo reticularis with ulceration is rare and also more common in women but in their third to fifth decades.[195]

Except for the rose, red, violet, or blue color of the lacelike reticular pattern and coldness of the extremities and sometimes the trunk, physical examination in benign livedo reticularis is normal. In livedo reticularis with ulceration, besides the reticular pattern, purpuric macular lesions and cutaneous nodules develop and progress to ulcers. These ulcers usually occur in the winter but some patients develop them in the summer.[187] Edema occurs in about half the patients often before ulcers appear. The ulcers are very painful and take months to heal. Most ulcers occur on the calves, ankles, and feet. Healed ulcers leave a smooth ivory-white plaque of atropic skin surrounded by hyperpigmented borders with telangiectatic blood vessels, which led to the name "atrophie blanche."

Secondary livedo reticularis occurs with diseases that cause decreased blood flow to the skin, for instance, connective tissue diseases, polyarteritis nodosa, hyperviscosity states, cryoglobulinemia, thrombocythemia, atheromatous emboli, obstructive arterial diseases, endocrine disorders, infections, and neurogenic diseases. Sneddon's syndrome is characterized by livedo reticularis with cerebrovascular lesions causing transient ischemic attacks or strokes.[196] Also groups of patients have been described with lupus erythematosus, arterial or venous thromboses, spontaneous abortions, livedo reticularis, and anticardiolipin antibodies.[197] Anticardiolipin antibodies may be the cause of these syndromes and precede other clinical and laboratory manifestations of lupus erythematosus by several years.[198]

Amantadine hydrochloride causes a benign form of livedo reticularis and is not a reason for stopping the medication.[199,200] It usually affects the legs of both sexes, and pedal edema may occur. It disappears 2 to 6 weeks after the drug is stopped.

There are no consistently abnormal laboratory tests in benign livedo reticularis or livedo reticularis with ulceration. The prognosis of the benign disease is excellent since it is only a cosmetic problem. Recurrent, painful ulcerations may occur for years in patients with livedo reticularis with ulceration.[186] Amputations have been rarely done for deep, unhealing ulcers or severe pain.[184,186]

No treatment is necessary in benign livedo reticularis. Treatment for livedo reticularis from underlying diseases is that of the associated disease. Many therapies have been recommended for patients with livedo reticularis with ulceration attesting to the fact that treatment is usually unsuccessful. Antiplatelet therapy with aspirin, dipyridamole, or triclopidine have benefited some patients[189,190] as has nicotinic acid[195] and sympathetic blocking drugs.[195,201] Fibrinolysis promoting agents have also sometimes been of benefit.[191] Some patients do not respond to any therapy and remissions often occur without treatment so that it is difficult to evaluate the uncontrolled studies. Controlled trials have not been performed because of the rarity of the disease.

REFERENCES

1. Raynaud M: On local asphyxia and symmetrical gangrene of the extremities, London, 1888, The Syndenham Society (Translated by T. Barlow).
2. Hines EA Jr and Christensen NA: Raynaud's disease affecting men, JAMA 129:1, 1945.
3. Blain A, Coller FA, and Carver GB: Raynaud's disease: a study of criteria for prognosis, Surgery 29:387, 1951.
4. Gifford RW Jr and Hines EA Jr: Raynaud's disease among women and girls, Circulation 16:1012, 1957.
5. Lewis T and Pickering GW: Observations upon maladies in which the blood supply to digits ceases intermittently or permanently and

upon bilateral gangrene of digits: observations relevant to so-called Raynaud's disease, Clin Sci 1:327, 1934.
6. Olsen N and Nielsen SL: Prevalence of primary Raynaud phenomena in young females, Scand J Clin Lab Invest 37:761, 1978.
7. Heslop J, Coggon D, and Acheson ED: The prevalence of intermittent digital ischaemia (Raynaud's phenomenon) in a general practice, J Royal Coll Gen Pract 33:85, 1983.
8. Maricq HR et al: Prevalence of Raynaud's phenomenon in the general population, J Chron Dis 39:423, 1986.
9. Lewis T: The pathological changes in the arteries supplying the fingers in warm-handed people and in cases of so-called Raynaud's disease, Clin Sci 3:288, 1938.
10. Burch GE, Harb JM, and Sun CS: Fine structure of digital vascular lesions in Raynaud's phenomenon and disease, Angiology 30:361, 1979.
11. Vajda K et al: Ultrastructural investigations of finger pulp biopsies: a study of 31 patients with Raynaud's syndrome, Ultrastruct Pathol 3:175, 1982.
12. Jeune R and Thivolet J: Etude arteriographique de la main au cours de 52 phenomenes de Raynaud d'etiologie diverse, Nouve Presse Med 7:2619, 1978.
13. Porter JM et al: The clinical significance of Raynaud's phenomenon, Surgery 80:756, 1976.
14. Laws JW, Lillie JG, and Scott JT: Arteriographic appearances in rheumatoid arthritis and other disorders, Br J Radiol 36:477, 1963.
15. Stevens MJ and Moulds RFW: Heterogeneity of post-junctional α-adrenoceptors in human vascular smooth muscle, Arch Int Pharmacodyn Ther 254:43, 1981.
16. Arneklo-Nobin B and Owman C: Adrenergic and serotonergic mechanisms in human hand arteries and veins studied by fluorescence histochemistry and in vitro pharmacology, Blood Vessels 22:1, 1985.
17. Coffman JD and Cohen RA: Role of alpha-adrenoceptor subtypes mediating sympathetic vasoconstriction in human digits, Eur J Clin Invest 18:309, 1988.
18. Coffman JD: Total and nutritional blood flow in the finger, Clin Sci 42:243, 1972.
19. Coffman JD and Cohen RA: Serotonergic vasoconstriction in human fingers during reflex sympathetic response to cooling, Am J Physiol 254:H889, 1988.
20. Coffman JD and Cohen AS: Total and capillary blood flow in Raynaud's phenomenon, N Engl J Med 285:259, 1971.
21. Peacock JH: A comparative study of the digital cutaneous temperatures and hand blood flows in the normal hand, primary Raynaud's disease, and primary acrocyanosis, Clin Sci 18:25, 1959.
22. Peacock JH: Vasodilatation in the human hand: observations on primary Raynaud's disease and acrocyanosis of the upper extremities, Clin Sci 17:575, 1957.
23. Lewis T: Experiments relating to the peripheral mechanism involved in spasmodic arrest of the circulation in the fingers, a variety of Raynaud's disease, Heart 15:7, 1929.
24. Jamieson GG, Ludbrook J, and Wilson A: Cold hypersensitivity in Raynaud's phenomenon, Circulation 44:254, 1971.
25. Edward JM et al: α_2-Adrenergic receptor levels in obstructive and spastic Raynaud's syndrome, J Vasc Surg 5:38, 1987.
26. Nielsen SL: Raynaud phenomenon and finger systolic pressure during cooling, Scand J Clin Lab Invest 38:765, 1978.
27. Olsen N, Petring OU, and Rossing N: Exaggerated postural vasoconstrictor reflex in Raynaud's phenomenon, Br Med J 294:1186, 1987.
28. Fagius J and Blumberg H: Sympathetic outflow to the hand in patients with Raynaud's phenomenon, Cardiovasc Res 19:249, 1985.
29. Downey JA and Frewin DB: The effect of cold on blood flow in the hands of patients with Raynaud's phenomenon, Clin Sci 44:279, 1973.
30. Kontos HA and Wasserman AJ: Effect of reserpine in Raynaud's phenomenon, Circulation 39:259, 1969.
31. Nielsen SL et al: Raynaud's phenomenon: peripheral catecholamine concentration and effect of sympathectomy, Acta Chir Scand 502:57, 1980.
32. Cohen RA and Coffman JD: Reduced fingertip arterial pressures in Raynaud's disease, J Vasc Med Biol 1:21, 1989.
33. Pringle R, Walder DM, and Weaver JPA: Blood viscosity and Raynaud's disease, Lancet 1:1086, 1965.
34. Goyle KB and Dormandy JA: Abnormal blood viscosity in Raynaud's phenomenon, Lancet 1:1317, 1976.
35. McGrath MA, Peck R, and Penny R: Raynaud's disease: reduced hand blood flows with normal blood viscosity, Aust N Z J Med 8:126, 1978.
36. Ayres ML, Jarrett PEM, and Browse NL: Blood viscosity, Raynaud's phenomenon and the effect of fibrinolytic enhancement, Br J Surg 68:51, 1981.
37. Halpern A et al: Raynaud's disease, Raynaud's phenomenon, and serotonin, Angiology 11:151, 1960.
38. Seibold JR and Terregino CA: Selective antagonism of S_2-serotonergic receptors relieves but does not prevent cold-induced vasoconstriction in primary Raynaud's phenomenon, J Rheumatol 13:337, 1986.
39. Miller D et al: Is variant angina the coronary manifestation of a generalized vasospastic disorder? N Engl J Med 304:763, 1981.
40. Coffman JD and Cohen RA: Vasospasm: ubiquitous? N Engl J Med 304:780, 1981.
41. Allen EV and Brown GE: Raynaud's disease: a critical review of minimal requisites for diagnosis, Am J Med Sci 183:187, 1932.
42. Carter SA, Dean E, and Kroeger EA: Apparent finger systolic pressures during cooling in patients with Raynaud's syndrome, Circulation 77:988, 1988.
43. Maricq HR et al: Diagnostic potential of in vivo capillary microscopy in scleroderma and related disorders, Arthritis Rheum 23:183, 1980.
44. Kallenberg CGM et al: Antinuclear antibodies in patients with Raynaud's phenomenon: clinical significance of anticentromere antibodies, Ann Rheum Dis 41:382, 1982.
45. Coffman JD: Evaluation of the patient with Raynaud's phenomenon, Postgrad Med 78:175, 1985.
46. Farmer RG, Gifford RW Jr, and Hines EA Jr: Raynaud's disease with sclerodactylia, Circulation 23:13, 1961.
47. Gerbracht DD et al: Evolution of primary Raynaud's phenomenon (Raynaud's disease) to connective tissue disease, Arthritis Rheum 28:87, 1985.
48. Wollersheim H et al: Influence of cold challenge on finger skin temperature during long-term use of beta-adrenoceptor blocking drugs in hypertensive patients, Int Angiol 6:307, 1987.
49. Marshall AJ, Roberts CJC, and Barritt DW: Raynaud's phenomenon as side effect of beta-blockers in hypertension, Br Med J 1:1498, 1976.
50. Feleke E et al: Complaints of cold extremities among patients on antihypertensive treatment, Acta Med Scand 213:381, 1983.
51. VandenBurg MJ et al: Is the feeling of cold extremities experienced by hypertensive patients due to their disease or their treatment? Eur J Clin Pharmacol 27:47, 1984.
52. Steiner JA, Cooper R, Gear JS, Ledingham JGG: Vascular symptoms in patients with primary Raynaud's phenomenon are not exacerbated by propranolol or labetalol. Br J Clin Pharmacol 7:401, 1979.
53. Coffman JD and Rasmussen HM: Effects of β-adrenoceptor blocking drugs in patients with Raynaud's phenomenon, Circulation 72:466, 1985.
54. Cameron EA and French EB: St. Anthony's fire rekindled: gangrene due to therapeutic dose of ergotamine, Br Med J 2:28, 1960.
55. Greene FL, Ariyan S, and Stansel HC Jr: Mesenteric and peripheral

vascular ischemia secondary to ergotism, Surgery 81:176, 1977.
56. Bagby RJ and Cooper RD: Angiography in ergotism, Am J Roent 116:179, 1972.
57. Carliner NH et al: Sodium nitroprusside treatment of ergotamine-induced peripheral ischemia, JAMA 227:308, 1974.
58. Dagher FJ et al: Severe unilateral ischemia of the lower extremity caused by ergotamine: treatment with nifedipine, Surgery 97:369, 1985.
59. Graham JR: Methysergide for prevention of headache, N Engl J Med 270:67, 1964.
60. Vogelzang NJ et al: Raynaud's phenomenon: a common toxicity after combination chemotherapy for testicular cancer, Ann Intern Med 95:288, 1981.
61. Teutsch C, Lipton A, and Harvey HA: Raynaud's phenomenon as a side effect of chemotherapy with vinblastine and bleomycin for testicular carcinoma, Cancer Treat Reports 61:925, 1977.
62. Birnstingl M: The Raynaud syndrome, Postgrad Med J 47:297, 1971.
63. Tuffanelli DL and Winkelmann RK: Systemic scleroderma: a clinical study of 727 cases, Arch Dermatol 84:359, 1961.
64. Fritzler MJ and Kinsella TD: The CREST syndrome: a distinct serologic entity with anticentromere antibodies, Am J Med 69:520, 1980.
65. Tuffanelli DL and Dubois EL: Cutaneous manifestations of systemic lupus erythematosus, Arch Dermatol 90:377, 1964.
66. Hochberg MC et al: Systemic lupus erythematosus: a review of clinico-laboratory features and immunogenetic markers in 150 patients with emphasis on demographic subsets, Medicine 64:285, 1985.
67. Scott JT et al: Digital arteries in rheumatoid disease, Ann Rheum Dis 20:224, 1961.
68. Laws JW, Lillie JG, and Scott JT: Arteriographic appearance in rheumatoid arthritis and other disorders, Br J Radiol 36:477, 1963.
69. Fox RI et al: Primary Sjögren syndrome: clinical and immunopathologic features, Semin Arthritis Rheum 14:77, 1984.
70. Boyland RC and Sokoloff L: Vascular lesions in dermatomyositis, Arthritis Rheum 3:379, 1960.
71. Sharp GC: Mixed connective tissue disease, Bull Rheum Dis 25:828, 1975.
72. Futatsuka M et al: Comparative study of vibration disease among operators of vibratory tools by factor analysis, Br J Ind Med 42.260, 1985.
73. Theriault G et al: Raynaud's phenomenon in forestry workers in Quebec, Can Med Assoc J 126:1404, 1982.
74. Hellstrom B and Andersen KL: Vibration injuries in Norwegian forest workers, Br J Ind Med 29:255, 1972.
75. Futatsuka M and Ueno T: Vibration exposure and vibration-induced white finger due to chain saw operation, J Occup Med 27:257, 1985.
76. Gurdjian ES and Walker LW: Traumatic vasospastic disease of the hand (white fingers), JAMA 129:668, 1945.
77. Ashe WF, Cook WT, and Old JW: Raynaud's phenomenon of occupational origin, Arch Environ Health 5:333, 1962.
78. Miyashita K et al: Epidemiological study of vibration syndrome in response to total hand-tool operating time, Br J Ind Med 40:92, 1983.
79. Ekenvall L and Carlson A: Vibration white finger: a follow up study, Br J Ind Med 44:476, 1987.
80. Matoba T, Ogata M, and Kuwahara H: Diltiazem and Raynaud's syndrome, Ann Intern Med 97:445, 1982.
81. Little JM and Ferguson DA: The incidence of the hypothenar hammer syndrome, Arch Surg 105:684, 1972.
82. Vayssairat M et al: Hypothenar hammer syndrome: seventeen cases with long-term follow-up. J Vasc Surg 5:538, 1987.
83. Millender LH, Nalebuff EA, and Kasdon E: Aneurysms and thromboses of the ulnar artery in the hand, Arch Surg 105:686, 1972.
84. Conn J Jr, Bergan JJ, and Bell JL: Hypothenar hammer syndrome: post-traumatic digital ischemia, Surgery 68:1122, 1970.
85. Pineda CJ et al: Hypothenar hammer syndrome, Form of reversible Raynaud's phenomenon, Am J Med 79:561, 1985.
86. Serra G, Migliore A, and Tugnoli V: Raynaud's phenomenon and entrapment neuropathies, Ann Neurol 18:519, 1985.
87. Stevens JC: The electrodiagnosis of carpal tunnel syndrome, Muscle Nerve 10:99, 1987.
88. Heller L et al: Evaluation of Tinel's and Phalen's signs in diagnosis of the carpal tunnel syndrome, Eur Neurol 25:40, 1986.
89. Taylor N: Carpal tunnel syndrome, Am J Phys Med 50:192, 1971.
90. Gelberman RH, Aronson D, and Weisman MH: Carpal-tunnel syndrome, J Bone Joint Surg 62A:1181, 1980.
91. Ellis JM et al: Survey and new data on treatment with pyridoxine of patients having a clinical syndrome including the carpal tunnel and other defects, Res Commun Chem Pathol Pharmacol 17:165, 1977.
92. Layton KB: Acroparaesthesia in pregnancy and the carpal tunnel syndrome, J Obstet Gynaec 65:823, 1958.
93. Beyer JA and Wright IS: The hyperabduction syndrome: with special reference to its relationship to Raynaud's syndrome, Circulation 4:161, 1951.
94. McGough EC, Pearce MB and Byrne JP: Management of thoracic outlet syndrome, J Thorac Cardiovasc Surg 77:169, 1979.
95. Banis JC Jr, Rich N, and Whelan TJ Jr: Ischemia of the upper extremity due to noncardiac emboli, Am J Surg 134:131, 1977.
96. Adson AW and Coffey JR: Cervical rib: a method of anterior approach for relief of symptoms by division of the scalenus anticus, Ann Surg 85:839, 1927.
97. Adson AW: Surgical treatment for symptoms produced by cervical ribs and the scalenus anticus muscle, Surg Gynecol Obstet 85:687, 1947.
98. Roos DB: The place for scalenectomy and first-rib resection in thoracic outlet syndrome, Surgery 92:1077, 1982.
99. Roos DB: Thoracic outlet syndromes: update 1987, Am J Surg 154:568, 1987.
100. Urschel HC Jr and Razzuk MA: Management of the thoracic-outlet syndrome, N Engl J Med 286:1140, 1972.
101. Rosati LM and Lord JW: Neurovascular Compression Syndrome of the Shoulder Girdle, New York, 1961, Grune & Stratton.
102. Brown GE and Griffin HZ: Peripheral arterial disease in polycythemia vera, Arch Intern Med 46:705, 1930.
103. Imhof JW, Boars H, and Verloop MC: Clinical haematologic aspects of macroglobulinaemia Waldenström, Acta Med Scand 163:349, 1959.
104. Invernizzi F et al: Secondary and essential cryoglobulinemias, Acta Haematol 70:73, 1983.
105. Ritzmann SE and Levin WC: Cryopathies: a review. Arch Intern Med 107:186, 1961.
106. McGrath MA and Penny R: Blood hyperviscosity in cryoglobulinemia: temperature sensitivity and correlation with reduced skin blood flow, Aust J Exp Biol Med Sci 56:127, 1978.
107. Ristow SC et al: Reversal of systemic manifestations of cryoglobulinemia, Arch Intern Med 136:467, 1976.
108. McLeod BC and Sassetti RJ: Plasmapheresis with return of cryoglobulin-depleted autologous plasma (cryoglobulinpheresis) in cryoglobulinemia, Blood 55:866, 1980.
109. Olesen H: The cold agglutinin syndrome, Dan Med Bull 14:138, 1967.
110. Marshall RJ, Shepherd JT, and Thompson ID: Vascular responses in patients with high serum titres of cold agglutinins, Clin Sci 12:255, 1953.
111. Markowitz SS et al: Occupational acroosteolysis, Arch Dermatol 106:219, 1972.
112. Ward AM et al: Immunological mechanisms in the pathogenesis of vinyl chloride disease, Br Med J 1:936, 1976.
113. Maricq HR et al: Capillary abnormalities in polyvinyl chloride pro-

duction workers, JAMA 236:1368, 1976.
114. Falappa P et al: Angiographic study of digital arteries in workers exposed to vinyl chloride, Br J Ind Med 39:169, 1982.
115. Hines EA Jr and Barker NW: Arteriosclerosis obliterans: a clinical and pathologic study, Am J Med Sci 200:717, 1940.
116. Goodman RM et al: Buerger's disease in Israel, Am J Med 39:601, 1965.
117. Drucker WR et al: Pathogenesis of post-traumatic sympathetic dystrophy, Am J Surg 97:454, 1959.
118. Gocke DJ et al: Association between polyarteritis and Australian antigen, Lancet 2:1149, 1970.
119. Kim WK and Koff RS: Coexistence of Raynaud's phenomenon and chronic active hepatitis and hepatitis B antigen, Digestion 11:152, 1974.
120. Cosgriff TM and Arnold WJ: Digital vasospasm and infarction associated with hepatitis B antigenemia, JAMA 235:1362, 1976.
121. Lappchen J et al: Raynaud-Phanomen bei dialysepatienten, Dtsch Med Wochenschr 102:521, 1977.
122. Nielsen SL and Lokkegaard H: Cold sensitivity and finger systolic blood pressure in hemodialysis patients, Scand J Urol Nephrol 15:319, 1981.
123. Gipstein RM et al: Calciphylaxis in man, Arch Intern Med 136:1273, 1976.
124. Shagan BP and Friedman SA: Raynaud's phenomenon in hypothyroidism, Angiology 27:19, 1976.
125. Nielsen SL, Parving H-H, and Hansen JEM: Myxoedema and Raynaud's phenomenon, Acta Endocrinol 101:32, 1982.
126. Andrasch RH et al: Digital ischemia and gangrene preceding renal neoplasm, Arch Intern Med 136:486, 1976.
127. Wytock DH, Bartholomew LG, and Sheps SG: Digital ischemia associated with small bowel malignancy, Gastroenterology 84:1025, 1983.
128. Celoria GC, Friedell GH, and Sommers SC: Raynaud's disease and primary pulmonary hypertension, Circulation 22:1055, 1960.
129. Winters WL, Joseph RR, and Learner N: "Primary" pulmonary hypertension and Raynaud's phenomenon, Arch Intern Med 114:821, 1964.
130. Walcott G, Burchell HB, and Brown AL: Primary pulmonary hypertension, Am J Med 49:70, 1970.
131. Fuster V et al: Primary pulmonary hypertension: natural history and the importance of thrombosis, Circulation 70:580, 1984.
132. Murray-Lyon IM et al: Scleroderma and primary biliary cirrhosis, Br Med J 3:258, 1970.
133. Sherlock S and Scheuer PJ: The presentation and diagnosis of 100 patients with primary biliary cirrhosis, N Engl J Med 289:674, 1973.
134. Smith CD and McKendry RVR: Controlled trial of nifedipine in the treatment of Raynaud's phenomenon, Lancet 2:1299, 1982.
135. Rodeheffer RJ et al: Controlled double-blind trial of nifedipine in the treatment of Raynaud's phenomenon, N Engl J Med 308:880, 1983.
136. Rhedda A et al: A double blind placebo controlled crossover randomized trial of diltiazem in Raynaud's phenomenon, J Rheumatol 12:724, 1985.
137. Kahan A, Amor B, and Menkes CJ: A randomized double blind trial of diltiazem in the treatment of Raynaud's phenomenon, Ann Rheum Dis 44:30, 1985.
138. Da Costa JT et al: Inefficacy of diltiazem in the treatment of Raynaud's phenomenon with associated connective tissue disease: a double blind placebo controlled study, J Rheumatol 14:858, 1987.
139. Kinney EL et al: The treatment of severe Raynaud's phenomenon with verapamil, J Clin Pharmacol 22:74, 1982.
140. Coffman JD and Cohen AS: Total and capillary fingertip blood flow in Raynaud's phenomenon, N Engl J Med 285:259, 1971.
141. LeRoy EC, Downey JA, and Cannon PJ: Skin capillary blood flow in scleroderma, J Clin Invest 50:930, 1971.
142. Kontos HA and Wasserman AJ: Effect of reserpine in Raynaud's phenomenon, Circulation 34:259, 1969.
143. McFadyen IJ, Housley E, and MacPherson AIS: Intra-arterial reserpine administration in Raynaud's syndrome, Arch Intern Med 132:526, 1973.
144. Nielsen SL, Vithing K, and Rasmussen K: Prazosin treatment of primary Raynaud's phenomenon, Eur J Clin Pharmacol 24:421, 1983.
145. Wollersheim H et al: Double-blind, placebo-controlled study of prazosin in Raynaud's phenomenon, Clin Pharmacol Ther 40:219, 1986.
146. Moser M, Prandoni AG, Orbison JA, Mattingly TW: Clinical experience with sympathetic blocking agents in peripheral vascular disease, Ann Intern Med 38:1245, 1953.
147. Hillestad LK: Dibenzyline in vascular disease of the hands, Angiology 13:169, 1962.
148. Varadi DP and Lawrence AM: Suppression of Raynaud's phenomenon by methyldopa, Ann Intern Med 124:13, 1969.
149. Strozzi G et al: Management of Raynaud's phenomenon with drugs affecting the sympathetic nervous system, Curr Therap Res 32:225, 1982.
150. Franks AG Jr: Topical glyceryl trinitrate as adjunctive treatment in Raynaud's disease, Lancet 1:76, 1982.
151. Nahir AM, Schapira D, and Scharf Y: Double-blind randomized trial of Nitroderm TTS® in the treatment of Raynaud's phenomenon, Isr J Med Sci 22:139, 1986.
152. Sovijarvi ARA, Siitonen L, and Anderson P: Transdermal nitroglycerin in the treatment of Raynaud's phenomenon: analysis of digital blood pressure changes after cold provocation, Curr Therap Res 35:832, 1984.
153. Mohrland JS et al: A multicenter placebo-controlled, double-blind study of prostaglandin E_1 in Raynaud's syndrome, Ann Rheum Dis 44:754, 1985.
154. Rademaker M et al: Prolonged increase in digital blood flow following Iloprost infusion in patients with systemic sclerosis, Postgrad Med J 63:617, 1987.
155. Belch JJF et al: Intermittent epoprostenol (prostacyclin) infusion in patients with Raynaud's phenomenon, Lancet 1:313, 1983.
156. Roald OK and Seem E: Treatment of Raynaud's phenomenon with ketanserin in patients with connective tissue disorders, Br Med J 289:577, 1984.
157. van de Wal HJCM et al: Quantitative study of the effects of ketanserin in patients with primary Raynaud's phenomenon, Microcirc Endothelium Lymphatics 2:657, 1985.
158. Brouwer RML et al: Does serotonin receptor blockade have a therapeutic effect in Raynaud's phenomenon? VASA (suppl 18):64, 1987.
159. Coffman JD et al: International study of ketanserin in Raynaud's phenomenon, Am J Med 87:264, 1989.
160. Lopez-Ovejero JA et al: Reversal of vascular and renal crisis of scleroderma by oral angiotensin-converting enzyme blockade, N Engl J Med 300:1417, 1979.
161. Tosi S et al: Treatment of Raynaud's phenomenon with captopril, Drugs Exp Clin Res 13:37, 1987.
162. Trubestein G et al: Behandling des Raynaud-Syndroms mit Captopril, Dtsch Med Wochenschr 109:857, 1984.
163. Talpos G et al: Plasmapheresis in Raynaud's disease, Lancet 1:416, 1978.
164. O'Reilly MJG et al: Controlled trial of plasma exchange in treatment of Raynaud's syndrome, Br Med J 1:1113, 1979.
165. Jobe JB et al: Induced vasodilation as treatment for Raynaud's disease, Ann Intern Med 97:706, 1982.
166. Surwit RS, Pilon RN, and Fenton CH: Behavioral treatment of Raynaud's disease, J Behav Med 1:323, 1978.
167. Keefe FJ, Surwit RS, and Pilon RN: Biofeedback, autogenic training and progressive relaxation in the treatment of Raynaud's disease, J Appl Behav Anal 13:3, 1980.

168. Freedman RR, Ianni P, and Wenig P: Behavioral treatment of Raynaud's disease, J Consult Clin Psych 51:539, 1983.
169. Gifford RW Jr, Hines EA Jr, and Craig WM: Sympathectomy for Raynaud's phenomenon, Circulation 17:5, 1958.
170. Tsur N et al: Upper thoracic sympathectomy, Isr J Med Sci 9:53, 1973.
171. Baddeley RM: The place of upper dorsal sympathectomy in the treatment of primary Raynaud's disease, Br J Surg 52:426, 1965.
172. Laroche GP et al: Chronic arterial insufficiency of the upper extremity, Mayo Clin Proc 51:180, 1976.
173. Felder DA et al: Evaluation of sympathetic neurectomy in Raynaud's disease, Surgery 26:1014, 1949.
174. Johnston ENM, Summerly R, and Birnstingl M: Prognosis in Raynaud's phenomenon after sympathectomy, Br Med J 1:962, 1965.
175. Janoff KA, Phinney ES, and Porter JM: Lumbar sympathectomy for lower extremity vasospasm, Am J Surg 150:147, 1985.
176. Crocq C: De l'acrocyanose, Semaine Med 16:297, 1896.
177. Stern ES: The aetiology and pathology of acrocyanosis, Br J Derm Syph 49:100, 1937.
178. Peacock JH: Vasodilatation in the human hand: observations on primary Raynaud's disease and acrocyanosis of the upper extremities, Clin Sci 17:575, 1957.
179. Jacobs MJHM et al: Nomenclature of Raynaud's phenomenon: a capillary microscopic and hemorheologic study, Surgery 101:136, 1987.
180. Bollinger A, Mahler F, and Meier B: Velocity patterns in nailfold capillaries of normal subjects and patients with Raynaud's disease and acrocyanosis, Bibl Anat 16:142, 1977.
181. Lewis T and Landis EM: Observations upon the vascular mechanism in acrocyanosis, Heart 15:229, 1930.
182. Peacock JH: A comparative study of the digital cutaneous temperatures, and hand blood flows in the normal hand, primary Raynaud's disease and primary acrocyanosis, Clin Sci 18:25, 1959.
183. Day R and Klingman WO: The effect of sleep on the skin temperature reactions in a case of acrocyanosis, J Clin Invest 18:271, 1939.
184. Barker NW, Hines EA Jr, and Craig W McK: Livedo reticularis: a peripheral arteriolar disease, Am Heart J 21:592, 1941.
185. Pearce LA, Waterbury LD, and Green HD: Amantadine hydrochloride: alteration in peripheral circulation, Neurology 24:46, 1974.
186. Cabbabe EB and Clift SD: Leg ulcerations in livedoid vasculitis, Plast Reconstr Surg 75:888, 1985.
187. Feldaker M, Hines EA Jr, and Kierland RR: Livedo reticularis with ulcerations, Circulation 13:196, 1956.
188. Cunliffe WJ and Menon IS: The association between cutaneous vasculitis and decreased blood fibrinolytic activity, Br J Dermatol 84:99, 1971.
189. Drucker CR and Duncan WC: Antiplatelet therapy in atrophie blanche and livedo vasculitis, J Am Acad Dermatol 7:359, 1982.
190. Yamamoto M et al: Antithrombic treatment in livedo vasculitis, J Am Acad Dermatol 18:57, 1988.
191. Milstone LM et al: Classification and therapy of atrophie blanche, Arch Dermatol 119:963, 1983.
192. Williams C and Goodman H: Livedo reticularis, JAMA 85:955, 1925.
193. Copeland PWM: Livedo reticularis, Br J Dermatol 93:519, 1975.
194. Heimans RLH, Rand MJ, and Fennessy MR: Some actions of amantadine on peripheral tissues, J Pharm Pharmacol 24:869, 1972.
195. Winkelmann RK et al: Clinical studies of livedoid vasculitis (segmental hyalinizing vasculitis), Mayo Clin Proc 49:746, 1974.
196. Sneddon IB: Cerebrovascular lesions and livedo reticularis, Br J Dermatol 77:180, 1965.
197. Hughes GRV: Autoantibodies in lupus and its variants: experience in 1000 patients, Br Med J 289:339, 1984.
198. Weinstein C et al: Livedo reticularis associated with increased titers of anticardiolipin antibodies in systemic lupus erythematosus, Arch Dermatol 123:596, 1987.
199. Shealy CN, Weeth JB, and Mercier D: Livedo reticularis in patients with Parkinsonism receiving amantadine, JAMA 212:1522, 1970.
200. Silver D, and Sahs AL: Livedo reticularis in Parkinson's disease patients treated with amantadine hydrochloride, Neurology 22:645, 1972.
201. Tindall JP, Whalen RE, and Burton EE Jr: Medical uses of intra-arterial injections of reserpine, Arch Dermatol 110:233, 1974.

Chapter 22

MISCELLANEOUS ARTERIAL DISEASES

Bruce H. Gray
Jess R. Young
Jeffrey W. Olin

Intermittent claudication is usually a warning symptom of arterial insufficiency induced by progressive arteriosclerosis obliterans (ASO). When intermittent claudication occurs in a younger individual, in whom the suspicion of ASO is low, other possible causes should be entertained, for instance, systemic emboli, thromboangiitis obliterans (TAO), popliteal artery entrapment syndrome (PAES), cystic adventitial disease (CAD), fibromuscular dysplasia (FMD), ergotamine ingestion, popliteal artery aneurysm, and vasculitis. PAES, CAD, and FMD will be discussed in this chapter.

POPLITEAL ARTERY ENTRAPMENT SYNDROME

Entrapment of a peripheral vessel as a mechanism of arterial insufficiency has been recognized for years. This is more frequently seen in younger individuals, although it can occur in all age groups. Entrapment can occur at a number of sites, including the axillary, brachial, celiac, common femoral, superficial femoral, and popliteal arteries. The most frequent and well-known site of entrapment is at the popliteal artery. Therefore the subsequent discussion will center on PAES.

Historical background

Popliteal artery entrapment was first described in 1879 by T.P. Anderson Stuart in an amputated gangrenous limb.[1] He described the abnormal path of the popliteal artery as it deviated medially around the medial head of the gastrocnemius muscle rather than coursing between the heads of the muscle. The involved muscle rose much higher on the femoral condyle than usual, allowing space for the artery to pass (Figs. 22-1 and 22-2).

In 1961 Hall reported a case in which the site of attachment of the medial head of the gastrocnemius muscle was more lateral than usual, separating the artery medially[4] (Fig. 22-3). In 1925 Chambardel-Dubreuil described a situation in which the popliteal artery and vein were separated by an accessory slip of the gastrocnemius muscle[2] (Fig. 22-4). It was not until 1959 that complications arising from this disease entity were successfully treated by Hamming in a 12-year-old boy.[3] Subsequent case reports then began to appear in the literature with greater frequency. Many of these had anatomic variants of the original type described by Stuart.

In 1964 Hall described another variant, coined "intervascular gastrocnemius insertion," in which the artery courses through the body of the muscle.[5] Later that same year, the concept of bilateral occurrence of these congenital anomalies was recognized by Carter and Eban.[6] In 1965 Love and Whelan labeled this disease popliteal artery entrapment syndrome.[7] They noted that entrapment could be caused by an abnormal popliteal muscle/popliteal artery relationship (Fig. 22-5). By 1967 the first case of entrapment of both the popliteal artery and vein was described by Rich and Hughes.[8] Since then at least 18 anatomical variants have been described.[9] Furthermore, cases with an isolated popliteal vein or popliteal nerve entrapment have also been reported.[10,11]

Pathogenesis

Popliteal artery entrapment has generally been regarded as a congenital aberration. Most frequently, the medial head of the gastrocnemius muscle has been the compressing structure, although the involvement of a concomitant compres-

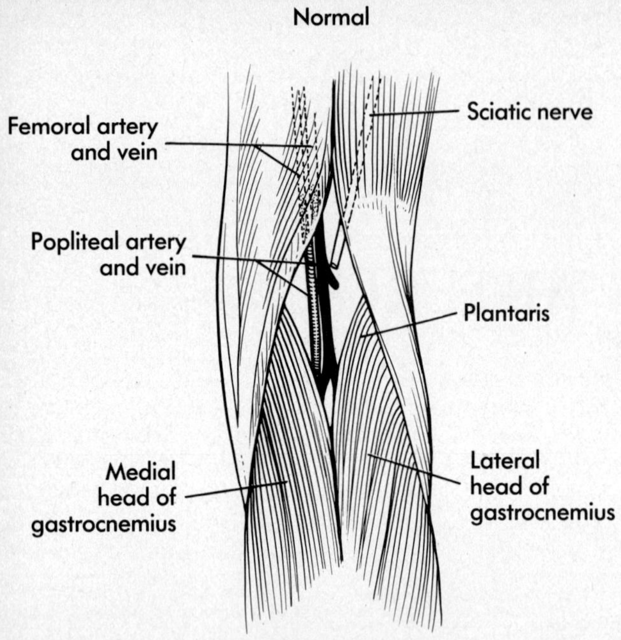

Fig. 22-1. Normal anatomic relationship (*posterior view*) of the right popliteal space. (From Insua JA et al: Arch Surg 101:771, 1970 [Copyright 1970, American Medical Association].)

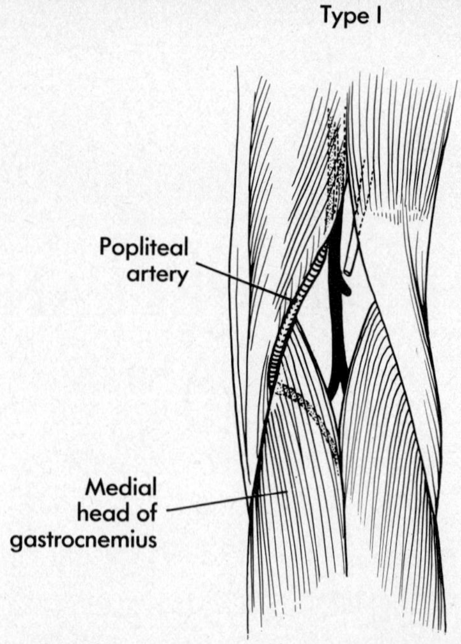

Fig. 22-2. Type I anomaly. The popliteal artery deviates medially around the medial head of the gastrocnemius muscle that arises close to its normal location. (From Insua JA et al: Arch Surg 101:771, 1970 [Copyright 1970, American Medical Association].)

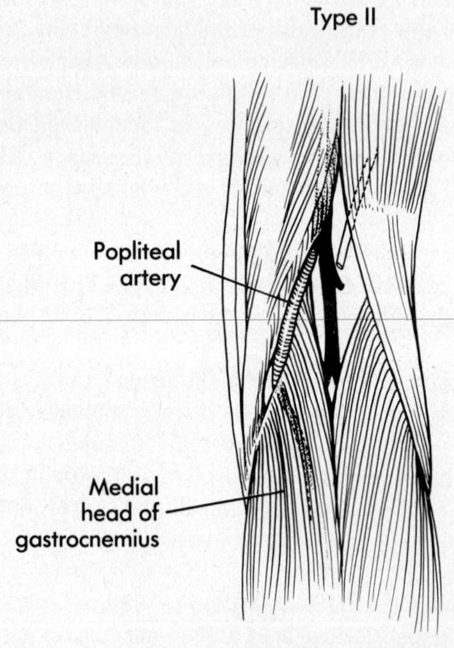

Fig. 22-3. Type II anomaly. The medial head of the gastrocnemius muscle arises more laterally on the femoral condyle, with a separation between the artery and vein. The artery may be minimally displaced on arteriogram. (From Insua JA et al: Arch Surg 101:771, 1970 [Copyright 1970, American Medical Association].)

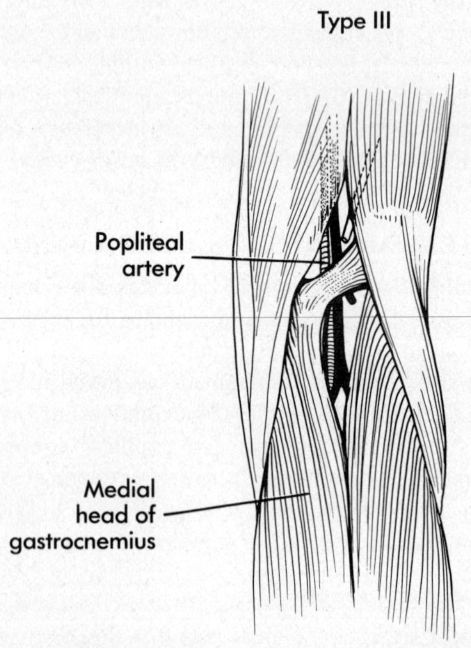

Fig. 22-4. Type III anomaly. The popliteal artery is entrapped by a lateral slip of the medial gastrocnemius muscle. The artery takes a normal course. (From Insua JA et al: Arch Surg 101:771, 1970 [Copyright 1970, American Medical Association].)

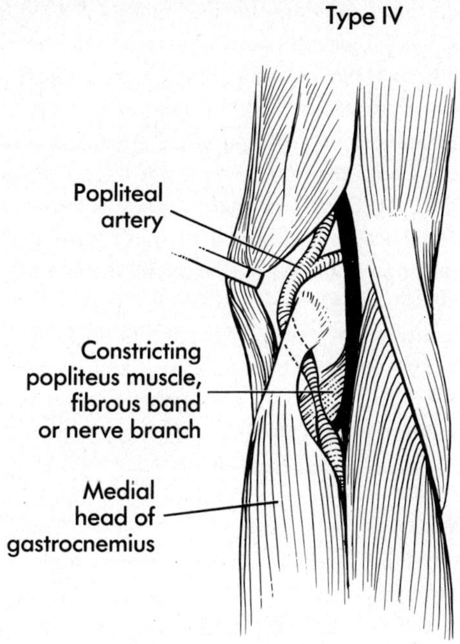

Fig. 22-5. Type IV anomaly. The popliteus muscle or a deep fibrous band compresses the popliteal artery. This anomaly can be accompanied by medial deviation of the artery around a normally arising medial head of the gastrocnemius muscle, but the site of entrapment is distal to this deviation. (Modified from Rich NM et al: Arch Surg 114:1377, 1979 [Copyright 1979, American Medical Association].)

sive popliteal muscle or band may be underestimated.[12] The actual ontogenic explanation for all the variants is incomplete.[13] Iatrogenic entrapment after placement of bypass grafts has also been described. This technical error usually has been the result of placing the graft medial to the medial head of the gastrocnemius muscle. Perhaps most of these resulted from a failure to recognize the underlying native artery entrapment.

Histologic examination of resected arterial segments has demonstrated the presence of abundant longitudinal muscle fibers in the tunica media.[14] The internal elastic lamina is disrupted with fibrous thickening of intima. It has been postulated that repetitive trauma to the arterial wall results in the development of these muscle bundles.[14,15] These muscular changes are generally seen on the arterial wall adjacent to the contracting muscle.[15] This can be a histologic feature distinguishing this condition from occlusive atherosclerotic disease.

Classification

Different classification schemes for PAES have appeared as regularly as new anatomic variants are recognized. The schemes have been based on anatomic or angiographic characteristics, because the same principles in treatment apply almost universally. Many of these classifications were proposed early in the era of clinical recognition of the disease, without the exposure to all the variants that have since been recognized.[9,16-18] There are many diverse anomalies in muscle, arterial, venous, and neural structures, making individual classification of each variant cumbersome. Therefore the specific classification schemes to date have limited usefulness in the management or prognosis of the entrapment phenomenon. A pictorial description of four of the most common types is seen in Figs. 22-1 to 22-5.

Clinical presentation

The clinical presentation is usually that of a healthy, "athletic-type" male complaining of typical claudication symptoms in the absence of evidence of premature atherosclerosis. It is not unusual for the onset of the claudication symptoms to be sudden. Patients may also describe nocturnal cramps, numbness, paresthesias, focal ischemia in the distal digits, worsening of symptoms with knee flexion, or the sudden development of a cold leg. The degree of stenosis and the presence of collateral flow will dictate the extent of circulatory compromise and the consequent symptoms. Acute thrombosis, distal embolization, or rupture can also occur if entrapment leads to poststenotic dilation and aneurysm formation.

The incidence in the general population is unknown, but reported incidences range from 0.165% in a study of 20,000 Greek army patients[18] to 3.5% in postmortem examinations of 86 patients.[19] Males are involved predominantly by a 15:1 ratio.[9] The patient age at the time of diagnosis has ranged from 12 to 64 years, with 60% being less than 30 years of age.[9] Bilateral popliteal artery involvement has been found to be about 22% in the older literature,[9] but a recent study reported bilateral anomalies in 67% (8 of 12 patients).[12] These higher figures could reflect a more consistent study of the contralateral side. The anatomic variant seen in bilateral disease may frequently vary from one side to another.[9]

Diagnostic testing

Palpation of the arteries in the involved limb is the cornerstone of the initial evaluation. The timing and the quality of the pulse may suggest the level of disease, the extent of involvement, and the presence of aneurysmal dilation. The disappearance of the pulse with passive dorsiflexion of the foot or active plantar flexion against resistance may suggest the diagnosis.[20] In patients with pulses that are difficult to palpate, Doppler ultrasound increases the diagnostic yield.

Plethysmographic tests such as pulse volume recordings have increased our diagnostic capabilities. A baseline waveform and blood pressure is established with the patient in the supine position. The foot is then put through flexion maneuvers, and changes in the flow tracing can be evaluated. Finally, the addition of stress testing with treadmill walking can elucidate not only symptoms, but also document the physiologic and functional alterations in blood flow.[21] The addition of treadmill testing should lower the false-negative rate associated with isolated supine testing. The mechanism for the change in flow characteristics with the foot put through flexion maneuvers can be explained either by direct compression of the entrapped artery or through an increase in runoff resistance secondary to contracting muscle beds.[21]

Confirmatory evidence for PAES can be provided by computed tomography (CT).[22] CT scanning can clearly delineate soft tissue, vascular, and bony structures, unlike ultrasound, which differentiates soft tissue structures less clearly. The relationship between the popliteal artery and vein, the architecture of the local osseus prominences, and the presence of interlying muscle can be documented. Furthermore, both popliteal spaces can be evaluated at the same time. This allows for direct comparison and screening for bilateral anatomic variances. Clinically, this is also useful in differentiating cystic adventitial disease of the popliteal artery from PAES. With better anatomic knowledge, the surgeon can prepare operative strategy.

Magnetic resonance imaging (MRI) may be a useful technique but has not been well studied to date.[22] Duplex ultrasonography of the arterial structures could provide functional as well as anatomic information, but the technique has been incompletely studied in this disease. Arteriography remains the gold standard for evaluation. A characteristic finding is medial deviation of the artery in the popliteal region, although the course of the artery may be normal (Fig. 22-6). Poststenotic dilation and aneurysmal dilation of the midpopliteal or distal popliteal artery are also highly suggestive of popliteal entrapment but have been found in only 27% of the cases.[23] Usually, atherosclerotic changes of the arterial tree are minimal in these patients, but the presence of angiographically documented atheroma should not exclude this diagnosis.

Other entities that cause midpopliteal occlusion include CAD, thrombosed popliteal aneurysm, and arteriosclerosis obliterans. When faced with a thrombosed popliteal artery, the combination of CT scanning and arteriography is usually sufficient to make the correct diagnosis.

Treatment

Once the diagnosis of PAES is made, surgical intervention is warranted regardless of symptoms. The prevention of thrombotic and embolic complications, coupled with highly successful surgical techniques, favor this approach. If the artery is already thrombosed or if emboli have occurred, the surgical procedure can be preceded by attempting intraarterial thrombolytic therapy.

The surgical approach is made either through a medial

A

B

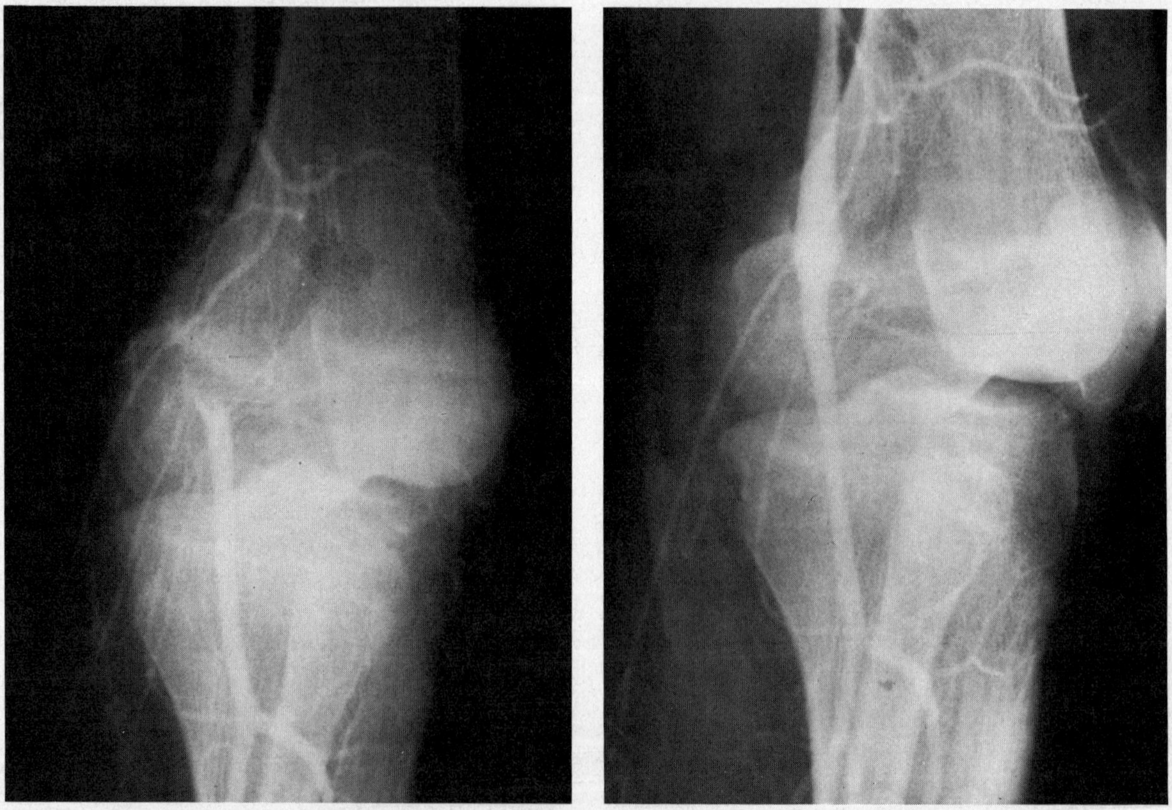

Fig. 22-6. A, Arteriogram of left superficial femoropopliteal artery in a 22-year-old man. Note medial deviation and occlusion in the midpopliteal region (Type I). **B**, Reversed saphenous vein interposition graft was performed with excellent angiographic results. The medial head of the gastrocnemius muscle was also transected.

or posterior incision. The medial approach is generally used in standard bypass surgery. However, the posterior approach offers a distinct advantage in the ability to visualize many of these anatomic variants.

Once entrapment is recognized, any surgical procedure should be tailored to the specific clinical situation. Transection of the offending structure is mandatory. The artery needs to be freely mobilized. The muscle or fibrous band need not necessarily be translocated for functional integrity. The condition of the underlying vessel dictates the need for thrombectomy, resection, patch angioplasty, or bypass procedure. Aneurysmal disease needs to be treated with excision or bypass and ligation. Presently, long-term success may best be accomplished with a saphenous vein interposition graft.

Operative complications can be minimized by correctly recognizing the anatomy and underlying pathology. Care must also be taken to avoid transection of the median cutaneous sural nerve in the posterior approach. Postoperative complications of infection, graft thrombosis, bleeding, and deep venous thrombosis have all been reported.[23]

CYSTIC ADVENTITIAL DISEASE

CAD most commonly affects the popliteal artery, although it can be associated with other upper or lower extremity vessels. The nomenclature proposed by Ishikawa separates the popliteal artery (CAD-PA) involvement from that of other vessels (CAD-non-PA).[24] This process has been referred to by many other names including cystic adventitial degeneration, cystic mucoid degeneration, cystic myxomatous adventitial degeneration, degenerescence colloide de l'adventice, mucinous cystic dissecting intramural degeneration, and subadventitial pseudocyst.

Historic background

Cystic adventitial disease was first reported in 1946 by Atkins and Key after finding during surgery a myxomatous tumor involving the left external iliac artery in a 40-year-old man.[25] In 1954 Ejrup and Hiertonn described a gelatinous-filled mass arising from the popliteal artery causing subtotal stenosis and calf claudication.[26] Hiertonn, Lindberg, and Rob had collected four cases of popliteal artery involvement in 1957 and noted that the process occurred particularly in young men.[27] By 1970 approximately 40 cases had been reported in the world literature, with most of them involving the popliteal artery and causing either stenosis or occlusion of the affected vessel.[28]

A group at Northwestern University developed a correspondence registry of all of the reported cases in the world literature and published these data in 1979.[29] They reported a total of 115 cases involving the popliteal artery, of which 105 were acceptable for inclusion. Of these 105 cases, 83 were men and 18 were women, and in 4 the patient's gender was not reported. The mean age was 42 years (range 11 to 70 years).

In 1987 Ishikawa added 91 additional cases of CAD-PA and presented 39 nonpopliteal artery cases (CAD-non-PA).[24] The other sites of involvement included vessels adjacent to joints such as the radial, ulnar, brachial, iliac, and femoral arteries. Of the cases recorded by Ishikawa 15% were documented to have an anatomic connection between the cyst and the adjacent joint capsule.[24] Sakamoto and others[30] reported a case of bilateral popliteal artery involvement and Ohta et al presented a case of ipsilateral iliofemoral artery and vein disease.[31] The sites of venous CAD include the femoral, external iliac, popliteal, and saphenous veins.

Pathophysiology

The cyst arises in the outer tunica media or subadventital layer with cyst expansion into the adventitia of the vessel wall. The rate of growth is unknown, but once the intracystic pressure exceeds that in the lumen of the vessel, stenosis (70%) or occlusion (30%) results.[24]

The exact pathophysiologic mechanism for the development of cystic adventitial disease is unknown. Several authors have supported the role of repeated microtrauma to the popliteal artery leading to degenerative changes and cyst formation.[24,27,29] A recent report describes two cases of CAD affecting the radial arteries two months after radial artery blood gas sampling.[32] The rarity of this disease and the fact that it is usually an isolated lesion detracts from the hypothesis of trauma as a sole factor. Another hypothesis tries to account for the disease involvement seen around adjacent joints. Robb proposed that synovial membrane from a tendon sheath or joint capsule became attached to the artery either developmentally or traumatically.[33] Ruppel recognized the chemical and structural similarity between vascular cysts and ganglia and proposed that these are true ganglia of the vessel wall.[34] Another theory suggests that pseudocyst formation occurred after hemorrhagic rupture of vasa vasorum. No one theory has received total support to explain the observed findings; possibly an interplay of more than one of the above mechanisms is responsible. As a rule CAD appears as an isolated lesion devoid of a systemic process. However, CAD-PA has been reported in a 32-year-old patient with the nail-patella syndrome.[35]

Analysis of pathologic specimens reveals a cyst arising from the subadventitial layer or the outer tunica media layer of the vessel. The cyst can be uniloculated or multiloculated and is lined by flattened cells, usually filled with clear fluid, although it can be hemorrhagic (currant jelly appearance) or even yellow in color. Mucoprotein and mucopolysaccharides, hyaluronic acid, and hydroxyproline have been reported as the major cystic components. Endo and others, through extensive chemical evaluation, concluded that the main component was proteohyaluronic acid.[36] The mechanism for the fluid accumulation in the cyst is unknown.

Clinical presentation

Initially, most case reports originated from Europe and Japan, but as recognition has increased, a global distribution

A

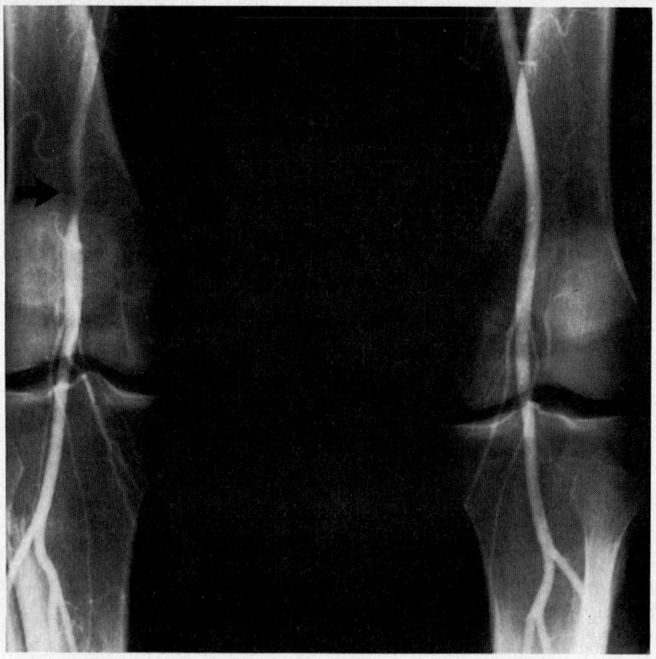

B

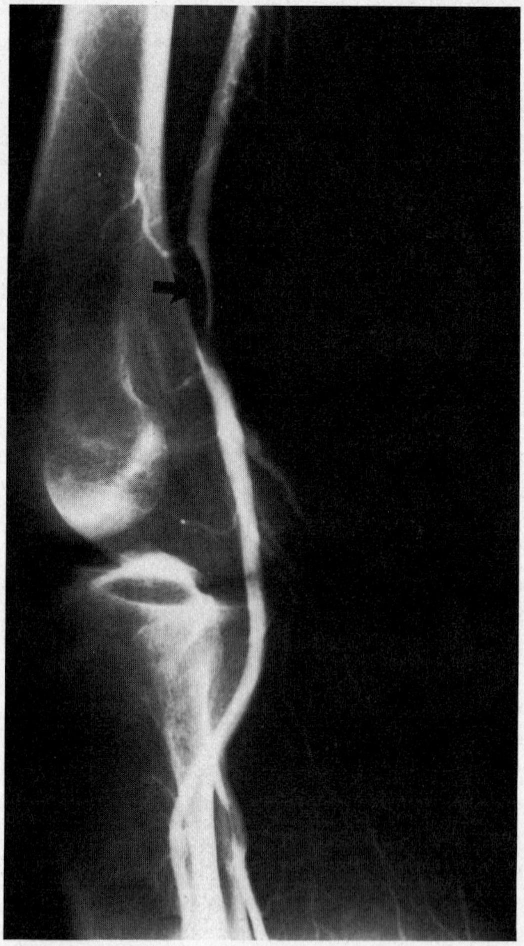

Fig. 22-7. **A**, Bilateral lower extremity arteriogram demonstrating smooth area of stenosis in right proximal popliteal artery (*arrow*). **B**, Lateral arteriogram of right leg shows the scimitar pattern (*arrow*) characteristic of cystic adventitial disease. (From Buonocore E: Cleve Clinic Q 50:46, 1982.)

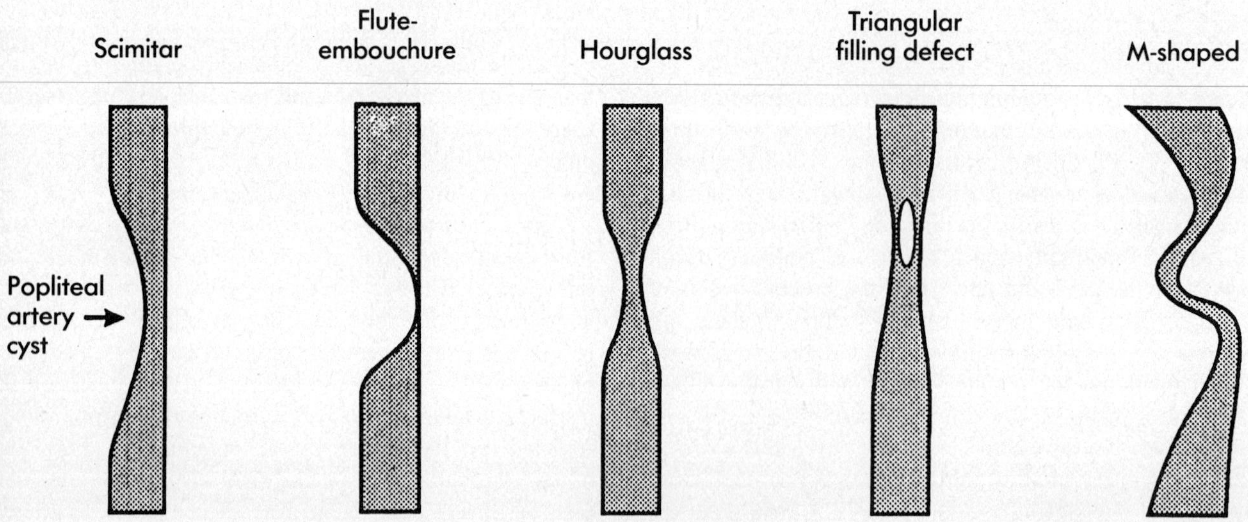

Fig. 22-8. Different arteriographic appearances of cystic adventitial disease (CAD) of the popliteal arteries. (Modified from Ishiwaka K: Jpn J Surg 17:227, 1987.)

has been seen. Men predominate by an approximate 5:1 ratio. The age ranges from 10 to 77 years, with a mean of 44.9 years. There is equal involvement of the right and left popliteal arteries.[24]

Claudication in a younger individual in the absence of atherosclerotic risk factors should heighten the clinical suspicion of CAD. Typically the symptoms develop over several months and can wax and wane. The degree of artery narrowing, as well as the degree of collateralization, dictates the severity of claudication. In the presence of stenosis, distal pulses are frequently present, but may disappear upon flexion of the knee joint (Ishikawa's sign).[24] A systolic bruit in the popliteal area has been suggested as a pertinent physical finding. Occlusion of the involved artery usually appears with absent distal pulses, but distal ischemia at rest or neurologic deficit secondary to ischemia is a rare finding.

Diagnostic testing

Frequently CAD can be diagnosed preoperatively. Pulse volume recordings may show the characteristic drop in blood pressure and change in waveform configuration at the affected level. These changes may not be evident at rest but can be brought out by exercise. The claudication distance depends on the degree of stenosis and the extent of collateralization.

Duplex ultrasonographic techniques can be helpful in recognizing the presence of a perivascular cystic structure. Ultrasound can demonstrate hypoechoic spaces that may be septated, while Doppler can show turbulence and an elevated shift frequency in the area of stenosis.[37] Computerized tomography (CT) scanning can provide direct evidence of adjacent masses, muscle insertions and the course of the artery.[22,38] On CT the cystic contents show no enhancement and the relative attenuation value is between those of water and muscle, thus clearly delineating the soft tissue structures.

Arteriography will demonstrate the degree of stenosis and is best done by including lateral and anterior-posterior projections. The arteriographic appearance is most frequently that of a scimitar, hourglass, or flute embouchure configuration but can also appear as an M-shaped or a triangular filling defect[24] (Figs. 22-7 and 22-8). Poststenotic dilation is not generally seen, and collateral channels may be well developed. Medial displacement of the artery is not seen in CAD-PA, and atherosclerotic changes of ASO are characteristically absent.

Treatment

An important factor in considering the best treatment option is the timing of the diagnosis. Treatment options differ on the basis of whether the artery is stenotic or occluded.[24] In the past most cases were diagnosed at the time of surgery, after the artery had occluded. Now, however, with increased awareness of the disease and with excellent noninvasive diagnostic studies available, early diagnosis allows wider therapeutic options. In the stenotic lesion, ultrasound or CT-guided needle aspiration of the cyst has been attempted.[39] The multiloculated lesion may not be totally evacuated by these methods, and the cystic structure left in place can lead to a higher recurrence rate. These techniques, however, can certainly improve the flow characteristics of the involved vessel, which may be the logical initial therapy in the stenotic lesion. Percutaneous balloon angioplasty has not proven to be a viable alternative.[40] With recurrent stenoses, persistent stenoses, or occlusive disease, a more definitive surgical technique can be performed. In the face of arterial occlusion intraarterial thrombolysis should be considered as the initial procedure to restore luminal patency. This can then be followed by the appropriate resectional or nonresectional technique to alleviate the underlying pathology.

Flanigan et al provide comparative data between resectional and nonresectional therapy.[29] Nonresectional therapy included simple evacuation, evacuation with vein patch, evacuation with synthetic patch, or simple aspiration. In this group an overall success rate of 85% (initial success 89%) was reported. This was compared with resectional techniques using vein graft, synthetic graft, end-to-end anastomosis, or homograft placement, which revealed an overall success rate of 91% (initial success 93%) (Table 22-1).[29] The patency of autogenous reversed saphenous vein graft after 27 to 30 years has been demonstrated in three patients who were originally operated on for complaints of intermittent claudication secondary to CAD-PA.[41] Long-term follow-up data on larger patient groups have not been available to date.

Table 22-1. Summary of resectional vs nonresectional techniques in CAD of the popliteal artery

	Initial success rate	
Category	**n**	**%**
Nonresectional		
1. Evacuation	38/42	90
2. Evacuation with vein patch	7/9	78
3. Evacuation with synthetic patch	3/4	75
4. Aspiration	2/2	100
TOTAL	49/56	89
Resectional		
1. Vein graft	28/30	93
2. Synthetic graft	6/7	86
3. End-to-end anastomosis	3/3	100
4. Homograft	2/2	100
TOTAL	39/42	93

(Modified from Flanigan DP et al: Summary of cases of adventitial cystic disease of the popliteal artery, Ann Surg 189:165, 1979.)

EXTRARENAL FIBROMUSCULAR DYSPLASIA

Fibromuscular dysplasia (FMD) is an uncommon, noninflammatory disease of the arteries. Exceedingly rare, venous FMD has been histologically documented in the renal, portal, mesenteric, and peripheral veins. FMD most commonly involves the renal arteries (60% to 75%) (see Chapter 15), but has been described in almost every arterial bed, including the cervicocranial (25% to 30%), visceral (9%), and extremity arteries (5%).[42-44] Histologic confirmation of FMD has been lacking in some of the reported cases.

Most types of FMD occur predominantly in females.[42] The clinical suspicion of FMD should be raised when a young woman develops hypertension. The workup should exclude FMD of the renal arteries. In 24% of patients with FMD there is involvement in more than one vascular territory.[42]

Table 22-2 summarizes several features of extrarenal FMD. The angiographic appearance can be very suggestive of FMD, but the diagnosis is based on histologic confirmation. The appearance of concomitant atherosclerosis may make the diagnosis more difficult, particularly in the older age groups; however, classic intimal or medial changes on arteriography are highly suggestive of FMD.[45] The lesions of FMD typically arise in the middle or distal arterial segments, sparing the orificial or bifurcation sites typical of atherosclerotic disease.[42]

The histologic classification system of renal artery FMD proposed by Harrison and McCormack is also used for extrarenal FMD.[46] The authors separated FMD into subtypes according to the layers of vessel wall involved. The classification includes intimal fibroplasia, medial *hyper*plasia, medial *fibro*plasia, perimedial fibroplasia, and periarterial fibroplasia. Whether spontaneous dissection is a complication of FMD or whether it is a separate category of FMD remains controversial.[42,46]

The pathogenesis of FMD remains unknown, although multiple theories exist. The genetic theory was used to explain the familial involvement seen particularly in whites. Rushton observed the inheritance pattern of FMD to be consistent with an autosomal dominant trait with variable penetrance.[47] In those patients without a prior family history of FMD, a new mutation was thought to have occurred.[42] The humoral theory relates the predilection of FMD in females to increased estrogen levels.[48] Mechanical factors such as local trauma, stretching, or vessel torsion have also been proposed to account for the anatomic location or topography of the disease.[49] Furthermore, some other injurious mechanisms may disrupt the vasa vasorum of the vessel wall leading to mural ischemia.[50] Other theories take into account the possibility of exogenous toxins such as smoking, ergotamine use, or rubella syndromes as causes.[42] A combination of these mechanisms may interact in the susceptible host.

The differential diagnosis of FMD should include vascular spasm, arterial hypoplasia, arteritis, or simply diminished flow leading to a decrease in the caliber of the visualized vessel. In the presence of arterial dilations, other considerations include aneurysmal disease, pseudoaneurysm, or atherosclerosis with poststenotic dilation.

Disease conditions that have been associated with FMD include coarctation of the aorta, neurofibromatosis,[51] pheochromocytoma,[52] Ehler-Danlos syndrome Type IV,[53] and Alport's syndrome.[54]

Cervicocranial FMD

In 1965 Connett and Lansche histologically confirmed that FMD can affect the cervicocranial arteries.[55] It can affect any or all of the arteries supplying the central nervous system (CNS) circulation.[55-60] The internal carotid artery is involved in approximately 90% of cases, with bilateral le-

Table 22-2. Characteristics of extrarenal fibromuscular dysplasia (FMD)

Artery involved	Predominant FMD subtype	Site of involvement	Associated lesions	Arteriograms
Internal carotid	Intimal and medial fibroplasia	Segment adjacent to C1-2	Intracranial aneurysms Renal FMD	String of beads Tubular stenoses Dissection
Vertebral	Medial fibroplasia	Segment adjacent C5	Carotid FMD	String of beads
Mesenteric and celiac	Intimal fibroplasia	Midvessel segment beyond orifice	Renal FMD Visceral aneurysms	Focal stenoses Long tubular stenoses
Upper extremity (subclavian, axillary)	Intimal fibroplasia	Middle or distal segments of vessel	Renal FMD	Long tubular stenoses
Lower extremity (external iliac, femoral, tibials)	Medial fibroplasia	Proximal segment of external iliac	Carotid FMD Renal FMD	String of beads

sions (60% to 85%) being more common.[57-59] Vertebral artery disease is seen in a minority of cases.[56] Associated FMD of the renal arteries is present in roughly one third of the cases.[42] There is also a high association of intracranial aneurysms with FMD, with estimates ranging from 21% to 50%.[56,57] In one series of patients with subarachnoid hemorrhage, 31 out of 102 (30%) had FMD.[61]

Females are predominant among individuals with cervicocranial FMD. The disease has been reported in all age groups (4 to 86 years, mean 58).[59,60]

Cervicocranial FMD can be symptomatic or asymptomatic. Asymptomatic carotid FMD disease is either found serendipitously or when searched for because of the presence of renal artery FMD. The symptoms associated with FMD depend on the location of the disease and the extent of ischemia induced. Strokes, transient ischemic attacks (TIAs), subarachnoid hemorrhage (SAH), Horner's syndrome, cranial nerve paresis, headache, vertigo, neck pain, nausea, vomiting, disorientation, drowsiness, seizure, or loss of consciousness can be among the associated symptoms.[48] Many of these symptoms arise from complications of FMD. The incidence of major complications, stroke, TIAs, and SAH in cervicocranial FMD is estimated between 29% and 44%.[58,60] On the other hand, many patients develop nonspecific symptoms (i.e., headache, tinnitus, dizziness), and FMD is diagnosed during the workup of these symptoms. The natural history of cervicocranial FMD is unknown.

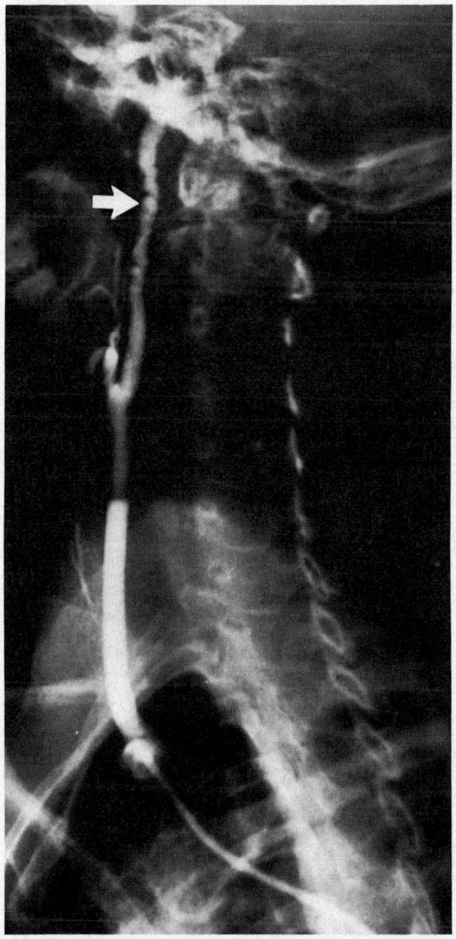

Fig. 22-9. Arteriographic demonstration of medial fibroplasia involving the right internal carotid artery in a 76-year-old woman. Note the "string-of-beads" appearance and the topographic location next to C1-2 (*arrow*).

All classic arteriographic and pathologic changes of FMD have been described in the cervicocranial arteries.[56] Subtypes of cervicocranial FMD reflect the same incidence as that in the renal circulation.[62] Topographically, the lesion in the internal carotid artery is usually adjacent to the C1-2 vertebral bodies and not at the proximal origin[58] (Fig. 22-9). A "string-of-beads" appearance next to C1-2 is quite suggestive of FMD. When the "beading" is larger than the proximal caliber of the vessel, it is indicative of medial fibroplasia. The "beads" are smaller than the proximal caliber of the vessel in perimedial fibroplasia. Not uncommonly, though, the changes of concomitant arteriosclerosis obliterans may be present (Fig. 22-10). The diagnosis of carotid FMD may be suspected with carotid duplex ultrasonography, but the examination is limited by the distal site of involvement in the internal carotid artery.

The treatment of cervicocranial FMD is quite variable, ranging from observation to surgical intervention. The natural history of the disease is uncertain, particularly in asymptomatic FMD. In general, asymptomatic FMD of the extracranial arteries should be observed. However, the presence of concomitant intracranial aneurysms may warrant surgical intervention.

Treatment options for symptomatic (TIAs, stroke) cervicocranial FMD include medical therapy (acetylsalicylic acid, coumarin), intraoperative graduated intraluminal dilation (GID), or surgical resection or bypass.[63-67] Percutaneous balloon angioplasty (PTA) has been tried in cervicocranial FMD but is not recommended based on unacceptable complication rates.[68] The expertise in the specific medical community should help dictate the procedure of choice. For symptomatic disease we favor intraoperative GID or surgical bypass. For asymptomatic disease we treat with aspirin.

Nonrenal visceral FMD

FMD of the visceral arteries other than the renal arteries is uncommon. The visceral arteries most frequently affected include (in descending order of prevalence) the celiac, superior mesenteric, hepatic, splenic, and coronary arteries. Estimates range from less than 0.1%, in unselected autopsy series, to 13% in patients with splenic artery aneurysms.[69,70]

Isolated visceral arterial involvement has been reported, but multiple visceral vessels are more commonly affected. Visceral artery involvement can also be associated with generalized hypoplasia of the aorta or coarctation of the

A

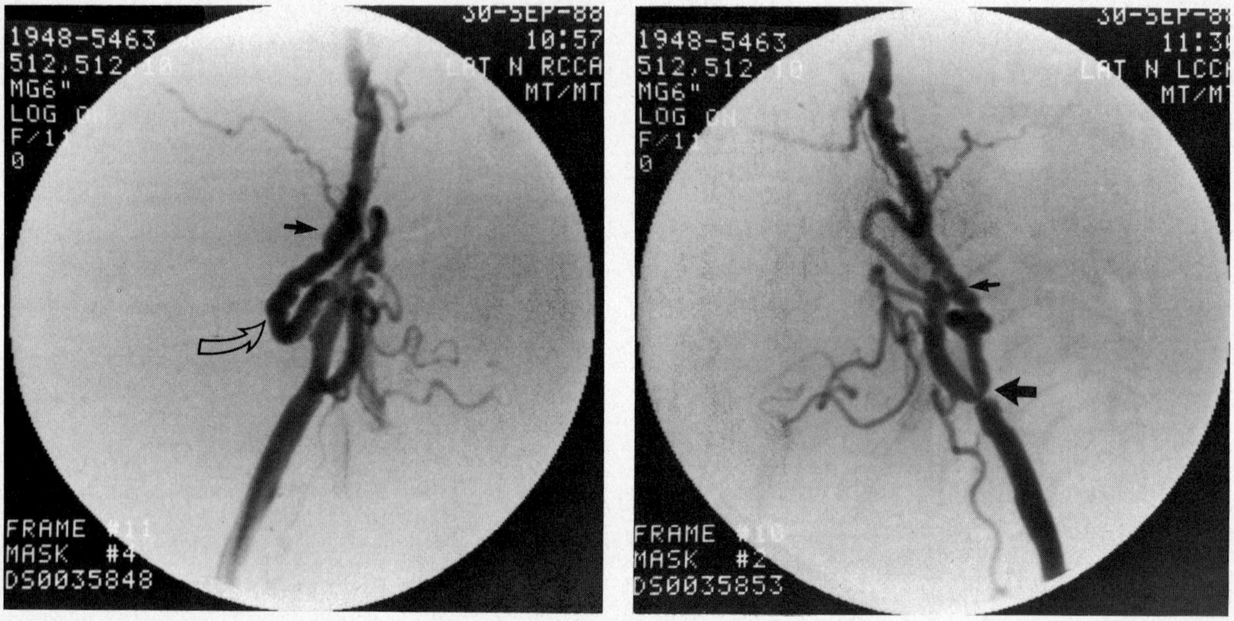

B

Fig. 22-10. Arteriogram of right (**A**) and left (**B**) carotid arteries in an 80-year-old woman. There appears to be arteriographic evidence of both medial fibroplasia (*small arrows*) and atherosclerosis (*large arrow*). Note the kinking of the right ICA (*open arrow*). She also had an asymptomatic 3 mm anterior communicating artery aneurysm (not seen). Left carotid endarterectomy was done with histologic confirmation of both medial fibroplasia and atherosclerosis.

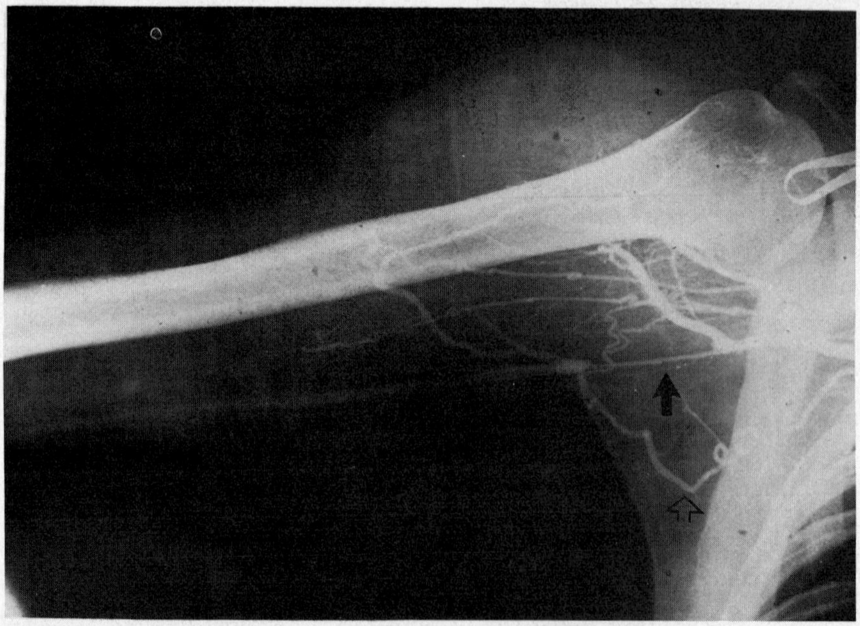

Fig. 22-11. Arteriogram of the right axillary artery with marked collaterals (*open arrow*) around an area of stenosis (*solid arrow*). This area of smooth narrowing (*solid arrow*) was histologically confirmed to be intimal fibroplasia.

aorta.[71] The coarctation may be thoracic, suprarenal, or infrarenal with concomitant involvement of the renal, mesenteric, or carotid circulation. Infrarenal coarctation is more commonly associated with FMD than is coarctation of the suprarenal or thoracic aorta. Frequently, the histologic specimens are consistent with those seen in neurofibromatosis; therefore, an extensive diagnostic workup should be performed to exclude this disease.[42,51]

Angiographically, nonrenal visceral FMD may reveal long areas of smooth narrowing rather than the classic "string-of-beads" appearance seen in FMD at other sites. This corresponds to the natural history in that arterial occlusion is a more common complication of nonrenal visceral FMD than aneurysm rupture or embolization. The histologic subtypes (intimal, medial, perimedial dysplasias) have all been described in the visceral circulation.[42-44] Intimal hyperplasia has been the predominant histologic form of FMD in the coronary circulation, but medial FMD with dissections has also been reported.[72] This exceedingly rare condition can affect all age groups, but only a handful of case reports exist.[73]

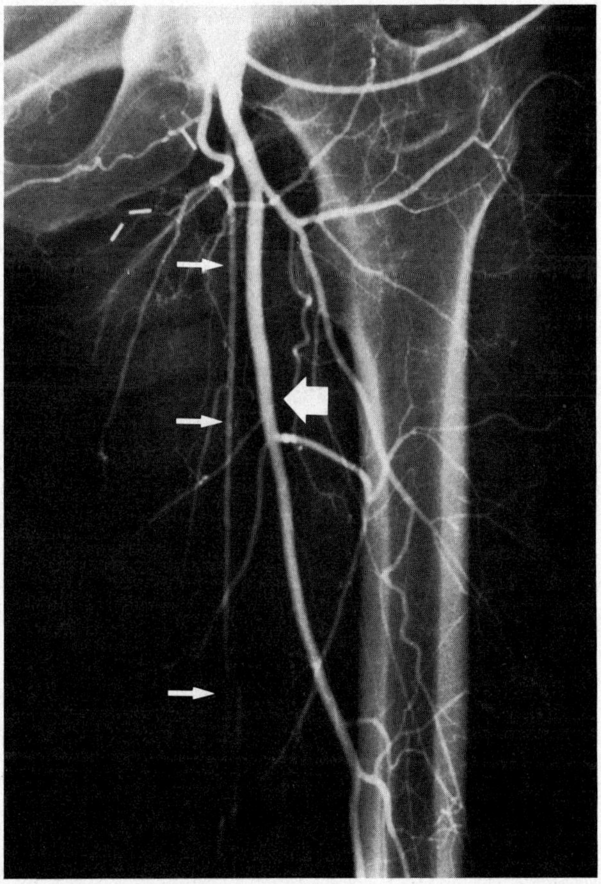

Fig. 22-12. Arteriogram of the left leg in a 58-year-old woman. Note the caliber of the superficial femoral (long smooth narrowing) (*small arrows*) compared to the normal appearing profunda femoris (*large arrow*). She also had internal carotid artery FMD that was confirmed to be intimal fibroplasia.

Because of the extensive collateralization normally available, mesenteric ischemia usually results only after 2 of the 3 main splanchnic vessels are occluded. Abdominal angina is usually accompanied by weight loss, cibophobia (fear of food) secondary to postprandial pain, and sometimes a change in stool formation. Aneurysm rupture and/or arteriovenous fistula formation can be manifested as hypotension, shock, or high output heart failure. Overall though, this is an asymptomatic disease and is most often found by chance in association with renal or carotid artery FMD. To date the primary treatment of symptomatic disease has been surgical intervention.[48] Percutaneous balloon angioplasty has been reported to be successful when technically feasible. It is the most viable alternative to surgery for patients with stenotic disease, but its applicability is limited by the presence of occlusive or aneurysmal disease.[74]

Extremities

FMD has been described in all of the peripheral arteries of the extremities (iliac, superficial femoral, popliteal, tibial, subclavian, axillary, radial, and ulnar) (Figs. 22-11 and 22-12). These lesions are typically asymptomatic but can produce signs and symptoms such as a difference in blood pressure, paresthesias, claudication, or frank ischemia.[42,48,75]

To date, most studies of FMD in the extremities demonstrate a female predominance. However, Estahani et al described 17 cases in Iranian men with upper and/or lower extremity occlusive disease (ages 22 to 45 years), but there was histologic confirmation in only 6 of these patients.[76] Arteritis, thromboangiitis obliterans, aneurysmal disease, or arteriosclerosis obliterans can masquerade as FMD and may have been overlooked in the study by Estahani et al. The symptomatic population has generally been older than 50 years of age, but complications of aneurysmal disease have been reported in the very young.[77] The older patients may have had predominantly asymptomatic FMD, but when the atherosclerotic process is superimposed on FMD, symptoms arise. Most cases have been diagnosed angiographically. Intimal fibroplasia seems to be the most frequent histologic subtype seen in peripheral FMD, although medial and perimedial fibroplasia have been described.[78]

The appropriate interventional therapy may be different, depending on the site, extent, and distal manifestations of the disease. Therapy should be reserved for symptomatic disease. The successful therapies reported to date include balloon dilation, graduated intraluminal dilation, surgical bypass and/or resection, and sympathetic blockade or transection.[79-81] If applicable, intervention with percutaneous balloon angioplasty should probably be the procedure of choice initially, with the surgical approach reserved for refractory or technically difficult disease. Minimal follow-up data are available to compare the efficacy of each approach.

ARTERIAL CALCIFICATION DISEASES

A heterogenous group of diseases, which share a common feature, calcification, are grouped together in this section. The four disease entities include arteriosclerosis obliterans (ASO); Mönckeberg's sclerosis, or medial calcinosis; idiopathic infantile arterial calcification; and arterial calcification associated with chronic renal failure. Arteriosclerosis obliterans is discussed in detail in other chapters and will not be considered further here.

The cellular mechanism of calcification is poorly understood and is probably dependent on the underlying disease process in which calcification is seen. Two theories help explain calcium phosphate complex formation in the arterial wall.[82] Intracellular uptake of excessive calcium at the mitochondrial level can lead to saturation and precipitation. This imbalance in calcium regulation intracellularly may account for metastatic calcification seen in end-stage renal failure patients with elevated calcium phosphate products. Selye proposed the term "calciphylaxis" to describe experimentally induced metastatic calcification.[83] The second theory describes an extracellular matrix vesicle as a common factor.[84] These membrane invested particles initiate calcification in a variety of sites, such as bone growth plates, cardiac prosthetic valves, and arterial vascular walls. This secondary process of dystrophic calcification usually results after ischemic or traumatic injury to the involved tissue.[85] The process or stimuli promoting vesicle formation is unknown.

Mönckeberg's sclerosis

In 1903 Mönckeberg described a condition of extensive calcification involving the tunica media of the large- and medium-sized arteries. This calcification can involve the lower extremities and the visceral and upper extremity vessels. The actual mechanism leading to calcification is unknown, but calcium, phosphate, and parathyroid hormone levels are usually normal.[86] The dense medial calcinosis produces a rigid conduit without encroachment on the vessel lumen. Therefore end-organ ischemia is not a complication. Mönckeberg's sclerosis is distinctly different from the intimal and medial calcification seen with ASO, where plaque progression leads to luminal narrowing and ultimately ischemia. The calcification secondary to ASO is often diffuse in distribution and frequently affects orificial and bifurcation arterial sites. Mönckeberg's sclerosis tends to spare these areas.

The cause of medial calcification is unknown; theories have tried to identify an insult to the medial wall such as infection or ischemia. Diabetics tend to have a higher incidence of medial arterial calcification.[87] This association is believed to be related to the duration of the metabolic derangement rather than the tightness of metabolic control. Some researchers suggest that diabetics with peripheral neuropathy have an even higher incidence of calcification than those without neuropathy.[88] Corticosteroids and immunosuppressant therapies have also been implicated in stimulating calcification. A link between Mönckeberg's sclerosis and metabolic bone disease such as osteoporosis has been suspected.

Histologic examination of affected arteries shows fibrotic and calcified replacement of the tunica media. The internal and external elastic lamina may be involved in the fibrotic process, whereas the intima is normal in pure Mönckeberg's.[86] The intimal changes of ASO can be superimposed on the medial disruption of Mönckeberg's sclerosis. This is usually present in patients over 50 years of age who may have had asymptomatic medial calcification for years.

The diagnosis of Mönckeberg's sclerosis is usually made by the classic radiographic appearance on plain roentgenograms. These changes are described as ringlike calcifications against a finely granular background.

Idiopathic infantile arterial calcification

Idiopathic infantile arterial calcification has been reported in less than 100 cases.[89-92] The diagnosis has been made by postmortem examination in most cases, but as awareness of the condition broadens, premortem and even prepartum diagnosis has been made.[89] Most newborns and infants develop cardiac or respiratory dysfunction, with myocardial ischemia being the primary mode of death early in life. Marked intimal proliferation sets this disease apart from the other calcification disorders, especially with the aggressive, progressive nature of the process. Calcification may be dramatic and affect all of the vessels including the heart, brain, mesentary, and extremities. The tunica media calcification may also be of a patchy distribution but is usually recognizable on plain roentgenograms of the extremities. An autosomal recessive transmission pattern is believed to account for the genetic familial occurrence of the disease.[89] Biochemical tests usually are normal in the disease with appropriate levels of calcium, phosphate, and parathyroid hormone.[90]

Treatment has consisted of strict blood pressure control with calcium channel blockers or angiotensin converting enzyme inhibitors.[89] Diphosphonates combined with a low-calcium diet have been shown to cause regression of the vessel calcification in some patients.[90,91] One survivor has reportedly lived to age 22 despite four myocardial infarctions,[92] whereas another is alive and well at 2 years of age with diphosphonate therapy.[91]

Arterial calcification associated with chronic renal failure

Arterial disease is common in patients with renal insufficiency, especially if they are also diabetic. Herman et al reported that 10% of the diabetic population in Rochester, Minnesota had peripheral vascular disease, whereas only 2.6% of the nondiabetic patients had similar symptoms.[93] The prevalence of arterial calcification is substantially greater in the dialysis population. At least one third of di-

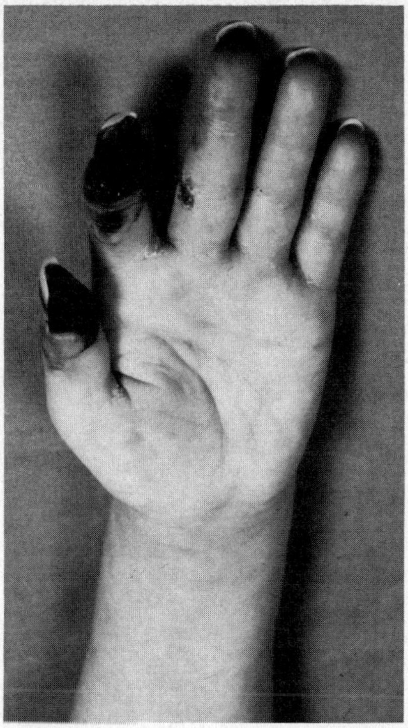

Fig. 22-13. Gangrene of several digits in a diabetic patient with end-stage renal disease.

alysis patients have arterial calcification, and this number escalates to 90% of diabetic predialysis patients.[94,95] These changes occur approximately 10 years earlier in the diabetic patient.

ASO and Mönckeberg's sclerosis are the two common arterial histopathologic features seen in renal insufficiency patients. Claudication, rest pain, and gangrene associated with extensive ASO can be seen in this population. Peripheral neuropathy can be a complicating factor in the masking of clinical signs of arterial insufficiency. Generally, the distribution of the disease includes a greater incidence of lower extremity arterial involvement especially of the profunda femoris and below-the-knee arterial sites. However, ASO can be diffuse and quite widespread. All these patients should be considered as having coronary artery disease, the clinical significance of which should be determined.

Arteriosclerosis obliterans usually does not occur in the distal portion of the arms or hands. An exception to this is patients with chronic renal failure, especially those with diabetes who undergo chronic dialysis treatment or who have undergone renal transplantation. The exact pathogenesis of this involvement of the arms and hands is unknown, but it cannot be solely explained on the basis of calcium-phosphorus imbalance or hyperparathyroidism. Accelerated atherosclerosis seems to be a more likely explanation. There is progressive systemic intimal proliferation. The smaller caliber vessels are most affected by the intimal proliferation, thus an acral distribution to the ischemia ensues.[96] There is usually calcification of the media. These patients can present in a dramatic fashion, have progressive gangrene of the fingers, and eventually lose the entire hand (Fig. 22-13). There is no known treatment for this complication.

Another severe form of calcification in end-stage renal disease patients is called systemic calcinosis, metastatic calcification, or calciphylaxis. This infrequent soft tissue and arterial deposition of calcium phosphate complex (hydroxyapatite) is a result of a high calcium-phosphorus product (>60 to 70).[97] The precipitation occurs in the connective tissue of organs such as the skin, lungs, kidneys, stomach, heart, and arteries. Most patients have elevated parathyroid hormone levels. Factors that exacerbate this calcification process include vitamin D, calcium carbonate, corticosteroids, immunosuppressants, and blood product therapies.[97,98]

The treatment is to lower the calcium phosphate product and remove any aggravating factors. Parathyroidectomy has been performed with successful reversal of the calcification process in some patients.[96] A vigilant approach to the control of infectious and septic complications should also be employed since this is a frequent complicating feature.

REFERENCES

1. Stuart TPA: Note on a variation in the course of the popliteal artery, J Anat Physiol 13:162, 1879.
2. Chambardel-Dubreuil L: Variations des arteres du pelvis et du membre inferieur, Paris, 1925, Masson and Cie.
3. Hamming JJ: Intermittent claudication at an early age, due to an anomalous course of the popliteal artery, Angiology 10:369, 1959.
4. Hall KV: Anomalous insertion of the medial gastrocnemic head with circulatory complications, Acta Path Microbiol Scand 148(suppl):53, 1961.
5. Hall KV: Intervascular gastrocnemic insertion, Acta Chir Scand 128:193, 1964.
6. Carter AE and Eban R: A case of bilateral developmental abnormality of the popliteal arteries and gastrocnemius muscles, Br J Surg 51:518, 1964.
7. Love JW and Whelan TJ: Popliteal artery entrapment syndrome, Am J Surg 109:620, 1965.
8. Rich NM and Hughes CW: Popliteal artery and vein entrapment, Am J Surg 113:696, 1967.
9. Cavallaro A et al: Popliteal artery entrapment: analysis of the literature and report of personal experience, Vasc Surg 20:404, 1986.
10. Connell J: Poplital vein entrapment, Br J Surg 65:351, 1978.
11. Podore PC: Popliteal entrapment syndrome: a report of tibial nerve entrapment, J Vasc Surg 2:335, 1985.
12. Collins PS, McDonald PT, and Lim RC: Popliteal artery entrapment: an evolving syndrome, J Vasc Surg 10:484, 1989.
13. Represa JAF et al: Popliteal artery entrapment syndrome, J Cardiovasc Surg 27:426, 1986.
14. Inada K et al: Popliteal artery entrapment syndrome: a case report, Br J Surg 65:613, 1978.
15. Iwai T et al: Diagnostic and pathological considerations in the popliteal artery entrapment syndrome, J Cardiovasc Surg 24:243, 1983.
16. Insua JA, Young JR, and Humphries AW: Popliteal artery entrapment syndrome, Arch Surg 101:771, 1970.
17. Delaney TA and Gonzalez LL: Occlusion of the popliteal artery due to muscular entrapment, Surgery 69:97, 1971.

18. Bouhoutsos J and Daskalakis E: Muscular abnormalities affecting the popliteal vessels, Br J Surg 68:501, 1981.
19. Gibson MHL et al: Popliteal artery entrapment syndrome, Ann Surg 185:341, 1974.
20. Hamming JJ and Vink M: Obstruction of the popliteal artery at an early age, J Cardiovasc Surg 6:516, 1965.
21. McDonald PT et al: Popliteal artery entrapment syndrome: clinical non-invasive and angiographic diagnosis, Am J Surg 139:318, 1980.
22. Rizzo RJ et al: Computed tomography for evaluation of arterial disease in the popliteal fossa, J Vasc Surg 11:112, 1990.
23. Whelan TJ: Popliteal artery entrapment. In Rutherford RB, ed.: Vascular Surgery, 1989, WB Saunders.
24. Ishikawa K: Cystic adventitial disease of the popliteal artery and of other stem vessels in the extremities, Jpn J Surg 17:221, 1987.
25. Atkins HJB and Key JA: A case of myxomatous tumour arising in the adventitia of the left external iliac artery, Br J Surg 34:426, 1946.
26. Ejrup B and Hiertonn T: Intermittent claudication: three cases treated by free vein graft, Acta Chir Scand 108:217, 1954.
27. Hiertonn T, Lindberg K, and Rob C: Cystic degeneration of the popliteal artery, Br J Surg 44:348, 1957.
28. Haid SP, Conn J Jr, and Bergan JJ: Cystic adventitial disease of the popliteal artery, Arch Surg 101:765, 1970.
29. Flanigan DP et al: Summary of cases of adventitial cystic disease of the popliteal artery, Ann Surg 189:165, 1979.
30. Sakamoto H et al: Bilateral cystic adventitial disease of the popliteal artery, J Jap Coll Angiol 16:607, 1976.
31. Ohta T et al: Cystic adventitial degeneration of the ilio-femoral artery and vein, Vasc Surg 18:119, 1984.
32. Durham JR et al: Adventitial cystic disease of the radial artery. J Cardiovasc Surg 30:517, 1989.
33. Robb D: Obstruction of popliteal artery by synovial cyst: report of a case, Br J Surg 48:221, 1960.
34. Ruppel V et al: Pathological anatomical observations in cystic adventitial degeneration of blood vessels, Beitr Path Bd 144:101, 1971.
35. Mark TM et al: Cystic adventitial degeneration of the popliteal artery, Arch Pathol Lab Med 107:186, 1983.
36. Endo M et al: Isolation and identification of proteohyaluronic acid from a cyst of cystic mucoid degeneration, Clin Chim Acta 47:417, 1973.
37. Bunker SR, Lauten GJ, and Hutton JE: Cystic adventitial disease of the popliteal artery, AJR 136:1209, 1981.
38. Jasinski RW et al: Adventitial cystic disease of the popliteal artery, Radiology 163:153, 1987.
39. Wilbur AC and Spigos DG: Adventitial cyst of the popliteal artery: CT-guided percutaneous aspiration, J Comput Assist Tomogr 10:161, 1986.
40. Fox RL et al: Adventitial cystic disease of the popliteal artery: failure of percutaneous transluminal angioplasty as a therapeutic modality, J Vasc Surg 2:464, 1985.
41. Hierton T and Hemmingsson A: The autogenous vein graft as popliteal artery substitute, Acta Chir Scand 150:377, 1984.
42. Luscher TF et al: Arterial fibromuscular dysplasia, Mayo Clin Proc 62:931, 1987.
43. Iwai T et al: Fibromuscular dysplasia in the extremities, J Cardiovasc Surg 26:496, 1985.
44. Palubinskas AJ and Ripley HR: Fibromuscular hyperplasia in extrarenal arteries, Radiology 82:451, 1964.
45. McCormack LJ et al: A pathologic-arteriographic correlation of renal arterial disease, Am Heart J 72:188, 1966.
46. Harrison EJ Jr and McCormack LJ: Pathologic classification of renal arterial disease in renovascular hypertension, Mayo Clin Proc 46:161, 1971.
47. Rushton AR: The genetics of fibromuscular dysplasia, Arch Intern Med 140:233, 1980.
48. Luscher TF et al: Fibromuscular hyperplasia: extension of the disease and therapeutic outcome, Nephron 44(suppl 1):109, 1986.
49. Rothfield NJH: Fibromuscular arterial disease: experimental studies, Australas Radiol 14:294, 1970.
50. Sottiurai VS, Fry WF, and Stanley JC: Ultrastructure of medial smooth muscle and myelofibroblasts in human arterial dysplasia, Arch Surg 113:1280, 1978.
51. Craddock GR, Challa VR, and Dean RH: Neurofibromatosis and renal artery stenosis: a case of familial incidence, J Vasc Surg 8:489, 1988.
52. Qunibi WJ et al: Pheochromocytoma and fibromuscular hyperplasia, South Med J 72:1481, 1979.
53. Schievink WI and Limburg M: Angiographic abnormalities mimicking fibromuscular dysplasia in a patient with Ehler-Danlos syndrome, type IV, Neurosurgery 25:482, 1989.
54. Hodgins LB and Limbacher JP II: Fibromuscular dysplasia in Alport's syndrome, J Tenn Med Assoc 75:733, 1982.
55. Connett MC and Lansche JM: Fibromuscular hyperplasia of the internal carotid artery: report of a case, Ann Surg 162:59, 1965.
56. Mettinger KL and Ericson K: Fibromuscular dysplasia and the brain: observations on angiographic, clinical and genetic characteristics, Stroke 13:46, 1982.
57. Mettinger KL: Fibromuscular dysplasia and the brain. II. Current concept of the disease, Stroke 13:53, 1982.
58. Houser OW et al: Cephalic arterial fibromuscular dysplasia, Radiology 101:605, 1971.
59. Osborn AG and Anderson RE: Angiographic spectrum of cervical and intra-cranial fibromuscular dysplasia, Stroke 8:617, 1977.
60. Corrin LS, Sandok BA, and Houser OW: Cerebral ischemic events in patients with carotid artery fibromuscular dysplasia, Arch Neurol 38:616, 1981.
61. George B et al: Vascular abnormalities in the neck associated with intracranial aneurysms, Neurosurg 24:499, 1989.
62. Sato S and Hata J: Fibromuscular dysplasia: its occurrence with a dissecting aneuyrsm of the internal carotid artery, Arch Pathol Lab Med 106:332, 1982.
63. Dublin AB, Baltaxe HA, and Cobb CA III: Percutaneous transluminal carotid angioplasty in fibromuscular dysplasia: case report, J Neurosurg 59:162, 1983.
64. Effeney DJ et al: Why operate on carotid fibromuscular dysplasia? Arch Surg 115:1261, 1980.
65. Ehrenfeld WK, Stoney RJ, and Wylie EJ: Fibromuscular hyperplasia of the internal carotid artery, Arch Surg 95:284, 1967.
66. Maiuri F et al: Fibromuscular dysplasia of the carotid arteries: clinical and radiographic considerations, Clin Neurol Neurosurg 90:57, 1988.
67. McNeill DH Jr, Dreisbach J, and Marsden RJ: Spontaneous dissection of the internal carotid artery: its conservative management with heparin sodium, Arch Neurol 37:54, 1980.
68. Hasso AN and Bird CR: Percutaneous transluminal angioplasty of carotid and vertebral arteries. In Jang GC, ed: Angioplasty, New York, 1986, McGraw-Hill Book Co.
69. Deterling RA: Aneurysm of the visceral arteries, J Cardiovasc Surg 12:309, 1971.
70. Kreel L: The recognition and incidence of splenic artery aneurysms: a historical review, Australas Radiol 16:126, 1972.
71. Connolly JE: Fibromuscular hyperplasia of the abdominal aorta, J Cardiovasc Surg 19:563, 1978.
72. Lie JT and Berg KK: Isolated fibromuscular dysplasia of the coronary arteries with spontaneous dissection and myocardial infarction, Hum Path 18:654, 1987.
73. James TN and Marshall TK: Multifocal stenoses due to fibromuscular dysplasia of the sinus node artery, Circulation 53:736, 1976.
74. Odurny A, Sniderman KW, and Colapinto RF: Intestinal angina: percutaneous transluminal angioplasty of the celiac and superior mesenteric arteries, Radiology 167:59, 1988.

75. Walter JF et al: External iliac artery fibrodysplasia, AJR 131:125, 1978.
76. Estahani F et al: Arterial fibrodysplasia: a regional cause of peripheral occlusive vascular disease, Angiology 40:108, 1989.
77. Stinnett DM, Graham JM, and Edwards WD: Fibromuscular dysplasia and thrombosed aneurysm of the popliteal artery in a child, J Vasc Surg 5:769, 1987.
78. van den Dungen JJAM, Boontje AH, and Oosterhuis JW: Femoropopliteal arterial fibrodysplasia, Br J Surg 77:396, 1990.
79. Parnell AP, Loose HW, and Chamberlain J: Fibromuscular dysplasia of the external iliac artery: treatment by percutaneous transluminal angioplasty, Br J Rad 61:1080, 1988.
80. Houston C et al: Fibromuscular dysplasia of the external iliac arteries: surgical treatment by graduated internal dilatation technique, Surgery 85:713, 1979.
81. Mashiah A, Pasik S, and David A: Phenol sympathectomy for symptomatic fibromuscular angiodysplasia of the lower limb, J Cardiovasc Surg 30:244, 1989.
82. Anderson HC: Calcific diseases, Arch Pathol Lab Med 107:341, 1983.
83. Selye H: Calciphylaxis, Chicago, 1962, University of Chicago Press.
84. Kim KM and Huang SN: Ultrastructural study of dystrophic calcification of human aortic valve, Lab Invest 26:481, 1972.
85. Tanimura A et al: Matrix vesicles in atherosclerotic calcification, Proc Soc Exp Biol Med 172:173, 1983.
86. Lachman AS et al: Medial calcinosis of Mönckeberg, Am J Med 63:615, 1977.
87. Goebel FD and Fuessl HS: Mönckeberg's sclerosis after sympathetic denervation in diabetic and non-diabetic subjects, Diabetologia 24:347, 1983.
88. Edmonds ME et al: Medial arterial calcification and diabetic neuropathy, Br Med J 284:928, 1982.
89. Juul S et al: New insights into idiopathic infantile arterial calcinosis, Am J Dis Child 144:229, 1990.
90. Moran JJ: Idiopathic arterial calcification of infancy: a clinicopathologic study, Pathol Annu 10:393, 1975.
91. Van Dyck M et al: Idiopathic infantile arterial calcification with cardiac, renal and central nervous system involvement, Eur J Pediatr 148:374, 1989.
92. Marrott PK et al: Idiopathic infantile calcification with survival into adult life, Pediatr Cardiol 5:119, 1984.
93. Herman WH et al: Closing the gap: the problem of diabetes mellitus in the United States, Diabetes Care 8:391, 1985.
94. Meema HE et al: Arterial calcifications in severe chronic renal disease and their relationship to dialysis treatment, renal transplant and parathyroidectomy, Radiology 121:315, 1976.
95. Meema HE and Oreopoulos DG: Arterial calcifications in patients undergoing chronic peritoneal dialysis: incidence, progression and regression, PD Bulletin Oct-Dec:241, 1985.
96. Wilkinson SP et al: Symmetric gangrene of the extremities in late renal failure: a case report and review of the literature, Q J Med 67:319, 1988.
97. Conn J Jr et al: Calciphylaxis: etiology of progressive vascular calcification and gangrene? Ann Surg 177:206, 1973.
98. Mallick NP and Berlyne GM: Arterial calcification after Vitamin D therapy in hyperphosphatemic renal failure, Lancet 2:1316, 1968.

Chapter 23

VASCULOGENIC IMPOTENCE

Ralph G. DePalma
Frederick J. Schwab

Penile erection requires adequate arterial inflow and closure of cavernosal outflow. Both are mediated by intact neural mechanisms and relaxation of the smooth muscle of the corpora cavernosa.[1] Increased arterial inflow conditions cavernosal closure of venous outflow; during erection intracavernous pressure increases to levels ranging from 80 to 99 mm Hg. Higher pressures contributing to penile rigidity are generated by contraction of the perineal muscles. There has been considerable recent progress in understanding the hemodynamics contributing to erectile failure.[2] The physiology of penile erection has been summarized recently.[3] This chapter reviews the diagnosis and treatment of vasculogenic impotence.

DIAGNOSIS

The accompanying box classifies causes of vasculogenic impotence. In general the origin of these causes may be arterial, cavernosal, or venous. The diagnosis of vasculogenic impotence is based on a sequence of noninvasive and invasive steps.[4] These include measurement of penile arterial pressure, penile plethysmography and waveform analysis, bulbocavernosal reflex time and measurement of pudendal evoked potentials, and observation of erectile response after intracavernous injection of papaverine or vasoactive agents such as phentolamine or prostaglandin E_1. For definitive anatomic diagnosis we now require selective arteriography, dynamic cavernosography, and cavernosometry after intracorporeal injections. Before proceeding to invasive tests, blood glucose, testosterone, and prolactin levels are obtained during the initial visit. Hypothyroidism may contribute to impotence, but in our experience this cause has not been encountered. Optimally, these tests would separate the various factors contributing to erectile failure and also help define hormonal or neural causes of impotence.

Classification of vasculogenic impotence

Arterial	
Large vessel:	Aorta and branches to internal iliac artery distribution
Small vessel:	Pudendal and penile arteries
Combined:	Emboli to pudendal or cavernosal arteries from aortic aneurysm or ulcerated plaques
Cavernosal	
Fibrosis:	Idiopathic or postpriapism
Peyronie's disease:	Deformity and/or venous leakage
Refractory states:	Diabetes, antihypertensive medications, hormonal
Venous	
Congenital:	Cavernous-spongious leak
Acquired:	Cavernosal leak syndrome

HISTORY AND PHYSICAL EXAMINATION

Both history and physical examination may contribute to better understanding of possible causes of arteriogenic impotence. Gradual erectile failure in the absence of traumatic life events and symptomatic lower extremity vascular disease suggest large vessel arteriogenic impotence. In men with these symptoms both the intensity and duration of atherosclerotic risk factors, mainly smoking, hypertension, diabetes, and hypercholesterolemia, contribute to arteriogenic impotence. This disease pattern may involve the aortoiliac segments and the first segment of the internal iliac artery. Abdominal aortic aneurysms or ulcerative atheromatous disease of the abdominal aorta can also cause embolic occlusions of the pudendal arteries. Traumatic arterial occlusions can be caused by perineal or pelvic injuries.

Urologic, vascular, or rectal operations can cause impotence. Thus a history of immediate onset of erectile failure following surgery is important. Under these circumstances postoperative erectile dysfunction can be the result of vascular or neural interruption. Alcohol and drug abuse contribute to erectile failure. Drugs used to treat hypertension and diabetes also commonly cause erectile failure because of both their neuropathic and metabolic effects.

On physical examination absence of leg pulses suggests large vessel disease. With normal femoral pulses femoral bruits suggest pelvic or internal iliac disease. Sensory testing of the extremities, perineum, or glans occasionally reveals neuropathies associated with impotence in diabetics. The prostate should be examined. Finally, palpation of the corpora cavernosa for Peyronie's plaques and estimation of testicular size completes specific examinations. Atrophy or absence of testicular mass leads to a diagnosis of primary hypogonadism. In these cases testosterone levels will be low. Often, however, physical examination is unrevealing.

NONINVASIVE VASCULAR TESTING

We require previsit noninvasive neurovascular tests in all patients referred for impotence. These tests help select patients for further studies or procedures—and have recently been summarized.[5] Because some of the tests involve intracavernous injections of vasoactive agents, an estimate of arterial perfusion is useful. Among 658 patients screened between September 1983 and January 1989, 46% were found to have abnormal penile arterial perfusion. These tests will be described in some detail.

Penile brachial indices (PBI)

PBI is a ratio between the systolic pressure detected by a Doppler probe placed distal to a penile cuff and systemic or brachial arm pressure. In an average-size penis a cuff of at least 2.5 cm is used. The cuff is inflated, then deflated. Reappearance of Doppler signals in the dorsal artery branches just proximal to the corona of the glans signals reflow. Normally this pressure is systemic. PBI above 0.75 suggests that no major obstacle exists between the aorta and the distal measurement point (Fig. 23-1). Generally PBI less than 0.6 relates to major vascular obstructions in the aortoiliac bed. PBI between 0.75 and 0.6 is abnormal and may occur with lesions involving the internal pudendal and the penile arteries.

Penile plethysmographic pulse volume recording (PVR)

Penile PVR is performed using a pneumoplethysmographic cuff with a contained transducer [6,7] on the penis in the flaccid state. The variables recorded are crest time, waveform, and the presence or absence of a dicrotic notch. Penile PVR measures total pulsation of all penile arteries as the cuff compresses the penile tissue. The cuff is applied and inflated to mean arterial pressure, which is calculated as diastolic pressure plus one third of systemic pulse pressure. Waveforms are recorded on a polygraph with a chart speed of 25 mm/sec and a sensitivity setting of 1. In normal patients the upstroke of the waveform is completed by 0.2 second (5 mm); normal waveform amplitudes vary from 5 to 6 to 30 mm in height. Examples of normal and abnormal waveforms are shown in Fig. 23-2. These tests help detect arteriogenic impotence. However, vasculogenic impotence caused by venous leak or Peyronie's disease is not detected.

Neurologic testing

Neural disorders frequently contribute to erectile failure. Among 290 patients evaluated in our laboratory using pudendal-evoked potentials and measuring bulbocavernosus reflex, 84 (28%) men exhibited at least one abnormality. Such subtle neurologic changes are not detected by ordinary physical examination. We have described the use of pudendal-evoked potentials in the evaluation of impotence[4,8] and have shown that reproducible responses can be obtained. Normal reference latencies for pudendal, lumbar, and cortical somatosensory-evoked potentials have been measured. Because many impotent patients are diabetic, pudendal responses are compared with spinal and cortical-evoked responses from posterior tibial nerve stimulation. Bulbocavernosus reflex time after dorsal penile nerve stimulation is measured. Mean normal bulbocavernosus reflex time in our laboratory is 28.3 to 37.5 ms. Grossly abnormal findings suggesting neurologic deficits contraindicate vascular operations for impotence.

Artificial erection

After completion of arterial and neural testing, clinical assessment of erectile function can be done. Injection of vasoactive agents into the corpora cavernosa causes a pharmacologic erection that can be observed clinically. We usually begin with an intracorporeal dose of papaverine ranging from 15 to 60 mg, depending on the results of arterial noninvasive testing. Alternatively, 10 μg of prostaglandin E_1 can be used. Phentolamine combined with papaverine has also been used. The discovery that these agents could cause erection added an important dimension to the diagnosis and treatment of erectile failure.[9,10] The major side effect of these agents is prolonged erection, which may require reversal; therefore we begin with smaller doses. On occasion leakage of papaverine may cause systemic hypotension. Therefore blood pressure must be monitored and a tourniquet applied to the penile base.

The erectile response after intracavernous injection helps separate arteriogenic from venogenic impotence. Normally, after intracavernous papaverine, erection occurs within 20 minutes and lasts 3 to 4 hours. With venous incompetence transient erection or tumescence occurs but is rapidly lost. In these cases PBI and penile PVRs are normal. With arterial insufficiency there will be delayed tumescence and refractoriness with increasing doses of papaverine.

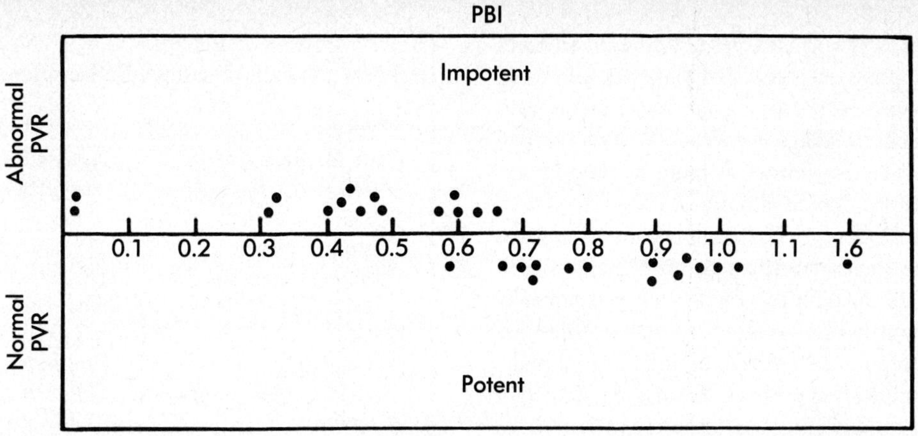

Fig. 23-1. Relationship between PBI and PVR in clinically potent and impotent men. Note zone of overlap at PBI of 0.6 to 0.7. (Recordings obtained with Buffington Plethysmographic Cuff, Buffington Clinical Systems, Inc., P.O. Box 24241, Cleveland, OH 44124.)

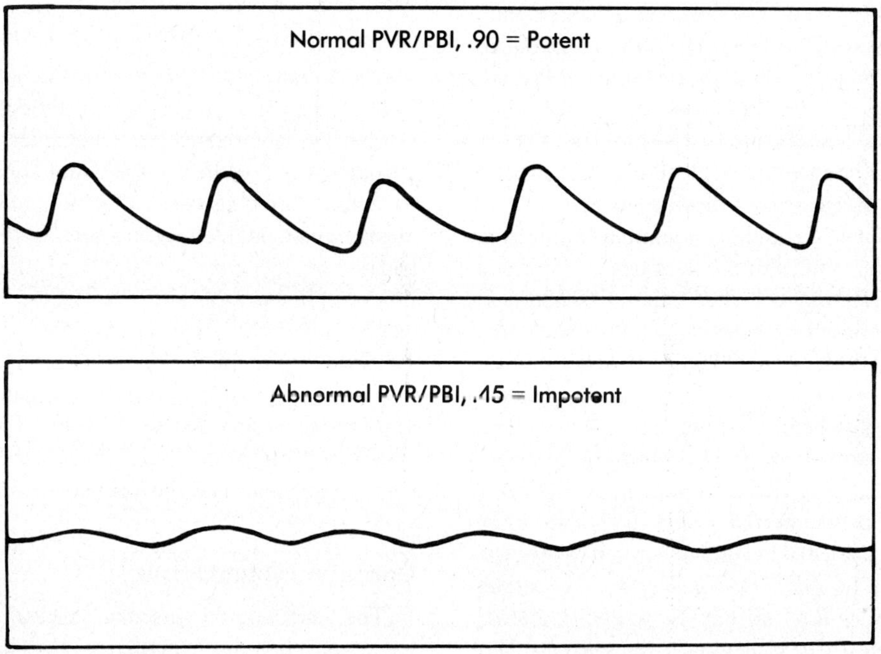

Fig. 23-2. Examples of pulse wave recordings in potent and impotent patients with arterial insufficiency.

We found it important to begin with smaller doses of papaverine, for instance, 15 to 30 mg. The patient is observed in the clinic until the erection subsides. Patients failing to have an erection after an injection of vasoactive agents are candidates for cavernosometry, cavernosography, and measurement of cavernosal artery occlusion pressure.

Cavernosometry and cavernosal artery occlusion pressure (CAOP)

While impotence can be caused by inadequate arterial supply, closure of the venous outflow system is also needed to achieve and maintain an erection. Arterial and venous function are thus closely related. Erection begins with cavernosal smooth muscle relaxation. This in turn decreases peripheral vascular resistance within the penis and increases arterial flow. Resulting dilation of the sinusoidal spaces then occludes the veins that pass through the tunica albuginea, dramatically reducing venous outflow. During maximal erection sinusoidal pressure at some point equilibrates with arterial inflow pressure; this value is called cavernosal artery occlusion pressure (CAOP).

During studies using fine needles inserted into the cavernous bodies, it is possible to measure CAOP with a Doppler probe. If arterial pressure is reduced by proximal occlusion, penile rigidity cannot occur. Cavernosal pressure also cannot rise when venous leakage is excessive. Such leakage can be caused by either congenital or more commonly acquired leaks through the tunica albuginea.

Techniques used at George Washington University have been modified from those described by Bookstein et al,[11] Goldstein,[12] and Lue et al.[13] To perform cavernosometry and cavernosography, two 21-gauge butterfly needles are placed into each corpora cavernosa for infusion of pharmacologic agents, saline, and pressure monitoring. Constant cavernosal pressure monitoring and an infusion pump are used. A 60 mg amount of papaverine and 1 mg of phentolamine, diluted to a total volume of 5 cc, are injected. After 15 minutes heparinized saline is infused at a rate of 20 ml/min. This rate is increased gradually until a rigid erection occurs. Cavernosal pressure then usually exceeds 100 mm Hg. The infusion rate is lowered to achieve steady state cavernosal pressure at this level. The flow rate to induce erection (FIE) and flow to maintain erection (FME) are recorded. Infusion rate is then further increased to produce a suprasystolic cavernosal pressure of 150 mm Hg, and the infusion is stopped. The rate of fall of cavernosal pressure over the succeeding 30 seconds is recorded.

To visualize venous leaks, a diluted nonionic contrast is injected, and spot filming in various obliquities is performed to identify specific abnormal opacified veins. FMEs of less than 12 ml/min have been proposed as normal, while a rate greater than 45 ml/min exceeds the ability of even a normal arterial system to compensate for increased venous leakage. Goldstein[12] suggests that the rate of pressure fall of greater than 1 mm Hg/sec strongly suggests cavernosal leakage. Following these procedures, CAOP is measured. CAOP, a physiologic index of penile arterial supply, is thought to be normal when greater than 90 mm Hg. However, a cavernosal brachial gradient must be taken into consideration. In certain cases a gradient greater than 30 mm Hg suggests arterial inflow reduction even if CAOP is greater than 90 mm Hg.

Duplex scanning and arteriography

Dorsal and deep cavernosal arteries can be examined by duplex scanning at intervals before and after papaverine injection.[14] To determine whether or not arterial occlusion exists, preoperative angiographic studies are needed. Conventional arteriography demonstrates large vessel occlusive disease and is selected when PBI is grossly abnormal. Highly selective internal iliac arteriography using artificial erection is required to display pudendal and penile arterial anatomy. We have now made it a policy to perform cavernosography, cavernosometry, CAOP, and selective arteriography at the same time in surgical candidates. All are needed to make a rational choice for specific surgical intervention.[15] We limit the use of duplex scanning to instances in which cavernosal disease is to be documented.

Treatment of vasculogenic impotence

Medical	*Surgical*
Risk factor interventions	***Arterial dysfunction***
Smoking cessation	Aortoiliac and/or internal iliac reconstruction
Control of diabetes	Dorsal artery bypass
Change of blood pressure medication	Dorsal vein arterialization
Drugs	***Cavernosal or neurogenic***
Isoxsuprine	Prostheses
Yohimbine hydrochloride	***Cavernosal leakage***
Injections	Vein resection and interruption
Intracorporeal papaverine	Transcatheter venous occlusion
Phentolamine	
Prostaglandin E_1	

TREATMENT OF VASCULOGENIC IMPOTENCE

The accompanying box summarizes treatment options. Medical treatment is generally tried first. For all patients it is wise to recommend risk factor intervention, particularly cessation of cigarette smoking and control of hypercholesterolemia. In some cases it is possible to alter antihypertensive treatment by weight control or changing drugs. After papaverine injection for artificial erection, some men resume function. In cases of mild arteriogenic impotence this effect can be enhanced by the addition of isoxsuprine 10 to 20 mg 4 times a day. In addition, yohimbine hydrochloride (Yocon) is effective in some cases. Its mechanism of action is unknown. In our experience, 10% to 15% of patients resume satisfactory function. Self-injection programs, with proper supervision, can also be offered to carefully selected patients.

Operative considerations

The candidate for vascular surgical correction of impotence must exhibit identifiable physiologic and anatomic vascular defects in the absence of neurogenic or hormonal causes of impotence. Arterial procedures for impotence are performed on the internal iliac arteries[15] and the small arteries, that is, the dorsal penile.[16] Deep dorsal vein arterialization is used for mixed impotence.[17] Venous ablation for cavernosal leak syndrome has been used in a variety of approaches depending on the demonstrated sites of venous leakage.[18] Small vessel arterial bypasses are still evolutionary.

Operations on large arteries. Operative methods in aortoiliac surgery to prevent postoperative sexual dysfunction and to restore sexual function have been described.[19] These operations provide flow to the internal iliac arteries and avoid neural arc disruption. Operations for arteriogenic impotence per se on the large arteries involve mainly those done for segmental internal iliac artery disease. Internal iliac endarterectomy or bypass have been effective. Restoration of normal blood flow with perfusion of one internal iliac artery is usually effective in restoring erectile function. In renal transplants the use of an end-to-side anastomosis to the external iliac artery avoids division of an internal iliac artery. This averts impotence after a second renal transplant.

Small vessel operations. Bypass of dorsal penile arteries requires retrograde flow into the deep cavernosal artery or the presence of an accessory deep cavernosal branch connecting the dorsal penile and cavernosal systems.[15] A penile vessel diameter of 1.5 mm is adequate for a standard microvascular technique. The inferior epigastric artery is our donor vessel of choice. If this is inadequate, a vein graft can be used. Deep dorsal vein arterialization for mixed vasculogenic impotence has been used with combined arterial and venous abnormalities. This method was pioneered by Virag et al.[17] The donor artery is anastomosed end-to-side with the centrally situated deep dorsal vein of the penis. To avoid glans hyperperfusion the distal dorsal vein should be ligated. Variations of this procedure include Hauri's,[20] where an arteriovenous fistula is fashioned between one dorsal artery and the dorsal vein and anastomosis of this aperture to the inferior epigastric artery.

The long-term results of all revascularizations require continual assessment. The operations on the large arteries, such as the aortoiliac axis, are quite secure. When adequate flow is restored, oftentimes the results are immediate and durable, depending mainly on the patient's age. Small vessel revascularization requires further observations for the long term. Virag et al[21] reported 201 men who underwent arterialization of the deep dorsal vein with 138 of these patients observed from 1 to 7 years. Of these men, 74 are reported presently to have good clinical results.

Venous interruption for cavernosal leak syndrome. Venous interruption operations of different types are evolving.[18] With appropriate cavernosometry and cavernosography, the results with resection of the dorsal penile vein from the penile hilum to the sulcus behind the glans are promising. Deep dorsal vein exposure and its proximal ligation of the hilum of the penis are facilitated by division of the suspensory ligament using a lateral penoscrotal incision. To assess the efficacy of venous interruption at surgery, we use intraoperative cavernosometry and cavernosography. To evaluate final results we use preoperative and postoperative cavernosometry and cavernosography to correlate the completeness of the venous interruption with reported functional results. Our recent approach for venous leakage has used the introduction of platinum flower coils to occlude abnormally draining veins. This was accomplished by passing a sheath into the surgically exposed dorsal vein or by a percutaneous femoral approach, introducing the catheter system into the femoral veins and into the distal internal pudendal veins.

The diagnosis and treatment of vasculogenic impotence has progressed remarkably in the past decade. Fig. 23-2 is a flow diagram outlining diagnostic and treatment methods described in this chapter. This approach, as in any evolving discipline, represents current state of the art considerations—these will undoubtedly change. In a recent clinical analysis of over 1000 men who received one or several treatments, including prostheses, Virag et al[21] described restoration of satisfactory function in 93% of cases. In cases

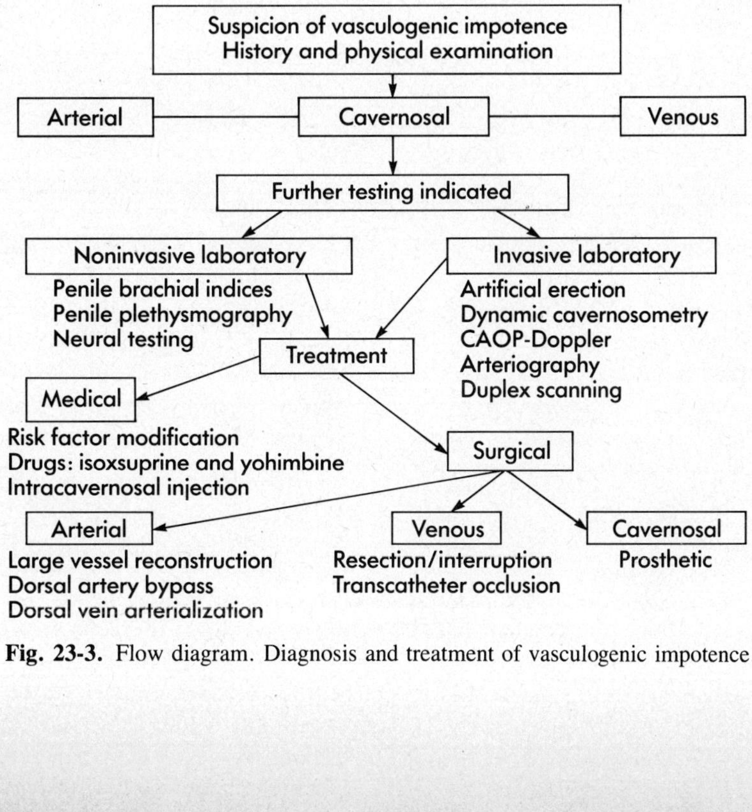

Fig. 23-3. Flow diagram. Diagnosis and treatment of vasculogenic impotence.

of postoperative impotence, late progression of vascular disease, neurogenic impotence, or failed small vessel bypass, a prosthesis is the logical option. However, once a prosthetic device is used, a prosthesis will always be required, and revascularization is no longer possible.

REFERENCES

1. DeTejada IS et al: Impaired neurogenic and endothelium-mediated relaxation of penile smooth muscle from diabetic men with impotence, N Engl J Med 320:1025, 1989.
2. Michal V: Arteriogenic impotence, Angio Archiv 8:4, 1985.
3. DePalma RG: Anatomy and physiology of male sexual function. In Giordano JM, Trout HH III, and DePalma RG, eds: The basic science of vascular surgery, Mt. Kisco, NY, 1988, Futura Publishing Co, Inc.
4. DePalma RG, Emsellem HA, Edwards CM et al: A screening sequence for vasculogenic impotence. J Vasc Surg 5:228, 1987.
5. DePalma RG et al: Noninvasive assessment of impotence, Surg Clin North Am 70:119, 1990.
6. DePalma RG, Kedia K, and Persky L: Surgical options in the correction of vasculogenic impotence, J Vasc Surg 14:92, 1980.
7. Merchant RF Jr and DePalma RG: The effects of femoro-femoral grafts on postoperative sexual functions: correlation with penile pulse volume recordings, Surgery 90:962, 1981.
8. Emsellem HA et al: Pudendal evoked potentials in the evaluation of impotence, J Clin Neuorphysiol 359:5, 1988 (abstract).
9. Virag R and Virag H: L'epreuve a la papaverine intracaverneuse dans l'ètude de l'impuissance, J Mal Vasc 8:293, 1983.
10. Brindley GS: Cavernosal alpha-blockade: a new technique for investigating and treating erectile impotence, Br J Psychiatry 143:332, 1983.
11. Bookstein JJ et al: Pharmacoangiographic assessment of the corpora cavernosa, Cardiovasc Intervent Radiol 11:218, 1988.
12. Goldstein I: Overview of types and results of vascular surgical procedures for impotence, Cardiovasc Intervent Radiol 11:240, 1988.
13. Lue TF et al: Functional evaluation of penile veins by cavernosography in papaverine-induced erection, J Urol 135:476, 1986.
14. Lue TF, Hricak H, and Marick KW: Evaluation of vasculogenic impotence with high resolution ultrasonography, Radiology 155:777, 1985.
15. DePalma RG and Olding MJ: Surgery for Vasculogenic Impotence. In Greenhalgh RM, ed: Vascular surgical techniques, London, 1989, WB Saunders Co.
16. Goldstein I: Penile revascularization, Urol Clin North Am 14:805, 1987.
17. Virag R et al: Possibilities chirurgicales dans l'impuissance vasculaire, Gaz Med France 90:2031, 1983.
18. Lewis RW: Venous surgery for impotence, Urol Clin North Am 14:115, 1987.
19. DePalma RG et al: Modern Management of Impotence Associated with Aortic Surgery. In Bergan JJ and Yao JST, eds: Arterial Surgery: new diagnostic and operative techniques, Orlando, 1988, Grune & Stratton.
20. Hauri D: Operative Moglichkeiten bei der vaskular bedingten Impotenz, Angio Archiv 8:25, 1985.
21. Virag R et al: Impuissance d'origine vasculaire, J Mal Vasc 14:112, 1989.

Part III

VENOUS DISEASES

Chapter 24

DEEP VEIN THROMBOSIS

Robert A. Graor
John R. Bartholomew

Deep vein thrombosis (DVT) is a common condition, especially among hospitalized patients.[1-5] Although most thrombi are small, asymptomatic, and confined to the deep calf veins, 20% extend into the proximal deep veins and can lead to fatal pulmonary embolism.[6] The frequency of venous thrombi in ambulatory patients is more difficult to estimate, but recent studies indicate that DVT is common if the individuals have been exposed to certain risk factors within the preceding 3 months[7,8] (see the accompanying box). Patients with venous thrombosis usually do not develop signs or symptoms until the thrombus has become large and occlusive.[7] Approximately 80% of thrombi in symptomatic patients are in or have extended into the popliteal and more proximal veins (Table 24-1).

The problems associated with diagnosing DVT were described by Horowitz and Tatter.[9] They analyzed the results of 11,000 autopsies and found that 2.8% (316 cases) had visible evidence of DVT, but only 11% of the 316 cases had an antemortem diagnosis of DVT.

Proximal thrombi rarely undergo spontaneous resolution and frequently remain occlusive. The patient's course can later be complicated by the postphlebitic syndrome, an important cause of chronic disability[10,11] (see Chapter 26).

Common risk factors associated with DVT

- Surgery and nonsurgical trauma
- Increasing age
- Malignancy
- Immobilization
- Heart failure or myocardial infarction
- Previous DVT
- Obesity
- Pregnancy and use of oral contraceptives
- Stroke with limb paresis or paralysis

Table 24-1. Clinical spectrum of DVT

Condition	Incidence (%)
Incidence of DVT/year	Unknown
Population with venous insufficiency	0.5-2
Actual DVT diagnosis in symptomatic patients	30-50
Proximal extension of calf DVT	20
Calf DVT with symptoms and signs	5
Above-calf DVT with symptoms and signs	40-50

THE PATHOGENESIS OF VENOUS THROMBI

Whether the presence of intimal lesions is a precondition for the pathogenesis of venous thrombosis is controversial. Hunter believed that inflammation of the "inner coat" (endothelium) caused thrombus formation, whereas Virchow believed that thrombi formed on normal endothelium and that the cellular reaction occurred after the thrombosis. The controversy led to the useless distinction between thrombophlebitis and phlebothrombosis; the former term indicates thrombus formation with inflammation, and the latter term indicates thrombus formation without wall inflammation. The distinction is not useful clinically or pathologically, and *thrombophlebitis* has been established as the accepted descriptive term because all thrombi eventually produce inflammatory reactions along the endothelial surface.

Many theories try to explain the complex interactions of the venous endothelium and the blood components in the development of venous thrombi. An intact layer of functioning endothelium appears to be necessary to inhibit clot formation. The spindle-shaped cells of the negatively charged endothelial layer are oriented along the long axis of the vessel and contain a high concentration of glycosaminoglycans, of which heparin forms a major component. In addition, the endothelium synthesizes and is rich in plasminogen activator, prostacyclin, antithrombin III, and various quantities of protein C. These surface agents interact with the flowing blood and other components of the vessel wall, including fibronectin and thromboxane, to maintain a normal balance that ensures the continuity of the layer and that prevents platelet deposition, leukocyte infiltration, and fibrin formation.

Venous thrombi are composed predominantly of fibrin and red cells, with variable amounts of platelets and leukocytes.[12] Thrombi frequently arise from the large venous sinuses of the calf and valve cusp pockets, either in the deep veins of the calf or thigh or in venous segments that have been exposed to direct trauma. The formation, growth, and dissolution of venous thrombi reflect the balance between the thrombogenic stimuli, the direction and velocity of venous flow, and the protective mechanisms that exist in vivo.

Several factors enhance the development of venous thrombi. These factors, often referred to as Virchow's triad, include vessel wall damage, venous stasis, and increased activation of clotting factors. Any one of these predisposing factors potentiates the others.

Sevitt and Gallagher have shown that no intimal damage or inflammation of the vein wall or valve cusps occurs at the site of small venous thrombi.[13] Later Stewart et al suggested that endothelial injury may be submicroscopic and not detectable by light microscopy.[14,15] They suggested that ischemia, chemotactic influences, or both, resulted in localized tissue response, increased vascular permeability, and the migration of leukocytes across the endothelial layer, all leading to endothelial damage and subsequent thrombosis. Subtle breaks in endothelial continuity might also be caused by stasis distention of the venous endothelial cell matrix and exposure of the subendothelial structures. The inactivation of activated coagulation factors by circulating inhibitors, the dissolution and clearance of activated coagulation factors by flowing blood, the removal of activated coagulation factors by the liver, the clearance of soluble fibrin complexes by reticuloendothelial cells, and the dissolution of fibrin by the fibrinolytic system are mechanisms that protect against thrombus formation.

Anatomic studies evaluating the development of early venous thrombi have confirmed that these thrombi are formed in areas of static blood flow and especially in valve pockets.[13,16] These thrombi may propagate in both directions as a result of slow venous flow, but they generally propagate in the direction of the venous flow. In larger veins, propagating thrombi are initially loosely attached to vessel walls, thus permitting detachment and embolization.

Experimental data using isolated venous segments and India ink indicate that blood flow through valvular structures results in eddy zones or zones of semistagnant accumulations.[17] Other experimental data indicate that turbulent flow enhances silting of formed elements and their deposition at eddy zones.[18] Therefore the likely sites of origin of venous thrombi are valve cusps, at bifurcations of vessels, and in the arcades of the soleal veins.

Careful venous dissection at autopsy has demonstrated that thrombi occur in a variety of locations in the leg. Thrombi in calf veins were often found to be independent of thrombi in thigh veins. Sevitt concluded that a variety of patterns of thrombosis can be explained on the basis that thrombi begin at one or more sites.[19] He also concluded that the concept of multiple independent sites of origin is supported by the presence of small isolated thrombi, most commonly occurring in the valve cusps. From his work, it is clear that the earliest and most frequent manifestation of DVT is the formation of a thrombus in a calf vein, whereas thrombi from the independent thigh vein form later.

Although these autopsy findings are not in question, they do not necessarily reflect the distribution of thrombi in the living patient. In a study of Browse and Thomas[20] that described 430 venograms, thrombi were most commonly confined to the muscle veins of the calf (42%). Continuous thrombus was seen extending from the calf to the thigh in 35% of the venograms, and in 23%, thrombi were located proximally in the thigh and were independent of the calf veins.[20]

Kakkar et al showed with ^{125}I fibrinogen scanning that, in surgical patients, venous thrombi began in the calf veins during the first week after the operation. In medical patients, they began within the first week of hospitalization. Most of these thrombi underwent local autolysis within approximately 72 hours or remained localized to the calf veins.[6] Most importantly, 20% of calf vein thrombi extended proximally into the popliteal vein.

Therefore the etiology of DVT suggested by in vivo studies differs from that suggested by postmortem studies. It remains unclear whether thrombi in the larger leg veins result from the contiguous spread of thrombi in the calf veins or whether they have an independent local origin.

When considering the risk for pulmonary embolism, the usual sites of thrombus formation in the lower extremities and the source of subsequent pulmonary emboli must be distinguished. The majority of such emboli come from the lower extremities, and fatal emboli are usually derived from the larger veins.[21] Other sources of emboli include the cardiac chambers on the right side; the pelvic veins and upper extremities are less commonly involved.

The outcome of venous thrombi is discussed in Chapter 26 (Venous Insufficiency). Occlusion or recanalization are probably the two most common outcomes of occlusive venous thrombi. Occlusive venous thrombi, in contrast to arterial thrombi, are often associated with recanalization. Occlusion usually results in a fibrotic plug that renders the vein impassable to blood flow.

Thrombogenic factors

Venous thrombi are generally thought to be secondary to blood coagulation and fibrin formation during venous stasis. Experimental and clinical studies demonstrate the role of the vessel wall, stasis, clotting factors and their inhibitors, and the fibrinolytic system in the pathogenesis of venous thrombosis (Table 24-2). An understanding of the pathogenesis of venous thrombosis at the vein surface is important in formulating a rational approach for the prevention and therapy of this disease.

Venous stasis. Static or altered blood flow in the deep veins of the lower limbs helps to initiate venous thrombi. Thermal dilution techniques can measure venous blood flow in femoral and iliac veins during surgery. Blood flow decreases by 50% during the induction of anesthesia, and this lower flow appears to remain constant throughout the operation.[17]

Venous stasis contributes to venous thrombosis by preventing activated coagulation factors from being diluted by nonactivated blood, by preventing activated coagulation factors from being cleared, and by preventing activated coagulation factors from mixing with their inhibitors.[22,23] Blood clearance from the lower extremities is enhanced by the contractions of calf muscles, which propels the blood from the calf toward the heart.

Venous stasis can be produced by immobility, venous obstruction, raised venous pressure, and increased blood viscosity. Autopsy findings suggest that immobility is a prominent risk factor, especially in patients confined to bed for more than a week (see the accompanying box).[24] Preoperative and postoperative immobility is also associated with an increased incidence of venous thrombosis.[25,26] Postoperative patients remain at risk during their entire period of immobility; postoperative thrombosis is not prevented if patients remain immobile after their period of prophylaxis.[27] Venous stasis and blood viscosity are also closely linked.[28] Blood viscosity increases in regions of slow blood flow. Blood viscosity is also increased in patients with polycythemia, erythrocytosis, or dysproteinemias and in some postoperative patients.

Injury to the vessel wall. Endothelial cells form a continuous, single layer of cells that are arranged longitudinally, parallel to the direction of flow. The luminal side of the cell is covered by a glycocalyx, consisting of glycoprotein and proteoglycans, (glycosaminoglycans), of which heparin sulfate forms 80%. The surface is negatively charged, which may prevent the adhesion of platelets and clotting factors. The endothelial cells can synthesize or bind with other components that inhibit thrombus formation (see Table 24-2). Thrombin inhibits the synthesis and the release of these factors.

Prostacyclin is a major component of the vessel-wall endothelium. It is a powerful inhibitor of platelet aggregation, as well as a potent vasodilator.

Table 24-2. Thromboresistant and thrombogenic factors at the endothelial surface

Thromboresistant	Thrombogenic
Cellular alignment	Mechanical trauma leading to:
Glycosaminoglycan surface (heparin-content surface)	Stasis
	Direct surgical trauma
Repulsive negative-charge surface	Thermal injury
	Burns
Avid surface binding of substances that inhibit thrombus:	Endotoxins
	Immune complexes
	Thrombin generation
Macroglobulin	
Protease inhibitors	
Plasminogen activator	
Prostacyclin	

Causes of venous stasis

Intrinsic

Immobilization
Outflow obstruction from previous DVT
Increased central venous pressure
Increased blood viscosity

Extrinsic

Extrinsic compression

Two theories have been proposed to explain the origin of venous thrombi. One suggests that the enzyme thrombin is generated in areas of stasis, which leads to local platelet aggregation and fibrin deposition. A second and more popular theory is that damage to a vessel wall exposes the subendothelial collagen, to which platelets then adhere (see Table 24-2).[29] The local accumulation of leukocytes, the activation of the intrinsic pathway through activation of factor XII by collagen, and the activation of factors XII and XI by activated platelets also occur during vessel-wall damage.[30-35]

Hypercoagulability, platelets in the vessel wall, and fibrinolytic activity. Platelets have a strong affinity to collagen. Their adhesion characteristics are enhanced with Factor VIII-related antigen, the factor ascribed to the classical von Willebrand's disease. As platelet adhesion occurs, platelet aggregates are formed and stabilized by fibrin that forms after the release of coagulation Factor V from platelet granules, by exposure of the platelet surface to phospholipoproteins (platelet factor III), and by platelet activation of the coagulation factors XII and XI after exposure to collagen.

The degree of spontaneous fibrinolytic activity must also regulate the amount of fibrin deposited in the area of an initial platelet nidus. The fibrinolytic activity of the vein wall under conditions of stasis is lower in the legs than in the arms. Perhaps this lower activity explains why DVT occurs more commonly in the legs. There is convincing evidence that the fibrinolytic activity of the blood is derived from plasminogen activators produced in the endothelium of small vessels and that activators are continuously in the bloodstream.

Therefore there may be an overactivity or underactivity of certain components of the coagulation system. Underactivity of the fibrinolytic system may produce hypercoagulable states. Known hypercoagulable states produce thrombosis, and the interplay of these pathologic states can disrupt the endothelium and consequently result in the formation of thrombi.

A number of inherited and acquired disorders that can cause a hypercoagulable state have now been identified. Under certain clinical situations, these disorders increase the patient's susceptibility to spontaneous thrombosis. These disorders are discussed in Chapter 4.

Certain coagulation factors are particularly relevant to the formation of venous thrombi. Although the final common pathway is a migration of polymorphonuclear leukocytes and the disruption of the continuity of the endothelium, the initial factors include a complex interplay of the exposed basement membrane, stasis, leukotaxins, and the altered balance between blood coagulation and thrombolysis. Endothelial hypoxia increases the production of thromboxane and decreases prostacyclin and antithrombin III, which increases the likelihood of thrombosis. Abnormalities of fibrinolysis may be an important factor in thrombosis formation but has been inadequately evaluated.[33,34]

Clinical risk factors in venous thrombosis

Some aspects of clinical practice may predispose patients to a higher incidence of venous thrombosis. Also, some patient characteristics function as risk factors for thromboembolic complications. These risk factors are shown in the box on p. 403.

Surgery and trauma. A number of well-recognized thrombogenic factors are associated with surgery and trauma. These include:

1. Increased blood coagulability resulting from the release of tissue thromboplastin into the blood
2. Venous stasis from immobilized limbs
3. Reduced fibrinolytic activity

The risk of venous thrombosis after surgery is related to the site and extent of surgical trauma, the duration and nature of the operation, and the length of time that the patient remains immobilized before and after surgery. Operative venography shows that the femoral vein is markedly twisted and distorted during total hip replacement. Endothelial damage likely occurs as a consequence of this distortion and is responsible for the unique localization of thrombi in the proximal venous segment in some patients. Patients undergoing orthopedic procedures involving the hip, knee, or pelvis; neurosurgery; and major pelvic or abdominal surgery for malignancy appear to be at the greatest risk (Table 24-3).

Age. Age is an important risk factor for venous thrombosis, but the underlying mechanism is unclear.[25,35] Possible explanations include increased immobility secondary to disease states and venous dilation that occurs in the elderly, which results in increased venous stasis. The fibrinolytic response also decreases in persons above the age of 65. Other unknown mechanisms undoubtedly also contribute to the high risk of venous thrombosis that occurs with advanced age.

Malignancy. Patients with malignancy can develop recurrent superficial DVT, venous thrombosis in unusual anatomic sites, thrombosis resistant to anticoagulant therapy and, rarely, phlegmasia cerulea dolens.[25,30,35] The risk of venous thrombosis after surgery for malignant conditions is two to three times greater than the risk for nonmalignant conditions.

A number of factors contribute to the increased risk of venous thrombosis in patients with malignant disease, including the elaboration of tissue thromboplastin-like active

Table 24-3. Risk of DVT according to surgical procedures

Author	Type of surgery	No. of patients	DVT (%)	Venography
Borgstrom et al (1965)	Hip fracture	29	56.5	Yes
Hamilton et al (1970)	Hip fracture	38	49	Yes
Hume et al (1973)	Elective hip	19	42	No
Evart et al (1971)	Elective hip	20	50	Yes
Hull et al (1979)	Elective knee	29	66	Yes
McKenna et al (1980)	Elective knee	22	75	Yes
Turpie et al (1980)	Neurosurgery	183	28	Yes
Skillman et al (1978)	Neurosurgery	199	25	Yes
Coe et al (1978)	Urologic	53	25	Yes
Kakkar et al (1972)	General	39	42	No
Nicolaides et al (1972)	General	122	29	No

substances from the tumor. Factor X activation is increased in malignant tissues.[30] In addition, patients with malignancies sometimes have reduced fibrinolytic activity. Malignant tumors may compress or infiltrate a vein and predispose the segment to thrombosis. Patients with malignant disease also have compounding risk factors, such as increasing age and an increased number of surgical procedures.

Heart failure. Heart failure is a well-established risk factor for venous thrombosis, presumably because of the raised central venous pressure and the immobility associated with heart failure.[22,36]

Previous venous thrombosis. Patients with a history of venous thrombosis have two to three times the risk of developing venous thrombi after elective abdominal surgery.[25,35] Patients with recurrent venous thrombosis also have a three to four times greater risk of developing a subsequent episode of venous thrombosis when anticoagulant therapy is discontinued 3 months after the initial event.

Obesity. Obesity is associated with venous thrombosis, probably because it impairs fibrinolytic activity and leads to greater immobility in some obese patients.[25,35]

Pregnancy and contraceptives. The evidence supporting pregnancy as a risk factor is imperfect. The evidence that the low-dose estrogen pill is a risk factor for venous thrombosis is also inconclusive.[37-38]

A number of humoral and mechanical events occurring during a normal pregnancy and delivery do, however, increase the risk of thrombosis during that period. These events include a decrease in the fibrinolytic activity that occurs during the third trimester and in the early stages of labor, before placental separation. The release of tissue thromboplastin into the circulation at the time of placental separation, venous stasis resulting from deep venous dilation, and the mechanical pressure of the uterus on the inferior vena cava during the third trimester of pregnancy and during delivery also play a role. In general, the levels of plasma fibrinogen and coagulation factors VII, VIII, and IX increase during pregnancy, but the relationship of these factors to an increase in the risk of venous thrombosis is unclear.

Estrogens and oral contraceptive pills produce many of the same changes that occur during pregnancy. They can produce venous dilation and, in some studies, estrogens have decreased functional levels of antithrombin III, as well as decreased fibrinolytic activity.

Miscellaneous risk factors. Other conditions reported to have a high association with venous thrombosis include thrombocytosis, polycythemia vera, systemic lupus erythematosus, and Behçet's syndrome.

NATURAL HISTORY OF VENOUS THROMBOSIS

Venous thrombi most commonly occur in the legs, probably because of the capacitance hemodynamics associated with these larger veins (stasis) and the effects of gravity. The outcome of venous thrombi is shown in the accompanying box. The mechanisms by which thrombi are removed include endogenous fibrinolysis, the digestion of fibrin by leukocytes, the organization of the thrombus, and embolization. Autolysis or spontaneous lysis of thrombi is uncommon, whereas occlusion or recanalization are the rule.

Natural history or outcome of venous thrombi

Extension
Lysis (autolysis)
Organization
Recanalization
Embolization

Table 24-4. Pulmonary emboli as the outcome of DVT

Clinical situation	Incidence (%)
Untreated above-knee—lower-extremity DVT resulting in pulmonary emboli	50-70
Pulmonary emboli in untreated patients with calf DVT	1-5
Patients with pulmonary emboli who have clinically overt DVT	30-40

Pulmonary emboli are commonly associated with venous thrombosis (Table 24-4). Clinically silent pulmonary embolism occurs in about 50% of patients with documented proximal vein thrombosis.[6] Pulmonary emboli occur more frequently and are larger in patients with proximal vein thrombosis than in patients with calf-vein thrombosis.[39]

Venous thrombi usually slowly undergo organization and occlusion or recanalization. The affected patients are predisposed to postphlebitic syndrome because of associated valvular damage or venous obstruction. These aspects of venous insufficiency are discussed in Chapter 26.

The thrombus is more likely to extend if the original thrombogenic stimulus persists, if marked endothelial damage or stasis occurs as a consequence of the original thrombosis, or if treatment is not instituted. A recent investigation using objective methods of diagnosis have shown that approximately 20% of asymptomatic calf thrombi extend into the popliteal vein, and when extension occurs, it is associated with a 40% to 50% risk of clinically detectable pulmonary embolism.[6] Hull et al also reported a 20% extension rate of symptomatic calf-vein thrombosis in ambulatory patients who remained untreated. In addition, they noted a 50% frequency of recurrent venous thrombosis over a 3-month period in patients with proximal venous thrombosis who were treated inadequately and a 20% frequency of recurrence over 12 months in patients with a history of recurrent venous thrombosis who are treated with anticoagulants for only 3 months.[40]

Lagerstedt et al reported a recurrence rate of more than 20% in patients with symptomatic calf-vein thrombosis who were treated with a 5-day course of intermittent IV heparin and no Coumadin.[41] They suggested that the short-term prognosis of patients with proximal DVT is good—a recurrent rate of less than 5%—provided that they are treated with adequate doses of heparin followed by oral anticoagulants for 3 months.

Clinically, the thrombus extends significantly in less than 5% of patients with proximal vein thrombosis during the initial period of heparin therapy and in only 2% during the subsequent 3 months of treatment with oral anticoagulants.[42-44] Recurrences occur in between 5% to 20% of patients in the year after the discontinuation of the 3 months of anticoagulant therapy.[43-50] The majority of these recurrences occur in patients who have idiopathic venous thrombosis, a continuing risk factor such as malignancy, or previous DVT.

The prognosis for patients with recurrent venous thrombosis is varied. They are often treated with anticoagulants for life and may suffer considerable mental anguish. In a recently completed prospective study of patients with clinically suspected acute recurrent DVT, almost two thirds did not have the diagnosis confirmed, when checked, by objective tests.[44] These patients did very well without anticoagulant treatment, a fact that stresses the importance of correct objective diagnosis.

Venography is less useful for the diagnosis of recurrent venous thrombosis, so confirming or refuting a clinical suspicion of acute recurrent venous thrombosis is difficult. The diagnostic process for this condition has been simplified by the application of the following noninvasive techniques:

1. Impedance plethysmography, which is sensitive and specific for proximal vein thrombosis if the results return to normal after the initial episode
2. Duplex scanning, which is sensitive for proximal extension
3. Radioactive fibrinogen scanning

DIAGNOSIS OF VENOUS THROMBI

Clinical diagnosis

Many potentially dangerous venous thrombi are clinically silent because they are nonobstructive and are not associated with inflammatory changes in the vessel wall or perivascular tissues. The symptoms of venous thrombi can also be caused by many nonthrombotic disorders, such as those shown in Table 24-5. Therefore the accuracy of the clinical diagnosis is low.

The unreliability of clinical diagnosis has been demonstrated by numerous studies that compare clinical findings with the results of objective testing. Hull et al evaluated more than 1000 patients with clinically suspected venous thrombosis by venography.[44] Approximately 70% of all patients did not have venous thrombosis. The prevalence of venous thrombosis was lower in patients who were hospitalized at presentation. Of those patients who had venous thrombosis, 90% were in the proximal venous segments and only 10% were confined to the deep-calf veins. The most common clinical findings were pain, tenderness, and swelling. Pain occurred in 50% of patients with thrombosis, whereas tenderness occurred in 75%. Other clinical features, including night cramps, redness, cyanosis, or dilated veins, were relatively rare and occurred with approximately equal frequency in patients with and without venous thrombosis.

Pain and tenderness are not related to the size or extent of venous thrombosis. Pain and tenderness associated with calf-vein thrombosis are usually localized to the calf but may extend along the anterior and medial aspects of the thigh and into the groin.

Swelling can be caused by obstructions in the large veins, increases in central venous pressure, or inflammation in the perivascular tissues. Swelling usually subsides when the leg is elevated; however, it frequently recurs during ambulation and may persist for weeks to months. Depending on the cause, it may never entirely subside. This is particularly true in patients with iliofemoral vein thrombosis.

Homans' sign, discomfort in the upper calf during forced dorsiflexion of the foot, is a time-honored sign of venous thrombosis. Unfortunately, it is insensitive and nonspecific.

Table 24-5. Differential diagnosis of venous thrombosis

Symptom/Sign	Differential diagnosis
Pain and tenderness	Muscle strain or trauma
	Muscle tear
	Muscle hematoma
	Direct muscle or leg trauma
	Arterial insufficiency
	Neurogenic pain
	Baker's cyst
	Arthritis or tendonitis
	Cellulitis or lymphangitis
	Vasculitis or myositis
	Long-bone disorders
	Fibrositis
Leg swelling	Postphlebitis syndrome
	Compartment syndromes
	Disuse
	Iliac vein compression
	Inflammatory conditions
	Lymphedema
	Lipedema
	Heart or liver failure
	Renal failure
	Factitial edema, (self-induced)
	Cancer

It is positive in less than one third of patients with documented DVT. In addition, more than 50% of patients with a positive Homans' sign do not have venous thrombosis.

Venous distention is a relatively uncommon and nonspecific manifestation of acute venous thrombosis. Prominent superficial veins have been recorded in up to 20% of patients with venography-proven venous thrombosis and in 20% of patients without thrombosis. When venous distention occurs, it is often a feature of major vein obstruction and usually disappears when the leg is elevated or when new collateral vessels form.

Patients with venous thrombosis may have pale, cyanotic, or reddish-purple legs. Cyanotic changes are caused by impaired venous return and stagnant anoxic blood in the cutaneous vessels. Cyanosis usually subsides in a few days. A pale or white leg, often called a *milk leg,* is caused by iliofemoral vein thrombosis. It is thought to result from an associated lymphatic obstruction. A mottled blue discoloration is associated with marked swelling and cyanosis and is frequently labeled *phlegmasia cerulea dolens,* but this term should be reserved for patients who have excessively high venous pressures resulting in signs of arterial insufficiency (Fig. 24-1). These pressures usually occur with the obstruction of the iliofemoral venous system and distal smaller vessels. Cyanosis is caused by severe extensive venous obstruction. The leg is usually very painful, swollen, and cyanotic and may have multiple petechial hemorrhages. The patient may be hypotensive as a result of blood pooling in the affected leg and may acquire thrombocytopenia as a result of platelet consumption in the thrombus. Half the patients with phlegmasia cerulea dolens may require amputation.

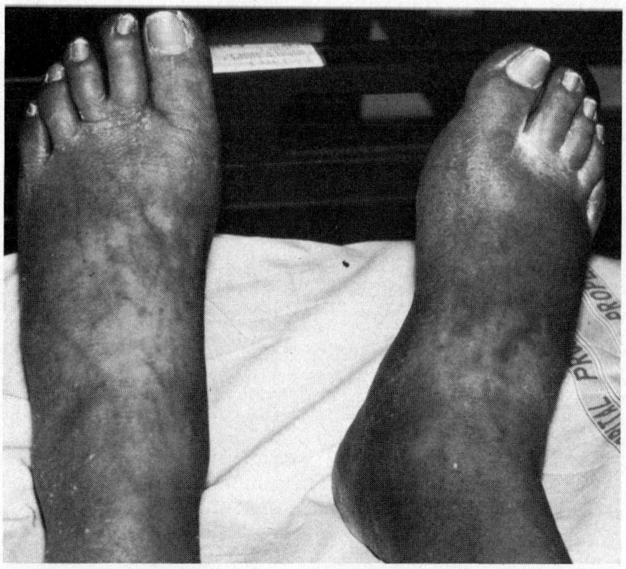

Fig. 24-1. Bilateral lower extremity phlegmasia. Ischemic tissue is noted in both lower extremities over the distal portion of the foot. These ischemic changes are characteristic of venous gangrene due to an extensive thrombotic process that involves the deep venous system, thus producing high postcapillary pressures that result in tissue ischemia.

Differential diagnosis

Approximately 70% of patients with clinically suspected DVT have negative results from objective tests.[6] Alternative diagnoses are shown in Table 24-5.

Muscle aches generally occur after strain or trauma from an unusual type or amount of activity with the extremities. Commonly, the patient has been jogging, hiking, or playing a vigorous sport 12 to 36 hours before the onset of pain. Generally the pain is of a crescendo-decrescendo nature. With most patients, the most important sign is tenderness during light palpation of the calf or thigh muscles. Edema is generally absent.

Muscle tears have a classic, sudden, severe pain in the back of the leg and may simulate direct trauma or gunshot wound to the calf. Typically, the muscles that tear are the medial head of the gastrocnemius and, less commonly, the plantaris muscle. The tear usually results from a sudden, strong stretch of the contracting calf muscles during plantar flexion. It is generally at the musculotendinous junction and is usually small and incomplete. Large tears, or even separation of the muscle from the tendon or avulsion of the tendon from the bone, may occur. The onset of severe pain may temporarily subside but is generally followed by a constant pain that becomes more severe as a hematoma forms. This further irritates the calf muscle and produces spasm. Physical examination reveals local tenderness, with fullness from the hematoma, in the region of the tear. After several days, a bruise may appear, either on the posterior medial aspect of the calf or along the posterior aspect of the medial malleolus.

Direct trauma to the leg can result in hematomas and subsequent inflammation. In general, this degree of insult occurs during vigorous sports activity or from trauma such as that from an automobile accident. The hematoma can confuse diagnosis because venous thrombosis is a well-recognized complication of leg trauma. In most cases, objective tests are necessary to exclude the possibility of DVT. Differentiation between hematomas and a venous thrombosis is critical because anticoagulation therapy for DVT can expand the hematoma and worsen the discomfort of the lower extremity, leading to a compartment syndrome.

Arterial insufficiency is seldom confused with venous thrombosis. The onset of pain in acute arterial occlusion is sudden and may be associated with some tenderness. Most often, the limb is cool and pale with nonpalpable pulses. Swelling is generally absent unless the leg has been in a dependent position to relieve ischemic rest pain.

Neurogenic pain can result from compression of the sciatic or lateral cutaneous nerve in the thigh, producing leg pain that is easily differentiated from venous thrombosis. There is no swelling, the onset is frequently sudden, and the pain is aggravated by maneuvers that cause elongation of the nerve. Neurologic deficits may be present, which can help in establishing the diagnosis.

Popliteal cysts or Baker's cysts are fluid-filled cavities that occur most commonly in the posterior aspect of the knee. These cysts can rupture and can track down the tissue planes between the calf muscles, producing inflammation. Symptoms of pain and warmth and signs of tenderness and swelling may simulate the clinical features of DVT. These cysts are commonly associated with arthritis or traumatic injury to the knee. On examination, there may be evidence of fullness in the popliteal fossa on the affected side. The diagnosis can be established with ultrasound or by arthrogram.

Arthritis and tendonitis can also mimic the signs and symptoms of DVT. However, a careful clinical history and physical examination generally reveal pain, tenderness, and swelling localized mainly to the affected area (joint or tendon); as a result, these conditions can be readily differentiated from DVT in most cases.

Other inflammatory conditions such as cellulitis, lymphangitis, vasculitis, myositis, fibrositis, fibromylagia, and panniculitis may cause pain and tenderness of the leg. These conditions can usually be differentiated from DVT on clinical grounds, although each may be slightly confusing at varying stages. Careful examination and a good history should distinguish them from DVT.

Patients with varicose veins frequently have pain and tenderness over the region of the varicosities. When superficial phlebitis occurs in a varicosity, it also becomes inflamed and tender, producing local edema in the perivenous tissues. Generalized diffuse discomfort is not usually associated with varicosities unless they are multiple or associated with venous insufficiency.

Conditions, described in other chapters, that may simulate DVT include:

1. Compression of the iliac vein by tumor, abscess, or other mechanical obstructing problems
2. Postphlebitic syndrome
3. Leg immobilization
4. Lymphedema
5. Lipedema
6. Factitial edema

Objective diagnostic tests

Venography is the "gold standard" for diagnosing venous thrombosis. With good technique, an ascending venogram should outline the entire deep venous system of the lower extremity, including the external and common iliac veins up to the distal portion of the inferior vena cava. However, because a perfect venogram is not always achieved, duplex scanning rivals the venogram as the preferred diagnostic method. Duplex scanning techniques have an excellent sensitivity and specificity for the diagnosis of proximal DVT (Table 24-6).

Table 24-6. Comparison of duplex ultrasound and venography for the diagnosis of DVT in selected studies

Study	No. of patients	Duplex studies*	
		Sensitivity†	Specificity†
Appelman, (1987)[45]	112	48/52 (93)	58/60 (97)
O'Leary (1988)[46]	50	22/24 (92)	25/26 (96)
Dauzat (1986)[47]	137	89/92 (97)	45/45 (100)
Vogel (1987)[48]	53	19/20 (95)	33/33 (100)
George (1987)[49]	50	23/24 (96)	26/26 (100)
TOTAL	402	201/212 (95)	187/190 (99)

*Confirmed by venogram.
†N/N (%).

Venography

Ascending venography is performed by injecting a radiopaque contrast medium into a dorsal vein in the foot. Several techniques have been described, but in general, the calf veins are filled in the dependent position under fluoroscopic monitoring.[50] A tourniquet at the ankle promotes filling of the deep veins by obstructing the superficial ones. Tilting the table further to a head-neutral or head-down position promotes more proximal filling of the deep venous system. If the common femoral and iliac system still cannot be well visualized, these veins can be injected and then viewed from the common femoral or retrograde cannulation of these venous segments. Interosseous injection can fill the more proximal segments, but it is painful and requires general anesthesia. It has also been associated with fatal fat pulmonary embolism.[50]

The normal venous system of the leg consists of three pairs of deep calf veins named in conjunction with the arterial supply to the area (the posterior tibial, the peroneal, and the anterior tibial veins). The soleal and the gastrocnemius plexus of veins is also found in the calf. The confluence of these deep veins forms the popliteal and superficial femoral veins. In general, the soleal veins drain into the posterior tibial veins, and the gastrocnemius plexus drains into the popliteal veins. The popliteal vein becomes the superficial femoral vein at the junction of the proximal part of the popliteal fossa and the adductor canal in the thigh. Ascending proximally, the superficial femoral vein is joined by the profunda femoris vein (or deep femoral vein) in the upper thigh to form the common femoral vein, which becomes the external iliac vein at the level of the inguinal ligament. The external iliac vein and its confluence with the internal iliac vein in the pelvis form the common iliac vein that converges with the contralateral side to form the inferior vena cava. The deep venous system has many variations. The most common is an accessory or duplicated popliteal and superficial femoral vein, commonly known as a *bifid system*.

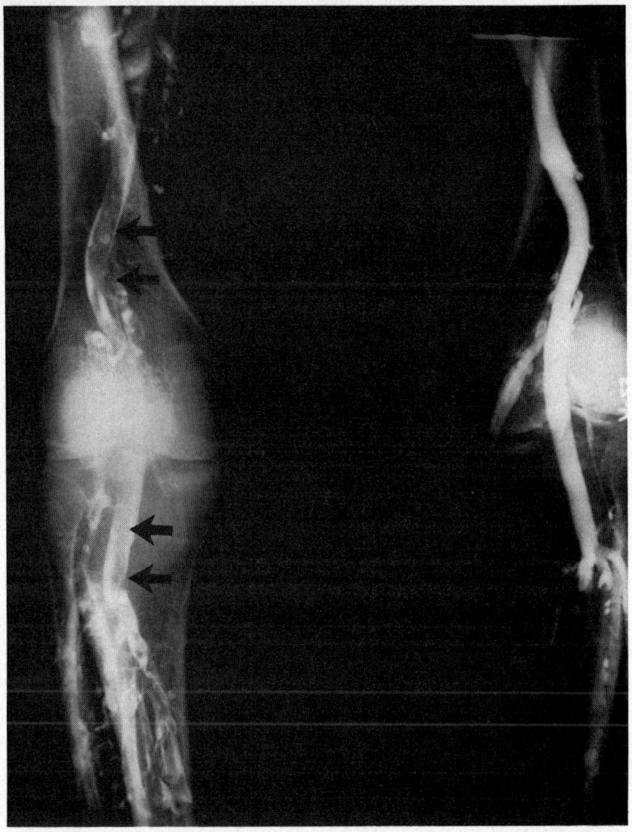

Fig. 24-2. The classic appearance of deep venous thrombosis shown by ascending venography. The right lower extremity demonstrates intraluminal filling defects with contrast streaming around the clot. The left lower extremity demonstrates a normal column of contrast within the deep venous system. The clot (*arrows*) extends from the calf veins into the popliteal and superficial femoral veins.

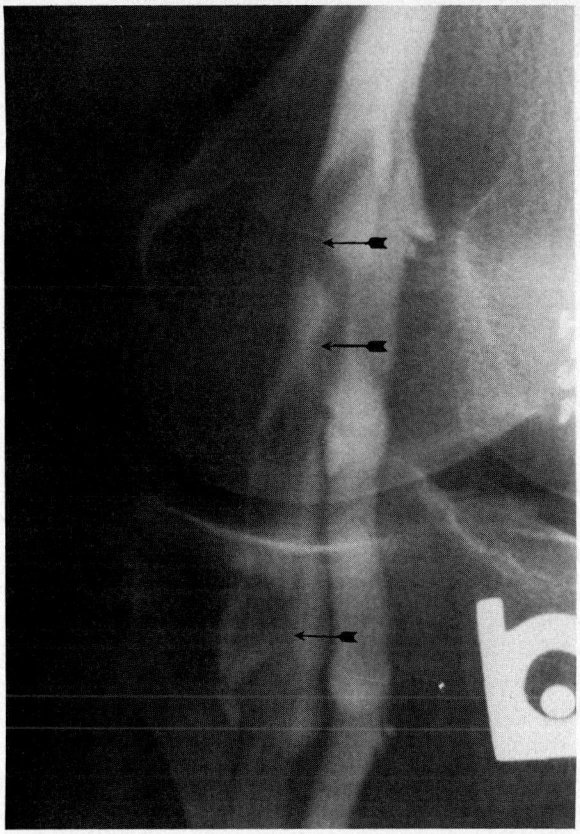

Fig. 24-3. The classic appearance of a coiled thrombus *(arrows)* in a popliteal vein. The duplicated popliteal system is a commonly occurring variant. The thrombus within the medial branch of the duplicated popliteal system appears to be free floating and extending to the level of the junction of the two channels.

The superficial system is composed of two major systems: the long and short saphenous veins or the greater and lesser saphenous veins. The veins drain into the common femoral and popliteal veins, respectively. Communicating veins connect the superficial venous system with the deep.

The most reliable criterion for confirming an acute venous thrombosis is an intraluminal filling defect consistent in multiple views (Figs. 24-2 and 24-3). Other criteria are less reliable and include nonfilling of a segment of the deep venous system with the abrupt termination of the contrast medium at a constant site above the segment or nonfilling of the deep venous system above the knee despite adequate venographic technique. The latter is the least reliable criterion.

Venography is invasive, and certain complications are associated with the injection of the contrast medium. In addition to the pain of injection, the hyperosmolar radiopaque contrast medium can damage endothelial cells and produce early and delayed pain. The injected medium may also produce a superficial phlebitis and DVT in a small percentage of patients who would otherwise have normal venograms. In our experience, approximately 0.5% to 1% of patients with negative venograms develop a DVT soon after venography. Perhaps 1% to 2% develop clinically significant venous thrombosis.[50] Other, less common complications include hypersensitivity reactions to the radiopaque dye, renal impairment, and local skin and tissue necrosis as a result of extravasation of the contrast medium at the site of injection.

Noninvasive tests for the diagnosis of venous thrombosis, including impedance plethysmography and duplex scanning, are discussed in Chapter 3.

TREATING DEEP VEIN THROMBOSIS

Anticoagulant therapy

Anticoagulant therapy is based on the premise that the initiation or extension of thrombi can be prevented by inhibiting the synthesis of clotting factors or by accelerating their inactivation. In contrast to thrombolytic agents, the anticoagulants, heparin and warfarin, do not induce thrombolysis but effectively prevent extension. The following characteristics of anticoagulation therapy must be understood before the therapy is prescribed:

1. Anticoagulation therapy is prophylactic; it prevents further extension and embolization of the thrombus.
2. Anticoagulation therapy has been proven to prevent recurrent pulmonary embolism and DVT.
3. Anticoagulation therapy should be given when the clinical suspicion for DVT is confirmed and when the therapy is not contraindicated.

Thrombolytic agents provide a more rapid return to the normal physiologic state and help prevent late sequelae of the disease. In general, thrombolytic agents are adjuncts to, rather than substitutes for, other therapies such as heparin and warfarin therapy. Their use should be monitored by clinicians experienced in the care of patients with venous or arterial thrombotic occlusive disease.

Heparin. Heparin is the drug of choice for the treatment of thromboembolic disease, despite renewed interest in thrombolytic therapy. Its action is through an anionic mucopolysaccharide that binds to antithrombin III or heparin cofactor II, enhancing the ability of antithrombin III to neutralize factors XIIa, XIa, IXa, and Xa and thrombin.

Treatment for venous thromboembolism should be initiated as soon as the diagnosis is suspected, unless treatment is contraindicated. An intravenous bolus of between 5000 and 10,000 units (usually 100 U/kg) can be given, followed by 500 U/kg every 24 hours, given by way of a continuous intravenous infusion. Peak plasma levels can be obtained almost instantaneously by parenteral administration. Intermittent intravenous and subcutaneous injections have also been advocated, but they increase the risk of bleeding. The efficacy of a subcutaneous injection during an acute event is questionable because of variable plasma levels.

Clinical trials have demonstrated that the recurrence of venous thromboembolism can be prevented by maintaining the activated partial thromboplastin time (APTT) at two to three times the laboratory control value, particularly during the first 24 hours after the acute thrombotic event.[51-53]

The APPT level should be checked approximately 4 to 6 hours after the bolus injection and then at least every 24 hours. Platelet counts should be obtained every 48 to 72 hours. Additional evidence from animal studies indicates that venous thrombosis can be prevented at heparin levels of 0.3 to 0.4 μL/L, even when the APTT is not prolonged to twice the normal control value.[54]

Heparin has a short half-life because it is transferred to the extravascular space and is probably cleared through the reticuloendothelial system. In patients with severe renal impairment, the half-life is prolonged, but this does not necessarily indicate that elimination is through the kidney. In addition, heparin may have either an increased or a decreased half-life in patients with liver disease. There is thus no solid evidence that the liver is the site of heparin metabolism.

Several studies have shown that the incidence of heparin-induced bleeding is affected by dose, route of administration (subcutaneous vs intravenous), type of infusion (continuous vs intermittent), patient's age, and associated comorbid factors.[42,51] Complications and other aspects of anticoagulation with heparin are described in Chapter 4.

Warfarin. Some aspects of therapy with warfarin (Coumadin) for venous thromboembolism are controversial. In particular, the point at which to initiate therapy, the duration of therapy for uncomplicated and recurrent venous thromboembolism, and the optimal dose for achieving adequate anticoagulation are debated.

The mean half-life of a single dose of Coumadin is 40 hours. In healthy volunteers the concentration in plasma is poorly correlated with its anticoagulant effect. Its metabolism and excretion can also vary greatly by individual. The absorption of Coumadin is influenced by diet, drugs, and the metabolism and excretion of drugs that can be significantly modified by a disease process.

Coumadin may be thrombogenic by inhibiting the synthesis of functional protein C (a potent anticoagulant) early in the initiation of oral anticoagulation therapy. The anticoagulant effect of Coumadin occurs from depleting factors II, VII, IX, and X. An early anticoagulant effect occurs in laboratory tests but not during in vivo anticoagulation, as a result of the suppression of factor VII. Factor VII is depleted rapidly, a fact reflected in the prothrombin time. The peak anticoagulant activity of Coumadin is delayed for 72 to 96 hours because of the longer half-lives of factors II, IX, and X.

Although many physicians do not initiate Coumadin therapy until the fifth day or later in patients receiving heparin, initiating Coumadin with heparin for uncomplicated documented venous thromboembolic events is recommended. For the patient with an initial thrombotic event, Coumadin treatment should last 3 to 6 months. In patients with a recurrent event, Coumadin from 6 months to 1 year is suggested, and in patients with three or more well-documented or defined events, life-long anticoagulation is recommended. Each event should be well documented with venograms, pulmonary angiograms, lung scans, or other reliable noninvasive studies.

The prothrombin time should be maintained between 1.25 and 1.8 times the control. These values are based on recently published findings that show less-intensive oral anticoagulation therapy to be as efficacious as more-intensive therapy.[55,56] The incidence of untoward bleeding has been greatly reduced with the newer, less-intensive therapy.[55] North American patients in the past were taking higher doses of oral anticoagulants than were patients in the United Kingdom. This difference in dose has been attributed to the source of thromboplastin used in the prothrombin time test. Rabbit brain has been used in North America, whereas human brain, which is more responsive to reductions in vitamin K–dependent coagulation factors, is used in the United Kingdom.

The mechanism of action, complications, and biochemical aspects of Coumadin therapy are discussed in Chapter 4.

Thrombolytic therapy

The ideal agent for treating DVT should reverse the thrombotic process and clear the thrombotic material from the veins, thereby preserving the anatomic and physiologic hemodynamic integrity of the venous system (Fig. 24-4). The clearance of thrombotic material from valvular structures and the restoration of normal venous hemodynamic function should be rapidly obtainable and durable. Although anticoagulation is the treatment of choice in most patients with venous thromboembolic disease and although the outlook for survival is excellent with this treatment, thrombus progression and embolization can occur. Therefore, although survival is nearly assured, there are problems: residual venous insufficiency and recurrent thrombosis as a result of residual damage from the initial thrombus.

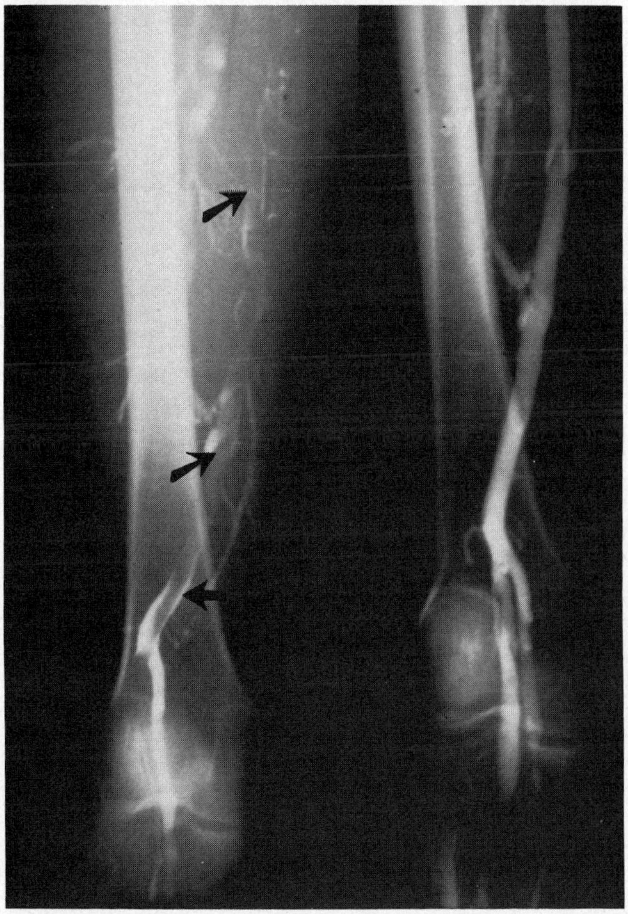

Fig. 24-4. The figure on the left is a diagnostic venogram of the left leg and demonstrates extensive clot *(arrows)* from the calf to the popliteal and superficial femoral veins. This venogram was taken before treatment with urokinase. The figure on the right demonstrates a posttreatment completion venogram after 18 hours of thrombolysis with urokinase. The clot has been dissolved, and contrast flows evenly through the venous channels.

Thrombolytic therapy may have many advantages over anticoagulant therapy, including clot dissolution that leads to the restoration of normal venous hemodynamics, the reduction or prevention of venous valvular damage, and the potential for preventing postphlebitic syndrome. Thrombolytic therapy for DVT has been evaluated in a small number of studies and has produced a greater effect on lysis of deep vein thrombi than heparin therapy. However, it has not yet been established whether thrombolytic therapy reduces the frequency of postphlebitic syndrome.

Six randomized trials comparing intravenous streptokinase to heparin in the treatment of DVT using venographic assessment have been reported.[57-62] None of the trials was large enough to determine the efficacy and safety of streptokinase. Goldhaber et al performed pooled analysis on these studies and demonstrated that thrombolysis was achieved approximately four times more often among patients treated with streptokinase than among those treated with heparin ($P < 0.001$).[63] Three of the six trials had sufficient data to compare bleeding complications, which occurred approximately three times more often in the streptokinase group than in the heparin group.[59,61,62]

A few properly designed clinical trials have evaluated urokinase for the treatment of venous thrombosis. These trials have found the rates of clot lysis to be similar to those of streptokinase, but urokinase improved safety and shortened the duration of infusion.[64,65]

Only a few studies report on the long-term effects of thrombolytic therapy in the treatment of DVT. In the studies of Elliot et al, Arnesen et al, and Common et al,[62,66,67] follow-up ranged from 7 to 76 months, and the results indicated that 24 of 62 (40%) patients treated with streptokinase had normal veins compared to only 1 of 58 (2%) of patients treated with heparin. The clinical evaluation of the trials indicated that none of the 62 patients treated with streptokinase had open leg ulcers, compared to 5 of 58 (9%) of patients treated with heparin. In addition, 35 of 62 (56%) patients treated with streptokinase were free of long-term symptoms, compared to only 14 of 58 (24%) of the patients treated with heparin.

Kakkar et al reported negative findings and found that postphlebitic syndrome was as common in patients treated with streptokinase as in patients treated with heparin after more than 5 years follow-up.[58] This, however, was not the experience of other trials.[64-67]

Johansson et al recently described their functional evaluation, using occlusion plethysmography, of the veins in patients initially treated with streptokinase for DVT.[68] The study had a mean follow-up of 2 years and found an excellent correlation between anatomically normal venograms and normal venous outflow capacity and valvular function. These normal outcomes occurred in 42% of patients treated with streptokinase. The authors concluded that an initial complete thrombolysis provides a good opportunity for obtaining a lasting restoration of deep venous anatomy and function without developing signs and symptoms of venous insufficiency.

In a study done at the Cleveland Clinic, we compared streptokinase and urokinase and found that both medications produced a high degree of clot lysis (80%) in patients who had DVT signs and symptoms for less than 7 days.[65] Urokinase had fewer major complications and was significantly safer ($P < 0.01$) than streptokinase. The safety advantage and the shorter infusion time of urokinase offset its higher cost; the cost is also offset by the more frequent complications of streptokinase resulting in longer hospital stays.

Few reports of experimental thrombolytic agents for the treatment of DVT are available. Case reports on the use of recombinant human tissue–type plasminogen activator (rt-PA) in patients with acute proximal venous thrombosis have been mixed. Turpie et al reported on 24 patients, 12 treated with rt-PA and 12 treated with heparin and placebo. Of the 12 patients who received rt-PA, 5 (42%) had greater than 50% lysis of thrombi, 4 (33%) had significant (but less than 50%) lysis, and 3 (24%) had no evidence of clot lysis.[69] In the heparin-placebo control group, 2 patients had less than 50% lysis, and 10 patients had no clot lysis at all. Two patients in the rt-PA group had overt hemorrhage, one had marked bruising, and one developed hemarthrosis 10 days after total hip replacement. Two other patients had a fall greater than 2.0 g/L in the hemoglobin level but without overt bleeding. One patient in the heparin-placebo group had spontaneous hemarthrosis of a shoulder.

In a follow-up study by the same investigator, rt-PA was given concomitantly with heparin in two, 8-hour infusion regimens given 24 hours apart. Twenty patients were studied: ten in the rt-PA-plus-heparin group and ten in the heparin-plus-placebo group. The thrombolytic and hemorrhagic results were similar to those of the first study. Six of the ten patients treated with rt-PA showed greater than 50% clot lysis, one showed less than 50%, and three showed no evidence of clot lysis. No patients in the heparin group showed evidence of lysis. Three of the ten patients in the rt-PA group had spontaneous hemorrhages, whereas none in the heparin group hemorrhaged. In contrast to the first study, the indices of thrombolysis were reduced only slightly.

Complications of thrombolysis. The major complication associated with thrombolysis is hemorrhage. This complication is to be expected because thrombolytic agents will lyse any hemostatic fibrin plug, regardless of its pathologic, morphologic, or anatomic characteristics.

The frequency with which major bleeding occurs is difficult to assess. Straub reviewed the literature to determine the frequency of bleeding in patients treated with streptokinase.[70] His review included 549 patients treated for DVT. Fatal bleeding occurred in 4 (0.73%) of these patients, and major nonfatal bleeding occurred in 63 (11.5%). The mean duration of treatment was extremely long (106 hours, or more than 4 days), and a uniform definition of major bleeding was not applied. The review indicates that the greatest risk for bleeding occurs when therapy is prolonged, perhaps for 3 to 4 days.

Interestingly, studies on bleeding complications with heparin therapy have similar findings. Holm gathered information on 710 patients treated for DVT with standard

Table 24-7. Characteristics of seven caval filters

Filter	Material	Caval patency/recurrent pulmonary embolism (%)	Migration	Advantage
Greenfield[72,73] Medi-Tech, Inc.	Stainless steel	95/5	<2%	First filter with good inferior vena caval patency
Bird's nest[74] Cook, Inc.	Stainless steel	97/3	<1%	Percutaneous placement
LGM[75] LG Medical	Eligiloy	92/2	>13%	None
Titanium Greenfield Medi-Tech, Inc.	Beta 3	Trials	Underway	
Simon nitinol[76]	Nickel-Titanium Titanium	91/2		Easy percutaneous placement
Gunther[77,78] William Cook, Inc.	Stainless steel	93/0	20%	None
Amplatz[79] William Cook, Inc.	Stainless steel	15-25/4		Retrievable

anticoagulation therapy.[71] Fatal bleeding occurred in 2 (0.3%) patients, and nonfatal major bleeding occurred in 52 (7.3%) patients.

Other complications of thrombolytic therapy include fever, nausea, vomiting, and allergic reactions, especially among patients treated with streptokinase.[65] These complications rarely occur with urokinase or rt-PA.

Vena cava interruption

Vena cava interruption is another option in the treatment of venous thromboembolism. Indications for this procedure include:

1. When anticoagulation is contraindicated (for example, in cerebral hemorrhage, active gastrointestinal bleeding, septic cerebral emboli, and major trauma)
2. The recurrence of documented pulmonary emboli, despite adequate anticoagulation
3. With surgical pulmonary embolectomy
4. Patients with chronic recurrent pulmonary embolization

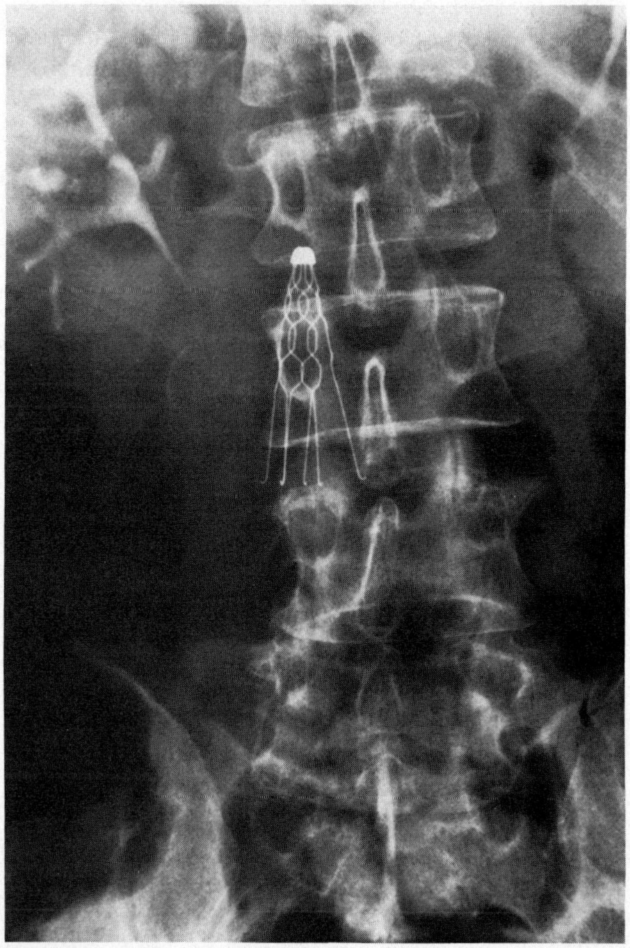

Fig. 24-5. This x-ray study shows a Greenfield filter properly situated in the inferior vena cava below the entry site of the renal veins. The nephrogram and draining ureters can be seen on both sides of the filter.

Several authors have recommended other, less accepted indications for caval interruption. These include (1) elderly patients with documented venous thromboembolic events who are at risk for anticoagulant therapy because of the danger of falling or because they are mentally unstable; (2) patients with free-floating thrombi; (3) a thrombus above a previously placed caval filter; (4) patients with low cardiopulmonary reserve or pulmonary hypertension; and (5) patients with massive pulmonary embolism who are hemodynamically unstable.[72-79]

The vena cava can be interrupted with a number of new products (Table 24-7) (Fig. 24-5). The newer products can be placed under local anesthesia with a venipuncture through the femoral, internal jugular, or subclavian veins. Other methods of caval interruption, including clips, ligation, or plication via a direct surgical approach while under general anesthesia, have become nearly obsolete.

Complications associated with caval devices include misplacement and migration (Fig. 24-6). In addition, procedural complications include hematoma, venous thrombosis, air embolism, perforation of the vascular wall, and filter thrombosis. These complications are often directly related to the experience of the physician inserting the device. A guide wire may minimize some complications. Recurrent emboli may develop despite filter insertion. These thrombi can embolize to the lungs through large venous collaterals of the epigastric, spermatic, or ovarian veins. In addition, thrombosis of the vena cava with subsequent postphlebitic syndrome may also occur.

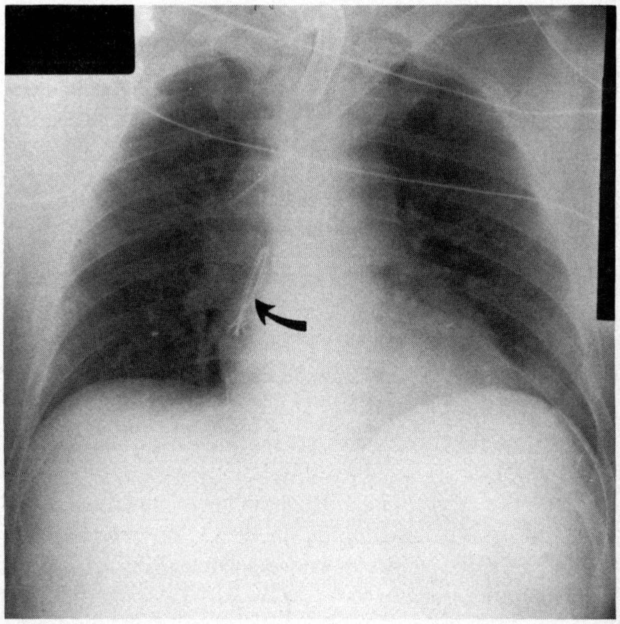

Fig. 24-6. Migration of a filter *(arrow)* into the right lower lobe pulmonary artery, one of the complications of filter placement in the inferior vena cava. Migration to the lung is not as common as migration laterally into the retroperitoneal space or into a venous structure branching from the inferior vena cava.

A filter can also be placed in other veins, such as the brachiocephalic or superior vena cava. Although a pulmonary embolism from the axillary, subclavian, or internal jugular vein is much less common than one from the deep venous system of the leg, it still can be a serious problem. The increased use of central venous catheters for hemodynamic monitoring and access for total parenteral nutrition, chemotherapy, and antibiotics may increase the chances of pulmonary embolism from these veins. In addition, Swan-Ganz catheters, pacemaker catheters, and pacemakers are other potential causes of venous thrombosis in the upper extremities.

Surgical venous thrombectomy

The three basic goals for venous thrombectomy are:

1. To avoid pulmonary embolism by removing the thrombus
2. To eliminate early morbidity by eliminating pain, swelling, and ischemic tissue loss of phlegmasia cerulea dolens
3. To minimize the late postthrombotic sequelae by preserving patency and retaining valvular function.

In the 1960s enthusiasm for venous thrombectomy was high as a result of reports of excellent initial patency and the absence of painful swelling and venous stasis.[80] Haller and Abrams claimed an 85% patency rate in patients undergoing surgery within 10 days of the onset of the thrombus and normal extremities with no edema in 81% of the survivors.[81] Soon, however, reports emerged of higher rates of rethrombosis, especially in phlegmasia cerulea dolens. In addition, venous stasis sequelae were often not prevented, in spite of patency, because valve competency had been destroyed.[81,82]

The most notable of these reports was a 5-year follow-up analysis by Lansing and Davis[82] of the same patients originally reported by Haller and Abrams.[81] In this follow-up study, 94% of the patients observed had sufficient edema and stasis changes to require elastic support and leg elevation consistent with the classical definition or description of venous insufficiency. The report also noted that two of the three postoperative deaths were from pulmonary embolism, that the wound complication rate was 30%, that 10% of the patients had pulmonary emboli, that the average blood transfusion was 1000 cc, and that the mean hospital stay was 12 days. This report essentially ended the enthusiasm for surgical thrombectomy. However, the report suffered from a selection bias, an incomplete follow-up (only 50% of the patients were seen), and a venographic documentation rate of less than 50%. In addition, there was no control group to compare these patients to patients who had not undergone surgical thrombectomy.

Subsequent reports indicated that from 82% to 88% of patients can undergo a thrombectomy successfully and that postoperative anticoagulation therapy was somewhat helpful in avoiding rethrombosis.[83,84] In selected patients and combined with postoperative anticoagulation therapy, venous thrombectomy had a limited but definite role in treating iliofemoral venous thrombosis, especially patients with phlegmasia cerulea dolens.

Although several trials have compared anticoagulant therapy with thrombolytic therapy, only one study has compared anticoagulant therapy with surgical thrombectomy.[85] No trials compare all three therapies.

The surgical thrombectomy literature suffers from the same problems of study design present in the thrombolysis and anticoagulation trials. For the most part, one is forced to compare reports that differ significantly in patient selection, time between the onset of symptoms and the beginning of treatment, technical differences (i.e., technique of thrombectomy and use of adjunctive arteriovenous fistula), extensiveness of thrombosis, type and duration of postoperative anticoagulation therapy, and duration and type of follow-up—in particular, the outcome criteria (clinical vs physiologic venous testing).

Venous thrombectomy can be performed, using local or regional anesthesia, through a groin incision without opening the abdomen, thereby reducing the operative risk. Operative mortality primarily reflects the seriousness of the underlying disease and the ability to avoid pulmonary embolism and to replace blood as fast as it is lost. Although the mortality in Haller and Abrams' series was 9% and two of the three fatalities were related to pulmonary embolism, the mortality risk has dropped steadily in the past 2 decades.[81] The choice of thrombectomy should be based primarily not on the risk but on its effectiveness relative to other therapies in reducing either early morbidity or the late sequelae of iliofemoral thrombosis.

Early morbidity. A prospective, randomized trial in Scandinavia, reported by Plate et al, showed no reduction in symptoms or the length of hospital stay among thrombectomy patients when compared with conservatively treated patients.[85] The increased cost of surgical treatment and the additional pain and risk of wound hematoma as a result of the incision in anticoagulated patients offset any immediate benefit of thrombectomy, except in patients with phlegmasia cerulea dolens. In these patients, the morbidity of surgical or nonsurgical treatment is high, but thrombolysis or thrombectomy can produce some dramatic early results.

Late sequelae. The major problem with reducing late sequelae is preventing rethrombosis, usually by continuing anticoagulation therapy for a longer postoperative period, by the surgical construction of a temporary arteriovenous fistula, or both. Late patency rates vary from 21% to 71%, and valve competency rates vary from 0% to 29%, with postphlebitic sequelae developing in 18% to 81% of patients. These rates explain the confusion regarding the efficacy of venous thrombectomy.

Thrombectomy performed more than 7 days after the development of symptoms is clearly inferior to early thrombectomy (that is, surgery performed 2 to 3 days after the onset of symptoms). Early thrombectomy in conjunction with postoperative heparin administration has improved early patency from 72% to 93% and late patency from 49% to 67%. The results with arteriovenous fistulae are less impressive. Early rethrombosis rates were reduced from 20% to 13% in the Scandinavian prospective trial,[85] and late patencies of 60% to 83%, with post phlebitic sequelae as low as 0% to 17%, have been achieved.

Indications and techniques. The patients most suitable for thrombectomy have phlegmasia cerulea dolens or phlegmasia alba dolens. A second, less well-documented group are young, active, healthy patients who have iliofemoral venous thrombosis and who have been symptomatic for less than 5 days. In both groups, thrombolysis also appears to be promising.

Surgical technique varies, but in general, it can be performed transfemorally under local, regional, or light general anesthetic. Adequate replacement blood must be available because blood loss commonly amounts to 1000 cc per patient.

An incision is made over the femoral venous system and systemic anticoagulation is continued or instituted during the procedure. To avoid pulmonary embolism, a balloon catheter can be inserted through the opposite saphenous vein to the vena cava, where a second ipsilateral catheter is introduced and advanced above the first. An alternative approach is the use of an inferior vena caval filter in this setting. The venous thrombectomy is performed using a Fogarty venous-catheter passed upward, ideally under fluoroscopic guidance.

After the proximal thrombectomy has been completed, treatment of the distal thrombus can be undertaken. As much clot as possible should be removed by extrusion, by stroking along the course of the distal veins or using a tight Esmarch's bandage wrapped upward. A Fogarty venous thrombectomy catheter can be introduced distally if the distal vein cannot be cleared by other mechanical methods. An arteriovenous fistula can then be created with a venous branch to the superficial femoral or profunda femoris artery.

Heparin, and in some cases dextran, should be used perioperatively. The patient should be started on Coumadin as soon as wound bleeding is eliminated as a problem, and the patient should remain on Coumadin for a minimum of 6 weeks, preferrably longer if the retained thrombus remains.

Venous thrombectomy has a limited but definite role in the clinical management of patients with lower extremity DVT. It is of little value in the management of patients who have recurrent thrombosis or thrombosis in the smaller vessels distal to the popliteal vein. The best results were achieved when selectively applied to patients with severe cases of venous thrombosis, including those with phlegmasia cerulea dolens and phlegmasia alba dolens, especially those with a contraindication to thrombolytic therapy.

AXILLARY-SUBCLAVIAN VEIN THROMBOSIS

Thrombosis of the axillary and subclavian veins accounts for 1% to 2% of all deep venous thrombi.[86] Recent data suggest that this incidence may be increasing, largely because of the increased use of the subclavian vein as an access site and for hemodynamic monitoring.

Although axillary-subclavian vein thrombosis is sometimes considered a benign disorder, the incidence of pulmonary embolism and postphlebitic syndrome suggests otherwise. The frequency of pulmonary embolism arising from axillary-subclavian vein thrombosis may be as high as 36%, although most authors suggest that this incidence approaches 12% to 15%.[86-90] The incidence of postphlebitic syndrome or residual disability resulting from upper-arm thrombosis varies between 7% and 74%, reflecting the various underlying causes for this syndrome.[86,90-92]

The pathogenesis of axillary-subclavian vein thrombosis is multifactorial but is generally similar to that of the lower extremity. Factors that may differ include the more common use of the subclavian vein for venous access and the use of irritating intravenous solutions or drugs, injury to the vascular endothelium directly related to venous puncture or catheter insertion, and the duration and size of catheter placement.

The causes for DVT involving the axillary-subclavian veins are diverse and are listed in the box. Axillary-subclavian vein thrombosis seen in young, muscular, healthy males may be related to unusual exercise, such as lifting, pulling, or hyperabduction of the arm, and is referred to as *effort thrombosis* or the *Paget-Schroetter's syndrome*.

Axillary-subclavian vein thrombosis also occurs with the use of central venous pressure (CVP) lines, pacemaker wires, Hickman or Broviac catheters, or intravenous drug abuse.

Signs and symptoms suggesting acute axillary-subclavian vein thrombosis include pain, local tenderness or warmth, edema, supraclavicular fullness, cyanosis, the presence of a palpable cord, or an increased venous pattern. The diagnosis is suggested by a thorough history and physical examination. Specific questions related to drug abuse, recent use of the subclavian vein for access or hemodynamic purposes, and types of physical activities should be queried. The diagnosis is established by venography, although duplex scanning is becoming widely acceptable as an alternative noninvasive approach.

Thrombosis of the axillary-subclavian veins is treated

Causes for axillary-subclavian vein thrombosis

Muscular effort of arms
Thoracic outlet syndrome
Trauma
Idiopathic
CVP lines
Intravenous drug abuse
Pacemaker wires
Tumor
Congenital venous malformation

like that of the leg: elevation, moist heat, and anticoagulants. The goal is to prevent pulmonary embolization and postphlebitic syndrome. Sympathetic ganglion blocks, conservative treatment with rest, and elevation without the concomitant use of anticoagulants have no role in modern therapy. Thrombolytic agents are also successfully used to treat acute, well-documented axillary-subclavian vein thrombi of less than 7 days duration.[87,92] These agents may be infused through a catheter directly into the thrombus or given systemically by a routine intravenous catheter.

Surgical approaches to axillary-subclavian vein thrombosis include the use of a superior vena caval filter, venous thrombectomy, or transaxillary first-rib resection. The use of superior vena caval filters is discussed elsewhere in this chapter. Venous thrombectomy is still advocated in many centers, although early rethrombosis is common. Transaxillary first-rib resection is probably helpful in the patient with thoracic outlet syndrome or with effort thrombosis after initial therapy with thrombolytic therapy or the more traditional use of anticoagulants.

SUPERIOR VENA CAVA SYNDROME

The superior vena cava syndrome was first recognized in 1757 by William Hunter who reported it as a complication of a syphilitic aortic aneurysm. Infectious diseases including syphilis and tuberculosis were the most common causes for this disorder; however, the large majority of cases now recognized are related to underlying malignancy.[93-96] These include bronchogenic cancer, lymphoma, or metastatic disease arising most often from the breast or testicles. Other less commonly reported causes include fibrosing mediastinitis secondary to histoplasmosis or radiation treatment, pericardial hematoma, aortic aneurysms, polyarteritis nodosa, and iatrogenic sources resulting from the use of the axillary-subclavian vein for hemodynamic monitoring including Swan-Ganz catheters, Hickman or Broviac catheters, CVP lines, or transvenous cardiac pacemakers.

The pathogenesis of this syndrome may involve an extrinsic compression or an intrinsic process. Most commonly, extrinsic compression is the result of a slowly progressive process, such as a tumor, that eventually obstructs the vessel. This may cause only minimal clinical findings. However, direct invasion of an aggressive tumor or an acute thrombosis causing acute obstruction occurs rapidly and produces a much more dramatic clinical picture.

Physical findings generally include upper-extremity and facial edema and occasionally conjunctival edema. Dilation of the superficial veins of the chest wall, neck, or arms is commonly observed. Patients may complain of cough, hoarseness, or shortness of breath and stridor due to laryngeal edema. Dysphagia secondary to esophageal edema may be present. Dizziness, headache, visual symptoms, somnolence, and changes in mental status (including stupor and coma) are reported. Symptoms are often aggravated by lying, bending, or stooping.

The diagnosis of superior vena cava syndrome can be confirmed by venography. Chest x-ray studies may help in identifying an underlying malignancy or other contributing causes. Computed tomography (CT) and venous duplex scanning are effective noninvasive studies. Biopsy diagnosis can be obtained by a percutaneous needle approach or through an endovascular procedure using a biopsy device or atherectomy catheter.[97-99]

Treatment has traditionally been the emergent use of radiation therapy based on the premise that the underlying disease process was cancer. This was often performed without confirming the diagnosis. Radiation therapy continues to play a major role in the treatment of this disorder; however, other modalities are now available and confirmation of the disease process is recommended before initiating treatment.

Medical measures including bed rest, diuretics and head elevation often help. Steroids have been advocated to reduce cerebral or laryngeal edema. The use of anticoagulants is imperative if thrombotic occlusion has occurred. Thrombolytic therapy has proved to be effective.[100] Surgical therapy to remove the thrombus or bypass to replace the superior vena cava has not been highly successful, and is not commonly used.

PREVENTING VENOUS THROMBOEMBOLISM

Pulmonary embolism is the most common preventable cause of in-hospital death. In the absence of prophylaxis, the frequency of postoperative fatal pulmonary embolism ranges from 0.1% to 0.8% in patients undergoing elective general surgery, 0.3% to 1.7% in patients undergoing elective hip surgery, and 4% to 7% in patients undergoing emergency hip surgery.[101-103] Other medical illnesses, such as stroke, myocardial infarction, and congestive heart failure, carry a risk of developing DVT, the precursor of pulmonary embolism, in 25% to 60% of patients.[104] Ideally, prophylaxis is most effective for preventing death and morbidity from pulmonary embolism. Therefore, the use of prophylaxis to lower the risk of DVT and subsequent pulmonary emboli is of great importance.

Effective prophylaxis is now available to most nonsurgical and surgical patients. Effective prophylactic measures in patients undergoing elective general surgery can prevent 4000 to 8000 postoperative deaths each year in the United States.

Despite convincing evidence that pulmonary embolism and DVT are largely preventable, many physicians and hospitals have no strategy for preventing venous thromboembolic disorders. This lack of strategy is explained, perhaps, by the fact that any given surgeon rarely has a patient die from pulmonary embolism and by the concern of physicians in all areas of practice that prophylaxis may not be as effective as some believe. In addition, hospitals have been reluctant to add prophylactic measures that may increase costs.[105-107] Many medical and surgical physicians rely solely

Table 24-8. Risk categories for postoperative venous thromboembolism

Risk category	Risk of venous thromboembolism (%)		
	Calf-vein thrombosis	**Proximal vein thrombosis**	**Fatal pulmonary embolism**
High risk			
General surgery in patients > 40 years with recent history of DVT or pulmonary embolism Extensive pelvic or abdominal surgery for malignant disease	40-80	10-20	1-5
Moderate risk*			
General surgery in patients > 40 years lasting 30 minutes or more Major medical illness including cardiac disease, chronic disease, inflammatory bowel disease, and malignancy	10-40	2-10	0.1-0.7
Low risk*			
Uncomplicated surgery in patients < 40 years with no additional risk factors Minor surgery (i.e., less than 30 minutes) in patients < 40 years with no additional risk factors	10	1	0.01

Summarized from Salzman and Hirsh.[102,107,110]
*Risk is increased by advancing age, malignancy, prolonged immobility, varicose veins, and cardiac failure.

on early ambulation and graded compression stockings to prevent thrombotic complications. These forms of prophylaxis are inadequate.

A number of clinical risk factors for venous thromboembolism have been identified and discussed in this chapter. By combining risk factors and procedures, one can establish whether a patient is at low, moderate, or high risk for developing venous thromboembolic problems. These risk factors are summarized in Table 24-8.

Various prophylactic strategies have been evaluated for patients in different risk categories.[108] Selecting the most appropriate strategy for different clinical settings is an important aspect of prescribing prophylaxis.

The most commonly used strategy is a low-dose heparin regimen that prevents thrombosis by enhancing antithrombin III and by inhibiting factor Xa, which triggers the conversion of prothrombin to thrombin. This enhancement and inhibition must occur before thrombin is activated; after thrombin is activated, low-dose heparin cannot prevent coagulation. As a result, low-dose heparin is not effective in the treatment of acute DVTs or for prophylaxis after a clot exists. In almost all of the randomized trials with nonorthopedic patients, low-dose heparin has been found to be more effective than other treatments in preventing thrombosis.[109]

Although low-dose heparin prophylaxis is effective in the general surgical and medical populations, its use has been limited by the fear that it will induce bleeding. This fear is unsupported. The administration of 5000 units of heparin every 12 hours has not been associated with a clinically or statistically significant increase in risk of bleeding among general surgical patients.[110] Bleeding is a possibility, of course, and low-dose heparin prophylaxis should not be given to patients undergoing cerebral, eye, or spinal surgery. Heparin is also relatively ineffective in patients undergoing emergency or elective hip surgery, prosthetic surgery, or knee replacement surgery.[110]

Anticoagulation monitoring is not required during low-dose, subcutaneous heparin therapy. However, platelet counts should be obtained weekly to warn of the rare occurrence of heparin-associated thrombocytopenia.

A popular and effective prophylactic strategy is intermittent pneumatic leg compression, which enhances blood flow in the deep veins of the legs and prevents venous stasis.[111-112] Leg compression also increases blood fibrinolytic activity, which may contribute to its antithrombotic properties. It is the strategy of choice for patients in whom low-dose heparin is contraindicated or has been proven to be ineffective (i.e., patients undergoing eye, spine, prostate, or orthopedic surgery, or neurosurgery). Intermittent pneumatic leg compression is virtually free of clinically important side effects and is a valuable alternative for patients who have a high risk of bleeding.

Several other prophylactic strategies are available, including low-dose oral anticoagulation, dextran, aspirin, dose-adjusted subcutaneous heparin, and combinations of strategies. Table 24-9 lists the recommended prophylactic strategies for the alternative risk patients. Although no pro-

Table 24-9. The common approach to prophylaxis in medical and surgical patients

Type of operation or condition	Usual-risk patient	High-risk patient (e.g. prior DVT or pulmonary embolism)
Abdominal or thoracic surgery	Fixed low-dose heparin, 5000 units SC q 12 h starting 2 hours preoperatively (per AHA guidelines) PLUS (Optional) Pneumatic compression stockings	Increase frequency of heparin dosage to 5000 units SC q 8 h and use intermittent pneumatic compression stockings
Eye or neurosurgery; open prostatectomy (Note: Bleeding must be minimized in these operations)	Pneumatic compression stockings	Pneumatic compression stockings
Orthopedic surgery; hip or knee replacement	Pneumatic compression stockings OR adjusted doses of heparin SC q 8 h to prolong APTT 1-3 seconds	Pneumatic compression stockings OR adjusted doses of heparin SC q 8 h to prolong APTT 1-3 seconds
General medical patients, including stroke and myocardial infarction patients	Fixed low-dose heparin 5000 units SC q 12 h OR Pneumatic compression stockings	Increased frequency of heparin dosage to 5000 units SC q 8 h OR "Full" dose-continous heparin
Hemorrhagic stroke	Pneumatic compression stockings	Pneumatic compression stockings

phylactic strategy has proved satisfactory for patients undergoing hip or knee replacement surgery, adjusted doses of heparin and pneumatic compression stockings are the most popular. In addition, the possibilities of using low-molecular-weight heparin in these patients are being investigated, and the early results are promising.

The most carefully documented guidelines for selecting prophylactic strategies are those proposed by the American Heart Association for thoracic and abdominal surgery patients. Combining the American Heart Association recommendations for fixed, low-dose subcutaneous heparin therapy with early ambulation and, in some situations, pneumatic compression stockings is a reasonable strategy (Table 24-9). For patients at higher risk of thrombosis, the dose of heparin can be increased, and intermittent pneumatic leg compression can be simultaneously used.

For patients undergoing eye surgery, neurosurgery, or prostatectomy, bleeding must be kept to an absolute minimum, and therefore the use of heparin is generally contraindicated. Intermittent pneumatic compression stockings are effective in preventing DVT in these patients and should be used as a primary strategy for prophylaxis.

Despite efforts at prophylaxis, DVT and pulmonary embolism will occur in some instances. To minimize the adverse impact of these complications, constant vigilance is required to establish an accurate diagnosis and provide effective treatment.

REFERENCES

1. Beswick W et al: Detection of deep venous thrombosis by scanning of 99m-technetium-labelled red-cell venous pool, Br Med J 1:82, 1979.
2. Gomes AS, Webber MM, and Buffkin D: Contrast venography vs radionuclide venography: a study of discrepancies and their possible significance, Radiology 142:719, 1982.
3. Ryo UY et al: Radionuclide venography: correlation with contrast venography, J Nucl Med 18:11, 1977.
4. Kakkar VV: The diagnosis of deep vein thrombosis using the ^{125}I fibrinogen test, Arch Surg 104:152, 1972.
5. Kakkar VV: Fibrinogen uptake test for detection of deep vein thrombosis—a review of current practice, Semin Nucl Med 7:229, 1977.
6. Kakkar VV et al: Natural history of postoperative deep vein thrombosis, Lancet 2:230, 1969.
7. Hull R et al: Combined use of leg scanning and impedance plethysmography in suspected venous thrombosis: an alternative to venography, N Engl J Med 296:1497, 1977.
8. Hull RD et al: Diagnostic efficacy of impedance plethysmography for clinically suspected deep-vein thrombosis: a randomized trial, Ann Intern Med 102:21, 1985.
9. Horowitz RE and Tatter D: Lethal pulmonary embolism. In Sherry S et al, eds: Thrombosis, Washington, DC, 1969.
10. O'Donnell TF et al: The socio-economic effects of an iliofemoral thrombosis, J Surg Res 22:483, 1977.
11. Strandness DE et al: Long-term sequelae of acute venous thrombosis, JAMA 250:1289, 1983.
12. Karinot K and Motomyia M: Flow through a venous valve and its implication for thrombus formation, Thromb Res 36:245, 1984.
13. Sevitt S and Gallagher N: Venous thrombosis and pulmonary embolism: a clinico-pathological study in injured and burned patients, Br J Surg 48:475, 1961.
14. Stewart GJ, Ritchie WGM, and Lynch PR: Venous endothelial damage produced by massive sticking and emigration of leukocytes, Am J Pathol 74:507, 1974.
15. Stewart GJ et al: The adhesion of leukocytes, erythrocytes, and noncellular material to the luminal surface of natural and artificial blood vessels in vivo, Ann NY Acad Sci 283:179, 1977.

16. Hamer JD, Malone PC, and Silver IA: The PO2 in venous valve pockets: its possible bearing on thrombogenesis. Br J Surg 68:166, 1981.
17. Cotton LT and Clark C: Anatomical localization of venous thrombosis, Ann R Coll Surg Engl 36:214, 1965.
18. Mustard JF et al: Factors influencing thrombus formation in vivo, Am J Med 33:621, 1962.
19. Sevitt S: Pathology and pathogenesis of deep vein thrombi. In Bergan JJ and Yao JST, eds: Venous problems, Chicago, 1978, Year Book Medical Publications Inc.
20. Browse NL and Thomas ML: Source of non-lethal pulmonary emboli, Lancet 1:258, 1974.
21. Mavor GE and Galloway JMD: The iliofemoral venous segment as a source of pulmonary emboli, Lancet 1:871, 1967.
22. Hirsh J and Genton E: Thrombogenesis. In Root WS and Hoffman FG, eds: Physiological pharmacology, New York, 1974, Academic Press Inc.
23. Wessler S and Yin ET: On the mechanism of thrombosis. In Brown EB and Moore CV, eds: Progress in hematology, New York, 1969, Grune & Stratton Inc.
24. Gibbs NM: Venous thrombosis of the lower limbs with particular reference to bedrest, Br J Surg 45:209, 1957.
25. Nicolaides AN and Irving D: Clinical factors and the risk of deep venous thrombosis. In Nicolaides AN, ed: Thromboembolism aetiology, advances in prevention and management, Lancaster, England, 1975, Medical and Technical Publishing.
26. Heatley RV et al: Preoperative or postoperative deep-vein thrombosis? Lancet 1:437, 1976.
27. Turpie AGG et al: Prevention of venous thrombosis in patients with intracranial disease by intermittent pneumatic compression of the calf, Neurology 27:435, 1977.
28. Leonard EF: Rheology of thrombosis. In Colman RW et al, eds: Hemostasis and thrombosis, Philadelphia, 1982, JB Lippincott Co.
29. Davies GS and Salzman EW: The pathogenesis of deep vein thrombosis. In Joist HJ and Sherman LA, eds: Venous and arterial thrombosis, New York, 1979, Grune & Stratton Inc.
30. Walsh PN and Griffin JH: Contributions of human platelets to the proteolytic activation of blood coagulation factors XII and XI, Blood 57:106, 1981.
31. Wilner GD, Nossel HL, and Leroy EC: Activation of Hageman factor by collagen, J Clin Invest 47:2608, 1968.
32. Zeldes SM et al: Tissue factor (thromboplastin): localization to plasma membranes by peroxidase-conjugated antibodies, Science 175:766, 1972.
33. Mellbring G et al: Fibrinolytic activity in plasma and deep vein thrombosis after major abdominal surgery, Thromb Res 32:575, 1983.
34. Wiman B et al: The role of the fibrinolytic system in deep vein thrombosis, J Lab Clin Med 105:265, 1985.
35. Kakkar VV et al: Deep vein thrombosis of the leg: is there a "high-risk" group? Am J Surg 120:527, 1970.
36. Anderson GM and Hull E: The effect of Dicumarol upon the mortality and incidence of thromboembolic complications in congestive heart failure, Am Heart J 39:697, 1950.
37. Bonnar J et al: Haemostatic mechanism in the uterine circulation during placental separation, Br Med J 2:564, 1970.
38. Bonnar J, McNicol GP, and Douglas AS: Fibrinolytic enzyme system and pregnancy, Br Med J 3:387-389, 1969.
39. Hume M, Sevitt S, and Thomas DP: Venous thrombosis and pulmonary embolism, New York, 1970, Cambridge University Press.
40. Hull R et al: Diagnostic efficacy of impedance plethysmography for clinically suspected deep-vein thrombosis: a randomized trial, Ann Intern Med 102:21, 1985.
41. Lagerstedt CI et al: Need for long-term anticoagulant treatment in symptomatic calf-vein thrombosis, Lancet 2:515, 1985.
42. Salzman EW et al: Management of heparin therapy: controlled perspective trial, N Engl J Med 292:1046, 1975.
43. Hull R et al: Warfarin sodium versus low-dose heparin in the long-term treatment of venous thrombosis, N Engl J Med 301:855, 1979.
44. Hull RD et al: Clinical validity of a negative venogram in patients with clinically suspected venous thrombosis, Circulation 64:622, 1981.
45. Appelman PT, DeJong TE, and Lampmann LE: Deep venous thrombosis of the leg: US findings, Radiology 163:743, 1987.
46. O'Leary DH, Kane RA, and Chase BM: A prospective study of the efficacy of B-scan sonography in the detection of deep venous thrombosis in the lower extremities, J Clin Ultrasound 16:1, 1988.
47. Dauzat MM et al: Real-time B-mode ultrasonography for better specificity in the noninvasive diagnosis of deep venous thrombosis, J Ultrasound Med 5:625, 1986.
48. Vogel P et al: Deep venous thrombosis of the lower extremity: US evaluation, Radiology 163:747, 1987.
49. George JE, Smith MO, and Berry RE: Duplex scanning for the detection of deep venous thrombosis of lower extremities in a community hospital, Curr Surg 44:202, 1987.
50. Rabinov K and Paulin S: Roentgen diagnosis of venous thrombosis in the leg, Arch Surg 104:134, 1972.
51. Glazier RL and Crowell EB: Randomized prospective trial of continuous vs intermittent heparin therapy, JAMA 236:1365, 1976.
52. Wilson JR and Lampman J: Heparin therapy: a randomized prospective study, Am Heart J 97:155, 1979.
53. Bentley PG et al: An objective study of alternative methods of heparin administration, Thromb Res 18:177, 1980.
54. Chiu HM, Hirsh J, and Yung WL: Relationship between the anticoagulant and antithrombotic effects of heparin in experimental venous thrombosis, Blood 49:171, 1977.
55. Hull R et al: Different intensities of oral anticoagulation therapy in the treatment of proximal vein thrombosis, N Engl J Med 307:1676, 1982.
56. Adar R and Salzman EW: Treatment of thrombosis of veins of the lower extremities, N Engl J Med 292:348, 1975.
57. Robertson BR, Nilsson IM, and Nylander G: The value of streptokinase and heparin in treatment of acute deep venous thrombosis: a coded investigation, Acta Chir Scand 134:203, 1968.
58. Kakkar VV et al: Treatment of deep vein thrombosis: a trial of heparin, streptokinase and arvin, Br Med J 1:806, 1969.
59. Robertson BR, Nilsson IM, and Nylander G: Thrombolytic effect of streptokinase as evaluated by phlebography of deep venous thrombi of the leg, Acta Chir Scand 136:173, 1970.
60. Tsapogas MJ et al: Controlled study of thrombolytic therapy in deep vein thrombosis, Surgery 74:973, 1973.
61. Porter JM et al: Comparison of heparin and streptokinase in the treatment of venous thrombosis, Am Surg 41:511, 1975.
62. Elliot MSW et al: A comparative randomized trial of heparin versus streptokinase in the treatment of acute proximal venous thrombosis: an interim report of a prospective trial, Br J Surg 66:838, 1979.
63. Goldhaber SZ et al: Pooled analyses of randomized trials of streptokinase and heparin in phlebographically documented acute deep vein venous thrombosis, Am J Med 76:393, 1984.
64. Sharma GVRK et al: Thrombolytic therapy in deep vein thrombosis. In Paoletti R and Sherry S, eds: Thrombosis and urokinase, New York, 1977, Academic Press Inc.
65. Graor RA et al: Comparison of cost-effectiveness of streptokinase and urokinase in the treatment of deep vein thrombosis, Ann Vasc Surg 1:524, 1987.
66. Arnesen H et al: A prospective study of streptokinase and heparin in the treatment of deep vein thrombosis, Acta Med Scand 203:457, 1978.
67. Common HH et al: Deep vein thrombosis treated with streptokinase or heparin: follow-up of a randomized study, Angiology 27:645, 1976.

68. Johansson L et al: Comparison of streptokinase with heparin: late results in the treatment of deep vein thrombosis, Acta Med Scand 206:93, 1979.
69. Turpie AGG et al: A randomized trial of recombinant tissue plasminogen activator for the treatment of proximal deep vein thrombosis, Circulation 72(abst):III, 1985.
70. Straub H: Letale komplikationen der fibrinolyse, Munch Med Wschr 124:17, 1982.
71. Holm HA: Trombosebehandling med heparin. in Hoechst, ed: Dyp venous trombose og lungeemboli, Oslo, 1981.
72. Greenfield LJ et al: Clinical experience with the Kimray Greenfield vena caval filter, Ann Surg 185:692, 1977.
73. Greenfield LJ et al: Greenfield vena caval filter experience, Arch Surg 116:1451, 1981.
74. Roehm JOF et al: The bird's nest inferior vena cava filter: progress report, Radiology 168:745, 1988.
75. Ricco JB et al: Percutaneous transvenous caval interruption with the "LGM" filter: early results of a multicenter trial, Ann Vasc Surg 2:242, 1988.
76. Simon M et al: Simon nitinol inferior vena cava filter: initial clinical experience, Radiology 172:99, 1989.
77. Fobbe F et al: Gunther vena caval filter: results of long-term follow-up, AJR 151:1031, 1988.
78. Yune HY: Inferior vena cava filter: search for an ideal device, Radiology 172:15, 1989.
79. Epstein DH et al: Experience with the Amplatz retrievable vena cava filter, Radiology 172:105, 1989.
80. Karp RB and Wylie EJ: Recurrent thrombosis after iliofemoral venous thrombectomy, Surg Forum 17:147, 1966.
81. Haller JA Jr and Abrams BL: Use of thrombectomy in the treatment of acute iliofemoral venous thrombosis in forty-five patients, Ann Surg 158:561, 1963.
82. Lansing AM and Davis WM: Five-year follow-up study of iliofemoral venous thrombectomy, Ann Surg 168:620, 1968.
83. Harris EJ and Brown WH: Patency after iliofemoral venous thrombosis, Ann Surg 167:91, 1968.
84. Lindhagen J et al: Iliofemoral venous thrombectomy, J Cardiovasc Surg 19:319, 1978.
85. Plate G et al: Thrombectomy with temporary arteriovenous fistula: the treatment of choice in acute iliofemoral venous thrombosis, J Vasc Surg 1:867, 1984.
86. Coon WW and Willis PW: Thrombosis of axillary and subclavian veins, Arch Surg 94:657, 1967.
87. Donayre CE et al: Pathogenesis determines late morbidity of axillosubclavian vein thrombosis, Am J Surg 152:179, 1986.
88. Harley DP et al: Pulmonary embolism secondary to venous thrombosis of the arm, Am J Surg 147:221, 1984.
89. Horattas MC et al: Changing concepts of deep venous thrombosis of the upper extremity—report of a series and review of the literature, Surgery 104:561, 1988.
90. Gloviczki P, Kazmier FJ, and Hollier LH: Axillary-subclavian venous occlusion: the morbidity of a nonlethal disease, J Vasc Surg 4:333, 1986.
91. Tilney NL, Griffiths HJG, and Edwards EA: Natural history of major venous thrombosis of the upper extremity, Arch Surg 101:792, 1970.
92. Demeter SL et al: Upper extremity thrombosis: etiology and prognosis, Angiology 33:743, 1982.
93. Lopez MI and Vincent RJ: Malignancy superior or vena cava syndrome. In Kapoor As, ed: Cancer and the heart, New York, 1986, Springer-Verlag.
94. Parish JM et al: Etiologic considerations in superior vena cava syndrome, Mayo Clin Proc 56:407, 1981.
95. Schraufnagel DE et al: Superior vena cava obstruction: is it a medical emergency? Am J Med 70:1169, 1981.
96. Lochridge SK, Knibbe WP, and Doty DB: Obstruction of the superior vena cava, Surgery 85:14, 1979.
97. Dake MD et al: The cause of superior vena cava syndrome: diagnosis with percutaneous atherectomy, Radiology 174:957, 1990.
98. Perez CA, Presant CA, and VanAmburg AL: Management of superior vena cava syndrome, Semin Oncol 5:123, 1978.
99. Armstrong P, Hayes DF, and Richardson PJ: Transvenous biopsy of carcinoma of bronchus causing superior vena caval obstruction, Br Med J [Clin Res] 1:662, 1975.
100. Gray BH et al: Safety and efficacy of thrombolytic therapy for superior vena cava syndrome, Chest (in press).
101. Dalen JE and Alpert JS: Natural history of pulmonary embolism, Prog Cardiovasc Dis 17:259, 1975.
102. Skinner DB and Salzman EW: Anticoagulant prophylaxis in surgical patients, Surg Gynecol Obstet 125:741, 1967.
103. Kakkar VV et al: Prophylaxis for post-operative deep-vein thrombosis, JAMA 241:39, 1979.
104. Fratantoni J and Wessler S: Prophylactic therapy of deep-vein thrombosis and pulmonary embolism, DHEW Publ No (NIH) 76-866, Washington, DC, 1975, US Government Printing Office.
105. Salzman EW and Davies GC: Prophylaxis of venous thromboembolism: analysis of cost-effectiveness, Ann Surg 191:207, 1980.
106. Hull R et al: Cost-effectiveness of primary and secondary prevention of fatal pulmonary embolism in high-risk surgical patients, Cereal Manuf Assoc J 127:990, 1982.
107. Carter C and Gent M: The epidemiology of venous thrombosis. In Coleman RW et al, eds: Hemostasis and thrombosis: basic principles and clinical practice, New York, 1982, JB Lippincott Co.
108. Salzman EW and Hirsh J: Prevention of venous thromboembolism. In Coleman RW et al, eds: Hemostasis and thrombosis: basic principles and clinical practice, New York, 1982, JB Lippincott Co.
109. Kakkar VV et al: Efficacy of low-doses of heparin in prevention of deep-vein thrombosis after major surgery: a double-blind randomized trial, Lancet 2:101, 1972.
110. Hull RD and Hirsh J: Preventing venous thromboembolism, J Cardiovasc Med 9:63, 1984.
111. Turpie ACG et al: Prevention of venous thrombosis in patients with intracranial disease by intermittent pneumatic compression of the calf, Neurology 27:435, 1977.
112. Skillman JJ et al: Prevention of deep-vein thrombosis in neurosurgical patients: a controlled, randomized trial of external pneumatic compression boots, Surgery 83:354, 1978.

Chapter 25

PULMONARY EMBOLISM

Robert A. Graor
John R. Bartholomew

Pulmonary embolism (PE) is one of the four most common causes of sudden death in the United States. Nearly 630,000 people develop pulmonary emboli each year, and approximately 67,000 (11%) of these individuals die in the first hour after symptoms appear.[1-5]

Retrospective studies show a high association between pulmonary embolism and venous thrombosis of the lower limbs, and prospective studies demonstrate that patients with venous thrombosis are at high risk for developing pulmonary embolism.[3,4] Most clinically significant and fatal emboli arise from thrombi in the proximal veins of the leg; occasionally, however, fatal emboli arise from large thrombi in calf veins.[4,6,7]

Autopsy studies published over the past decade indicate that major pulmonary emboli occur in as many as 25% of hospitalized patients.[8-11] Nevertheless, pulmonary emboli are not observed clinically in as many as 80% of patients, and they are accurately diagnosed in only about 50% of patients.[12,13]

The inability to recognize and diagnose emboli probably is responsible for the lack of improvement in the fatality rate for pulmonary embolism. Goldhaber in 1988 reported that the fatality rate for pulmonary embolism did not change from 1979 to 1985 (Fig. 25-1).[12] The importance of establishing a prompt diagnosis is shown by the difference in mortality rates for treated and untreated pulmonary embo-

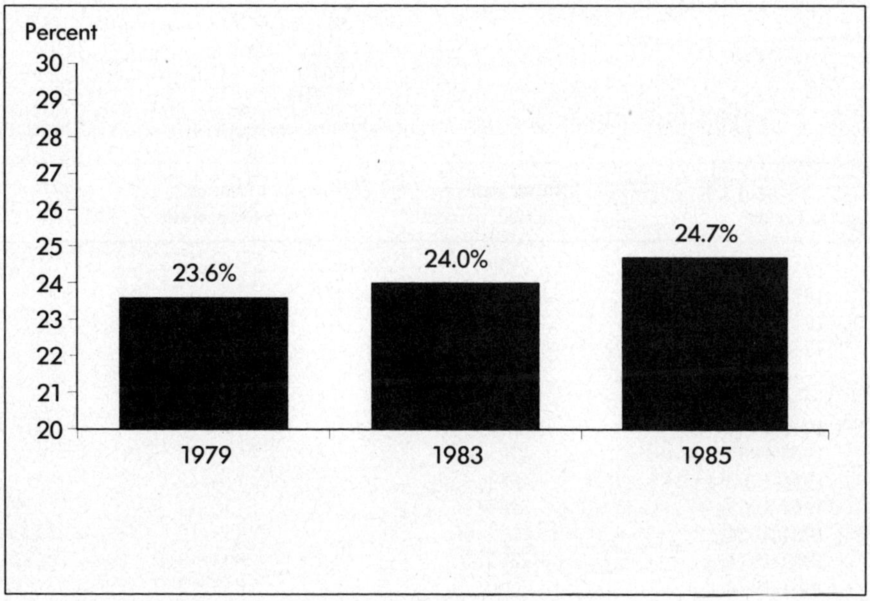

Fig. 25-1. Ratio of all death certificates to hospital discharge diagnosis citing pulmonary embolism as the cause of death.

lism. The mortality rate for untreated pulmonary embolism is between 20% and 35%; it is 8% when the condition is recognized and appropriately managed.[11,13-15]

Studies of the clinical factors associated with failure to establish the diagnosis of pulmonary embolism stress the vagueness of the patient's clinical picture. None of the symptoms or signs of pulmonary embolism is unique, and all may be associated with other cardiorespiratory disorders.[15,16] The Urokinase Pulmonary Embolism Trial (UPET) published in 1973 shows that 49% of 3986 patients had clinical signs and symptoms of pulmonary embolism; however, the diagnosis of pulmonary embolism was excluded because of negative perfusion lung scan findings.[17] Other studies indicate that the diagnosis of pulmonary embolism is confirmed in less than half of all patients with clinical signs and symptoms of the condition.[18,19]

INCIDENCE OF PULMONARY EMBOLISM

The incidence of pulmonary embolism is not easy to determine because of problems in distinguishing between clinically significant and incidental pulmonary emboli at autopsy, in coding pulmonary emboli on death certificates, and in correlating clinical signs and symptoms of pulmonary embolism with objective evidence of the diagnosis.

At autopsy pathologists do not routinely conduct extensive dissection of the leg veins to search for thrombophlebitis. Most pathologists externally milk the blood back through the transected iliac vein and examine the effluent for thrombi. Most autopsy series attempt to differentiate between major pulmonary emboli that cause or significantly contribute to the patient's death and minor emboli that are clinically incidental. However, many autopsy series show a wide variation in the proportion of patients who had major pulmonary emboli and those who had minor emboli. Autopsy series published from 1919 to 1982 report proportions ranging from 8% to 52% (Table 25-1). These series suggest that the more meticulous the dissection of the lungs, the more pulmonary emboli are found.[6,20-33]

Studies that rely on death certificates may grossly underreport the clinical impression of pulmonary embolism at the time of death because of improper coding of death certificates. Rossman reviewed 6385 death certificates filed in New York City during a single month and found that 207 (3.2%) listed pulmonary embolism as a major or a contributing cause of death.[34] Closer review of these death certificates demonstrated that coding methods used to identify pulmonary embolism were not appropriate. As a result, the number of death certificates listing pulmonary embolism as a cause of death was reduced to 31 (0.05%).

When autopsy findings are correlated with findings in medical records, the proportion of patients who were suspected of having major pulmonary emboli before death can be determined.[28,29,31,32] However, some of these studies indicate that pulmonary embolism is being underdiagnosed, while others suggest that it is being overdiagnosed.

In studies conducted between 1928 and 1981 the proportion of patients who were thought to have pulmonary embolism before death varied from 16% to 38% (Table 25-1). These studies show that other pulmonary and cardiac conditions mislead clinicians.[29-32] Although pneumonia may occur concomitantly with pulmonary embolism, frequently only pneumonia is recognized clinically. Other medical conditions that hinder the diagnosis of pulmonary embolism are congestive heart failure and cancer. Increasing age also is associated with less frequent detection of pulmonary embolism.

In studies published from 1965 to 1972 the proportion of patients who had a clinical diagnosis of pulmonary em-

Table 25-1. The prevalance of pulmonary embolism found at autopsy and percent of major pulmonary embolism

Study	Period	No. of patients autopsied/percent	No. of PEs/percent	Percent with massive PE
Belt[20]	1929-1934	567	56/10	7
Collins[21]	1928-1935	10,950		2
McCartney[22]	1919-1938	25,771	2603/10	3
Roe[23]	1930-1947	5906	464/8	4
Ochsner[24]	1938-1950	10,946/34		4
Fowler[25]	1930-1953	2457/37		4
Towbin[26]	1949-1954	512/58	132/26	14
Coon[27]	1945-1954	4391/69	606/14	9
Uhland[28]	1956-1960	981	118/12	7
Morrell[7]	1964-1965	263/76	136/52	14
Modan[29]	1961-1964	2107/66	353/17	11
MacIntyre[30]	1967-1971	2291/40	303/13	9
Coon[31]	1964-1974	4600/70	567/12	7
Goldhaber[32]	1973-1977	1455/61	216/15	4
Mossey[33]	1969-1981	2255	731/32	10

bolism that was confirmed at autopsy ranged from 38% to 68%.[29,35,36] These studies imply that pulmonary embolism is mistaken for other conditions.

More recent data suggest that better diagnosis rates are occurring. This improvement should reduce the fatality rate associated with pulmonary embolism. In 1982 the United States National Hospital Discharge Survey found that pulmonary embolism was being diagnosed with increasing frequency and that the case fatality rate was decreasing. This study, which surveyed 400 hospitals and 216,000 acute care medical records, reported that the case fatality rate for pulmonary emboli decreased from 20% in 1971 to 13% in 1978 and that the greatest decrease in the overall frequency of pulmonary emboli and in the proportion of fatal emboli occurred in patients aged 65 and older. However, the study did not suggest whether the decline in the fatality rate was from the presence of fewer massive pulmonary emboli, the diagnosis of greater numbers of minor pulmonary emboli, the improvement in treatment methods and prophylaxis, or a combination of these factors.[37]

Potential long-term risk factors for major pulmonary embolism

Information on the risk factors that predispose individuals to pulmonary embolism over the long-term has been gathered only on a small cohort of patients in the Framingham Heart Study. This study did not obtain information prospectively on pulmonary embolism or venous thrombosis, but it did collect information on potential long-term risk factors for pulmonary embolism from a group of patients who had autopsy-confirmed pulmonary emboli. Data on these patients were compared with data on all patients in the Framingham Heart Study who died within the study's 26-year period. Multiple regression analysis of the comparative data showed that only overweight women were significantly at risk for pulmonary embolism over the long-term.

PATHOLOGY AND PHYSIOLOGY OF PULMONARY EMBOLISM

The first description of thrombotic occlusion of the pulmonary arteries was reported by Tulpius in 1641. However, it was not until the mid-1800s that factors leading to the occlusion of pulmonary blood vessels were discovered. In 1856 Virchow found that stagnant blood was predisposed to coagulation. In 1889 Cohnheim and Ribbert demonstrated that injury to the lining of blood vessels led to the development of thrombi. Subsequently, others showed that the danger of thrombi increased after surgery because the number of platelets and other blood coagulation factors commonly increased.

The realization that most pulmonary emboli originate from the deep veins of the legs as well as the discovery of concepts relevant to the current understanding of venous thrombosis emerged later in the nineteenth century. Finally, in 1940 classic studies by Hampton and Castleman defined the pathologic changes and clinical correlates of pulmonary emboli.[38]

Structure of pulmonary emboli

Pulmonary emboli usually have the characteristic structure of thrombi that are found in the deep veins of the legs.[39] They are red, contain large amounts of trapped red cells, and are laminated with both circumferentially and longitudinally added thrombus. Pulmonary emboli discovered before death can be differentiated from those found after death. Clots found after death are red or yellow. Red clots generally are soft and rubbery and have no internally constituted lamination. Yellow clots sometimes are called chicken fat clots. The cast of the vein, which has produced indentations in the thrombus by means of its valves, is often detected in thrombi removed at autopsy.

Sites of thrombi formation

Thrombi form in the pockets of valve cusps, in saccules in the vein wall, and at vein junctions. Six primary sites of thrombophlebitis have been described: the iliac vein, the common femoral vein, the termination of the deep femoral vein, the popliteal vein, the posterior tibial veins, and the intramuscular veins of the calf, particularly the soleal veins.[40] Although thrombi within calf veins are common, they are less likely to cause significant emboli than thrombi from other larger and more proximal veins.

Most pulmonary emboli originate as thrombi in the large deep veins of the legs.[2,5,18,41] Thrombi in the superficial varicosities rarely embolize. Other venous sites of thrombi that may produce pulmonary emboli include the prostatic plexus, the veins of the broad ligaments, the periovarian and the uterine veins, and subclavian and axillary veins.

Distribution of thrombi in the lung

Most pulmonary emboli lodge in the lower lobes of the lungs, particularly in the posterobasilar and apical segments of the lower lobes.[42,43] Two reasons have been suggested for this distribution: (1) The lower portions of the lungs have much greater blood flow than the upper portions and (2) the main axial artery that supplies blood to the lower lobes terminates in these segments. Emboli also occur more commonly in the right lung than in the left. The reason for this distribution is unclear, although it is probably related to blood flow patterns.

Large venous thrombi sometimes form a "saddle embolus" at a bifurcation of the pulmonary artery. More commonly, however, a packed thrombus occludes a major pulmonary vessel (Fig. 25-2).

Physiologic responses

The physiologic response to acute pulmonary emboli depends on the degree of pulmonary arterial blood flow obstruction, the nature of a patient's preexisting cardiopulmonary status, and the type of vasoactive humoral factors

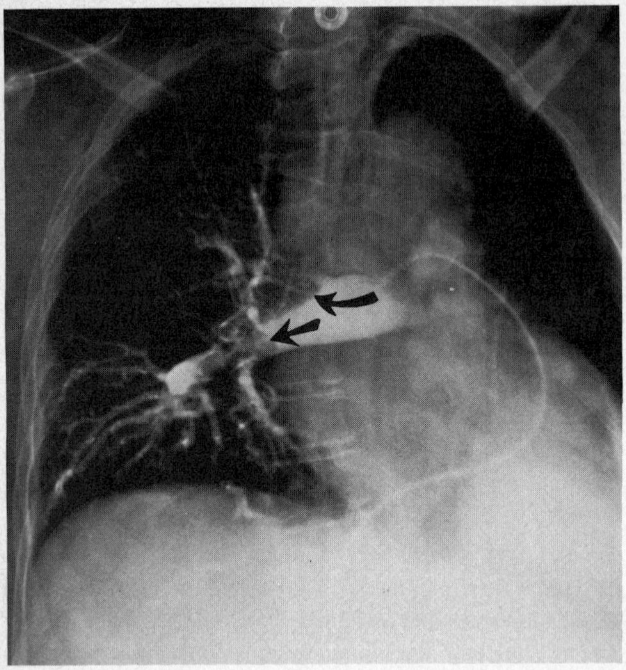

Fig. 25-2. A pulmonary angiogram demonstrating a right main pulmonary artery embolus *(arrows)* with occlusion of arteries supplying all lobes of the right lung.

that are released from activated platelets at the site of the clot.

Pulmonary arterial obstruction. Physiologic decompensation arises from an increase in right ventricular and pulmonary arterial pressures. In a patient who has no history of pulmonary disease and no right ventricular hypertrophy, right ventricular afterload increases when obstruction of the pulmonary artery reduces the pulmonary vascular bed by 25% or more.[44] Normally, the right ventricle generates a maximum systolic pressure of 30 mm Hg to 40 mm Hg in the pulmonary artery. The increase in pressure is linearly related to the amount of embolic obstruction of the pulmonary artery. As pulmonary artery pressure increases, right ventricle chamber dilation may occur, leading to tricuspid regurgitation and hypokinesis of the free wall of the ventricle.

Come has demonstrated by echocardiography that right ventricular dilation and hypokinesis occur with pulmonary emboli.[45] She has also shown that a modest elevation of pulmonary arterial systolic pressure causes a mild tricuspid regurgitant jet. Even with only a mild increase in pulmonary arterial pressure, the right ventricle generally appears diffusely hypokinetic and slightly dilated. As pulmonary arterial pressures increase, the dilation and hypokinesis worsen linearly. Systolic and diastolic septal flattening, compatible with combined right ventricular pressure and volume overload, are observed unless the pulmonary embolus is small. As the right ventricle fails, right atrial pressure rises, and cardiogenic shock ensues.

Preexisting cardiopulmonary disease. Hemodynamic decompensation occurs with smaller emboli that obstruct fewer branch vessels in patients with preexisting cardiopulmonary disease. In individuals who have antecedent pulmonary hypertension, right ventricular dysfunction is not directly related to the extent of thrombotic pulmonary arterial obstruction.[45,46]

In patients who have primary pulmonary hypertension caused by a chronic lung disease, pulmonary arterial changes progress slowly. The gradual evolution of pulmonary arterial changes leads to the development of right ventricular hypertrophy, which, in turn, allows the right ventricle to generate high systolic pressures in the pulmonary artery. Sometimes these pressures exceed systemic arterial pressure levels. Pulmonary arterial changes are reflected on echocardiography as a hypertrophied right ventricle and an increase in the tricuspid regurgitant jet. Because the relationship between the degree of right ventricular dysfunction and the extent of embolic obstruction is not significant, right ventricular wall motion may be normal, or it may show varying degrees of hypokinesis.[47]

In addition to preload, afterload, heart rate, and contractility, which are the standard determinants of left ventricular function or left ventricular systolic performance, acute increases in right ventricular pressure also affect left ventricular function. Experimental data have proven that the anatomic position of the two ventricles during pressure overload of the right ventricle creates ventricular interdependency.[45] This interdependency causes decreased left ventricular diastolic filling and volume and an apparent change in left ventricular distensibility by increasing the size and pressure of the right ventricle.

Come et al have demonstrated by Doppler echocardiography that cardiopulmonary abnormalities associated with pulmonary emboli resolve quickly.[71] They have shown that significant and early reversal of right ventricular dilation and hypokinesia, tricuspid regurgitation, and decreased left ventricular cavity dimension follow thrombolysis. These changes occur simultaneously with a decrease in pulmonary arterial pressure, and they correlate with angiographic evidence of reperfusion. The early reversal of the cardiopulmonary abnormalities suggests that the right ventricle is not "stunned"; rather, it is capable of recovering in response to a decrease in afterload of the right ventricle.

Neurohumoral factors. In addition to changes in right and left heart hemodynamics, the release of neurohumoral factors may cause vasoconstriction and bronchospasm that adversely affect the physiologic outcome of embolization. The two most important vasoactive humoral factors are serotonin and thromboxane A_2. Serotonin, which is stored primarily in platelets, mediates a potent neural and smooth muscle agonistic process that produces bronchospasm. Thromboxane A_2, which is secreted by activated platelets, is also a potent vasoconstrictor and bronchoconstrictor.

To summarize, the right ventricle of an individual who has no prior heart or lung disease cannot generate mean pulmonary arterial pressures greater than 30 mm Hg to 40 mm Hg, presumably because of the absence of right ventricular hypertrophy. With progressive increases in pulmonary vascular resistance, the right ventricle of such an individual begins to fail. Failure of the right ventricle causes elevation of right atrial pressure and symptoms and signs of right heart failure. The relationship between the mean pulmonary arterial pressure and the mean right atrial pressure is significant.

Some patients maintain stroke volume and consequently cardiac output on the basis of increased sympathetic drive and the Frank-Starling mechanism (the ventricular response to an increase in either volume load or pressure by diastolic distention and increased energy release). Other patients, especially those with massive pulmonary emboli, fail to maintain stroke volume, and this failure may cause decreased cardiac output, cardiogenic shock, and death. In patients with prior heart or lung disease, right ventricular hypertrophy usually generates higher pulmonary arterial pressures.

In patients with antecedent pulmonary hypertension, right ventricular dysfunction is not related to the extent of embolic obstruction observed angiographically. In patients with pulmonary embolism whose right ventricular function has been impaired, mortality is increased.

DIAGNOSIS OF PULMONARY EMBOLISM

Clinical diagnosis

Most pulmonary emboli are clinically silent, and the correlation between signs and symptoms of thromboembolic disease and the documented presence of pulmonary emboli is poor.[48] When pulmonary emboli do produce clinical manifestations, the manifestations vary widely. They may include (1) transient dyspnea and tachypnea; (2) pulmonary infarction with atelectasis; (3) right-sided heart failure with severe dyspnea and tachypnea; (4) cardiovascular collapse with hypotension, syncope, and even coma; and (5) confusion, pyrexia, wheezing, resistant heart failure, and unexplained arrhythmias or other nonspecific findings such as diaphoresis, cyanosis, edema, gallop, or murmurs.

In the UPET symptoms and signs of thromboembolic disease were described in 327 patients with angiographically documented pulmonary emboli (Table 25-2).[17] These patients' most common symptoms were chest pain (74%), dyspnea (84%), apprehension (59%), and cough (53%). The most common signs in these patients were tachypnea (92%), rales (58%), an accentuated P_2 second heart sound (53%), tachycardia (44%), and temperature greater than 37.8° C (43%). However, thrombophlebitis was clinically diagnosed in only 32% of the patients.

Although chest pain is the most common symptom of pulmonary embolism, it is not diagnostic of the condition. The type of pain that is most often associated with pulmonary embolism is pleuritic. Pleuritic pain is caused by an inflammatory reaction of the lung parenchyma and the overlying pleura or by pulmonary infarction or ischemia caused by obstruction of small pulmonary arterial branches. Pleuritic chest pain typically is sudden in onset, and it is aggravated by breathing; however, it usually does not occur in the first 24 hours following the onset of pulmonary embolism.

Table 25-2. Symptoms and signs in 327 patients with pulmonary embolism

Signs and symptoms	Percent of patients
Symptoms	
Dyspnea	85
Pleuritic chest pain	74
Apprehension	59
Cough	53
Hemoptysis	30
Diaphoresis	36
Syncope	13
Signs	
Tachypnea (RR > 16/min)	92
Rales	58
Accentuated second heart sound	53
Tachycardia (HR > 100/min)	44
Fever (Temp > 37.8° C)	43
Phlebitis	32
Cyanosis	19

Central, substernal chest pain also may be associated with pulmonary embolism; however, it is often indistinguishable from angina pectoris. The cause of this type of pain may be a transient decrease in stroke volume and increase in heart rate resulting in decreased diastolic phase time and decreased filling of the coronary arteries.

Although hemoptysis is a hallmark of pulmonary embolism, it occurs infrequently; for example, 30% of patients in the UPET study had hemoptysis.[17] The presence of hemoptysis indicates that pulmonary infarction or atelectasis has produced alveolar hemorrhage. As a result, hemoptysis does not occur in the acute period of pulmonary embolism but several days afterward. Pulmonary hemorrhage is unusual, and it usually is not aggravated by anticoagulant therapy.

Certain triads of symptoms and signs are considered to be classic manifestations of pulmonary embolism, such as hemoptysis, cough, and sweating; hemoptysis, chest pain, and dyspnea; or dyspnea, chest pain, and apprehension. However, Allen's sign (the triad of fever, tachypnea, and tachycardia) was present in only 23% of patients in the UPET.[17]

A report by Goodall and Greenfield reviewed the clinical pictures of 73 patients who had undergone angiography to search for pulmonary emboli and found that symptoms do not help discriminate between the patients who do have pulmonary emboli and those who do not.[49] Angiography confirmed the diagnosis of pulmonary embolism in only 29% of patients who had clinical signs and symptoms suspicious of pulmonary embolism. Of note, chest pain and hemoptysis occurred more often in patients who did not have angiographic evidence of pulmonary emboli. Dyspnea and sweating occurred with virtually identical frequency in both groups of patients.

This study also demonstrated that signs detected during physical examination are not useful in discriminating between those patients who do have pulmonary emboli and those who do not. In fact, 21% of the patients who had angiographic evidence of pulmonary emboli had a heart rate of fewer than 100 beats per minute, and all the patients had a respiratory rate greater than 16 breaths per minute.

Unfortunately, pulmonary embolism is often overlooked because the signs and symptoms are typical of other conditions, such as pneumonia, congestive heart failure, or myocardial infarction.

History of preexisting cardiopulmonary diseases

Common preexisting conditions in patients in the UPET study included venous thrombi (50%) and congestive heart failure or chronic lung disease (38%).[17] However, 50% of patients in this study had no apparent preexisting conditions. This finding may reflect bias in the selection of patients who were sufficiently healthy to withstand angiography and thrombolytic therapy.

Other characteristics, including medical or surgical conditions and medication usage, may predispose patients to the development of pulmonary embolism. These characteristics include surgery and trauma, malignancy, advanced age, obesity, pregnancy, cardiac disease, varicose veins, and use of oral contraceptives. Other characteristics are less well recognized as factors that predispose patients to pulmonary embolism. These include nationality (e.g., the incidence of pulmonary embolism in the United States is 24% while it is only 5% in Japan) and a non-O blood group.

Clinical syndromes

Several clinical syndromes are associated with pulmonary embolism, and they vary with the size of the emboli.

Massive pulmonary emboli are large enough to obstruct the pulmonary arterial blood flow and cause an increase in right ventricular afterload and a consequent elevation of the pulmonary arterial systolic pressure. Patients with massive pulmonary emboli are at highest risk for sudden death and chronic pulmonary hypertension because of their thromboembolic disease when emboli fail to lyse within the pulmonary arteries.

Common signs and conditions associated with massive pulmonary emboli include syncope, cor pulmonale, cardiogenic shock, and cardiac arrest, especially with electromechanical dissociation. When syncope occurs, it may be associated with a brief period of vagal bradyarrhythmia followed by tachycardia, tachypnea, and cyanosis along with distended neck veins and evidence of cardiogenic shock.

Other conditions may be confused with massive pulmonary emboli, including septic shock, superior vena caval syndromes, pericardial tamponade, constrictive pericarditis, and right ventricular infarction.

Submassive pulmonary emboli cause embolization in one or more pulmonary arterial segments, which is not accompanied by significant elevations in the right ventricular and pulmonary arterial systolic pressures. Patients with submassive pulmonary emboli frequently have dyspnea and pleuritic chest pain. A single submassive pulmonary embolus usually does not cause death; however, recurrent submassive emboli that are undiagnosed and untreated may be fatal. Recurrent pulmonary emboli also may cause chronic thrombotic pulmonary hypertension.[50]

A pulmonary embolus that occludes a small peripheral pulmonary arterial branch and interrupts collateral blood flow in the bronchial arteries may cause pulmonary infarction. The diagnosis of pulmonary infarction is based on chest x-ray findings of an infiltrate, the presence of pleuritic chest pain, and evidence of a pulmonary embolus on a lung scan or arteriogram. Hemoptysis may be present in varying degrees, but virtually all patients experience intense pleuritic chest pain that begins 1 to 5 days following the onset of pulmonary embolism and that subsides gradually with supportive treatment.

A single pulmonary embolus that does not totally resolve and therefore continues to interfere with normal pulmonary hemodynamics may cause chronic thromboembolic pulmonary hypertension.[51-53] Several recurrent emboli also may produce chronic thromboembolic pulmonary hypertension by following an aberrant path of organization or recanalization, which leaves residual obstructive narrowing of major pulmonary arteries. Chronic thromboembolic pulmonary hypertension tends to develop insidiously in patients who have undiagnosed or inadequately treated pulmonary embolism. Similarities and differences for thrombotic and primary pulmonary hypertension are shown in Table 25-3.[35] The diagnosis is based on physical findings of new or changing heart murmurs, dyspnea, cyanosis, peripheral edema, or ascites in the presence of clear lung fields. The degree of dyspnea appears to correlate with the degree of elevation of pulmonary arterial pressure.[50] Chronic pulmonary hypertension caused by recurrent pulmonary emboli carries a poor prognosis; only such surgical procedures as thromboendarterectomy of the pulmonary vasculature, lung transplantation, or heart-lung transplantation are treatment options.

PRELIMINARY DIAGNOSTIC TESTS

Electrocardiogram

Electrocardiograms (ECGs) of patients with pulmonary embolism show certain signs; however, at best, they merely exclude cardiac causes of a patient's symptoms.

ECGs of the majority of patients with pulmonary em-

Table 25-3. Primary pulmonary hypertension (PPH) vs recurrent pulmonary embolism (PE)

	Similarities	
Symptoms	Fatigue, dyspnea on exertion—most common Chest pain, syncope, hemoptysis, cyanosis—also common	
Clinical course	Progressive dyspnea, right ventricular heart failure	
Hemodynamics	Elevated right ventricular heart pressures, normal pulmonary capillary wedge pressure	
	Differences	
	PPH	**Recurrent PE**
Age	20 to 40 yr	>50 yr
Female/male ratio	4:1	1:1
Clinical course	Continued deterioration	Deterioration with stabilization between episodes
Lung scan	No segmental perfusion defects	Segmental or larger perfusion defects
Pulmonary artery systolic pressure	>60 mm Hg	<60 mm Hg
Pulmonary arteriogram	"Pruning"	Intraluminal filling defects
Confounding problems with arteriogram	Thrombi may occur on or distal to PPH lesions	"Pruning," a common angiographic finding in PPH, can also indicate PE. Arteriogram may not show emboli late in clinical course.
Diagnostic alternatives	Open lung biopsy	Pulmonary angioscopy
Therapy	Isoproterenol Hydralazine Nifedipine Anticoagulation	Anticoagulation IVC interruption Thromboendarterectomy

bolism show sinus tachycardia. ECGs also may show arrhythmias, including premature ventricular contractions, premature atrial contractions, and atrial fibrillation, which are consistent with changes in the electrical activity of the heart caused by pulmonary embolism. However, none of these findings is diagnostic of pulmonary embolism.

Although ECGs of patients with submassive emboli are few and variable, ECGs of patients with massive pulmonary emboli may show characteristic abnormalities such as an $S_1Q_3T_3$ pattern, complete right bundle branch block, P pulmonale, or right axis deviation. However, the ECGs of many patients with massive pulmonary emboli may not exhibit these abnormalities. In the UPET study, for example, ECGs of only 26% of the patients had these changes.

Chest x-ray examination

The chest x-ray examination is insensitive as a screening test for pulmonary emboli. However, it can provide valuable information to support a preliminary diagnosis of the condition.

Important clues to the diagnosis of acute pulmonary embolism may be found on a routine chest x-ray examination, especially when a previous x-ray film is available for comparison. A zone of hyperlucency and markedly diminished vascular markings (an engorged major hilar artery or an engorged "plump" or "sausagelike" right pulmonary artery) indicate occlusion of a lobar or segmental artery caused by an embolus.[54] Abrupt termination of a vessel, called the "knuckle sign," is highly suggestive of pulmonary emboli, but it occurs rarely. Pleural effusion is found in approximately 50% of the chest x-ray films of patients with pulmonary emboli, nevertheless, pleural effusion is not specific for the diagnosis.[55] Displacement of the major fissure, elevation of a hemidiaphragm, and atelectasis are other nonspecific chest x-ray findings of acute pulmonary embolism.

X-ray findings of right-sided cardiomegaly, mosaic oligemia, or enlargement of the right descending pulmonary artery are clues to the diagnosis of chronic recurrent pulmonary embolism.

A chest x-ray film showing an infiltrative radiographic density suggests pulmonary infarction. The classic radiographic configuration of infarction is a wedge-shaped infiltration whose convex portion points toward the hilum, which is occasionally called "Hampton's hump" (Fig. 25-3).[41]

Arterial blood gases

An arterial blood gas study is a traditional screening test for pulmonary emboli; however, the diagnosis of pulmonary embolism should not be excluded or confirmed on the basis of arterial blood gas studies alone. Many patients with pulmonary embolism have hypoxemia and hypocarbia, although in one series 14% of the patients with angiographically documented pulmonary emboli had a Po_2 value greater than 85 torr, and one patient had a Po_2 of 108 torr.[36] Un-

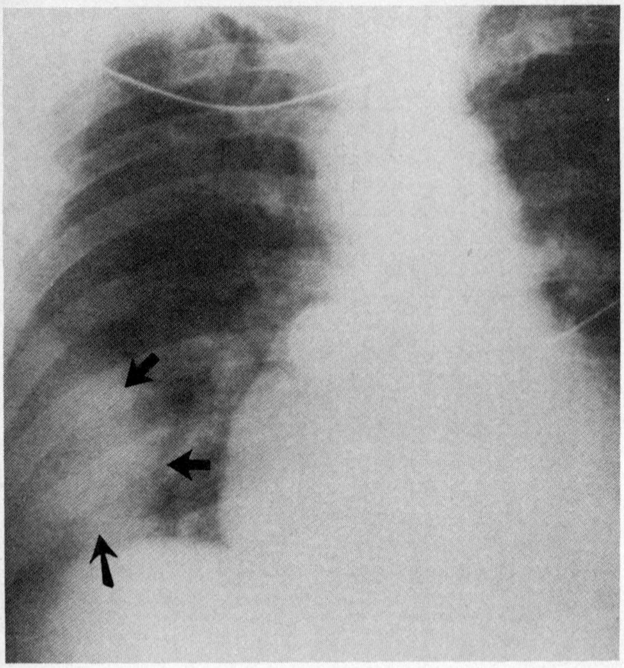

Fig. 25-3. The standard chest x-ray film shows a triangular infiltrate in the right lower lung lobe, which represents a pulmonary infarct *(arrows)*. The base of the triangle is located along the pleura with the apex pointing toward the heart. This is the characteristic appearance of Hampton's hump.

fortunately, Po_2 and Pco_2 values such as these may mistakenly dissuade a physician from further testing for pulmonary emboli.

MORE DEFINITIVE DIAGNOSTIC STUDIES

Lung scanning

Lung scanning, originally described by Taplin and Poe in 1965, currently is an effective means of detecting pulmonary emboli; however, in some cases it does not provide a definitive diagnosis of pulmonary embolism.[57]

Perfusion lung scanning. Perfusion lung scanning detects pulmonary emboli as small as 1 to 2 mm in diameter. In general, however, this type of lung scanning also identifies defects that are caused by conditions other than pulmonary embolism. Perfusion lung scanning detects interruptions in blood flow or a paucity in blood flow to the segment of the lung that is being visualized. These defects usually are secondary to abnormalities in ventilation, such as regional hypoxia and hypoxic pulmonary arterial constriction, or to the loss of a vascular bed from diseases such as emphysema.

Several studies confirmed the inability of perfusion lung scanning to accurately establish a diagnosis of pulmonary embolism. Pulmonary embolism was confirmed by angiography in only 40% of 167 patients in one study and 34% of 146 patients in another study who had an abnormal perfusion scan and clinical signs suggestive of pulmonary embolism.[16,58] Pulmonary embolism was confirmed by angiography in only 95 of 305 patients (31%) in another study, who had clinically suspicious signs and an abnormal perfusion lung scan.[18,59] Excluding patients who had had an abnormal chest x-ray examination did not improve the diagnostic sensitivity of perfusion lung scanning in any of these studies.

Ventilation lung scanning. Ventilation lung scanning was introduced as an adjunct to perfusion lung scanning to aid in the diagnosis of pulmonary embolism. This form of lung scanning is based on the premise that ventilation is preserved in areas of the lung that have reduced perfusion caused by pulmonary embolism. It improves the clinician's ability to diagnose pulmonary embolism by differentiating embolic occlusion of the pulmonary vasculature from defects in perfusion that are secondary to ventilatory disorders. Nevertheless, ventilation lung scanning by itself has not been as effective a diagnostic tool as hoped.

Ventilation-perfusion scanning. In an effort to improve the clinician's ability to diagnose pulmonary embolism, ventilation and perfusion scanning have been combined. Criteria for diagnosing pulmonary embolism on the basis of ventilation-perfusion ($\dot{V}/\dot{Q}$) lung scanning interpretations have not been consistent or practical. These criteria have evolved on the basis of results from retrospective studies.[16,60,61] Although few prospective studies have examined the criteria, a recent prospective study uses scan interpretation criteria that appear to be feasible (see the accompanying box).[62] In the Prospective Investigation of Pulmonary Embolism Diagnosis (PIOPED) study, 102 of 251 (41%) patients with thromboemboli on angiography had $\dot{V}/\dot{Q}$ scan findings classified by PIOPED as highly probable for pulmonary emboli (Table 25-4).[62] $\dot{V}/\dot{Q}$ scan findings classified as highly probable for pulmonary embolism therefore had a sensitivity rate of 41% (95% confidence interval). When $\dot{V}/\dot{Q}$ scan findings classified as having an intermediate probability for pulmonary embolism were included, the sensitivity for thromboemboli increased to 82% (95% confidence interval). When all abnormal scan findings were considered, the sensitivity for thromboemboli was 98% (95% confidence interval) (Table 25-5).[59]

When clinical assessments of patients were compared with the PIOPED lung scanning diagnostic categories, the chance of reaching a correct diagnosis of acute pulmonary embolism improved. Clinical findings that were highly suspicious and $\dot{V}/\dot{Q}$ lung scan findings that were highly probable for pulmonary emboli yielded a 96% probability for pulmonary embolism. According to statistical analysis, clinical assessment was more often correct in excluding pulmonary embolism than in identifying the condition.

In an attempt to establish the proper place for ventilation-perfusion lung scanning, Hull et al conducted the largest prospective study to date that compared abnormal ventilation-perfusion lung scan findings with the results of pulmonary arteriography in patients suspected of having pulmonary emboli.[60] Patients with clinically suspected pulmonary embolism underwent ventilation-perfusion lung

PIOPED lung scan interpretation categories and criteria

High probability

>2 Large (>75% of a segment) segmental perfusion defects without corresponding ventilation or roentgenographic abnormalities or substantially larger than either matching ventilation or chest roentgenogram abnormalities
>2 Moderate segmental (>25% and <75% of a segment) perfusion defects without matching ventilation or chest roentgenogram abnormalities and 1 large mismatched segmental defect
>4 Moderate segmental perfusion defects without ventilation or chest roentgenogram abnormalities

Intermediate probability (indeterminate)

Not falling into normal, very low, low, or high-probability categories
Borderline high or borderline low
Difficult to categorize as low or high

Low probability

Nonsegmental perfusion defects (e.g., very small effusion causing blunting of the costophrenic angle, cardiomegaly, enlarged aorta, hila and mediastinum, and elevated diaphragm)
Single moderate mismatched segmental perfusion defect with normal chest roentgenogram
Any perfusion defect with a substantially *larger* chest roentgenogram abnormality
Large or moderate segmental perfusion defects involving no more than four segments in one lung and no more than three segments in one lung region with matching ventilation defects either equal to or larger in size and chest roentgenogram either normal or with abnormalities substantially smaller than perfusion defects
>3 Small segmental perfusion defects (<25% of a segment) with a normal chest roentgenogram

Very low probability

<3 Small segmental perfusion defects with a normal chest roentgenogram

Normal

No perfusion defects present
Perfusion outlines exactly the shape of the lungs as seen on the chest roentgenogram (hilar and aortic impressions may be seen, chest roentgenogram and/or ventilation study may be abnormal)

Table 25-4. Comparison of scan category with angiographic findings

Scan category	PE present	Angiographic diagnosis	PE uncertain
High probability	102	14	1
Intermediate probability	105	217	9
Low probability	39	199	12
Near normal/normal	5	50	2
TOTALS	251	480	24

Table 25-5. Comparison of scan category with angiographic findings, sensitivity, and specificity

Scan category	Sensitivity (%)	Specificity (%)
High probability	41	97
High or intermediate probability	82	52
High, intermediate, or low probability	98	10

scanning, pulmonary angiography, and venography. The results of the ventilation-perfusion lung scanning did not influence the decision to perform pulmonary angiography or venography.

In this study 59 patients with large perfusion defects and a ventilation-perfusion mismatch were considered to have a high probability of pulmonary embolism, and 51 of them (86%) had pulmonary emboli detected by angiography. Patients with a ventilation-perfusion match and those with small perfusion defects were considered to have a low probability of pulmonary embolism. However, the frequency of pulmonary embolism was not low enough to exclude the diagnosis. Angiography confirmed the presence of pulmonary emboli in 16 of 40 (40%) patients with small perfusion defects and a ventilation-perfusion mismatch. Angiography confirmed the diagnosis of pulmonary embolism in 6 of 24 (25%) patients with small perfusion defects and a ventilation-perfusion match.

This study indicates that the common clinical strategy of using low probability lung scan findings to exclude pulmonary embolism is incorrect. The frequencies of occurrence of venous thromboembolism associated with low-probability lung scan findings ranged from 29% to 46%. The use of improved methods of ventilation scanning in this study did not increase the specificity of ventilation-perfusion

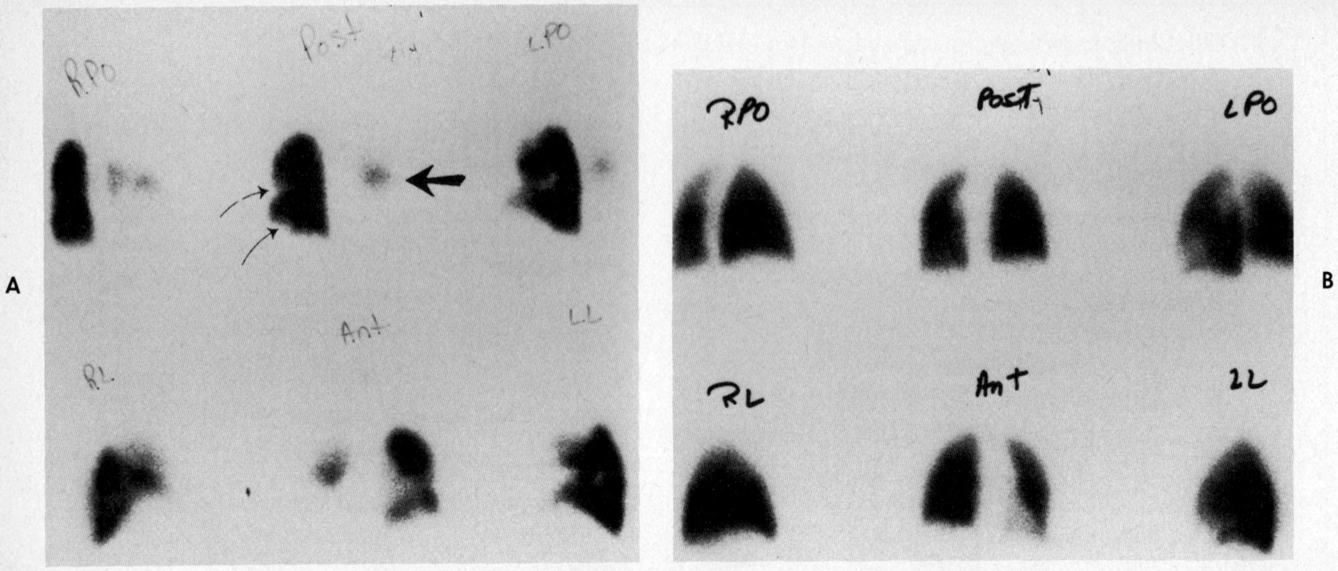

Fig. 25-4. A, A perfusion lung scan with a typical triangular perfusion defect *(small arrow)* and an almost complete absence of perfusion to the right lung *(large arrow)*. These defects were caused by multiple pulmonary emboli. **B,** The perfusion after thrombolysis with urokinase. Reperfusion to the entire right lung has occurred, and only a minor defect remains in the left lower lobe.

lung scanning, which suggests that the diagnostic dilemma probably will not be resolved by refinement of ventilation imaging techniques.

Applying the data from research studies of lung scanning to clinical practice is difficult. In general, intermediate or low-probability lung scan findings provide little additional helpful information when clinical signs of pulmonary embolism are present and further tests such as a venogram or duplex scanning of the leg veins must be done. High-probability lung scan findings in conjunction with a highly suspicious clinical situation or test results that identify a thromboembolic source provide a highly accurate diagnosis of pulmonary embolism. Normal lung scan findings and a clinical situation that is not suspicious of pulmonary embolism indicate that the possibility of pulmonary embolism is exceedingly low.

Although $\dot{V}/\dot{Q}$ lung scanning may follow any one of a number of protocols, ventilation studies generally use ^{133}Xe-labeled gas and a gamma camera with a 20% symmetric window set over the 80-keV energy peak. Ventilation studies take a first breath image in the posterior view for over 100,000 counts. The studies then take posterior equilibrium images for two consecutive 120-second periods and three serial washout views. Perfusion scans use a radiolabeled material, technetium-99m macroaggregated albumin, that contains 100,000 to 700,000 particles. They use a gamma camera with a 20% symmetric window set over the 140-keV energy peak. The radioactive material is injected into the antecubital vein during five to ten respiratory cycles while the patient is lying supine or is sitting up at a 45-degree angle. Perfusion scans take anterior and posterior, both oblique and lateral, view images with 750,000 counts per image for each (Fig. 25-4).

In all situations lung scanning must be done within hours of the onset of pulmonary embolism. A lung scan done after 24 hours may be falsely negative because the clot is lysed.

Pulmonary angiography

Pulmonary arteriography is an underutilized procedure. Its use is increasing, however, because the limitations of lung scanning and clinical signs and symptoms in establishing the diagnosis of pulmonary embolism are becoming more widely appreciated.[60-64]

Indications. Pulmonary angiography is the diagnostic reference standard for pulmonary embolism. However, the indications for pulmonary arteriography have waxed and waned throughout the years.

When Hull et al prospectively studied patients with clinical signs of pulmonary embolism and an abnormal lung scan, they found that the ability of ventilation-perfusion scanning to predict pulmonary embolism was high when patients had one or more perfusion defects involving a lung segment or lobe and normal ventilation scans. However, they found that the predictive value of ventilation-perfusion lung scanning was low for other categories of patients, such as those with one or more segmental defects and a ventilation scan that showed matching defects. The predictive value of scanning also was low for patients with one or more subsegmental perfusion defects or those with a perfusion scan defect that matched a radiographic abnormality. When Hull et al examined the association between angiographically demonstrated pulmonary emboli and venographically demonstrated venous thrombosis, they found that only 12 of 41 patients (29%) with positive pulmonary arteriograms had negative venograms, and they concluded that substituting venography for pulmonary angiography can be misleading.[60] An interesting study done by Marsh, Glynn, and Torman suggested that a pulmonary arteriogram should be performed when lung scan results differ markedly from clinical impressions.[65] Of 30 patients who underwent angiography despite having low-probability lung scan findings, 10 (30%) had positive pulmonary angiograms. Marsh, Glynn, and Torman also showed that of 18 patients who underwent pulmonary angiography despite having high-probability lung scans, 10 had negative pulmonary angiograms. These patients were distinctly unusual, and they underwent angiography because their clinical status was particularly perplexing. Because this study was highly selective, its results must be interpreted with caution.

Although pulmonary angiography is diagnostic of pulmonary embolism, it generally should be reserved for patients who have low, moderate, or indeterminate lung scan findings and highly suspicious clinical signs of pulmonary embolism.[56,65-67] Pulmonary angiography also should be performed on patients who may undergo thrombolytic therapy, vena caval interruption, or pulmonary embolectomy.

Contraindications. Pulmonary arteriography has been used sparingly because of the perceived risk of complications. Clinically significant complications of pulmonary angiography include tachyarrhythmia and bradyarrhythmia, endocardial and myocardial injury, cardiac perforation, cardiac arrest, and hypersensitivity to contrast media. These complications occur, however, in only approximately 3% to 4% of patients, and they have an associated mortality of 0.2%.[68] A recently described hazard of pulmonary angiography occurs in patients with amiodarone-induced pulmonary toxicity, which reportedly causes rapidly progressive and fatal adult respiratory distress syndrome.[69]

Pulmonary arteriography is contraindicated for patients who have had an anaphylactic reaction to contrast media or who have an end-stage disease whose treatment will not be affected by the results of the pulmonary arteriogram. For patients who have a right ventricular end diastolic pressure exceeding 20 mm Hg, low osmolarity, angiography may be performed using non-ionic contrast agents and selective and subselective angiographic techniques.[70]

Diagnosis. The angiographic diagnosis of pulmonary embolism is based on the presence of a consistent intraluminal filling defect or a sharp cutoff of blood flow in vessels greater than 2.5 mm in diameter shown on several films (Fig. 25-5). In most situations multiple segmental or lobar perfusion defects in areas of normal ventilation correspond angiographically with pulmonary embolism. Any other abnormality, such as oligemic areas, vessel pruning, and loss of filling of smaller vessels, is nonspecific. Such abnormalities may be found in patients with pneumonia, atelectasis, bronchiectasis, primary and thrombotic pulmonary hypertension, emphysema, or pulmonary neoplasia.

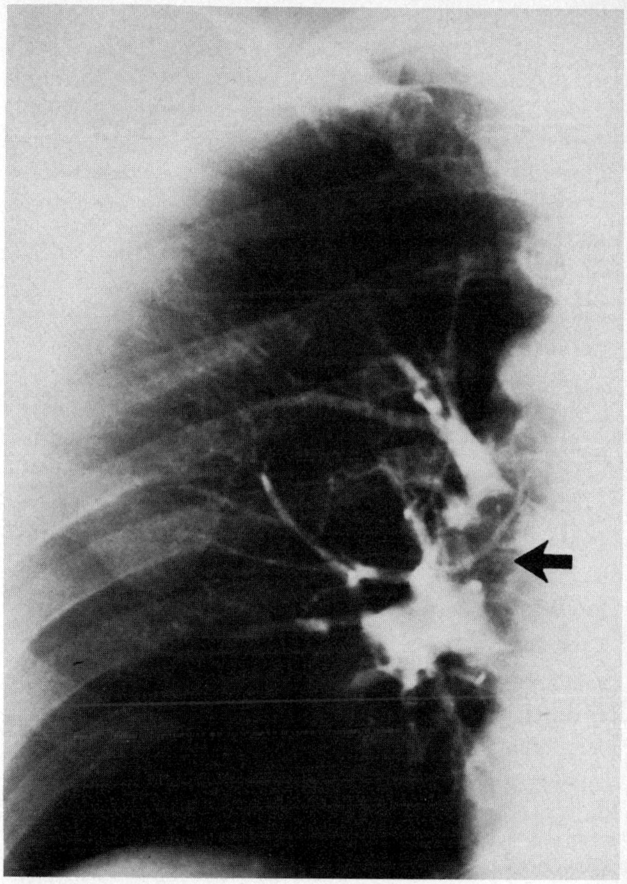

Fig. 25-5. A standard pulmonary angiogram with selective injection of the right pulmonary artery, demonstrating an intraluminal filling defect in the proximal portion of the pulmonary artery *(arrow)*. Smaller defects are seen in branches of the lobar pulmonary arteries. This represents a typical appearance of an intraluminal filling defect and occlusion of smaller branch pulmonary arteries.

Performance. Although other access routes to the pulmonary vasculature are available, including the median basilic, internal and external jugular, and axillary veins, most often clinicians performing pulmonary arteriography insert a catheter with multiple side holes into the right femoral vein. After injecting small amounts of contrast material to check the patency of the inferior vena cava, the clinician manipulates the catheter first into the main pulmonary artery of the lung and then selectively into the right or left main pulmonary artery for filming. Initial filming of both right and left main pulmonary arteries is in the anterior-posterior projection, with magnification if it is available; however, other views may be obtained without magnification.

Although angiography should be done within 24 hours of the onset of pulmonary embolism, it does not need to be done on an emergency basis unless the patient is hemodynamically unstable or cannot receive heparin. When pulmonary embolism is the primary consideration, pulmonary angiography should not be replaced solely by lower extremity noninvasive venous studies or venography because other veins and the right side of the heart may be responsible for pulmonary embolism.[18] Angiography also should not be replaced by serial lung scanning. Although serial lung scanning may demonstrate improved perfusion or the resolution of a defect, these findings still can be misleading, especially when the scan is low, intermediate, or of indeterminate probability.[60] It is also noteworthy that lung scan interpretability is not as reliable as the reading of pulmonary angiograms. Reading agreement in the PIOPED study was as follows:

Lung scan	
Probability	*Percentage agreement*
High	90
Normal	94
Low or indeterminant	70
Pulmonary angiogram	
Thrombus	
Present	95
Absent	92

Doppler echocardiography

Standard two-dimensional echocardiography and transesophageal echocardiography have produced images of proximal pulmonary emboli.[45] Right ventricular morphologic information, which is suggestive or supportive of the diagnosis of pulmonary embolism, also may be obtained through echocardiography.

Come has described the use of M-mode, two-dimensional, and pulsed Doppler echocardiographic studies in patients with pulmonary emboli.[45] She obtained two-dimensional scans in the standard long-axis and short-axis planes and graded right ventricular wall movement as normal, mildly, moderately, or severely hypokinetic on the basis of parasternal, apical, and subcostal views. Then she generated M-mode echocardiograms by placing a two-dimensional directed cursor on the left ventricle at the upper chordal level on patients in the supine position. She then took M-mode tracings from the parasternal long axis view or from the subcostal four chamber view and measured right ventricular dimensions from the leading edge of the right ventricular wall to the leading edge of the right septal surface at the onset of the QRS complex.

Pulse Doppler echocardiography, using a high pulse repetition frequency, determined the presence of tricuspid regurgitation and quantitated its flow velocity. Maximal flow velocity in the tricuspid regurgitant jet was compared with the right atrial pressure gradient and was calculated using the modified Bernoulli equation, which subtracts right atrial pressure from right ventricular pressure (Δ P) to arrive at the maximal flow velocity ($\Delta P = 4V^2$).

In patients with pulmonary embolism Doppler echocardiography shows a dilated hypokinetic right ventricle in the absence of right ventricular hypertrophy. In patients with acute right ventricular pressure overload that occurs with pulmonary embolism, echocardiography shows a nonhypertrophied ventricle and a mild increase in flow velocity in the tricuspid regurgitant jet, which can be caused by even a modest elevation in pulmonary arterial systolic pressure. Despite only a mild increase in estimated pulmonary arterial pressure, the right ventricle generally appears to be diffusely hypokinetic with systolic and diastolic septal flattening, which is compatible with combined right ventricular pressure and volume overload. These findings rapidly subside following thrombolysis and the reversal of pulmonary hemodynamic abnormalities, and improvement or normalization of the right ventricular wall movement follows a decrease in the tricuspid regurgitant jet and a resolution of systolic septal flattening (Tables 25-6[71] and 25-7).

Digital subtraction pulmonary angiography

Although digital subtraction pulmonary angiography detects proximal pulmonary emboli, it is frequently not able to identify peripheral emboli. For the most part, therefore,

Table 25-6. Echocardiographic findings differentiating acute PE from chronic pulmonary hypertension and Eisenmenger's syndrome

Cardiac structure	Acute pulmonary embolism (n = 4)	Chronic pulmonary hypertension (n = 5)	Eisenmenger's syndrome (n = 1)
RV size, supine (cm)	6.0, 4.2 3.2, 3.33	3.0, 3.8 4.8, 5.4 4.8	3.2
RV wall thickness (mm)	5, 5, 5, 3	7, 9, 14, 6 10	10
RV hypokinesis	Marked (2 patients) Moderate (2 patients)	Marked (3 patients) Moderate (1 patient)	Mild
RV-RA pressure gradient from tricuspid regurgitant jet (mm Hg)	28, 36, 28 in three assessed	69, 44, 44 58, 105	Not assessed
Evident shunt	None	None	Atrial septal defect, right-to-left
Systolic septal flattening	All 4 patients	All 5 patients	Yes

RV, Right ventricular.
RA, Right atrial.

it is an experimental technique for the detection of pulmonary emboli. Technologic modifications that reduce respiratory motion artifacts may improve the technique and the ability to detect peripheral emboli.

Computed tomography

Computed tomography identifies chronic pulmonary emboli in patients with pulmonary hypertension. However, it has not been used as a diagnostic modality for acute pulmonary emboli because it is unable to distinguish intravascular thrombi from other motion artifacts.

TREATMENT

Anticoagulation

Anticoagulation allows the body's natural thrombolytic mechanisms to dissolve emboli, and it prevents these autolytic mechanisms from being overwhelmed by recurrent venous thromboembolism. Although Dalen et al demonstrated that pulmonary emboli persist weeks after anticoagulants have been given, at least to some extent, the emboli usually lyse in sufficient numbers to restore right heart pressures to normal or near-normal levels in the first week after anticoagulation.[53]

Heparin therapy. The rationale for instituting heparin therapy is to prevent thrombus propagation and pulmonary emboli from recurring during the first few days after onset of pulmonary embolism. Alpert et al demonstrated that mortality could be kept low by administering heparin to avert recurrent pulmonary emboli. They reported 144 consecutive patients with angiographically documented pulmonary emboli who received heparin. A total of 124 (86%) of the patients survived. Only 12 patients died of pulmonary embolism, and the most important factor contributing to their death was shock caused by acute right ventricular failure, which had been precipitated by massive emboli.[72]

A number of studies indicate that heparin is useful in the treatment of venous thromboembolism. Its primary effect is to halt the extension of previously formed thrombi and thereby reduce the incidence of recurrent pulmonary emboli. In a study of 12 patients with venous thromboembolism, venography showed that after 5 days of treatment with therapeutic doses of heparin three patients had only a minor extension of the thrombus; five patients exhibited no change in the thrombus; and four patients had a decrease in the extent of the thrombus.[73] The UPET study disclosed similar pulmonary angiographic findings for patients treated with heparin.[17]

However, a recent study of 24 patients with acute deep venous thrombosis showed that thrombi extended even though the patients appeared to have been adequately anticoagulated. Nine of the patients (38%) in the study had duplex ultrasound scans showing progression of the thrombus, and six of these patients were consistently anticoagulated, which was defined as elevation of the baseline partial thromboplastin time (aPTT) by 150%. Fifteen patients (62%) had duplex scans showing stability or improvement in the thrombus, and nine of these patients were consistently anticoagulated.[74]

After ensuring that a patient has no history or physical signs of a bleeding disorder, the clinician may administer heparin in a dosage regimen that will elicit optimal anticoagulation as determined by the aPTT. Anticoagulation is considered to be optimal when the aPTT is two to three times greater than the patient's baseline level, although some studies suggest that anticoagulation therapy that achieves aPTT 1.5 times greater than the baseline level will prevent recurring pulmonary emboli.[16,75]

Generally, adequate anticoagulation may be obtained by administering heparin in an initial dose of 500 U/kg/24 hours and by adjusting the dosage according to the patient's response. Continuous intravenous administration of heparin is safer and more effective than either subcutaneous or intermittent intravenous administration of the anticoagulant.[74-79]

The risk of hemorrhage in patients who are receiving heparin does not correlate with the degree of elevation of aPTT.[72-74] This risk is influenced by a number of variables,

Table 25-7. Echocardiographic features suggestive of pulmonary arterial disease

Diagnosis	Echocardiographic features
Acute pulmonary hypertension (e.g., in acute pulmonary embolism)	Absence of significant left heart pathologic conditions (unless embolism occurred in the setting of left side of the heart pathologic lesion)
Chronic pulmonary hypertension	Dilated +/− hypokinetic right ventricle; right ventricular hypertrophy; tricuspid regurgitation with increased flow velocity, usually compatible with moderate to severe elevation of pulmonary arterial systolic pressure
Secondary pulmonary hypertension	Significant aortic or mitral valve disease of myocardial dysfunction; chronic pathologic condition in the left side of the heart
Chronic lung disease	Abnormal pulmonary function; absence of significant left heart pathologic condition (unless unrelated left ventricular heart disease)
Eisenmenger's syndrome	Right-to-left shunt (atrial septal defect, ventricular septal defect, patent ductus arteriosus) evident by imaging, contrast or Doppler echocardiography
Primary pulmonary hypertension	Absence of a detectable right-to-left shunt or evidence for mild atrial shunting only (such as might occur via a patent foramen ovale); no evidence for chronic lung disease; no evident pathologic condition in the left side of the heart (unless unrelated left ventricular heart disease)

including (1) the dose of heparin, (2) the method of heparin administration, (3) the patient's health status and comorbid conditions, and (4) the concurrent administration of antiplatelet agents.

Warfarin therapy. Regulation of warfarin therapy for patients who have complications from venous thromboembolism has been simplified by the use of prothrombin time (PT) to determine the optimum amount of anticoagulation in vitro. Based on clinical studies, it has been found that warfarin levels that raise the PT between 1.2 and 1.5 times the patient's baseline level adequately protect against the propagation of thrombus and embolization and minimize bleeding complications.

As stated previously, the optimal duration for oral warfarin therapy is unknown. Patients who are at continuous risk for thrombosis may require chronic anticoagulation. However, patients who are at risk for thrombosis because of a transient problem may require only 3 months of anticoagulation. Any patient who has recurrent venous thromboembolism or pulmonary emboli should undergo anticoagulation for at least 6 months, even if he or she has no specific risk factor.

Anticoagulation during pregnancy. The use of anticoagulation during pregnancy is a problem because both heparin and warfarin commonly cause maternal bleeding, and they may adversely affect the fetus.

Warfarin derivatives cross the placenta and, when given in the first trimester, may produce warfarin embryopathy, which consists of nasohypoplasia and stippled epiphyses.[80] Warfarin derivatives also may produce fetopathic effects when administered during the second and third trimesters, although the risks are not as great.

Although heparin does not cross the placenta, and therefore should not adversely affect the fetus, Hall, Pauli, and Wilson reported that heparin therapy was associated with adverse outcomes in approximately one third of the pregnancies studied.[81] Critical review of these data suggests that the high rate of adverse fetal outcomes in the heparin-treated patients may be the result of maternal comorbid conditions such as preeclampsia and renal failure.

Heparin is the anticoagulant of choice during pregnancy. Although warfarin may be instituted during the second and early portions of the third trimester, heparin usually is reinstituted just before delivery.

Thrombolytic therapy

Because thrombolytic agents actually dissolve existing thrombi, they can quickly move cardiopulmonary function toward normal. These agents relieve obstruction to the pulmonary arterial blood flow, thereby improving right ventricular function, reducing pulmonary arterial pressures, and improving pulmonary tissue perfusion (Fig. 25-6). Throm-

A

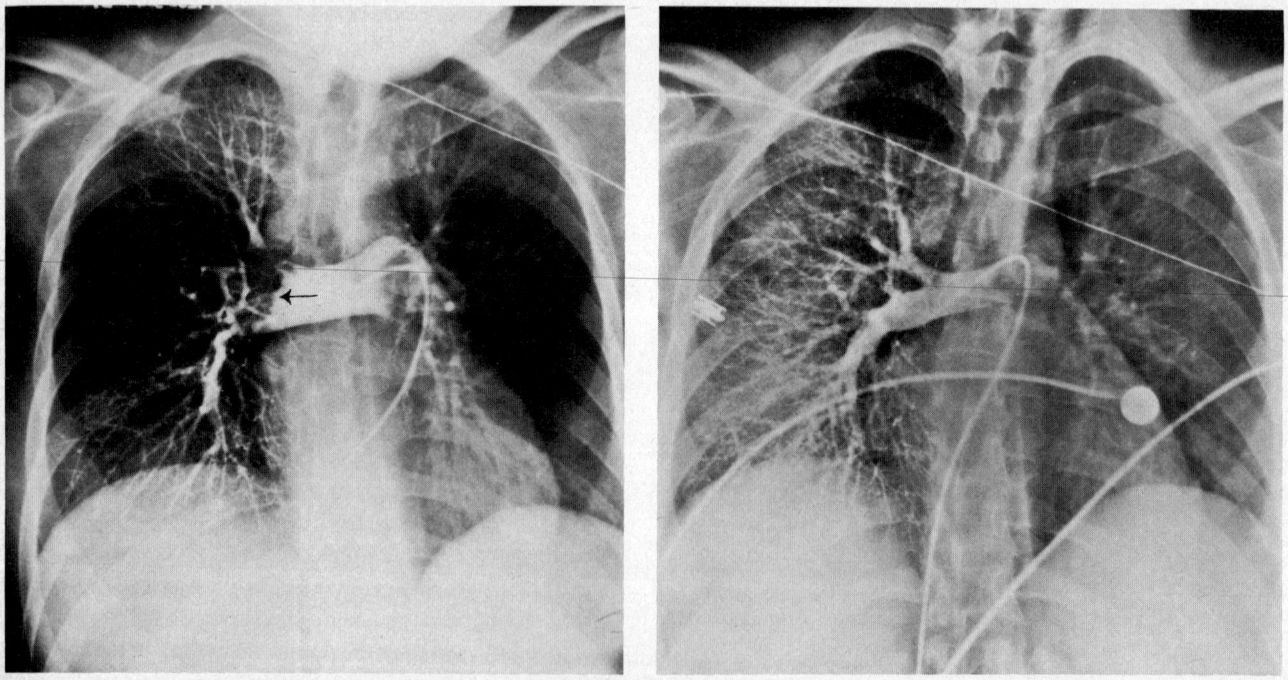

B

Fig. 25-6. A, A standard pulmonary arteriogram with the pulmonary artery injection from the main pulmonary artery indicating a large right main pulmonary artery embolus *(small arrow)*. There is a suggestion of a defect in the left main pulmonary artery in addition. This represents a large pulmonary embolus in the right main pulmonary artery before thrombolysis. **B,** A selective right main pulmonary artery injection with resolution of the previously demonstrated pulmonary embolism. This resolution occurred following 12 hours of urokinase infusion. Even flow with no intraluminal filling defects are now seen.

bolytic agents also may reduce the frequency of chronic thrombotic pulmonary hypertension, venous insufficiency, and recurrent pulmonary emboli.

The use of anticoagulation therapy alone to treat major pulmonary emboli results in complete thrombus resolution in less than 25% of patients after 1 to 4 weeks and in only 50% of patients after 4 months.[13,16,80] Four randomized and controlled clinical studies that included a total of 390 patients demonstrated that patients who were treated with thrombolytic agents exhibited more rapid anatomic and physiologic improvement than did patients who were treated with heparin.[82-85] However, none of the studies found a significant difference in mortality between the treatment and the control groups, perhaps because of the low mortality rate among both groups of patients and the small sample sizes.

The well-known Phase I portion of the UPET study compared heparin and urokinase treatment in 160 patients who had angiographically documented pulmonary emboli and who underwent hemodynamic, angiographic, and lung scan examinations.[17] Twenty-four hours after the initiation of therapy, the urokinase-treated patients exhibited significantly greater clinical, hemodynamic, and anatomic improvement than did the heparin-treated patients. However, after 5 to 7 days of therapy, urokinase-treated patients and heparin-treated patients had similar anatomic findings on lung scanning. In the 2 weeks following therapy urokinase-treated patients had fewer recurring pulmonary emboli (17%) than heparin-treated patients did (23%), but this difference was not statistically significant.

The USPET study examined three treatment groups (1) patients who received urokinase for 12 hours, (2) patients who received urokinase for 24 hours, and (3) patients who received streptokinase for 24 hours.[83] This study revealed that 12 hours of urokinase therapy produced the same degree of thrombolysis as 24 hours of urokinase therapy or 24 hours of streptokinase therapy. The study also showed that 12 hours of urokinase treatment produced greater thrombolysis than 24 hours of streptokinase therapy, although the difference was not statistically significant. Data from the UPET and USPET studies indicate that urokinase and perhaps streptokinase yield more consistent angiographic and lung scan improvement than heparin does.

In addition, Sharma, Folland, and McIntyre showed that patients who had been treated with urokinase or streptokinase had greater pulmonary capillary blood volume and pulmonary diffusion capacity at 1 week and 1 year after treatment than did patients who had received standard anticoagulation therapy.[86] Five-year follow-up of this study group demonstrated that the thrombolytic-treated group had better functional capacity and pulmonary hemodynamics than the anticoagulation-treated patients.[87] This study also suggested that thrombolytic-treated patients had better lower extremity venous hemodynamic function and had a decreased incidence and severity of venous insufficiency.

Although 27% of the urokinase-treated patients in the UPET Phase I study had severe bleeding (defined as a fall in hematocrit of greater than 10% or the requiring of a blood transfusion of two or more units), only 12% of urokinase-treated patients in the UPET Phase II study had severe bleeding. The reduction in the frequency of bleeding problems in the second trial indicates that either investigators had gained greater experience in managing patients receiving thrombolytic agents or that fewer transfusions were given to patients. More recently, different regimens of urokinase for PE (e.g., bolus administration) have been studied with excellent results.[88-90]

Data concerning the effectiveness of thrombolytic agents and the reduced incidence of bleeding problems associated with their administration convinced the National Institutes of Health Consensus Development Conference in 1980 that thrombolytic agents could be used more often for patients with pulmonary embolism.[11] The conference participants further suggested that thrombolytic agents should be used in those patients who have obstruction of blood flow to an entire lobe or to several lung segments as well as to those patients who are hemodynamically compromised, regardless of the size of the pulmonary embolus. Despite these recommendations, the use of thrombolytic therapy for pulmonary embolism has progressed slowly, whereas lytic therapy for acute myocardial infarction and other vascular diseases has increased.

Although the U.S. Food and Drug Administration approved the use of urokinase and streptokinase for pulmonary embolism in 1977, these agents have been used in fewer than 10% of patients with acute pulmonary embolism because of questions concerning contraindications to thrombolytic therapy. During a recent 1-year period, investigators in 44 clinical centers in the United States treated 2539 patients who had lung scan findings that were highly probable for pulmonary embolism or who had angiogram results that were positive for pulmonary embolism.[91] After reviewing the records of these patients for possible contraindications to thrombolytic therapy, the researchers found that overall 53% of the patients would have been acceptable candidates for thrombolytic therapy, a proportion higher than is generally accepted (Table 25-8).[91]

Tissue plasminogen activator. Recombinant tissue plasminogen activator (rt-PA) has achieved encouraging results in the treatment of patients with pulmonary emboli. An initial report by Goldhaber et al demonstrated that 28 of 30 patients had angiographic evidence of clot lysis after 2 hours of treatment with rt-PA.[92] The study also showed marked or moderate hemodynamic improvement in thrombolysis in 83% of patients. Quantitative angiographic scoring of pulmonary emboli before and after therapy showed a 48% overall improvement in clot lysis following a brief period of rt-PA infusion. Patients with a pretreatment angiographic score of 6.1 (which represented large pulmonary emboli involving two or more lobes) had an angiographic score of 4.7 after 2 hours of rt-PA infusion and a score of 3.2 after 6 hours of infusion, indicating a significant re-

Table 25-8. Exclusion criteria for thrombolysis in pulmonary embolism (n = 2,539)

Characteristic	Frequency no. (%)
Risks of blood loss	
Bleeding (internal or significant within 6 mo)	255 (10.1)
Internal surgery or organ biopsy within 20 days	410 (16.2)
Hematocrit <30%	283 (11.2)
Occult blood in stool	165 (6.5)
Liver function tests abnormal	178 (7.0)
CNS risk	
CVA or TIA	234 (9.2)
Intracranial or intraspinal surgery	148 (5.8)
Intracranial or intraspinal disease	226 (8.9)
Infective endocarditis	9 (0.4)
Arterial hypertension (severe)	7 (0.3)
Special risks	
Hemorrhagic retinopathy	6 (0.2)
Open heart surgery within 2 wk	63 (2.5)
Pregnancy	7 (0.3)
Survival	
Expected (<1 mo)	116 (4.6)

duction in clot mass. Average pulmonary arterial pressures decreased significantly after rt-PA therapy from a mean pressure of 21 mm Hg to 18 mm Hg ($P = 0.003$). The average mean pulmonary arterial pressure decreased from 24 mm Hg to 20 mm Hg ($P = 0.001$) in patients who had pulmonary hypertension defined as pulmonary arterial pressure greater than 17 mm Hg before treatment. Right ventricular dysfunction and tricuspid valve regurgitation resolved rapidly after therapy in a subset of patients.

In a more recent double-blind prospective investigation, nine patients received 40 mg to 80 mg rt-PA plus heparin, and four patients received a placebo plus heparin.[93] The patients who received rt-PA showed modest improvement in total pulmonary resistance. Arteriograms reflected no significant changes after 2 hours of therapy. Although lung scans showed greater improvement in the rt-PA group than in the placebo group after 24 hours, the rate of improvement was not statistically significant. Massive bleeding occurred in one patient. The observations from this study suggest that 2 hours of rt-PA treatment has little effect on the angiographic clot burden but does produce at least some hemodynamic improvement. No final conclusions can be drawn from this study, however, because patient enrollment was small, and the dose of rt-PA was smaller than the dose tested in other protocols. Further investigation of rt-PA as well as the use of higher doses of urokinase will be important in the future evaluation of thrombolytic treatment of pulmonary emboli.

Pulmonary embolectomy

Pulmonary embolectomy is performed in the following two clinical situations: (1) during the acute phase of embolization when the patient is in a life-threatened state, and (2) when treating the disabled dyspneic patient who has chronic pulmonary hypertension caused by occult or recurrent pulmonary emboli. Because of the high mortality rate (20% to 50%) associated with embolectomy of pulmonary emboli during the acute period, this procedure should be reserved for patients who are the most gravely ill and for whom thrombolytic therapy is contraindicated.

The incidence of chronic thromboembolic pulmonary hypertension is unknown. Early studies suggested that chronic thromboembolic pulmonary hypertension was rare among patients who had had acute pulmonary embolism; however, more recent investigations have concluded that the condition is more common than anticipated and that it affects a broad spectrum of patients.

Nevertheless, not all patients with chronic thromboembolic pulmonary hypertension require surgical correction. Criteria for selecting patients with chronic thromboembolic pulmonary hypertension for surgery are evolving. Moser, Auger, and Fedullo propose the following criteria for surgical repair of patients with this disease entity: (1) a resting pulmonary vascular resistance of at least 300 dynes/sec/cm-5, (2) accessible thrombi as defined by angiography and angioscopy, and (3) the patient's willingness to accept the morbidity and risk of mortality associated with the procedure.[50]

Thromboendarterectomy is performed while the patient is undergoing cardiopulmonary bypass with hypothermia and cardioplegia. It requires adequate visualization of lobar and segmental branches of the pulmonary arteries and meticulous dissection. It also requires presurgical placement of a filter to protect the patient from emboli arising from thrombi in the lower extremities.

Pulmonary thromboendarterectomy may be preferable to heart-lung or lung transplantation because its immediate postoperative mortality rate is low, its long-term outcomes are excellent, and it does not require continuous immunosuppressive therapy. Unfortunately, not all patients with this condition will improve with endarterectomy alone, especially those patients with extensive small pulmonary vessel involvement. In these patients, transplantation is a better alternative. If thromboendarterectomy can be performed before patients with chronic thromboembolic pulmonary hypertension fall into the functional class IV of the New York Heart Association, the mortality rate from the procedure should be significantly reduced.

Vena caval interruption

Inferior vena caval interruption is indicated for patients with venous thromboembolic disease when (1) anticoagulation is contraindicated; or (2) anticoagulation has failed. It also is occasionally performed for prophylaxis.

The Greenfield filter* is the most carefully studied intraluminal filter for the prevention of pulmonary embolism. Up to 70% of the Greenfield filter can be filled by thrombi without reducing the filter's effective cross-sectional area more than 50%.[94-96]

This device consists of six 0.15-inch stainless steel wires that are fashioned into a cone and that extend from a central hub. The filter is inserted percutaneously by the transfemoral or internal jugular route.

The main disadvantage of this filter is its large introducer sheath. As transfemoral placement of filters has grown in popularity and caused a 10% to 24% incidence of clinically symptomatic femoral vein thrombosis, the large stainless steel Greenfield filter has become less attractive. However, a smaller-size Greenfield titanium filter is being developed.[97]

The Gianturco-Roehm bird's nest filter has been tested in clinical trials since 1982.[98] These trials showed that the filter reduced the rate of recurrent pulmonary emboli to 2.7% and produced vena caval occlusion in only 2.9% of patients. Four occlusions of the filter have been attributed to the massive volume of embolic material that has been trapped within the wire mesh, which attests to the filter's efficacy and efficiency.

The filter wire mesh consists of a set of four 25-cm long, 0.18-inch stainless steel wires that have preshaped random bends. The mesh is affixed to proximal and distal V-struts that attach to the vena caval wall.

The bird's nest filter has several advantages over the Greenfield filter. Its introducer sheath is significantly smaller, which avoids the need to handle the filter during placement; its free-form mesh of filtration wire can be placed within the vena caval lumen without tilting or centering, and its structure can accommodate inferior vena cavae up to 40 mm in diameter.

*Manufactured by MediTech, Watertown, Massachusetts.

REFERENCES

1. McLachlin J and Paterson JC: Some basic observations on venous thrombosis and pulmonary embolism, Surg Gynecol Obstet 93:1, 1951.
2. Sevitt S and Gallagher NG: Venous thrombosis and pulmonary embolism: a clinicopathological study in injured and burned patients, Br J Surg 48:475, 1961.
3. Hunter WC et al: Thrombosis of deep veins of the leg: its clinical significance as exemplified by three hundred and fifty-one autopsies, Arch Intern Med 68:1, 1941.
4. Browse NL and Lea Thomas M: Source of nonlethal pulmonary emboli, Lancet 1:258, 1974.
5. Corrigan TP et al: Phlebography in the management of pulmonary embolism, Br J Surg 61:484, 1974.
6. Kakkar VV et al: Natural history of postoperative deep vein thrombosis, Lancet 2:230, 1969.
7. Morrell MP and Dunhill MS: The postmortem incidence of pulmonary embolism in a hospital population, Br J Surg 55:347, 1968.
8. Henderson EF: Fatal pulmonary embolism: a statistical review, Arch Surg 15:231, 1927.
9. Smith GT, Dammin GJ, and Dexter L: Postmortem arteriographic studies of the human lung in pulmonary embolization, JAMA 188:143, 1964.
10. Freiman DG, Suyemoto J, and Wessler S: Frequency of pulmonary thromboembolism in man, N Engl J Med 272:1278, 1965.
11. NIH Consensus Development Conference: Prevention of venous thrombosis and pulmonary embolism, JAMA 256:744, 1986.
12. Goldhaber SZ: Pulmonary embolism death rates, Am Heart J 115:1342, 1988.
13. Dalen JE and Alpert JS: Natural history of pulmonary embolism, Probl Cardiovasc Dis 171:259, 1975.
14. Coon WW, Willis PW, and Keller JB: Thromboembolism and other venous disease in the Tecumseh Community Health Study, Circulation 48:839, 1973.
15. Barritt DW and Jordan SC: Anticoagulant drugs in the treatment of pulmonary embolism: a controlled trial, Lancet 1:309, 1960.
16. McNeil B: Ventilation-perfusion studies and the diagnosis of pulmonary embolism: concise communication, J Nucl Med 21.319, 1980.
17. The Urokinase Pulmonary Embolism Trial: A National Cooperative Study, American Heart Association Monograph, No. 39, circulation 47 (suppl 2) 47:II-1-108, 1973.
18. Hull R et al: Pulmonary angiography, ventilation lung scanning, and venography for clinically suspected pulmonary embolism with abnormal perfusion lung scan, Ann Intern Med 98:891, 1983.
19. Szucs MM et al: Diagnostic sensitivity of laboratory findings in acute pulmonary embolism, Ann Intern Med 71:161, 1971.
20. Belt TH: Thrombosis and pulmonary embolism, Am J Path 10:129, 1934.
21. Collins DC: Pulmonary embolism, based on a study of 271 instances, Am J Surg 33:210, 1936.
22. McCartney JS: Postoperative pulmonary embolism, Surgery 17:191, 1945.
23. Roe BB and Goldthwait JC: Pulmonary embolism: a statistical study of postmortem material at the Massachusetts General Hospital, N Engl J Med 241:679, 1949.
24. Ochsner A et al: Thromboembolism: an analysis of cases at the Charity Hospital in New Orleans over a 12-year period, Ann Surg 134:405, 1951.
25. Fowler EF and Bollinger JA: Pulmonary embolism: a clinical study of ninety-seven fatal cases, Surgery 36:650, 1954.
26. Towbin A: Pulmonary embolism: incidence and significance, JAMA 156:209, 1954.
27. Coon W and Coller FA: Clinicopathologic correlation in thromboembolism, Surg Gynecol Obstet 109:259, 1959.
28. Uhland H and Goldberg LM: Pulmonary embolism: a commonly missed clinical entity, Dis Chest 45:533, 1964.
29. Modan B, Sharon E, and Jelin N: Factors contributing to the incorrect diagnosis of pulmonary embolic disease, Chest 62:388, 1972.
30. MacIntyre IMC and Ruckley CV: Pulmonary embolism: a clinical and autopsy study, Scott Med J 19:20, 1974.
31. Coon WW: Risk factors in pulmonary embolism, Surg Gynecol Obstet 143:385, 1976.
32. Goldhaber SZ and Hennekens CH: Time trends in hospital mortality and diagnosis of pulmonary embolism, Am Heart J 104:305, 1982.
33. Mossey RT et al: Pulmonary embolism: low incidence in chronic renal failure, Arch Intern Med 142:1646, 1982.
34. Rossman I: True incidence of pulmonary embolization and vital statistics, JAMA 230:1677, 1974.
35. Goldhaber SZ et al: The predictive value of the antemortem diagnosis of pulmonary embolism, Unpublished observations.
36. Smith GT, Dexter L, and Dammin GJ: Postmortem quantitative studies in pulmonary embolism. In Sasahara AA and Stein M, eds: Pulmonary embolic disease, New York, 1965, Grune & Stratton.
37. Goldhaber SZ et al: Factors associated with correct antemortem diagnosis of major pulmonary embolism, Am J Med 73:822, 1982.
38. Hampton AO and Castleman B: Correlation of post mortem chest

roentgenograms with autopsy findings with special reference to pulmonary embolism and infarction, AJR 43:305, 1940.
39. Sevitt S: The structure and growth of valve pocket thrombi in femoral veins, J Clin Pathol 27:517, 1974.
40. Macleod JG and Grant IWB: A clinical radiographic and pathological study of pulmonary embolism, Thorax 9:71, 1954.
41. Pryce DM and Heard BE: The distribution of experimental pulmonary emboli in the rabbit, J Path Bact 71:15, 1956.
42. Sevitt S: Pathology and pathogenesis of deep vein thrombi. In Moser KM and Stein M, eds: Pulmonary thromboembolism, Chicago, 1973, Year Book Medical Publishers.
43. Hume M, Sevitt S, and Thomas DP: Venous thrombosis and pulmonary embolism, New York, 1970, Cambridge Harvard University Press.
44. McIntyre KM and Sasahara AA: The hemodynamic response to pulmonary embolism in patients without prior cardiopulmonary disease, Am J Cardiol 28:288, 1971.
45. Come PC: Echocardiographic recognition of pulmonary arterial disease and determination of its cause, Am J Med 84:384, 1988.
46. McIntyre KM and Sasahara AA: Determinants of right ventricular function and hemodynamics after pulmonary embolism, Chest 65:534, 1974.
47. McIntyre KM and Sasahara AA: Hemodynamic and ventricular responses to pulmonary embolism, Prog Cardiovasc Dis 17:175, 1974.
48. Stein PD, Willis PW III, and DeMets DL: History and physical examination in acute pulmonary embolism in patients without preexisting cardiac or pulmonary disease, Am J Cardiol 47:218, 1981.
49. Goodall RJR and Greenfield LJ: Clinical correlations in the diagnosis of pulmonary embolism, Ann Surg 191:219, 1980.
50. Moser KM, Auger WR, and Fedullo PF: Chronic major-vessel thromboembolic pulmonary hypertension, Circulation 81:1735, 1990.
51. Benotti JR and Dalen JE: The national history of pulmonary embolism, Clin Chest Med 5:403, 1984.
52. Sutton GC, Hall RJC, and Kerr IH: Clinical course and late prognosis of treated subacute massive, acute minor, and chronic pulmonary thromboembolism, Br Heart J 39:1135, 1977.
53. Dalen JE et al: Resolution rate of acute pulmonary embolism, N Engl J Med 280:1194, 1969.
54. Kerr IH, Simon G, and Sutton GC: The value of the plain radiograph in acute massive pulmonary embolism, Br J Radiol 44:751, 1971.
55. Bynum LJ and Wilson JE III: Radiographic features of pleural effusions in pulmonary embolism, Am Rev Respir Dis 117:829, 1978.
56. Robin ED: Overdiagnosis and overtreatment of pulmonary embolism: the emperor may have no clothes, Ann Intern Med 87:775, 1977.
57. Taplin GV and Poe ND: A dual lung scanning technique for evaluation of pulmonary function, Radiology 85:365, 1965.
58. Denardo G et al: The ventilatory lung scan in the diagnosis of pulmonary embolism, N Engl J Med 282:1334, 1974.
59. The PIOPED Investigators: value of the ventilation/perfusion scan in acute pulmonary embolism, JAMA 263:2753, May 23, 1990.
60. Hull R et al: Diagnostic value of ventilation-perfusion in patients with suspected pulmonary embolism and abnormal perfusion lung scans, Chest 88:819, 1985.
61. Dalen JE and Alpert JS: Natural history of pulmonary embolism, Probl Cardiovasc Dis 17L:259, 1975.
62. Alderson PO et al: The role of 133Xe ventilation studies in the scintigraphic detection of pulmonary embolism, Radiology 120:633, 1976.
63. Cheely R et al: The role of non-invasive tests versus pulmonary angiography in the diagnosis of pulmonary embolism, Am J Med 70:17, 1981. Review, Arch Surg 15:231, 1927.
64. Williams O et al: Ventilation-perfusion lung scanning for pulmonary emboli, Br Med J 600, 1974.
65. Marsh JD, Glynn MA, and Torman HA: Pulmonary angiography: application in a new spectrum of patients, Am J Med, 75:763, 1983.
66. Dalen JE: Pulmonary angiography. In Grossman W, ed: Cardiac catheterization and angiography, ed 2, Philadelphia, 1974, Lea & Febiger.
67. Bookstein JJ and Silver TM: The angiographic differential diagnosis of acute pulmonary embolism, Radiology 110:25, 1974.
68. Mills SR et al: The incidence, etiologies, and avoidance of complications of pulmonary angiography in a large series, Radiology 136:295, 1980.
69. Wood DL et al: Amiodarone pulmonary toxicity: report of two cases associated with rapidly progressive fatal adult respiratory distress syndrome after pulmonary angiography, Mayo Clin Proc 70:601, 1985.
70. McCracken S and Bettmann M: Current status of ionic and non-ionic intravascular contrast media, Postgrad Radiol 3:345, 1983.
71. Come PC et al: Early reversal of right ventricular dysfunction in patients with acute pulmonary embolism after treatment with intravenous tissue plasminogen activator, J Am Coll Cardiol 10:971, 1987.
72. Alpert JS et al: Mortality in patients treated for pulmonary embolism, JAMA 236:1477, 1976.
73. Marder VJ et al: Quantitative venographic assessment of deep vein thrombosis in the evaluation of streptokinase and heparin therapy, J Lab Clin Med 89:1018, 1972.
74. Krupski C et al: Propagation of deep venous thrombosis identified by duplex ultrasonography, J Vasc Surgery 12(4):467, 1990.
75. Basu D et al: A prospective study of the value of monitoring heparin treatment with the activated partial thromboplastin time, N Engl J Med 287:355, 1972.
76. Deykin D: Regulation of heparin therapy, N Engl J Med 287:355, 1972.
77. Glazier RL and Crowell EB: Randomized prospective trial of continuous vs intermittent heparin therapy, JAMA 236:1365, 1976.
78. Salzman EW et al: Management of heparin therapy, N Engl J Med 292:1046, 1975.
79. Wilson JE, Bynum LJ, and Parkey RW: Heparin therapy in venous thromboembolism, Am J Med 70:808, 1980.
80. Shaul WL and Hall JG: Multiple congenital anomalies associated with oral anticoagulants, Am J Obstet Gynecol 127:191, 1977.
81. Hall JG, Pauli RM, and Wilson KM: Maternal and fetal sequelae of anticoagulation during pregnancy, Am J Med 68:122, 1980.
82. Korn D et al: Pulmonary arterial bands and webs: an unrecognized manifestation of organized pulmonary emboli, Am J Pathol 40:129, 1962.
83. Urokinase Streptokinase Embolism Trial: Phase II results—a cooperative study, JAMA 229:1606, 1974.
84. Tibbutt DA et al: Comparison by controlled clinical trial of streptokinase and heparin in treatment of life-threatening pulmonary embolism, Br Med J 1:343, 1974.
85. Ly B et al: A controlled clinical trial of streptokinase and heparin in the treatment of major pulmonary embolism, Acta Med Scand 203:465, 1978.
86. Sharma GVRK, Burleson VA, and Sasahara AA: Effective thrombolytic therapy on pulmonary capillary blood volume in patients with pulmonary embolism, N Engl J Med 303:842, 1980.
87. Sharma GVRK et al: Long-term benefit of thrombolytic therapy in pulmonary embolic disease, J Am Coll Cardiol 15:65A, 1990.
88. The UKEP Study Research Group: the UKEP study—multicentre clinical trial on two local regimens of urokinase in massive pulmonary embolism, Eur Heart J 8:2, 1987.
89. Petitpretz P et al: Effects of a single bolus of urokinase in patients with life-threatening pulmonary emboli: a descriptive trial, Circulation 70:861, 1984.
90. Cella G, Palla AL, and Sasahara AA: Controversies of different regimens of thrombolytic therapy in acute pulmonary embolism, Semin Thromb Hemost 13:163, 1987.
91. Thrombolysis in Pulmonary Embolism Investigators: selection of patients with acute pulmonary embolism for thrombolytic therapy—Thrombolysis in pulmonary embolism (TIPE) patient survey, Chest 95:279S, 1989.

92. Goldhaber SZ et al: Acute pulmonary embolism treated with tissue plasminogen activator, Lancet 2:886, 1986.
93. Goldhaber SZ et al: Randomized controlled trial of tissue plasminogen activator in proximal deep venous thrombosis, Am J Med 88:235, 1990.
94. Wingerd M et al: Comparison of caval filters in the management of venous thromboembolism, Arch Surg 113:1264, 1978.
95. Greenfield LJ et al: Greenfield vena caval filter experience: late results in 156 patients, Arch Surg 116:1451, 1981.
96. Greenfield LJ, Stewart JR, and Crute S: Improved technique for insertion of Greenfield vena caval filter, Surg Gynecol Obstet 156:217, 1983.
97. Greenfield LJ, Cho KJ, and Tauscher JR: Limitations of percutaneous insertion of Greenfield filters, J Cardiovasc Surg 1991 (in press).
98. Roehm JOF et al: The bird's inferior vena cava filter: progress report, Radiology 168:745, 1988.

Chapter 26

CHRONIC VENOUS INSUFFICIENCY AND VARICOSE VEINS

Thomas F. O'Donnell, Jr.

Although arterial occlusive disease has received more attention than chronic venous insufficiency (CVI), CVI affects as much as a quarter of the population and also a younger segment. CVI is a significant problem in the United States. This process can lead to significant morbidity as a result of venous ulceration, edema, or leg pain. Loss of work and frequent hospitalizations may occur. In the following sections, I will review the pathophysiology, clinical findings, classification, diagnosis, and treatment of CVI.

In a discussion of the prevalence of venous disease in the population, simple varicose veins must be distinguished from advanced CVI with venous ulcer. Browse, Burnand, and Lea[1] have reviewed this subject and summarized the results of the following four national surveys on the prevalence of varicose veins: the U.S. National Survey of 1935-1936,[2] The Survey of Sickness conducted in the United Kingdom in 1950,[3] The Sickness Survey of Denmark, 1952-1953,[4] and The Canadian Sickness Survey, 1950-1951.[5] These summaries revealed a prevalence that ranged from 1.53% of the population in the Canadian study to 2.25% in the U.S. and U.K. studies (Table 26-1). These national surveys, however, probably underestimate the true prevalence of varicose veins in the population because the data were gathered from questionnaires and the surveys were conducted by nonmedical personnel. Therefore local or regional studies may provide a truer definition of varicose vein prevalence. Widmer's[7] survey typifies the true prevalence in an industrialized society. He conducted a clinical study that included physical examinations and photographs of the extremities of over 4000 chemical workers. Varicose veins affected men more frequently than women (5.2%/3.2%). The incidence of varicose veins increased with age, so that patients under the age of 35 had a 10% incidence, while 50% of those over the age of 65 were affected. In any event if 2% of the population are affected by varicose veins, it represents a substantial health problem.

The prevalence of venous ulceration is more difficult to determine than the prevalence of varicose veins. The earliest studies on this subject by Dickson-Wright[8] and Linton[9] appear to be extrapolations. Linton estimated that 300,000 to 400,000 patients in the United States had venous ulcers. A Swedish study demonstrated a prevalence of less than 0.1%.[11] Specific studies of a defined population perhaps provide the best data on venous ulcer. Widmer's[7] study of chemical workers uncovered a 1.3% incidence of venous ulcer. Callam's et al[12] West Lothian leg ulceration survey, which was conducted in the form of mailed questionnaires to nurses, physicians, and hospital outpatient facilities, demonstrated an incidence of 0.15%—quite similar to that described by Hellgren[11] in his Swedish study. A compilation of these studies suggests that nearly 1% of the population have experienced or currently have an active leg ulceration.[1] Like varicose veins, the incidence of venous ulcer increases with age but, unlike varicose veins, appears to be more common in females.

NORMAL VENOUS ANATOMY

Superficial veins

To understand the anatomic classification of CVI, one must appreciate the anatomy of a normal venous system. The long, or greater, saphenous vein is the main superficial vein in the lower extremity and begins anterior to the medial malleolus, rising obliquely and posteriorly to this boney

Table 26-1. Prevalence of chronic venous insufficiency

Study	Location	Type	Years	Prevalence (%)
Varicose veins				
U.S. National Survey[2]	US	Interview	1935-1936	2.25
U.K. Survey of Sickness[3]	UK	Interview	1950	2.25
Denmark Sickness Survey[4]	Denmark	Hospital	1953	—
Canadian Sickness Survey[5]	Canada	Interview	1951	1.53
Bobeck (regional)[6]	Czechoslovakia	Medical examination	over 15	
Widmer[7]	Switzerland	Medical examination	1974	4.2
Venous ulcer				
Dickson-Wright[8]	UK	?	1931	0.5
Linton[9]	US	? Extrapolation	1948	300-400K*
Lockhart-Mummery[10]	UK	Derivation	1951	0.2-0.5
Hellgren[11]	Sweden	Survey	1967	0.1
Widmer[7]	Switzerland	Medical examination	1974	1.3
Callam[12]	UK	Survey district hospital	1985	0.15

*An estimation of the total number of people in the United States with venous ulcers.

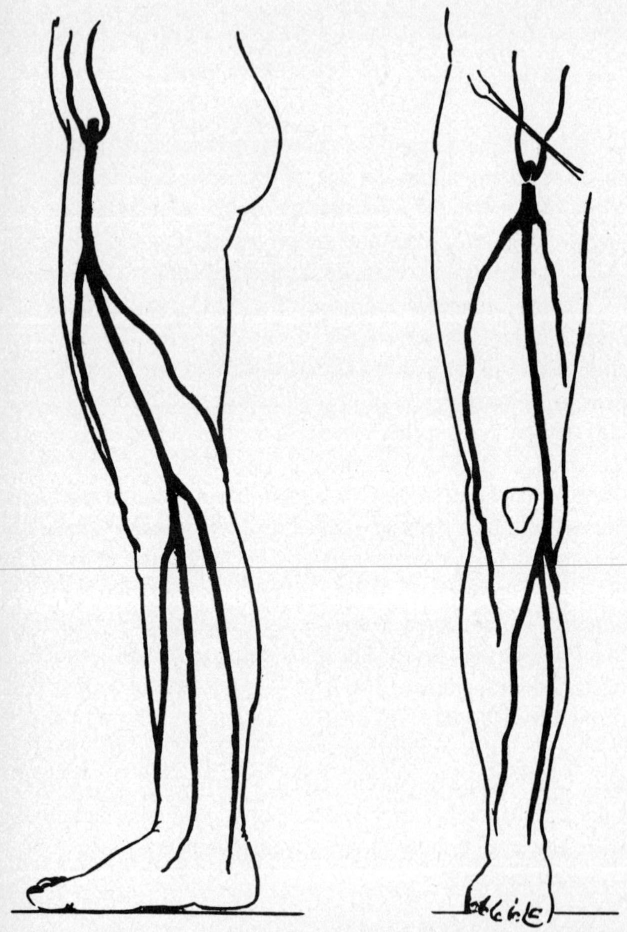

Fig. 26-1. Anatomy of the greater saphenous vein. The major trunk of the greater saphenous vein lies superficial to the deep fascia. At the thigh level the greater saphenous has an anterior and a posterior branch that run in a more superficial plane, while at the knee, the saphenous trifurcates with both anterior and posterior branches. Varicosities usually occur in the branches and lie more superficial in the loose areolar subcutaneous tissue.

prominence as it crosses the anteromedial surface of the tibia (Fig. 26-1). Below the knee joint the saphenous vein is joined by the posterior arch vein. This anterior branch of the saphenous vein also crosses the tibia anteriorly and joins the main trunk of the saphenous vein at a variable distance below or at the knee. The long saphenous vein usually lies on top of the deep fascia and joins the common femoral vein at the foramen ovale. The anterolateral and posteromedial veins of the thigh enter the saphenous vein at variable distances in the upper third of the thigh. In approximately 10% or more of instances there may be reduplication of the long saphenous vein between the knee and the foramen ovale. Studies using B-mode duplex scanning have suggested that this duplication may be more common than previously recognized.[13]

The short, or lesser, saphenous vein typically lies posterior to the lateral malleolus and courses upwards, lateral to the Achilles tendon (Fig. 26-2). As the lesser saphenous vein reaches the lower and middle third of the calf, it becomes midline and lies on the deep fascia. The vein then penetrates the deep fascia of the calf at the upper third so that it enters the popliteal space between the heads of the gastrocnemius muscles. Although in approximately two thirds of the cases the lesser saphenous vein enters the popliteal vein *above* the level of the knee joint, in one third of the cases the lesser saphenous vein may join with the greater saphenous vein or even with the deep muscular veins in the upper thigh.[14]

Perforating (communicating) veins

The perforating, or communicating, veins provide the bridges between the superficial and deep system. Blood flows through one-way valves from the superficial to the deep system (Fig. 26-3). Perforating veins are classified as either *direct,* when they permit the superficial venous sys-

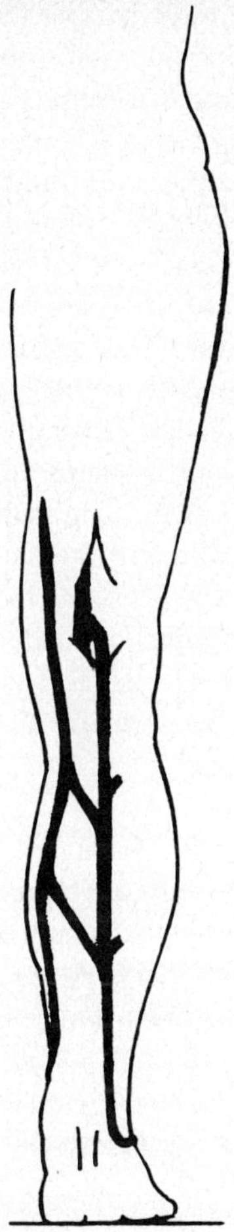

Fig. 26-2. Anatomy of the lesser saphenous vein. This posterior view of the lower extremity shows the lesser saphenous vein with its intercommunication to the greater saphenous (located medially). The lesser saphenous vein originates posterior to the lateral malleolus and courses proximally to enter the popliteal vein, above the popliteal crease.

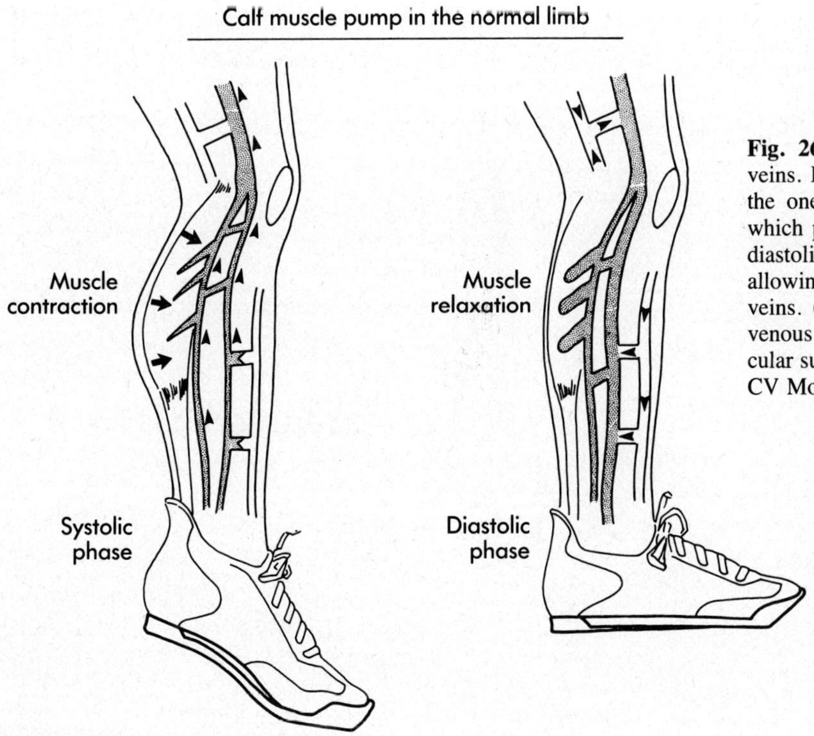

Fig. 26-3. Anatomy of the perforating (communicating) veins. During the systolic phase of calf muscle contraction the one-way valves of the perforating veins are closed, which prevents deep to superficial blood flow. During the diastolic phase the valves of the perforating veins are open, allowing superficial to deep blood flow to refill the deep veins. (From O'Donnell TF Jr and Shepard AD: Chronic venous insufficiency. In Jarrett F and Hirsch SA, eds: Vascular surgery of the lower extremities, St Louis, 1985, The CV Mosby Co.)

tems to communicate directly with the main veins, or *indirect,* when the perforating veins connect with the deep veins by way of a muscular vein. The direct perforating veins are generally constant in anatomic location. The greatest number are located posterior to the medial malleolus in an area overlying the posterior tibial vein—the lower perforating vein.[15] By contrast, the middle perforating vein is found approximately 7 to 10 cm above the medial malleolus and posterior to the tibia. This perforating vein communicates directly with the posterior tibial vein. Finally, the most superior of the three medial perforating veins is located in the upper third of the calf, posterior to the tibia. While this vein usually connects with the long saphenous vein by means of a tributary, it drains directly into the posterior tibial vein. The thigh perforating vein is usually located within Hunter's canal, from which it derives its name. This vein communicates with a superficial vein and enters either the long saphenous vein directly or indirectly through one of its branches.

Deep veins

In the calf the deep veins are paired and usually accompany the named arteries with venous tributaries intertwining over the surface of the artery. At the knee joint the veins usually join to form a single trunk, which is the popliteal vein. The deep veins transport blood from the muscles of the limb and provide an important carrier function for the calf muscle pump. The soleal sinusoids and the calf muscle veins are encased within a tight muscle-fascial envelope, similar to an elastic support stocking. This may prevent dilation of the deep veins in contrast to the superficial veins, which are contained within loose nonsupportive areolar tissue.[14] These veins communicate in a latticework manner with the posterior tibial and peroneal veins. Although most textbooks imply that the anatomy of the popliteal and superficial veins are single trunks, this anatomic situation is observed in less than 20% of limbs. The most frequent anatomic finding is one main trunk, which is interlinked with a plexus of venae comitantes. In about 10% of cases the profunda femoris vein communicates directly with the popliteal vein.

NORMAL VENOUS PHYSIOLOGY

To understand the altered physiology of CVI, normal venous physiology should first be reviewed. The calf muscles and deep veins of the calf act like the cardiac ventricles so that the phasic changes in the calf veins, which occur with walking, can be compared to systole and diastole of the cardiac cycle.[16] During the *systolic phase* of the ambulatory venous calf muscle pump cycle, contraction of the calf muscles compresses the blood contained within the venous sinuses and deep calf veins, thereby pumping the blood toward the heart. Valves in the communicating (perforating) veins, which link the deep with the superficial system, are closed to prevent retrograde flow of venous blood from the deep veins to the superficial system (Fig.

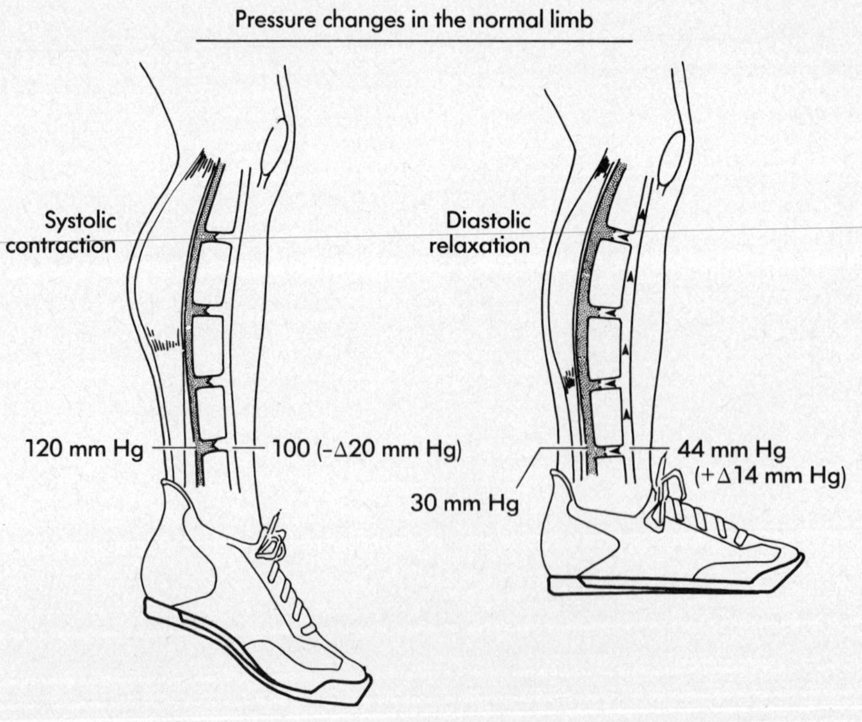

Fig. 26-4. Venous pressure changes in the normal limb. (From O'Donnell TF Jr and Shepard AD: Chronic venous insufficiency. In Jarrett F and Hirsch SA, eds: Vascular surgery of the lower extremities, St Louis, 1985, The CV Mosby Co.)

26-3). The pressure within the deep system at this point may reach 120 mm Hg during peak systolic contraction (Fig. 26-4). During the *diastolic phase* of the venous calf muscle pump, the relaxation of the calf muscle allows the soleal sinuses and deep calf veins to refill, thus recharging the pump and allows blood to flow from the superficial to the deep venous system through the perforating veins whose valves are now open. At this point, the higher pressure in the superficial venous system favors flow to the deep system.

CHRONIC VENOUS INSUFFICIENCY

Pathophysiology

In the limb with CVI the systolic phase of the calf muscle pump is altered, while the diastolic phase is similar to that of the normal limb. During the systolic phase, blood flows conversely from the deep to the superficial venous system through the damaged valves of the perforating veins (Fig. 26-5).[17] Thus the high pressure generated within the deep venous system during the systolic phase may be transmitted directly to the superficial venous system. Venous pressure measurements in CVI in our laboratory have shown peak systolic pressures of 150 to 160 mm Hg during calf muscle compression.[18] Venous pressure may increase even further in limbs with either proximal deep venous obstruction caused by thrombotic occlusion or valvular dysfunction of the deep venous system. Segmental occlusion in the deep venous system increases resistance to venous outflow and concomitantly elevates venous pressure. Destruction of the valves of the deep venous system permits an uninterrupted column of blood under the influence of gravity in the upright position to exert additional hydrostatic pressure on the deep venous system. These two mechanisms, valvular insufficiency and obstruction, may further increase superficial venous system pressure. Thus the increased venous pressure within the superficial venous system during the systolic phase of the calf muscle pump plays a major role in the development of CVI.[19]

Our understanding of the pathophysiology of CVI, particularly at the cellular level, has been expanded greatly by the work of several investigators, most notably the group at St. Thomas' Hospital, headed by Professors Norman Browse and Kevin Burnand.[20] Using data derived from a series of both human and animal studies, these investigators formulated a cellular mechanism for the pathophysiologic changes observed in CVI. They conducted a series of experiments in a canine model with surgically induced CVI, which paralleled clinical studies. In these studies the histologic changes found in the skin and subcutaneous tissue were correlated with hemodynamic alterations, such as ambulatory superficial venous pressures. Histologic studies

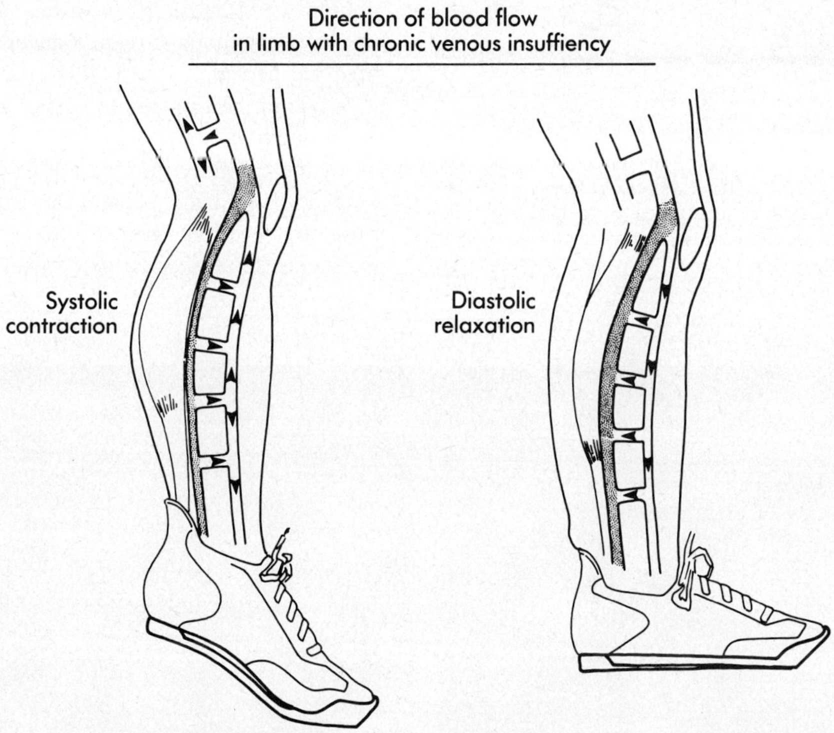

Fig. 26-5. Venous blood flow in chronic venous insufficiency. In contrast to flow direction in the normal limb (Fig. 26-3) with chronic venous insufficiency, blood flows paradoxically from the deep to the superficial system across the incompetent valves of the perforating veins during the systolic phase of the calf muscle pump. High pressure, as shown in Fig. 26-4, is, therefore, introduced from the deep system into the superficial system during this phase of the cycle. (From O'Donnell TF Jr and Shepard AD: Chronic venous insufficiency. In Jarrett F and Hirsch SA, eds: Vascular surgery of the lower extremities, St Louis, 1985, The CV Mosby Co.)

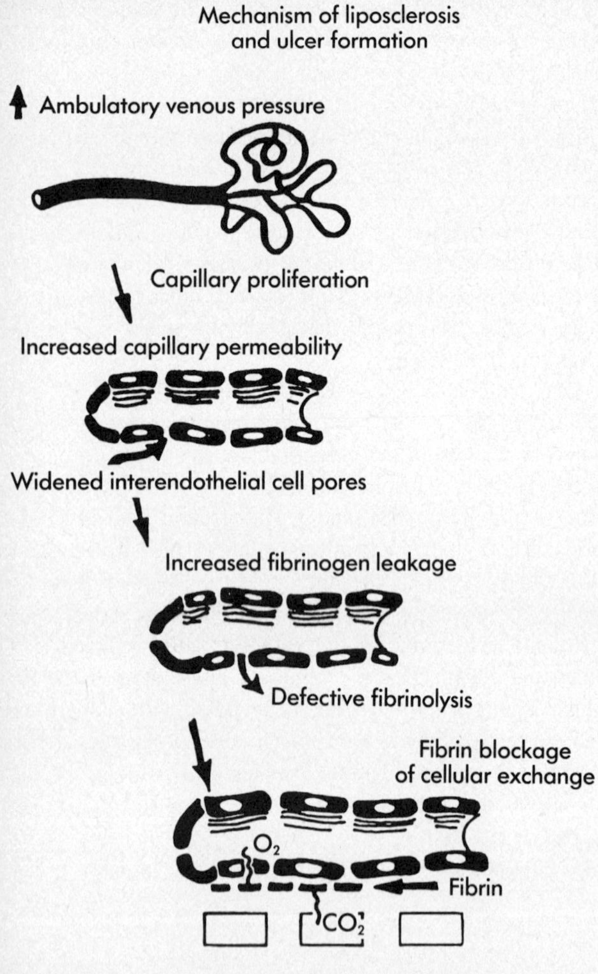

Fig. 26-6. Proposed sequence of events in the pathophysiology of advanced chronic venous insufficiency. (From O'Donnell TF Jr and Shepard AD: Chronic venous insufficiency. In Jarrett F and Hirsch SA, eds: Vascular surgery of the lower extremities, St Louis, 1985, The CV Mosby Co.)

showed that CVI is characterized by a proliferation of venous capillaries, which develop secondary to elevated superficial ambulatory venous pressure. The degree of capillary proliferation correlates directly with the level of superficial ambulatory venous pressure—the higher the pressure, the greater the degree of capillary proliferation (Fig. 26-6).

In addition to capillary redundancy, the capillaries had increased permeability, which, on electron microscopic examination, was ascribed to widened interendothelial cell pores. The altered capillary permeability permitted fibrinogen and other osmotically active particles to leak into the interstitial space. The normal vein wall usually possesses sufficient fibrinolytic activity to break down the extravascular fibrin, so that it is reabsorbed. By contrast, in the limb with CVI, the fibrinolytic capability of the vein wall is defective, and fibrin accumulates around the capillary wall.[21] Histologically, the vessel resembles the perivascular fibrin capping of the Kimmelstiel-Wilson syndrome seen in diabetics. The fibrin coating around the capillary wall prevents normal exchange of oxygen, carbon dioxide, and other nutrients across the capillary wall (Fig. 26-6). Normal cellular metabolism is altered, and cell death can ensue. This mechanism accounts for the subcutaneous fibrosis (liposclerosis) and skin breakdown observed in advanced cases of CVI.

Limb swelling, a characteristic early finding in the limb with CVI, develops through a disturbance in at least one of three mechanisms.[16] First, hydrostatic pressure on the venous side of the capillary is increased because of the mechanisms previously discussed, and this favors transfer of fluid out of the capillary into the interstitial space. Second, the lymphatics in many patients have been damaged and fibrosed by recurrent skin infections, thereby preventing the normal transport of water and protein by the lymphatics out

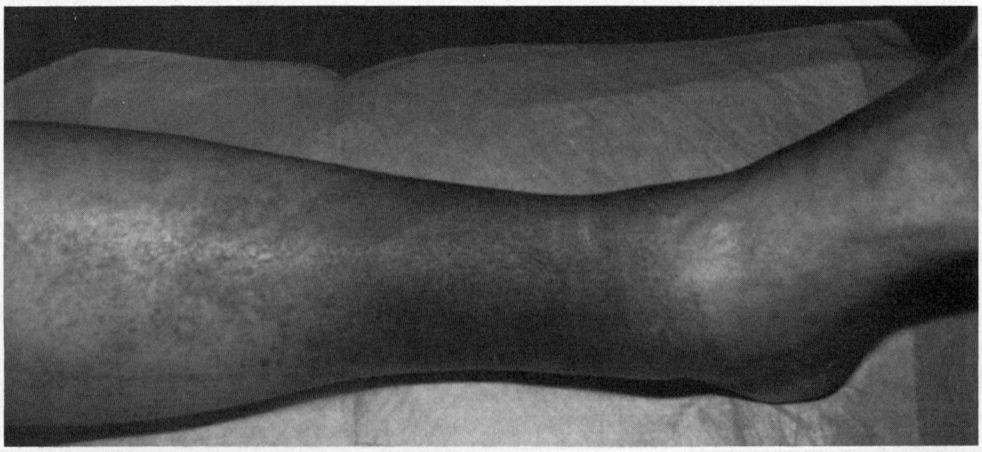

Fig. 26-7. Clinical findings in long-standing and advanced chronic venous insufficiency. Edema to the supramalleolar level and pronounced pigmentary changes are observed, which are indicative of stage II disease. (From O'Donnell TF Jr: Clinical diagnosis and classification of chronic venous insufficiency. In Rutherford RB, ed: Vascular surgery, ed 3, Philadelphia, 1989, WB Saunders Co.)

of the interstitial space. Third, edema formation in the limb with CVI is favored by the increased protein content within the interstitial space, which develops because of leaky capillary walls. These mechanisms are associated with the transfer of osmotically active particles from the intravascular to the interstitial space and produce a phenomenon called "water-trapping."

Clinical findings

The chief clinical manifestations of CVI are dilated veins, leg pain, edema, and cutaneous changes, and their frequency is related to both the site of anatomic involvement (superficial or deep system) and to the severity of disease.

Before the clinical classification is discussed, the individual symptoms and physical findings will be discussed separately. It is somewhat artificial to discuss each one of these clinical manifestations individually because they usually occur together.

Edema. Edema may be the first manifestation of early CVI. The patient usually notes that the swelling is mild and limited to the area just above the shoe line around the malleoli. The edema usually resolves with bed rest, particularly if the legs are elevated during sleep. In the early phases of CVI the distribution of the edema is limited to the perimalleolar area, but with long-standing CVI the edema may progress to involve the midcalf (Fig. 26-7). As opposed to limb swelling associated with lymphedema (Fig. 26-8) the metatarsal area usually is not involved in the early phases of CVI. Initially, the edema may be pitting, but with chronic edema formation subcutaneous fibrosis occurs so that the edema may fail to pit. This fibrosis is probably related to deposition of protein within the subcutaneous tissue and the subsequent inflammatory process. While it has been taught that only lymphedema fails to pit, the critical factor that determines pitting is the degree of subcutaneous fibrosis, irrespective of a venous or lymphatic cause.

Venous dilation. With involvement of the superficial venous system, the most common initial sign, in addition to mild edema, may be cosmetically displeasing dilated superficial veins. Initially, the venous dilation may be most apparent in the dependent portion of the limb, particularly on the medial aspect of the lower calf. The patient may observe dilation of small veins underneath the medial malleolus, the so-called "ankle flare" sign, pathognomonic of CVI. As with edema formation, the veins may become most prominent following prolonged standing or in women at the time of menses. With progression of CVI the veins become more tortuous and larger, and the patient will note their appearance in the proximal portion of the limb (Fig. 26-9). While some mild varicosities may develop in women during adolescence, they usually progress rapidly in size and number during pregnancy. With each successive pregnancy, the number and width of these varicosities usually increase.

Leg pain. Although not all patients with CVI experience pain, several distinct types of pain are commonly associated with CVI. The most frequent type is limb heaviness or ache, which occurs after prolonged standing. The pain is usually experienced in the calf area, and, as opposed to the calf pain associated with arterial insufficiency, this ache may be eased by walking. Lying down, particularly with elevation of the limb, relieves limb heaviness within a short period. The aching sensation may be worse in warm, humid weather or for women during their menses, because both conditions

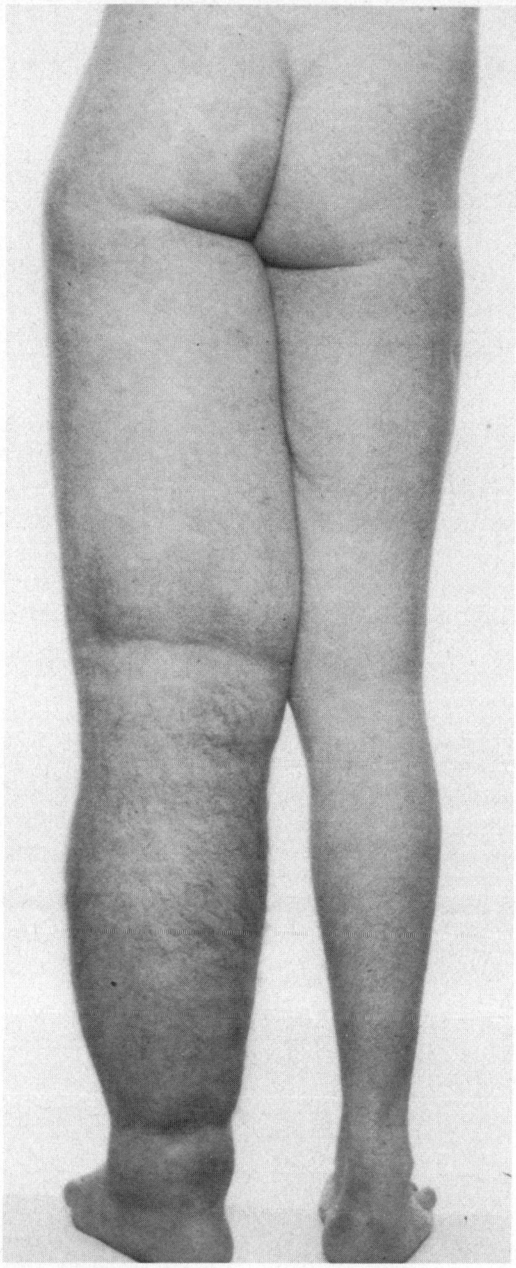

Fig. 26-8. Nonvenous causes of leg edema. The enlarged left limb of this patient with lymphedema has no significant pigmentary changes or prominent varices, which is in striking contrast to the patients with chronic venous insufficiency shown in Figs. 26-9 to 26-13.

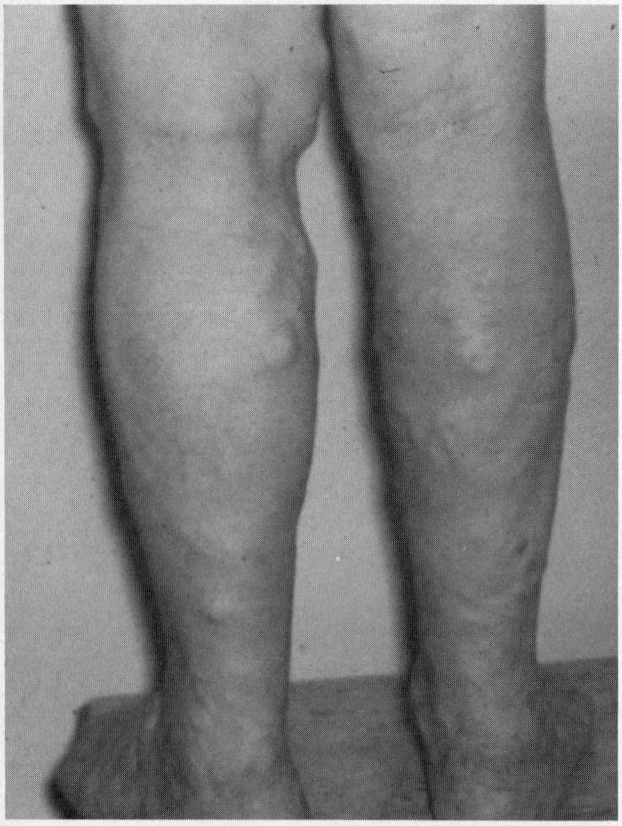

Fig. 26-9. Early stage II venous disease. Posterior view of patient with stage II chronic venous insufficiency—characteristically prominent bilateral varicosities involving both calves and the right thigh. Mild bilateral edema is present.

are associated with greater salt and water retention, which worsens the edema. Edema presumably produces the pain by increasing both intracompartmental and subcutaneous tissue volume and pressure. Mild calf pain or ache after prolonged standing is usually characteristic of CVI involving the superficial system. In addition, patients may experience pain along the course of dilated varicose veins after prolonged standing, which is probably a result of venous stasis within the varicosity and distention of the vein wall.

The pain associated with deep venous insufficiency is related to the cause of deep system disease. Patients with obstruction of the deep venous system may experience "venous claudication." While mild aching sensation is experienced at rest, ambulation produces an intense bursting cramping sensation in the calf. As with the patient with arterial insufficiency, the patient with venous claudication may have to stop and allow the venous congestion to resolve. Studies by Negus and Cocket[22] and recent investigations by Killewitch et al[23] have shown that venous claudication is caused by a rapid increase in both superficial and deep venous pressure. The increased resistance to venous blood flow out of the limb, which is usually related to iliofemoral occlusion, sharply elevates venous pressure. Patients with inadequate venous collateral flow around an iliofemoral occlusion usually experience venous claudication.

The second type of pain experienced by a patient with chronic deep venous insufficiency is related to valvular incompetence. On standing, the patient may note the sudden development of leg heaviness. My patients have described it as similar to the sensation of water being poured into the leg to fill it up. After standing for awhile, this sensation may be followed by a bursting type of heaviness in the calf, which can be quite incapacitating.

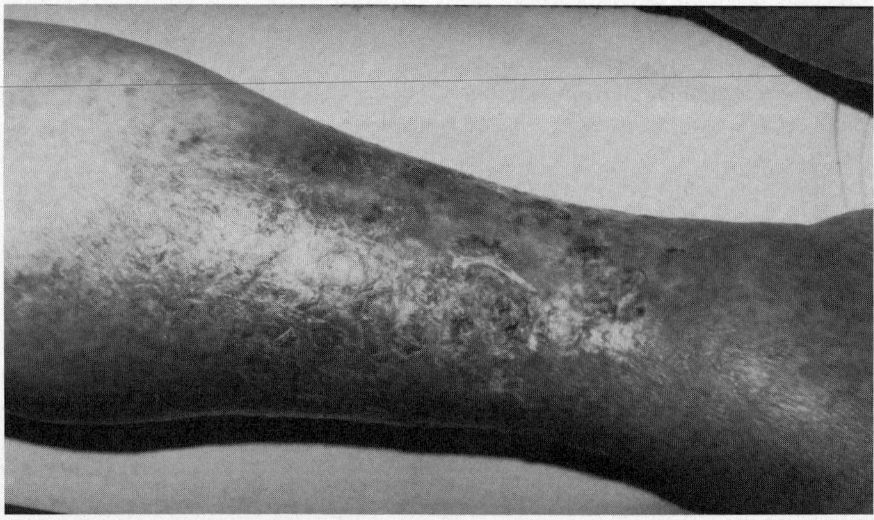

Fig. 26-10. Advanced stage II venous disease. Scaling eczematous dermatitis and skin changes characteristic of long-standing disease. (From O'Donnell TF Jr: Clinical diagnosis and classification of chronic venous insufficiency. In Rutherford RB, ed: Vascular surgery, ed 3, Philadelphia, 1989, WB Saunders Co.)

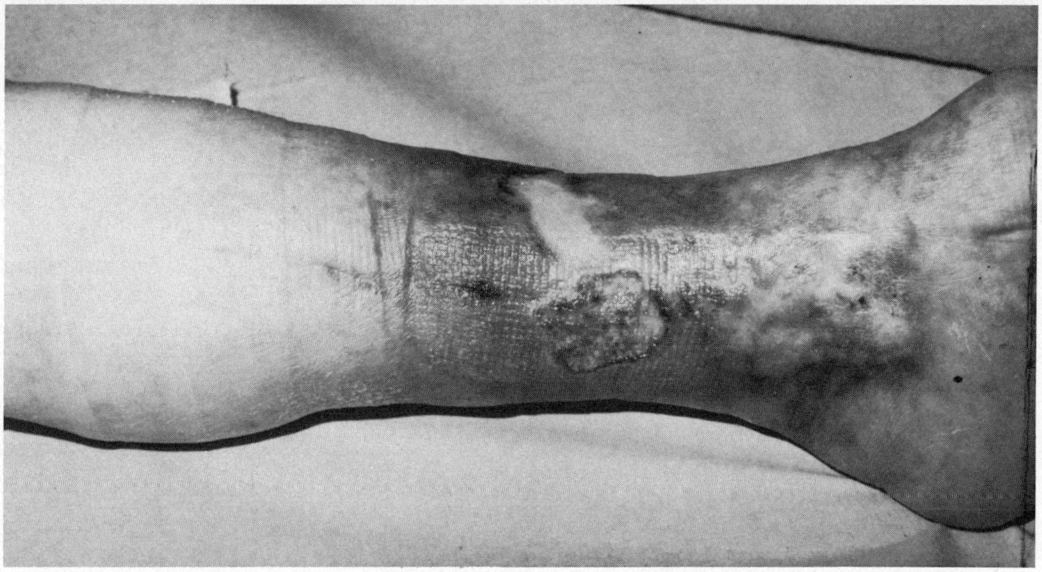

Fig. 26-11. Stage III venous disease. The medial view of limb with end stages of venous disease as characterized by a chronic venous ulcer *(above the medial malleolus)* and marked cutaneous pigmentary changes. (From O'Donnell TF Jr: Clinical diagnosis and classification of chronic venous insufficiency. In Rutherford RB, ed: Vascular surgery, ed 3, Philadelphia, 1989, WB Saunders Co.)

Classifications of chronic venous insufficiency

I. Anatomic

A. System(s) involved: superficial or deep
B. Segment(s) involved: proximal or distal

II. Clinical

A. Severity: stage I (mild) to stage III (severe)

III. Hemodynamic

A. Extent
B. Severity

Cutaneous infection, secondary to dermatitis or, alternatively, an open ulcer, can produce pain in the limb with CVI, but this pain is related to the primary process rather than to actual venous involvement (Fig. 26-10).

Cutaneous manifestations. Finally, the patient may observe skin pigmentary changes, usually characterized by brownish hemosiderin deposits in the skin (see Fig. 26-7). Frequently, the eczematous dermatitis associated with advanced CVI may prompt referral to a skin specialist for treatment (Fig. 26-11). In general, such skin changes are manifestations of long-standing venous insufficiency.

Classification

CVI is classified broadly into three areas (see the accompanying box). The first is *anatomic*—where the system(s) involved are described (superficial and deep levels) or segments involved are defined (proximal-iliofemoral or distal popliteal and calf veins). The second is *clinical*—where the severity of the disease is estimated. The third is *hemodynamic*—where the extent and severity of the disease is determined objectively by noninvasive vascular laboratory testing.

Anatomic. The anatomic classification of CVI is important because it relates directly to the causes of the clinical manifestations of CVI, and it influences the type of therapy. CVI can involve the superficial venous system alone (greater and lesser saphenous veins) or can combine with involvement of the deep venous system as is usual in more advanced cases. The perforating veins are included with the superficial venous system in the classification system used in this chapter (see the box on p. 453). Finally, deep venous system involvement alone, without involvement of the perforating (communicating veins) or segments of the superficial venous system, is unusual.

Fig. 26-12 illustrates schematically the major anatomic components of the superficial and deep venous systems of the lower extremity in the normal limb. CVI of the superficial venous system includes the most frequently encountered form of CVI, varicose veins. In a clinical, phlebographic, and Doppler study of nearly 600 consecutive patients who went to a venous clinic, Darke[24] demonstrated that 78% were related to varicose veins and therefore involved predominantly the superficial venous system. Traditionally, involvement of the superficial venous system alone has been termed *primary varicose veins,* which im-

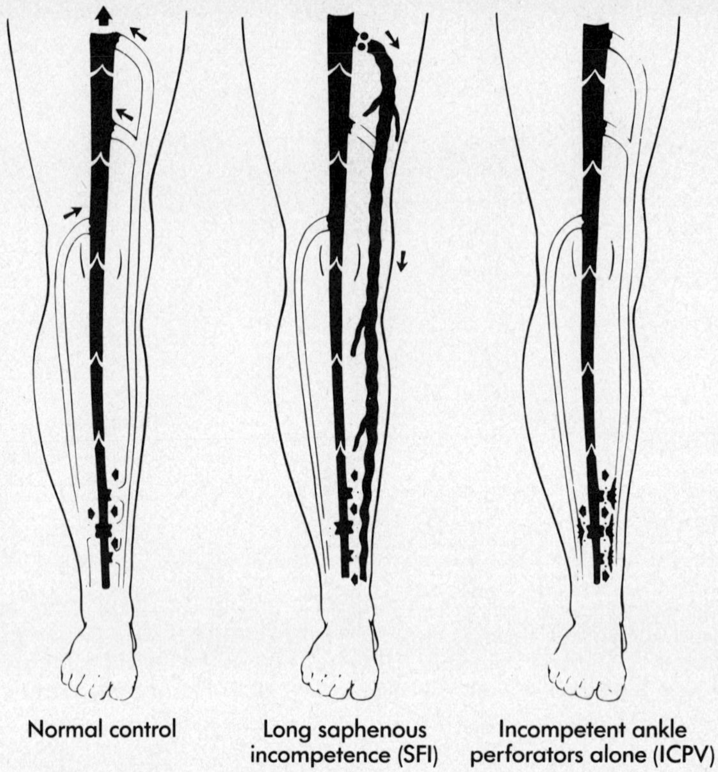

Fig. 26-12. Blood flow alterations in superficial venous insufficiency. Normal limb *(left)* is contrasted to limb with long saphenous incompetence *(middle)* where valvular damage in superficial system alters flow. Similar changes are observed in the limb with incompetent ankle perforators alone *(right)*. (From O'Donnell TF Jr: Clinical diagnosis and classification of chronic venous insufficiency. In Rutherford RB ed: Vascular surgery, ed 3, Philadelphia, 1989, WB Saunders Co.)

Table 26-2. Clinical classification of chronic venous insufficiency

Grade	Symptoms	Physical findings
I	Mild swelling Heaviness Vein dilation	Ankle edema <1 cm Dilated superficial veins Normal skin and subcutaneous tissue
II	Moderate to severe swelling Heaviness Varicosities Skin changes	Edema >1 cm Multiple dilated veins Incompetent perforating veins (mild) Pigmentation (mild) Liposclerosis (mild)
III	Severe swelling Calf pain with or without claudication	Edema >2 cm Multiple dilated veins Incompetent perforating veins (severe) Multiple vein varicosities Marked skin pigmentation Severe liposclerosis Ulcer

plies a congenital or inherited cause rather than an acquired one. The congenital cause of varicose veins is strengthened by the strong family history of varicose veins in over 75% of the patients who have them.[16,25]

The deep system may be involved in approximately one quarter of all patients with CVI[24] (Fig. 26-13). Although deep venous insufficiency is usually attributed to the sequelae of acute deep venous thrombosis, a history of documented deep venous thrombosis may be elicited in only 40% to 50% of patients.[26,27] Bauer[28] demonstrated nonthrombotic valvular incompetence in 30 of 55 limbs with typical postthrombotic clinical changes. Subsequently, Kistner[29] described primary valvular incompetence in approximately 50% of "postthrombotic" limbs examined by phlebography, because none of these 22 limbs had typical phlebographic evidence of previous deep venous thrombosis. Recently Darke[24] performed descending phlebographic studies in a series of patients with characteristic clinical changes of the postthrombotic limb, but the venograms showed anatomic alterations typical of the postthrombotic limb in only 15 out of 65 limbs (23%) with grade II reflux and in 7 out of 32 limbs (21%) with grade III or IV reflux. As in Kistner's

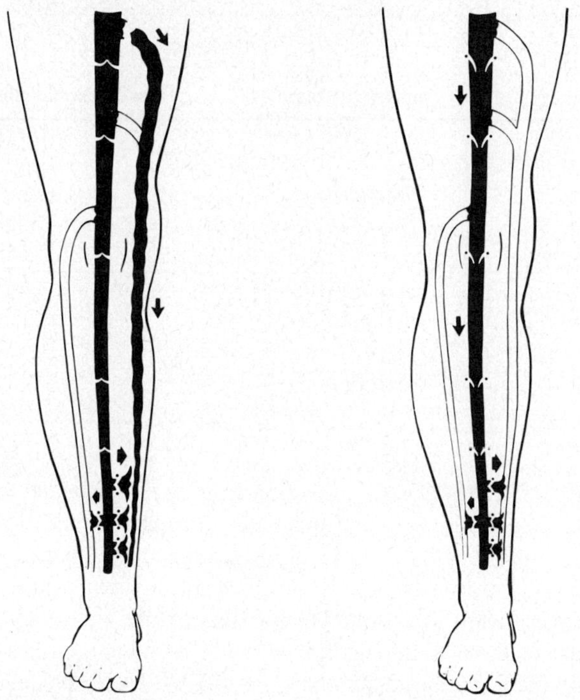

Fig. 26-13. Blood flow alterations in combined saphenous and perforating vein incompetence *(left)* are contrasted to patient with deep venous valvular incompetence and obstruction *(right)*. (From O'Donnell TF Jr: Clinical diagnosis and classification of chronic venous insufficiency. In Rutherford RB, ed: Vascular surgery, ed 3, Philadelphia, 1989, WB Saunders Co.)

Anatomic classification

I. System(s) involved
- A. Superficial
  1. Saphenous (greater or lesser)
  2. Perforating (communicating) veins
- B. Deep
- C. Combination of A and B

II. Segment(s) involved
- A. Deep veins
  1. Calf veins
  2. Femoral veins: iliofemoral
  3. Iliac veins: iliofemoral
  4. Cava
- B. Superficial veins
  1. Greater
  2. Lesser
  3. Perforating

III. Morphology
- A. Obstruction
- B. Valve incompetence

study, these data imply that a congenital cause or acquired weakness in the vein from causes other than an episode of deep venous thrombosis may be more common than the postthrombotic state as a cause of deep venous insufficiency.[30]

I have observed that patients with typical postthrombotic changes on phlebography in their calf or popliteal veins distally may have floppy and redundant valve leaflets in the femoral vein at a more proximal level. Thus the dual cause may confound simple ascription to either post deep venous thrombosis or primary valvular incompetence.

The anatomic distribution of CVI is further subdivided by the specific location within the superficial or deep venous systems (see the accompanying box). In the superficial system, varicose veins may involve the greater or lesser saphenous veins or perforating veins (Figs. 26-12 and 26-13). In chronic deep venous insufficiency the iliac, superficial femoral, profunda femoris, popliteal, and calf veins may be affected. Chronic deep venous insufficiency can be further classified anatomically as to whether obstruction, valvular incompetence, or a combination of both is present. The anatomic finding has important clinical implications for the subsequent pathophysiology, as discussed previously in this chapter. Traditionally, authors have divided the anatomic involvement of the deep system into central (iliofemoral) or peripheral (popliteal-tibial) disease (see the accompanying box). This distinction is somewhat artificial, and it is perhaps better to specify the actual site involved and whether the process is caused by obstruction or valvular incompetence.

Clinical. The Subcommittee for Standards in Vascular Surgery formulated a classification of CVI that could be based on the clinical evaluation of the patient.[31]

There are three clinical categories that are related to the severity of the disease. The various symptoms and physical findings previously described help classify the disease. Tables 26-2 and 26-3 show the three grades of CVI.

Grade I CVI is characterized by symptoms of mild swelling, limb heaviness after prolonged standing, and dilation of the superficial veins, particularly underneath the medial malleolus. On physical examination the ankle girth is usually increased by less than 1 cm when compared to the contralateral limb. Superficial venous dilation usually involves the greater saphenous system, particularly at the lower thigh and calf areas. Incompetent perforating veins are unusual. The skin has normal pigmentation and the subcutaneous tissue lacks fibrosis.

By contrast, grade II CVI indicates a more extensive anatomic process. The greater saphenous system is extensively involved with varicosities and the perforating (communicating) veins are usually incompetent. Varicosities are

Table 26-3. The three grades of chronic venous insufficiency

Clinical	Vascular laboratory study			Pathology report	
Grade	VRT (Sec)	VE (%)	MVO* =/−	Capillary increase	Extravascular fibrin
I	20-25	40-60*	NL-28	0	0
II	10-20	15-39	27-20	Moderate	Moderate
III	<10	<15	<20	Gross	Gross

*If obstructive component available.
VRT, Venous refill time.
VE, Venous emptying.
MVO, Maximum venous outflow.

quite numerous and easily observable. The patient complains of moderate to severe swelling and limb heaviness and observes mild skin pigmentary changes. On physical examination the edema is usually greater than 1 cm in girth. There are multiple dilated tributaries of the greater saphenous vein in the calf and thigh. Incompetent perforating veins are palpated. Cutaneous changes are limited to mild pigmentary deposition—brownish-red streaks, particularly in the gaiter or supramalleolar area. The subcutaneous tissue is slightly indurated secondary to liposclerosis.

Finally, with grade III CVI the swelling is severe and extends up from the ankle area to involve the calf. The patient complains of calf ache and heaviness, which occur earlier in the day or after short periods of standing. If iliofemoral involvement is present, venous claudication may occur. An active ulcer is observed or it may have recently healed. Physical findings include more significant edema of greater than 2 cm in girth at the ankle level, multiple dilated superficial veins, and evidence of incompetent perforating veins. There is marked dark brown-black skin pigmentation with brawny edema. Eczematous changes of the skin are observed. Severe induration of the subcutaneous fat is palpated, which reflects more advanced liposclerosis. An active or healed ulcer is usually present.

Diagnosis

The physician diagnosing CVI relies on a thorough history and physical examination, the use of bedside maneuvers and the assistance of the noninvasive vascular laboratory.

Physical examination. The physical examination of the limb with CVI may play a more important role in guiding therapy than it does for the limb with arterial insufficiency. The patient should be examined in the upright position, preferably standing on a stool or bench. The use of a nonfluorescent lamp is quite helpful to allow the varicosities, if present, to cast shadows. The four traditional stages of the physical examination—inspection, palpation, percussion, and auscultation—are followed in succession with particular emphasis on the first two. The patient's limb is inspected in a standing position from the front, side, and rear. Specially prepared anatomic diagrams of the lower extremity for CVI are helpful for making clinical notations. I usually examine the limb from the ankle up to the abdomen in a standard fashion. The presence of the ankle venous flare underneath the medial malleolus is sought and is usually found as one of the first signs of CVI. Next, the degree of edema formation and its extent are assessed at the foot, ankle, and lower calf levels. Limb girths should be measured at specified anatomic points to document objectively the extent of edema. The presence of skin pigmentary changes, particularly in the supramalleolar area, should be observed (see Fig. 26-7). An associated scaling dermatitis may be present (see Fig. 26-10).

The location of a venous ulcer is charted. The size and depth of the ulcer as well as the degree of granulation tissue should be described (see Fig. 26-11). Venous ulcers usually occur over the gaiter area (medial supramalleolar area), the site of the lower three major perforating veins, and also the area that is under the maximum influence of hydrostatic pressure. As opposed to arterial ulcers, venous ulcers are superficial and do not frequently penetrate through the fascia. The location of incisions from previous venous surgery should be sought for anterior to the medial malleolus, in the inguinal area, or over the perforating vein area. Finally, the distribution of dilated superficial veins should be charted.

Next the limb is palpated. The compliance of the subcutaneous tissue edema is assessed. Does the edema pit easily? And at what level? What is the extent of subcutaneous fibrosis? The limb with more advanced CVI will feel woody and resilient to palpation. The skin temperature is assessed, and an increased temperature may indicate underlying cellulitis. The saphenofemoral junction should be palpated for valvular incompetence. The fingers are placed over the foramen ovale (Fig. 26-1), and the patient is instructed to cough or to perform Valsalva's maneuver. In the limb with saphenofemoral incompetence a definite expansile impulse will be felt at the origin of the greater saphenous

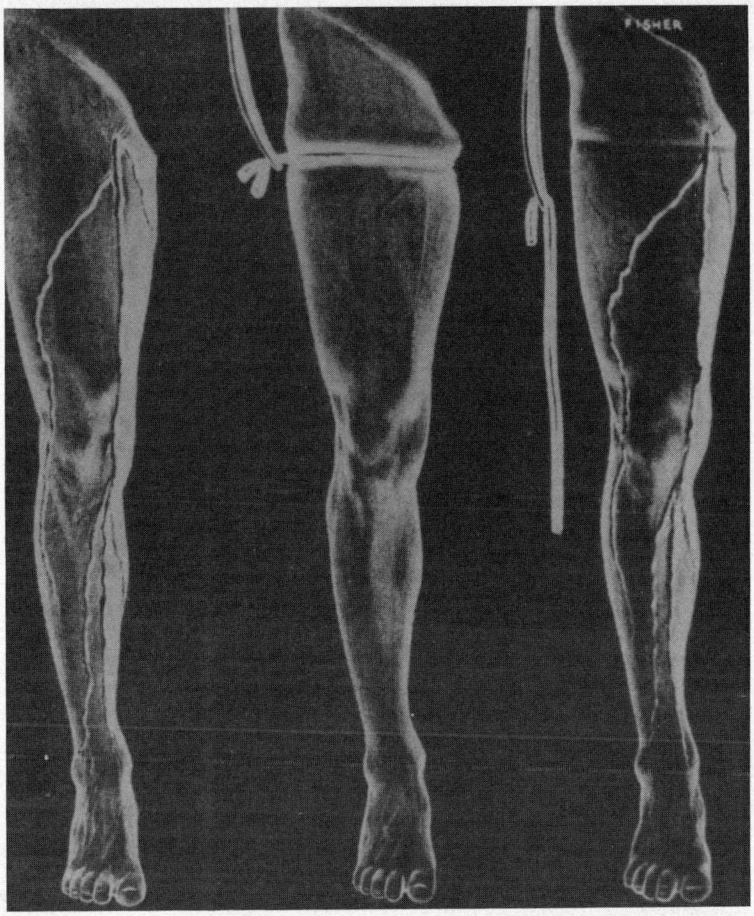

Fig. 26-14. Sequence of findings in tourniquet test showing incompetence of the greater saphenous vein. (From O'Donnell TF Jr: Clinical diagnosis and classification of chronic venous insufficiency. In Rutherford RB, ed: Vascular surgery, ed 3, Philadelphia, 1989, WB Saunders Co.)

vein, which is caused by reflux of blood in an antegrade direction. Since some veins will not be readily visible in patients with moderate obesity, palpation may be the best method to locate dilated superficial varicosities of the thigh and calf. In the calf region, palpation of circular defects in the subcutaneous tissue usually reveals the site of incompetent dilated perforating veins.[15] These sites should be marked on the skin before surgery or noted on the diagram what their distance is from the malleoli.

The physical examination is not complete without auscultation. While it is an unusual occurrence, arteriovenous fistulae can be associated with the development of prominent lower extremity varicosities. Auscultation over the varicosities will usually reveal a continuous murmur. A pulsatile arterial component will be heard if a Doppler probe is placed over the varicose veins. In addition, there will be increased skin temperature.

Tourniquet tests. While tourniquet tests, originally developed by Brody and subsequently by Trendelenburg, have confused generations of medical students, their purpose is twofold: to determine the level of valvular incompetence in the superficial system and to ascertain whether deep venous system involvement is present. I prefer to use a multilevel tourniquet test. The patient should be in a supine position with the limb elevated for at least a minute before the examination is begun. This latter maneuver empties the veins by reducing venous congestion in the superficial venous system. Tourniquets (½ inch Penrose drains) are then placed at several levels: (1) at the upper thigh just below the origin of the greater saphenous vein, (2) at the lower thigh below the adductor canal, (3) at the upper calf below the level of the lesser saphenous vein, and (4) at the upper ankle level above the malleoli (Fig. 26-14). The patient is then instructed to stand. If the superficial veins of the calf segment fill, then perforating vein incompetence is usually present. The tourniquets are usually removed from the bottom upward (Fig. 26-15). As previously stated, if removing the ankle tourniquet fills the superficial venous system, then perforating vein incompetence is suspected. If, after removal of the below-knee tourniquet, the lesser saphenous system fills, then lesser saphenous incompetence is most likely. Next the above-knee tourniquet is removed to assess

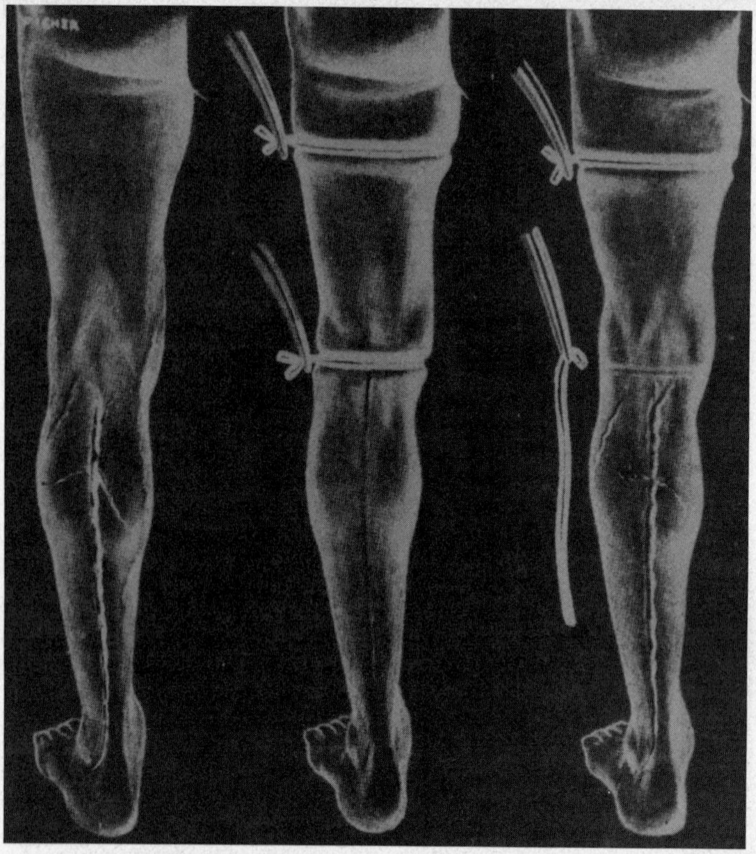

Fig. 26-15. Tourniquet test demonstrating lesser sapheneous incompetence. (From O'Donnell TF Jr: Clinical diagnosis and classification of chronic venous insufficiency. In Rutherford RB, ed: Vascular surgery, ed 3, Philadelphia, 1989, WB Saunders Co.)

the competence of the Hunter's canal perforator. Finally, if the superficial venous system remains empty, then the high thigh tourniquet is removed to detect whether saphenofemoral incompetence is present (Fig. 26-14).

Different sequences of tourniquet removal will help to define the level of valvular incompetence. The tourniquet test is used similarly with quantitative photoplethysmography by light reflection rheography (LRR) to document the level of incompetence.[32]

In addition to observation and direct palpation of incompetent perforating veins, a tourniquet test with exercise is helpful in establishing the condition of perforating veins. The patient should exercise in place by elevating the heels, and the extent of superficial venous congestion should be observed. Next a tourniquet is applied to the upper calf to compress the superficial venous system. This tourniquet prevents filling of the greater and lesser saphenous system from above. The patient then reexercises to activate the calf muscle pump. Various responses may be observed. If the superficial calf veins become less congested with exercise, the perforating veins are usually competent, because of the normal direction of venous flow from the superficial to deep venous systems. Alternatively, if the calf veins fail to decompress or if congestion increases, this is indicative of incompetent perforating veins. In addition to the tourniquet tests for perforator incompetence, digital control of the perforating veins can be carried out. The physician's fingers are placed over the sites of the perforating veins, and the limb is elevated to decompress the superficial venous system. The patient is then instructed to stand and the physician's fingers are removed from the perforating veins individually as if he or she were playing notes on a piano keyboard. Veins will bulge at the sites of incompetent perforators, when the fingertip is removed.

Noninvasive assessment. The purpose of the noninvasive assessment of CVI is to answer three questions:

1. What *systems* are involved—deep, communicating veins, or superficial venous system?
2. What is the *pathologic process*—valvular incompetence, obstruction, or a combination of both?
3. What *anatomic level* is involved by the pathologic changes?

Like the noninvasive assessment of arterial occlusive disease, the present methods for evaluation of CVI can be divided into those that provide hemodynamic or functional information and those that provide anatomy. A full discus-

A

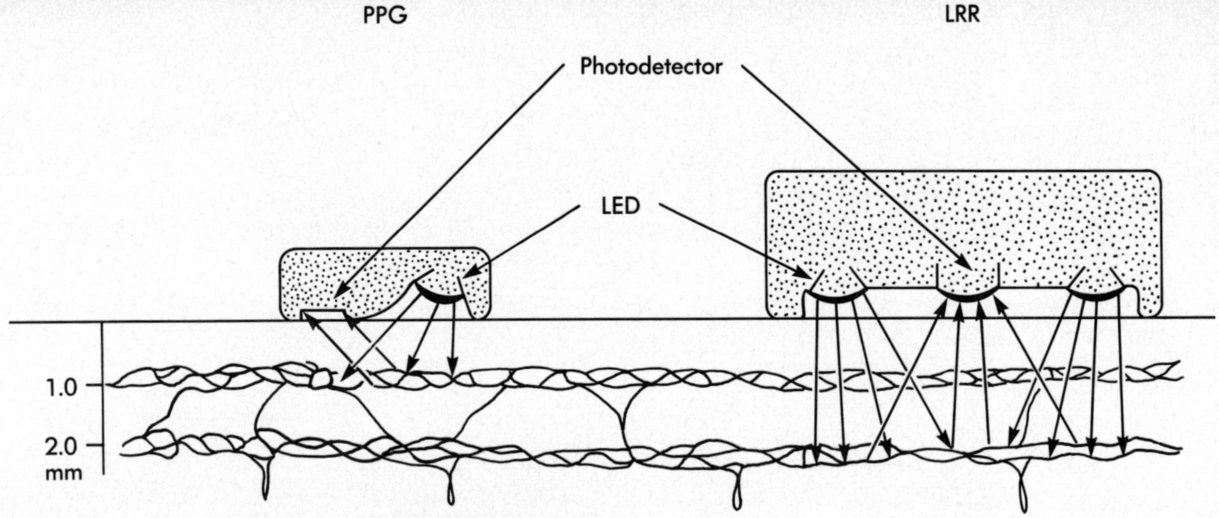

B

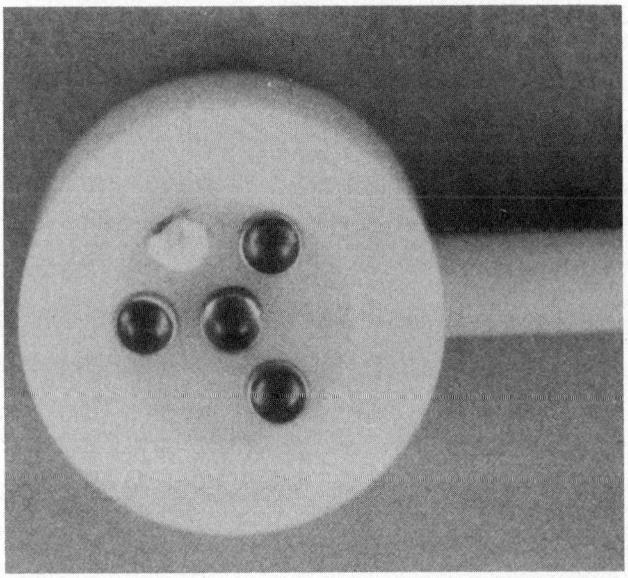

Fig. 26-16. Schematic of photoplethysmographic determination of venous refill time. **A,** Comparison of photoplethysmography *(PPG)* to light reflection rheography *(LRR)*. The latter has greater skin depth penetration and three light emitting sources. **B,** Actual LRR probe demonstrating central photodetector. (From O'Donnell TF Jr, McEnroe CS, and Heggenick P: Surg Clin North Am 70:159, 1990.)

sion of these techniques is beyond the scope of this chapter, and the reader is referred to lengthier reviews by McEnroe and O'Donnell.[33,34] The various noninvasive devices will be described in the sequence in which they are used in my diagnostic evaluation of the patient with CVI.

Plethysmography. I find quantitative photoplethysmography (light reflection rheography) an indispensable tool for the routine evaluation of the patient with CVI and use it in the same manner that I use Doppler pressure measurements in patients with arterial occlusive disease. This method allows quantitative and objective assessment of both the severity of CVI and the systems that are involved. In photoplethysmography light is emitted from a cell through the skin to the subdermal plexus and is reflected back to sensors by red blood cells. The amount of light reflected is related to the content of blood cells in the subdermal venous plexus (Fig. 26-16, *A*). The reflected light is recorded by the sensing head (Fig. 26-16, *B*) and translated into an electrical signal (Fig. 26-17), thus providing a continuous recording of dermal venous blood volume.[32] Quantitative photoplethysmography by light reflection rheography (LRR) has several advantages over pulsed photoplethysmography. LRR quantifies both venous emptying and venous refill time (VRT) without having to use cumbersome and time-consuming calibration maneuvers. It is not subject to alterations by heavily pigmented skin. Several studies have shown that LRR correlates directly with simultaneously performed direct invasive pressure measurements of the ambulatory venous pressure[23,35] (Fig. 26-18, *A* and *B*).

In the performance of the test the subject is seated comfortably with both feet flat on the floor, and the probe is applied with a double-faced adhesive tape 10 cm above the medial malleolus. The patient is instructed in a standard exercise program of 10 foot dorsiflexions over 15 seconds with the audible aid of a metronome. The examination is generally repeated three to five times with a 2- to 3-minute rest period in between studies to minimize the effect of exercise-induced hyperemia. Manual calf compression can be used for patients who are unable to dorsiflex their legs or who have obviously poor calf muscle pump function. Skin temperatures are obtained to exclude patients who may produce false positive results because of alterations in cutaneous blood flow with skin temperatures of 28° C to 32° C. The sensing probe should be placed away from localized regions of active inflammation such as dermatitis, cellulitis, or skin ulceration.

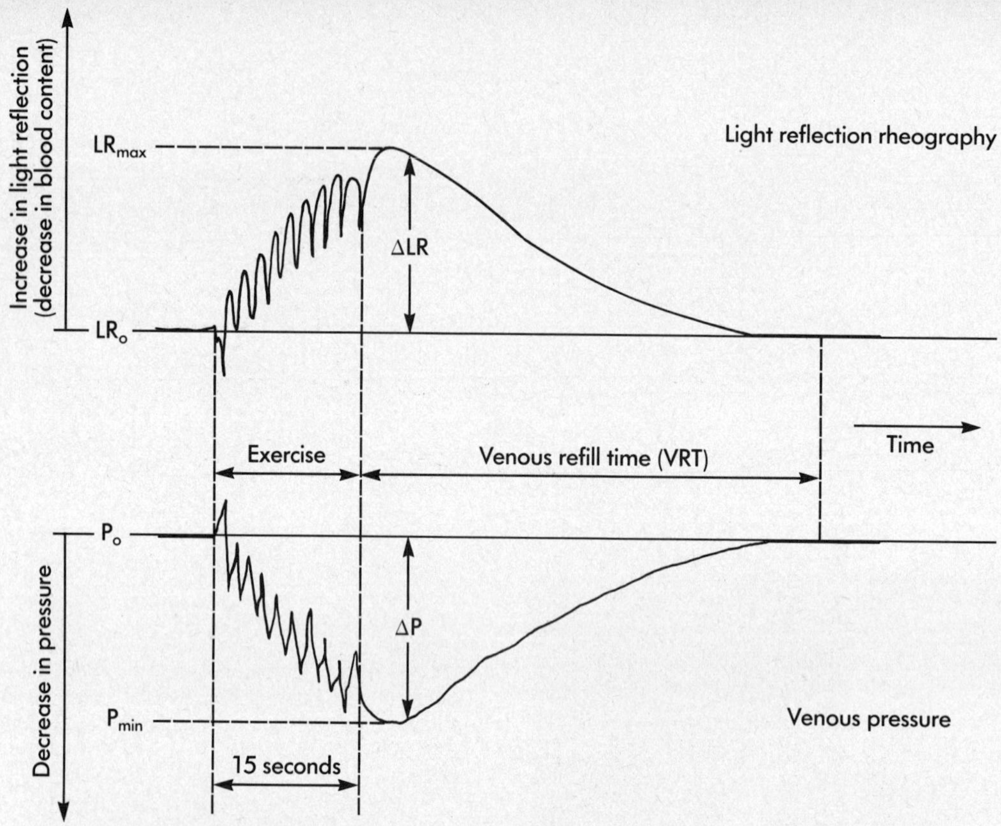

Fig. 26-17. Normal tracing from quantitative photoplethysmography by light reflection rheography. The venous refill time *(VRT)* is determined in the horizontal axis, while the change in light reflection, which correlates with venous emptying, is determined in the vertical axis. Following cessation of exercise, venous refill time is in excess of 30 seconds in the normal limb. (From O'Donnell TF Jr, McEnroe CS, and Heggenick P: Surg Clin North Am 70:159, 1990.)

In the normal limb the blood content of the skin, which is located predominantly in the subdermal venous plexus, decreases in response to calf muscle exercise and recovers to baseline after 25 seconds (Fig. 26-17). Many healthy young patients have VRTs of 35 to 45 seconds.[32] If the VRT is less than 25 seconds, then tourniquets are placed around the ankle, above and below the knee, so that the test can be repeated with sequential removal of these tourniquets. Complete normalization of VRT following tourniquet application is diagnostic of superficial venous insufficiency alone (primary varicosities) (Fig. 26-19). If there is no improvement in the VRT, then isolated deep venous insufficiency should be suspected (Fig. 26-20). The location of the tourniquets responsible for the improvement in VRT indicates the main source of superficial venous reflux. For example, if application of a thigh tourniquet corrects VRT, then saphenofemoral valve incompetence is suggested. If tourniquet application to the superficial venous system improves VRT by approximately 5 seconds, but VRT is not completely normalized, then *combined* deep and superficial venous insufficiency is most likely present. Recent studies by Mitrani[36] have shown that the venous outflow volume can be quantitated to determine venous outflow obstruction. The upslope of the LRR curve is used as a sensitive method for detecting DVT.

As an example of the usefulness of LRR, 850 limbs of patients with CVI were evaluated in our noninvasive laboratory.[37] A clear relationship was demonstrated between VRT as determined by LRR and clinical severity of CVI (Fig. 26-21). Of patients with stage III venous disease (active or healed ulcerations), 80% had VRTs of less than 15 seconds. Thus LRR appears useful not only for determining the anatomic level of venous valvular insufficiency but also for providing important information on the severity of CVI.

Bidirectional Doppler velocity probe. Venous survey with a bidirectional Doppler velocity probe appears most valuable for the detection of valvular incompetence or obstruction of the superficial and deep venous systems.[38,39] This instrument is less reliable for detecting incompetence or obstruction below the knee. While incompetent perforating veins can be identified in approximately 60% to 70% of patients with CVI,[40] many investigators, including myself,[15] consider such findings at times confusing, inconclusive, and difficult to interpret. Since only a relatively short

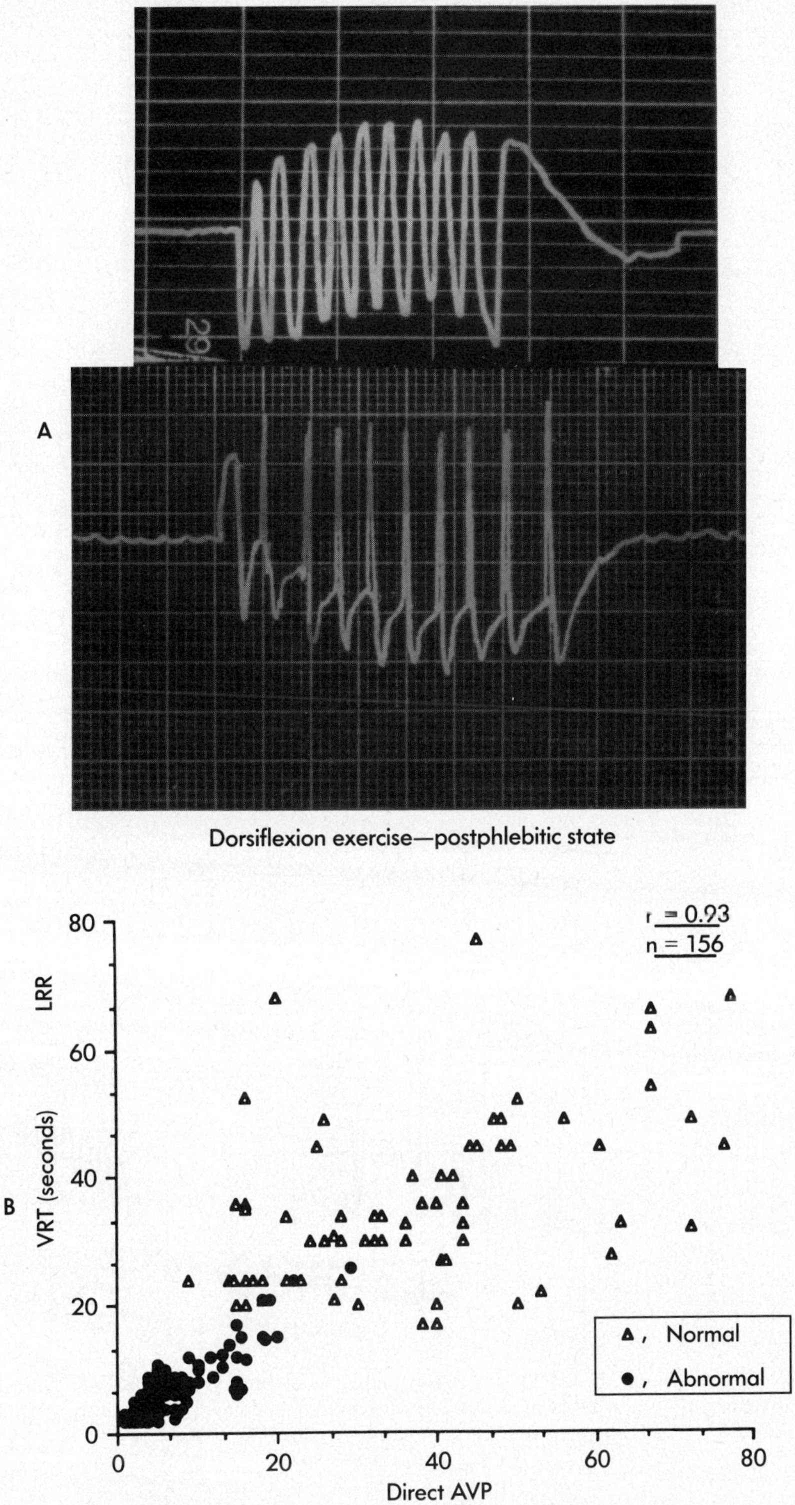

Fig. 26-18. A, Simultaneous quantitative photoplethysmograph. Light reflection rheography *(top)* and direct invasive venous pressure measurement *(bottom)* in patient with postthrombotic state. Both studies show poor venous emptying, as indicated by the flat pressure and photoplethysmographic curve. **B,** Correlation of venous refill time as determined by light reflection with venous pressure measurements. R value shows excellent correlation. (From O'Donnell TF Jr, McEnroe CS, and Heggenick P: Surg Clin North Am 70:159, 1990.)

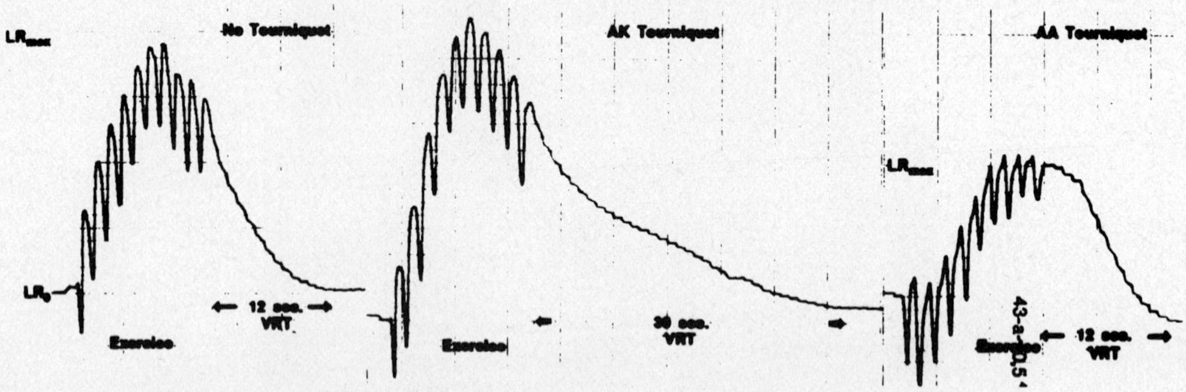

Fig. 26-19. Light reflection rheography tracing in patient with primary varicose veins. The shortened venous refill time and poor emptying on the left is improved by the placement of an above-knee *(AK)* tourniquet, which corrects the saphenofemoral incompetence. An above ankle *(AA)* tourniquet has no effect. (From O'Donnell TF Jr, McEnroe CS, and Heggenick P: Surg Clin North Am 70:159, 1990.)

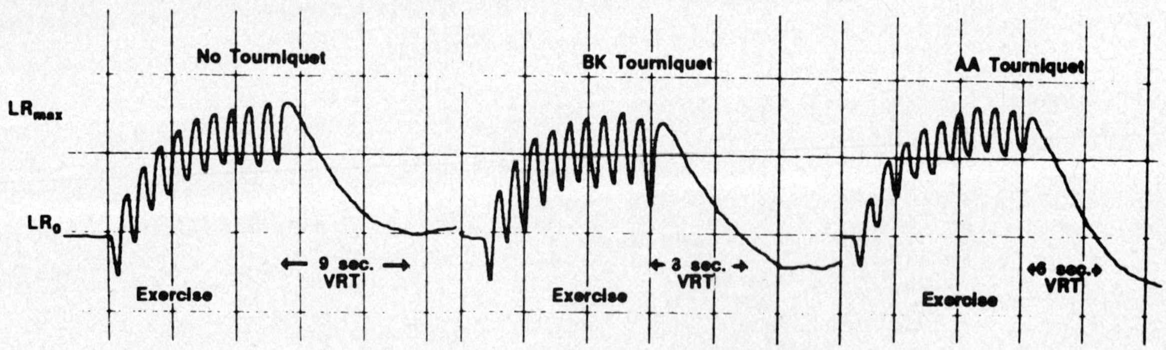

Fig. 26-20. Light reflection rheography tracing in patient with deep venous disease. This study shows rapid venous refilling without improvement with tourniquet compression. (From O'Donnell TF Jr, McEnroe CS, and Heggenick P: Surg Clin North Am 70:159, 1990.)

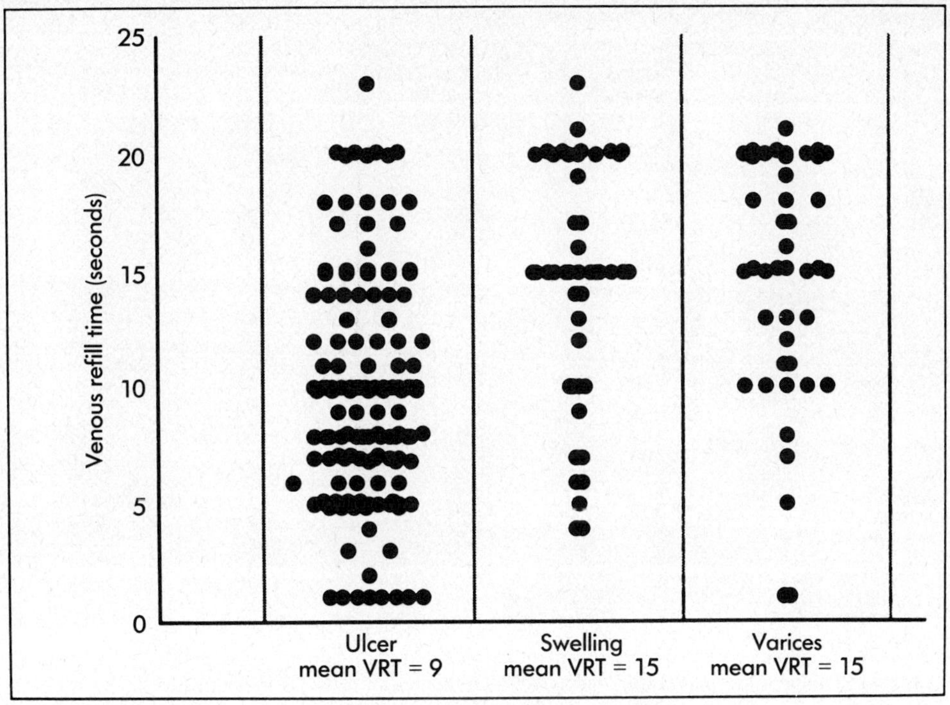

Fig. 26-21. Three characteristic symptoms of chronic venous insufficiency ulcer swelling and varices correlated with the hemodynamic state of the disease. Venous ulcer is associated with a markedly shortened venous refill time. (From O'Donnell TF Jr, McEnroe CS, and Heggenick P: Surg Clin North Am 70:159, 1990.)

segment of vein can be studied at a time, incompetence of an entire vein should not be based on retrograde flow through a single venous segment.[41]

The patient is placed in the supine position with the leg slightly dependent for this examination. A 10-MHz probe is used for examination of the superficial venous system, while a 5-MHz probe is used for evaluation of the deep venous system. Audible venous signals and flow direction is ascertained at rest, during abdominal compression, during Valsalva's maneuver, or following calf and thigh compression maneuvers. The probe is sequentially positioned over the posterior tibial, femoral, and greater saphenous veins. The patient is then placed in the prone position for examination of the popliteal vein. Proper assessment of this vein requires the placement of a below-knee tourniquet to occlude the short saphenous vein. Valvular incompetence in the examined vein segment is indicated by retrograde flow regardless of the maneuver used to elicit this change. For example, incompetence of the popliteal vein is demonstrated in Fig. 26-22. This finding is critical because of the known importance of this vein valve as a "gatekeeper" to the calf muscle pump.[26,42,43] An occluded venous segment either proximal to or distal to the examining probe is suggested by absence of spontaneous flow, loss of the normal respiratory variation, or diminished augmentation during distal compression maneuvers. Finally, incompetent perforating veins may be suggested by compression proximal to a below-knee tourniquet with reflux toward the probe from deep to superficial venous systems.

While the Doppler examination is simple in methodology and extremely portable, this technique requires significant examiner experience. This test is subjective and highly operator dependent. Furthermore, it may be insensitive to minor venous anatomic abnormalities that do not influence overall venous flow patterns.

Duplex imaging. While duplex imaging has been an important noninvasive technique for the evaluation of arterial occlusive disease, particularly carotid stenosis, this technique recently has been applied to diagnose acute deep venous thrombosis with equally superior results.[44] Duplex scanning provides not only functional hemodynamic information but also anatomic morphology on the status of both the superficial and deep venous systems.[45] Like the Doppler examination, duplex scanning is highly operator and interpreter dependent. Thus considerable experience with this technique is required. Duplex imaging permits examination of the greater and lesser saphenous veins as well as the perforating veins of the superficial system.[46] The femoral, popliteal, and calf veins of the deep system are well imaged. In our vascular laboratory the inguinal region is assessed first. The saphenous and saphenofemoral junction are examined, then the common femoral, superficial femoral, and profunda femoris veins. The examiner next proceeds to the lower thigh where the superficial femoral vein is imaged at

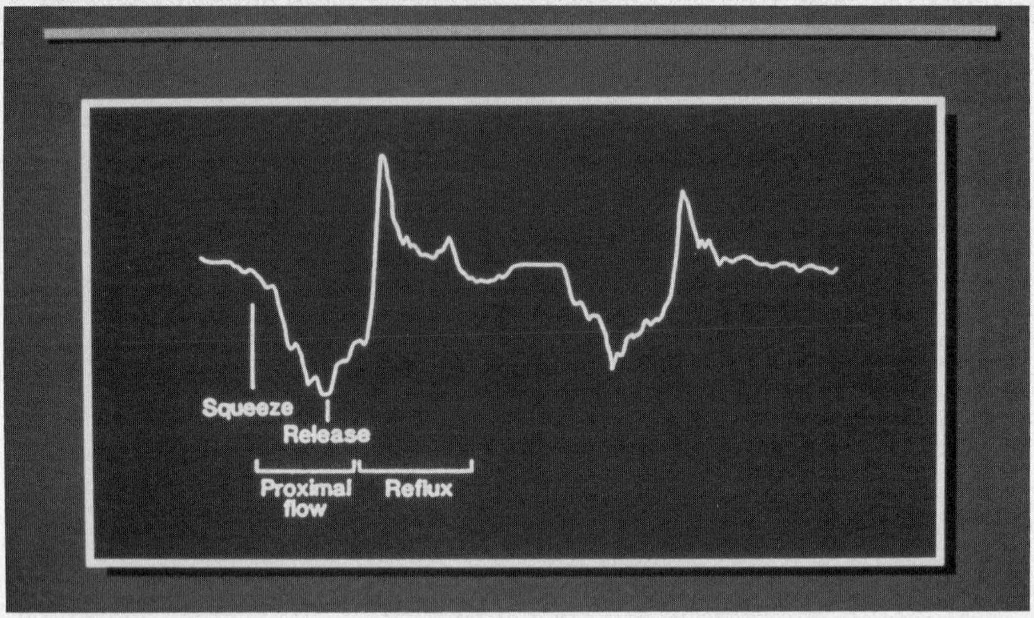

Fig. 26-22. Doppler ultrasound assessment of popliteal vein hemodynamics. Reversal of flow on proximal compression or Valsalva maneuver—an abnormal test—is indicative of an incompetent popliteal vein valve. (From O'Donnell TF Jr, McEnroe CS, and Heggenick P: Surg Clin North Am 70:159, 1990.)

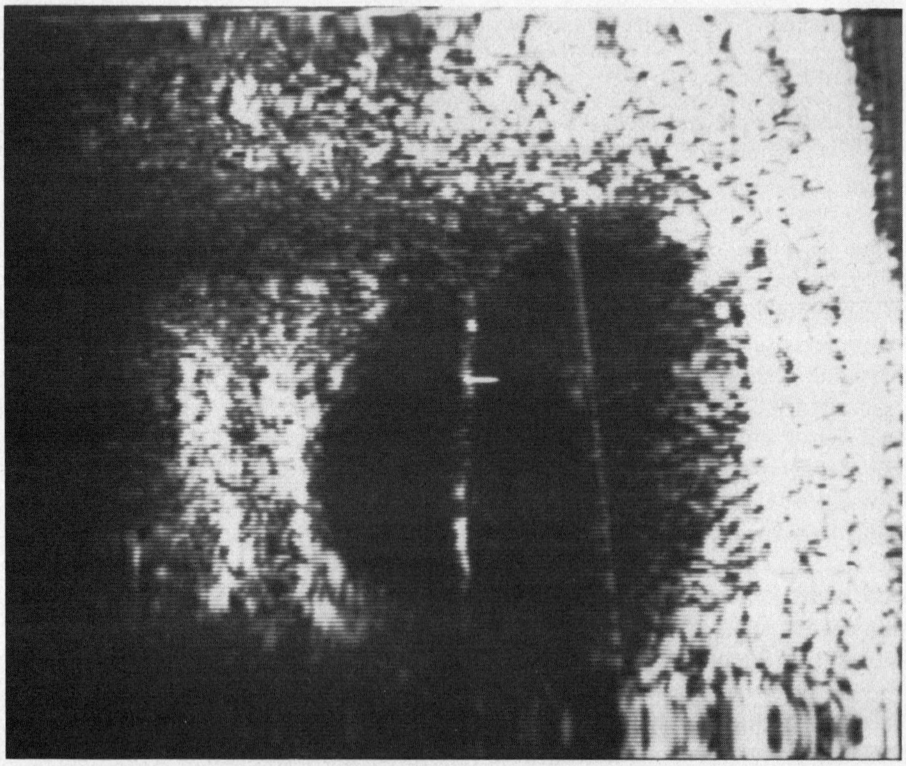

Fig. 26-23. Duplex assessment of saphenofemoral junction. The large dilated greater saphenous vein is seen to the right with wispy incompetent saphenofemoral valve *(near center by cursor)*. (From O'Donnell TF Jr, McEnroe CS, and Heggenick P: Surg Clin North Am 70:159, 1990.)

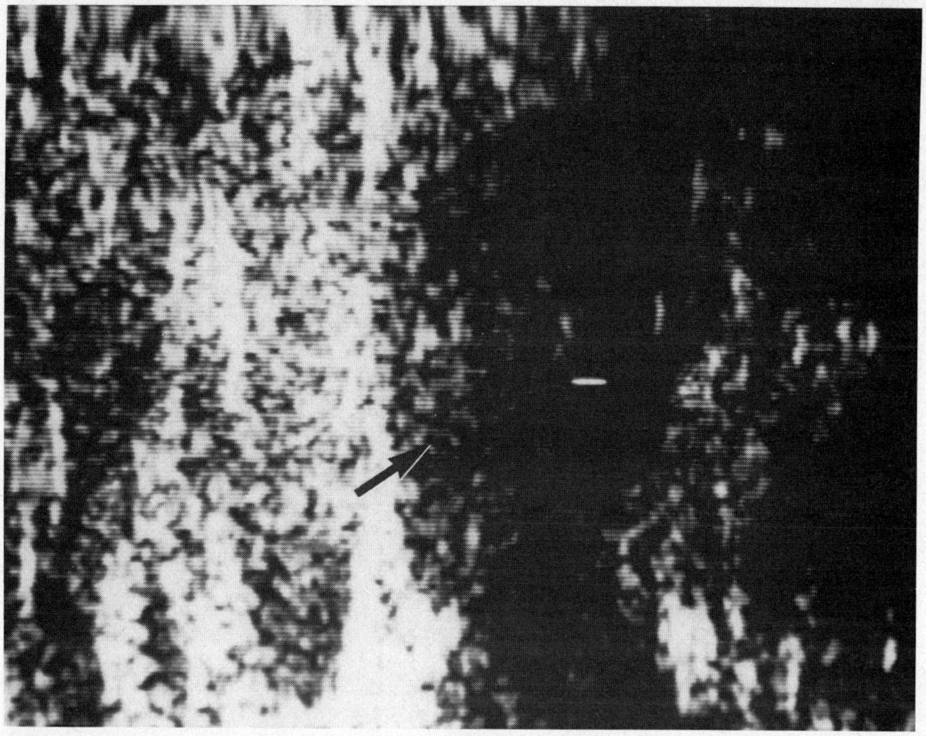

Fig. 26-24. Occluded vein segment. Lumen of vein is filled by echoic substance representative of mature thrombus *(to left of cursor, arrow)*, as seen in this transverse view. Spectral analysis showed absence of flow.

the adductor canal. Then the entire saphenous and perforating veins are visualized. Finally, the calf and popliteal veins are imaged.

Superficial venous system: Saphenofemoral competence, saphenous vein diameter, wall thickness, the diameter of the saphenous tributaries, and valvular competence within the remaining saphenous veins should be assessed by duplex scanning.[46] Before surgery on the superficial venous system, the status of perforating (communicating) veins also should be established, so that concomitant perforating vein ligation can be performed with saphenectomy. Fig. 26-23 demonstrates a transverse B-mode image of an incompetent saphenofemoral junction. In addition to the image, spectral analysis reveals reflux during Valsalva's maneuver. The addition of color to this examination provides visual evidence of reflux.

Deep venous system: Chronic venous occlusion on duplex imaging demonstrates a relatively echoic, white, and highly reflective homogeneous material that occupies the lumen of the vessel[44] (Fig. 26-24). The degree of echogenicity is determined by the collagen content of the thrombus and, therefore, its age. Long-standing deep venous occlusion presents a highly echoic image. The vein wall is also noncompressible and collateral vessels are visualized proximally and distally to the occluded venous segment.[45] Finally, no flow is auscultated in the vessel. The infrainguinal deep veins can usually be visualized for changes characteristic of occlusion. Occlusion of the iliac segment can be indirectly suggested by increased collateral flow and abnormal velocity signals at the femoral level, while direct visualization of iliac vein occlusions can be achieved by the use of the deep Doppler probe. Recanalization of a vein represents a common sequela of deep venous thrombosis (Fig. 26-25). The thrombus incompletely resolves so that a thickened nondilatable venous wall results. A recanalized vein typically appears with an irregular lumen and highly echoic and thickened walls. Flow is present on auscultation.

Detection of valvular incompetence by duplex scanning of the deep venous system relies on three phenomena: (1) direction of blood flow, (2) valve thickness, and (3) valve coaptation. Studies by Rollins et al[47] have shown that 96% of venous valves demonstrated on phlebography can be accurately identified by a prior B-mode examination. These investigators found that anatomic definition of incompetent venous valves was superior to standard phlebography. In approximately 1000 lower extremity examinations Flanagan, Sullivan, and Cranley[45] showed that 90% to 100% of lower extremity veins could be visualized in a longitudinal survey conducted over a 20-month period. These investigators visualized thigh communicating veins and even soleal sinuses in nearly one half of their subjects. A typical vein segment with venous valvular incompetence is shown in

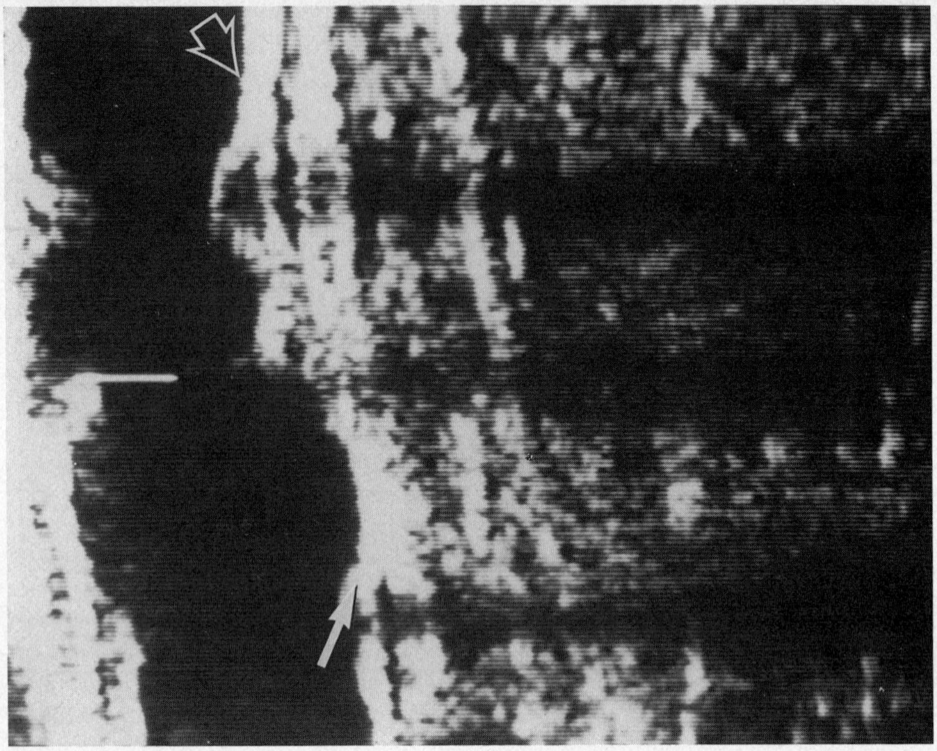

Fig. 26-25. Recanalized vein segment. Highly echoic wall with irregular lumen is indicative of previous thrombosis. No valve leaflets are visualized. Note intense scarring at valve sites *(arrows)*.

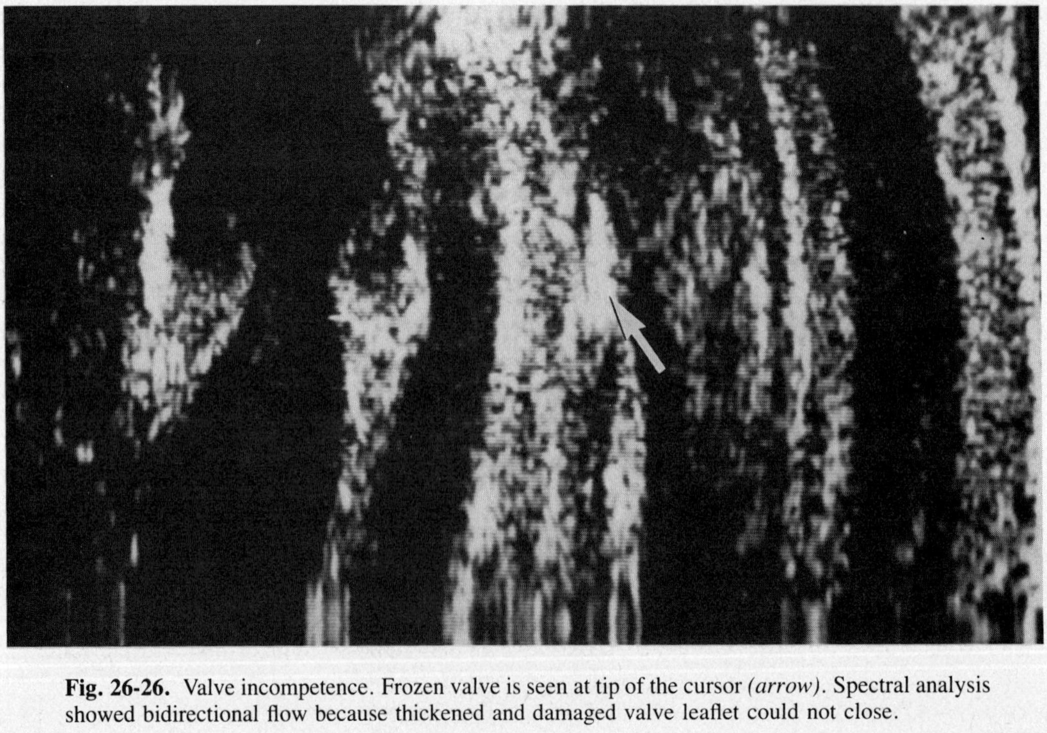

Fig. 26-26. Valve incompetence. Frozen valve is seen at tip of the cursor *(arrow)*. Spectral analysis showed bidirectional flow because thickened and damaged valve leaflet could not close.

Fig. 26-26. The vein valves appear thickened. On dynamic scanning they do not move, so that they fail to coapt. Doppler auscultation showed bidirectional flow across the valve with Valsalva's and proximal pressure maneuvers. As stated earlier, special attention should be paid to the competence of the popliteal vein valve because of its important role as a gatekeeper to the calf muscle pump. Shull et al[42] and others[26] have shown that competence of the popliteal vein valve is closely associated with the presence of venous ulcer.

Overall diagnostic approach (Fig. 26-27)

My patients first undergo quantitative photoplethysmography to determine the degree of venous insufficiency. With the use of tourniquets the relative involvement of the superficial and deep system can be ascertained. In general, patients with severe (grade III) disease have a VRT that is less than 10 seconds, and the VRT is not improved by tourniquet compression of the saphenous or perforating veins. It is not unusual for a patient with a shortened VRT and moderate to severe clinical stigmata of CVI to obtain significant improvement of the VRT with tourniquet compression of the greater saphenous vein.[39] This signifies that greater saphenous incompetence contributes in a major way to the hemodynamic abnormalities and, presumably, the overall clinical status. In this situation ligation and stripping of the greater saphenous vein should be the initial surgical procedure.

The great proportion of patients, however, have advanced clinical disease and a shortened VRT that is not improved by tourniquet compression. In these patients B-mode ultrasonographic examination is carried out as the next diagnostic step to determine the presence of obstruction or valvular incompetence within the deep system. Direct signs of *proximal* venous obstruction on B-mode examination include actual visualization of the occluded venous segment, which is occasionally possible even with iliac vein thrombosis. The occluded segment is usually highly echoic with absence of velocity signals indicating no blood flow. Indirect signs of proximally located iliac vein occlusion include multiple dilated collateral channels at the femoral level and altered velocity flow patterns. Next the valves in the superficial femoral veins, profunda femoris vein, and popliteal vein are examined for anatomic evidence of incompetence, that is, "frozen valve." Finally, Doppler signal analysis following proximal compression is used to substantiate the valvular insufficiency by demonstrating reversed flow or reflux.

Based on the anatomic and functional characterization of patients' CVI, and of course, the clinical symptoms and their response to nonoperative management, certain patients would be considered potential candidates for operative intervention. Such patients would then undergo ascending phlebography, wherein tourniquets would be used to occlude the filling of the superficial venous system. Visualization of contrast media within the superficial venous system usu-

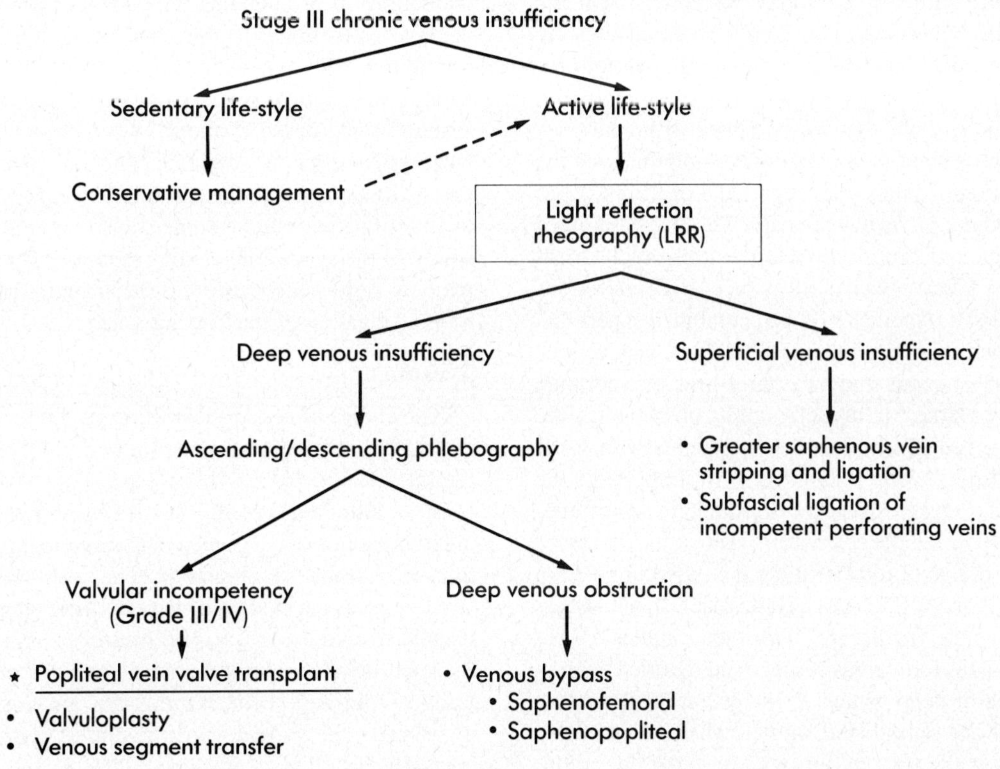

Fig. 26-27. Overall diagnostic approach to chronic venous insufficiency.

ally indicates flow from the deep system via incompetent perforating veins. Their level (site) can be determined by fluoroscopy.[15] Specific anatomic details of the deep venous disease, such as recanalization, occlusion, or avalvular segments, are sought. If the deep system shows no major (bypassable) obstruction, the patient then will undergo descending phlebography. With the patient on the tilt table, which is positioned at 70 degrees to 90 degrees, the rate and level of dye descent within the deep venous system permits categorization of the degree of deep venous valvular incompetence.[48] Surgery for valvular incompetence is usually reserved for those in which dye promptly refluxes to the below-knee popliteal or calf vein segments.

This overall method (Fig. 26-27) of evaluation allows more definitive selection of the patient for superficial venous surgery, such as ligation, stripping, and interruption of incompetent perforating veins, or deep venous reconstructive surgery, to correct valvular incompetence or to bypass obstruction.

Epidemiology

The incidence of superficial vs deep venous system disease. The relative proportion of limbs with involvement of the superficial venous system alone is important, because this incidence reflects the number of patients who may benefit from relatively straightforward surgery. Several biases, however, enter into the assessment of the relative proportion of superficial and deep venous system involvement. Many reports originate in large teaching hospitals, where patients with more severe forms of CVI may be referred. On the other hand, other reports are based only on candidates for surgery and, therefore, may be biased toward a greater proportion of limbs with more severe disease, or, alternatively, concern only those limbs that would benefit from surgery. Allowing for these limitations, Table 26-4 summarizes the relative proportion of limbs with superficial or deep CVI in several series. Our own review of nearly 720 limbs[37] showed that the proportion of limbs with deep venous involvement was three times greater than those with superficial venous insufficiency (21%). Another 14% had combined superficial and deep venous disease. The incidence of deep venous involvement (65%) in our study was three times greater than that reported by Darke[24] in his series of a comparable size. Like Darke we studied a full range of patients with CVI, in contrast to Raju,[49] who examined only limbs with the classic clinical changes of the postthrombotic syndrome. The relatively high incidence of deep venous insufficiency in our study is probably related to the increased proportion of limbs with advanced CVI (stage III disease). In our series, 142 limbs had stage III disease. Two other studies[50,51] focused on candidates for venous surgery and reported a much lower incidence of deep venous involvement. This finding may be related not only to the surgical character of these series but also to the type of surgery under consideration, namely ligation and stripping of the saphenous vein or subfascial ligation of incompetent perforating veins. This would bias toward a greater proportion of superficial venous involvement.

As can be seen from Table 26-5, obstruction of the deep system is an infrequent cause of deep venous disease. In our series only 5% of patients with deep venous disease had outflow obstruction. While Shanzer and Peirce's[52] smaller series had an incidence of venous obstruction comparable to ours, Moore, Himmel, and Sumner[43] and Raju[49] reported double our frequency of obstructive venous disease. However, the majority (85%) of limbs had valvular insufficiency as the cause of their CVI.

Several studies have used descending phlebography to determine the anatomic location of deep venous valvular incompetence. They indicate that the popliteal vein segment was incompetent in over 80% of the 300 limbs examined (Table 26-5). Alternatively, other studies, which utilize a bidirectional Doppler instrument for assessment of deep venous valvular function, demonstrated a comparable proportion of limbs (80%) with popliteal vein valve incompetence. From this, one would conclude that (1) valvular incompetence is the chief cause of chronic venous insufficiency and (2) the popliteal vein valve is usually incompetent in significantly symptomatic patients.

Spectrum. There are few studies that have correlated the clinical stages of CVI in a large unselected population. Our recent study showed that 40% of limbs had advanced stage III disease,[37] which is twice the proportion observed by Darke.[24] In his study only 20% of limbs had venous ulceration. These patients with an open or recently healed venous ulcer represent the most challenging management problem in CVI. Since the major proportion of patients with venous ulcer have valvular incompetence of the deep venous system as the cause of their CVI, there exists a relatively large population of potential candidates for deep venous reconstruction. Of additional interest, however, is the 13% to 15% of patients with venous ulcers who have involvement solely of the superficial venous system.[35] By contrast, these patients may benefit from ligation and stripping with or without ligation of perforating veins.

Treatment

The choice of nonsurgical vs surgical treatment is usually dictated by the severity of symptoms and the anatomic system(s) affected by the disease process. My approach has been to define the severity of CVI by clinical examination, aided by noninvasive objective measurements such as quantitative photoplethysmography. The latter may also suggest what systems are involved. Patients with stage I disease are usually treated by nonsurgical means unless involvement of the superficial venous system has produced moderate symptoms or the superficial varicosities are cosmetically displeasing to the patient. I use a similar approach for early stage II disease. For advanced stage II and stage III CVI (venous ulcer), a full workup including phlebography is

Table 26-4. Incidence of deep venous disease

Study	No. of limbs	Criteria for entry	Methods of diagnosis				System involved (%)	
			Clin	Dop	AVP	Phleb	Superficial	Deep
Darke and Andress[24]	594	CVI	+	+		+	78	22
NEMCH[37]	346	CVI	+	+	+		35	65
Moore et al[43]	174	PT	+	+			65	38
Raju and Fredericks[50]	147	PT	+		+	+	27*	73
St. Thomas Hospital[51]	119	Surg	+		+	+	66	37
Schanzer and Peirce[52]	52	Surg	+		+	+	65	35

*Combined with superficial.
Clin, Clinical.
Dop, Bidirectional Doppler.
AVP, Venous pressure.
Phleb, Ascending or descending phlebogram.
CVI, Chronic venous insufficiency.
PT, Postthrombotic syndrome.
Surg, Candidate for surgery.

Table 26-5. Type and location of deep venous insufficiency

Study	No. of limbs	Criteria for entry	Methods of diagnosis				Obstruction (%)	Valvular incompetence	
			Clin	Dop	AVP	Phleb		Proximal	Distal (popliteal)
Darke and Andress[24]	100	Ulcer	+	+		+	0	19	88
NEMCH[37]	346	CVI	+	+	+		5	11	80
Moore et al[43]	113	PT	+	+			12	22	78
Raju and Fredericks[50]	100	PT	+		+	+	13		
Schanzer and Peirce[52]	17	Surg	+		+	+	7		
Pearce et al[53]	48	PT	+		+	+	0	47	14
Bruns-Slot et al[54]	194	PT	+	+			0	14	86
Gooley and Sumner[55]	74	PT	+	+	+		0	54	46

CVI, Chronic venous insufficiency.
Surg, Candidate for surgery.
Clin, Clinical.
Dop, Bidirectional Doppler.
AVP, Venous pressure.
Phleb, Ascending or descending phlebogram.
PT, Postthrombotic Syndrome.

undertaken. The patient's age, medical risks, and preferences for therapy dictate the form of treatment. If isolated superficial venous insufficiency is defined, surgery is the preferred option. By contrast, if both deep venous and superficial venous system involvement is present and the quantitative photoplethysmographic examination shows little improvement with tourniquet testing, then conservative measures are recommended as the initial treatment plan.

Nonsurgical therapy. The goals of nonsurgical therapy are reduction of ambulatory superficial venous hypertension by external compression and improvement of skin nutrition.[16] Wound healing is obviously a focus in the treatment of stage III disease.

External compression. The benefits of external compression were recognized by the Romans. A compression linen bandage was recommended by Celsus[56] to treat venous ulcers, while Wiseman[57] developed a forerunner of today's elastic stocking—a laced leather stocking. This garment was contoured to fit the lower extremity—a remarkable feature in 1676.

Three forms of external compression presently are available: compression wraps, elastic stockings, and intermittent pneumatic compression devices. The theoretical advantages of external compression is that it blocks transcapillary fluid flow during the ambulatory venous pressure cycle. The pressure required to achieve this effect at the ankle varies with the clinical state of the limb. Starling[58] has shown that approximately 40 to 50 torr are required at the ankle in patients with stage III disease to reduce transcapillary fluid flow. External compression has also been shown not only to increase the fibrinolytic activity of veins[59] but also to improve deep venous blood flow.

Compression bandages: Compression bandages are the simplest and least expensive form of external compression. Unfortunately, they are associated with poor patient compliance because of difficulty in consistently applying the correct pressure, loss of elasticity with repeated washing, and problems in maintaining the wrap in the correct position. Many have commented that the wrapping of a leg is an art form and great variability has been noted from physician to physician or nurse to nurse.

Despite these disadvantages the Ace wrap bandage is helpful for the elderly patient who cannot pull on an elastic stocking, or it is useful in instances where there is a weeping wound and bulky dressings that require frequent dressing changes are used. Finally Ace wraps are useful in abnormally contoured limbs. I generally avoid an elastic stocking when there is an ulcer requiring treatment so that an Ace wrap is used. Before wrapping the leg an ABD pad or sanitary napkin can be placed over an area requiring special compression, such as large varices or incompetent perforating veins. The wrap is started at the malleoli for the first turn and then continued distally to the forefoot from ankle to forefoot. The wrap is continued back up over the leg in a medial to lateral direction, with the outside of the roll applied to the leg.

Elastic stockings: Specially, custom-fitted elastic compression stockings are the standard for treatment of CVI. Like compression bandages, elastic stockings should employ graduated pressure with the highest pressure placed at the ankle level and the lowest pressure at the calf level. Below-knee stockings are usually prescribed while thigh-high or other forms of above-knee stockings are to be avoided because they bind in the popliteal fossa, and, theoretically, high pressures are really not needed above the knee but rather at the ankle area. The graduated elastic compression stocking reduces superficial venous volume and prevents transcapillary leakage of fluid into the interstitium. In a study assessing the effects of elastic stocking on ambulatory venous pressure measurements in the postthrombotic limb we showed that the major hemodynamic effect of these stockings was to reduce the peak systolic pressure achieved during the ambulatory walking cycle (Fig. 26-28).[18] All patients had ascending phlebography that showed extensive postthrombotic involvement of the deep venous system. All patients had advanced stage II or stage III disease. Neither venous refill time nor percent reduction in ambulatory venous pressure was altered by elastic compression. A recent study by Kerstein and Fox[60] demonstrated a reduction in venous refill time, as measured by photoplethysmography. This benefit appeared to be present

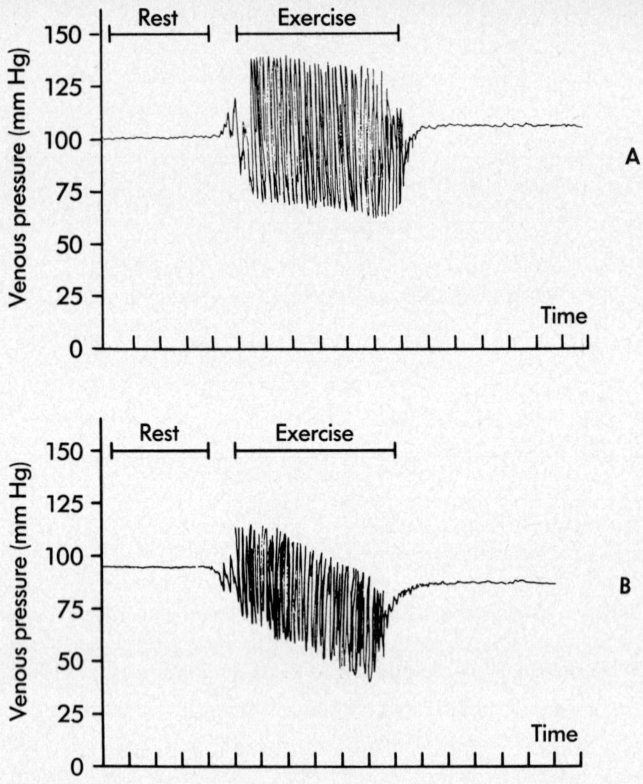

Fig. 26-28. A, Ambulatory venous pressure study in limb with postthrombotic syndrome without elastic compression. Note the high peak systolic pressure, which rises to nearly 150 mm Hg, mostly with exercise and rapid refilling. **B,** Ambulatory venous pressure study in limb **(A)** with elastic compression. The effect of elastic compression is to lower the peak systolic pressure. Venous emptying and refill time are unaffected.

even without application of the elastic stocking. The reason for this improvement without external compression is difficult to explain. Unfortunately, in contrast to our study Kerstein and Fox did not have any anatomic definition of the extent of involvement of either the superficial or the deep venous system. In addition, no clinical classification was mentioned.

Assessment of the tension produced by an elastic stocking is beyond the scope of this chapter, but the British Standards Commission has tested various elastic stockings and measured the pressure at contact points underneath the elastic stocking.[61] Certainly, the choice of the brand of stocking is up to the physician, who should be guided by the reliability of fit, durability, comfort, and finally, patient acceptance, which usually arises from the previous factors. Stockings come in several varieties of compression, 20 to 30 torr, 30 to 40 torr, and 40 to 50 torr. For mild venous disease, stage I, I prescribe the 20 to 30 torr seamless, double-weave stocking (Sigvaris), while for patients with stage II or stage III (healed ulcer) I prefer the 40 to 50 torr stocking. The life of a pair of elastic stockings is from 4 to 6 months, depending on the brand. I prefer that the patient purchase two pairs so he or she can alternate them with washing. Generally four stockings per limb per year will be required. The patient is instructed to put the stocking on before he or she arises from bed, because presumably this is the time of maximal edema reduction. I regularly check the tension of the elastic stockings on office visits, but instruct the patient to notify me if the stocking feels easy to apply. At this time it has obviously lost its elasticity.

Circ-Aid: A novel approach to elastic compression has been the use of individual circumferential rubber bands that are secured by Velcro. This device allows the patient to adjust the tension of each strip and to fit the compression device to an abnormally contoured leg. Circ-Aid also allows dressing changes to be carried out in a more facile manner. Recent trials have shown improved hemodynamic benefits with the use of this device.[62]

Intermittent pneumatic compression: Intermittent pneumatic compression devices have been used extensively for the prevention of deep vein thrombosis.[63] These devices have been shown by controlled trials to prevent DVT by promoting increased deep venous blood flow. In addition, the fibrinolytic activity of veins has been enhanced.[59] There are various forms of intermittent pneumatic compression, the single-cell unit (Venodyne or Flowtron), the two- or three-cell unit (Kendall), and finally the multiple-cell sequential pneumatic compression device (Lympha-Press). Recent early trials have shown improved ulcer healing in patients who have used these devices.[64] Intermittent pneumatic compression devices are reserved for patients with stage III ulcers or marked edema. Lymphatic involvement may make venous edema worse, so that these devices are helpful in such limbs.

Skin care. Patients with stage I and early stage II disease should be encouraged to use skin cream to improve skin nutrition. A water-based, soluble cream or lotion is preferred. Since Polysorb Hydrate is not oil-based, it does not act on the overlying elastic compression stocking. Its lack of greasy feeling improves patient compliance. Patients with advanced stage II disease and eczematous skin changes complain bitterly of pruritus. Topical steroid cream is helpful in reducing this symptom and, therefore, preventing scratching. Excoriations may convert a stage II limb to a stage III limb. The addition of an oral antihistamine supplements the topical application of the steroid in such patients. Patients with acute infection should be treated vigorously to prevent damage to the lymphatics. Lymphatic obliteration compounds the edema of CVI. In general, the cellulitic infection is related to group B streptococci and, therefore, penicillin or erythromycin are appropriate treatment. Fungal infection should not be overlooked in patients with scaling dermatitis. If fungal infection is suspected, a skin scraping should be obtained for microscopic examination and oral antifungal agents prescribed.

Ulcer care. Venous ulcer represents the end stage of CVI. Unfortunately, most studies gauge the effect of any treatment modality for venous ulcer by the incidence of ulcer healing, but few provide follow-up data on ulcer *recurrence*. It is important to focus on ulcer recurrence as the gold standard rather than on the initial healing of the venous ulcer, because as Browse has stated, "Almost all venous ulcers can be healed with good medical treatment, but universal prevention of recurrence cannot yet be achieved."[1] Therefore the true measure of success for any treatment method should be determined by its prevention of ulcer recurrence rather than ulcer healing alone. Implicit in the assessment of ulcer recurrence is a long-term follow-up program similar to the reporting of arterial reconstructive procedures or survival with antineoplastic medicines. We have used a life table method for assessing the results of ulcer healing.[65] This method is similar to that used for determining the graft patency of arterial grafts. This measure of ulcer recurrence has been termed *the ulcer-free interval rate* (Fig. 26-29).

External compression is essential to promote ulcer healing. I prefer a frequently changed, high-tension elastic compression bandage or the Circ-Aid device to complement wound care. Occasionally patients will be able to wear an elastic compression stocking over the dressing, but this is difficult to apply over bulkier dressings. These external compression methods may be supplemented by the nightly use of an external pneumatic compression device. While considered a form of external compression, the Unna boot will be addressed subsequently as a form of wound care.

The goal of ulcer treatment is to prevent recurrence and frequent hospitalizations with lost time from work, which has a significant socioeconomic impact.

Ulcer care should reduce the bacterial population of the ulcer, arrest periulcer infection, and promote epithelialization of the ulcer. Three types of dressings are currently available to treat venous ulcers: (1) absorbent dressings, (2) occlusive dressings, and (3) impregnated bandages. I do not use dressings impregnated with antibiotic cream, another form of wound care, because of the danger of sensitization.

Absorbent dressings, such as gauze sponges, should "blot" or "sponge up" the ulcer exudate. In ulcers with exudate I prefer Betadine-soaked gauze sponges thoroughly wrung out to achieve a wet-to-dry effect. These dressings are changed every 6 hours and are initially monitored by a visiting nurse once daily. The dressings are changed by the patient or the patient's family. These gauze bandages should not be filled with paper and should be of the wide-mesh type to allow the interstices of the gauze to débride the ulcer when dried and removed. Once the ulcer is no longer purulent and granulation tissue is observed, then saline wet-to-dry gauzes are employed. There are a variety of other absorbent dressings such as Telfa, but because of their poor absorptive capacity I do not use them.

Occlusive wound dressings are a newly developed form of ulcer treatment that absorb transudate from the ulcer, but remain moist and nonadherent. Because of the lack of evap-

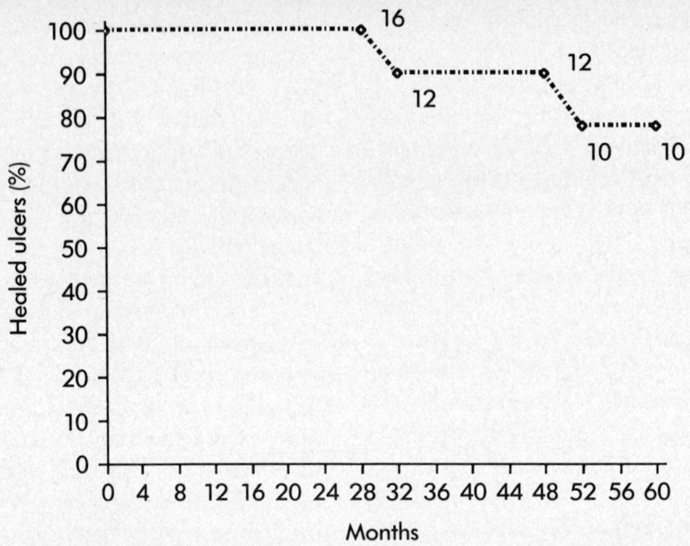

Fig. 26-29. Life table analysis of 32 patients treated by surgery for recurrent venous ulcer. The curve shows the ulcer-free interval following surgery.

Medical therapy for chronic venous insufficiency

I. External compression

- A. Elastic stockings: custom fitted
- B. Ace wrap or variant
- C. "Circ-Aid"
- D. Intermittent external pneumatic compression

II. Skin care

- A. Lanolin
- B. Water-based lotion: Polysorb Hydrate
- C. Topical antifungal agent

III. Ulcer care

- A. Absorbent
  - 1. Wide-mesh gauze
    - a. Purulent: half strength Betadine
    - b. Nonpurulent: saline wet to dry
- B. Occlusive dressing
  - 1. Hydrogels: Synthaderm
  - 2. Hydrocolloids: DuoDerm
  - 3. Polyurethane: "Opsite"
  - 4. Foam: Lyofoam
- C. Impregnated compression bandages
  - 1. Unna boot

oration from the dressing the occlusive wound dressings do not stick to the ulcer. Examples of these types are Sorbsan, a biodegradable hydrophilic gel made from an alginate; hydrocolloids, such as a methylcellulose base with a foam backing; polyurethane sheets, such as Opsite; and finally, foam dressings, such as Polyurethane foam dressings (Synthaderm, Armer Pharmaceuticals) (see the accompanying box).

Impregnated bandages, such as the Unna boot, are widely used in the management of venous ulcer. The term *Unna boot* is used in a generic sense, because the medication, developed by a dermatologist, is a mixture of gelatin, zinc oxide, sorbitol, gelatin magnesium, aluminum silicate and calamine. Unna boots represent a popular form of bandage and are used in many large outpatient clinics in urban hospital settings. The advantages of an Unna boot are that both wound care and external compression are contained in one unit; the boot can be changed on a twice or once weekly basis depending on the amount of exudate; and the boot prevents the patient from doing damage to the skin by scratching. The disadvantages of this treatment are the obvious personal hygiene problem, sensitization to the paste, and exudate forming underneath the boot, which could further macerate the skin.

Results of treatment: Cranley[66] has shown that 86% of 18,055 ulcerated extremities, monitored from 1952 to 1987, could be healed by a combination of pressure bandage applications and wound care alone. Similarly, Browse, Burnand, and Lea[1] found that over 80% of leg ulcers would heal within the first year after treatment in a special venous clinic when treated by a combination of paste bandages and elastic compression. Recently, occlusive hydrocolloid dressings, such as Duoderm,[67] have been used in conjunction with external compression. A randomized, prospective, comparative study by Kikta et al[68] showed superiority of the Unna boot regimen (70% healing rate) (Table 26-6) over that of the hydrocolloid dressing treatment (38% healing rate). While the hydrocolloid dressing was more acceptable to the patient with respect to comfort and convenience, 10 patients in the hydrocolloid dressing group required cessation of therapy because of complications. Ericksson[69] showed diametrically opposite results in a comparative study

Table 26-6. Results of ulcer healing with nonsurgical treatment

Study	No. of cases	Method	Ulcers healed (%)
Cranley[66]	18,055	Pressure bandage and wound care	86
Browse[1]	>100	Elastic compression	80
		Paste bandage	
Kikta[68]	30	Unna boot	70
	39	Hydrocolloid dressing	38
Ericksson[69]	17	Hydrocolloid and elastic compression	53
Van Rijswijk[70]	152	Hydrocolloid	62

(see Table 26-6). The incidence of healing was comparable between the hydrocolloid group and the Unna boot group. Rubin et al[71] recently reported a comparative trial of Unna boot vs polyurethane foam dressings (PFD). During a 12-month period 36 consecutive ambulatory patients with lower extremity chronic venous ulcer were randomized into the two treatment programs. Of the patients treated with PFD, 52% withdrew from the study because of wound odor, while conversely there was 100% compliance in the Unna boot group. In addition, the overall wound healing rate was better in the Unna boot group (95% vs 41% of the PFD group). Finally the healing rate was superior in the Unna group (0.5 cm^2/day) than in the PFD group (0.07 cm^2/day). This most recent study suggests that the old standby Unna boot should not be abandoned as a form of therapy. Unfortunately, little data are available on subsequent ulcer recurrence. In the most extensive series reported on conservative therapy, Cranley[66] observed a 21% incidence of recurrent ulcers with documented deep venous disease in patients treated in his clinic. This rate is similar to the 18% recurrence rate noted in patients with superficial venous disease who were treated with wound care and compression bandages. For a review of medical therapy see the box on p. 470.

Sclerotherapy. Sclerotherapy is an important adjunct to the treatment of CVI (Table 26-7). There is some debate as to the proper role of sclerotherapy but most physicians use this method in selected circumstances. Sclerotherapy had developed a poor reputation in the United States principally because of indiscriminant application and improper patient selection. European physicians have greatly contributed to the clinical development of sclerotherapy. Sclerotherapy depends on producing a limited inflammatory response in a segment of vein. Subsequent external compression of that vein segment produces adherence of the vein walls. Fibrosis and possible reabsorption eventually ensue. Fegan[72] demonstrated that only a small amount of sclerosing solution entered the deep venous system and was rapidly diluted if the patient exercised.

As stated previously, patient selection is critical. Hobbs'[73] prospective study, which compared sclerotherapy with surgery, showed that sclerotherapy was most useful for the treatment of incompetent perforating veins and for recurrent veins after surgery. Long saphenous incompetence was associated with a high incidence of recurrence in the sclerotherapy-treated group. Saphenopopliteal and saphenous vein high thigh incompetence had poor results with sclerotherapy, usually caused by the difficulty in obtaining compression in the large volume of sclerosant required. Hobbs suggested surgery for these groups to avoid such problems. With sclerotherapy, however, some physicians use high ligation of the vein with sclerotherapy or with stripping to the knee. Sclerotherapy of the calf varices is also carried out.

Table 26-7. Results with sclerotherapy

Study	No. of patients	Years of follow-up care	Recurrence (%)
Fegan[72]	760	6	15
Hobbs*[73]		1	18
		5	93
Strother[74]	348	1-3	11
		>4	32
Dejode[75]	146	1-5	17
Reid[76]	1080	1	10
Chant[77]	155	3	22

*Greater saphenous vein.

In many cases cosmetic improvement is an important factor leading one to decide on treatment for varicosities. Although surgical and injection treatment options are available for varicose veins, spider telangiectasias respond only to injection therapy, and the response may be quite variable. Surgical removal is inappropriate and nearly impossible.

Sclerotherapy for venous telangiectasia is best accomplished using 23% saline and a 30-gauge needle to enter the vein (Fig. 26-30). Complete filling of the telangiectatic area should be easily accomplished with the injection, and extravasation should be avoided. Compression following injection is of limited value in our experience. Resolution of the veins following adequate injection should occur within 2 to 6 weeks. This technique is ideal for cosmetic management of venous telangiectasias.

Various sclerosing solutions are available for larger veins. Sodium tetradecyl (STD) (3%) is FDA approved and widely used. Alternatively, hypertonic saline can be used, but the

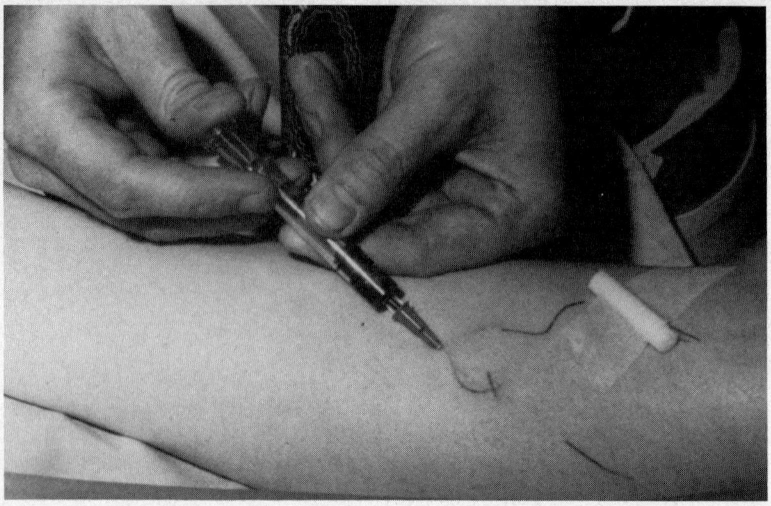

Fig. 26-30. Sclerotherapy for superficial calf varicosities. A 25 + -gauge needle has aspirated blood before injection of sclerosant. A dental roll is placed over the vein for direct compression of leg. Elastic stockings or Ace wraps are then worn.

solution may be painful to the patient. Some of the discomfort of hypertonic saline can be avoided by mixing a regional anesthetic agent, such as Xylocaine or Marcaine, with the solution. The concentration of the sclerosant depends on the size of the vein sclerosed. For smaller veins I prefer to dilute 3% STD in half or in quarter with saline. While the patient is standing his or her veins are marked, and a 25- or 30-gauge needle can be inserted attached to the end of a tuberculin syringe and taped into place. Five to six syringes may be required. Alternatively, the vein may be entered with the patient in the horizontal position. If carried out with the patient lying down, I prefer a 25- or 30-gauge scalp vein. The leg is elevated to empty the vein. A small amount of air is injected first to be sure that the needle is in the vein and to prevent extravasation of the sclerosant solution. Next, 0.5 to 0.75 ml of the sclerosing solution is injected. The physicians' index and ring fingers are placed a few centimeters above and below the site of injection to maintain the sclerosing solution in the proper location. I generally milk the sclerosing solution within the vein segment with my index finger. A dental roll provides compression over the vein segment. Care should be taken to avoid tension on the skin with the tape holding the dental rolls, because the tape may cause traction burns. I prefer to incorporate the dental rolls into the Ace wrap to avoid traction burns. The patient is instructed to walk at least a mile or two a day following sclerotherapy to dilute the sclerosing solution in the deep venous system. There is argument over how long the Ace wrap should stay in place. Personal hygiene demands a shorter period than the usual 4 to 6 weeks originally recommended. European specialists suggest a period of at least 3 weeks. I generally restrict sclerotherapy to the cooler months so that the patient is more comfortable wearing the Ace wraps. After a week of compression the patient may remove the Ace bandage and take a bath, or, alternatively, the Ace wrap limb may be placed in a large garbage bag to allow showering. The patient should be seen 10 to 14 days after injection. If thrombus is present in a vein segment, it can be evacuated with a No. 11 blade and compression. This decreases unsightly pigmentation.

Complications such as extravasation may lead to skin sloughing in a small percentage of patients. This can be avoided by absolute assurance that the needle is in the vein and by the use of dilute sclerosing solution for small veins. Thrombophlebitis is unusual with this technique. Pigmentation along the vein will fade by 4 to 6 months if present.

Surgical treatment. Until recently, the patient with advanced CVI was treated according to the regimen outlined by John Hunter in 1642: "The sores of poor people are often mended by rest in the horizontal position, fresh provisions, and warmth in hospitals."[78] Now, however, as an alternative to medical therapy, direct reconstruction of the deep venous system may be offered to selected patients with advanced chronic venous disease. The candidates for such surgery are few, as Darke's study[24] implied, numbering less than one quarter of patients with chronic venous disease. To determine the site and degree of valvular dysfunction or obstruction in potential candidates, a thorough diagnostic evaluation is performed preoperatively (as summarized previously).

Ligation and stripping. Burnand et al have previously shown that ligation and stripping of the greater saphenous system restores hemodynamics to normal where ambulatory pressure and VRT are normalized.[51] I use flush ligation of the greater saphenous vein at its junction with the femoral vein. For patients with only a few (less than 3) incompetent perforating veins, small calf incisions can be made directly over the site of the suspect perforating vein, which is then ligated through this incision. For patients with multiple incompetent perforating veins I usually use the posterior stocking seam approach in preference to the standard medial

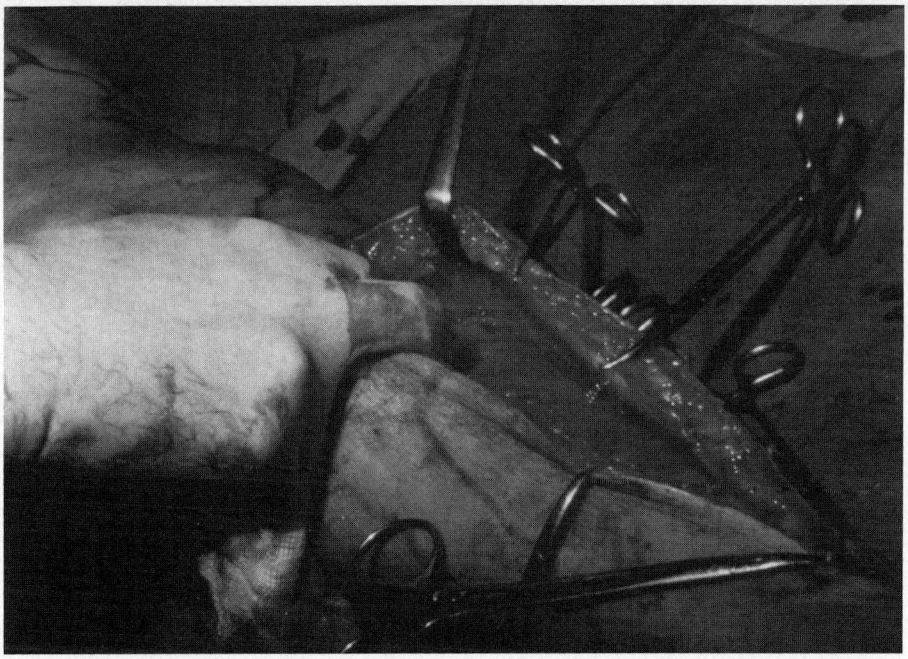

Fig. 26-31. Subfascial vein ligation. Incompetent perforating veins are exposed through the medial or posterior subfascial approach. They are then ligated and interrupted. Perforating veins are seen at the top of the scissors and underneath the retractor *(right)*.

subfascial calf incision (Fig. 26-31). The latter approach places the lower portion of the incision over the supramalleolar area, which usually contains the most severely affected tissue. Like ligation and stripping, this procedure usually normalizes altered hemodynamics. Table 26-8 summarizes the results with superficial venous surgery.

Venous reconstructive surgery. Burnand et al[81] showed that recurrence of venous ulcer was common following ligation of incompetent perforating veins in patients with concomitant deep venous disease, as demonstrated by phlebography. By contrast, recurrence of ulcer was unusual if the perforating veins and the superficial system were involved, but there was no evidence of deep venous disease, and hemodynamics improved. Direct venous reconstruction is designed to either bypass isolated obstruction within the deep system or to interpose a functioning valvular segment in a patent, but incompetent deep venous system. Surgical procedures for obstruction or valve incompetence are outlined in Fig. 26-32.

Crossover-saphenofemoral venous bypass: The natural history of deep venous thrombosis is recanalization of the involved vein with destruction of valves. If the recanalization process is incomplete and collateral vessel formation is inadequate, functional venous obstruction may result. When anatomic obstruction is limited to a short segment of vein, such as the iliac, and severe symptoms of edema or venous claudication are present, the patient may be a candidate for a venous bypass procedure. The number of postthrombotic patients who fall into this category appears limited and has been estimated to be between 2% and 4%.[82]

Table 26-8. Surgical results with varicose veins

Study	No. of patients	Length of follow-up care (yrs)	Recurrence (%)
Lofgren[7]	1000	10	15
Haeger[25]	578	5	8
Rivlin[80]	2000	>6	7
Hobbs[73]	170	10	29
Chant[77]	100	3	14

In the crossover-saphenofemoral bypass, initially described by Palma and Esperson in 1958,[83] the saphenous vein from the nonaffected limb is mobilized to the level of the distal thigh, ligated distally and tunneled suprapubically to the inguinal region of the obstructed side. The saphenous vein is anastomosed to either the common femoral or superficial femoral vein to bypass the obstructed ipsilateral iliac vein (Fig. 26-33). Methods to increase venous blood flow in the transposed saphenous segment appear important to prevent graft thrombosis. An arterial-venous fistula may be created distal to the anastomosis, or intermittent pneumatic compression devices may be applied postoperatively. In addition, I generally employ carefully monitored heparin therapy with conversion to warfarin in these patients. Table 26-9 summarizes the results of several series. While clinical criteria have been used to judge the success, only two series report follow-up care with anatomic and functional studies.[26,82] Our smaller series has used B-mode ultrasound as

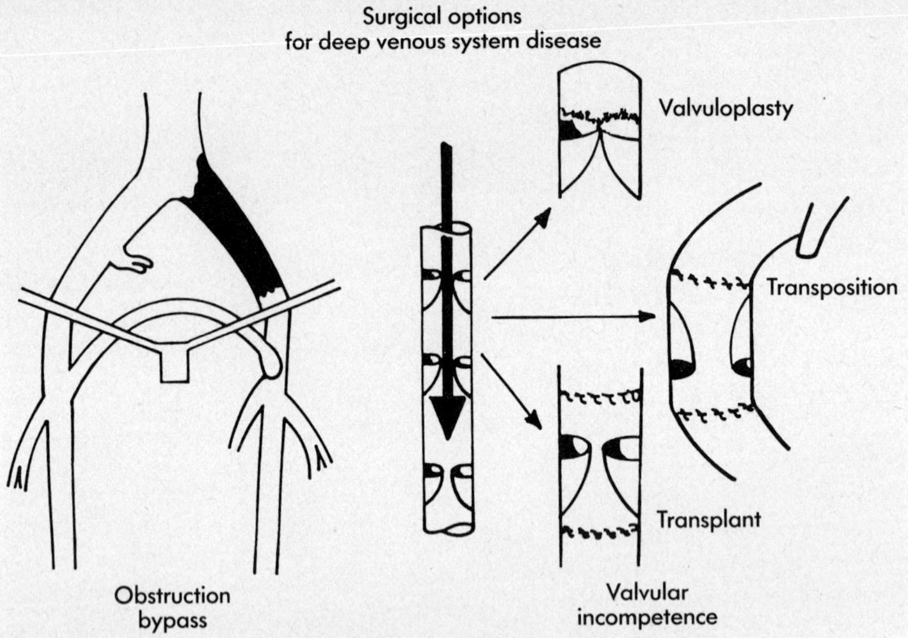

Fig. 26-32. Range of deep venous reconstructive surgery. Surgery is carried out in a selected group of patients for advanced venous disease. Procedures are either for obstruction or valve incompetence.

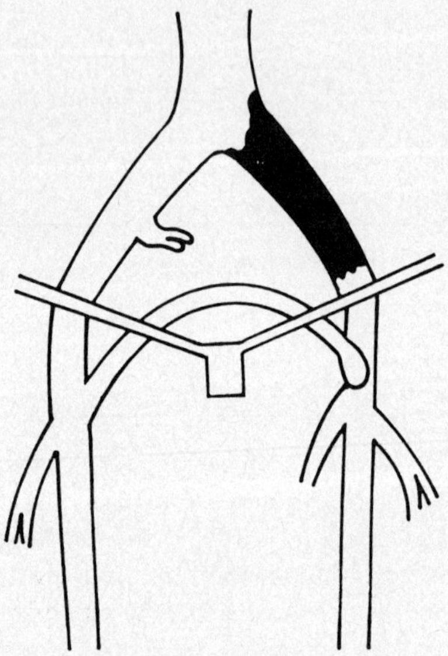

Fig. 26-33. Saphenofemoral bypass (Palma procedure). This procedure uses the contralateral saphenous vein, which is anastomosed to the ipsilateral femoral vein to bypass an iliac obstruction.

a method for demonstrating late anatomic and functional patency of the bypass.[26] Long-term follow-up study has shown adequate patency.

Saphenous bypass: The greater saphenous vein has been used to bypass an isolated obstruction of superficial femoral vein as popularized by Husni.[86] The early experience of Linton[9] showed little sequelae to ligation of the superficial femoral vein. Indeed, this vein has even been used as a conduit for arterial bypass without any deleterious consequences. It is unusual to find a patient in this situation who has not undergone a previous saphenectomy or whose saphenous vein is unaffected by the same disease process. Therefore this procedure is rarely used.

Venous valvuloplasty: In the patient with primary venous valvular incompetence, Kistner[48] has used venous valvuloplasty of the highest valve within the superficial femoral vein. The redundant valve is repaired by reefing up excess leaflet tissue to the vein wall with interrupted sutures, either through a longitudinal or transverse venotomy (Fig. 26-34). Table 26-10 summarizes the results of several series. Following surgery, few patients had completely normal venous pressure patterns, but most were improved. Kistner believes this procedure placed them in a "compensated" state. This procedure is not applicable for the large majority of patients with deep system incompetence secondary to the sequelae of acute deep venous thrombosis, because the valve is destroyed and thickened by the process. However, this should be the first procedure attempted because of its results, durability, and restriction to one vein segment without transplantation.

Venous segment transfer (Table 26-11): This procedure is used for patients in whom the valves of the superficial and comon femoral venous system have been destroyed. A competent valve-bearing venous segment is transposed into the main deep venous system at the groin level (Fig. 26-35). Several varieties of transposition have been used, either the ipsilateral saphenous vein or competent profunda femoris vein. While Ferris and Kistner's studies showed ex-

Table 26-9. Crossover saphenofemoral venous bypass for postthrombotic syndrome

Study	No. of patients	Clinical results (percent of patients)		
		Excellent	Good	Unimproved
Palma (1960)[83]	7	57	29	14
Dale (1969)[84]	23	43	43	14
May (1981)[85]	66	73	0	27
Husni (1981)[86]	82	61	15	24
Halliday (1985)[82]	50*	76	0	24
O'Donnell (1986)[26]	6†	83	17	0

*Patent by phlebography.
†Patent by late B-mode ultrasound.

Table 26-10. Valvuloplasty: clinical, hemodynamic, and phlebographic results

Study	No. of limbs	Preoperative ulcer (%)	Ulcer healing		Pain relief		VRT improved		AVP improved		Patent and functioning segment by phlebography	
			Short-term (%)	Long-term (%)	Short-term (%)	Long-term (%)	Short-term (%)	Long-term (%)	Short-term (%)	Long-term (%)	Short-term (%)	Long-term (%)
Kistner[48]	32	7	83	—	—	—	—	—	86		88	—
Raju[50]	61	66	85	63	90	87	64	—	100	—	—	—

VRT, Venous refill time.
AVP, Ambulatory venous pressure.

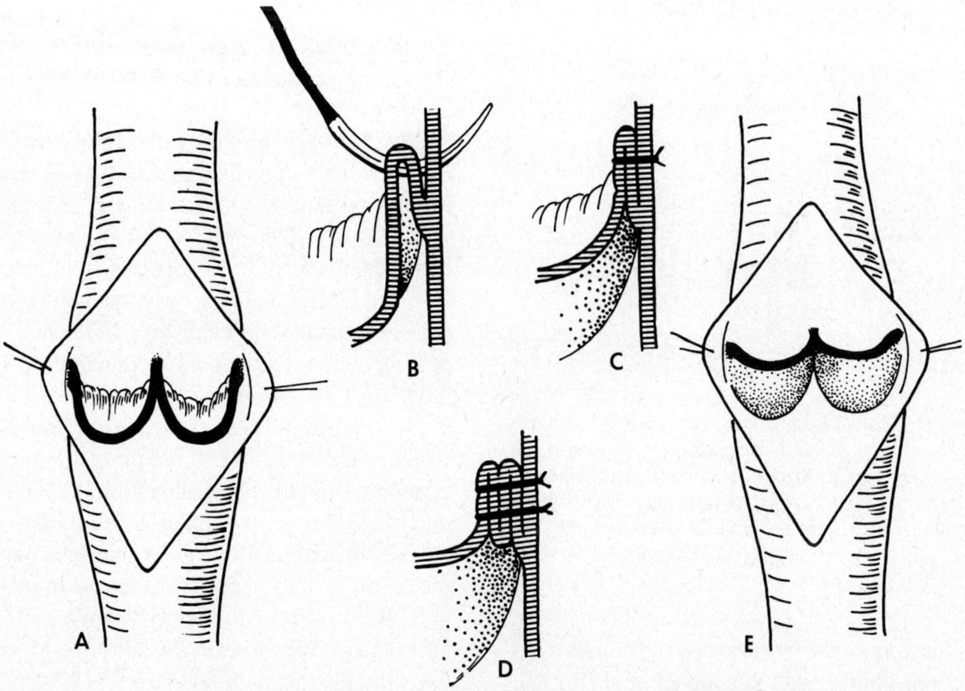

Fig. 26-34. Valvuloplasty for primary valvular incompetence. This procedure corrects the floppy redundant valve edges **(A)** by "reefing" the valve up **(B-D)** so that valves now coapt **(E).** (From O'Donnell TF Jr: The clinical management of deep venous valvular incompetence. In Rutherford RB, ed: Vascular surgery, ed 3, Philadelphia, 1989, WB Saunders Co.)

Table 26-11. Venous segment transfer: clinical, hemodynamic, and phlebographic results

Study	No. of limbs	Preoperative ulcer (%)	Ulcer healing		Pain relief		VRT improved		AVP improved		Patent and functioning segment by phlebography	
			Short-term (%)	Long-term (%)	Short-term (%)	Long-term (%)	Short-term (%)	Long-term (%)	Short-term (%)	Long-term (%)	Short-term (%)	Long-term (%)
Kistner[87]	14	?	80	—	64	—	—	—	92	—	100	57
Queral[89]	12	33	100	—	75	—	92	—	50	—	75	—
Johnson[88]	12	33	0	0	—	25	—	25	0	0	—	—

VRT, Venous refill time.
AVP, Ambulatory venous pressure.

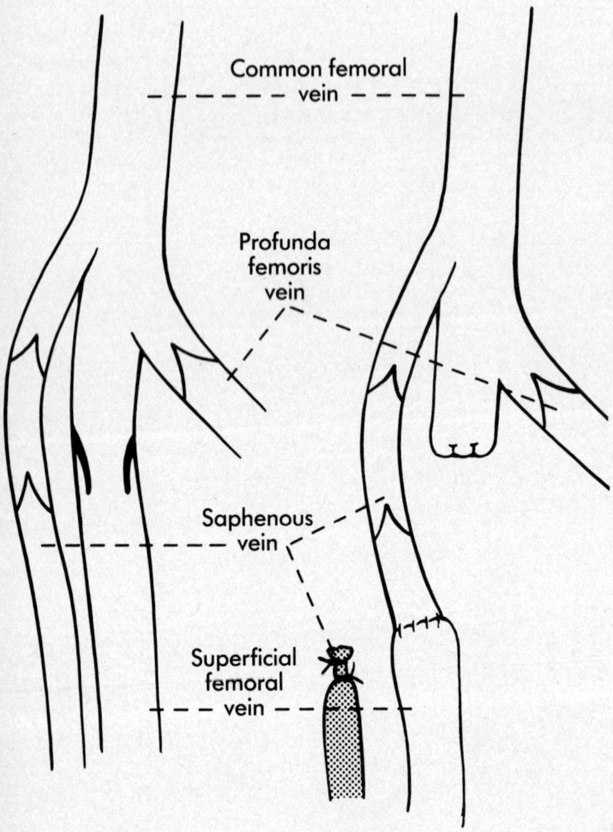

Fig. 26-35. Venous segment transposition. This procedure interposes a normal valve from saphenous or preferably profunda femoris vein into the deep venous circuit to correct incompetence of a superficial femoral vein valve. (From O'Donnell TF Jr: The clinical management of deep venous valvular incompetence. In Rutherford RB, ed: Vascular surgery, ed 3, Philadelphia, 1989, WB Saunders Co.)

cellent results,[87] the work of the Northwestern group showed degeneration of both clinical and functional state by one year.[88,89] In contrast to Ferris and Kistner's patients, the Northwestern group did not treat incompetent perforating veins and found that patients with the most significant clinical and hemodynamic recurrence following venous segment transfer had concomitant perforator vein disease.[88]

Vein valve transplantation: The use of venous autografts has been discussed experimentally for several decades and has been reviewed by Haimovici et al.[70] Taheri et al[71] deserve the credit for introducing and popularizing the use of vein valve transplantation in the treatment of CVI. Taheri et al's concept is similar to Ferris and Kistner's venous segment transposition, namely to ameliorate deep system reflux by placing a competent valve in the main deep system at the level of the thigh. Initially, Taheri et al used a short segment of superficial femoral vein just below the femoral bifurcation and replaced that segment with a 2 to 2.5-cm valve-bearing segment of the brachial vein (Fig. 26-36). Raju and Fredericks[50] have used the superficial femoral vein level, but they used the large-caliber axillary vein as the valve-containing segment. Table 26-12 summarizes the results of these two series.

My approach to vein valve transplantation differs from the previously described approaches in that I use the larger caliber axillary vein and transpose it to the popliteal level (Fig. 26-37). I do this for two reasons. First, the larger caliber axillary vein is a better size match for the popliteal vein, which theoretically may prevent eventual dilation of the transplanted segment and secondary valvular incompetence. A second benefit to placing the valve at the popliteal vein level is suggested in the work of Bauer,[28] Shull et al,[42] and more recently Moore, Himmel, and Sumner,[43] which showed that the function of the popliteal vein valve is important in avoiding ulceration. Table 26-13 summarizes our long-term follow-up of a small, but carefully studied series.[26] In contrast to the two other reported series, all of our patients had venous ulceration preoperatively and all underwent objectively hemodynamic and anatomic follow-up studies. We believe, in addition to correcting venous valvular insufficiency, incompetent perforating veins should be ligated before, or concomitant with, deep venous reconstruction.

Patients with the obstructive form of chronic venous dis-

Table 26-12. Superficial femoral vein valve transplant

Study	No. of limbs	Preoperative ulcer (%)	Ulcer healing		Pain relief		VRT improved		AVP improved		Patent and functioning segment by phlebography	
			Short-term (%)	Long-term (%)	Short-term (%)	Long-term (%)	Short-term (%)	Long-term (%)	Short-term (%)	Long-term (%)	Short-term (%)	Long-term (%)
Taheri[91]	13		n = 10	60	—	100	—	—	88	—	—	100
Taheri[92]	43		n = 17	94	—	75	—	—	n = 18	89	n = 29	90
Raju[50]	24		79	42	77	50	63	—	46	13	—	—

VRT, Venous refill time.
AVP, Ambulatory venous pressure.

Table 26-13. Popliteal vein valve transplant: clinical, hemodynamic, and anatomic results

Study	No. of limbs	Preoperative ulcer (%)	Ulcer healing		Pain relief		VRT improved		AVP improved		Patent and functioning segment by phlebography	
			Short-term (%)	Long-term (%)	Short-term (%)	Long-term (%)	Short-term (%)	Long-term (%)	Short-term (%)	Long-term (%)	Short-term (%)	Long-term (%)
O'Donnell[26]	10	100	100	100	100	100	30	30	—	—	100	90

VRT, Venous refill time.
AVP, Ambulatory venous pressure.

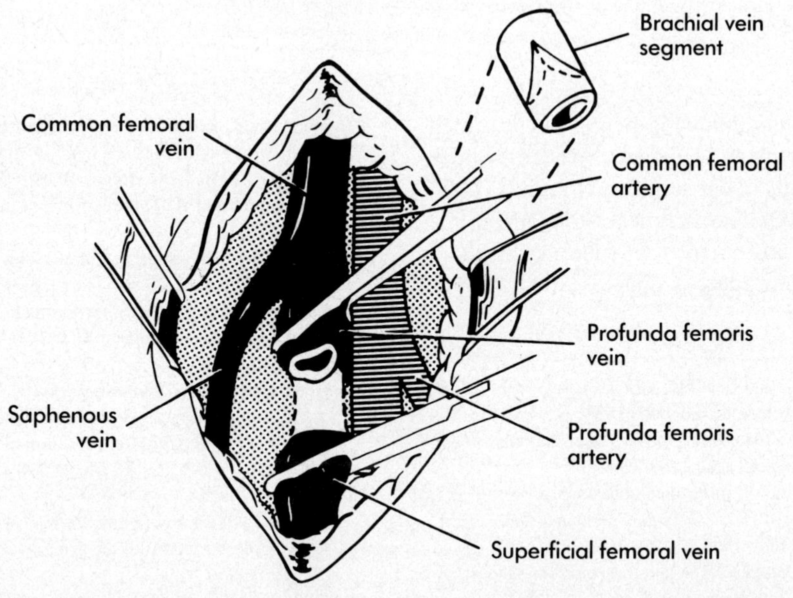

Fig. 26-36. Femoral vein valve transplant. Brachial vein segment is transplanted with competent valve as an interposition graft into the superficial femoral vein. (From O'Donnell TF Jr: The clinical management of deep venous valvular incompetence. In Rutherford RB, ed: Vascular surgery, ed 3, Philadelphia, 1989, WB Saunders Co.)

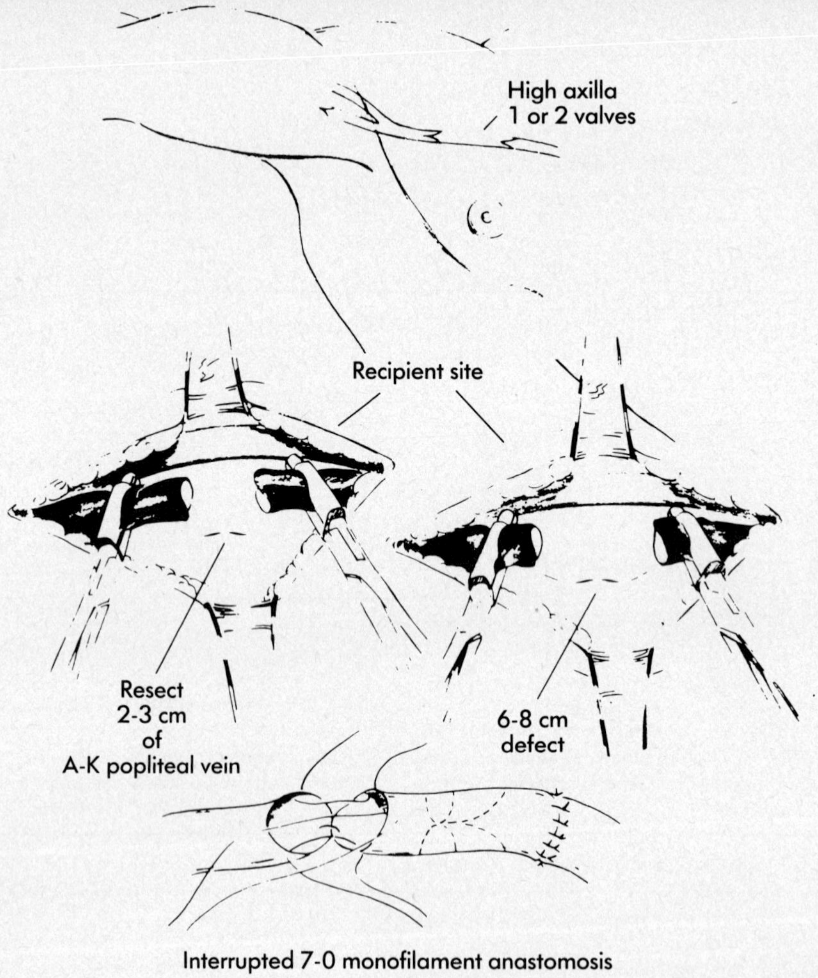

Fig. 26-37. Popliteal vein valve transplant. Axillary vein valve whose competence has previously been confirmed by B-mode ultrasound is transplanted to the above-knee popliteal vein as an interposition graft.

ease enjoy excellent results following bypass. Less settled is the management of valvular insufficiency. We are cautious about extending the results of our series and those of Taheri et al,[76] but they do show relief of clinical symptoms in the majority of patients with postthrombotic syndrome on whom a valve transplantation procedure is done.

REFERENCES

1. Browse NL, Burnand KG, and Lea TM, eds: Diseases of the veins: pathology, diagnosis and treatment. London, 1988, Edward Arnold.
2. US Department of Health, Education, and Welfare: National health survey 1935-1936, Washington, DC, 1938.
3. General Register Office: Studies on medical and population subjects, #12. The survey of sickness 1943-52, Logan WPD and Brooke EM, London, H.M. Stationery Off, 1957.
4. The Sickness Survey of Denmark: The committee on the Danish national morbidity survey, Copenhagen, 1960.
5. Illness and Health Care in Canada: Canadian Sickness Survey 1950-1951. The Department of National Health and Welfare and the Dominion Bureau of Statistics, Ottawa, 1960.
6. Bobek K. et al: The study of the frequency of venous disorders and the influence of several etiologic factors, Phlebologie 19:217, 1966.
7. Widmer LK: Peripheral venous disorders: prevalence and sociomedical importance—observations in 4529 apparently healthy persons, Basle III Study, Bern Hans Huber, 1978.
8. Dickson-Wright A: The treatment of indolent ulcer of the leg, Lancet 1:457, 1931.
9. Linton RR: The communicating veins of the lower leg and the operating techniques for their ligation, Ann Surg 107:582, 1938.
10. Lockhart-Mummery HE and Smithan JH: Varicose ulcer: a study of the deep veins with special references to retrograde venography, Br J Surg 38:284, 1951.
11. Hellgren L: An epidemiology survey of skin diseases, tatooing and rheumatic diseases, Ups Linquist Wiksel, 1967.
12. Callam MJ et al: Chronic ulceration of the leg: extent of the problem and provision of care, Br Med J 290:1855, 1985.
13. Leather RP and Kupinski AM: Preoperative evaluation of the saphenous vein as a suitable graft, Semin Vasc Surg 1:51, 1988.
14. Kosinski C: Variations of the external saphenous vein, J Anat (London) 60:131, 1926.
15. O'Donnell TF et al: Doppler examination versus clinical and phlebographic detection of the location of incompetent perforating veins, Arch Surg 112:31, 1977.
16. O'Donnell TF and Shepard AD: Chronic venous insufficiency. In Jarrett F and Hirsh J, eds: Vascular surgery of the lower extremity, St. Louis, 1985, The CV Mosby Co.

17. Negus D: Perforating vein interruption in the postphlebitic syndrome. In Bergan JJ and Yao JST, eds: Surgery of the veins, New York, 1985, Grune & Stratton, Inc.
18. O'Donnell TF et al. Effect of elastic compression on venous hemodynamics in the postphlebitic limb, JAMA 242:2766, 1979.
19. Haeger K: Leg ulcers. In Hobbs JT, ed: The treatment of venous disorders, Lancaster, England, 1977 MPT.
20. Browse NL and Burnand KG: The cause of venous ulceration, Lancet 2:243, 1982.
21. Burnard KG et al: The relationship between the number of capillaries in the skin of the venous ulcer bearing area of the lower leg and the fall in foot vein pressure during exercise, Br J Surg 68:297, 1981.
22. Negus D and Cocket FB. Femoral vein pressures in postphlebitic iliac vein obstruction, Br J Surg 54:522, 1967.
23. Killewitch LA et al: Pathophysiology of venous claudication, J Vasc Surg 1:502, 1984.
24. Darke SG: Reconstructive surgery for chronic venous insufficiency in the lower limbs. In Greehalgh RA, Jamieson CW, and Nicolaides AN, eds: Vascular surgery issues in current practice, London, 1986, Grune & Stratton.
25. Haeger K: Five-year results of radical surgery for superficial varices with or without coexisting perforator insufficiency, Acta Chir Scand 131:38, 1966.
26. O'Donnell TF et al: Clinical, hemodynamic, and anatomic follow-up of direct venous reconstruction, Arch Surg 122:474, 1987.
27. Negus D, Friedgood A: The effective management of venous ulceration, Br J Surg 70:623, 1983.
28. Bauer G: The etiology of leg ulcers and their treatment by resection of popliteal vein, J Int Chir 8:937, 1948.
29. Kistner RL: Primary venous valve incompetence of the leg, Am J Surg 140:218, 1982.
30. Lodin A and Lindvall N: Congenital absence of valves of the deep veins of the leg: a factor in venous insufficiency, Arch Derm Venereol 41(suppl 45):1, 1961.
31. Porter JM et al: Reporting standards in venous disease—venous subcommittee, J Vasc Surg 8:172, 1988.
32. Shepard AD et al: Light reflection rheography: a new non-invasive test of venous function, Bruit 8:266, 1984.
33. McEnroe CS and O'Donnell TF: Noninvasive evaluation of chronic venous insufficiency. In Rutherford RB, ed: Seminars in vascular surgery, Philadelphia, 1988, WB Saunders Co.
34. O'Donnell TF, McEnroe CS, and Heggerick P: Chronic venous insufficiency, Surg Clin North Am 70:159, 1990.
35. Abramowitz HB, Queral LA, and Flinn WR: Use of photoplethysmography in the assessment of chronic venous insufficiency: a comparison to venous pressure measurements, Surgery 86:434, 1979.
36. Mitrani A: The use of light reflection rheography in the diagnosis of DVT, Clin Res 37:8A, 1989.
37. McEnroe CS, O'Donnell TF, and Mackey WC: Correlation of clinical findings with venous hemodynamics in 396 patients with chronic venous insufficiency, Am J Surg 156:148, 1988.
38. Barnes RW: Noninvasive tests for chronic venous insufficiency. In Bergan JJ and Yao JST, eds: Surgery of the veins, Philadelphia, 1985, Grune & Stratton, Inc.
39. Sigel B et al: A Doppler ultrasound method for diagnosing lower extremity venous disease, Surg Gynecol Obstet 127:339, 1986.
40. Miller SS and Foote AV: The ultrasonic detection of incompetent perforating veins, Br J Surg 61:653, 1974.
41. Folse R and Alexander RH: Directional flow detection for localizing venous valvular incompetence, Surgery 67:114, 1970.
42. Shull KS et al: Significance of popliteal reflux in relationship to ambulatory venous pressure and ulceration, Arch Surg 114:1304, 1979.
43. Moore EJ, Himmel PD, and Sumner DS: Distribution of venous valvular incompetency in patients with the post-phlebitic syndrome, J Vasc Surg 3:49, 1986.
44. Talbot SR: Use of real time imaging in identifying deep venous obstruction: a preliminary report, Bruit 6:41, 1982.
45. Flanagan LD, Sullivan ED, and Cranley JJ: Venous imaging of the extremities using real time B-mode ultrasound. In Bergan JJ and Yao JST, eds: Surgery of the veins, Philadelphia, 1985, Grune & Stratton, Inc.
46. Buchbinder D et al: B-mode imaging in the preoperative evaluation of saphenous vein, Am Surg 53:368, 1987.
47. Rollins DL et al: Use of ultrasound venography with evaluation of venous valve function, Am J Surg 154:189, 1987.
48. Kistner RL: Surgical repair of the incompetent femoral vein valve, Arch Surg 110:1336, 1975.
49. Raju S: Venous insufficiency of the lower limb and stasis ulceration: changing concepts and management, Ann Surg 197:688, 1983.
50. Raju S and Fredericks R: Valve reconstruction procedures for non-obstructive venous insufficiency: rationale, techniques and results in 107 procedures, J Vasc Surg, 1991 (in press).
51. Burnand KG et al: The relative importance of incompetent communicating veins in the production of varicose veins in venous ulcer, Surgery 82:9, 1977.
52. Schanzer H and Peirce EC: A rational approach to surgery: the chronic venous stasis syndrome, Ann Surg 195.25, 1982.
53. Pearce WH et al: Hemodynamic assessment of venous problems, Surgery 93:715, 1983.
54. Bruns-Slot V, Vermeiden I, and VanDam R: The detection of deep venous incompetence in 980 legs using the Doppler in combination with a spectral analysis, London, Sept 1986, Second International Vascular symposium.
55. Gooley NA and Sumner DS: Relationship of venous reflux to the site of venous valvular incompetence: implications for venous reconstructive surgery, J Vasc Surg 7:50, 1988.
56. Celsus AC: Of medicine in eight books, London, 1756, Wilson (translated by J Grieve).
57. Wiseman R: Eight surgical treatises, London, 1676, Meridon.
58. Starling EH: On the absorption of fluid from the connective tissue spaces, J Physiol (Lond) 19:312, 1986.
59. Clark RL, Orandi A, and Cliffton EE: Tourniquet induction of fibrinolysis, Angiology 11:367, 1960.
60. Kerstein M and Fox L: Changes in venous hemodynamics with elastic stocking surgery, Surgery 106:114, 1989.
61. Burnand KG and Layer G: Graduated elastic stockings, Br Med J 293:224, 1986.
62. Vilavicencio JL et al: Leg ulcers of venous origin. In Cameron JL, ed: Current surgical therapy-three, Toronto, 1989, BC Decker.
63. Hills NH et al: Prevention of deep vein thrombosis by intermittent compression of calf, Br Med J 1:131, 1972.
64. Wilkinson GE and MacLaren IF: Long-term review of procedure for venous perforator insufficiency, Surg Gynecol Obstet 163:117, 1986.
65. O'Donnell TF, McEnroe CS, and Mackey CS: Long-term follow-up on the management of venous ulcer, Arch Surg, 1991 (in press).
66. Cranley J: The management of venous disorders. In Rutherford R, ed: Vascular surgery, Philadelphia, 1989, WB Saunders Co.
67. Friedman SJ and SU WDD: Management of leg ulcers with hydrocolloid occlusive dressings, Arch Dermatol 120:1329, 1984.
68. Kikta MJ et al: A prospective randomized trial of Unna's boots versus hydroactive dressing in the treatment of venous stasis ulcers, J Vasc Surg 7:478, 1988.
69. Ericksson G: Comparison of two occlusive bandages in the treatment of leg ulcers, Br J Dermatol 114:227, 1986.
70. van Rijswijk L, Brown D, and Friedman S: Multicenter clinical evaluation of a hydrocolloid dressing for leg ulcers, Cutis 35:173, 1985.
71. Rubin JR et al: Unna's boots and polyurethane foam dressing for the treatment of venous ulceration, Arch Surg 125:489, 1990.
72. Fegan WG. Continuous compression treatment for injecting varicose veins, Lancet 2:109, 1963.
73. Hobbs JT: Surgery and sclerotherapy in the treatment of varicose veins: a randomized trial, Arch Surg 109:793, 1974.
74. Strothen IG, Bryson H, and Alexander S: Treatment of varicose veins by compression sclerotherapy, Br J Surg 61:387, 1974

75. Dejode LR: Injection compression treatment of varicose veins, Br J Surg 57:285, 1970.
76. Reid RG and Rothnie NG: treatment of varicose veins by compression sclerotherapy, Br J Surg 55:889, 1968.
77. Chart ADB, Jones HO, and Weddel JM: Varicose veins: a comparison of surgery and injection/compression sclerotherapy, Lancet 2:1188, 1972.
78. Hunter J: Of specific diseases, tumours, hydatids, etc. In Palmer JF, ed: The works of John Hunter, London, 1837, Longman, Reese, Orme, Brown, Green and Longman.
79. Lofgren KA: Post phlebotic syndrome (chronic deep venous insufficiency): In Haimovici H, ed: Vascular surgery principles and techniques, ed. 1, New York, McGraw-Hill, 1971.
80. Rivlin, S: The surgical core of primary varicose veins, Br J Surg 62:913, 1975.
81. Burnand KG et al: Relationship between post-phlebitic changes in the deep veins and results of surgical treatment of venous ulcers, Lancet 1:936, 1976.
82. Halliday P, Harris J, and May J. Femoral-femoral cross-over grafts (Palma operation): a long-term follow-up study. In Bergan JJ and Yao JST, eds: Surgery of the veins, New York, 1985, Grune & Stratton, Inc.
83. Palma ED and Esperson R: Vein transplants and grafts in the surgical treatment of the post-phlebitic syndrome, J Cardiovasc Surg 1:94, 1960.
84. Dale WA: Crossover vein grafts for relief of iliofemoral block, Surgery 57:608, 1965.
85. May R: Späkergebnissr nach venosom femoralis bypass, Vasa 8:67, 1974.
86. Husni EA: Issues in venous reconstruction, Vasc Diagn Ther 2:37, 1981.
87. Ferris ED and Kistner RL: Femoral vein reconstruction and the management of chronic venous insufficiency: a 14-year experience, Arch Surg 117:1571, 1982.
88. Johnson ND et al: Late objective assessment of venous valve surgery, Arch Surg 116:1461, 1981.
89. Queral LA et al: Surgical correction of chronic deep venous insufficiency by valvular transposition, Surgery 87:685, 1980.
90. Haimovici H et al: Experimental and clinical evaluation of the grafts in the venous system, Surg Gynecol Obstet 131:1173, 1970.
91. Taheri SA et al: Surgical treatment of post-phlebitic syndrome with vein valve transplant, Am J Surg 144:221, 1982.
92. Taheri SA: Pendergast DR, and Lazar E: Vein valve transplantation, Am J Surg 150:201, 1985.

Part **IV**

LYMPHEDEMA

Chapter 27

LYMPHEDEMA

Alexander Schirger
Peter Gloviczki

The term *lymphedema* describes accumulation of fluid in a part of the body—most commonly in the extremities but also in the lower part of the abdomen, the scrotum, the external genitalia, and the face. Lymphedema is caused by the inability of the lymphatic system to carry lymph, which causes stasis of the lymph. Lymphedema must be distinguished from other forms of edema of systemic, venous, or allergic origin.

Lymphatic vessels develop from mesenchymal cells. Their existence was first recognized by Gasparo Aselli (1581-1626), an Italian anatomist and surgeon at the University of Milan.[1] During an operation on a dog, designed to study the action and innervation of the diaphragm, Aselli discovered enlarged lymphatic vessels in the dog's mesentery. When he incised one of these structures, a whitish fluid was released. In a similar experiment on a second animal no such vessels were noted. Aselli realized that the difference between the two experiments was that the second animal had not been fed before the operation, and he concluded that the structures observed in the first experiment represented channels in which some substance was carried from the intestine.

Although the clinical entity of lymphedema has been recognized since ancient times, and the similarity of the grossly disfigured human extremities to the legs of an elephant has led to the term *elephantiasis*, the correlation of these disfiguring conditions with Aselli's discovery of the lymphatic system some three centuries earlier did not occur until Milroy[2] in 1928 and Allen[3] in 1934 described lymphatic malfunction. Both of these clinicians published accurate descriptions of the clinical entities of idiopathic lymphedema. The introduction of lymphangiography into clinical medicine by Kinmonth et al[4] has aided in establishing the link between the areas of knowledge for which Aselli laid the foundation 300 years earlier and the conclusions derived from the astute clinical observations and vast bedside experience of eminent clinicians such as Milroy and Allen.

ANATOMY AND PATHOPHYSIOLOGY

Lymph is collected from the interstitial space by the initial or terminal lymphatic capillaries and then transported through major collecting lymph channels. In the lower extremity, major collecting channels are located both in the deep compartments and subcutaneously. The deep lymphatic system follows the tibial, popliteal, and femoral vessels. The more significant superficial lymphatic system carries 80% of the lower extremity lymph fluid. This system consists of 10 to 15 large lymphatic channels that are located mostly along the greater saphenous vein. The two systems join in the inguinal nodes, and the lymph then is transported through iliac and paraaortic lymph channels and nodes into the thoracic duct. The duct, which also carries chyle from the mesenteric lymph vessels, has an average output of 1.5 L daily, which is emptied into the venous system at the left jugulosubclavian junction. The lymphatic system of the left upper extremity and the left side of the neck and head drains into the thoracic duct, but that of the right upper extremity and the right side of the head and neck drains through the right cervical trunk directly into the right subclavian vein.

Unidirectional flow in the collecting lymphatic channels is ensured by the presence of fine valves. Congenital or acquired obstruction of lymphatic flow results in accumulation of protein-rich fluid in the subcutaneous space. Because lymphatic capillaries of the dermis do not contain valves, the lymph refluxes through these dermal lymphatics, a phenomenon called *dermal reflux*. This can be demonstrated in patients with lymphedema by intradermal injection of blue dye. If collateral lymphatic circulation is not satisfactory and the function of the tissue macrophages is exhausted, lymphedema develops. The mechanism of the de-

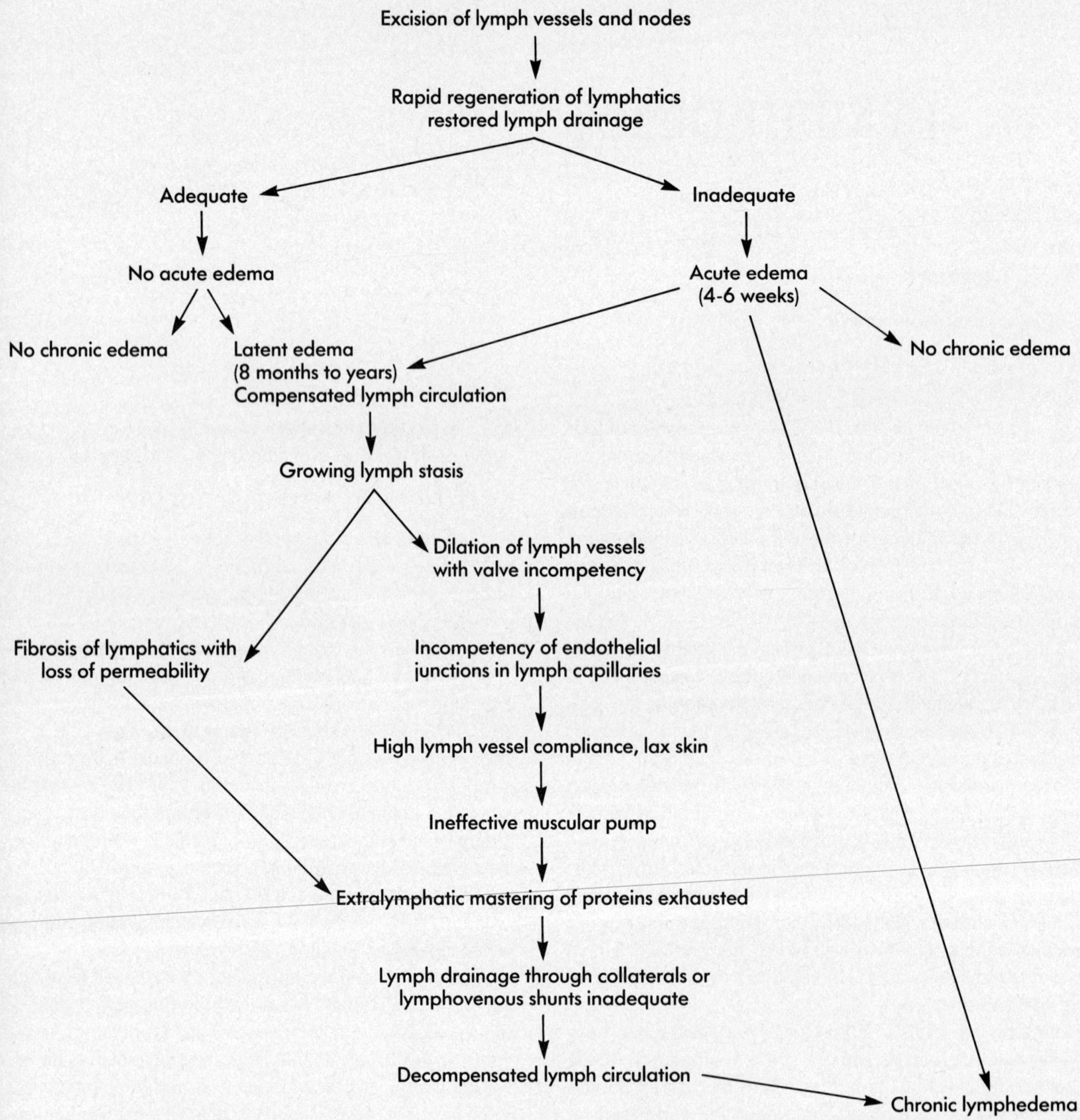

Fig. 27-1. Stages in development of postoperative lymphedema. (From Gloviczki P and Schirger A: Lymphedema. In Spittell JA Jr, ed: Clinical medicine, Philadelphia, 1985, Harper & Row, Publishers.)

> **Classifications of lymphedema**
>
> ***Primary (idiopathic)***
>
> ***Congenital***
> Simple
> Hereditary or familial (Milroy's disease)
> ***Lymphedema praecox***
> ***Lymphedema tarda***
>
> ***Secondary***
>
> ***Obstructive***
> Malignant occlusion by metastasis or invasion
> Interruption of lymphatic channels or nodes by surgery or radiation therapy
>
> ***Inflammatory***
> Nontropical
> Tropical

velopment of acute and chronic lymphedema after surgical excision of lymph vessels and lymph nodes is outlined in Fig. 27-1. It is not unusual for chronic lymphedema to develop several months or even years after interruption of the lymphatic transport system.

CLASSIFICATION

Lymphedema can be classified as primary (idiopathic) or secondary (see the accompanying box). Primary lymphedema may be present at birth or make its appearance later in life. When present at birth, it may occur in a single patient or cluster in a family. It is to this form of congenital familial lymphedema that the eponym "Milroy's disease" is properly applied because it corresponds to the description by Milroy[2] in 1928. When primary lymphedema makes its appearance later in life, it is usually at the time of menarche or in the late teens or early 20s. It was because of this temporal relationship that Allen[3] assigned the term *lymphedema praecox* to the noncongenital type of primary lymphedema.

Experience has taught clinicians that when lymphedema does make its appearance later in life, most commonly it is because of an identifiable cause and is therefore secondary in nature. Nevertheless, one occasionally may see an older patient with truly primary lymphedema. To this group of cases Kinmonth et al[4] applied the term lymphedema tarda.

Secondary lymphedema may result from obstruction of, interruption in, or replacement* of lymphatic channels and nodes.

*By a mechanical process such as trauma, surgical intervention, invasion by tumor, or a fibrosing process including radiation fibrosis.

The other form of secondary lymphedema is caused by an inflammatory process in which lymphatic channels are obstructed by acute or recurrent lymphangitis and cellulitis. In the Western world the most common cause of inflammatory lymphedema is streptococcal infection, usually via a portal of entry caused by trichophytosis, but in many other parts of the world, Bancroft's filariasis and other parasitic infections account for this form of lymphedema.

CLINICAL PICTURE

Primary lymphedema

The clinical picture of *congenital lymphedema,* that of a child born with lymphedema, whether familial or nonfamilial, is identical. There is a visible enlargement of the extremity or extremities or affected parts of the body. The swelling is painless and is more resistant to pitting than venous edema; the extremity color is normal. There are no signs of venous insufficiency or venous malformations. Although congenital lymphedema may involve only one extremity, we have seen it in both lower extremities and in the hands and arms as well. External genitalia and parts of the face also may be affected. During the first year of life, when the child is supine most of the time, gravity does not play a significant role, and the swelling may not become apparent until the child is fully ambulatory.

Association of congenital lymphedema with other congenital abnormalities—such as Turner's syndrome,[5,6] congenital absence of the nails,[7] bilateral pleural effusion, and the presence of yellow nails (referred to as "the yellow nail syndrome")—has been described.[8] In rare instances children with the congenital familial type of lymphedema have been noted to have an extra row of eyelashes.[9]

Lymphedema praecox is the form of lymphedema that makes its appearance around puberty (during the mid or late teens) or, rarely, at the beginning of the third decade. In his description of 300 such patients, Allen et al[3,10] coined the term "lymphedema praecox." Data from Allen's series and from a later series[11] at the Mayo Clinic revealed a preponderance of cases in women with a female-to-male ratio of approximately 10:1. In congenital lymphedema, by definition, the swelling is detected by family members or attendant physicians or nurses. In lymphedema praecox it is the patient who most commonly calls the condition to the attention of his or her physician. The first thing that may be noted is a painless, spontaneously occurring swelling, usually on the dorsum of the foot and gradually involving the ankle and lower leg and the remainder of the forefoot and toes, which are often squared (Figs. 27-2 and 27-3).

Characteristically, ulceration is absent, and there are none of the hallmarks of deep venous insufficiency, such as increased pigmentation, evidence of enlarged collateral veins, or ulceration. The swelling is painless and is more resistant to pitting than venous edema. In a Mayo Clinic series[11] in about one third of the cases there was an antedating trau-

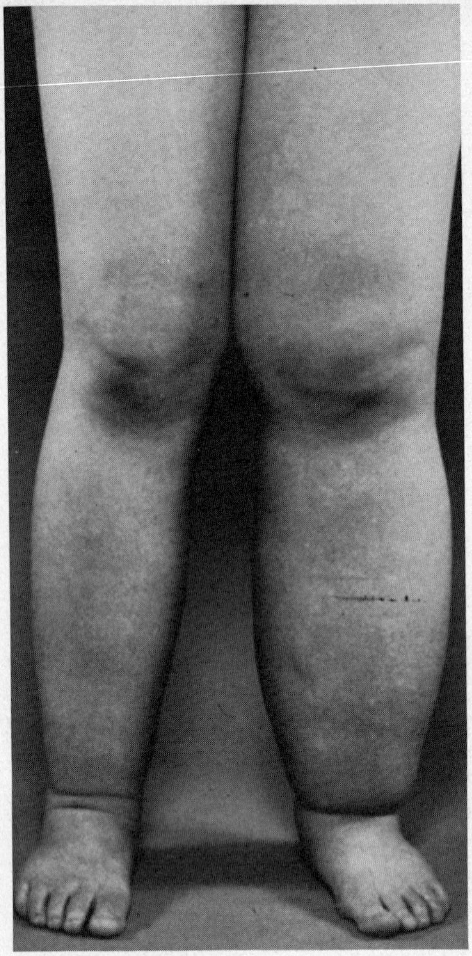

Fig. 27-2. Idiopathic lymphedema (praecox type) in a 19-year-old woman.

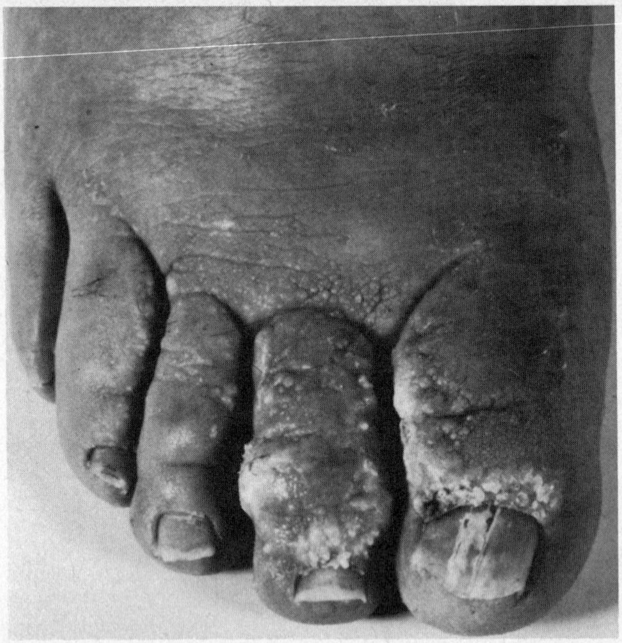

Fig. 27-3. Squaring of toes in a 47-year-old man with secondary lymphedema (obstructive type). (From Gloviczki P and Schirger A: Lymphedema. In Spittell JA Jr, ed: Clinical medicine, Philadelphia, 1985, Harper & Row, Publishers.)

matic event such as a contusion. At first the swelling in the extremity will disappear after a night's rest in the horizontal position, but if allowed to persist, only prolonged periods of bed rest (often with mechanical attempts to resolve the swelling) will result in its disappearance. In Allen's original series 13% of the patients had a history of complicating lymphangitis and cellulitis. The swelling may be unilateral or bilateral and, as in primary lymphedema of the congenital type, may be associated with other congenital abnormalities such as yellow nails[12] or with pleural effusions,[13] primary pulmonary hypertension, unequal breasts, bronchiectasis,[14] and pes cavus.[15] In children the lymphedema of the extremities may be associated with intestinal lymphangiectasia and accompanying gastrointestinal symptoms, resulting in failure to grow.[16] In rare instances hereditary intermittent cholestasis may be associated with lymphedema praecox.[17]

In the series of cases of primary and secondary lymphedema reported from the Mayo Clinic, the majority of patients with primary lymphedema had onset of swelling before the age of 39. However, there are genuine cases of primary lymphedema in which onset of swelling occurs later in life, and no cause can be identified. Thus the appearance of lymphedema before age 39, in the absence of signs and symptoms of acute lymphangitis and cellulitis, indicates an idiopathic process in all likelihood.

Secondary lymphedema

Secondary lymphedema may be caused by obstruction of the lymphatic pathways by trauma, surgery, irradiation, or replacement of lymph channels or lymph nodes by metastatic tumor, or it may be caused by inflammatory changes (Fig. 27-4). The hallmark of obstructive lymphedema is the fairly abrupt onset, usually the unilateral nature of the swelling initially, and the absence of inflammatory changes. Onset after age 39 distinctly points to this possibility. In a Mayo Clinic series[18] in men, carcinoma of the prostate was the most common cause of secondary obstructive lymphedema; in women, carcinoma of the ovary was high on the list of the cancerous tumors, but lymphoma appeared to be more common. Lymphedema of an upper extremity after radical or modified radical mastectomy is a distinct form of secondary obstructive lymphedema. The swelling may appear at variable intervals postoperatively (Fig. 27-5).

The hallmarks of inflammatory lymphedema are recurrent episodes of lymphangitis and cellulitis, characterized by acute onset, shaking chills, a temperature up to 40.6° C, and either de novo onset of swelling or intensification

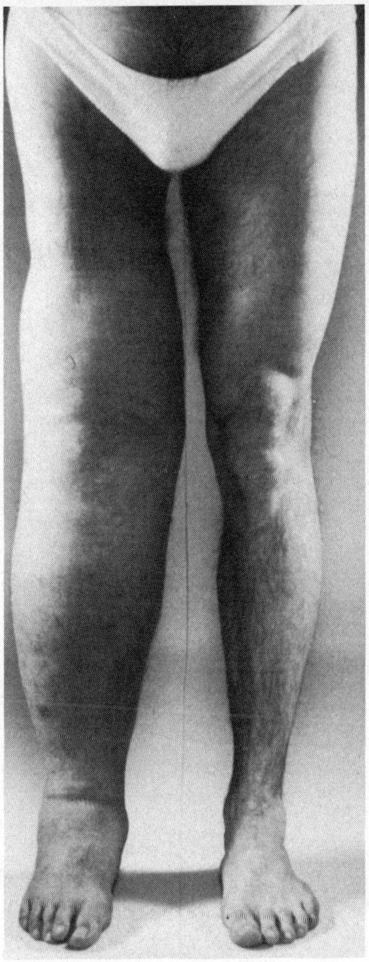

Fig. 27-4. Secondary lymphedema of lower extremities in a 55-year-old man. (From Gloviczki P et al: J Vasc Surg 7:647, 1988. By Permission of the Society for Vascular and the North American Chapter of the International Society for Cardiovascular Surgery.)

Fig. 27-5. Lymphedema of left upper extremity after mastectomy.

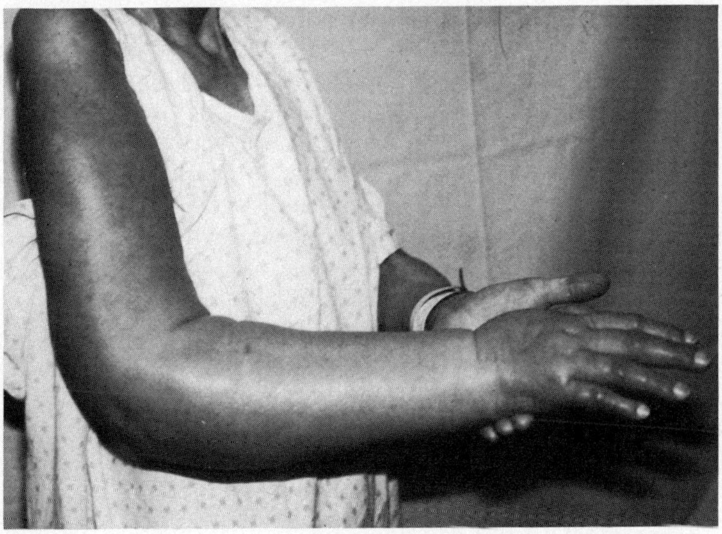

A

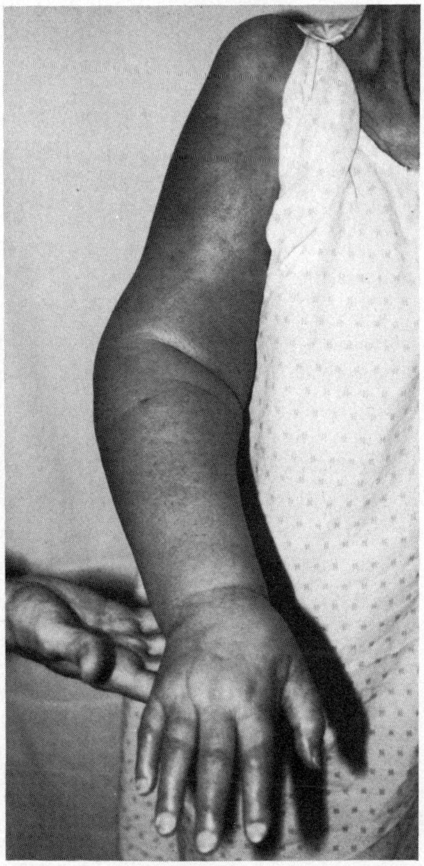

B

of swelling already present. There usually are red streaks on the feet, lower extremities, and thighs along the course of lymphatic channels and palpable, enlarged, tender lymph nodes in the retropopliteal space and groin. In addition, there may be a diffuse cellulitis involving the entire leg. Frequently, the portal of entry for the offending organism, most commonly a streptococcus, can be detected as dermal fissures in the web spaces between the toes, indicating trichophytosis. The systemic symptoms of fever and chills may be accompanied by an intense malaise, headaches, nausea, vomiting, and diffuse sweats. Although acute thrombophlebitis may be accompanied by an increase in body temperature, the degree of increase seen in acute lymphangitis and cellulitis is seldom encountered in a thrombophlebitis, with the exception of pelvic septic thrombophlebitis. In Third World countries filariasis still is a frequent and important cause of secondary inflammatory lymphedema.

DIAGNOSIS

Diagnosis of lymphedema is based on the history, the characteristic appearance of the involved extremity, and the absence of symptoms and signs indicating a systemic cause for the swelling or arterial or deep venous insufficiency. Arterial pulses characteristically are normal unless the swelling is excessive. The venous pattern is not prominent, and there is no tenderness along the course of the deep veins of the calf and thigh.

The age at onset is of great aid in the differential diagnosis of primary or secondary lymphedema, even though a swelling that is idiopathic may develop late in life. Of the tests found helpful in confirming the diagnostic impression of either primary or secondary lymphedema, the ultrasonographic examination of the pelvis and prostate is valuable, as is computed tomographic examination of the abdomen and pelvis. Although lymphangiography, introduced by Kinmonth[19] and widely used, has aided in the diagnosis and the pathophysiologic understanding of lymphedema, we seldom find it necessary to use this procedure. If it is necessary to ascertain the lymphatic flow, we prefer lymphoscintigraphy, a less invasive examination.

Lymphoscintigraphy uses technetium-99m (^{99m}Tc) as a radioactive label and antimony trisulfide for labeling particles. We inject 400 to 500 μCi of ^{99m}Tc-labeled antimony trisulfide colloid (Cadema Medical Products, Inc., Middletown, NY) subcutaneously into the second interdigital space in the foot or the hand (0.3 to 0.6 mL). We ask the patient to squeeze a rubber ball or to perform toe stands for 3 minutes after the injection. In the first hour 12-minute images are obtained with the gamma camera (Fig. 27-6). At 1 and 3 hours additional 5-minute images are made. In selected cases, images are recorded at 6 and 24 hours.

Semiquantitative evaluation of the lymphatic drainage and visual interpretation of the different image patterns in 190 lymphoscintigraphic examinations at the Mayo Clinic

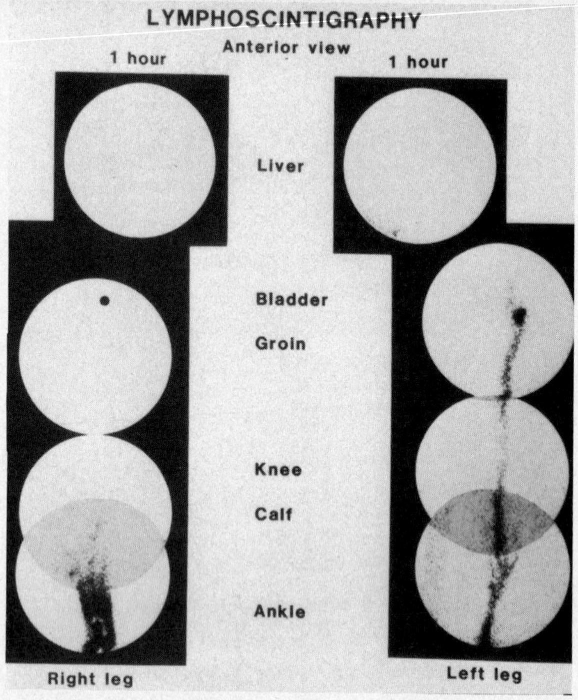

Fig. 27-6. Lymphoscintigram (*anterior view*) in patient with right lower extremity lymphedema.

showed a sensitivity of 92% and a specificity of 100% for distinguishing lymphedema from edemas of other origin.[20] We could not distinguish primary from secondary lymphedema consistently by using this method. Because lymphoscintigraphy is a reliable and safe method and has no side effects, it has replaced contrast lymphangiography in our institution for the routine evaluation of a swollen extremity. For a differential diagnosis of the swollen limb see Chapter 36.

TREATMENT

Medical therapy

There is no known cure for lymphedema once the swelling appears. At present, with few exceptions, we have no way of restoring lymphatic flow. The aim of treatment thus should be to remove as much fluid as possible from the affected extremity and to maintain an edema-free state.

In our experience the removal of fluid is best done in the hospital. The extremity is elevated in a lymphedema sling. A diuretic, such as furosemide, is administered by mouth while the patient is being protected from the hazards of venous thromboembolism by subcutaneous injection of heparin in doses of 5000 to 10,000 units twice daily. Because a vigorous diuresis may ensue, attention needs to be focused on potassium losses and, if necessary, on potassium replacement. This becomes more imperative in patients who are prone to cardiac arrhythmias or who are on a digitalis regimen. However, diuresis does not change the protein content of the subcutaneous space, and its effect on edema of lymphatic origin is temporary.

The drainage of the fluid from the affected extremity is aided by the use of the lymphedema sling, which allows the patient to keep the extremity elevated without flexing the back. It also affords periods of rest, which provide comfort and will not jeopardize the gains already made by having the extremity elevated for several hours. In some patients maximal fluid drainage can be obtained in 24 to 48 hours; in others several days are necessary in the hospital setting.

Once all the fluid that can be removed has been, the patient is measured for an elastic stocking. If the lymphedema involves only the leg, a knee-length stocking suffices. If it involves the thigh, thigh-length stockings or a pantyhose type of support may be necessary. It usually is best for the patient to remain in the hospital with this treatment continued until the made-to-measure stocking is delivered and tested by ambulation.

Edema can also be removed from lymphedematous limbs by mechanically pumping the limbs for 2 to 8 hours to make them edema free. Of the different intermittent pneumatic compression devices available, we prefer those that have several cells for sequential compression.

The hope is that early drainage of the fluid and use of an elastic stocking will prevent accumulation of lymphedematous fluid and avoid the resulting overgrowth of tissue, induration, fibrosis, and eventual disfiguring distortion of the extremity. The intermittent use of a thiazide diuretic, 3 days a week, will aid in maintaining the decrease in fluid accumulation in the lymphedematous extremity. If more than one episode of lymphangitis and cellulitis occurs, the intermittent use of antibiotic prophylaxis is indicated. We prescribe penicillin VK, 500 mg orally four times daily for 7 to 10 days, or, in patients allergic to penicillin, erythromycin, 250 mg four times daily for 7 to 10 days[21] each month for a minimum of 12 months. Good skin and nail care, and especially the early treatment of tinea pedis, are important to prevent portals of entry for bacterial invasion.

Some patients find it helpful to have a period of rest at midday with their extremities elevated. Others use an intermittent pneumatic compression device during the night to massage the fluid out of the affected extremity.

The goal of treatment of lymphedema is the achievement and maintenance of as normal-appearing an extremity as possible. This is particularly important for children during their period of physical, social, and emotional growth. We try not to interdict in young patients those activities that clearly will not aggravate the lymphedema. All forms of exercise involving the legs, other then contact sports, are encouraged. Swimming seems to be ideally suited as a disciplined, regular, repetitive activity because the water exerts pressure on the extremity during the time that the muscle pump is being used.

Surgery

Despite the best efforts medical therapy will fail in some patients. Then, surgical consultation needs to be obtained to determine whether an operation will help to control the swelling. In general, there are two types of operations—excisional or debulking operations, and the so-called physiologic operations, which include microvascular reconstruction of the lymph drainage with lymphovenous anastomosis or lymph vessel transplantation. No procedure currently available is going to cure the disease.

In the excisional or debulking operations first introduced by Sir Havelok Charles, some or most of the edematous subcutaneous tissue and the underlying fascia are resected. The skin of the extremity may be so diseased that it cannot be used for coverage, and skin grafting to the entire excised area has to be performed. Wound healing can be a significant problem, and additional skin grafting frequently is needed. There may remain a difference in circumference between the edematous and excised areas, at the ankle or at the knee, creating a cosmetic deformity. Joint stiffness, secondary skin changes, hypesthesia or burning sensation, or hyperesthesia at and distal to the operated area may occur. For us, the only indication for excisional operation is disabling severe lymphedema—that is elephantiasis. We favor the staged excisional procedure[22] originally described by Homans[23] and modified by several other authors.[19,24,25] We make every attempt to use local skin flaps for coverage after excision.

Thompson's buried dermal flap operation is partly excisional and partly a physiologic operation. Thompson[26] claimed to improve lymphatic drainage of the superficial tissue to the deep compartments by suturing one of the skin flaps down to the muscles. Although the improvement probably is only the result of excision of some of the edematous tissue,[27] we have had patients who were pleased with the outcome many years afterward. Because of persisting lymphedema, these patients need continuous, conservative treatment, but problems with healing the incision are less than with other excisional operations.

The enteromesenteric bridge operation was suggested by Kinmonth.[19] He reported decreased edema in several patients with primary lymphedema who had proximal pelvic lymphatic obstruction. Postoperative lymphangiography in three patients confirmed good lymphatic drainage from the inguinal lymph nodes to the mesenteric lymphatic circulation.

Perfection of microsurgical techniques has made direct reconstructions of the lymph vessels possible. Lymph node-to-vein and lymph vessel-to-vein anastomoses have been performed for more than 20 years now, but long-term effectiveness and patency have yet to be demonstrated with objective tests. O'Brien and Shafiroff[28] reported an improvement in two thirds of their patients treated surgically; how-

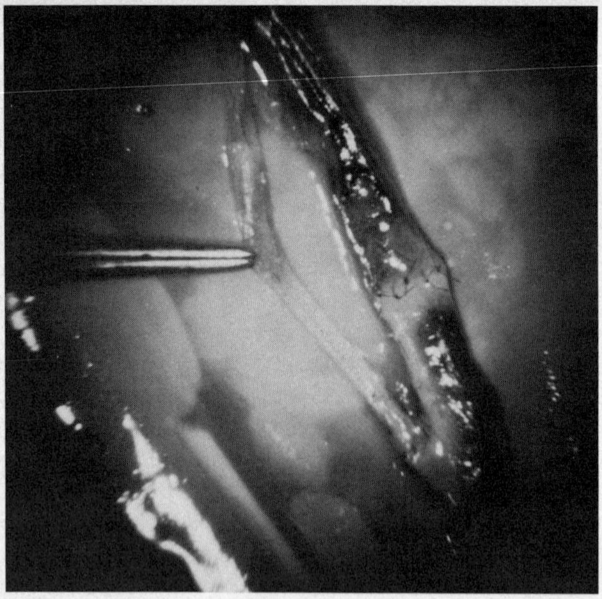

Fig. 27-7. Lymphaticovenous anastomosis in patient with secondary lymphedema.

ever, in many cases an additional excisional operation also was performed.

In our laboratory we found patency of lymphovenous anastomoses in dogs up to 8 months after the operation by using contrast cinelymphangiography.[29] Our experience with 18 patients treated surgically has been reported;[30] 14 underwent successful lymph vessel-to-vein anastomosis. Decrease in limb circumference, frequency of postoperative cellulitis, patient satisfaction, and lymphoscintigraphic findings were used to assess the results. Only one of seven patients with primary lymphedema and four of seven with secondary lymphedema showed improvement at a mean of 36 months after the operation (Figs. 27-7 and 27-8). However, lymphoscintigraphy can only provide indirect evidence of patency. We continue to perform this operation in selected patients with secondary lymphedema who have no history of cellulitis. We admit that contrast lymphangiography could be the only test that proves late patency. However, this procedure is invasive and is uncomfortable for the patient, and we are reluctant to advise it unless it has definite therapeutic consequences. Worsening of lymphedema has been described after lymphangiography.[28]

A

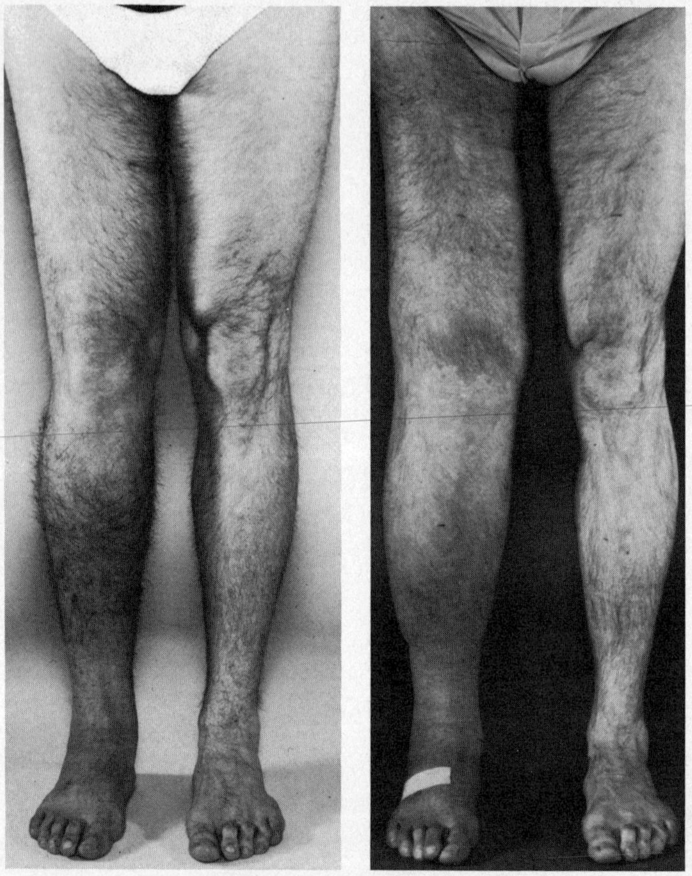

B

Fig. 27-8. At 3 (**A**) and 12 (**B**) months after lymphaticovenous anastomosis (same case as in Fig. 27-4). (**A** from Gloviczki P et al: J Vasc Surg 7:647, 1988. By Permission of the Society for Vascular and the North American Chapter of the International Society for Cardiovascular Surgery.)

Baumeister et al[31] performed lymph vessel transplantation from the thigh to the arm to treat patients with postmastectomy lymphedema. Two years after the operation, objective improvement was found in 22 of the 23 patients. The same group performed suprapubic lymph vessel transplantation to treat unilateral secondary lower extremity lymphedema, with similar good result. This operation currently is under evaluation by other centers, including ours.

Results of surgical interventions for chronic lymphedema are far from satisfactory at this time. Because the number of patients needing surgical attention is not large, we believe that surgical treatment for lymphedema should be performed only by those who have special interest and expertise in this field.

LATE COMPLICATIONS

In lymphedema the deleterious sequelae generally are only esthetic and emotional. In some cases there may be loss of working time because of acute increases in swelling such as when acute lymphangitis and cellulitis develop. Occasionally, a late and serious life-threatening complication may occur—the appearance of a malignant lymphangiosarcoma originating from the distorted, enlarged lymphatic channels. This was first described in postmastectomy lymphedema by Stewart and Treves.[32] It also may be seen, although rarely, in patients with idiopathic lymphedema of long duration. The eponym "Stewart-Treves syndrome" has been applied to the former circumstance, and in the latter the eponym "Kettle syndrome" has been used.[33] The clinical picture is that of a new lesion appearing in the skin of the affected extremity (Figs. 27-9 to 27-11). The patient at first identifies the bluish flat lesion as a bruise, even though being unable to recall a trauma that would have caused such a bruise. Despite the absence of original trauma and of any further trauma, the bruise seems to enlarge, and eventually satellite lesions appear. The central or primary lesion eventually may ulcerate.

Such a sequence of events should lead the clinician to

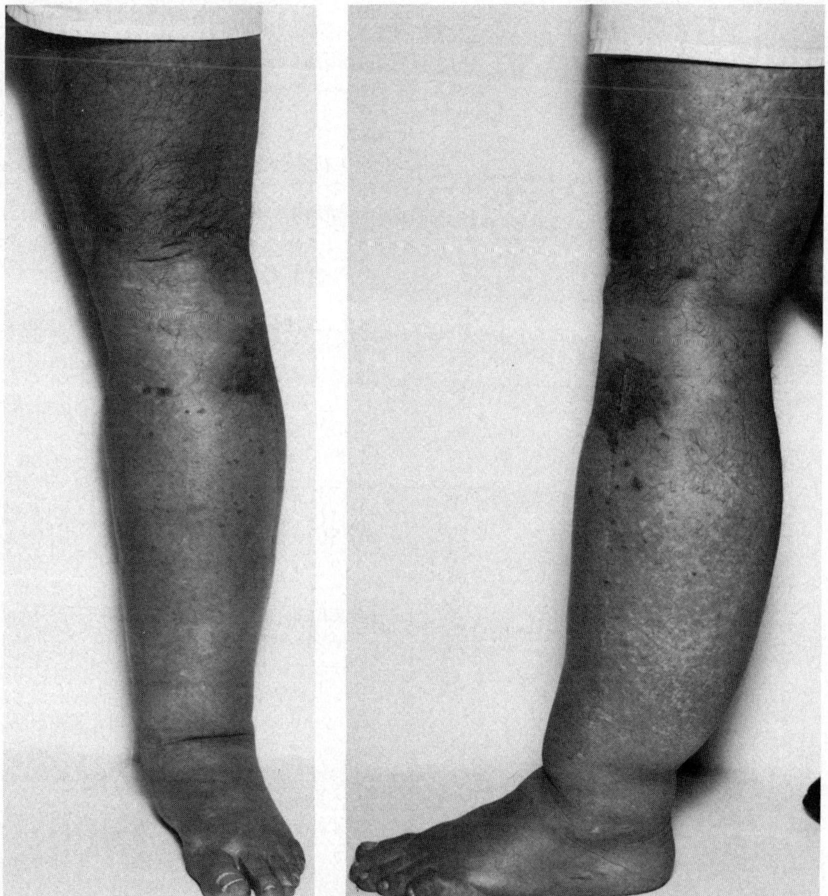

Fig. 27-9. Idiopathic lymphedema of 25 years' duration and early appearance of lymphangiosarcoma in a 52-year-old man. (From Schirger A and Peterson LFA: Lymphedema. In Juergens JL, Spittell JA Jr, and Fairbairn JF II, eds: Allen-Barker-Hines peripheral vascular diseases, ed 5, Philadelphia, 1980, WB Saunders Co. By permission of Mayo Foundation.)

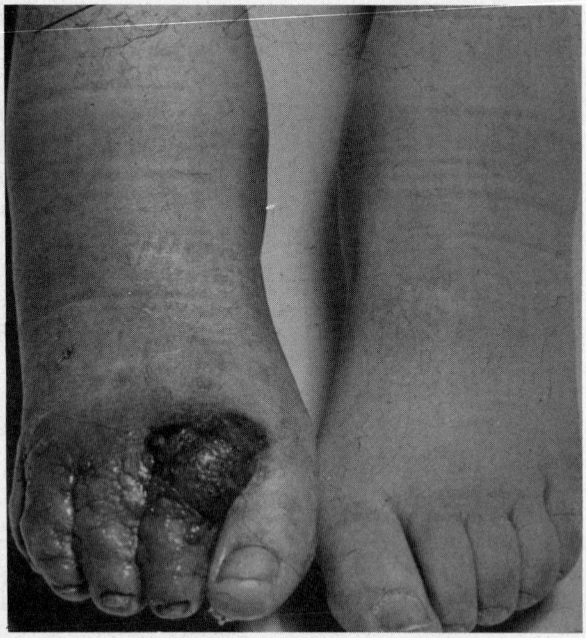

Fig. 27-10. Early lymphangiosarcoma in a 24-year-old man with idiopathic lymphedema. (From Schirger A: Cardiovasc Clin 13(2):293, 1983. By permission of FA Davis Co.)

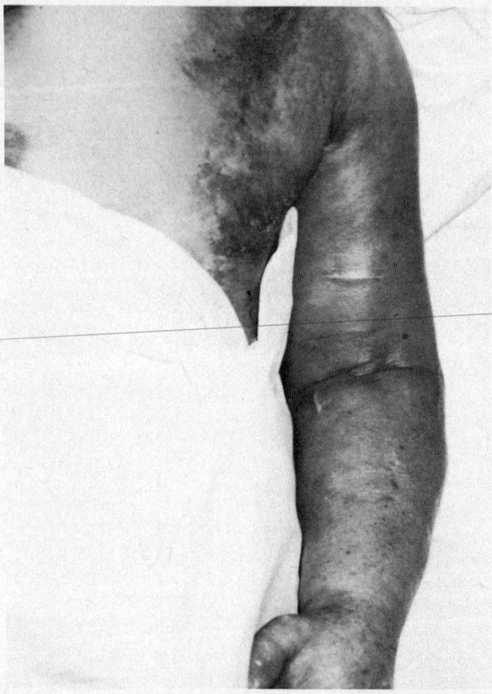

Fig. 27-11. Postmastectomy lymphedema of 9 years' duration in an 82-year-old woman, complicated by lymphangiosarcoma.

suspect lymphangiosarcoma and mandates immediate biopsy and appropriate therapy.[34] Unfortunately, this therapy involves fairly radical surgery, because wide excision is insufficient and blood-borne metastasis occurs early. Because of this, an appropriate high amputation, sometimes followed by radiation therapy, usually is favored. At the present time there is no proven method of chemotherapy. We have observed one patient for over 20 years who was cured by a high amputation of a lymphangiosarcoma of many years' duration that occurred in a lymphedematous extremity.

REFERENCES

1. Juergens JL, Spittell JA Jr, and Fairbairn JF II: Gaspare Aselli. In Allen-Barker-Hines peripheral vascular diseases, ed 5, Philadelphia, 1980, WB Saunders Co.
2. Milroy WF: Chronic hereditary edema: Milroy's disease, JAMA 91:1172, 1928.
3. Allen EV: Lymphedema of the extremities: classification, etiology and differential diagnosis; a study of three hundred cases, Arch Intern Med 54:606, 1934.
4. Kinmonth JB et al: Primary lymphoedema: clinical and lymphangiographic studies of a series of 107 patients in which the lower limbs were affected, Br J Surg 45:1, 1957.
5. Benson PF, Gough MH, and Polani PE: Lymphangiography and chromosome studies in females with lymphoedema and possible ovarian dysgenesis, Arch Dis Child 40:27, 1965.
6. Courtecuisse V et al: Lympoedeme tardif dans le syndrome de Turner, Arch Fr Pediatr 35:988, 1978.
7. Maisels DO: Anonychia in association with lymphoedema, Br J Plast Surg 19:37, 1966.
8. Siegelman SS, Heckman BH, and Hasson J: Lymphedema, pleural effusions and yellow nails: associated immunologic deficiency, Dis Chest 56:114, 1969.
9. Robinow M, Johnson GF, and Verhagen AD: Distichiasis-lymphedema: a hereditary syndrome of multiple congenital defects, Am J Dis Child 119:343, 1970.
10. Allen EV and Ghormley RK: Lymphedema of the extremities: etiology, classification and treatment; report of 300 cases, Ann Intern Med 9:516, 1935.
11. Schirger A, Harrison EG Jr, and Janes JM: Idiopathic lymphedema: review of 131 cases, JAMA 182:14, 1962.
12. Yellow nails and oedema, Br Med J 4:130, 1972.
13. Runyon BA, Forker EL, and Sopko JA: Pleural-fluid kinetics in a patient with primary lymphedema, pleural effusions, and yellow nails, Am Rev Respir Dis 119:821, 1979.
14. Bowers D: Unequal breasts, yellow nails, bronchiectasis and lymphedema, Can Med Assoc J 100:437, 1969.
15. Jackson BT and Kinmonth JB: Pes cavus and lymphoedema: an unusual familial syndrome, J Bone Joint Surg 52B:518, 1970.
16. Vardy PA, Lebenthal E, and Shwachman H: Intestinal lymphangiectasia: a reappraisal, Pediatrics 55:842, 1975.
17. Aagenaes Ø: Hereditary recurrent cholestasis with lymphoedema—two new families, Acta Paediatr Scand 63:465, 1974.
18. Smith RD, Spittell JA Jr, and Schirger A: Secondary lymphedema of the leg: its characteristics and diagnostic implications, JAMA 185:80, 1963.
19. Kinmonth JB: The lymphatics: surgery, lymphography and diseases of the chyle and lymph systems, London, 1982, Edward Arnold.
20. Gloviczki P et al: Noninvasive evaluation of the swollen extremity: experiences with 190 lymphoscintigraphic examinations, J Vasc Surg 9:683, 1989.

21. Babb RR et al: Prophylaxis of recurrent lymphangitis complicating lymphedema, JAMA 195:871, 1966.
22. Sakulsky SB et al: Lymphedema: results of surgical treatment in 64 patients (1936-1964), Lymphology 10:15, 1977.
23. Homans J: The treatment of elephantiasis of the legs: a preliminary report, N Engl J Med 215:1099, 1936.
24. Miller TA: A surgical approach to lymphedema, Am J Surg 134:191, 1977.
25. Servelle M: Pathologie vasculaire, vol 3, Pathologie lymphatique, Paris, 1975, Masson.
26. Thompson N: Buried dermal flap operation for chronic lymphedema of the extremities: ten-year survey of results in 79 cases, Plast Reconstr Surg 45:541, 1970.
27. Sawhney CP: Evaluation of Thompson's buried dermal flap operation for lymphoedema of the limbs: a clinical and radioisotopic study, Br J Plast Surg 27:278, 1974.
28. O'Brien BM and Shafiroff BB: Microlymphaticovenous and resectional surgery in obstructive lymphedema, World J Surg 3:3, 1979.
29. Gloviczki P et al: The natural history of microsurgical lymphovenous anastomoses: an experimental study, J Vasc Surg 4:148, 1986.
30. Gloviczki P et al: Microsurgical lymphovenous anastomosis for treatment of lymphedema: a critical review, J Vasc Surg 7:647, 1988.
31. Baumeister RGH et al: Experimental basis and first application of clinical lymph vessel transplantation of secondary lymphedema, World J Surg 5:401, 1981.
32. Stewart FW and Treves N: Lymphangiosarcoma in postmastectomy lymphedema: a report of six cases in elephantiasis chirurgica, Cancer 1:64, 1948.
33. Kettle EH: Tumours arising from endothelium, Proc R Soc Med 11(part 3):19, 1918.
34. Taswell HF, Soule EH, and Coventry MB: Lymphangiosarcoma arising in chronic lymphedematous extremities: report of thirteen cases and review of literature, J Bone Joint Surg 44A:277, 1962.

Part V

VASCULAR DISEASES OF DIVERSE ORIGIN

Chapter 28

THORACIC OUTLET SYNDROMES

Edwin G. Beven

The thoracic outlet syndromes are a group of disorders that produce symptoms affecting the neck, shoulder, and upper extremity by compression or mechanical irritation of the brachial plexus, subclavian artery, or subclavian vein as these structures pass through the thoracic outlet (Fig. 28-1). The syndromes are divided into three types: neurologic, arterial, and venous, based on the predominant structure compromised.

The neurologic type is the most common type, accounting for 95% of all thoracic outlet patients, and results from compression of elements of the brachial plexus. It occurs mainly in young to middle-aged adults from their second to fifth decade with a 3:1 predominance in women.

The arterial type is the least common, accounting for 1% to 2% of all thoracic outlet patients, but it is the most serious. It can produce arterial lesions with thromboembolic complications that can jeopardize the viability of the upper extremity.

The venous type is caused by compression of the subclavian vein and accounts for about 3% to 4% of all thoracic outlet patients. It is most commonly observed from the third to the fourth decade and is more prevalent in men.

A small number of patients have symptoms of compression of more than one of these structures, exhibiting a combination of neurologic and vascular symptoms.

The thoracic outlet syndrome has been surrounded by confusion, misconceptions, and controversy in regard to etiology, diagnosis, and methods of treatment.[1-6] Thus depending on the offending structure or maneuver thought to cause compression of the neurovascular structures in the cervical-axillary canal, the thoracic outlet syndrome has been known in the past as *cervical rib syndrome*[7]; *scalenus anticus syndrome*, *Naffziger's syndrome*[8,9]; *first thoracic rib syndrome*[10]; *costoclavicular syndrome*[11-13]; and *hyperabduction syndrome*.[14] Peet et al, in 1956, recommended that all of these clinical entities be grouped together as the *thoracic outlet syndrome*.[15] Two years later Rob and Standeven referred to it as the *thoracic outlet compression syndrome* in describing arterial complications of the syndrome.[16] During the last three decades the term *thoracic outlet syndrome* has become the accepted name, but its plural, *thoracic outlet syndromes*, is probably a better term because it denotes more than one group or subdivision.[4]

The treatment of thoracic outlet syndromes has also been controversial. Paralleling the historic development of the differently named syndromes that describe the cause of the compression of the neurovascular bundle, surgical treatment was directed at the corresponding offending anatomic structure by excision of the cervical rib,[17] first thoracic rib,[18] or by division of the anterior scalene muscle[19] or the pectoralis minor tendon.[20]

Finally, much controversy has centered around the diagnosis of the neurologic type of thoracic outlet syndrome, which paradoxically is the most common type. The difficulty in diagnosing this type of thoracic outlet syndrome lies in the lack of objective signs and thus the lack of confirmatory diagnostic tests. Problems also arise from the diffuse distribution of pain and paresthesias experienced by patients, causing them considerable difficulty in describing their symptoms and their location. Because of these problems, some authors have even questioned the existence of the neurologic type of thoracic outlet syndrome.

NEUROLOGIC TYPE

Etiology

The anatomic abnormalities in the thoracic outlet that can cause neurologic symptoms are various skeletal or soft tissue anomalies that compress, displace, or irritate the brachial

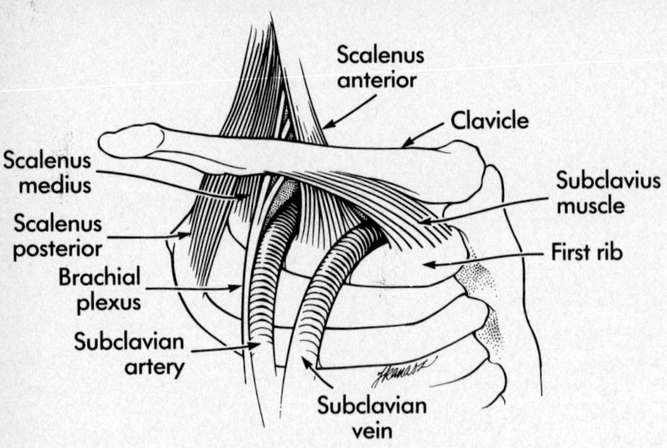

Fig. 28-1. Schematic drawing of the right thoracic outlet. The subclavian artery and brachial plexus exit through the scalene triangle, bordered by the anterior and middle scalene muscles and the first rib. The subclavian vein crosses the first rib between the anterior scalene and subclavius muscles anteriorly.

plexus as it exits between the anterior and middle scalene muscles (see Fig. 28-1). Although the most obvious and easily detected of these are diverse osseous abnormalities (i.e., cervical ribs, elongated transverse process of C7 vertebra with its fibrous band that functionally acts as a cervical rib, hypoplasia or anomalies of the first thoracic rib, and abnormal callous formation or angulation from clavicular or first rib fractures), these anomalies account for only 8% of all causes of thoracic outlet syndrome (Fig. 28-2). In contrast, the more common soft tissue structural changes in the thoracic outlet, such as various congenital myofascial bands or anomalies of the scalene muscles[21,22] that compress the brachial plexus, are more elusive since their contribution to the clinical syndrome can only be inferred from the symptoms they produce and can only be recognized by the surgeon at operation.

Roos[23] has identified 10 different congenital fibromuscular bands that compress the brachial plexus at its lower C8 and T1 nerves and 7 other anomalies of the anterior scalene muscle that encroach on the brachial plexus at its upper C5, C6, and C7 nerves. Undoubtedly, there are factors other than congenital anomalies that trigger the symptoms of thoracic outlet syndrome. This must be so since the onset of symptoms often occurs during a patient's third and fourth decades. Postural changes, such as drooping shoulders and those associated with activities involving arm elevation above the shoulders, are probably important. The fact that a significant number of patients develop symptoms of thoracic outlet syndrome following hyperextension injuries of the neck may be attributed to stretch injury of the anterior scalene muscle with resultant edema, hemorrhage, and spasm. Eventually, muscle fibrosis may occur, which, in turn, can entrap the brachial plexus and cause symptoms of thoracic outlet syndrome.[8,24]

Clinical manifestations

Pain and paresthesias of the neck and upper limb are the most prominent symptoms. The pain is variously described as aching or throbbing, but rarely as burning. It is of variable intensity and commonly insidious in onset with various degrees of progression and severity. The pain is frequently aggravated by activity, especially that involving arm elevation above the shoulders. It may last for hours after the physical activity has ceased.

Roos has described two separate patterns of distribution of pain.[25] The more common pattern is that associated with compression of the *lower* nerves of the brachial plexus (C8 and T1) that eventually form the ulnar nerve. The pain is described in the infraclavicular and supraclavicular areas; in the posterior aspect of the neck, down the upper back medial to the scapula and down the medial aspect of the arm; and in the forearm and hand to the fourth and fifth fingers. The intensity of the pain may vary in different areas. Paresthesias along the ulnar nerve distribution to the hand and medial two fingers are frequently associated with this neurologic type. The paresthesias at times can affect all the fingers. Weakness of the arm and hand can also accompany this pattern. These symptoms are commonly aggravated by arm activity and especially with activity above the head. Nocturnal exacerbation of pain or numbness is common.

The second pattern of pain distribution is that attributed to compression or irritation of the *upper* nerves of the brachial plexus (C5, C6, and C7). The pain is commonly described in the anterolateral aspect of the neck, extending at times from the upper anterior chest to the mandible, face, and temporal and occipital areas of the head. It can also extend to the scapular and deltoid regions and down the lateral aspect of the arm and forearm to the dorsal surface of the hand between the thumb and index fingers.

A third pattern of pain distribution involves a combination of the *upper and lower* brachial plexus involvement. From a therapeutic point of view it is important to identify each of these patterns so that appropriate surgical treatment can be tailored specifically to each group.[25-27]

In more than half the patients with thoracic outlet syndrome, the symptoms appear to follow an injury to the neck or upper back, commonly of the hyperextension type.[23,26-28] Pain and neck stiffness, often accompanied by headache, become severe. After a variable period of days to weeks, pain and paresthesia of the upper limb appear with all the features of thoracic outlet syndrome. An asymptomatic interval between injury and symptoms is frequently described. Many patients are involved in litigation for work-related accidents or motor vehicle "whiplash" injuries, which may lead the physician to label the patient a "malingerer."

Headache is not an unusual symptom of thoracic outlet syndrome and can be severe enough to incapacitate the patient. It is commonly occipital, radiating from the posterior part of the neck, and may extend to affect the ipsilateral hemicranium. It is not unusual for the diagnosis of thoracic outlet syndrome to be seriously questioned for patients in whom headache is a prominent part of the symptom complex, especially in nervous and tense patients prone to psychosomatic complaints.

Generally, most patients with thoracic outlet syndrome have had symptoms for months or even years and have sought repeated medical attention with little relief because of misdiagnosis.

Physical examination should include a careful evaluation of the neck, supraclavicular area, shoulder, and the entire upper extremity, as well as a complete neurologic examination, in order to exclude other causes of pain. Palpation of the supraclavicular fossa and neck may demonstrate the presence of a cervical rib or prominent C7 transverse process. Tenderness of the upper nerves of the brachial plexus or the anterior scalene muscle is a common finding. Spasm and tenderness of the trapezius and paraspinal muscles are frequently observed in patients with a history of trauma. Radicular pain may be elicited by rotation and extension of the head or by axial cervical spine compression, indicating cervical disk disease. Pain and tenderness of the shoulder joint may be caused by rotator cuff injury or tendonitis.

All muscle groups should be tested for strength. Patients with upper brachial plexus involvement may exhibit objective weakness of the deltoid and trapezius musles, demonstrated by the patient's inability to keep the arms extended in the abduction position, especially against mild resistance.[23] Other compression syndromes, such as entrapment of the ulnar nerve at the elbow and median nerve at the wrist (carpal tunnel syndrome), can coexist with thoracic outlet syndrome and should be excluded by percussion at the elbow and over the volar carpal ligaments (Tinel's sign), respectively. Hand weakness, associated with wasting of the intrinsic muscles of the hand and the presence of an ipsilateral cervical rib or its analog, is seen in an extremely rare form of thoracic outlet syndrome.[29,30]

Sensation in all dermatomes is usually intact in thoracic outlet syndrome, although a mild decrease in pinprick sensation can be observed over the ulnar nerve distribution in patients with lower brachial nerve involvement. However, major sensory changes with decreased deep tendon reflexes may be caused by nerve root compression from a herniated cervical disk, spinal cord tumor, or superior pulmonary sulcus tumor.

The thoracic outlet, or compression, maneuvers initially described for testing for what was mistakenly attributed to the arterial type of thoracic outlet syndrome contribute little to the diagnosis of neurologic thoracic outlet syndrome. They simply indicate arterial compression, a common finding in over 50% of normal individuals[14] and in 30% to 50% in the asymptomatic, contralateral arm of patients with unilateral thoracic outlet syndrome.[31,32] The thoracic outlet maneuvers include Adson's maneuver,[19] performed by rotation and extension of the head of the seated patient with the arms resting on his or her lap; the costoclavicular maneuver (exaggerated military position)[11]; and the hyperabduction maneuver.[14] These are considered positive when reduction or obliteration of the radial pulse is obtained and therefore reflect only compression of the subclavian or axillary artery in these extreme positions. They do not necessarily identify the patient with thoracic outlet syndrome.

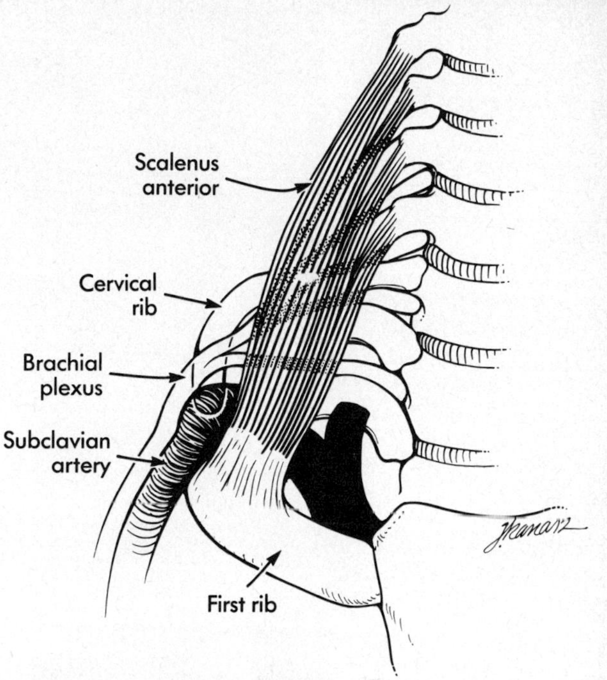

Fig. 28-2. Schematic drawing of the right cervicoaxillary region, demonstrating the usual anatomic position of a cervical rib coursing underneath the lower trunks of the brachial plexus and compressing the subclavian artery against the anterior scalene muscles. Note the presence of poststenotic dilation of the subclavian artery.

Roos has described the Elevated Arm Stress Test (EAST) as a reliable test for diagnosing neurologic thoracic outlet syndrome.[23] It is performed by holding the arms at 90-degree abduction and external rotation while the patient opens and closes the hands for 3 minutes. It is considered positive when the symptoms of thoracic outlet syndrome are reproduced.

Vascular examination should be complete with evaluation of all pulses and blood pressure determination in both arms to exclude arterial stenoses, obstructions, or aneurysms.

Roentgenograms of the chest and cervical spine should be performed routinely. These may demonstrate skeletal abnormalities, such as a cervical rib, C7 transverse process, anomalous first rib, or remote fractures of the clavicle, that could be the cause of thoracic outlet symptoms (Figs. 28-3 and 28-4). If significant degenerative cervical spine dis-

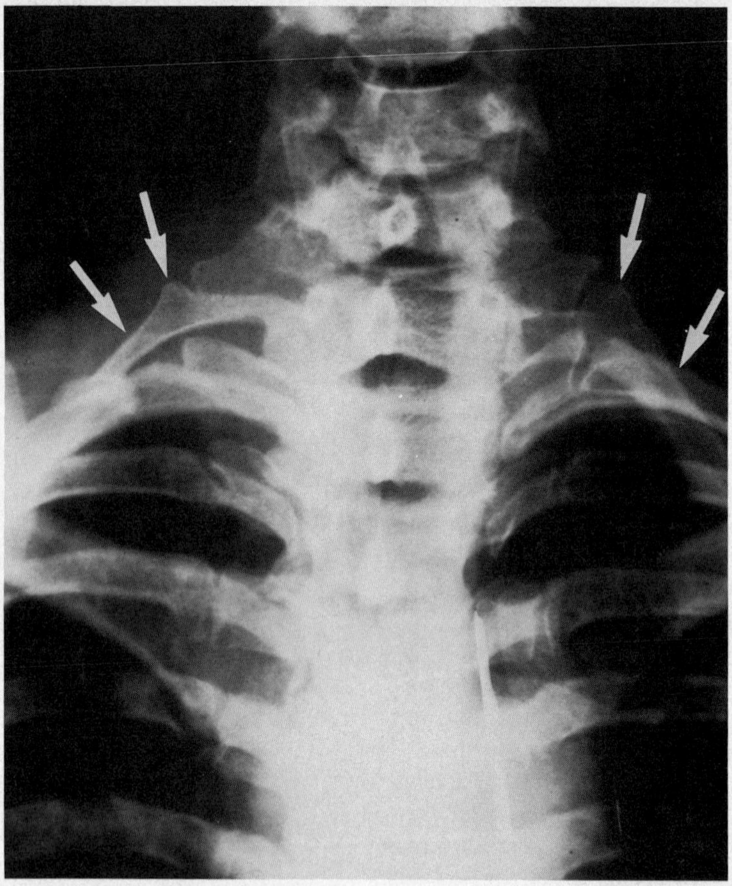

Fig. 28-3. Chest roentgenogram demonstrating well-formed and ossified bilateral cervical ribs (*arrows*). The patient had severe bilateral neurologic type of thoracic outlet syndrome.

ease is present, and if clinically indicated, further evaluation can be done with oblique views of the cervical spine, myelography, computed tomography, or magnetic resonance imaging.

After an initial enthusiasm for neuroelectric testing, such as electromyograms, nerve conduction times, and somatosensory evoked potentials, researchers have found these tests to be nonspecific. The tests add little to the evaluation of patients with thoracic outlet syndrome, except for those patients with suspected carpal tunnel syndrome.[33-35]

Similarly, arteriography and phlebography have no role in the routine evaluation of patients with neurologic symptoms but are indispensable for those patients with vascular complications of thoracic outlet syndrome. Arteriography should also be considered for patients with a supraclavicular bruit, diminished upper limb pulses, or a blood pressure differential in the arms. The noninvasive vascular studies should likewise be confined to patients with obvious vascular symptoms, since the tests add little to the diagnosis of neurologic thoracic outlet syndrome.

Management

Conservative treatment in the form of physical therapy should be the initial management for all patients with neurologic thoracic outlet syndrome. There is no risk involved in this treatment, and most patients with mild to moderate symptoms show enough improvement that no further treatment is necessary.

Physical therapy is directed at strengthening the suspensory muscles of the shoulder girdle by specific exercises for the trapezius, levator scapulae, and rhomboid muscles. These should be supplemented with stretching exercises and correction of any abnormal posture. Patients with severe associated muscle spasm of the back and neck may need initial management with a variety of treatments including heat; massage; ultrasound; and the administration of muscle relaxants, analgesics, and antiinflammatory drugs. After initial improvement patients are instructed to avoid prolonged periods with the arm elevated or in positions that reproduce their symptoms. This program should be tried for a minimum of 3 months to properly evaluate its effectiveness. A small number of patients, especially those with severe symptoms, are either unaffected by this treatment or cannot tolerate it because their symptoms are aggravated by the exercises.

Surgical treatment for neurologic thoracic outlet syndrome should be restricted for those patients with severe, intolerable symptoms unchanged by conservative therapy or for those who consider their symptoms unacceptable be-

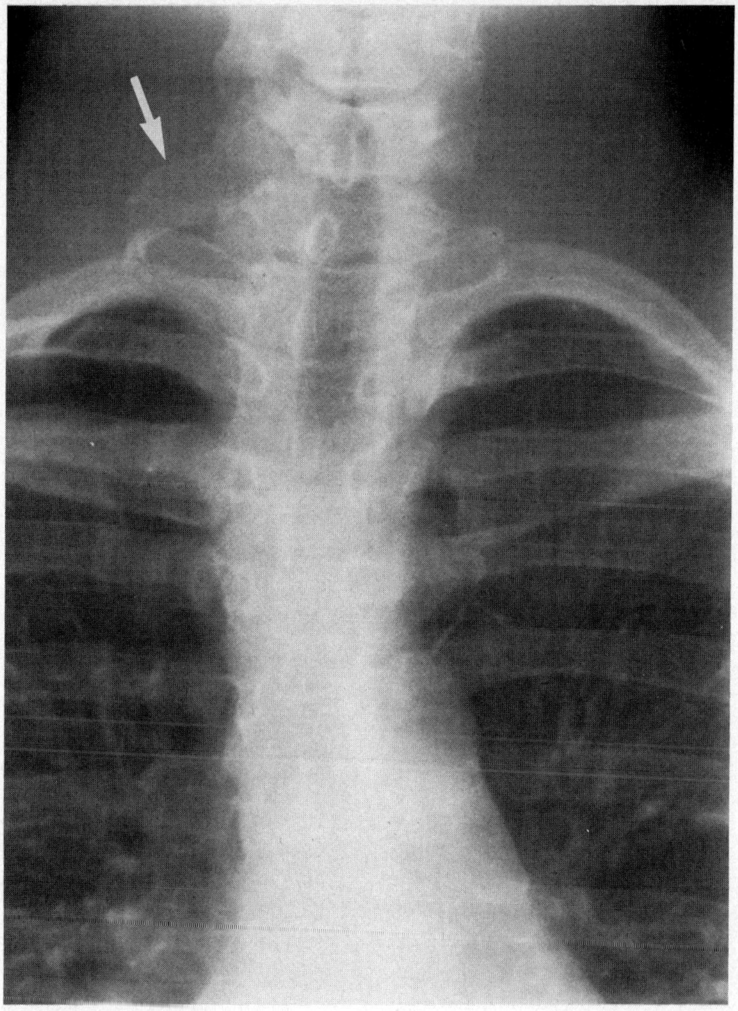

Fig. 28-4. Chest roentgenogram of a patient with elongated C7 transverse process (*arrow*) and symptoms of thoracic outlet syndrome on the right. An operation revealed a tight fibrous band stretched from the tip of the C7 transverse process to the inner aspect of the first rib, elevating the T1 nerve and inferior trunk of the brachial plexus.

cause they interfere with their occupation or their normal daily activities. Mere failure of conservative treatment does not warrant surgical treatment as long as the symptoms are tolerable to the patient. It is estimated that 15% to 30% of patients require surgical treatment.[21,26,36]

Treatment is based on the concept that excision or division of the structure or structures causing the neurovascular compression will result in the relief of the neurologic symptoms. Thus historically the procedures described have been the excision of a cervical rib, the first operation for thoracic outlet syndrome, performed by Coote in 1861[17]; excision of the normal, first thoracic rib via the supraclavicular approach, performed by Murphy in 1910[18]; division of the anterior scalene muscle or "scalenotomy," performed by Adson and Coffey in 1927[19]; excision of the clavicle, performed by Rosati and Lord in 1968[37]; excision of the pectoralis minor tendon, performed by Lord in 1953[20]; and excision of the scalene muscles or "scalenectomy," performed by Sanders, Monsour, and Gerber in 1979.[26]

Although first rib resection effectively decompresses the thoracic outlet, the operation never became popular. It was the scalenotomy that became the preferred operation for over three decades because of its simplicity, lack of complications, and immediate positive results. It was not until 1962 when Clagett,[38] because of the disappointing long-term results of scalenotomy with a 50% to 60% recurrence rate,[38,39] revived interest in first rib resection for thoracic outlet syndrome. The common denominator in the compression mechanism is the first rib, and he advocated its excision through a posterior parascapular approach, an operation that never gained much popularity because of its magnitude.

In 1966 Roos revolutionized the surgical treatment of thoracic outlet syndrome when he described a new technique for first rib resection through the transaxillary approach. This method was less traumatic, safer, and easier to perform.[40] Although other approaches to first rib resection (i.e.,

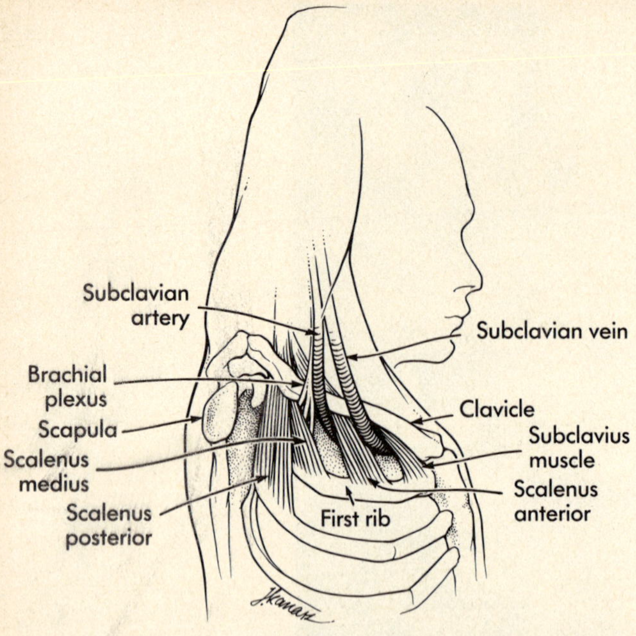

Fig. 28-5. Schematic drawing of the right thoracic outlet as viewed from the axillary approach. Note that excision of the first rib and division of the scalene and subclavius muscles would amply decompress the thoracic outlet.

the supraclavicular,[13] the posterior,[38] and the anterior subclavicular[41]) had been described, Roos's transaxillary approach was the one that became widely adopted.[25,42-44] This approach allows for wide decompression of the thoracic outlet since it permits complete excision of the first rib, and the cervical rib when present, as well as division and partial excision of the scalene muscles and congenital fibromuscular bands (Fig. 28-5). This technique was a major factor in the improved results of surgical management with 85% to 92% positive results reported in large representative series.[25,42-44]

During the last 12 years, for various reasons, there has been a trend by many surgeons toward performing supraclavicular operations. There have been concerns regarding the safety of the transaxillary route for first rib resection because of the incidence of brachial plexus traction injuries.[45] In addition, recurrence of symptoms has been reported by some in up to 15% of patients following first rib resection.[26,27] Others have found that most patients are relieved of symptoms by excision of supraclavicular soft tissue structures, without the need for first rib resection,[46] while still others have found the supraclavicular approach to first rib resection technically easier to perform.[31]

Roos uses transaxillary first rib resection for patients with lower brachial plexus involvement (the majority of patients) and anterior scalenectomy for those with upper brachial plexus compression. In his experience this latter group accounts for only 2% of all primary operations for thoracic outlet syndrome.[25] Sanders, Monsour, and Gerber prefer anterior and middle scalenectomy without rib resection for both groups of patients because of the observed lower incidence of complications with this technique.[26]

It is obvious that there is still no agreement among surgeons with respect to the choice of operation for thoracic outlet syndrome.

Complications associated with all thoracic outlet operations include injuries to the subclavian artery or vein, brachial plexus, phrenic nerve, or long thoracic nerve. Fortunately, these occur infrequently and seldom result in long-term sequelae. Pneumothorax, although observed more commonly, is easily managed with needle aspiration or, occasionally, with a chest tube. Sensory disturbance in the inner aspect of the arm caused by injury to the intercostal brachial nerve occurs in 35% of patients who undergo transaxillary surgery.[26]

Following transaxillary first rib resection, recurrence of symptoms within 2 years after an initial positive result occurs in 5% to 20% of operations.[25-27] Recurrent symptoms of thoracic outlet syndrome are caused by scalene muscle reattachment to the bed of the first rib and dense scar formation, which can entrap the brachial plexus. At times, retained periosteal cells can regenerate another rib, which, when associated with scar tissue, can again result in brachial plexus compression with recurrence of symptoms.

Reoperation for recurrent symptoms is recommended for those patients who had an initial positive result following transaxillary first rib resection and whose recurrent symptoms are severe. The operation of choice is scalenectomy with neurolysis of the brachial plexus through the supraclavicular approach.[25,26,28] Roos obtained positive results in 79% of 72 operations for recurrent symptoms.[25]

Patients whose symptoms are unchanged following operations for thoracic outlet syndrome may have been misdiagnosed and therefore should be completely reevaluated so that the true cause of their symptoms can be established.

ARTERIAL TYPE

Arterial complications of thoracic outlet syndrome are the least common but have the most serious implications because they frequently result in severe ischemia of the upper extremity.[47] They usually occur in adults from the third to the sixth decade with equal incidence in men and women. In contrast to the more common neurologic thoracic outlet syndrome, these patients almost always have a congenital bony abnormality in the thoracic outlet.

Etiology

The basic pathophysiologic mechanism is chronic compression of the subclavian artery with resultant arterial changes, leading to the formation of intimal and mural thrombus and eventually peripheral embolization. The compression site is usually in the scalene triangle where a cervical rib compresses and angulates the subclavian artery from behind against the anterior scalene muscle and first rib (see Fig. 28-2). A fully developed cervical rib appears to be the most common mechanism for arterial compression, being present in 50% of cases.[4,47] Congenital anomalies of the first rib, exostosis of the first rib, and, less commonly, malunion following fracture of the clavicle are other causes of arterial compression. Arterial complications are rarely seen in the absence of osseous abnormalities. Although soft tissue structures, such as congenital fibromuscular bands or abnormalities of the anterior scalene muscle, commonly produce neurologic symptoms, they rarely lead to arterial complications.[21,48,49]

The arterial compression eventually causes thickening of the arterial wall, with inflammation and periarterial fibrosis. Poststenotic dilation then follows, secondary to blood flow turbulence just beyond the constricted segment.[50] In time a true aneurysm may form from the long-standing effects of flow disturbance.

Thromboembolic events can result from either an intimal lesion formed at the site of compression or from mural thrombus layered in the subclavian aneurysm. Platelet aggregates tend to deposit on intimal lesions and can dislodge, resulting in microembolization of the hand and fingers. Embolization from a mural thrombus usually causes occlusion of larger, more proximal arteries. Thrombosis of the subclavian artery is an infrequent event.[51] Retrograde subclavian artery thrombosis with cerebral embolization is extremely rare.[52]

The severity of the ischemic symptoms depends on the site and extent of the arterial occlusion. Microembolization of the fingers and hand can result in Raynaud's phenomenon as the only initial symptom. Repeated embolization may eventually obliterate the distal arterial bed, resulting in severe ischemia, which can progress to irreversible changes and gangrene. Larger emboli that lodge in the proximal arteries tend to result in milder ischemic symptoms because of the available collateral vessels around the shoulder girdle.

Clinical manifestations

The earliest manifestation of arterial thoracic outlet syndrome is an ischemic episode of the affected upper extremity resulting from embolic occlusion. Depending on the size and number of emboli, and on the site of occlusion, this may appear as Raynaud's phenomenon, secondary to microemboli of the digital arteries and palmar arch. It can also appear as distinct ischemia of one or more digits, as a single event, or in "showers" with repeated and varied episodes of ischemia. Ischemia of the hand and forearm, or even the entire arm, occurs with larger emboli.

The diagnosis of arterial thoracic outlet syndrome is rarely made before thromboembolic events occur. On occasion, early diagnosis is possible in patients examined for asymptomatic subclavian aneurysm or in those patients with neurologic symptoms associated with a cervical rib or other bony abnormality.[53]

Diagnosis is easily made if all patients with upper limb ischemia are investigated for possible sources of emboli. The diagnosis should be suspected in young patients with unilateral arm, hand, or finger ischemia. A history of cervical rib or trauma with healed fractures of the clavicle or upper ribs should alert the physician to the possibility of thoracic outlet syndrome.

Since most patients with thoracic outlet syndrome develop ischemia of the upper extremity, physical examination will reveal the usual characteristics of tissue ischemia with pallor, cyanosis, and coldness, depending on the severity and level of the arterial occlusion. A complete vascular examination should be performed to search for a proximal source of emboli. Examination may reveal a subclavian aneurysm, or a prominent subclavian artery that has been displaced anteriorly and superiorly by a cervical rib may be detected. A supraclavicular bruit is frequently audible with the arm in the neutral position, indicating a subclavian stenosis at the point of compression. Examination of the contralateral arm and lower extremities should be carefully performed to exclude evidence of other embolic occlusions from a cardiac source. Upper thoracic and cervical roentgenograms are critical, since a bony abnormality is almost always present.

Noninvasive vascular studies are important in the evaluation with respect to the level of the arterial occlusion, as well as the degree of collateral circulation present. Duplex scanning of the subclavian and axillary arteries may reveal the presence of a subclavian aneurysm or poststenotic dilation with the presence of mural thrombus.

Arteriography is the most specific diagnostic test and should be obtained routinely in any patient with ischemic symptoms that could be of embolic origin. It should include the entire upper extremity from the aortic arch to the digital arteries. In most cases the arteriographic changes are obvious, demonstrating severe angulation of the subclavian artery with poststenotic dilation or a subclavian artery aneurysm (Fig. 28-6). Careful examination of the films is necessary for those arteries with more subtle findings such as minor intimal changes or small intravascular filling defects (Fig. 28-7). Evaluation of the more distal arteries is crucial in patients with severe ischemia in order to plan surgical treatment, which may include distal embolectomy or bypass to improve perfusion (Fig. 28-8).

Management

The treatment for arterial complications of thoracic outlet syndrome is always surgical and is frequently performed as an emergency because of the common development of an acute embolic or thrombotic event with severe ischemia.

Surgical management consists of three specific steps: (1) excision of the anatomic abnormality responsible for the arterial compression, (2) removal of the source of the emboli by arterial reconstruction, and (3) improvement in distal perfusion by appropriate thromboembolectomy.

Thoracic outlet decompression is performed through the supraclavicular approach, which allows for adequate access to the cervical rib or other anomalies, as well as control of the subclavian artery for the subsequent arterial reconstruction. The thoracic outlet should be fully decompressed with

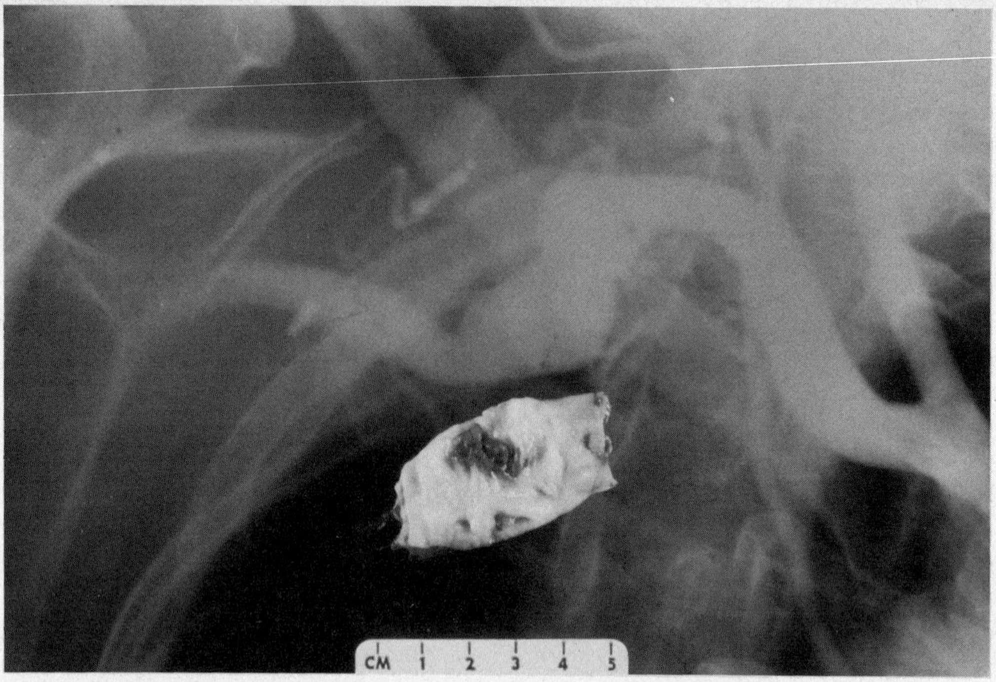

Fig. 28-6. Right subclavian arteriogram showing an aneurysm secondary to thoracic outlet syndrome. Superimposed is the surgical specimen demonstrating the intimal thrombus that was the source of distal emboli.

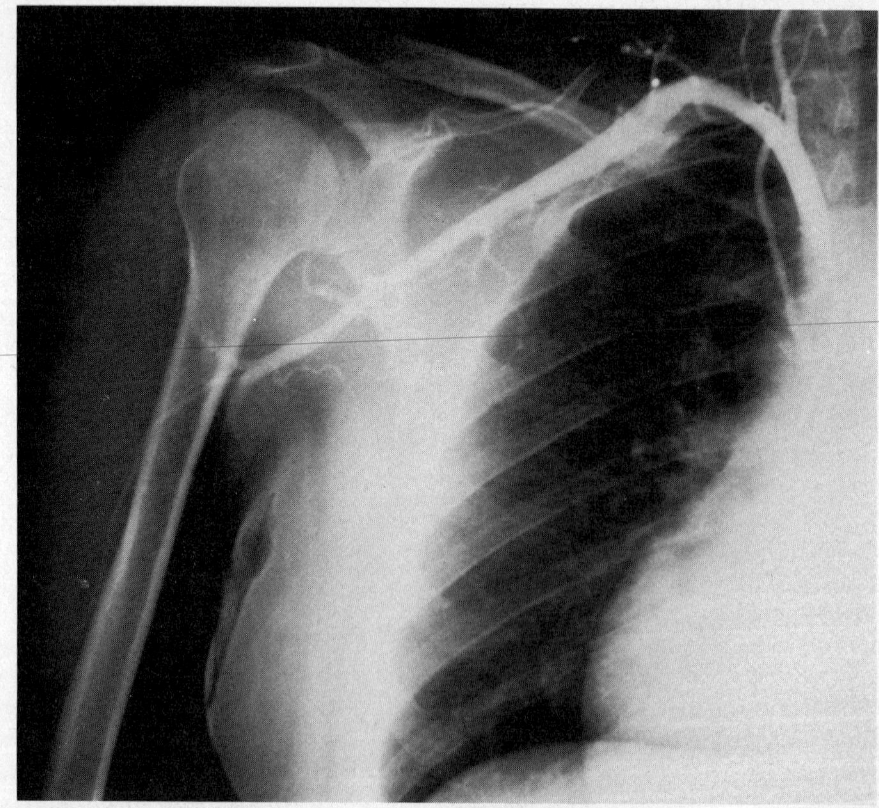

Fig. 28-7. Right subclavian arteriogram in a patient with thoracic outlet syndrome showing mild poststenotic dilation.

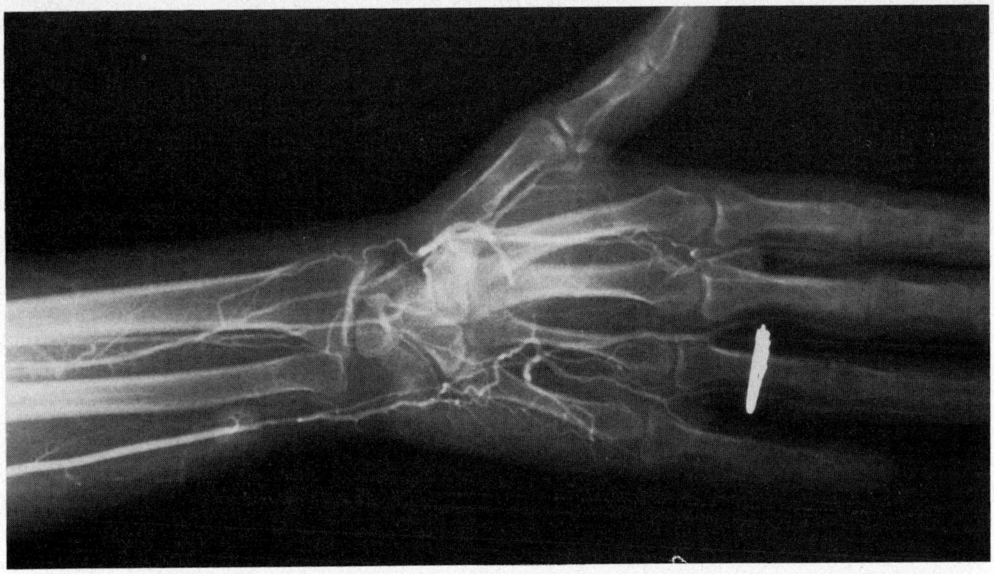

Fig. 28-8. Arteriogram of the left forearm and hand showing embolic occlusion of the proximal radial and distal ulnar arteries from a subclavian intimal thrombus caused by thoracic outlet syndrome secondary to cervical rib.

excision of the first rib and all anomalous osseous elements and the scalene muscles.[53]

After decompression the subclavian-axillary artery becomes more accessible and mobile, and thus the arterial component of the operation can be performed through the same incision. For extensive aneurysms, however, an infraclavicular counterincision will improve the surgical exposure for arterial reconstruction. This may entail excision of the subclavian aneurysm with end-to-end anastomosis when this is feasible, or replacement of the aneurysm with a saphenous vein or prosthetic graft. In lesser intimal lesions an endarterectomy or intimectomy may be all that is required.[53,54]

For most patients with mild chronic ischemia, removal of the source of emboli is all that is necessary. For patients with recent thromboembolic episodes affecting the arteries proximal to the hand, thromboembolectomy will be necessary to improve arm perfusion. With severe distal ischemia caused by digital artery and palmar arch embolization, without proximal obstructions, cervical sympathectomy may improve perfusion. It can be performed after completion of the subclavian artery reconstruction.

Patients with repeated embolization and severe obliteration of the distal vascular bed of long-standing duration are frequently not amenable to embolectomy. These patients should have revascularization with a vein bypass to the interosseous, other forearm, or wrist artery.[53,54] From a technical standpoint some patients may not be candidates for these reconstructions and may require a major amputation for rehabilitation.[47,49,54]

The results of surgery for arterial complications of thoracic outlet syndrome are excellent when early diagnosis is made and treatment is instituted before multiple emboli occlude the distal arterial runoff with resultant irreversible ischemia. Therefore early diagnosis and treatment cannot be emphasized enough.

VENOUS TYPE

Extrinsic compression of the subclavian vein in the thoracic outlet has been implicated as one of the common causes of spontaneous axillosubclavian vein thrombosis. It is known as *Paget-von Schröetter syndrome* from the first two authors who described it.[55,56] It is also commonly referred to as "effort" thrombosis because of its temporal relationship between vigorous physical activity of the arm and shoulder and the development of symptoms. It is more prevalent in men in their third and fourth decades. The right side is affected in two thirds of the patients, probably because the physical activity or "effort" is generally concentrated in the dominant arm.[57,58] Sanders and Haug postulate that the acute angle at the junction between the right subclavian vein and innominate vein may be another factor in the higher incidence of right-side symptoms, compared with the left side.[59]

Etiology

The most accepted etiologic factor in primary thrombosis of the axillosubclavian vein is external compression resulting from anatomic structures in the anterior portion of the thoracic outlet (see Fig. 28-1). These include a large costoclavicular ligament or subclavius muscle, a more anterior insertion of the anterior scalene muscle to the first rib, or congenital fibromuscular bands.[21] The pectoralis muscle tendon can also compress the axillary vein more laterally.[60] Repetitive arm and shoulder movements then lead to chronic intermittent compression of the vein, which eventually results in its damage with reactive inflammation and fibrosis and finally culminates in thrombosis.

Other factors that have been incriminated are intrinsic abnormalities such as malformation or hypertrophy of the subclavian vein valves.[61,62]

Clinical manifestations

The symptoms of axillosubclavian vein thrombosis are swelling, pain, and cyanosis of the upper extremity. The onset is usually sudden and dramatic. Occasionally, some patients develop slowly progressive or intermittent symptoms. The severity of the symptoms depends on the extent of the thrombotic process and the degree of collateralization that develops. Pulmonary emboli rarely occur.[63]

Physical examination reveals a swollen, cyanotic arm with distended superficial veins around the shoulder and anterior chest. Depending on the severity of the symptoms, the arm may be tender to palpation. A thickened cord is sometimes palpable in the axilla.[64]

Diagnosis is confirmed with upper extremity phlebography. The study should demonstrate occlusion of the axillosubclavian vein for several centimeters (Fig. 28-9). In patients with intermittent symptoms, venograms should be obtained with the arm in the neutral position and with the arm abducted to 90 degrees to demonstrate subclavian vein compression.

Duplex scanning may be helpful but can be misleading because collateral veins may be erroneously mistaken for the axillary vein.

Management of acute obstruction

There are three options in the treatment of acute subclavian vein thrombosis: conservative therapy, surgical thrombectomy, or thrombolytic therapy.

Conservative therapy is indicated for patients with mild symptoms and for those whose thrombosed segment is limited in extent so that collateral pathways are expected to be ample and effective. The treatment consists of arm elevation and anticoagulation. The upper extremity should be elevated in a forward position, thus avoiding any possible venous compression in the thoracic outlet by some degree of abduction, which invariably occurs when the arm is elevated to the patient's side. Anticoagulation is instituted by administering heparin by the continuous intravenous route and is continued with warfarin therapy for 3 to 6 months.

The results of conservative treatment vary widely in reported series. Sanders and Haug, in their collective review, found that disabling arm swelling occurred in 49% of 185 patients who received anticoagulant therapy alone.[59] Because of these results, Rutherford and Piotrowski recommend early thrombectomy for this group.[65]

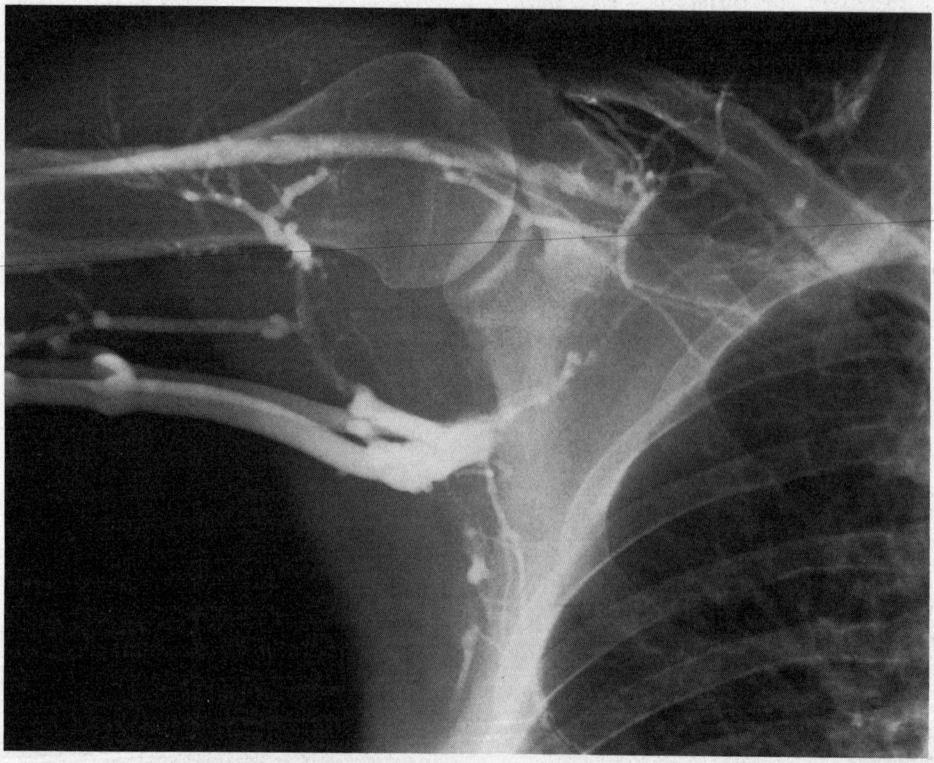

Fig. 28-9. Right arm phlebogram showing axillary vein thrombosis.

Thrombectomy is indicated for patients with severe symptoms of pain and swelling of no more than 3 or 4 days duration. The operation can be performed through the infraclavicular, supraclavicular, or transclavicular approach.[58,59] After removal of the thrombus and closure of the venotomy, decompression of the thoracic outlet should follow. This is accomplished by excision of the first rib and division of the costoclavicular ligament and the subclavius and anterior scalene muscles. If the transclavicular approach is used, claviculectomy amply decompresses the thoracic outlet. The results reported on 33 patients in 5 published series showed that subjective improvement in symptoms occurred in 94%.[59]

The indications for thrombolytic therapy are similar to the indications for thrombectomy: acute onset of moderately severe symptoms of short duration. Streptokinase, urokinase, and tissue plasminogen activator (t-PA) are the common agents available for thrombolytic therapy. The first two have been used most frequently. They can be administered either systemically or locally via a catheter into the thrombus. The number of published reports of patients receiving thrombolytic therapy is still too small to draw any conclusions about the relative effectiveness of each agent. Venography is performed at the completion of the treatment to check for possible extrinsic compression of the subclavian vein at the thoracic outlet (Fig. 28-10). If extrinsic compression is noted, transaxillary first rib resection should be considered shortly after thrombolysis, or else it should be staged 2 to 3 months later. Anticoagulation therapy with warfarin should be instituted during that interval to prevent recurrent thrombosis of the subclavian vein. A review of published results of combined thrombolytic therapy with surgical decompression since 1983 by Sanders and Haug show a success rate of 74% in 62 patients.[59]

Patients with symptoms of intermittent obstruction of the subclavian vein, who demonstrate extrinsic compression on positional venography, should be considered for elective decompression to prevent subclavian vein thrombosis.

Although experience with balloon angioplasty as a method to dilate stenotic subclavian vein segments is meager, it is doubtful that it can be effective in permanent decompression of the subclavian vein at the thoracic outlet.

Management of chronic obstruction

Patients who seek medical help too late after the onset of symptoms of axillosubclavian vein occlusion, or those patients in whom thrombolytic therapy or thrombectomy has failed, may reach a chronic stage in their clinical course

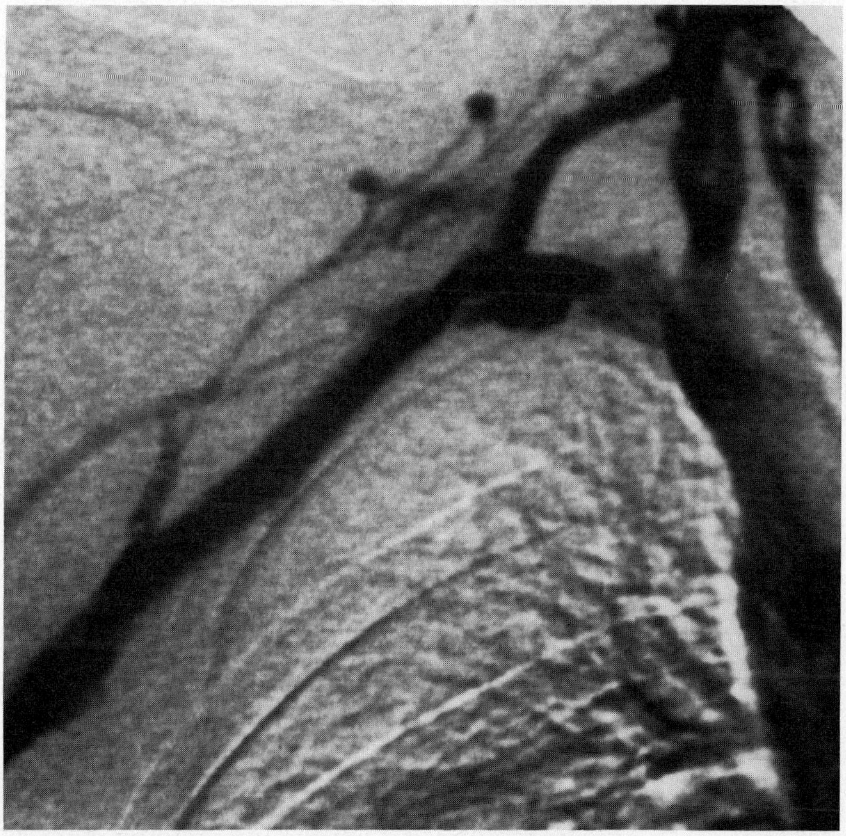

Fig. 28-10. Right arm venous digital subtraction angiogram following dissolution of the axillary vein thrombus with thrombolytic therapy.

when the collateral development is not adequate enough to keep their symptoms at an acceptable level. Some patients may report only mild symptoms at rest but develop severe pain and swelling with moderate physical activity. Since most of these patients are young and active, other treatment options must be considered.

Thoracic outlet decompression by transaxillary first rib resection has been reported to result in symptomatic improvement in patients with chronic axillosubclavian occlusion.[54] The authors theorize that first rib resection decompresses the functioning venous collateral vessels with resultant improvement in symptoms.

From a flow dynamic point of view, subclavian vein reconstruction by endovenectomy[66] or venous bypass[67-69] is probably the only effective method available for correction of the resultant venous hypertension in patients with poor collateral vessels. Because of the relatively high incidence of thrombosis following venous reconstructions, the operation should be combined with the construction of a temporary arteriovenous fistula to increase flow and improve patency.[70]

In general, because of the small number of patients with venous complications of thoracic outlet syndrome and because of the variety of the treatments used, there are insufficient data available for use as guidelines in determining the best possible therapeutic approach for treating patients with the difficult venous complications of thoracic outlet syndrome.

REFERENCES

1. Barker WF: An historical look at the thoracic outlet compression syndrome, Ann Vasc Surg 3:293, 1989.
2. Wilbourn AJ and Porter JM: Thoracic outlet syndromes. SPINE: State of the Art Reviews, 2:597, 1988.
3. Gilliatt RW: Thoracic outlet syndromes. In Dyck PJ et al, eds: Peripheral neurology, ed 2, Philadelphia, 1984, WB Saunders Co.
4. Lord JW: Thoracic outlet syndromes: real or imaginary? N Y State J Med 81:1488, 1981.
5. Porter JM et al: Thoracic outlet syndrome: a conservative approach, Vasc Diagn Ther 3:35, 1982.
6. Dale A: Thoracic outlet compression syndrome. In Management of vascular surgical problems, New York, 1985, McGraw-Hill, Inc.
7. Todd TW: Posture and the cervical rib syndrome, Ann Surg 75:105, 1922.
8. Ochsner A, Gage M, and DeBakey M: Scalenus anticus (Naffziger) syndrome, Am J Surg 28:669, 1935.
9. Naffziger HC and Grant WT: Neuritis of the brachial plexus mechanical in origin, Surg Gynecol Obstet 67:722, 1938.
10. Hvoslef J: Abnormal first thoracic rib simulating cervical rib, J Minn State Med Assoc and NW Lancet, 31:251, 1911.
11. Keen WW: The symptomatology, diagnosis and surgical treatment of cervical ribs, Am J Med Sci 133:173, 1907.
12. LeVay AD: Costoclavicular compression of brachial plexus and subclavian vessels, Lancet 2:164, 1945.
13. Falconer MA and Li FW: Resection of first rib in costoclavicular compression of brachial plexus, Lancet 1:59, 1962.
14. Wright IS: The neurovascular syndrome produced by hyperabduction of the arms, Am Heart J 29:1, 1945.
15. Peet PM et al: Thoracic outlet syndrome: evaluation of a therapeutic exercise program, Mayo Clin Proc 31:281, 1956.
16. Rob CG and Standeven A: Arterial occlusion complicating thoracic outlet compression syndrome, Br Med J 2:709, 1958.
17. Coote H: Exostosis of the left transverse process of the seventh cervical vertebra, surrounded by blood vessels and nerves: successful removal, Lancet 1:360, 1861.
18. Murphy T: Brachial neuritis caused by pressure of first rib, Aust Med J 15:582, 1910.
19. Adson AW and Coffey JR: Cervical rib: a method of anterior approach for relief of symptoms by division of the scalenus anticus, Ann Surg 85:839, 1927.
20. Lord JW: Surgical management of shoulder girdle syndromes, Arch Surg 66:69, 1953.
21. Roos DB: Congenital anomalies associated with thoracic outlet syndrome: anatomy, symptoms, diagnosis and treatment, Am J Surg 132:771, 1976.
22. Thomas GI et al: The middle scalene muscle and its contribution to the thoracic outlet, Am J Surg 145:589, 1983.
23. Roos DB: Thoracic outlet nerve compression. In Rutherford RB, ed: Vascular surgery, Philadelphia, 1989, WB Saunders Co.
24. Urschel HC and Razzuk MA: Thoracic outlet syndrome. In Sabiston DC and Spencer FC, eds: Gibbon's surgery of the chest, Philadelphia, 1989, WB Saunders Co.
25. Roos DB: The place for scalenectomy and first rib resection in thoracic outlet syndrome, Surgery 92:1077, 1982.
26. Sanders RJ, Monsour JW, and Gerber WF: Scalenectomy versus first rib resection for treatment of thoracic outlet syndrome, Surgery 85:109, 1979.
27. Qvarfordt PG, Ehrenfeld WK, and Stoney RJ: Supraclavicular radical scalenectomy and transaxillary first rib resection for the thoracic outlet syndrome: a combined approach, Am J Surg 148:111, 1984.
28. Reilly LM and Stoney RJ: Supraclavicular approach for thoracic outlet decompression, J Vasc Surg 8:329, 1988.
29. Gilliatt RW et al: Wasting of the hand associated with a cervical rib or band, J Neurol Neurosurg Psychiatry 33:615, 1970.
30. Wilbourn AJ: Case Report No.7: True neurogenic thoracic outlet syndrome. American Association of Electromyography and Electrodiagnosis, Rochester, Minnesota, 1982.
31. Hempel GK et al: Supraclavicular resection of the first rib for thoracic outlet syndrome, Am J Surg 14:213, 1981.
32. Sallstrom J and Gjores JE: Surgical treatment of thoracic outlet syndrome, Acta Chir Scand 149:555, 1983.
33. Jerrett SA, Cuzzone LJ, and Pasternak BM: Thoracic outlet syndrome: electrophysiological reappraisal, Arch Neurol 41:960, 1984.
34. Cherington M: Ulnar conduction velocity in thoracic outlet syndrome, N Engl J Med 294:1185, 1976.
35. Raskin NH, Howard MN, and Ehrenfeld WK: Headache as the leading symptom of thoracic outlet syndrome, Headache 25:208, 1985.
36. Pretre R, Spiliopoulos A, and Megevand R: Transthoracic approach in the thoracic outlet syndrome: an alternative operative route for removal of the first rib. Surgery 106:856, 1989.
37. Rosati LM and Lord JW: Neurovascular compression syndromes of the shoulder girdle. In Modern surgical monographs, New York, 1968, Grune & Stratton, Inc.
38. Clagett OT: Presidential address: research and prosearch, J Thorac Cardiovasc Surg 44:153, 1962.
39. Raaf J: Surgery for cervical rib and scalenus anticus syndrome, JAMA 157:219, 1955.
40. Roos DB: Transaxillary approach for first rib resection to relieve thoracic outlet obstruction, Ann Surg 163:354, 1966.
41. Nelson RM and Davis RW: Thoracic outlet compression syndrome: collective review, Ann Thorac Surg 8:437, 1969.
42. Urschel HC and Razzuk MA: Thoracic outlet syndrome, N Engl J Med 286:1140, 1972.
43. Dale WA and Lewis MR: Management of thoracic outlet syndrome, Ann Surg 181:575, 1975.

44. Kelly TR: Thoracic outlet syndrome: current concepts of treatment, Ann Surg 190:657, 1979.
45. Dale WA: Thoracic outlet compression syndrome: critique in 1982, Arch Surg 117:1437, 1982.
46. Stallworth JM, Quinn GJ, and Aiken AF: Is rib resection necessary for relief of thoracic outlet syndrome? Ann Surg 185:581, 1977.
47. Judy KL and Heymann RL: Vascular complications of thoracic outlet syndrome, Am J Surg 123:536, 1974.
48. Dorazio RA and Ezzet F: Arterial complications of the thoracic outlet syndrome, Am J Surg 138:246, 1979.
49. Short DW: The subclavian artery in 16 patients with complete cervical ribs, J Cardiovasc Surg 16:135, 1975.
50. Pairolero PC et al: Subclavian axillary artery aneurysms, Surgery 90:757, 1981.
51. Bouhoutsos J, Morris T, and Martin P: Unilateral Raynaud's phenomenon in the hand and its significance, Surgery 82:547, 1977.
52. DeVillers JC: A brachiocephalic vascular syndrome associated with cervical rib, Br Med J 2:140, 1966.
53. Kieffer E and Ruotolo C: Arterial complications of thoracic outlet compression. In Rutherford RB, ed: Vascular surgery, Philadelphia, 1989, WB Saunders Co.
54. Etheredge S, Wilbur B, and Stoney RJ: Thoracic outlet syndrome, Am J Surg 138:175, 1979.
55. Paget J: Clinical lectures and essays, London, 1875, Longmans, Green & Co.
56. von Schröetter L: Erkrankungen der Gefossl. In Nathnogel, Handbuch der Pathologie und Therapie, 1884, Wein, Holder.
57. Adams JT et al: Intermittent subclavian vein obstruction without thrombosis, Surgery 63:147, 1968.
58. DeWeese JA, Adams JT, and Gaiser DL: Subclavian venous thrombectomy, Circulation 16 (suppl 2):158, 1970.
59. Sanders RJ and Haug C: Subclavian vein obstruction and thoracic outlet syndrome: a review of etiology and management, Ann Vasc Surg 4:397, 1990.
60. Daskalakis E and Bouhoutsos J: Subclavian and axillary compression of musculoskeletal origin, Br J Surg 67:573, 1980.
61. Cucci CE, Bottino CG, and Ciampa V: Venous obstruction of the upper extremity caused by a malformed valve of the subclavian vein, Circulation 27:275, 1963.
62. Wilder JR, Haberman ET, and Nach RL: Subclavian vein obstruction secondary to hypertrophy of the terminal valve, Surgery 55:214, 1964.
63. Tilney NL, Griffiths HJG, and Edwards EA: Natural history of major venous thrombosis of the upper extremity, Arch Surg 101:792, 1970.
64. Hughes ESR: Venous obstruction in the upper extremity, Br J Surg 36:155, 1948.
65. Rutherford RB and Piotrowski JJ: Axillary-subclavian vein thrombosis. In Rutherford RB, ed: Vascular surgery, Philadelphia, 1989, WB Saunders Co.
66. Gloviczki P, Kazmier FJ, and Hollier LH: Axillary subclavian venous occlusion: the morbidity of a nonlethal disease, J Vasc Surg 4:333, 1986.
67. Rabinowitz R and Goldfarb D: Surgical treatment of axillosubclavian venous thrombosis: a case report, Surgery 70:703, 1971.
68. Hashmonai M, Schramek A, and Farbstein J: Cephalic vein crossover bypass for subclavian vein thrombosis: a case report, Surgery 80:563, 1976.
69. Jacobson JH and Haimov M: Venous revascularization of the arm: report of three cases, Surgery 81:599, 1977.
70. Sanders RJ, Rosales C, and Pearce WH: Creation and closure of temporary arteriovenous fistulas for venous reconstruction or thrombectomy: description of technique, J Vasc Surg 6:504, 1987.

Chapter 29

REFLEX SYMPATHETIC DYSTROPHY AND CAUSALGIA

Jess R. Young

THE REFLEX SYMPATHETIC DYSTROPHIES

Reflex sympathetic dystrophy (RSD) and causalgia represent a family of overlapping disorders, and a number of terms have been used to describe them (see the accompanying box). Although many of these terms are descriptive, their use has confused clinicians and has obscured the clinical features of these disorders. Confusion is not surprising since RSD occurs in different forms at different times during its course. The various names given in the past have mainly been used to describe separate clinical aspects of this syndrome.

RSD can be defined as an excessive or exaggerated response of an extremity to some form of internal or external trauma. The response to this trauma usually includes rather constant characteristics including intense or unduly prolonged pain, delayed functional recovery, and, frequently, vasomotor disturbances and associated trophic changes.

Causalgia is a type of RSD. This term should be used to define a syndrome of burning pain. There is often sympathetic overactivity with coldness and sweating, and the syndrome is associated with allodynia (aggravation of pain by normally nonpainful stimuli such as light touch and movement) and hyperalgesia (increased sensitivity to noxious stimuli) after a major nerve trunk injury. The discomfort does not respond well to narcotics but does respond to sympathetic nerve blocks or sympathectomy.

Most authorities do list causalgia as a type of RSD. This is logical since there is evidence of sympathetic overactivity associated with this condition and the pain can be stopped by sympathetic blocks or sympathectomy. RSDs can therefore be divided into two major types, one associated with

Terms used to describe RSD syndromes

Algodystrophy
Algoneurodystrophy
Disuse phenomenon
Posttraumatic dystrophy
Reflex neurovascular dystrophy
Causalgia
Mimo-causalgia
Minor causalgia
Major causalgia
Sudeck's osteodystrophy
Osteoporosis with disability
Painful osteoporosis
Posttraumatic osteoporosis
Posttraumatic fibrosis
Shoulder-hand syndrome
Posttraumatic sympathalgia
Postinfarctional sclerodactyly
Acute atrophy of bone
Traumatic angiospasm
Traumatic vasospasm
Posttraumatic pain syndrome
Posttraumatic neurovascular pain syndrome
Posttraumatic spreading neuralgia
Peripheral trophoneurosis
Disability after real or alleged venous thrombosis
Posttraumatic neurovascular pain syndrome

RSD syndromes

With no major nerve injury

RSD stage 1
RSD stage 2
RSD stage 3

With major nerve injury

Causalgia

Disorders associated with RSD syndromes

Traumatic (60%)

Fractures
Sprains
Contusions
Muscle strains
Crush injuries
Peripheral nerve injuries
Burns
Iatrogenic injuries
Dislocations
Lacerations

Nontraumatic (15%)

Cerebrovascular accident with hemiplegia
Myocardial infarction
Thrombophlebitis
Prolonged bed rest
Neoplasm
Metabolic bone disease
Cervical osteoarthritis
Herpes zoster

Idiopathic (25%)

major nerve injury (causalgia) and the other not associated with major nerve injury (RSD) (see the accompanying box).

Causes of the RSD syndromes can be grouped under three categories: traumatic (after an injury), nontraumatic (after a noninjurious condition), and idiopathic (see the box at the top right).

In the past, patients with causalgia and RSD were often misdiagnosed and mistreated by physicians because confusing and conflicting descriptions made diagnosis and treatment difficult. With a better understanding of these conditions, physicians no longer need to be confused and frustrated. Increased awareness of the clinical pictures, knowledge of the wide array of predisposing events, and prompt initiation of proper therapy will prevent protracted cases with persistent limitation of function of the extremity.

Reflex sympathetic dystrophy

The term *reflex sympathetic dystrophy* in this discussion will be applied to patients with a persistent pain syndrome in an extremity, usually after an injury or an insult to the extremity. It is not associated with major nerve injuries, and there may be clinical evidence of sympathetic overactivity. RSD is a common, frequently misdiagnosed condition characterized by pain, tenderness, limitation of motion, and a favoring of one limb. It is the result of a failure of a patient to become rehabilitated normally.

Although RSD has been known for a long time, knowledge of it is still quite limited. Mitchell et al[1] wrote the first clinical description of causalgia based on cases of gunshot wounds to the nerves and blood vessels during the Civil War. Sudeck[2] described cases of painful joint involvement giving rise to the term *Sudeck's syndrome* after injury. Leriche[3] called attention to the role of the sympathetic nervous system in these disorders. Evans[4] coined the term *RSD* to describe posttraumatic pain syndromes that were not related to major nerve damage.

Etiology. As mentioned, the precipitating causes for RSD can be discussed under three headings: traumatic, nontraumatic, and idiopathic (see box). In reviewing the literature, about 60% of cases of RSD are posttraumatic, about 25% are associated with nontraumatic conditions, and 15% are idiopathic.

Most cases of RSD are posttraumatic secondary to sprains, fractures, crush injuries, burns, and injuries to minor peripheral nerves. The injury can be iatrogenic (e.g., after surgical procedures on the hand including carpal tunnel release or palmar fasciotomy). Transaxillary resection of the first rib for thoracic outlet syndrome has also been complicated by RSD. Nontraumatic causes of RSD include failure to rehabilitate after a stroke, myocardial infarction, or thrombophlebitis. RSD has also been associated with metabolic bone diseases, neoplasm, cervical osteoarthritis, and herpes zoster.

Plewes[5] estimated that RSD occurred in 0.05% of patients seen in a trauma unit, although others suggest that it may be present in up to 5% of patients with injuries. It has been reported in 0.2% to 11% patients with a Colles' fracture,[6] in 5% to 20% of patients with myocardial ischemia,[7] and in 12% to 20% of patients with hemiplegia.[8] Its presence in myocardial ischemia appears to be decreasing, probably because of the tendency to mobilize and discharge patients from the hospital earlier. The prevalence in hemiplegia remains high.

In a comprehensive review by Kozin,[6] RSD was found to occur most frequently after fractures. In 25% to 30% of the cases, no specific precipitating event could be identified. In a review by Pak[9] of 140 cases, the precipitating cause was not recognized in 15%.

Psychogenic factors such as emotional or psychiatric problems can play a large part in the development of symptoms of RSD. In Pak's review,[9] psychiatric problems or emotional disturbances existed before the onset of RSD in 37% of the patients.

The syndrome can be aggravated and prolonged by incorrect diagnosis on the part of the physician. The physician may keep the patient in bed or immobilized for an unreasonably long period of time. When the patient finally does become active, the tender, painful limb is often misdiagnosed as thrombophlebitis, and an additional period of bed rest and immobilization is prescribed. This furthers the development of RSD.

Pathophysiology. The exact mechanism by which the initial trauma and tissue damage results in a chronic irritation of the peripheral sensory nerves is unknown. It may be enzymatic, biochemical, or bioelectric in nature. Regardless of the mechanism, the result is a prolonged stimulation of pain impulses.

Most investigators have proposed that RSD is caused by an abnormal activity in the sympathetic nervous system. The cause and nature of this abnormality is unclear, although a number of hypotheses have been proposed. In general these can be grouped into two categories, one favoring a peripheral mechanism and the other a central mechanism. Some theories propose a combination of the two mechanisms.

DeTakats[10] argued the peripheral injury theory. He proposed that impulses originating at the site of a peripheral injury could alter the vasomotor tone of the skin, thus enhancing nociceptor activity. Doupe et al[11] also favored the peripheral injury theory. They proposed that RSD results from an artificial synapse between fibers of an injured nerve at the point of injury. As a result of these artificial synapses, efferent sympathetic impulses can produce afferent impulses in the sensory fibers back to the spinal cord. This would explain why interruption of the efferent sympathetic portion of the cycle by nerve block or surgery can be curative.

Devor,[12] another proponent of the peripheral injury theory, presented experimental evidence to support his theory that any form of nerve injury or inflammation damages Schwann cells or the axones themselves. This damage results in local sprout outgrowths or demyelination, further leading to the acquisition of chemosensitivity by the demyelinated segment or nerve sprout and the acquisition of ectopic pacemaker activity. The pacemaker then discharges spontaneously and in response to any depolarizing stimulus. Circulating catecholamines and those released from sympathetic efferent fibers also activate the ectopic pacemaker and augment the discharge. Devor's theory is backed by the experimental evidence indicating abnormal increased firing of the peripheral nerves after nerve injury.[12-14]

The theory supporting central neurologic dysfunction was first developed by Livingston[15] in 1943. He proposed a theory of reverberating circuits in the spinal cord to explain RSD. According to this theory, the initial factor was injury and tissue damage resulting in chronic irritation of a peripheral sensory nerve. The exact mechanism of this chronic irritation, whether bioelectric, biochemical, or enzymatic, was unknown. The painful stimuli initiate reverberating circuits in the internuncial neuron pools of the spinal cord. Once established, these reverberating circuits can also be triggered by normal stimuli and are centrally interpreted as pain. Increased activity in the internuncial pools also results in a continuous cross stimulation of efferent motor and sympathetic nerves. This produces various responses in the extremity and results in increased afferent impulses to the spinal cord. As a result of all of these activities, some synapses include the sympathetic motor neuron cells in the lateral horn, affecting vasomotor tone and the sweat glands. Spasm in the arteriolar and venule ends of the capillary loops raises filtration pressure, and edema and swelling result. Cyanosis and anoxemia increase capillary permeability, further worsening the edema. Other synapses may involve the anterior horn cells, leading to muscle cramps and spasms.

Clinical picture. RSD is a dynamic process that has just one common denominator to all forms and all stages: pain. Changes in bones, blood vessels, muscles, tendons, connective tissue, and skin may occur.

The pain of RSD is usually described as an aching or throbbing discomfort that is aggravated by weight bearing or by use of the extremity. Pain at rest, if present, is usually mild. Because of the pain with weight bearing, limping and the use of a cane, crutch, or wheelchair are common. If an arm is involved, it is often carried in a sling. RSD is found twice as often in the lower extremities as the upper, and a dominant extremity is most often affected.

Steinbrocker and Argyros[16] suggested dividing RSD into three stages. This classification has proven to be of great help to us clinically and is as follows:

Stage 1 (see box on p. 514), the *acute stage,* is characterized by pain, tenderness, varying degrees of swelling, increased temperature, and excessive sweating of the extremity. This stage may persist for 3 to 6 months. Roentgenograms may reveal patchy osteoporosis. Evidence of sympathetic overactivity is not present. This stage has also been described as the *disuse syndrome stage*.

Stage 2 (see box on p. 514), the *dystrophic stage,* may last another 3 to 6 months. In this stage, pain, tenderness, and edema are more pronounced. Evidence of sympathetic overactivity is present. Skin temperature is usually cool, and excessive sweating may be present. More marked patchy osteoporosis may be seen roetgenographically.

Stage 3 (see box on p. 514), the *atrophic stage,* evolves gradually as pain and tenderness diminish. Atrophy of skin and subcutaneous tissues appears. Wrinkling may be lost, and the skin may have a tight, shiny appearance suggestive of scleroderma. The fascia becomes thickened, and flexion contractures may occur. Muscle wasting and weakness are prominent. Evidence of sympathetic overactivity is usually not present, whereas skin temperature and sweating become normal. Roentgenograms demonstrate more severe osteo-

Clinical features of RSD

Stage 1 (acute stage)

Pain
Tenderness
Edema
Increased temperature
No evidence of sympathetic overactivity
Roentgenograms may reveal patchy osteoporosis

Stage 2 (dystrophic stage)

Pain
Tenderness
Increased edema
Evidence of sympathetic overactivity with coolness, hyperhydrosis, cyanosis
Roentgenograms may reveal more marked patchy osteoporosis

Stage 3 (atrophic stage)

Pain and tenderness may diminish
Less or no evidence of sympathetic overactivity
Atrophy of skin and subcutaneous tissues
Ankylosis and contractures may develop
Roentgenograms may reveal more severe osteopenia with diffuse, ground glass appearance

penia and ankylosis. The patchy features may give way to a diffuse, ground-glass appearance.

These stages appear sequentially but with great variability. The groupings should be used only as a rough clinical classification since there is considerable overlapping between the various stages. This may cause difficulty in diagnosis and classification.

It is important to recognize that there is a stage of RSD after an injury or insult to the extremity, stage 1, that is not associated with any clinical evidence of sympathetic overactivity. Because of this lack of evidence of sympathetic dysfunction, clinicians often miss the diagnosis. They think that there must be evidence of sympathetic overactivity to qualify for the diagnosis of RSD. There are more patients with RSD who do not have evidence of sympathetic dysfunction than those who do.

RSD can occur in any age-group. The series of 140 patients reported by Pak[9] and the series of 61 patients reported by Drucker et al[17] were evenly distributed among all age-groups, with a female-to-male ratio of 4:2. It was originally thought that RSD was rare in children, but there have been increasing numbers of reports in children with this disorder.[18-22] RSD in children appears to differ somewhat from that in adults. The children do not appear to be as disabled, there usually are few or no roentgenographic or bone scan changes, vasomotor disturbances are mild, and the children usually respond well to conservative therapy.

Osteoporosis can develop in any of the stages of RSD and is termed *Sudeck's atrophy*. It is a later development and should never be considered an antecedent to RSD or a cause of RSD. Osteoporosis developed in 31% of the patients described by Drucker et al.[23]

Although Lexer et al[24] described four types of osteoporosis, most authors simply describe the bone changes as acute or chronic. In the acute form, there are numerous small, round lucent areas in the juxtaarticular bone. In the chronic form the trabeculae are very fine and difficult to see, and patchy areas of rarification are seen. In severe cases the next stage is marked with diffuse demineralization.

Patients with RSD often appear to be emotionally unstable and anxious. Chronic invalidism, drug addiction, psychiatric commitment, and suicide can occur. Disparity between the degree of pain reported by the patient and the physical examination findings, combined with the patient's anxiety, leads many physicians to think that the pain is psychogenic. Some observers believe that emotional instability is a result of chronic pain and report that emotional disturbances are usually resolved with successful treatment of the condition.[25] However, Pak's[9] review of 140 patients with RSD revealed that emotional disturbances and psychiatric problems were thought to be present before the onset of RSD. Julsrud[26] and Owens[27] believe that patients with RSD are "sympathetic reactors" with a background of emotional and vasomotor instability that make them more prone to develop the syndrome of RSD.

A classic case history demonstrating the three stages of RSD would be a patient with disability after deep venous thrombosis. Typically, this involves an anxious patient with a low pain threshold who is treated for deep thrombophlebitis with abnormally prolonged bed rest for weeks or even months. When ambulation is attempted, the leg becomes swollen, feels tight and stiff, and hurts on weight bearing. The patient limps, producing more discomfort because of abnormal weight bearing. The muscles become increasingly sore and tender, and a wrong diagnosis of recurrent phlebitis is made. Additional bed rest and immobilization only worsens the condition. The leg continues to ache and throb constantly. The patient cannot bear much weight on the extremity and resorts to a cane or crutches. On examination, a full-blown picture of RSD is seen with mild-to-moderate swelling, generalized tenderness in the muscle and bones, and limitation of motion of the toes and ankles. In this first stage, there may be increased skin blood flow with increased warmth and rubor. After 2 or 3 months the skin becomes cool, sweaty, and frequently cyanotic. X-ray films show osteoporosis. These are typical signs and symptoms of sympathetic overactivity found in the second stage. In the third stage symptoms include increased stiffness, muscle atrophy, tight skin, diffuse osteoporosis, and rigid joints.

Diagnosis. The diagnosis of RSD is primarily clinical. A history of persistent pain, usually after an injury or insult to an extremity, is of primary importance in making an accurate diagnosis. If pain is out of proportion to that expected from the initial incident, a diagnosis of RSD must be seriously entertained. RSD is initially misdiagnosed in approximately 70% of all cases.[28]

The criteria used to identify RSD vary widely. Some authors require only the presence of the typical pain syndrome, whereas others insist that evidence of sympathetic overactivity be present. As discussed, evidence of sympathetic overactivity is usually absent in stage 1 RSD.

Kozin[7] has proposed criteria for a diagnosis of definite, probable, possible, and doubtful RSD. Patients would be considered to have definite RSD when pain, tenderness, swelling, and vasomotor and sudomotor changes are present. Probable RSD would be present if pain, tenderness, and vasomotor and sudomotor changes are present, but swelling is absent. Possible RSD would be diagnosed if only vasomotor or sudomotor changes are present and doubtful RSD if only unexplained pain and tenderness are present. These criteria may be of some help in evaluating the patient with persistent pain.

Many believe that the failure of a lumbar sympathetic nerve block to relieve pain excludes the diagnosis of RSD, providing that the block was properly done. Although relief is usually obtained, this is not invariably seen.

Laboratory tests are generally helpful only to exclude other causes of painful limbs (e.g., collagen vascular diseases or bone or soft tissue infections). Radiologic features are important in the diagnoses of RSD. Standard roetgenograms may show some other cause for the persistent pain in the extremity such as a stress fracture. With the use of fine-detail roetgenography, osteoporosis can be found in 90% of patients with definite RSD.[29] It may take 4 to 8 weeks to develop. The acute form is characterized by an irregular mottled appearance, usually marked most in the tarsal bones and heads of the metatarsals. In the chronic form of osteoporosis, the trabeculae of the bones are very fine and sometimes difficult to recognize, and a diffuse osteopenia may be present.

Abnormal bone scans using technetium-99m are present in over 80% of patients with RSD.[30] Asymmetrical blood flow is typically present. In most patients, increased flow and uptake are noted, but diminished flow and uptake can also be seen. The delayed images generally show increased uptake in periarticular tissues, although a few patients have reduced uptake in the entire affected extremity. Holder and Mackinnon[31] have suggested specific criteria for judging the bone scan in patients suspected of having RSD.

Kozin et al[30] compared the sensitivity and specificity of roetgenography and bone scan in patients with RSD. The sensitivity was found to be 69% in roetgenography and 60% in bone scans, whereas the specifities were 71% and 86% respectively. Bone scans may also be helpful in predicting prognosis in RSD. Kozin et al[30] reported that 90% of the patients identified by positive bone scan had a good response to corticosteroid treatment.

Differential diagnosis. The differential diagnosis of RSD depends on the major clinical features at the time of presentation. The list of conditions that can cause pain, tenderness, swelling, and heat or coldness of an extremity is long. This list would include: tendinitis, myositis, tenosynovitis, septic or inflammatory arthritis, collagen vascular disorders, metabolic arthropathy, chondromalacia, digital sheath infections or abscesses, muscle strains, sprains, senile or postmenopausal osteoporosis, unrecognized fracture (e.g., stress fractures), thrombophlebitis, arterial insufficiency, osteomyelitis, compartment syndrome, fascial hernias, overstretched sensory nerves, severe fibromyalgia (fibrositis), peripheral neuropathy, radiculitis, and hysterical conversion reaction. The clinician must also consider false presentation by a patient who is thereby anticipating compensation, disability, or physician attention. In stage 3, the atrophic stage of RSD, the tight skin and joint contractures may suggest scleroderma.

Erythermalgia, also called erythromelalgia, is a uncommon condition with a typical triad of symptoms: erythema, heat, and burning pain of the involved part. Symptoms are intermittent and are related to increases in environmental temperature or to exercise. Relief can be obtained by administering aspirin or by cooling the environment. These features should make the condition easy to distinguish from RSD.

A careful check of the pulses should be made to exclude the possibility of arterial ischemia in the patient with a painful, tender, cool extremity. If the pulses are not easily felt, assessment of the arterial status by Doppler pressure determination or by referring the patient to a noninvasive vascular laboratory will be helpful.

If nerve involvement is suspected as a cause of a painful extremity, electromyogram with nerve conduction studies may be helpful. Laboratory tests should help exclude other conditions such as infections of bone or soft tissue and collagen vascular diseases.

The bone changes of Sudeck's atrophy appear radiographically similar to those found in hyperparathyroidism, Cushing's syndrome, Paget's disease, metastatic cancer, or multiple myeloma. These diagnoses should be considered when evaluating roetgenograms in patients with painful extremities.

If malingering is suspected, the physician may test the affected extremity while distracting the patient to see if symptoms occur when the patient is not focused. Malingering should also be suspected if the patient is noncompliant to a treatment program.

Treatment. The most effective treatment for RSD is prevention. The importance of early mobilization of an injured extremity, after even minor trauma, must be emphasized. Early mobilization is essential for patients known to be predisposed to RSD, such as those with hemiplegia, myocardial infarction, fracture, or trauma. This is especially true if these conditions occur in a patient with a severe anxiety state or a low pain threshhold.

Once RSD is established, the most important factor in successful treatment is early diagnosis and treatment. The goal is to restore the normal use of the disabled extremity. This may be accomplished in the early stages of RSD by a careful explanation of the disorder, along with copious reassurance and encouragement. An attempt should be made to convince a patient that it is not a serious disease and that a full recovery is expected. A patient should be instructed to walk without aid and to make a real effort to avoid limping. The use of crutches or canes is strictly avoided. The patient should be cautioned that there may be increased discomfort in the limb for the first days or even weeks of rehabilitation.

If the patient is not responding adequately and rapidly to these simple measures, an intensive physical therapy program should be started. The role of physical therapy in the treatment of patients with RSD is well established and should be tried before proceeding to more complicated forms of treatment. Trudel et al[32] reported good-to-excellent results in 44 of 50 RSD patients treated with physical therapy.

The physical therapy program should include full range of motion exercises, stretching of taut muscles and tendons, gait training for normal weight bearing, and exercises in a whirlpool bath. Active exercises are encouraged. Desensitization massage may help some patients. Contrast baths of the affected extremity often help, alternating four minutes at 40.6° C (105° F) with 4 minutes of melting ice water at 0° C (32° F) until hot and cold baths total 32 minutes. The final bath should be hot water, immediately followed by range of motion exercises. Intensive physical therapy may be sufficient, especially early in the course of the disease (i.e., stage 1 or stage 2). Patients with too much pain to participate in physical therapy should initially be treated with pain medications or sympathetic blocks.

Transcutaneous electrical nerve stimulation (TENS) can be useful in some patients with RSD.[33] The TENS unit is postulated to relieve pain by the electrically generated barrage of nerve impulses in large axons. Although there have been mixed results reported in the use of this form of therapy, recent experiences with TENS have been encouraging. Since this method is rapid and safe, it should be tried before more invasive treatments are used. It was reported effective as the only treatment in a child with RSD.[22] TENS may be a useful adjunct to sympathetic blockade, providing analgesia between intermittent blocks. It may also help control pain in chronic cases that do not respond to other modes of therapy.

For the patient who is not responding to reassurance, physical therapy, and TENS, the next step should be a trial of high-dose corticosteroids. Several reports have indicated that this treatment may be of benefit to RSD patients. Fair-to-excellent responses have been reported in 63% to 67% of patients.[30,34,35] Most patients were started on 60 to 200 mg of prednisone daily, with gradual tapering over 2 to 6 weeks. A typical regimen would start with a daily dose of 60 mg of prednisone or equivalent doses of related preparations. This is tapered every 3 days by 5 mg, for a total therapy duration of about 5 weeks. Few side effects are noted with this regimen. If the symptoms increase too much during tapering, therapy may have to be extended.

In the past, paravertebral sympathetic ganglion blockade has been one of the most widely recommended treatments for RSD.[36-39] Good-to-excellent results have been reported in 50% to 80% of patients, though improvement may not be permanent. When the sympathetic block is indicated, the sooner the treatment is initiated, the better the prognosis. A block performed within the first 4 weeks of symptoms may give long-term or permanent relief. When symptoms have been present longer than 6 to 8 weeks, a series of blocks over several days or weeks may be needed. If no significant improvement has appeared after three to five sympathetic blocks given daily or every other day, this approach should be abandoned. Loh and Nathan[36] stressed the importance of hyperpathia in predicting the response to sympathetic blocks. Most patients with hyperpathia responded well to blocks, and only a small percentage without that symptom responded.

Paravertebral ganglionectomy should be considered for patients whose relief with sympathetic blocks is only temporary and whose overall course shows little improvement. In elderly or poor-risk patients, chemical sympathectomy using an injection of phenol or alcohol into the sympathetic chain is an alternative to surgery. This approach cannot be used in the upper extremity because of the proximity of the brachial plexus to the cervical sympathetic chain.

Several authors have reported the results of paravertebral ganglionectomy in patients with RSD.[39-43] Complete relief of symptoms was obtained in 58% to 100% of patients during a follow-up period of 6 months to 17 years. Results were better when surgery was done within 6 months of the onset of symptoms. Failures of treatment were seen most often in patients with severe, long-standing disease or in those with incomplete sympathetic denervation.

Bier blocks have been successfully used in RSD patients. A Bier block is a method used for regional anesthesia. The limb is elevated, a tourniquet applied, and an anesthetic or other substance injected into the limb intravenously for up to 15 minutes. The tourniquet is then removed. Success has been reported[44-46] using Bier blocks with 10 to 20 mg of guanethidine sulfate, with pain relief lasting from hours up to 6 months. This treatment seemed to be most effective in patients with hyperesthesia or hyperpathia. Poplawski et al[47] used Bier blocks with lidocaine hydrochloride (Xylocaine) and methylprednisolone sodium succinate (Solu-Medrol) for

28 patients with RSD. Excellent results were obtained in 16 patients, 5 had some improvement, and 7 had no response. All patients had been symptomatic for more than 9 months. The exact role of Bier blocks in the treatment of RSD is not clear. This method of treatment should be considered when symptoms recur after ganglionectomy or when the patient refuses ganglionectomy.

RSD has been treated by direct infusion of reserpine (Serpasil)[48,49] or guanethidine monosulfate (Ismelin)[50] into the affected limb followed by physical therapy. Neither of these agents has been approved by the Food and Drug Administration for intravenous use, and IV reserpine is no longer commercially available. Both deplete the peripheral nerves of noradrenaline, the primary agent for vasoconstriction, thus producing a chemical sympathectomy that may last 4 to 5 days or longer.

Steinberg[51] found that the use of periarterial blocks with any anesthetic agent was effective in the treatment of RSD. Severe cases were treated with daily blocks. An average of 3 to 12 treatments were required to resolve the condition.

Antiinflammatory agents may help patients with RSD. Other agents, including oral vasodilating agents such as guanethidine,[52] reserpine, and hydralazine, have been reported to be effective. Beta blockers such as propranolol have also been used.[53] Other agents include griseofulvin 3 g orally per day[54] and calcitonin 100 to 160 MRC units intramuscularly daily.[55]

Portwood et al[56] reported on three patients with lower extremity RSD who responded dramatically to daily, low-dose ultrasound therapy to the tarsal tunnel and plantar nerve distribution of the foot and the use of a shoe insert. Several weeks of daily treatments were required to bring about significant improvement. Another measure employed in the treatment of RSD is acupuncture.[57]

In the past, one frequent suggestion was to immobilize the affected part with a cast or splint. Casting or immobilization is not recommended since this procedure not only exacerbates the problem[18,58] but also can cause the problem.

Treatment of patients with chronic, stage 3, atrophic RSD, with symptoms enduring a year or more, is difficult, and the recovery rate is small. High-dose corticosteroids, sympathetic blocks, and sympathectomy should be considered, but most patients do not respond well. Manipulation of the joints with the patient anesthetized may be necessary for severe contractions. Therapy should also include reducing drug dependency by psychiatric pain therapy units when available and the use of psychotrophic agents such as tricyclic antidepressants. Amitriptyline is one of the more potent tricyclics. Vocational guidance and rehabilitation may also be helpful.

This great variety of treatment modalities proposed in the literature attests to the fact that the management of RSD is controversial. The main point regarding therapy is that the degree of disability and response to treatment depend greatly on the time between the onset of the problem and initiation of proper treatment. Problems arise because of difficulties in diagnosis and great variability of the disease expression and course. There are few controlled trials to judge the relative value of the different proposed treatment methods.

Based on a review of the literature and experience with this condition, the following broad guidelines for treatment are suggested for treatment (see the accompanying box):

1. *Stage 1 RSD* (acute stage). In this stage, there is no clinical evidence of sympathetic overactivity. Success is often achieved by education and reassurance of the patient and a vigorous physical therapy program. The TENS unit may also be useful at this stage. A local nerve block or sympathetic block may be necessary to facilitiate these exercises. For patients unresponsive to these measures, a course of corticosteroid therapy should be given.
2. *Stage 2 RSD* (dystrophic stage). Education, reassurance, and physical therapy should be combined with corticosteroid therapy in this patient with clinical evidence of sympathetic overactivity. Steroid therapy should not be delayed. For those patients unresponsive to this course of therapy, sympathetic blocks and sympathectomy should be considered.
3. *Stage 3 RSD* (atrophic stage). Corticosteroid therapy should be tried but may be unsuccessful. Sympathetic

Suggested treatment programs for RSD syndromes

RSD stage 1 (acute stage)

Education and reassurance of patient
Intensive physical therapy
Transcutaneous electrical nerve stimulus (TENS)
If not responding in reasonable amount of time, proceed to modalities outlined for stage 2

RSD stage 2 (dystrophic stage)

Try steps outlined for stage 1 (usually not too effective)
If not responding, try oral corticosteroid course of therapy
If not responding, try sympathetic blocks and sympathectomy

RSD stage 3 (atrophic stage)

Try steps outlined for stages 1 and 2 (usually not too effective)
Free adhesions under general anesthesia
Tricyclic antidepressants
Referral to pain therapy unit
Vocational rehabilitation

Causalgia

Trial course of phenoxybenzamine
If not responding, try sympathetic blocks and sympathectomy

blocks and sympathectomy should also be considered but likewise may not be greatly successful. Manipulation of the joints under general anesthesia may be necessary for severe contractures. Pain therapy units, antidepressants, and vocational guidance may be helpful.

Prognosis. RSD may follow a benign course, causing moderately severe symptoms and resolving with minimal therapy, or it may be severe, lasting years with chronic pain and disability. In general, the earlier the treatment, the more effective the result.

The majority of patients with RSD respond dramatically to nonsurgical therapy. In a series of 75 patients reported by Trudel et al[32] 44 had good-to-excellent results with encouragement, reassurance, and physical therapy. An additional 16 had good-to-excellent results with lumbar sympathetic blocks and physical therapy. Another 8 patients had good results with physical therapy, sympathetic blocks, and sympathectomy. Only 7 of 75 patients had poor results after all forms of therapy.

Pak,[9] in his review of 140 patients, reported that, of those receiving physical therapy for more than 3 days, 80% showed subjective or objective improvement. In a follow-up of 68 patients, 92% showed continued improvement.

Bonica,[59] reviewing his own and others' data, reported that over 80% of patients achieved lasting benefits from sympathetic blocks. Wang et al[60] found that 40% of their patients obtained good-to-excellent results from sympathetic blocks, 22% had partial relief, and 38% had a poor outcome. Lower success rates occur if treatment has been postponed for several months.

Although high-dose corticosteroid therapy has been used only in recent years, there are several series of patients with fair-to-excellent responses in 63% to 76% of cases.[30,34,35] Patients with RSD whose symptoms have been present for a year or more are much less likely to respond to corticosteroid therapy, nerve blocks, or sympathectomy. Irreversible muscle, tendon, and joint dysfunction develop making rehabilitation difficult.

Secondary-gain motives or negative feedback from family members aggravate the situation in a patient with RSD. If litigation is pending, drawn-out legal proceedings may markedly slow rehabilitation efforts. The use of tranquilizers, hypnotics, and narcotics further complicate the situation. The recovery rate in this group of chronic patients is small.

Causalgia

Although causalgia is a form of RSD, it seems advantageous to separate it from the other clinical states already described (i.e., stages 1, 2, and 3 of RSD). Causalgia has sufficiently different diagnostic criteria to be separated from these other conditions. In addition, patients with causalgia fail to respond to physical therapy, whereas practically 100% respond to sympathectomy.

Causalgia is usually easily recognized clinically (see the accompanying box). It is characterized by a severe burning pain and hyperesthesia after a peripheral nerve injury. It is also associated with hyperalgesia (increased sensitivity to noxious stimuli) and allodynia (increased pain due to nonnoxious stimuli) in the painful area. It is a distressing condition that should be diagnosed and treated promptly.

Clinical features of causalgia

- Severe sustained burning pain in distribution of injured nerve or distal to it
- Often associated with hyperalgesia (increased sensitivity to noxious stimuli)
- Often associated with allodynia (increased sensitivity to nonnoxious stimuli)
- Sympathetic overactivity usually present with coolness, hyperhidrosis, cyanosis

Causalgia is derived from two Greek words that translate into "burning" and "pain." The International Association for the Study of Pain has defined causalgia as "sustained burning pain after a traumatic nerve lesion combined with vasomotor and sudomotor changes (sweating and piloerection) and late trophic changes."

In 1813 Denmark[61] described an agonizing pain in the arm of a soldier after a battle injury. In 1838 Hamilton[62] reported on patients with painful extremities after nerve injuries. In 1864 Mitchell, Morehouse, and Keen[1] described a painful syndrome in soldiers suffering from gunshot wounds during the Civil War. Mitchell[63] later introduced the term *causalgia* to describe the most striking feature of this condition: a persistent, severe, burning pain. His vivid description remains unsurpassed in describing the clinical picture of causalgia.

Causalgia is a strictly defined syndrome and represents a subcategory of RSD itself. Terms such as *causalgia-like states, mimo-causalgia, major causalgia,* and *minor causalgia* are inaccurate and should not be used.

Etiology. Causalgia may occur after a wide spectrum of injuries in both military and civilian populations. It is most frequently seen in wartime after penetration of the body by a high-velocity projectile, usually a bullet or shell fragment, that causes an incomplete lesion of the peripheral nerve. Other nerve injuries can occur from knife wounds, motor vehicle accidents, falls, athletic accidents, and iatrogenic injuries. Although most injuries are partial nerve injuries, causalgia occasionally is associated with total transection. Shumacker[64] found complete transection lesions in 10% of patients that he saw with causalgia. There appears to be no clinical correlation between the severity of the nerve injury and the intensity of the symptoms.

Pathogenesis. The exact neurophysiologic explanation of causalgia remains uncertain. Theories proposed to explain this syndrome are the same outlined in the pathogenesis section of RSD. Three theories are commonly proposed.

The first is that artificial synapses are produced by the nerve injury so that sensory afferent fibers are activated by efferent sympathetic fiber impulses. The second theory is that nerve impulses from the site of injury alter the vasomotor status of the skin in the painful areas, thus increasing afferent nociceptor activity. The third theory is that increased spinal cord neuronal activity occurs secondary to changes in the peripheral nervous system. There is little available evidence to fully support any of these theories.

Clinical manifestations. The discomfort of causalgia is usually so severe that the clinical presentation is characteristic. The patient keeps the extremity constantly protected and immobile. In addition the patient is tense, nervous, and apprehensive and devises all sorts of measures to lessen the pain, including moist towels to protect the extremity from drafts of air.

The discomfort of causalgia is usually described as an intense, agonizing burning or aching. It is usually present along the distribution of a major peripheral nerve (e.g., the median, ulnar, femoral, or sciatic nerve) distal to the site of injury. The pain can be diffuse and spread to the proximal and distal portions of the limb without following specific dermatome patterns.

The pain usually begins soon after the injury and reaches peak intensity within a few days to weeks. Onset can be delayed as long as 3 weeks. The pain is usually spontaneous and persistent but subject to exacerbations by various sensory or emotional stimuli. The slightest sensory stimulus, whether tactile, auditory, visual or emotional, may greatly increase the severity of the pain. Examples of this annoyance are moving or touching the involved part, touching slick objects, touching dry objects, feeling the slightest breeze, hearing certain words, feeling vibrations, experiencing upsetting emotional situations, or just gazing upward or downward. Bandages, towels, stockings, or gloves are often worn by the patient to limit sensory stimuli. Causalgia frequently is associated with hyperalgesia and allodynia in the painful area, but these characteristics are not essential for the diagnosis.

Because of the unrelenting burning pain and frequent hyperesthesia, most patients cannot continue working or carry out regular daily activities. They tend to become extremely irritable and withdrawn and may even exhibit psychotic behavior. Severe depression, drug addiction, and suicide have been reported.[65-67] Because of these reactions, patients suffering from causalgia may be thought to be malingering or hysterical. However, these personality disorders are a result of the condition and not the cause of it. The personality disorders usually clear after pain relief with suitable treatment. Psychological studies done after successful treatment have failed to show any predisposing personality disturbances.[68,69]

The distribution of the pain is a point of controversy. Some authors state that the pain should be restricted to the skin distribution of the involved nerve. Others state that the pain is not restricted to this segment and is usually distal in the hand or foot. Mitchell[63] wrote that "the seat of burning is very various, but it never attacks the trunk, rarely the arm or thigh, and not often the forearm or leg. Its favorite site is the foot or hand." All 20 patients reported by Jebara and Saade[70] had pain distally in the hand or foot. Patients with causalgia may have such severe pain that they have difficulty describing the exact distribution, and this may account for the discrepancies in reported series. In Kirklin et al,[71] pain was not limited to the exact distribution of one nerve in 43% of patients.

Altered sympathetic activity is usually present in causalgia. Shumacker et al,[72] in a study of 54 patients, found a cooler than normal limb in 10 patients and a warmer than normal limb in 25. Other signs of altered sympathetic activity may be present, including edema, increased or decreased sweating, and erythema or cyanosis. If the syndrome has been persistent for months to years, dystrophic changes can occur such as skin or muscle atrophy, muscle fibrosis, demineralization of bone, flexion contractures, and joint ankylosis.

Most patients with causalgia have nerve injuries proximal to the knee or elbow.[66] The tibial division of the sciatic nerve, the median nerve, and the medial cord of the brachial plexus are frequent sites of involvement. Upper limbs are more frequently involved than lower limbs with a 5:4 ratio.[1]

Diagnosis. Physicians, especially those dealing with acute trauma patients, should recognize the possibility that a nerve injury, usually a penetrating nerve injury, can be followed by causalgia. Early diagnosis and treatment are important for a favorable outcome. Without proper treatment, long suffering neurotic tendencies and narcotic dependency can develop in many patients.

Since causalgia is most often seen in wartime, it is unfamiliar to most physicians whose training and experience are limited to civilian practice. As a result, when it is seen in a nonwartime setting, the diagnosis is frequently missed, causing needless protracted suffering and disability.

Although not in agreement, most authorities believe that the criteria for diagnosis of causalgia should include the presence of a continuous burning pain distal to the site of an injury, hyperalgesia and allodynia in the painful area, a traumatic event occurring proximal to the painful area (either immediately or within a few weeks before the onset of pain), and the relief of symptoms with a sympathetic nerve block (see the accompanying box). Clinical evidence of nerve

Proposed criteria for diagnosis of causalgia

Traumatic event, often a penetrating wound, occurring proximal to the painful area, either immediately or within a few weeks before onset of pain
Continuous burning pain distal to site of injury
Hyperalgesia and allodynia often present
Relief with a sympathetic block

injury, sympathetic dysfunction, and trophic changes are not required for the diagnosis.

Differential diagnosis. The clinical picture is so striking and unique that causalgia should not be confused with other clinical conditions. It should easily be differentiated from the three stages of classical RSD, Sudeck's atrophy, painful osteoporosis, and a painful amputated stump (with or without neuroma).

Treatment. Spontaneous remission of causalgia is rare. Treatment should be started as early as possible to prevent contractures, atrophy, and psychological disturbances. Although physical therapy is the cornerstone of treatment for other forms of RSD, it is ineffective in causalgia. Manipulations and other modalities of therapy only serve to aggravate the suffering.

Narcotic analgesics may relieve causalgia pain, especially when given in large doses, but the danger of addiction is great. Oral medications, including sympatholytic agents and β-adrenergic blocking agents, have been sporadically reported to be useful in causalgia, but medications do not adequately control symptoms. TENS has occasionally been reported to be effective,[33] but it is usually not helpful and can aggravate symptoms.

Sympathetic blocks will relieve the pain of causalgia only temporarily, and the pain will return to the preinjection levels within hours. Some authors[66,73,74] have advocated neurolysis or resection of the damaged section of nerve with suture sealing of the proximal and distal stumps, but others[68,71] have reported failures of this treatment. Another procedure that has been attempted but abandoned is periarterial sympathectomy.

In the past the best method of treatment has been paravertebral ganglion sympathectomy. The first documented cure of a patient with causalgia was reported in 1930 by Spurling, a neurosurgeon who performed a successful cervical thoracic sympathectomy.[75] Although some surgical series may confuse causalgia with other forms of RSD, the success rate for complete relief from symptoms of causalgia after surgical sympathectomy range from 84% to 91%, and only 4% to 5% fail to improve.[76,77] The failure of some patients to improve may be related to incomplete sympathectomy or to severe dystrophic changes in muscles and joints in prolonged causalgia.

Jebara and Saade[70] described 20 patients with causalgia resulting from war injuries by high-velocity missiles. All patients were treated with sympathectomy and had complete dramatic relief in the immediate postoperative period. The follow-up period ranged from 4 months to 10 years, with a mean of 5.3 years. No return of symptoms was found.

Chemical sympathectomy using an injection of phenol or alcohol into the sympathetic chain is an alternative to surgical sympathectomy, especially in elderly or poor-risk patients with lower-extremity causalgia. It is not applicable in the upper extremity because of the proximity of the cervical sympathetic chain to the brachial plexus.

In 1984 Ghostine et al[78] reported a method of treatment that should be seriously considered before sympathetic blocks or sympathectomy. They treated a series of 40 causalgia patients with a postsynaptic α-1 blocker and presynaptic α-2 blocker, phenoxybenzamine (Dibenzyline). Although none of the patients had a sympathetic block to test the diagnosis of causalgia, all fulfilled the criteria of a deep burning pain, which was exacerbated by physical or emotional stimuli, was associated with partial nerve injury to a major peripheral nerve, and often followed the cutaneous innervation of the injured nerve. The drug was given in a daily dose of 40 to 120 mg for 6 to 8 weeks. Total resolution of pain was achieved in all patients, with a follow-up period from 6 months to 6 years. Thus, this regimen appears to be highly successful and should be tried as the initial treatment in patients with causalgia (see box on p. 519).

Prognosis. Left untreated, the pain of causalgia may gradually subside in a number of patients. According to Echlin et al,[79] there was a gradual improvement of discomfort within 2½ months in 38% of patients and within 6 months in an additional 20%. Other authors report patients whose pain persisted for many years.[42,80] With phenoxybenzamine treatment or sympathectomy the prognosis is excellent.

REFERENCES

1. Mitchell SW, Morehouse CR, and Keen WW: Gunshot wounds and other injuries of nerves, Philadelphia, 1864, JB Lippincott Co.
2. Sudeck P: Über die akute (reflecktorische) Knochenatrophie nach Entzündungin und Verletzungin an den Extremitäten und ihre Klinichen Erscheinungen, Fortschr Geb Röntgenstra 5:277, 1901-1902.
3. Leriche R: The surgery of pain, Baltimore, 1939, Williams & Wilkins (Translated and edited by A. Young).
4. Evans J: Reflex sympathetic dystrophy: report on 57 cases, Ann Intern Med 26:417, 1947.
5. Plewes LW: Sudeck's atrophy in the hands, J Bone Joint Surg (Br) 38:195, 1956.
6. Kozin F: The painful shoulder and reflex sympathetic dystrophy syndrome. In McCarty DJ, ed: Arthritis and allied conditions, ed 10, Philadelphia, 1985, Lea & Febiger.
7. Kozin F: Reflex sympathetic dystrophy syndrome, Bull Rheum Dis 36:1, 1986.
8. Davis SW: Shoulder-hand syndrome in a hemiplegic population: 5 year retrospective study, Arch Phys Med Rehabil 58:3553, 1977.
9. Pak TJ: Reflex sympathetic dystrophy: a review of 140 cases, Minn Med 53:507, 1970.
10. DeTakats G: Nature of painful vasodilation in causalgic states, Arch Neurosurg Psychiatr 50:318, 1943.
11. Doupe J, Cullen CH, and Chance GQ: Post-traumatic pain and the causalgia syndrome, J Neurol Neurosurg Psychiatr 7:33, 1944.
12. Devor M: Nerve pathophysiology and mechanisms of pain in causalgia, J Auton Nerv Syst 7:371, 1983.
13. Blumberg H and Janig W: Changes in unmyelinated fibers including sympathetic postganglionic fibers of a skin nerve after peripheral neuroma formation, J Auton Nerv Sys 6:173, 1982.
14. Wall PD and Devor J: The effect of peripheral nerve injury on dorsal root potentials and on transmission of afferent signals into the spinal cord, Brain Res 209:95, 1981.
15. Livingston WK: Pain mechanisms, New York, 1943, Macmillan Publishing Co.

16. Steinbrocker O and Argyros TG: The shoulder-hand syndrome: present status as a diagnostic and therapeutic entity, Med Clin North Am 42:1538, 1958.
17. Drucker WR et al: Pathogenesis of post-traumatic sympathetic dystrophy, Am J Surg 97:454, 1959.
18. Bernstein BH et al: Reflex neurovascular dystrophy in childhood, J Pediatr 93:211, 1978.
19. Bermaglich DR: Reflex sympathetic dystrophy in children, Pediatrics 60:881, 1977.
20. Ruggeri SB et al: Reflex sympathetic dystrophy in children, Clin Orthop 163:225, 1982.
21. Silber TJ and Majd M: Reflex sympathetic dystrophy syndrome in children and adolescents: report of 18 cases and review of the literature, Am J Dis Child 142:1325, 1988.
22. Kesler RW et al: Reflex sympathetic dystrophy in children: treatment with transcutaneous electric nerve stimulation, Pediatrics 82:728, Nov 1988.
23. Drucker WR, Hubay CA, and Holden WB: Pathogenesis of post-traumatic sympathetic dystrophy, Am J Surg 97:451, 1959.
24. Lexer E, Kuliga R, and Turk W: Untersuchgen über Knochenarterien, Berlin, 1904, Hirschwald.
25. Echlin F, Owens FM, and Wells WL: Observations on "major" and "minor" causalgia, Arch Neurol 62:183, 1945.
26. Julsrud ME: A review of reflex sympathetic dystrophy, J Am Podiatr Med Assoc 70:512, 1980.
27. Owens JC: Causalgia, Am Surg 23:636, 1957.
28. DeTakats G: Sympathetic reflex dystrophy, Med Clin North Am 49:117, 1965.
29. Kozin R et al: The reflex sympathetic dystrophy syndrome. II. Roentgenographic and scintigraphic evidence of bilaterality and of periarticular accentuation, Am J Med 60:332, 1976.
30. Kozin F et al: The reflex sympathetic dystrophy syndrome. III. Scintigraphic studies, further evidence for the therapeutic efficacy of systemic corticosteroids and proposed diagnostic criteria, Am J Med 70:23, 1981.
31. Holder LE and Mackinnon SE: Reflex sympathetic dystrophy in the hands: clinical and scintigraphic criteria, Radiology 152:517, 1984.
32. Trudel J et al. Disuse phenomenon of the lower extremity: diagnosis and treatment, JAMA 186:1129, 1963.
33. Meyer GA and Fields HL: Causalgia treated by selective large fibre stimulation of peripheral nerve, Brain 95:163, 1972.
34. Glick EN: Reflex dystrophy (algoneurodystrophy): results of treatment by corticosteroids, Rheumatol Rehabil 12:84, 1973.
35. Rosen PS and Graham W: The shoulder-hand syndrome: historical review with observations on 73 patients, Can Med Assoc J 77:86, 1957.
36. Loh L and Nathan PW: Painful peripheral states and sympathetic blocks, J Neurol Neurosurg Psychiatry 41:664, 1978.
37. Subbarao J and Stillwell GK: Reflex sympathetic dystrophy syndrome of the upper extremity: analysis of total outcome of management of 125 cases, Arch Phys Med Rehabil 62:549, 1981.
38. Betcher AM, Bean G, and Casten DF: Continuous procaine block of paravertebral sympathetic ganglions, JAMA 154:288, 1953.
39. Shumacker HB and Abramson DI: Postraumatic vasomotor disorders: with particular reference to late manifestations and treatment, Surg Gynecol Obstet 88:417, 1949.
40. Patman RD, Thompson JE, and Persson AV: Management of post-traumatic pain syndrome: report of 113 cases, Ann Surg 177:780, 1973.
41. Holden WD: Sympathetic dystrophy, Arch Surg 57:373, 1948.
42. Barnes R: The role of sympathectomy in the treatment of causalgia, J Bone Joint Surg (Br) 35b:172, 1953.
43. Evans JA: Sympathectomy for reflex sympathetic dystrophy: report of 29 cases, JAMA 172, 1946.
44. Glynn CJ, Basedow RW, and Walsh JA: Pain relief following post-ganglionic sympathetic blockade with IV guanethidine, Br J Anaesth 53:1297, 1981.
45. Tabira T, Shibasaki H, and Kuroiwa Y: Reflex sympathetic dystrophy (causalgia) treatment with guanethidine, Arch Neurol 40:430, 1983.
46. Loh L et al: Effects of guanethidine infusion in certain painful states, J Neurol Neurosurg Psychiatry 43:446, 1980.
47. Poplawski ZJ, Wiley AM, and Murray JF: Post-traumatic dystrophy of the extremities, J Bone Joint Surg (Am) 65:642, 1983.
48. Chuinard RG et al: Intravenous reserpine for treatment of reflex sympathetic dystrophy, South Med J 74:1481, 1981.
49. Benzon HT, Chomka CM, and Brunner EA: Treatment of reflex sympathetic dystrophy with regional intravenous reserpine, Anesth Analg 59:500, 1980.
50. Bonnelli S et al: Regional intravenous guanethidine vs stellate ganglion block in reflex sympathetic dystrophies: a randomized trial, Pain 16:297, 1983.
51. Steinberg MD: Gout and Sudeck's atrophy: a simplified office approach to treatment, J Am Podiatr Med Assoc 65:379, 1975.
52. Headley B: Historical perspective of causalgia: management of sympathetically maintained pain, Phys Ther 67:1370, 1987.
53. Visitsunthorn U and Prete P: Reflex sympathetic dystrophy of the lower extremity—a complication of herpes zoster with dramatic response to propranolol, West J Med 135:62, 1981.
54. Doury P: Reflex sympathetic dystrophy (algodystrophy), Int Med for the Specialist 6:67, 1985.
55. Doury P and Pattin S: Treatment of algodystrophy with cacitonin, Rhumato 32:111, 1980.
56. Portwood MM, Lieberman JS, and Taylor RG: Ultrasound treatment of reflex sympathetic dystrophy, Arch Phys Med Rehabil 68:116, 1987.
57. Chan CS and Chow SP: Electroacupuncture in the treatment of post-traumatic sympathetic dystrophy (Sudeck's atrophy), Br J Anaesth 53:899, 1981.
58. Kim HJ et al: Reflex sympathetic dystrophy syndrome of the knee following meniscectomy, Arthritis Rheum 22:177, 1979.
59. Bonica JJ: Causalgia and other reflex sympathetic dystrophies, Postgrad Med 53:143, 1973.
60. Wang JK, Johnson KA, and Ilstrup DM: Sympathetic blocks for reflex sympathetic dystrophy, Pain 23:13, 1985.
61. Denmark A: An example of symptoms resembling tic douloureux produced by a wound in the radial nerve, Med Chir Trans 4:48, 1813.
62. Hamilton J: On some effects resulting from wounds of nerves, Dublin J Med Sci 13:38, 1838.
63. Mitchell SW: Injuries of nerves and their consequences, Philadelphia, 1872, JB Lippincott Co.
64. Shumacker HB Jr: Causalgia. III. A general discussion, Surgery 24:485, 1948.
65. Horowitz SH: Brachial plexus injuries with causalgia resulting from transaxillary rib resection, Arch Surg 120:1189, 1985.
66. Richards RL: Causalgia: a centennial review, Arch Neurol 16:339, 1967.
67. Shumacker HB Jr: A personal overview of causalgia and other reflex dystrophies, Ann Surg 201:278, 1985.
68. Mayfield FH and Devine JW: Causalgia, Surg Gynecol Obstet 80:631, 1945.
69. DeTakats G: Causalgic states in peace and war, JAMA 128:699, 1945.
70. Jebara VA and Saade B: Causalgia: a wartime experience-report of twenty treated cases, J Trauma 27:519, 1987.
71. Kirklin JW, Chenoweth AI, and Murphey F: Causalgia: a review of its characteristics, diagnosis, and treatment, Surgery 21:321, 1947.
72. Shumacker HB, Spiegel LL, and Upjohn RH: Causalgia, Surg Gynecol Obstet 86:76, 1948.
73. Allbritten FF Jr and Maltby GL: Causalgia secondary to injury of the major peripheral nerves, Surgery 19:407, 1946.

74. Paget J: Effects from a wound to the radial nerves, Med Times 612:1, 1864.
75. Spurling RG: Causalgia of the upper extremity: treatment by dorsal sympathetic ganglionectomy, Arch Neurol and Psychiatr 23:784, 1930.
76. Bonica JJ: Causalgia and reflex sympathetic dystrophies. In Bonica JJ and Albe-Fessard D, eds: Advances in pain research and therapy, vol. 3, New York, 1979, Raven Press.
77. Mayfield FH: Causalgia, Springfield, Ill., 1951, Charles C Thomas.
78. Ghostine SY et al: Phenoxybenzamine in the treatment of causalgia: report of 40 cases, J Neurosurg 60:1263, 1984.
79. Echlin F, Owens FM Jr, and Wells WL: Observations on major and minor causalgia, Arch Neurol Psychiatr 62:183, 1949.
80. Abram SE and Lightfoot R: Treatment of long-standing causalgia with prazosin, Reg Anesth 6:79, 1981.

Chapter 30

VASCULAR ANOMALIES

Earl Z. Browne, Jr.

In no area of peripheral vascular disease is there more confusion than in the etiology and pathophysiology of vascular anomalies. A bewildering classification exists, contrasting numerous eponyms and lengthy Latin descriptions with the tendency to describe all types of vascular malformations as hemangiomas.[1-3] This has been especially true in the British literature, where the term *cavernous hemangioma* is applied to a wide variety of pathologic variants.[4] The use of syndromes often adds to the confusion. Although there are some syndromes associated with relatively uniform manifestations, others are not so clear. For example, Ollier's disease, that of multiple congenital enchondromatosis, is referred to as Maffucci's syndrome when vascular malformations are present, and the actual malformations have been described in many different ways.[5]

GENERAL CONSIDERATIONS

Classification

As with all diseases, it is best to minimize the use of long Latin names and base classification on pathophysiology. Common to all vascular lesions is the presence of endothelial cells. Studies of the characteristics of these cells in various vascular lesions indicate that the lesions fall into two major categories. These include lesions with proliferative endothelium and lesions with static endothelium (or vascular malformations) (see the accompanying box).

Lesions with proliferative endothelium. The normal process of healing is a form of vascular proliferation. Angiogenesis is one of the earliest histologic activities in healing, leading to granulation tissue formation in the open wound. Proliferative vascular masses, primarily the true hemangiomas, are vascular tumors with increased endothelial cell turnover during an early phase of proliferation.[6] Although not true neoplasms, capillary hemangiomas demonstrate increased mast cell activity, angiogenesis, and capillary migration.[7] These lesions characteristically enlarge rapidly in the initial stage, then stabilize, and usually regress. Other lesions with proliferative endothelium include pyogenic granuloma and neoplasms of vascular origin.

Lesions with static endothelium. Lesions with static endothelium are most appropriately called vascular malformations. Depending on the structures that are present, vascular malformations may be arterial, venous, lymphatic, capillary, or any combination of those forms. Since they do not have increased endothelial cell turnover, their increased size represents enlargement of previously existing vascular channels.[8] A misnomer in the group is the cavernous hemangioma. This is not a proliferative lesion like the capillary,

I. ***Lesions with proliferative endothelium***
   - A. True hemangiomas (strawberry nevus)
   - B. Pyogenic granulomas
   - C. Neoplasms (hemangiopericytoma, angiosarcoma)

II. ***Lesions with static endothelium (vascular malformations)***
   - A. Capillary malformations (port-wine stains)
   - B. Lymphatic malformations (cystic hygromas and lymphangiomas)
   - C. Venous malformations (cavernous hemangiomas)
   - D. Arteriovenous malformations
     1. Congenital
     2. Acquired
        a. Trauma (penetrating injuries, fractures)
        b. Iatrogenic (surgery)
        c. Spontaneous

III. ***Syndromes in which vascular lesions are present***
   - A. Sturge-Weber syndrome (port-wine stain)
   - B. Klippel-Trenaunay syndrome (port-wine stain)
   - C. Kasabach-Merritt syndrome (true hemangiomas, venous malformations)
   - D. Maffucci's syndrome (Ollier's disease)

or true hemangioma, although it usually enlarges with time because of hemodynamic changes.[9] Vascular malformations are generally congenital lesions but can be caused by penetrating trauma such as a stab wound.

A study of the embryology of the vascular system provides insight into how these abnormalities, and the various combinations, might occur.[10] The vascular system in the early embryo initially consists of blood spaces forming a diffuse network in the mesenchyme. There is then a coalescence of these spaces into a primitive capillary network. At that stage there is no differentiation of the type of vessel. In the second so-called "retiform" phase there is a coalescence of this primitive capillary network into large plexiform structures, which appear to be separate from one another. It appears that the collateral vessel system is established during this phase, especially in the extremities, and regions of the body develop their own autonomous microcirculation. In the third stage large blood vessels grow out from the great vessels, and communications develop between these vessels and the preexisting retiform plexuses. Arterial, venous, and lymphatic systems are thus established. Depending on the phase in which an embryologic insult occurs, failure of any of these systems to evolve or to involute may occur, causing excessive or faulty development of one or more elements destined to develop during that time of the embryologic differentiation. Therefore there can be nests of capillaries, veins, or arteries, persistence of arteriovenous connections from the retiform stage, lymphatic accumulations, or any combinations of these. Common to all of these malformations, however, is the presence of mature endothelial cells, which do not proliferate to a greater extent than normal cells.[9] Enlargement to "cavernous" structures is a manifestation of blood inherently following the path of least resistance and dilating existing structures.

The classification of these lesions is therefore best done by naming them all vascular malformations, and then subclassifying them according to the most predominant element present.[6] Thus the term malformation is more descriptive than cavernous hemangioma, and a capillary malformation might be considered to be venous, lymphatic, or mixed. Only if it can be demonstrated that definite shunting is present should a structure be called an arteriovenous malformation. It is also convenient from a clinical standpoint to subcategorize lesions as high flow or low flow. Clearly, no matter what type of lesion is present, those which have high flow are more apt to enlarge and to require consideration for treatment.

Diagnosis

Although sophisticated tests may sometimes be necessary to determine the extent of a vascular lesion, the diagnosis can almost always be made on physical examination. Those lesions that are characterized by proliferation of endothelium will grow and increase in size over a period of time out of proportion to the surrounding part of the body. Lesions that are static may slowly increase in size but will do so by becoming more engorged with blood and will not truly grow. In addition to obtaining this history it is possible to determine whether there is a high or low degree of blood flow in the lesion on physical examination. High-flow lesions are characterized by warmth and evidence of increased metabolic activity in the area of the lesion. There may be obvious overgrowth in the area. If there is an arterial component, a thrill may be felt on palpation, a bruit heard when listening to the lesion with a stethoscope, and characteristic sounds of either arterial or venous flow can be heard with the Doppler. Plain radiographs can be helpful in determining the presence of localized increased metabolic activity, and in lesions with large venous spaces phleboliths can also be seen. Arteriography and computerized imaging can sometimes be of value and will be discussed in relation to the individual lesions.

Treatment

In general, large vascular lesions are diffuse and are not often symptomatic. Many times the patient or family members are primarily concerned about the appearance of the lesion and its potential for worsening. The physician must first be very accurate in establishing the pathophysiology of the lesion, and then he or she must consider which is worse, the treatment or the disease. For the most part symptomatic treatment and psychologic reassurance are the best approaches for diffuse lesions. Only if it can be determined that a small localized lesion can be easily treated, or that a large lesion has a significant potential for threatening life or limb, should specific treatment measures be considered for relatively asymptomatic lesions.

LESIONS WITH PROLIFERATIVE ENDOTHELIUM

True hemangioma

The true hemangioma is the so-called "strawberry nevus" of infancy. This classically appears during the second to fourth week of life, having sometimes been noted at birth as a small red cutaneous spot.[10] By 1 year of age approximately 12% of children will have developed a hemangioma, and it is more commonly found in white female infants.[11] The hemangioma characteristically grows very rapidly and is most commonly found in the head and neck region. There is an initial bright red swelling that becomes raised and rapidly shows signs of involution on the surface[12] (Fig. 30-1). After growing rapidly for the first 8 to 10 months of life, significant involution occurs, and a large number of the lesions have completely involuted by 2 years of age. Many studies have indicated that complete resolution occurs in at least 50% of patients by the age of 5 years and in 90% by 7 years.[13,14] The involution, which occurs on the surface, generally starting at the center, causes lighter areas of scarring, which gives this lesion its characteristic appearance of a strawberry. Although they are usually small, occasionally the lesion will proliferate to an enormous size and can cause problems by encroachment on important structures such as the eyelid (Fig. 30-2). They may also ulcerate and bleed. The syndrome of disseminated intravascular coagulation (DIC) in association with extensive, rapidly growing hemangioma in the young infant has been named Kasabach-Merritt syndrome.[15] Although this is rare, it can be associated with a profound bleeding diathesis, and there is a high mortality rate in untreated cases.[16]

In general, these lesions are best left alone, since they will typically involute with time.[12,13] The results of treatment are often worse in terms of scarring than the subsequent results of the involution. Occasionally the lesion will not completely involute and surgical excision is warranted, but this is generally reserved for those circumstances where involution of very large lesions has left redundancy of the skin and subcutaneous tissue. The results of cryotherapy, sclerotherapy, and laser ablation are fraught with excessive scarring, so in general they are less desirable than complete surgical excision. These measures, however, may be of value in helping to reduce the size of massive lesions.[9] Sometimes because of excessively rapid growth, airway obstruction can develop, which may require treatment. One specific problem requiring intervention is extensive involvement of the eyelid. Amblyopia will develop if obstructed vision is left untreated. Encouraging results with early surgical excision in these circumstances have been reported.

Systemic steroid therapy is used to treat infants with large

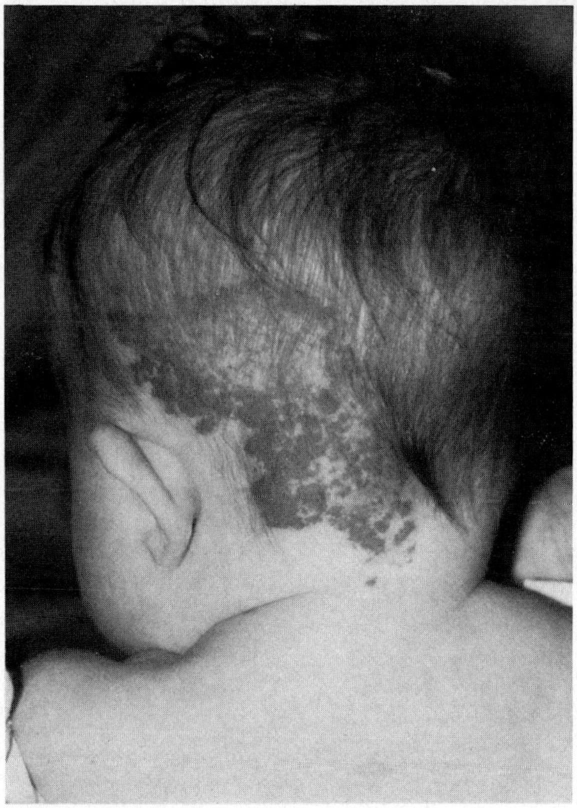

Fig. 30-1. Hemangioma of recent onset, which is already undergoing involution in scattered areas.

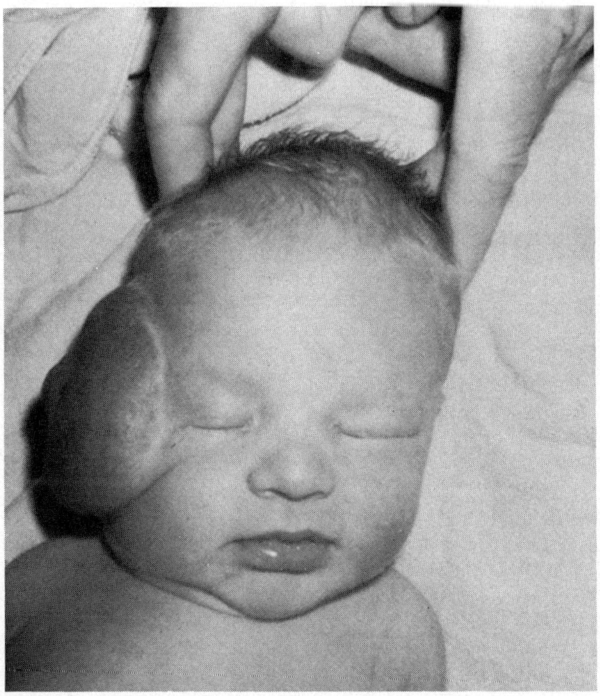

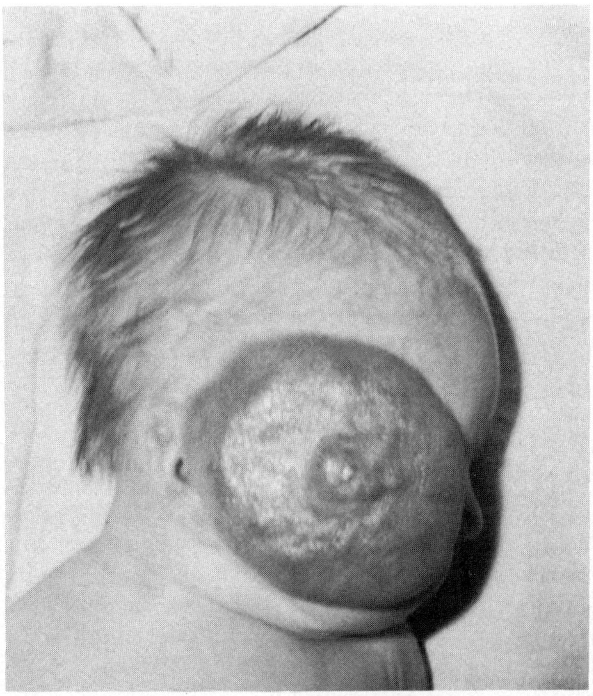

Fig. 30-2. Rapidly growing hemangioma in infant.

A 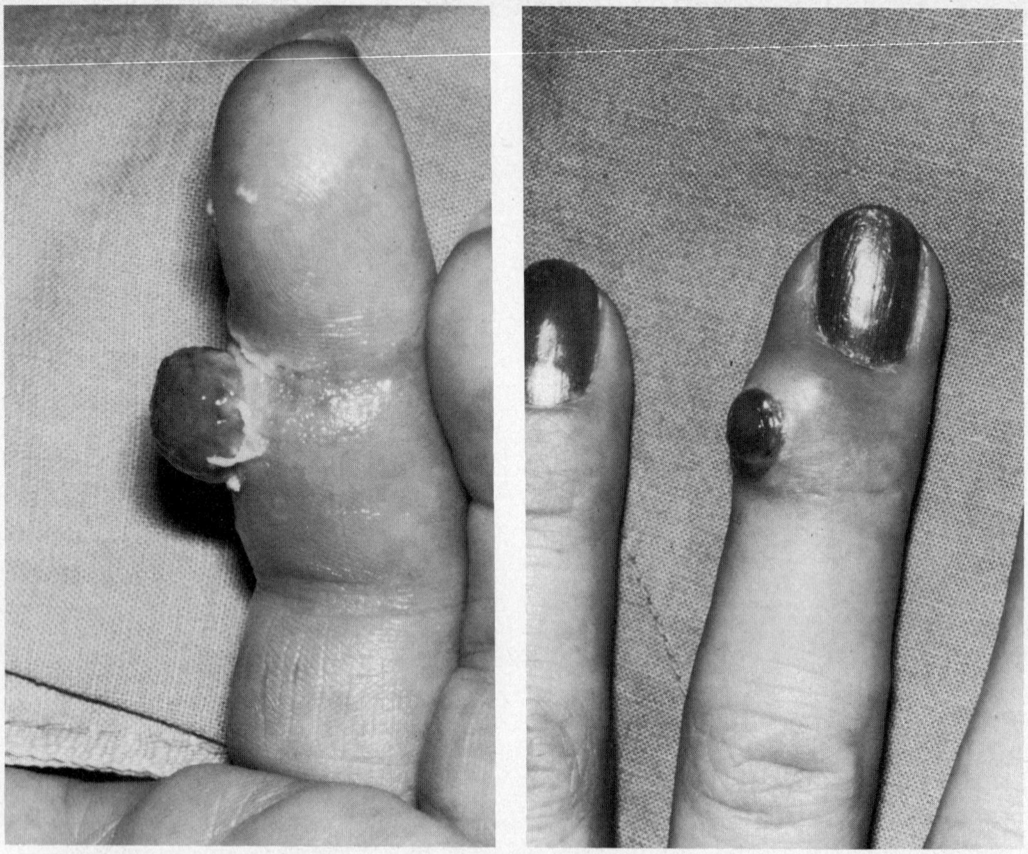 B

Fig. 30-3. Two different pyogenic granulomas occurring after penetrating injury. **A** is polypoid, resembling granulation tissue. **B** is tumorous, involving adjacent normal tissue, resembling a hemangioma.

hemangiomas, especially if there is significant bleeding or ulceration, encroachment on an important structure such as the eye, or such widespread involvement that there is concern about cardiac failure.[16] Hemorrhage associated with the coagulopathy of the Kasabach-Merritt syndrome usually responds to steroids. It appears that steroids accelerate the beginning of involution in these large lesions, but it is important that treatment begin at a very early age. Edgerton maintains that this treatment must begin before the age of 6 months for the hemangioma to be responsive to steroids.[17] If the lesion is sensitive, a response will occur within a few weeks with a dosage of 2 to 3 mg/kg/day.

Pyogenic granuloma

An interesting proliferative vascular lesion is the pyogenic granuloma. This is a localized tumorous growth appearing in small wounds, which often appear to have been chronically infected.

Histologically similar to the capillary hemangioma, the pyogenic granuloma is a small polypoid growth that generally develops in the area of trauma (Fig. 30-3). Often there is a small laceration that appears to become chronically infected, although these lesions may arise de novo, as well as in apparently well-healed wounds. Although an infectious cause is indicated by its name, seldom is there bacterial growth present unless the lesion ulcerates and becomes secondarily infected.[9] These lesions may spontaneously regress, though many of them have a history of repeated episodes of ulceration and bleeding. Because of that they are generally treated either by excision or electrodesiccation and seldom have the opportunity to proliferate to a very large size.

Vascular neoplasms

Although quite rare, there are true neoplasms of vascular origin such as hemangiopericytoma or angiosarcoma, which also have cells that proliferate to a greater than normal extent. These are discussed in Chapter 34.

LESIONS WITH STATIC ENDOTHELIUM

Capillary malformations (port-wine stains)

The most common lesion is the purplish cutaneous staining, commonly seen on the face along the distribution of one of the trigeminal nerves (Fig. 30-4). These are always low-flow lesions that characteristically thicken over the years, developing a raised nodular surface.[18] Histologically,

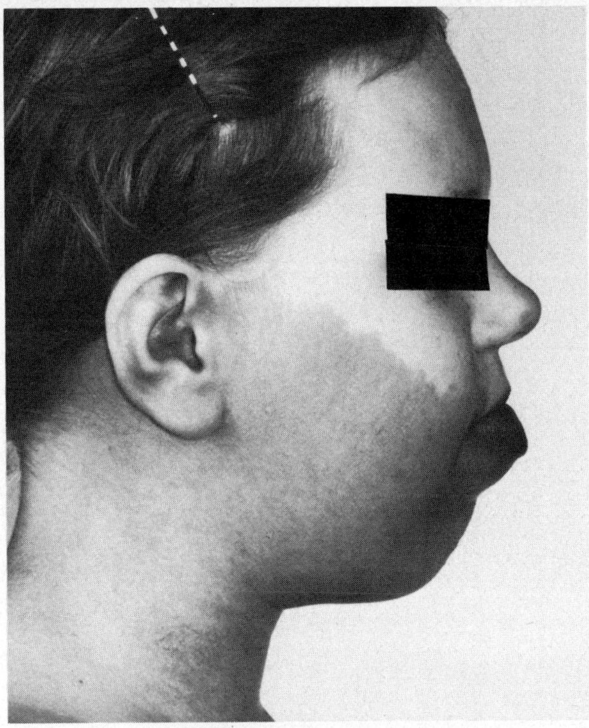

Fig. 30-4. Port-wine stain of face.

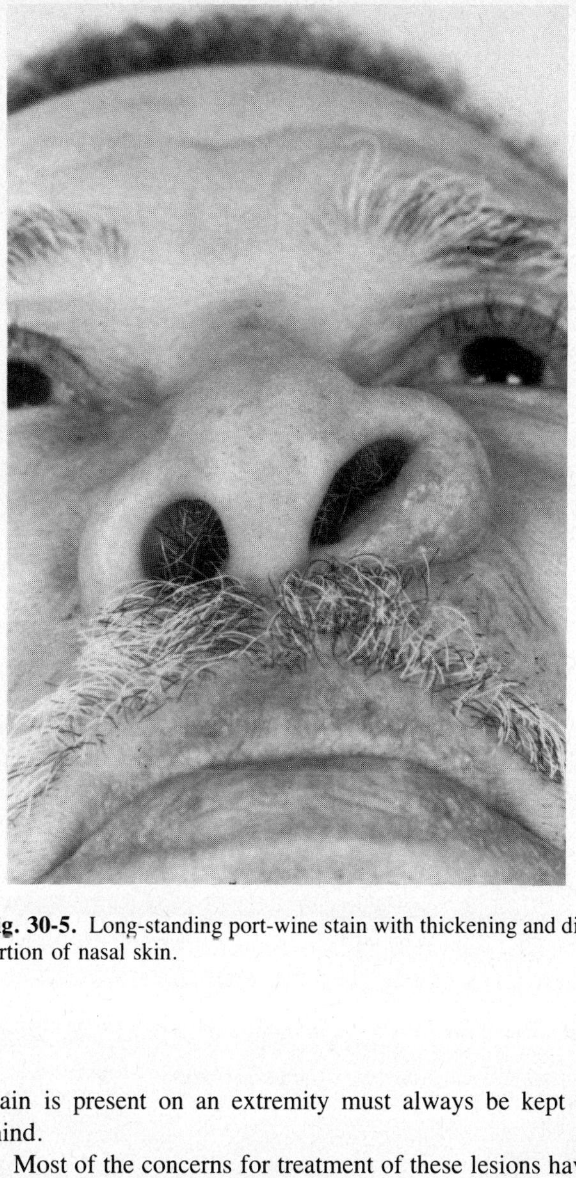

Fig. 30-5. Long-standing port-wine stain with thickening and distortion of nasal skin.

there are numerous dilated capillary- or venule-size structures present in the dermis. They are always present at birth, although they never appear to be as extensive as the network eventually becomes. Especially in the lower extremities, not only does the surface of the skin become much thicker and involved with dilated vessels, but also more and more of these vessels open in the collateral bed with time, so that the lesion has the appearance of spreading centripetally (Fig. 30-5). There is no evidence at all of endothelial proliferation in these lesions, however.[6]

There are two fairly characteristic syndromes associated with port-wine stains. The presence of a stain in the trigeminal nerve distribution may be associated with an underlying venous or arteriovenous malformation of the leptomeninges. This is referred to as the Sturge-Weber syndrome.[19] The Klippel-Trenaunay syndrome is a port-wine stain of the trunk and/or extremities, associated with muscular hypertrophy and varicose veins.[20] Congenital venous malformations may be present. Often very large tortuous vascular channels develop in the leg (Fig. 30-6). There is characteristically increased warmth of the extremity and often overgrowth, especially if it involves the lower extremity.

Port-wine stains are always permanent defects; the color usually darkens with age, and in adults the surface becomes raised and irregular. The possibility of an underlying vascular malformation such as the Sturge-Weber syndrome with a facial stain or the Klippel-Trenaunay syndrome when a stain is present on an extremity must always be kept in mind.

Most of the concerns for treatment of these lesions have to do with appearance, since they can be quite psychologically disturbing. Over the years there have been many techniques used such as electrical desiccation, cryotherapy, tattooing, serial excision, and skin grafting, but although helpful in extreme cases, most of these result in such excessive scarring that the appearance is worse than the lesion itself.[21] There are several very good camouflage makeups that can be used, and skillful application of one of these is probably the best form of therapy available.

There is considerable interest in the use of lasers to treat port-wine stains.[21,22] The principle of this is the absorption by hemoglobin of energy in a relatively narrow wavelength. Theoretically, if the lesion is purely capillary, it would be possible to deliver enough localized energy in a small focused beam that the treated area could be vaporized, not harming adjacent tissue. This is only applicable to very small vessels and not dilated channels. By the use of multiple treatments, using a grid pattern, which is changed for each

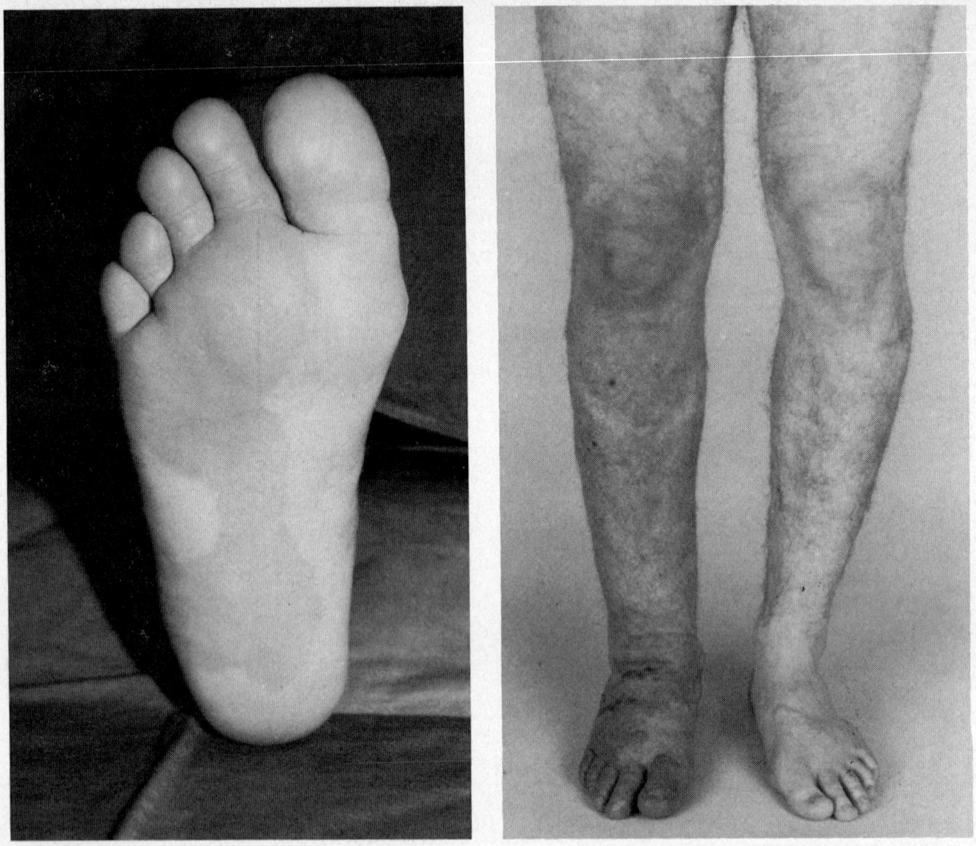

Fig. 30-6. Features of Klippel-Trenaunay syndrome, showing port-wine stain, tortuous venous channels, and hypertrophy of the extremity.

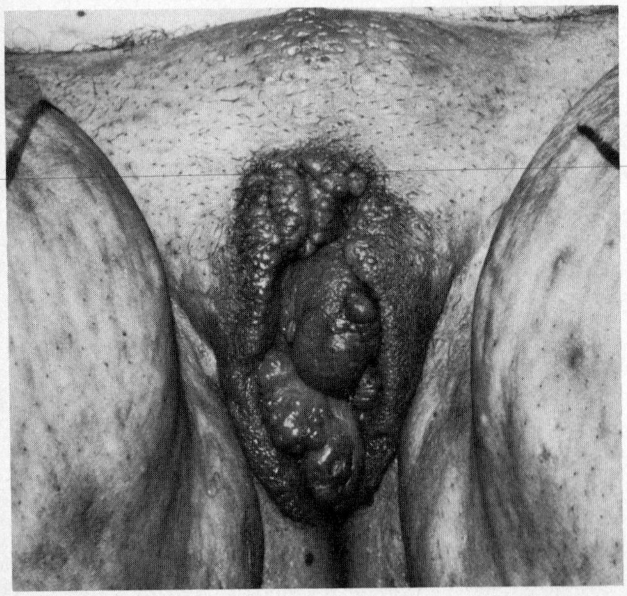

Fig. 30-7. Chronically inflamed, painful, lymphatic malformation of vulva.

successive treatment, the lesion can be obliterated over a period of time. The Argon laser has been used for this purpose in many instances, but, unfortunately, there is a tendency towards hypertrophic scarring, especially in very young children.[21] Tunable dye lasers, which allow adjustable wavelengths, are now being used experimentally and may prove to be of much greater value.[22]

Lymphatic malformations

Lymphatic malformations are almost always low-flow vascular lesions, although they may become quite large because of increased resistance. Two characteristic forms are seen, lymphangioma and cystic hygroma. A lymphangioma most commonly involves the extremity. It might involve only superficial vessels in the skin, which characteristically become nodular over a period of years. It may also develop into quite large diffuse cystic channels, causing extensive swelling of the entire extremity. Cystic hygromas are always much larger and more diffuse than they appear. They usually appear as spongy-feeling swellings in the neck, which may enlarge with straining or crying. These lesions consist of large dilated cystic spaces filled with lymphatic fluid. If located in areas that are frequently traumatized,

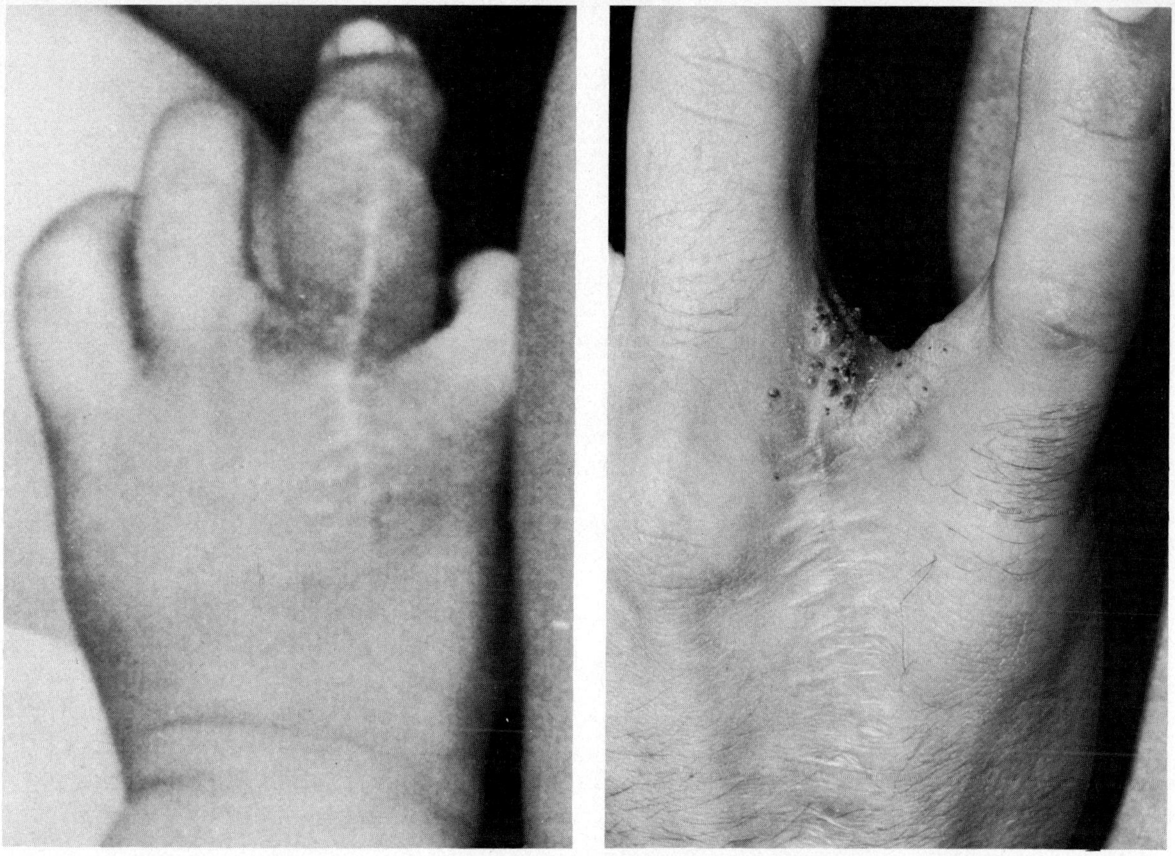

Fig. 30-8. A, Digital lymphatic malformation requiring amputation in a child. **B,** Symptomatic ulceration of residual lesion in a teenager, which was subsequently excised and skin grafted.

they may increase and become chronically inflamed and scarred (Fig. 30-7).

Lymphatic malformations are all low-flow lesions and are best treated only if complications develop. Often surface irregularities develop, leading to cracking and scaling, and over a period of years cutaneous infections may develop. This, just as in the case with lymphedema, can become a significant problem with recurrent bouts of cellulitis and lymphangitis. Because of this, excision and skin grafting may sometimes be necessary for cutaneous lesions (Fig. 30-8). Although well-localized deeper lesions can be totally excised, these lesions typically are much more extensive than they appear, and recurrence after excision is the rule rather than the exception. This is especially true in the cervical cystic hygroma. Prevention of infection with good skin care and compression with elastic garments to help prevent subsequent lymphedema are the primary methods of treatment. Bouts of cellulitis should be treated vigorously with antibiotics to help prevent scarring and progressive lymphatic obliteration in adjacent areas.

Venous malformations

Clinical picture. Venous malformations are lesions that have been commonly called cavernous hemangiomas. They may be low flow, relatively localized, and appear only as a cystic dilated nest of blood vessels (Fig. 30-9). Venous malformations may also be quite diffuse and involve a very large portion of the body as in the Klippel-Trenaunay syndrome. These lesions may expand with trauma and frequently enlarge around the time of puberty or hormonal change. Thrombosis often occurs within these channels because of sluggish flow and may lead to intermittent localized pain and tenderness. Phleboliths can be palpated as lumps in the affected areas and are always seen on radiographic evaluation. There can also be a low-grade DIC present, a form of the Kasabach-Merritt syndrome.[15]

Small, localized lesions are generally asymptomatic. Large diffuse lesions involving the extremities may slowly enlarge to the point where significant problems can occur because of the size of the dilated vessels. Skin changes of stasis, ulceration, and hemorrhage can occur, and may become quite painful. Pain may also be produced by pressure on deep structures, especially nerves passing through confined spaces. Nerve deficit may be present because of direct involvement of the nerve by the malformation, but symptoms of nerve entrapment may develop as well. One frequent manifestation is carpal tunnel syndrome caused by compression of the median nerve either in the carpal tunnel or the

A

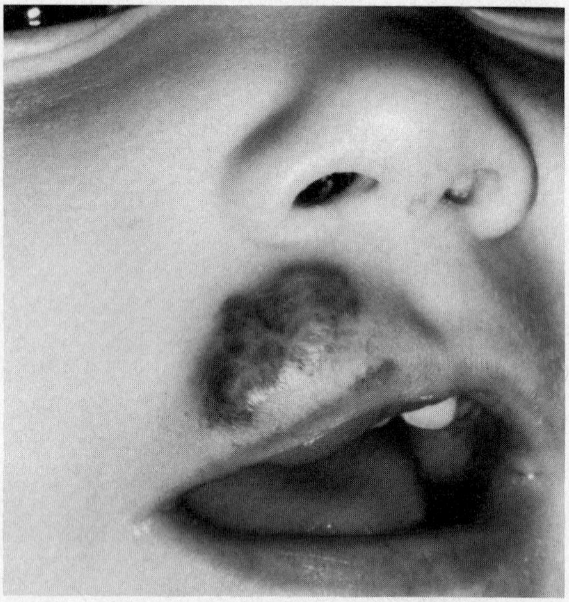

Fig. 30-9. **A-C,** Localized venous malformations. Although erroneously referred to as "cavernous hemangiomas," these are not proliferative lesions.

B

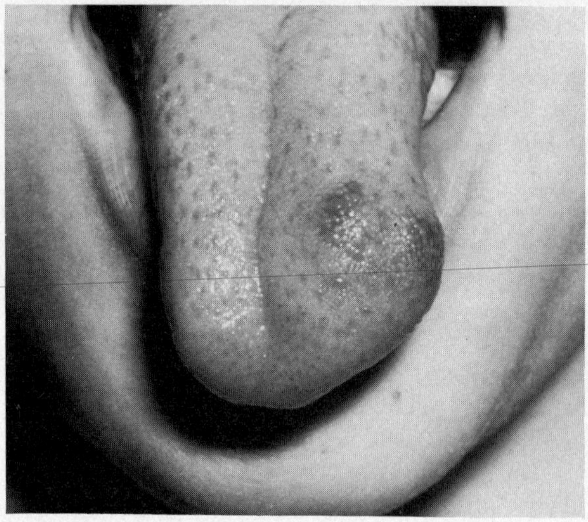

C

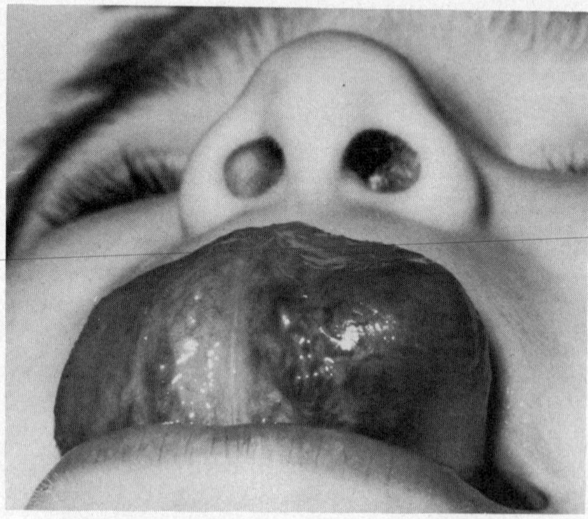

A

B

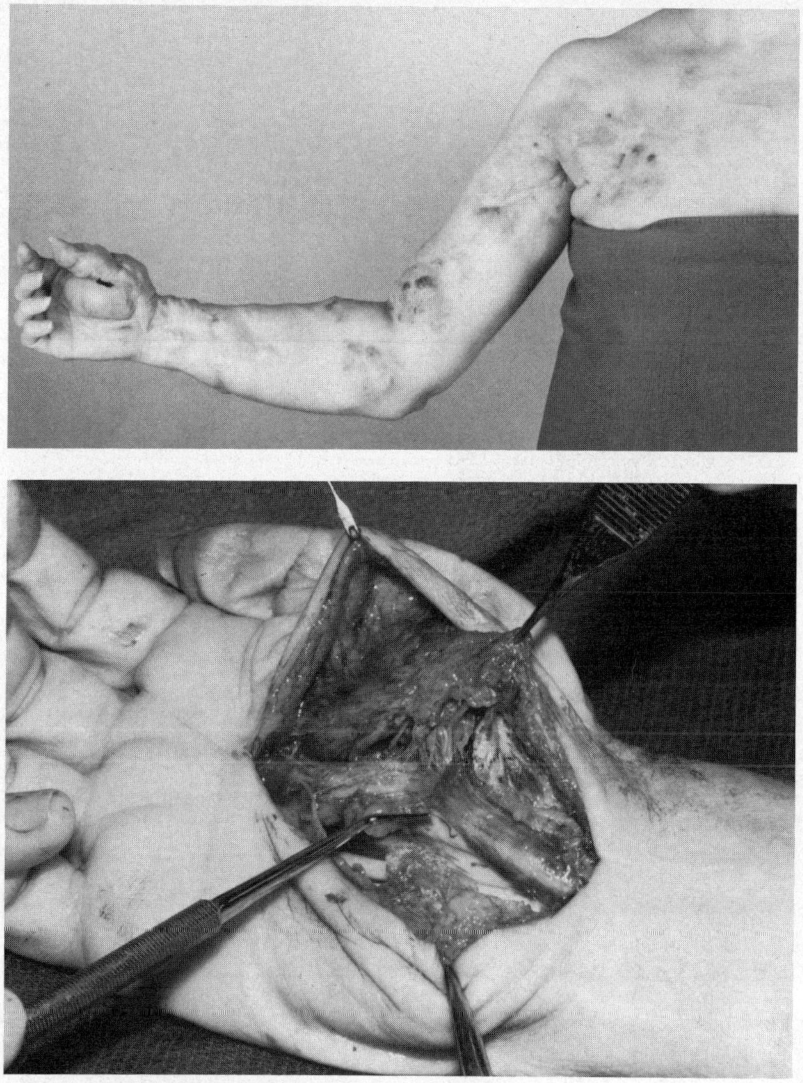

Fig. 30-10. A, Diffuse venous malformation of upper extremity causing severe compression of median nerve in carpal tunnel (**B**).

distal forearm. If allowed to persist for a long time, permanent nerve deficit may result from degeneration from localized pressure (Fig. 30-10).

Diagnosis. On physical examination there may be very few findings except for a soft compressible mass. Since there is no arterial component, there are no thrills or bruits present, although there is generally a diffuse continuous nondirectional venous sound heard over the involved area when listening with the Doppler. Larger lesions imply not only a more diffuse network of vessels, but also a higher flow causing increased resistance and opening up of more channels. In this circumstance, the involved area is often warmer than the rest of the body, and there may be evidence of hypertrophy (see Fig. 30-6). Skeletal overgrowth of the involved extremity is a classic finding in the Klippel-Trenaunay syndrome.[9,24] Hypertrophy can be seen on radiographic examination as well as on physical examination (Fig. 30-11).

Plain radiographs almost always demonstrate phleboliths present in the involved area (Fig. 30-12). This is generally a sign of stasis and subsequent thrombosis within the lesion, connoting that it is a relatively stable lesion.[24] With higher flow, especially in arteriovenous malformations, phleboliths seldom develop. Arteriography is not especially useful in purely venous malformations. The arterial phase is characteristically normal, demonstrating normal caliber arteries and no evidence of shunting.[25] Small puddles of contrast medium can be seen on late phase follow-up films during the venous phase but are seldom valuable in determining the entire extent of the lesion (Fig. 30-13). CT scans and MRI studies are of much greater value in helping to determine the size and extent of involvement (Fig. 30-14).

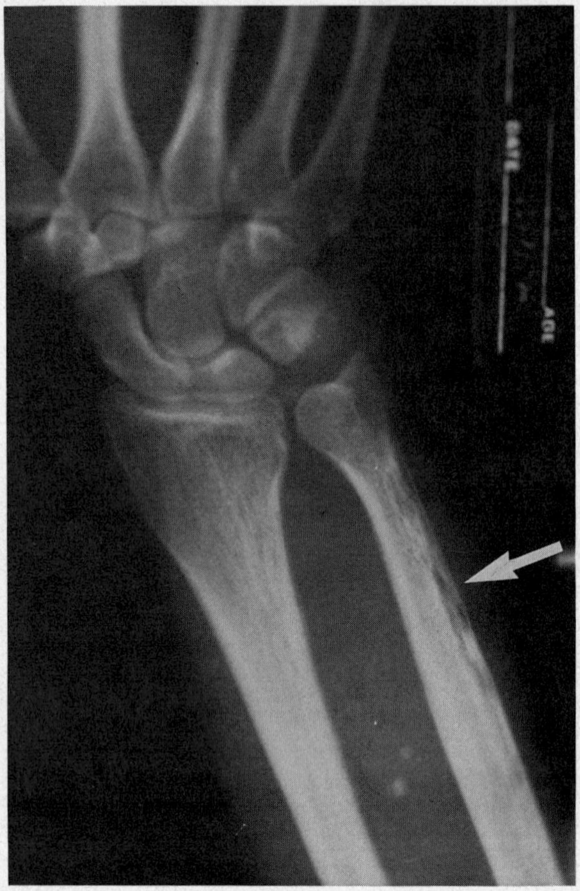

Fig. 30-11. Arrow points to venous malformation centered over ulna in forearm with bony overgrowth seen on radiograph.

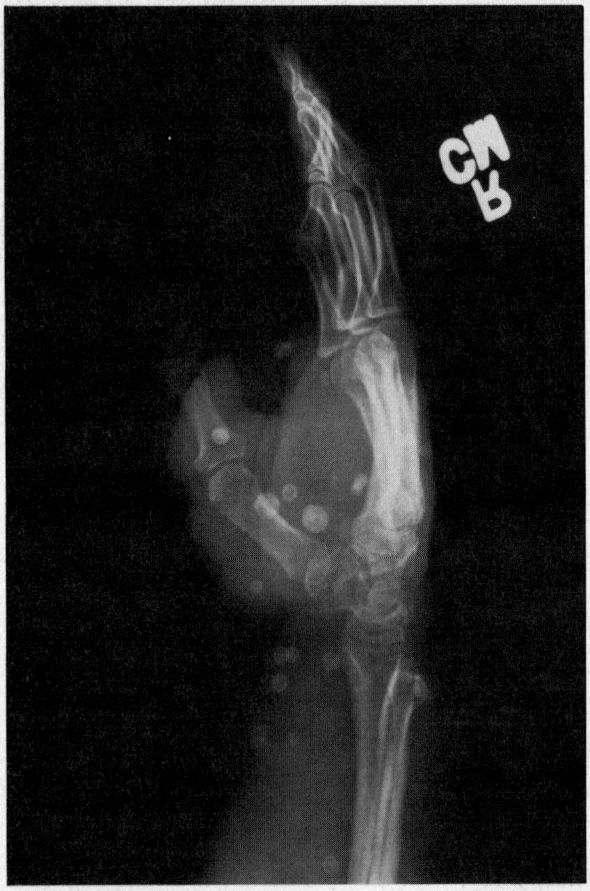

Fig. 30-12. Phleboliths scattered throughout a venous malformation of upper extremity.

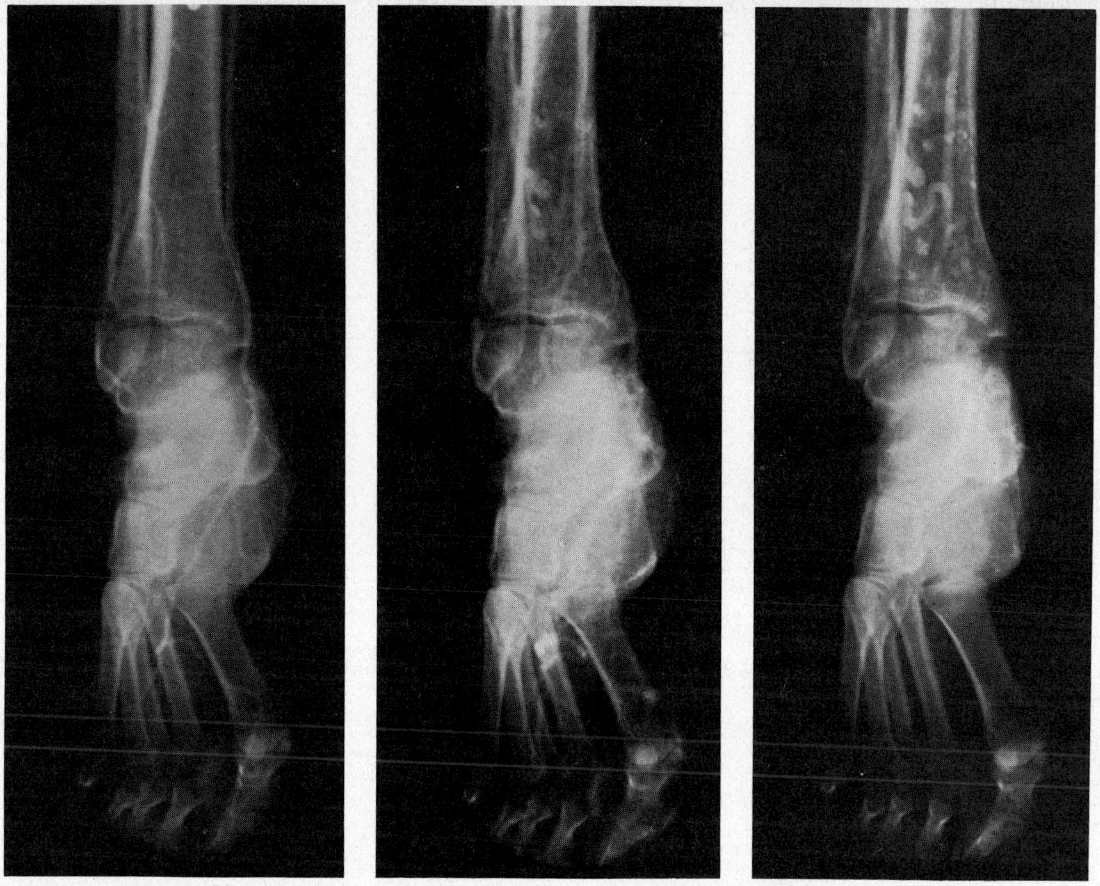

A B C

Fig. 30-13. A, Normal arteriogram of venous malformation of lower extremity. B, Shows "puddling" of contrast medium in early venous phase. C, Residual tortuous venous channels seen in later phase.

Treatment. Venous malformations, like the deeper lymphatic lesions, are more diffuse than they appear to be and are best treated symptomatically with elastic compression. Although occasionally DIC can develop as part of the Kasabach-Merritt syndrome, it is unusual for these purely venous conditions to require specific therapy. Small lesions may respond to injection of thrombosing agents. The obvious limitation of this technique is the ability to confine the agent only to the lesion. Although in the past Klippel-Trenaunay syndrome was treated by excision of varicosities, this form of therapy has not been especially successful.[26] Surgical excision is best done for lesions in which ulcerations or bleeding develop. This does happen occasionally in chronically traumatized areas, such as the foot, and may require excision of the involved area and skin grafting (Fig. 30-15). No attempts should be made to excise the entire involved area unless it is small and localized.

One specific indication for consideration of surgical treatment of venous malformations is the presence of pain. This in itself should raise the possibility of an arterial component, but pain caused by compression by the enlarging malformation can occur. This is most common in the upper extremity, and partial excision of the lesion or decompression may be necessary for pain relief. Compression of nerves can occur, especially in the forearm and in the carpal tunnel. These nerve entrapments are slow in onset, and the symptoms can be subtle. It is easy to overlook these symptoms, blaming the pain on vascular engorgement. It is very important for the physician to make the distinction between entrapment and engorgement. Simple decompression of the nerve, while leaving the malformation alone, can afford marked symptomatic relief of entrapment. Complete resection of the lesion can sometimes be done, providing this will not compromise function (Fig. 30-16).

Arteriovenous malformations

Pathophysiology. Arteriovenous malformations can be congenital or acquired. Acquired arteriovenous fistulas are usually caused by penetrating injuries or fractures. They have also been reported after many types of surgical procedures and may occur spontaneously as a result of arteriosclerotic or mycotic aneurysms.[19]

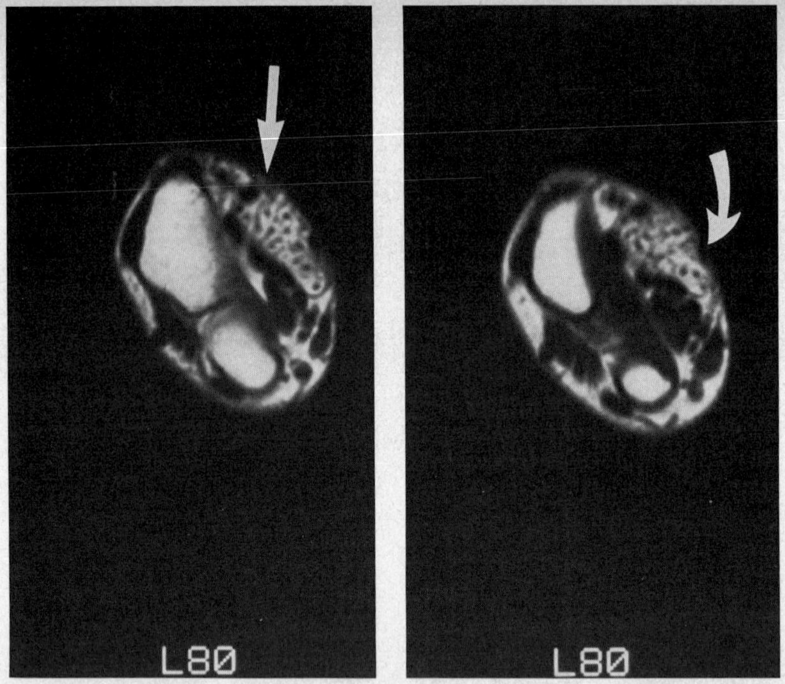

Fig. 30-14. **A** and **B,** Two sections of an MRI of a venous malformation at the level of the distal forearm, showing that the lesion is confined to skin and subcutaneous tissue *(arrows).*

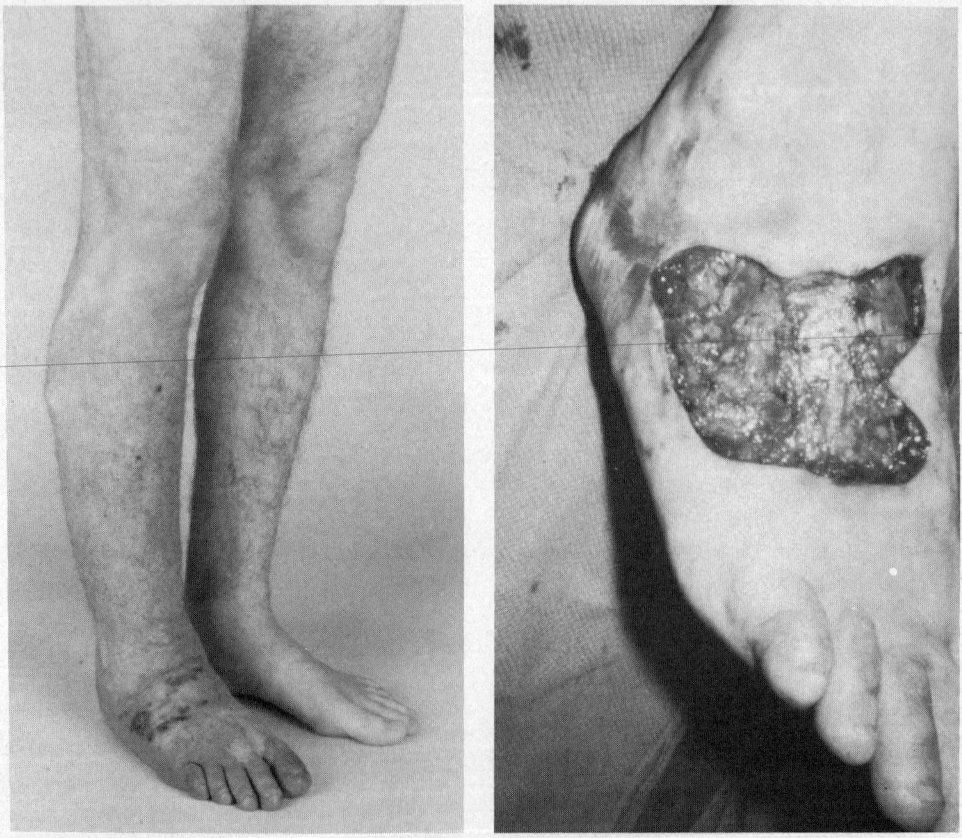

Fig. 30-15. **A,** Chronic ulceration over dorsum of foot in Klippel-Trenaunay syndrome. **B,** Extent of excision and skin grafting.

A B

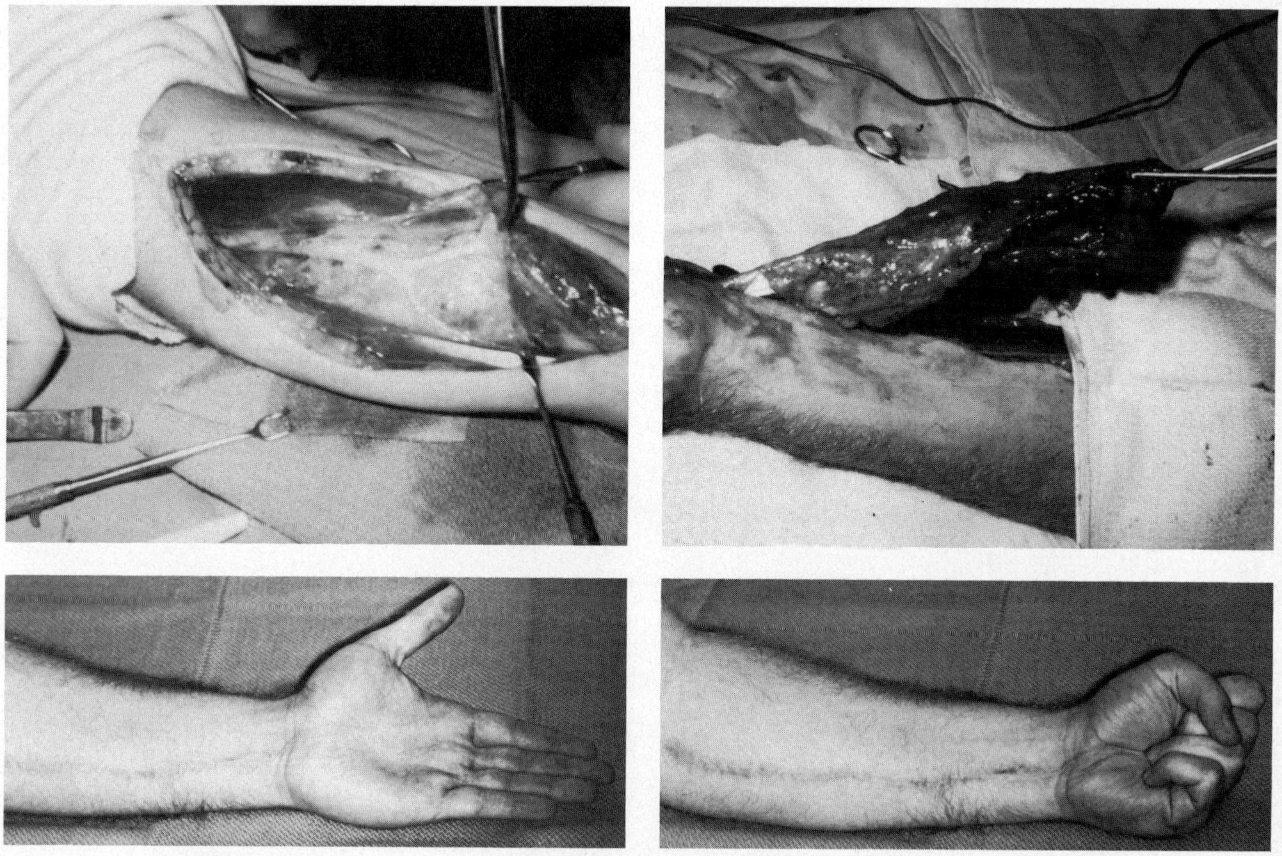

C D

Fig. 30-16. A, Painful venous malformation caused by compression of the median nerve. After complete resection of involved muscle (**B**) and tendon transfer, complete function is preserved (**C** and **D**).

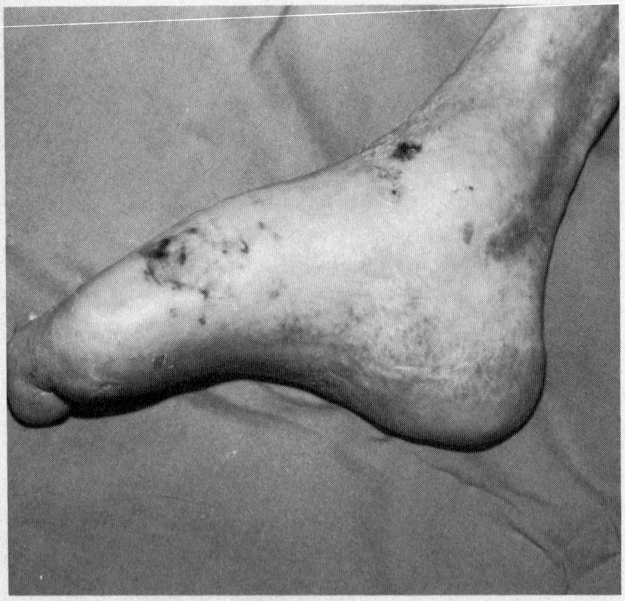

Fig. 30-17. Vascular insufficiency and ulceration of the foot distal to an arteriovenous malformation.

The pathophysiologic changes occurring in congenital lesions are the same as those in acquired fistulas. The basic principle is that blood follows the path of least resistance.[27] The arteriovenous malformation is an abnormal connection between a high-pressure arterial system and a low-pressure venous system with high capacity. Because of the difference in resistance, blood flows preferentially through the fistula rather than continuing along the artery into the normal capillary bed. This causes decreased flow in the artery distal to the fistula and increased flow in the venous system. In addition to causing a steal of blood from the distal bed, the hemodynamic changes that are present lead to the development of increased collateral circulation around the fistula.

Clinical picture. Many small congenital arteriovenous malformations are relatively asymptomatic, but acquired lesions often cause such significant shunting that they can become a danger to life or limb. Blood volume, heart rate, and stroke volume can increase, progressing to pulmonary hypertension and even cardiac failure in extreme conditions.[27] This almost never happens in congenital arteriovenous malformations of the extremities, but it is not uncommon for them to become painful, and for ulceration and bleeding to take place (Fig. 30-17). As is the case with large venous malformations, vascular engorgement of an

A

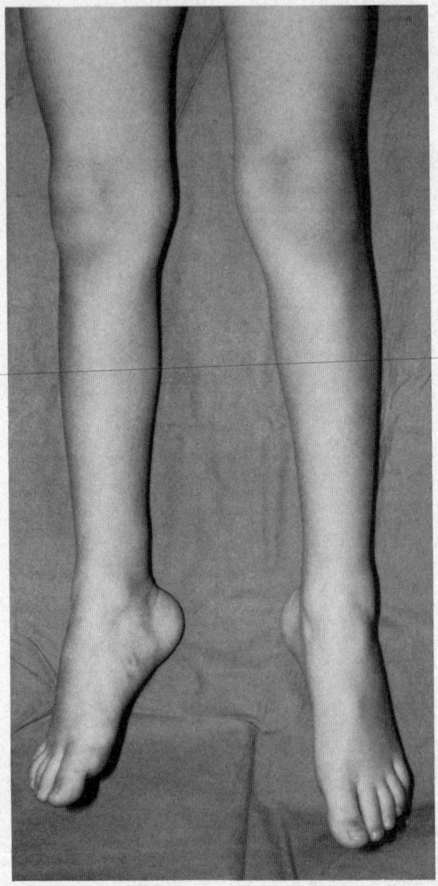

B

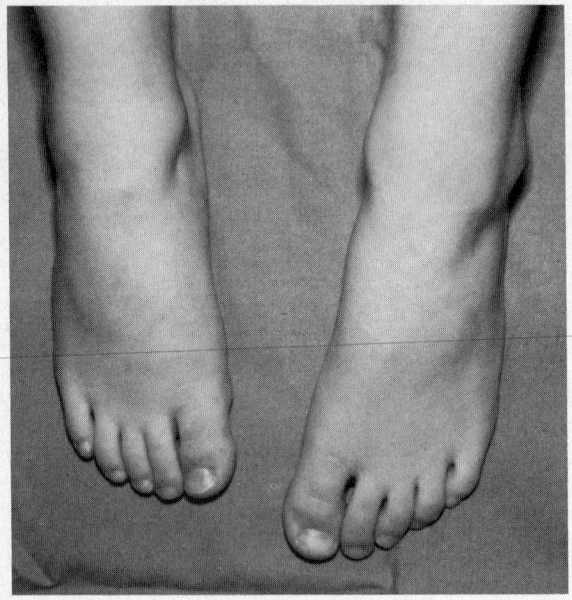

Fig. 30-18. **A** and **B,** Decreased growth of foot distal to arteriovenous malformation at level of the ankle.

extremity can be a cause of nerve entrapment such as carpal tunnel syndrome.

Acquired arteriovenous malformations often appear as emergent problems. They characteristically tend to worsen fairly rapidly and cause problems because of distal ischemia as well as proximal overload. Even vascular access in the forearm for dialysis can cause significant ischemia of the hand, which can be painful and threaten the survival of the digits.

With an early lesion it is often difficult to determine on physical examination whether or not a malformation is venous or if there is an arterial component. As changes progress, however, visible signs of shunting will become apparent.[25] Characteristically, the area of the malformation will be enlarged and warm, and there will be a palpable thrill present over the fistula. Veins may appear pulsatile, and there will be signs of atrophic changes in the extremity distal to the lesion (Fig. 30-18). Decreased growth occurs distal to the shunt.[28] A bruit is heard with the stethoscope, and marked prominence of both arterial and venous sounds is heard diffusely over the area with the Doppler. It is usually possible to identify several unidirectional feeding arteries with this instrument. The classic sign on physical examination is the Nicoladoni-Branham sign. In this the heart rate slows with compression of the arterial venous communication.[29] This is a reliable sign in acquired fistulas, but if there are many diffuse feeding vessels present in congenital malformations, this sign is not always present.

Diagnosis. The most important consideration in evaluation of a vascular malformation is whether or not the lesion is a true arteriovenous malformation. If it can be determined that this is not the case, treatment is generally only supportive. True arteriovenous malformations are considered to be unstable lesions because of their tendency to progressively enlarge and because of their potential life- or limb-threatening nature.[19,27] If the diagnosis is very plausible on a clinical basis, it is probably wise to confirm by selective arteriography even though no specific therapy is indicated at that time. An angiogram serves not only to confirm the diagnosis but also to indicate the extent of involvement. In addition, it serves as a baseline for comparison should subsequent deterioration take place in the future.

While plain radiographs may show skeletal changes of decreased growth and even atrophy, the most important imaging technique is angiography.[25] Selective angiograms show almost immediate shunting with blood present in veins before the contrast medium has progressed any appreciable distance past the fistula (Fig. 30-19). In addition, many tortuous channels are demonstrated, and the largest of the feeding vessels are identified. In congenital lesions, however, there are usually multiple feeding channels, and only the largest ones can be identified angiographically. A very good estimation of the size of the malformation can be gained with angiography, but sometimes CT or MRI scanning can also be of value in determining the extent of the lesion, especially if there is concern that bony involvement may be present[30] (Fig. 30-20).

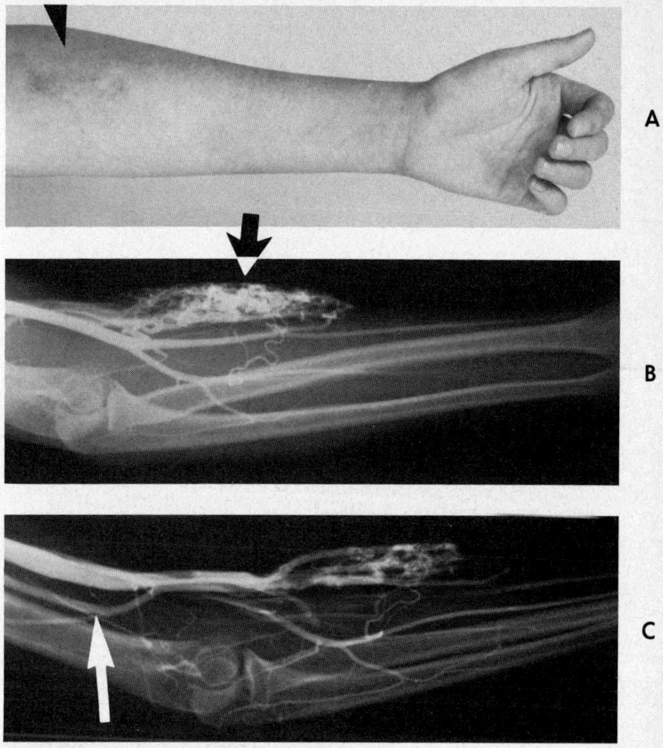

Fig. 30-19. A, Small but symptomatic congential arteriovenous malformation of proximal volar forearm (*arrow*). **B,** Rapid filling of lesion through multiple feeders from radial and ulnar arteries (*arrow*). **C,** Prominent venous return seen before contrast has reached the hand (*arrow*).

Treatment of congenital lesions

General remarks. Congenital arteriovenous malformations are usually slowly progressive in nature but may enlarge rapidly following trauma, during growth spurts, or during periods of hormonal or vascular changes such as adolescence or pregnancy. In the absence of life- or limb-threatening problems, treatment must be determined on the basis of whether or not it is possible to completely eradicate the lesion. Any form of treatment other than complete eradication is doomed to failure because of the presence of multiple feeding vessels.[9,19,27]

If the lesion is threatening life or limb, there is no choice and the lesion must be treated. On the other hand, if it is small and relatively asymptomatic, especially a congenital lesion, then probably no treatment is indicated. As most cases will fall somewhere in between, consideration must be given not only for the problem that the patient has at the time but also for the potential of it becoming worse. For example, even though a small localized lesion may not be terribly symptomatic, it might be that the potential for com-

A B C

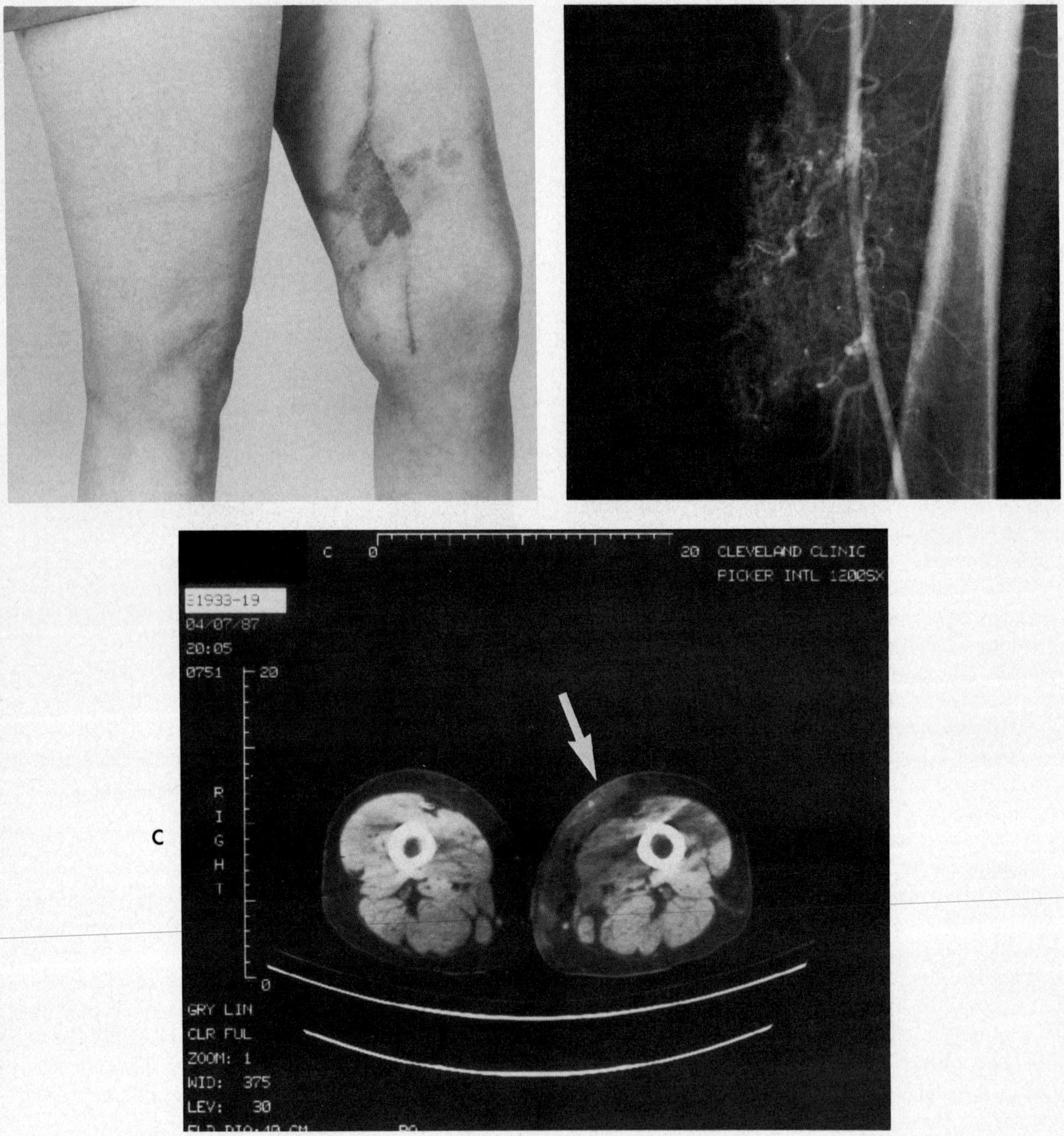

Fig. 30-20. A, Recurrent arteriovenous malformation of inner thigh. **B,** Arteriogram shows lesion with multiple feeders and early venous phase. **C,** Section of CT scan showing extent of involvement of subcutaneous tissue onto surface of muscle (*arrow*).

plete eradication would be quite good. In that circumstance, treatment might be justified on the basis that if the lesion significantly enlarged, the consequences would be much worse—either in terms of the extent of treatment necessary for eradication, or the problems that the lesion itself might cause. An example of this could be decreased growth in a hand or foot distal to an arteriovenous malfunction. If it would be possible to remove the lesion without sacrificing function, then this seemingly more radical approach would end up more conservative in the long run. In general, however, consideration of treatment in marginal cases depends on the presence of complications such as ulceration, bleeding, and pain.

Embolization. Once the decision is made to treat a congenital arteriovenous malformation, embolization with super selective angiography has become an increasingly important form of therapy.[31-33] Theoretically it should be possible to inject material into the feeding vessels, which would then cause occlusion at the capillary level. Small particles of many materials such as absorbable Gelfoam sponge or various nonabsorbable polymers have been used for this purpose. These particles are small enough to pass into minute feeding vessels but too large to pass through the capillary bed.[32-34] The obvious drawback with this technique is not only the ability to successfully do this but also to prevent systemic spread of the embolizing material. Especially in the case of congenital lesions, it also means being able to identify all of the feeding vessels so that the entire structure can be brought under control. This requires very careful planning and an extremely high level of competence in very selective catheterization.

Two obvious problems exist with this technique. The first is the significant incidence of recurrence of arteriovenous malformation, especially the congenital malformations. The second is the potential for severity of complications, such as stroke, if the embolizing material cannot be confined to the lesion. Consequently, at present this technique is seldom used as the only mode of therapy except in those instances where surgical eradication of the lesion would not be considered feasible, and yet the condition is deemed life threatening.[34,35] So far, the most valuable use for this technique is in combination with surgical excision. By preoperatively embolizing the main trunks with a substance such as a gelatin sponge or collagen, the mass of the arteriovenous malformation can be temporarily reduced so that the operative blood loss can be markedly reduced.

Surgical treatment. Two problems are encountered in attempting only to eradicate the feeding vessels of an arteriovenous malformation. Because the fistula results in reduced peripheral blood flow, ligation of proximal inflow serves only to decrease the perfusion in the distal extremity. It has been known for years that gangrene is a common result of ligation of proximal vessels for acquired fistula.[19] The second problem is that ligation of only some of the feeders, by causing anoxia in the peripheral bed, will serve as a potent stimulus for opening up of collaterals. This establishes many more feeders for the fistula, which results in the arteriovenous malformation growing larger and larger.

Ligation of vessels is not usually feasible in congenital lesions, since they represent a mass of collaterals with multiple malformed vessels in the given area. When it is feasible to remove this entire mass and still preserve function, then total excision is carried out. When combined with preoperative embolization two or three days before the operation, blood loss is minimized. It has been difficult in the past to excise some of these lesions even though they were relatively localized because of the subsequent tissue defect (Fig. 30-21). With the advent of free tissue transfer by microsurgical means, however, it is now possible to replace these defects with tissue that can be spared from another part of the body. One of the most common of these procedures is the use of part or all of a relatively expendable muscle such as the latissimus dorsi or rectus abdominus. The muscle is removed as a free graft with its vascular pedicle and placed into the surgical defect, then circulation is reestablished by microvascular anastomosis (Fig. 30-22). This accomplishes two functions. The first is to resurface the defect and make appearance and function better. The second is to make this microsurgically revascularized tissue healthy with good blood supply. One of the most potent stimuli to angiogenesis is local tissue ischemia. Radical excision of large amounts of tissue, combined with poor wound coverage such as skin grafting, result in scarred, locally anoxic wound beds (Fig. 30-23). In these wound beds collaterals open up and new arterial feeders develop, resulting in recurrent arteriovenous malformations. In addition to the vascular problem, resulting scar contracture may markedly limit function (Fig. 30-24). If the arteriovenous malformation is excised and replaced by healthy, well-vascularized tissue, minimal stimulus for collateralization will be present. This provides the best chance of all for reducing the possibility of recurrence as well as preservation of function.[36] Therefore when treatment is necessary, the combination of preoperative embolization to reduce blood loss and complete excision of the lesion, combined with replacement of the tissue with a well-vascularized free tissue transfer, is recommended as the treatment of choice.

Treatment of the acquired lesion. In the acquired fistula the so-called quadruple ligation method can be effective, especially in the distal extremity.[27] In this procedure ligation of both artery and vein above and below the fistula, along with ligation of any significant collateral, is employed. A more effective method, however, is eradication of the fistula itself with reconstruction of flow in both artery and vein.

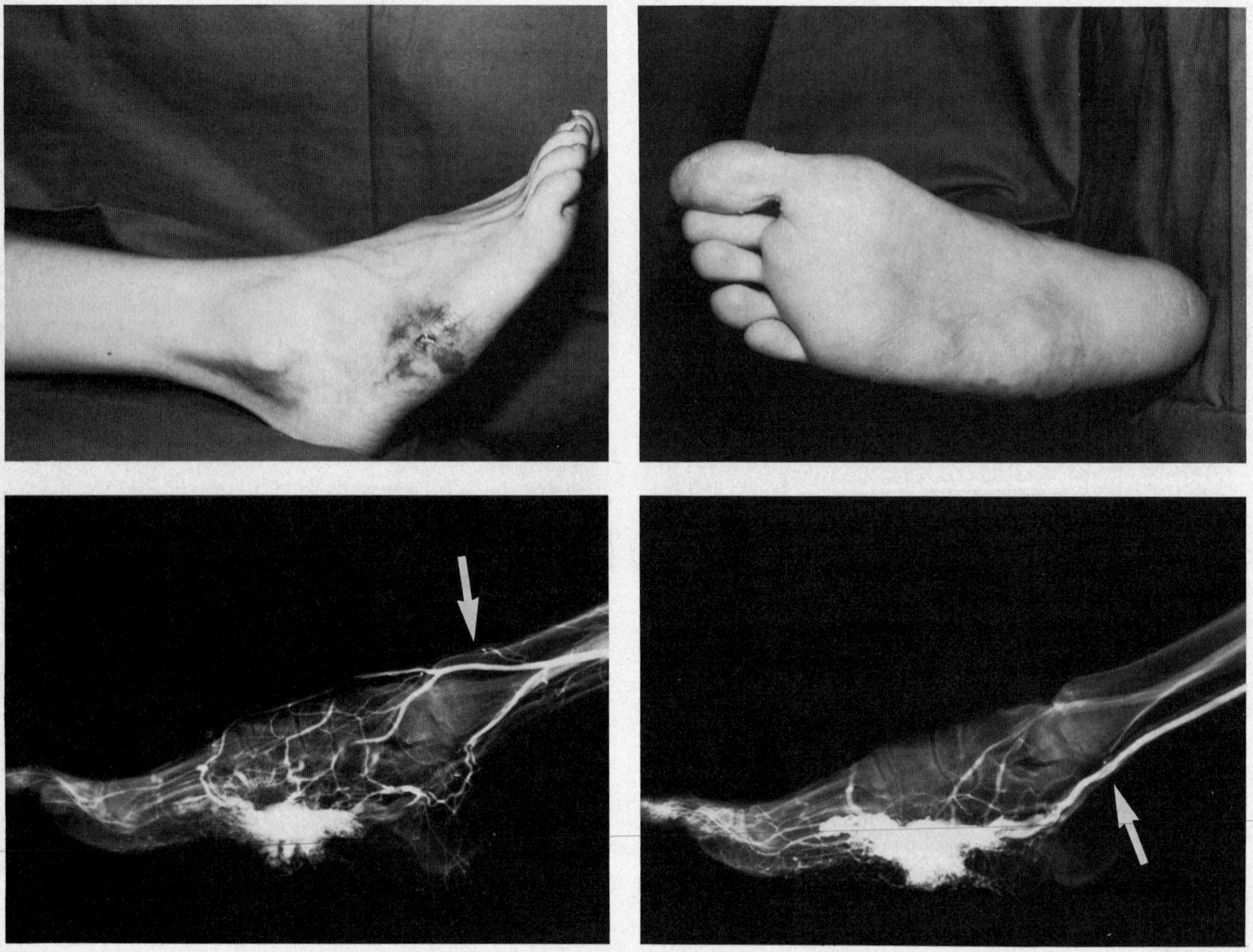

Fig. 30-21. A and **B,** Arteriovenous malformation with ulceration and pain involving lateral and plantar surface of foot. **C** and **D,** Angiograms show multiple feeders from both anterior (*arrow*) and posterior (*arrow*) tibial systems. Resection will create a significant functional defect.

A

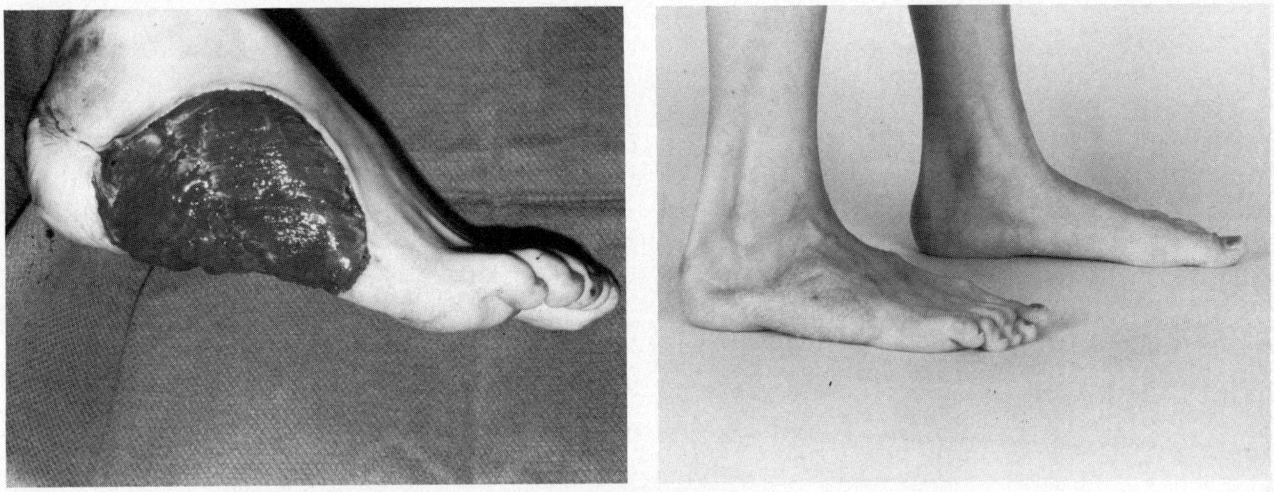

B

Fig. 30-22. A, The patient in Fig. 30-21 has had total resection of lesion and defect replaced with latissimus dorsi microvascular flap and skin graft. **B,** Function is normal with no pain or ulceration 3 years later.

A

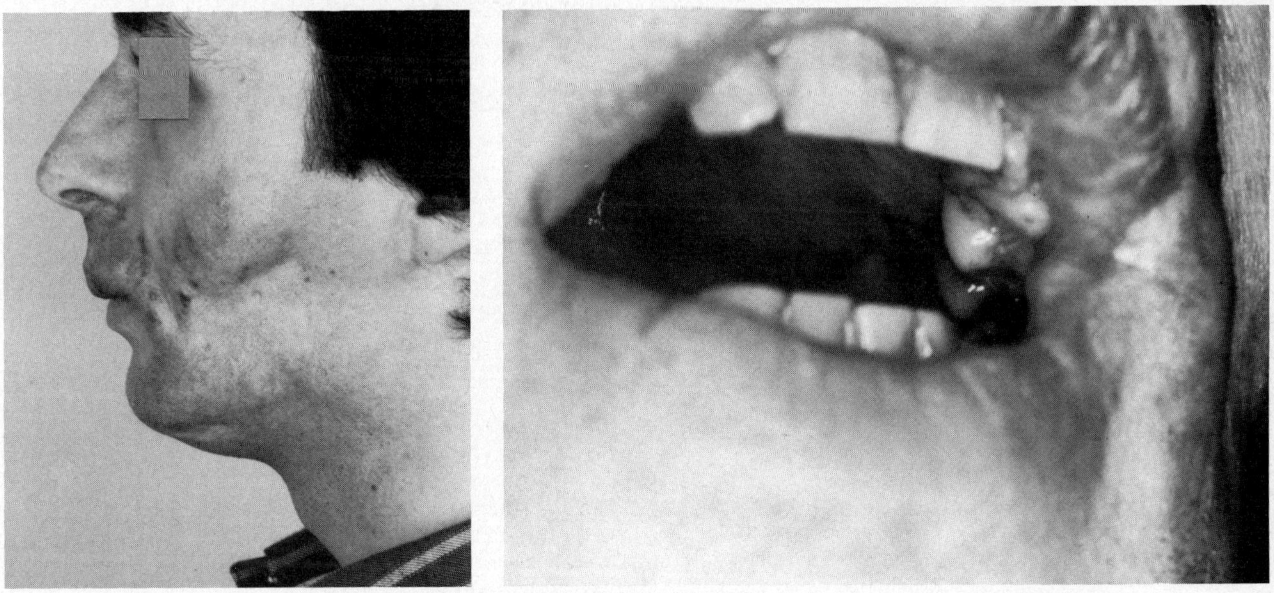

B

Fig. 30-23. A, Scarring. **B,** Limited ability to open mouth after resection of vascular malformation.

A

B

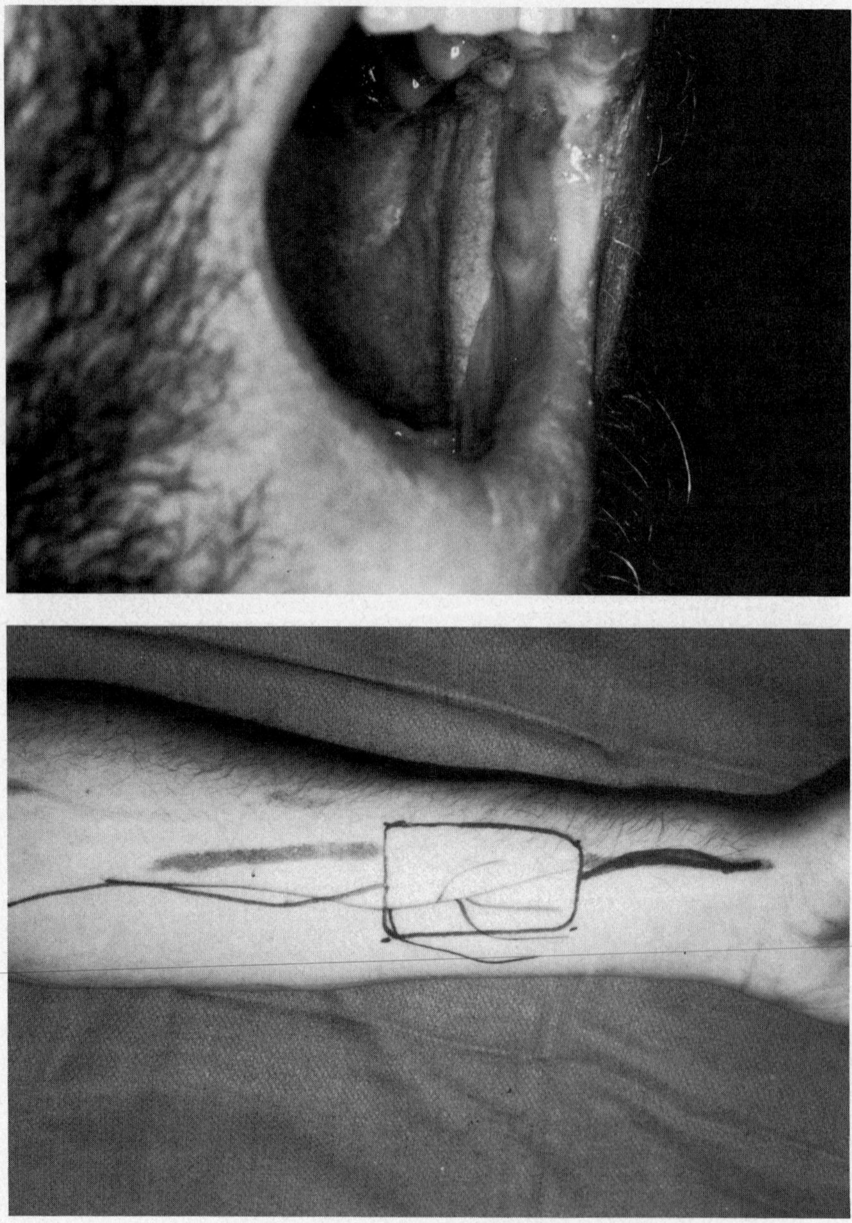

Fig. 30-24. A, Marked improvement in function seen in patient shown in Fig. 30-23 after resection and replacement of intraoral tissue with a free microvascular flap from the forearm (**B**).

REFERENCES

1. South DA and Jacobs AH: Cutis marmorata telangiectatica (congenital generalized phlebectasia), J Pediatr 93:944, 1978.
2. Malan E and Puglionisi A: Congenital angiodysplasia of the extremities. I: Generalities and classification: venous dysplasia, J Cardiovasc Surg 5:87, 1964.
3. Malan E and Puglionisi A: Congenital angiodysplasia of the extremities. II: Arterial, arterial and venous, and haemolymphtic dysplasis, J Cardiovasc Surg 6:255, 1965.
4. Simpson JR: The natural history of cavernous hemangiomata, Lancet 2:1057, 1959.
5. Loewinger RJ et al: Maffucci's syndrome: a mesenchymal dysplasia and multiple tumour syndrome, Br J Dermatol 96:317, 1977.
6. Mulliken JB and Glowacki J: Hemangiomas and vascular malformations in infants and children: a classification based on endothelial characteristics, Plast Reconstr Surg 69:412, 1982.
7. Azizkhan RG et al: Mast cell heparin stimulates migration of capillary endothelial cells in vitro, J Exp Med 152:931, 1980.
8. Mulliken JR, Zetter BR, and Folkman J: In vitro characteristics of endothelium from hemangiomas and vascular malformations, Surgery 92:348, 1982.
9. Mulliken JB: Cutaneous vascular lesions of children. In Serafin D and Georgiade NG, eds: Pediatric plastic surgery, St Louis, 1984, The CV Mosby Co.
10. Woollard HH: The development of the principal arterial stems in the forelimb of the pig, Cont Embryol 14:65-71, 139-154, 1922.
11. Holmdahl K: Cutaneous hemangiomas in premature and mature infants, Acta Paediatr 44:370, 1955.
12. Hidano A and Nakajima S: Earliest features of the strawberry mark in the newborn, Br J Dermatol 87:138, 1972.
13. Bowers RE, Graham EA, and Tomlinson KM: The natural history of the strawberry nevus, Arch Dermatol 82:667, 1960.
14. Lister WA: The natural history of the strawberry naevi, Lancet 1:1429, 1938.
15. Kasabach HH and Merritt KK: Capillary hemangioma with extensive purpura: report of a case, Am J Dis Child 59:1063, 1940.
16. Zarem HA and Edgerton MT: Induced resolution of cavernous hemangiomas following prednisolone therapy, Plast Reconstr Surg 39:76, 1967.
17. Edgerton MT: The treatment of hemangiomas, with special reference to the role of steroid therapy, Ann Surg 183:517, 1976.
18. Mulliken JB and Murray JE: Natural history of vascular birthmarks. In Williams HB.: Symposium on vascular malformations and melanotic lesions, St Louis, 1982, The CV Mosby Co.
19. Gloviczki P and Hollier LH: Arteriovenous fistulas. In Haimovici H, ed: Vascular surgery: principles and techniques, ed 3, New York, 1989, Appleton & Lange.
20. Klippel M and Trenaunay P: Du naevus variqueux osteohypertrophique, Arch Gen Med (Paris) 3:641, 1900.
21. Noe JM et al: Port wine stains and the response to argon laser therapy: successful treatment and the predictive role of color, age, and biopsy, Plast Reconst Surg 65:130, 1980.
22. Hayashi H, Yasuda Y, and Tsukada S: Tunable dye laser treatment of port wine stains, Jpn J Plast Reconstr Surg, 8:38, 1988 (Japanese). (Abstract in Plast Reconstr Surg 84:384, 1989.)
23. Clodius L: Excision and grafting of extensive facial hemangiomas, Br J Plast Surg 30:185, 1977.
24. Rosen RJ, Riles TS, and Berenstein A: Congenital vascular malformations. In Rutherford RB, ed: Vascular surgery, ed 3, Philadelphia, 1989, WB Saunders Co.
25. Sumner DS and Rutherford RB: Diagnostic evaluation of arteriovenous fistulas. In Rutherford RB, ed: Vascular surgery, ed 3, Philadelphia, 1989, WB Saunders Co.
26. Gloviczki P et al: Surgical implications of Klippel-Trenaunay syndrome, Ann Surg 197:353, 1983.
27. Sumner DS: Hemodynamics and pathophysiology of arteriovenous fistulas. In Rutherford RB, ed: Vascular surgery, ed 3, Philadelphia, 1989, WB Saunders Co.
28. Boyd JB et al: Skeletal changes associated with vascular malformations, Plast Reconstr Surg 74:789, 1984.
29. Branham HH: Aneurysmal varix of the femoral artery and vein following a gunshot wound, Int J Surg 3:250, 1890.
30. Berquist TH: Bone and soft tissue tumors. In Berquist TH, ed: Magnetic resonance of the musculoskeletal system, New York, 1987, Raven Press.
31. Merland JJ et al: Les malformations vasculaires cervico-cephaliques protocole actuel de tratement. À propos de 230 cas. Phelbologie 33:95, 1980.
32. Rosen RJ: Embolization in the treatment of arteriovenous malformations. In Goldberg HI, Higgins CB, and Ring EJ, eds: Contemporary imaging, San Francisco, 1985, University of California Press.
33. Gomes AS, Mali WP, and Oppenheim WL: Embolization therapy in the management of congenital arteriovenous malformations, Radiology 144:41, 1982.
34. Forbes G et al: Therapeutic embolization angiography for extra-axial lesions in the head, Mayo Clin Proc 61:427, 1986.
35. Stanley P et al: Therapeutic embolization of infantile hepatic hemangioma with polyvinyl alcohol, Am J Roent 141:1047, 1983.
36. Hurwitz DJ and Kerber CW: Hemodynamic considerations in the treatment of arteriovenous malformations of the face and scalp, Plast Reconstr Surg 67:421, 1981.

Chapter 31

TRAUMA AND PERIPHERAL VASCULAR DISEASE

Malcolm O. Perry

Trauma ranks overall as the fourth leading cause of death in the United States, but in the first four decades of life, it is first.[1] Over 140,000 people die each year from accidents, and injuries lead to more than 140,000,000 bed days of annual disability.

Most major arterial injuries are the result of aggressive acts of violence, and although few communities are spared, these events are more likely to occur in urban areas, where violence is endemic and drug abuse is common. In fact, recent government studies indicate that most violent crimes now are drug related.[2,3]

ETIOLOGY

Penetrating wounds caused by bullets and knives are usually seen, but accidental stab wounds resulting from motor vehicle accidents or industrial mishaps also may be encountered[4,5] (see the accompanying box). Stab wounds are seen more frequently than gunshot wounds; many of them are not serious, and vital organs may be spared. Gunshot wounds usually penetrate deeply and often involve the trunk as well as the extremities. Many of the patients with bullet wounds of the abdomen and chest do not survive long enough to reach the hospital. Multiple vascular wounds are often encountered in these patients, and although any major vascular wound can lead to lethal bleeding, death is more common with injuries of major vessels in the chest or abdomen, where early detection and rapid control of hemorrhage are more difficult (see the accompanying box).

Those injuries that are the result of substance abuse present particularly difficult problems.[6,7] The patients generally do not seek medical aid until complications of the arterial punctures have occurred, usually false aneurysms, infection, and occasionally sepsis. In many of these people thromboembolism has already supervened, and viability of the extremities is in doubt at the time they are first seen. Moreover, a major threat at anytime is rupture of an infected artery.[8]

With the increasing use of transarterial procedures for various studies, and balloon dilation of stenotic arteries, there are more iatrogenic injuries of major vessels.[9] The incidence of complications varies a great deal depending on the indication for the arterial procedure.[10,11] Transfemoral catheter studies are often uncomplicated, even in patients with atherosclerosis. One recent study reported an overall

Distribution of arterial injuries in 665 patients

Extremity	501
Aorta	31
Visceral	37
Cervical	96
TOTAL	665

From Perry MO: The management of acute vascular injuries, Baltimore, 1981, Williams & Wilkins.

Associated injuries (%) in 665 patients with arterial injuries

Large vein	34
Major nerve	18
Separate artery	7
Lung, abdominal viscera	39

From Perry MO: The management of acute vascular injuries, Baltimore, 1981, Williams & Wilkins.

complication rate of only 1%.[12] If the common femoral artery is used for balloon dilation of stenotic arteries, the problems are more numerous, probably related to the length and complexity of the procedures.[13] Intraaortic assist procedures and transfemoral cardiac valve operations, such as valvuloplasty, are even more risky; complications are seen in 5% to 11% of patients.[12]

Most angiographers and cardiologists try to use the femoral artery rather than the brachial or axillary arteries. These routes also carry a higher risk, not only of arterial damage, but also of major nerve problems. Although these problems can be severe, the complications usually are identified early since the patient is under direct observation in the hospital.[14] An accurate diagnosis and expedient repair is usually feasible, and therefore the results generally are satisfactory. If initial arterial repairs are not undertaken, delayed complications can occur, even after months or years.[15]

PATHOPHYSIOLOGY

Penetrating injuries, producing direct vascular wounds, are usually caused by knives or bullets traveling at a low velocity, and most of the damage is confined to the wound tract. Lacerations of the artery are the most common finding, but contusions, punctures, and transections are also encountered. High-velocity bullets can produce severe damage to the structures in their path, and the blast effect can cause more remote injuries. Contusion or even vessel transection can follow the cavitation effect associated with bullets traveling at velocities of 2000 to 3000 ft/sec. Even if immediate arterial disruption does not occur, mural contusions can result in delayed thrombosis or wall necrosis, late hemorrhage, and false aneurysm formation.

Although unusual in the civilian environment, a high-velocity bullet or metal fragment can produce a great deal of damage because of its high energy. Secondary missiles consisting of bullet or shell fragments or bone splinters also may be created, and they in turn produce other wounds. There is a powerful suction effect as the blast cavity collapses, and surface structures such as clothing and dirt can be drawn into the wound. Such widespread destruction may not be suspected from inspection of the skin surface where, in some cases, rather small entrance and exit wounds are seen, despite the extent of the interior damage.

Motor vehicle accidents also result in vascular trauma, and usually the victims have multiple injuries. Direct injury to the arteries can occur, but often vascular wounds are the result of fractures. This is especially likely to occur to vessels located near the joints; there they are relatively fixed and more vulnerable to shear forces.

The break of large, heavy bones such as the femur or the tibia releases tremendous amounts of energy. The damage to the soft tissues in the area can be extensive, and the effects are similar to those produced by high-velocity bullets. After the bones fall back to a near-normal position, the magnitude of the injuring forces may not be appreciated, and the severity of the damage is easily underestimated.

DIAGNOSIS

Clinical diagnosis

Injuries of large arteries usually can be identified readily because of severe hemorrhage, large hematomas, and pulse deficits[5] (see the accompanying box). Less extensive injuries may not be as obvious. Ischemia distal to the area of the arterial injury may not be present, especially when intervening collateral vessels are adequate and hypotension is absent. The assessment of the adequacy of blood flow based on the detection of distal extremity pulses is limited by specific hemodynamic features. The pulse wave is a pressure wave that attains velocities of up to 10 m/sec, while the flow wave of blood has a velocity of 40 cm/sec. The phys-

Clinical features of arterial injuries

Diminished or absent pulse
Enlarging hematoma
Pulsatile arterial bleeding
Symptoms of ischemia
Injury of anatomically related nerves
Major hemorrhage with hypotension

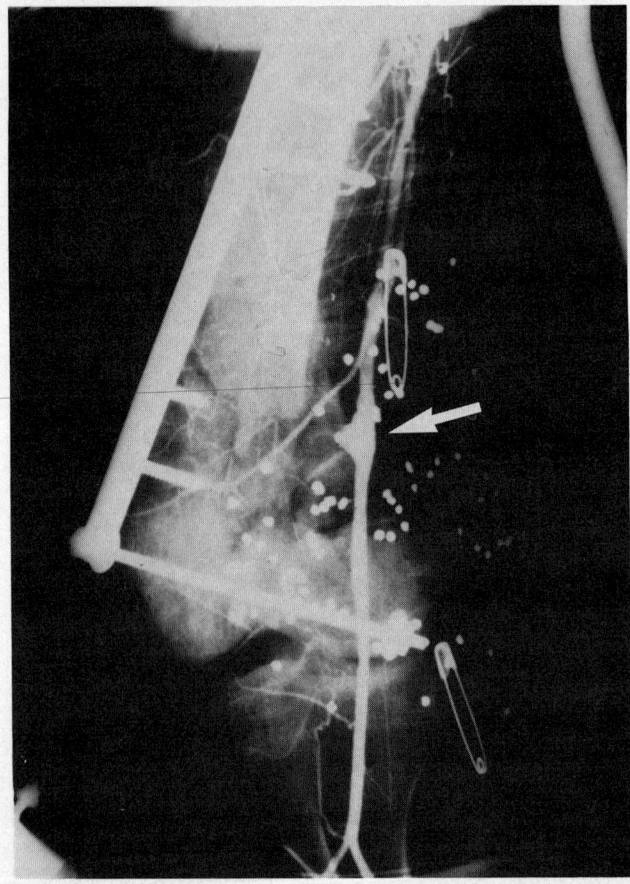

Fig. 31-1. This injury from shotgun pellets shattered the femur, but the patient had palpable pedal pulses, despite the injury to the superficial femoral artery (*arrow*).

ical examination must take this fact into account because the pulse wave can be transmitted past intimal flaps, through collateral arteries, or even beyond limited areas of fresh soft clot. Moreover, if the injuries are limited only to damage of the vessel wall, then distal pulses usually will be unimpaired (Fig. 31-1). One series reported that up to 18% of patients with operatively proven major arterial injuries in the extremities had normal distal pulses at the time of the initial examination.[5,16] Such a combination of findings is especially likely to be seen in patients who have penetrating wounds near the hip or shoulder where the collateral circulation is abundant.

Injuries of the great vessels in the chest and abdomen present special problems in diagnosis since they are inaccessible for direct evaluation. A hemopneumothorax or mediastinal bleeding is common with penetrating injuries to the chest even in patients who do not have major vascular wounds. These patients may initially be stable and are thought only to have parenchymal lung damage or minor arterial injuries, and sudden hemodynamic collapse may be the first sign of more severe problems. In such patients a wide mediastinum, cardiac arrest, persistent shock, cardiac tamponade, and recurring hemothorax strongly suggest the presence of major vascular injuries.[5,16] Patients with penetrating or blunt trauma to the abdomen also are vulnerable to vascular injuries although not with as great a frequency as in the extremities. The diagnosis of a vascular wound in these patients rests primarily on the detection of continued bleeding.[17]

Adjunctive diagnostic methods

Although ordinary radiographs rarely establish the diagnosis of an arterial injury, they are of value in evaluating these patients since such studies may disclose the presence of subcutaneous or mediastinal air, collections of fluid or blood, and displacement of viscera. The wound tract of a bullet is not usually a straight line, but x-ray film studies may offer some assistance in determining the nature and the extent of the wound, and thus suggest a need for other studies. An assessment of the vulnerable structures between the entry site and exit site (or final resting place) of the bullet should be undertaken.

Computerized tomography (CT) is of benefit in the examination of injured patients, and even without the administration of contrast medium, soft tissue distortion, hematomas, and some injuries of solid organs can be detected.[16] Magnetic resonance imaging (MRI) promises to be of even greater value in the evaluation of trauma patients. Specialized adjustments, which change the resonance frequency, can generate images of the blood vessels even without radiopaque contrast material. Although these methods are not sufficiently refined so as to permit them to be used exclusive of other techniques, they do offer valuable data in the evaluation of vascular injuries.

Doppler techniques may be helpful in detecting vascular injury, and also in assessing the adequacy of arterial blood flow in the extremities. The measurement of distal arterial systolic blood pressure is helpful, but specificity of these methods suffers from hemodynamic limitations, which also govern arterial pulses. Subtle abnormalities in the Doppler-derived measurements are common, but relatively normal values are also seen. This may be a particular problem in the patient with multiple injuries who is hypotensive. These techniques are of considerable value as an extension of the physical examination in the initial evaluation of the patient, and they offer a great deal of assistance postoperatively, but none can be relied on to exclude an arterial injury.[5]

Arteriography

In the management of trauma patients preoperative arteriography is used for three main reasons: (1) to exclude the presence of a vascular injury in a patient who otherwise has no indications for operative exploration, (2) to detect a lesion that was not exposed by other diagnostic techniques, and (3) to plan the operative management of a patient with a major vascular injury.

In patients who have penetrating trauma to the lower extremity a simple needle puncture of the common femoral artery and single plane arteriograms may be quite useful in excluding the need for operation when other indications for exploration do not exist (Fig. 31-2). Feliciano et al have clearly demonstrated that this is a safe and reliable technique, and although their follow-up series was relatively short, no serious immediate complications were seen.[4] Snyder et al have emphasized that high-grade biplane arteriography is reliable, although not infallible, in detecting arterial injuries.[18] In a prospective study of 183 patients with penetrating trauma of the extremity, biplane arteriography was evaluated. All of the patients had arteriograms and then were operated on for the listed indications regardless of the arteriographic findings. There were 28 false-positive studies, 32 true-positive studies, one false-negative examination, and the rest were true negatives in this series, thus confirming the usefulness of this technique in establishing the diagnosis of major vascular injuries in the extremities. Recent studies have suggested that in those patients who have no firm indications for operation, if arteriography is performed solely because of the proximity of the injury to a vessel, it is likely to have a positive yield of less than 10%.[19] In such situations a careful selection of patients must be undertaken to avoid performing unnecessary studies, but arteriography, particularly the abbreviated procedures, can be of considerable assistance in excluding the need for operation in such patients.

Although direct punctures are possible, more often than not transfemoral Seldinger catheter techniques have been used for these studies. They enable the angiographer to examine many portions of the arterial tree via a single arterial entry. In the unstable patient it is best not to undertake these prolonged procedures but to go directly to the operating room. In such situations sudden hemodynamic collapse may occur; it often will have a lethal outcome if the

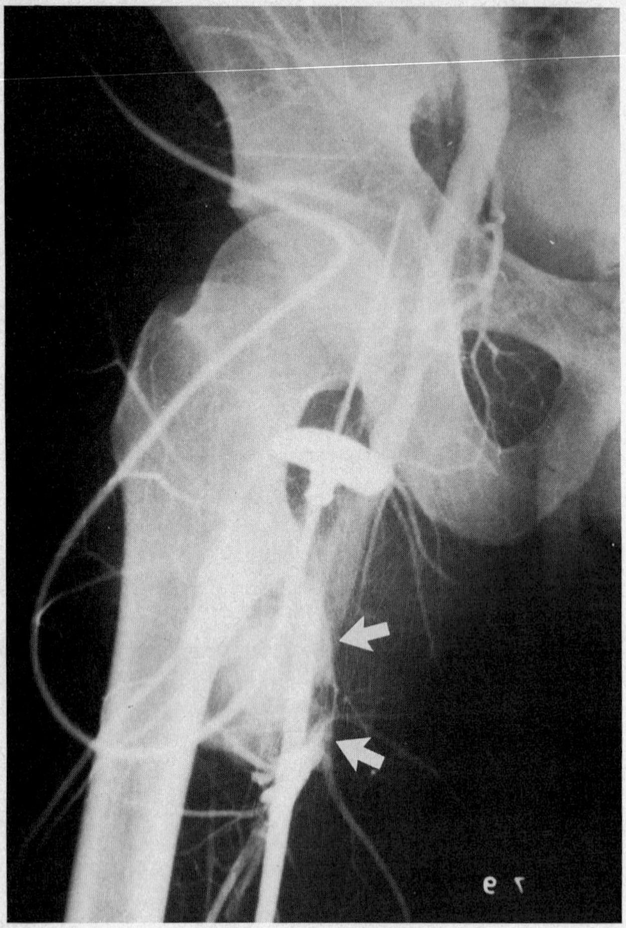

Fig. 31-2. A stab wound of the profunda femoris artery caused this false aneurysm (*arrows*). The patient had normal pedal pulses.

patient is not in a position where bleeding can be controlled immediately. Diagnostic studies in a hemodynamically unstable patient should be performed in the operating room so the surgical team may intervene immediately if necessary.

Special problems are presented when drug abuse patients with arterial wounds are seen.[6] Since these wounds are invariably infected, arteriography may be particularly valuable in planning the operative procedure. Remote bypass techniques using subcutaneous grafts may be required to maintain viability of the extremities in such patients, since direct repairs in the grossly contaminated field are not safe.[20] A careful and complete evaluation of the vascular system in the involved area must be undertaken in these patients, and that usually means biplane arteriography as well as CT or MRI scans.

For people in whom injuries to the internal carotid artery at the base of the skull or at the root of the neck are suspected, preoperative arteriography is of considerable value in planning the operation (Fig. 31-3). Moreover, if the patient has a neurologic deficit, biplane intracranial films should be obtained at the same time to determine if distal thromboembolism has already supervened. Specialized surgical procedures for exposure and vascular repair may be required in these patients, and it is best to have this knowledge before beginning the operation.[5]

A special situation also exists in the evaluation of patients who are thought to have renal artery or kidney injury.[16] In a patient with hematuria an intravenous pyelogram (IVP) is performed, and if there was a prior disturbance in renal function, this is followed by an arteriogram. In such a patient if the major vascular architecture to the kidney is intact,

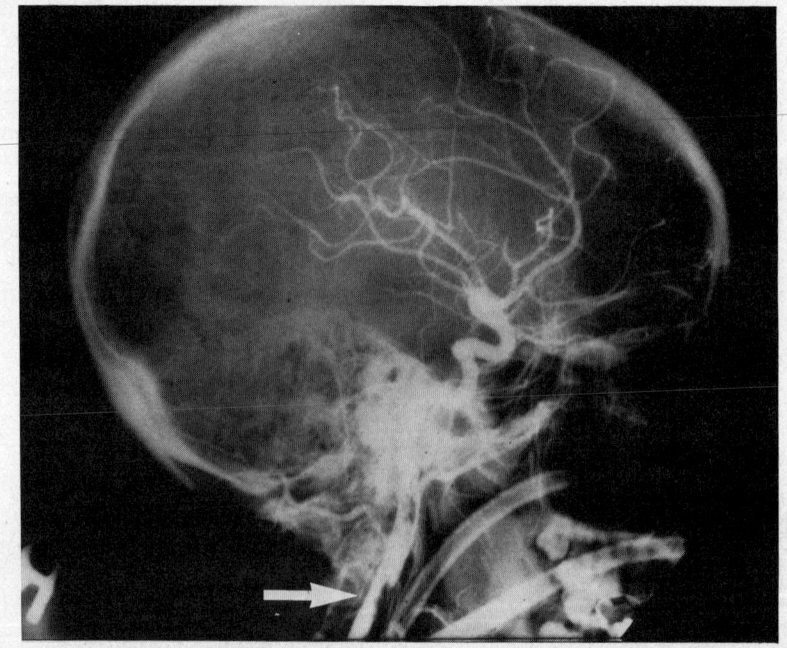

Fig. 31-3. Injuries to the internal carotid artery can be difficult to diagnose. This mural damage and intraluminal clot resulted from blunt trauma (*arrow*).

and if there is no disruption of the collecting system, observation rather than exploration is preferred. In such people injuries to the kidney cortex can be expected to heal if Gerota's fascia is left intact. On the other hand, if major arterial injury or collecting system disruption is identified, then surgical repair is required.

Arteriography also may be of use when patients are suspected of having injuries to other major visceral arteries, again primarily to identify the area of injury and to accurately plan the operation. If these patients are unstable, however, abbreviated arteriographic studies can be performed in the operating room during the course of the procedure; this offers considerable assistance both in identifying other lesions and in planning the repairs. The intraoperative method is not as satisfactory as the more sophisticated studies available in the radiology suite, but it is the preferred solution for an unstable patient.

MANAGEMENT

General principles

A patient with a major vascular injury usually has dramatic symptoms—bleeding, pallor, shortness of breath, and often hypotension. Successful resuscitation requires that certain priorities be established and specific plans for treatment be formulated. In all of these people initial attention to the airway and stopping the bleeding is first. Once control of the airway has been obtained and the vital signs assessed, an overall evaluation can be completed and proper priorities assigned. If external bleeding is present, it is usually controlled with direct finger pressure, pressure dressings, or pressure on proximal vascular structures. Blind attempts to clamp bleeding vessels located deep in the wound are ineffective and often dangerous, and should not be done. Tourniquets are rarely necessary.

After control of the airway is secured and respiratory assistance initiated, ventilation and pulmonary function are evaluated. Chest trauma is not uncommon in these patients and a hemothorax or pneumothorax must be treated initially. If chest tubes are needed, these should be inserted early during the resuscitation before pressure-assisted ventilation causes more severe mechanical problems by increasing the air leak and perhaps producing a tension pneumothorax.

Since these patients often require large amounts of fluid and blood, large catheters are placed into uninjured upper and lower extremity veins and carefully secured. One line is committed only for fluid replacement and is not used for drug administration or anesthetic manipulations.

In most cases these patients require a combination of a balanced electrolyte solution and whole blood to replace losses. As described by Shires and Shires, trauma and shock cause internal shifts of interstitial fluid that are best treated with appropriate infusions of electrolyte solutions and blood.[1] It is wise not to overtransfuse, especially if cardiopulmonary disease is present, since this may lead to cardiac overload. It appears that a whole blood hematocrit of approximately 30% is optimum; further increases in hemoglobin are unneeded and may increase blood viscosity unnecessarily. There are little convincing data showing that the infusion of a colloid solution such as albumin or dextran is of any additional value, and some studies suggest that colloid solutions may be harmful.[1]

During the initial examination if there is a need for special monitoring techniques, this is usually obvious. Hemodynamically stable patients with minor wounds of the extremities require only routine procedures, especially if they are young and free of intercurrent illnesses. In contrast, the patient who has multiple injuries or shock, or someone with preexisting cardiopulmonary problems, is almost certain to need continuous monitoring of vital signs, pulmonary mechanics, and cardiac function. Some estimate of cardiac filling and output is needed in these patients. A venous catheter to measure central venous pressure is helpful, but most of these people will benefit from a Swan-Ganz balloon catheter for direct evaluation of pulmonary artery pressure and cardiac function.

Control of bleeding

Most bleeding wounds can be controlled with direct digital pressure. In the majority of instances brisk hemorrhage has stopped in patients who have survived to reach the emergency room, but often large hematomas are present, and some bleeding may persist. If the wound is not bleeding it is best not to disturb it during the initial resuscitation; no attempt should be made to remove foreign bodies, or to evacuate clots until a general assessment has been completed and measures for obtaining proximal control are underway. Penetrating objects that are in the wound must be protected during transportation because they are capable of causing further damage, and it is best not to extract these foreign bodies until the patient reaches the operating room.

If fatal hemorrhage appears likely to occur in the emergency room, the wound can be extended and vascular clamps applied under direct vision. In large trauma centers even thoracotomy can be performed rapidly and safely in the emergency room, and in some hospitals patients have been placed on cardiopulmonary bypass in the emergency pavilion before being transported to the operating room.[21] These are unusual requirements, and they should be approached with caution, especially by those who are not experienced in such operations. A separate indication for emergency thoracotomy may exist when patients are admitted in profound hypovolemic shock from penetrating trauma. In such people open cardiac massage can be lifesaving, and an aggressive approach is needed.

Operative management

The patients are usually placed supine in the anatomic position and prepared to allow access to the thorax and abdomen as well as the involved extremities. Vertical incisions are preferred since they parallel the neurovascular structures and can be extended in either direction if required. Generous incisions are made to permit proximal and distal

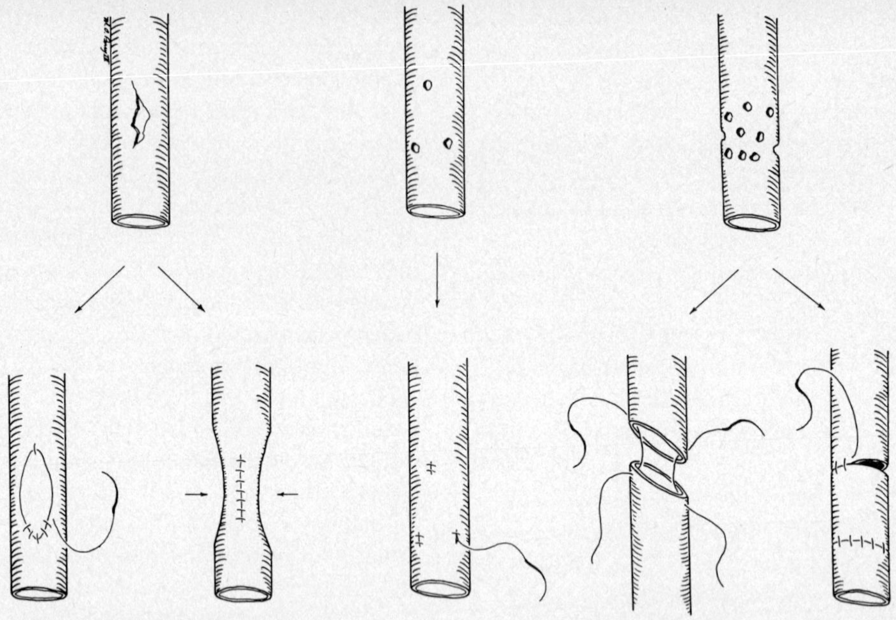

Fig. 31-4. Although lateral repair of injuries of large arteries is possible without narrowing, smaller ones require either patch-graft angioplasty or perhaps an interposition graft after resection of the damaged artery.

control of major vessels above and below the area suspected of being injured. Once the wound has been exposed and the clot carefully evacuated, the extent of the damage is ascertained. Every effort is made to avoid fragmenting and dislodging intraluminal clots, which can result in thromboembolism. In patients with atherosclerosis the arteries are often fragile, and it is easy to extend the damage by a hasty and rough exposure. Specific arterial repairs are not begun until hemorrhage has been arrested, all the injuries are identified, and priorities set.

Methods of repair

Lacerations of large vessels are easily repaired with lateral suture techniques if wide debridement is not required, but in patients who have sustained wounds as a result of medium- or high-velocity bullets, or have associated blunt trauma, it is often necessary to resect the damaged area and perform an end-to-end anastomosis if sufficient mobility can be obtained[16] (Fig. 31-4). If it is not possible to restore vascular continuity directly, then interposition grafts are chosen, usually using the saphenous vein if it is an appropriate size, although in some cases the hypogastric artery or other grafts may be used. In injuries involving the aortoiliac system autogenous grafts of suitable size are not available, and it will be necessary to employ plastic grafts.

Although autogenous tissue is preferred in the repair of vessels, both for patch-graft angioplasty and interposition grafts, in large arteries such as the aorta or iliac vessels plastic prostheses are needed. Special problems exist if the patient has associated injuries of the colon that have resulted in widespread bacterial contamination. In these patients rather than insert a plastic prosthesis into a severely contaminated field, the surgeon can oversew the ends of the arteries, cover them with viable tissue, and construct remote subcutaneous bypass grafts (axillary-femoral, femoral-femoral, obturator).[4,16] When the threat of infection has passed, a direct reconstruction can be considered.

Special problems

Although most arterial injuries can be repaired directly, once identified, particular difficulties are encountered in patients who have arterial damage as a result of substance abuse and repeated arterial punctures.[6] The usual complications of untreated vascular injuries such as thrombosis, delayed bleeding, arteriovenous fistulas, and false aneurysms are more likely to be seen in these people than in the normal trauma patient. Moreover, these arterial lesions are invariably associated with infection, both local and remote, and, in many patients, inanition and other illnesses as well.

A false aneurysm is the result of an incomplete injury of an artery, usually tangential, that permits continued bleeding. Transection of an artery is customarily followed by retraction and clotting, and in the case of small vessels, cessation of bleeding. The tangential laceration of an artery permits the blood to escape into the surrounding tissues, and sometimes to form a tamponading clot. In other cases it continues to bleed, resulting initially in what is called a "pulsating hematoma," and then subsequently a false aneurysm. If there is a contiguous tangential wound of an

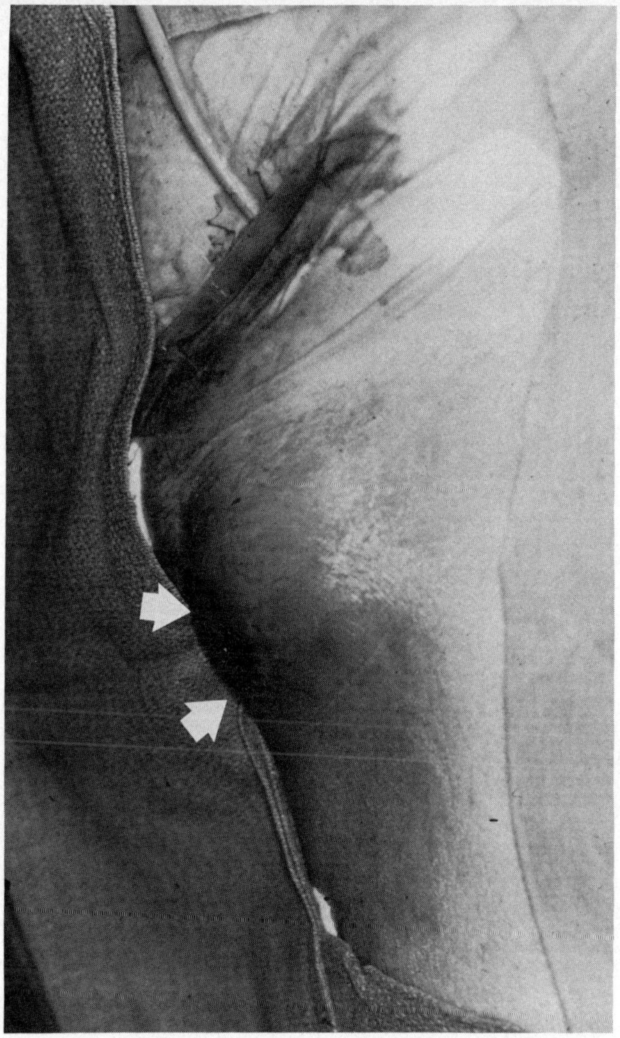

Fig. 31-5. This large, infected false aneurysm of the profunda femoris artery is eroding through the skin of the thigh (*arrows*). The Rummel tourniquet is around the distal external iliac artery, placed there to obtain proximal control of bleeding.

artery and vein an arteriovenous (AV) fistula can accompany the false aneurysm.

These lesions are easily diagnosed; there is a pulsatile mass, commonly in the groin, following a penetrating wound. There may be a bruit over the mass as a result of the blood escaping into the cavity of the false aneurysm, or if there is an AV fistula, there can be a continuous "machinery-like" murmur at and proximal to the area of injury.

False aneurysms and AV fistulas can heal only by thrombosis. In many patients thrombosis of a major artery will not be tolerated without severe distal ischemia. Previous studies by Shumacker and Wayson demonstrated that spontaneous cure is unlikely, occurring in only 3% of posttraumatic AV fistulas and less than 6% of posttraumatic false aneurysms.[22] The incidence of spontaneous cure in infected aneurysms following substance abuse is likely to be even lower. Many of these patients are first seen when there is threatened or overt erosion of the skin as a result of expansion of the aneurysm and invasive infection. Thus a patient may require an emergency operation to control bleeding (Fig. 31-5).

Although the diagnosis of false aneurysms and AV fistulas can be made on physical examination, a B-mode ultrasonic scan or CT scan is of assistance in determining the exact size and extent of the lesions. Preoperative arteriography is recommended in the hemodynamically stable patient to plan the operative repair.

There is no unanimity of opinion about how these lesions should be handled when infection is present. Recent studies suggest that even when the common femoral artery is involved, repair may be possible by using techniques of remote revascularization, bringing the graft through the obturator foramen, or perhaps via a lateral approach to reach uninvolved vessels distal to the area of infection.[23] A study by Johnson, Ledgerwood, and Lucas and a study by Reddy suggest that in many patients the extent of arterial infection is such that a direct repair is not safe.[20,24] In some patients it may be feasible to control the bleeding by direct suture of the artery, then follow-up on extremity viability carefully, perhaps with the patient receiving heparin. If the limb is not viable, the patient is returned to the operating room for a remote bypass graft. Other surgeons have suggested that an initial direct repair can be performed if properly staged, with an amputation rate no higher than 15%.[23] All of these series contain relatively small numbers of patients, and the types of cases that have been studied, although similar, vary somewhat. It is not possible to state with finality which procedure usually is safer. It is clear that direct reconstruction in the infected field is not likely to be successful. If some type of vascular repair is required, it must be remote, and placed in uninfected tissues.

Even if the initial repair is successful and the infection is controlled, recidivism is high, and many of the patients return. If the newly placed graft is accessible, it is often used for the injection of additional drugs by the addict. Clearly there is no single answer to the management of these serious problems, and a variety of reconstructive techniques will be required.

Operative evaluation

In most situations the success of the operation is easily validated by the restoration of distal pulses and the return of function. In patients with multiple injuries the adequacy of the repair can be difficult to ascertain, and intraoperative Doppler techniques may confirm the return of arterial blood flow. In other people completion arteriography may be required, and in many trauma centers this is considered almost a routine, especially in patients who have had repairs of carotid or lower extremity arteries.[16] If there is any question as to the adequacy of the repair, completion arteriography is indicated.

Postoperative care

If the vascular repair has been successful, only routine care is needed during the patient's recovery. The adequacy of the vascular repair is evaluated by repeated evaluations of neuromuscular function. The sine qua non for continued viability of the extremities includes the normal perception of light touch and the maintenance of intrinsic motor function. If there are disturbances in these neuromuscular modalities, then repeat arteriography is usually required, regardless of limb blood pressures, distal pulses, skin temperature, or appearance.

In the evaluation of patients who have had repairs of the visceral or splanchnic vessels repeated assessment of organ function is necessary. Disturbances in the function of the kidney, for example, suggest the need for repeat arteriography, and perhaps retrograde urography.

RESULTS

The overall results of repairing major vascular wounds are quite good, as shown in the accompanying box. If the initial repair is successful, and viability of the extremity has been gained, postoperative disability is usually a result of nerve injury, fractures, or soft tissue problems.

When evaluating the results of treating injuries of specific arteries, there is clearly a difference depending on the vessel involved. Injuries of the abdominal aorta, for example, particularly at the diaphragm, are often lethal; over half of these patients die.[17] In contrast, it is unusual for a patient with a penetrating wound distal to the knee or to the elbow to die. As seen in Table 31-1 the results of repairing penetrating wounds of the carotid artery are good if the patient does not have a neurologic deficit before surgery. It is unusual for complications to occur postoperatively if a successful repair has been performed. Most neurologic disability associated with these injuries is present before the operation. Although any vascular repair can clot, it is rare. Many trauma patients are young and have relatively normal arteries. Once the initial recovery is completed, the majority of patients have no further problems related to the vascular injury.

Arterial injuries: results of repair in 665 patients (%)

Failure of repair	5.2
Bleeding	2.0
Infection	3.1
Amputation	1.8
Death	10.4

From Perry MO: The management of acute vascular injuries, Baltimore, 1981, Williams & Wilkins.

Table 31-1. Penetrating carotid artery injuries: results of repair

Preoperative status	Number	Mortality
Group 1 —no neurologic deficit	61	0
Group 2 —mild neurologic deficit	9	1
Group 3 —severe neurologic deficit	15	5
TOTALS	85	6 (7%)

(From Perry MO: The management of acute vascular injuries, Baltimore, 1981, Williams & Wilkins.)

REFERENCES

1. Shires GT III and Shires GT: Trauma. In Schwartz SI, Shires GT, and Spencer FC, eds: Principles of surgery, ed 5, New York, 1989, McGraw-Hill, Inc.
2. The New York Times, January 6, 1986.
3. The Tennessean, January 1, 1989.
4. Feliciano DV et al: Civilian trauma in the 1980's, Ann Surg 199:717, 1984.
5. Perry MO: The management of acute vascular injuries, Baltimore, 1981, Williams & Wilkins.
6. Carey JP and Penn I: Cardiovascular complications of parenteral drug abuse, Contemp Surg 27:59, 1985.
7. Wright CB, Hobson RW, and Hollis HW: Acute vascular insufficiency due to drug abuse. In Rutherford RB, ed: Vascular surgery, ed 3, Philadelphia, 1989, WB Saunders Co.
8. Maxwell TM, Olcott C, and Blaisdell FW: Vascular complications of drug abuse, Arch Surg 105:875, 1972.
9. Natali J and Benhamou AC: Iatrogenic vascular injuries, J Cardiovasc Surg 20:169, 1979.
10. McFadden PM, Ochsner JL, and Mills N: Management of thrombotic complications of invasive arterial monitoring of the upper extremity, J Cardiovasc Surg 24:35, 1983.
11. Shield CF et al: Pseudoaneurysm of the brachiocephalic arteries: a complication of percutaneous internal jugular vein catheterization, Surgery 78:190, 1975.
12. Skillman JJ, Kim D, and Baim DS: Vascular complications of percutaneous femoral cardiac interventions: incidence and operative repair, Arch Surg 123:1207, 1988.
13. Orcutt MB et al: Iatrogenic vascular injury, Arch Surg 120:384, 1985.
14. Soderstrom CA et al: Infected false femoral artery aneurysm secondary to monitoring catheters, J Cardiovasc Surg 24:63, 1983.
15. Mills JL et al: Minimizing mortality and morbidity from iatrogenic arterial injuries: the need for early recognition and prompt repair, J Vasc Surg 4:22 1986.
16. Snyder WH, Thal ER, and Perry MO: Peripheral and abdominal vascular injuries. In Rutherford RB, ed: Vascular surgery, Philadelphia, 1984, WB Saunders Co.
17. Lim RC, Trunkey DD, and Blaisdell FW: Acute abdominal aortic injury, Arch Surg 109:706, 1974.
18. Snyder WH et al: The validity of normal arteriography in penetrating trauma, Arch Surg 113:424, 1978.
19. Reid JDS et al: Assessment of proximity of a wound to major vascular structures as an indication for arteriography, Arch Surg 123:943, 1988.
20. Johnson JR, Ledgerwood AM, and Lucas CE: Mycotic aneurysm, Arch Surg 118:557, 1983.
21. Baker CC, Thomas AN, and Trunkey DD: The role of emergency room thoracotomy and trauma, J Trauma 20:848, 1980.
22. Shumacker HB and Wayson EE: Traumatic arteriovenous fistulas and false aneurysms, Am J Surg 79:532, 1950.
23. Patel KR, Semel L, and Clauss RH: Routine revascularization with resection of infected femoral pseudoaneurysms from substance abuse, J Vasc Surg 8:321, 1988.
24. Reddy DJ: Treatment of drug related infected false aneurysm of the femoral artery: is routine revascularization justified? J Vasc Surg 8:344, 1988.

Chapter 32

COMPARTMENT SYNDROME

J. Tracy Watson

HISTORICAL DEVELOPMENT

Volkmann's classic paper in 1881 described ischemic contractures resulting from excessively tight bandages.[90] Compartment syndrome as a clinical finding has thus been well known for more than a century, although the exact pathophysiology has been less well understood. Volkmann concentrated primarily on changes in the muscular compartments, primarily paralysis and contractures, occurring after occlusive bandaging. He differentiated these from contractures resulting strictly from nerve palsies, noting that nerve paralysis contractures undergo gradual development, whereas ischemic contractures have a more temporal relationship with a close onset of paralysis and contracture. Associated with this temporal relationship is the fact that as time progresses, so does the severity of the contracture. Volkmann surmised that the paralysis and subsequent contracture had their origin in the muscle as a result of occlusive tight bandaging causing arterial insufficiency.

The early 1900s saw many proponents of the pressure theories, that is, compromise of the arterial supply by constricting bandages, and the emphasis remained on the contracture itself, not on the diagnosis or treatment.

In 1914 Murphy[67] pointed out that following a fracture, "blood and serum (effusion) follows and the tension in the subfascial zone in the forearm can be so great as to cause cyanosis of the whole forearm and hand." It was the pressure that caused the cell destruction. He described releasing the forearm fascia if symptoms persisted. Also during this period, Rowlands suggested the concept of postrevascularization of limbs as a potential cause in the development of compartment syndrome.[61] He stated that following the rapid return of blood flow to an extremity, congestion and edema could occur, thus causing subsequent muscle cell death. Vascular causes were subsequently proposed, but in 1926 Jepsen[38,39] became the first investigator to reproduce ischemic compartment syndrome in animals and document the results following prompt surgical decompression.

Griffith's article in 1940 established the classic "four *p*'s" for the diagnosis of compartmental syndrome.[22]

1. Pain
2. Paralysis
3. Pallor
4. Pulselessness

These signs were based on the concept of arterial injury or, at the very least, "spasm" of the artery caused by antecedent injury. Because of this "spasm," extensive surgical exploration was often performed to discover and excise the area of the artery in spasm.

Most of the experience of ischemic necrosis was derived from the war years during the 1940s when physicians dealt with many high-velocity injuries and major arterial disruption. During the 1960s and 1970s, the concept of increased intracompartmental pressures arose as the unifying feature in the development of compartment syndromes and Volkmann's ischemic necrosis. Contributing to our current knowledge of compartment syndrome was the work of Rorabeck in 1975.[76] He showed a decrease in the clearance of technetium-99m after intramuscular injection into the tibialis anterior muscle of dogs. This clearance was directly related to an increased compartmental pressure created in dogs by IM injection of serum into that compartment. Thus anatomic intracompartmental pressures were felt to be a major determining factor in the normal physiology of the compartment musculature. In 1975 Sheridan and Matson[81] determined experimentally that the closer the compartmental pressure is to the mean arterial blood pressure, the greater the decrease in the blood flow to that compartment. Mildly elevated compartmental pressures resulted in a marked muscular inflammatory necrosis, and with markedly elevated pressures, the muscle underwent ischemic necrosis.

CAUSES OF COMPARTMENT SYNDROME

Current authors agree that the "unifying concept" of compartment syndrome is a condition in which increased tissue

A

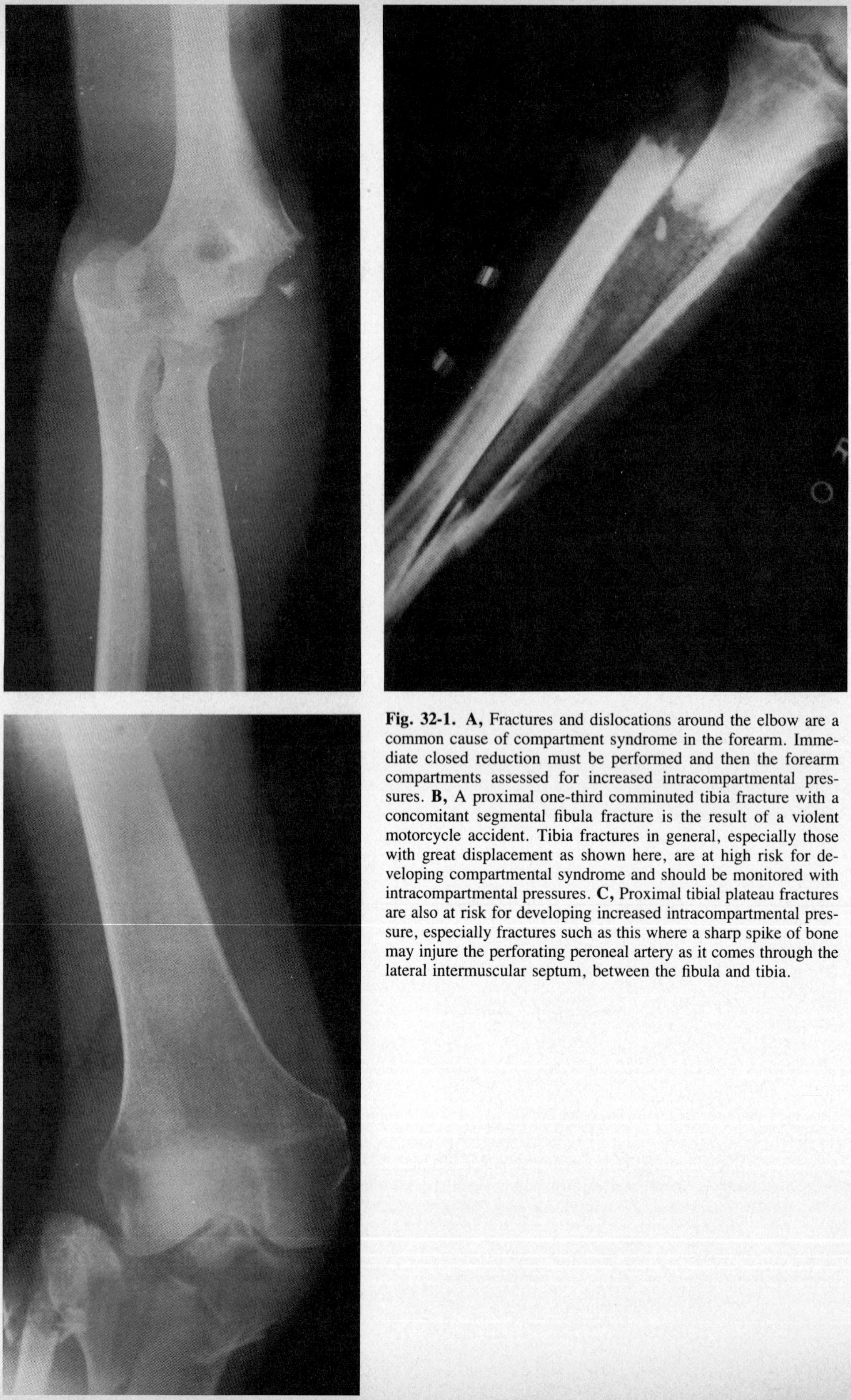

B

C

Fig. 32-1. A, Fractures and dislocations around the elbow are a common cause of compartment syndrome in the forearm. Immediate closed reduction must be performed and then the forearm compartments assessed for increased intracompartmental pressures. **B,** A proximal one-third comminuted tibia fracture with a concomitant segmental fibula fracture is the result of a violent motorcycle accident. Tibia fractures in general, especially those with great displacement as shown here, are at high risk for developing compartmental syndrome and should be monitored with intracompartmental pressures. **C,** Proximal tibial plateau fractures are also at risk for developing increased intracompartmental pressure, especially fractures such as this where a sharp spike of bone may injure the perforating peroneal artery as it comes through the lateral intermuscular septum, between the fibula and tibia.

pressure develops in a fascial envelope, restricting the volume available to the enclosed tissue. This, in turn, can cause ischemia sufficient to compromise myoneural structures.[31,49]

The origin of this abnormally high tissue pressure can occur in many ways. Most commonly, fluid accumulation originates from hemorrhage, extracellular edema, intracellular edema, or a combination of these mechanisms.[61] As internal compartmental tissue swells, this causes an increase in the compartmental content and raises the pressure, thereby decreasing the relative compartmental size with the resultant effect of increasing the compartment pressure.

Fractures

Fractures are probably the most common cause of an acute compartment syndrome. Tibial fractures are followed closely by forearm fractures in children and adults, and these are the two fractures in which one must have a high index of suspicion regardless of the energy expenditure causing the fracture (Fig. 32-1). Following a fracture, hemorrhage from bone ends occurs as does edema from the trauma itself. This accumulation of hemorrhage and edema combines to increase the tissue pressure within a closed fascial envelope.

One must be aware that soft tissue injury without a concomitant fracture may also lead to an increase of intracompartmental contents with the accumulation of edema and hemorrhage, especially following a crush type of injury. Compartment syndromes resulting from fractures or soft tissue trauma have now been described in virtually every anatomic compartment in the human body. They have been noted to occur in the thigh,[89] upper arm,[8] hand,[44] buttock,[74] foot,[4] and even in the extraocular muscles following a blowout fracture to the orbital region.[84] Open fractures do not preclude the development of increased tissue pressure occurring from hemorrhage and the edema of trauma itself (Fig. 32-2).

One must also be aware of the potential for arterial injury to coexist with the fracture (Fig. 32-3). Injury to a major

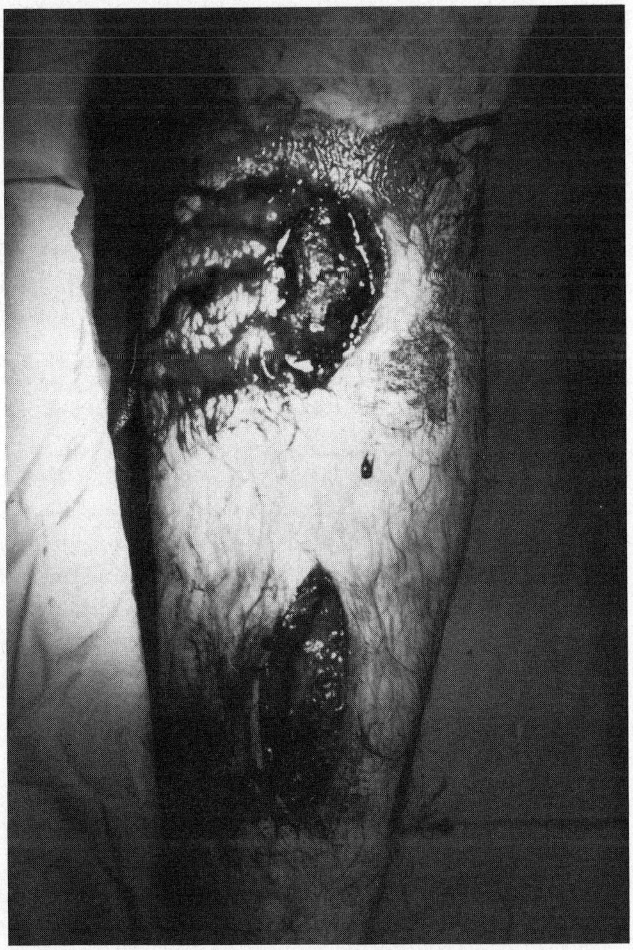

Fig. 32-2. Open fractures do not preclude the occurrence of compartmental syndrome. Even though the wound was open in two regions, note the massive swelling and bulging of the muscle through the open wounds. Intracompartmental pressures were elevated in this tibia fracture.

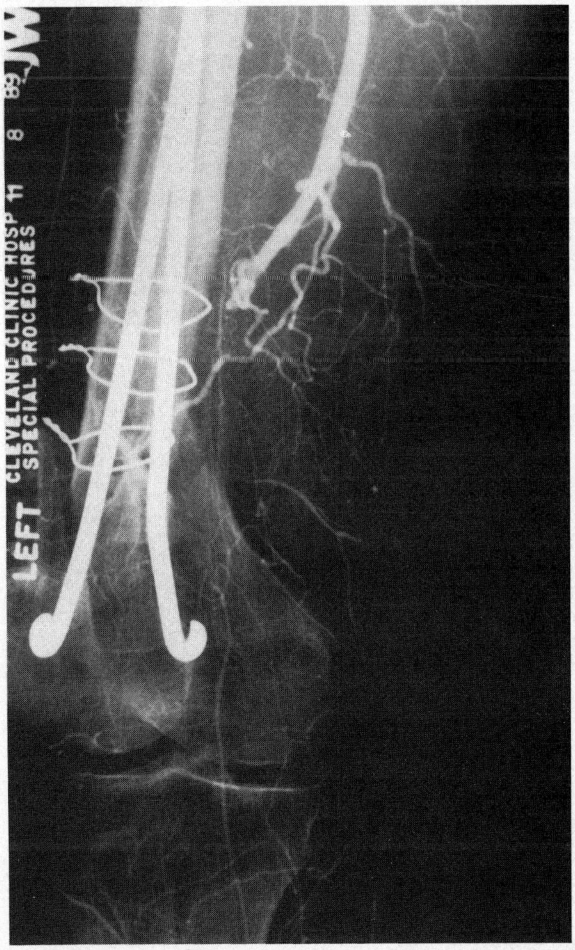

Fig. 32-3. This patient was transferred to our institution with unrecognized arterial occlusion of the femoral artery resulting from the original injury or the operative fixation. Ischemic time was well over 6 hours and the patient went on to full-blown lower extremity compartment syndrome with ischemic necrosis and contracture, even though arterial repair was performed.

artery can also cause compartment syndrome. If the injury has caused complete occlusion of the artery, ischemic changes may occur. Temporary ischemia produces edema by two mechanisms. Extracellular edema is first produced by elevated capillary permeability[91] caused by temporary ischemia. This is followed by the generation of intracellular edema as a result of postischemic swelling associated with muscle membrane depolarization and intracellular water accumulation.[82] As the edema accumulates and increases tissue pressure, the pressure may be able to reduce the local arteriovenous gradient as well as the local blood flow. This in turn will prolong the period of ischemia to muscles and nerves of the compartment, thus producing more and more swelling within the compartment. Restoration of circulation, either by reduction of the fracture or direct repair to the artery itself, will result in postischemic swelling.

The incidence of postischemic compartment syndrome in elective revascularization procedures is extremely low, approximately 0.45%. However, after repair of arterial injuries, acute postischemic compartment syndrome occurs over 30% of the time.[70] Total time of arterial ischemia is crucial. Experimentally elevated compartment pressures have been generated within 4 to 6 hours of tourniquet ischemia.[61] It is recommended that routine fasciotomy be performed following arterial repair if the ischemic period has been greater than 6 hours. Unless fasciotomy is carried out, the resulting postischemic compartment syndrome will prolong the period of ischemia.

Blood dyscrasia and systemic disease

Various blood dyscrasias and bleeding diatheses can also be the cause of acute or chronic compartment syndromes. Hemorrhage can occur in hemophiliacs and cause an increase in intracompartmental volume. Compartment syndrome has been described in the hand and forearm.[44,46] Iliacus syndrome with femoral neuropathy caused by bleeding into the iliacus muscle compartment has also been described in hemophilia.[6] A similar cause, that of increased compartmental volume with hemorrhage, can occur in anticoagulated patients. This may occur in many ways such as blunt trauma causing hemorrhage, or more commonly iatrongenic hemorrhage produced from venipuncture or arterial puncture for diagnostic blood work.

Sickle cell trait has also been shown to have a causal relationship to the development of compartment syndrome.[34] Sickling is known to occur in areas of low-oxygen tension, and it is suggested that in a muscle compartment with a minimally elevated pressure to begin with, such as following vigorous exercise, this elevated pressure results in decreased capillary perfusion and thus longer oxygen diffusion gradients. If the sickle cell trait is present, this could cause enough hemoglobin saturation to precipitate sickling. Sickling would, in turn, impede capillary flow, resulting in further ischemic swelling and a spiraling of this effect. Hence, sickle cell trait, though not the direct cause, can increase the tendency for a syndrome to develop.[34,98]

Various systemic diseases have also produced acute or chronic compartment syndromes. Hughes[37] described a patient who developed bilateral compartment syndrome during a febrile event associated with vasculitis. Browne,[7] in 1962, presented examples of patients with bilateral compartment syndrome resulting from generalized leprosarial panniculitis. Metabolic complications resulting from disease as varied as malaria and heat stroke have been reported in connection with the development of compartment syndrome.[73,98]

Purpura fulminans, a rare catastrophic illness of childhood, has also been implicated in the development of acute compartment syndrome. It begins as a seemingly benign infectious process that progresses to high fever, purpuric ecchymoses of the skin, hypotension, and disseminated intravascular coagulation. This is followed by muscle necrosis and, if pressures are allowed to progress, full-blown gangrene of the extremity.[83]

Exercise-initiated compartment syndrome

Chronic compartment syndrome can occur from exercise-initiated activity. The pathogenesis is similar to that seen in sickle cell trait. This condition is primarily caused by a relative inadequacy of the musculofascial compartment size that is further compromised by an increase in muscle volume resulting from strenuous activity. This increased pressure interferes with the micromuscular capillary blood flow leading to decreased oxygen uptake by the muscle cells. Ischemia and pain then follow. This condition contrasts with an acute compartment syndrome in that the symptoms in the chronic syndrome will usually resolve with rest.[37,48,77]

In athletes, particularly runners, there is a variety of causes of pain occurring during and after exercise. Most commonly these are entities such as stress fractures, tenosynovitis or a nerve entrapment syndrome. For most of these patients, workup should include whole body bone scans with 99m Tc-labeled pyrophosphate to exclude the possibility of stress fractures in either the tibia or the fibula. In addition, electromyographic studies can also be done in the distribution of the tibial or common peroneal nerve to rule out nerve entrapment syndromes. Occasionally venography can be performed to exclude an occult thrombophlebitis. Most of these pain syndromes can be treated successfully by conservative means. However, there are entities that may become chronic in spite of adequate nonsurgical therapy. These are exercise-related chronic compartment syndromes and are called shin splints, march synovitis, anterior tibial pain syndrome, and medial tibial syndrome. These entities all describe a chronic exertional compartment syndrome picture.

The clinical symptoms of exertional compartment syndrome may involve any of the four compartments of the lower extremity. Most commonly, patients experience a recurrent aching and cramping of the anterior or lateral aspect of the leg brought on by exercise. Usually the onset of the pain is within 5 to 10 minutes after exercise. The patient may complain of swelling in the anterior aspect of the leg and occasionally dysesthesia will be described along the terminal branch of the deep peroneal nerve into the first webspace or along the lateral border of the foot. If the compartment syndrome involves the deep posterior compartment, pain is usually located posteromedially in the calf and invariably radiates into the posterior aspect of the leg on to the medial sole of the foot. Numbness and dysesthesia along the plantar aspect of the sole is associated with this pain. There are usually no positive physical findings with these patients other than vague local discomfort occurring with pressure over the anterior or posterior compartments. The neurologic examination is usually negative.

Numerous nonoperative modalities have been used in an attempt to treat this condition. Avoidance of activity followed by a return to activity in a supervised graduated fashion is usually recommended to all patients. Various types of prescription footwear as well as orthoses have also been prescribed, as have physiotherapy programs including ice, stretching, isotonic, and isometric muscle exercises. These measures usually fail after the patient's return to sports activity.[91]

The clinical symptoms of the patients should alert the physician to a diagnosis of an exertional form of chronic anterior compartment syndrome. In the absence of clinical signs, which is the rule, compartment pressure measurements should be performed to confirm the diagnosis. While most of these patients will have slightly elevated resting compartment pressures, this measurement alone is not enough to confirm the diagnosis. Rorabeck[73-77] suggests continuous pressure monitoring with exercise. First resting pressures should be measured with the slit catheter technique with the patient in a supine position. This is followed by continuous pressure measurements while the patient exercises on a treadmill at a recommended speed of 6.4 km/hr for 15 minutes, with the catheter in place. The patient then remains supine for approximately 30 minutes while the compartment pressures are monitored continuously until a final measurement is obtained. The compartment chosen for measurement is guided by the patient's clinical symptoms and the pain location. The average resting compartment pressure is ± 4 mm Hg. After a period of enforced and controlled exercise, the compartment pressure should return to its normal resting value within 15 minutes. Most patients with chronic exertional compartment syndromes will have persistently elevated pressures 30 minutes after cessation of exercise. The clinical signs combined with the elevated compartment pressure measurements after exercise support the diagnosis of chronic exertional compartment syndrome.[77,87,91] These patients should undergo fasciotomy since conservative measures are not successful in the treatment of this entity. Fasciotomy will relieve symptoms in patients with chronic exertional compartment syndrome, will normalize the intramuscular pressure, and will increase the functional capacity of the involved compartment.

Crush syndrome

Compartment syndrome has also been described in relationship to the *crush syndrome*. This is a term popularized after World War II, used to describe the syndrome that developed following crush injuries to the extremities caused by bombing debris.[9] Classically described, crush syndrome is a prolonged compression to the extremities that results in muscle necrosis, followed by myoglobinuria, third space fluid loss, shock, acidosis, hyperkalemia, and renal failure. This full-blown syndrome is rarely seen today, although a lesser form of the syndrome has been described in patients who suffer from drug overdose[80] with compression of the individual's extremities by the head and torso. It also occurs because of abnormal posturing such as a hyperflexion of knees in a prolonged crouch position for spine surgery.[41] Other abnormal patient positions for surgery have been found to cause compartment syndrome. Prolonged use of the lithotomy position for orthopedic, urologic, and vascular procedures has been reported as the cause of lower extremity compartment syndrome.[42] The key here is the time interval involved. This complication of the lithotomy position has been seen only in procedures lasting longer than 6½ hours.[14] Crush syndrome has been described in patients who have attempted suicide through carbon monoxide poisoning in which prolonged periods of unconsciousness have resulted in abnormal pressures resulting from body positioning.[36,85]

Whatever the cause, the prolonged pressure to regional body areas causes localized muscle and capillary ischemia. If the pressure is prolonged, with the development of more extensive local injury, sufficient edema may be produced to initiate a compartment syndrome via the edema/ischemia cycle.[69] As more muscle becomes infarcted, systemic manifestations of hypovolemia from third space fluid loss occur. Myoglobinuria is the result of muscle cellular breakdown, which is followed by renal failure. Mubarak and Owen[64] were able to correlate the severity of the crush syndrome with the number of compartments involved.

External factors

The preceding section discussed various internal volumetric changes that can precipitate acute compartment syndrome. There are many external factors that can produce compartment syndrome by decreasing the compliance of a compartment, or by reducing the overall size of the compartment, which can increase the pressure within the compartment itself.

Dressings and casts. The volume restricting effect of casts and circular dressings was first incriminated as the cause of compartmental ischemia by Volkmann in 1872 and 1881.[60] A cast or rigid dressing lowers tissue compliance and also lowers the threshold of fluid accumulation that will elevate the pressure to ischemic levels. However, most bony injuries require a cast or dressing to supply circumferential pressure to maintain a reduction of the fracture. A potential dilemma exists if there is a question of compartment syndrome in a freshly casted fracture. Is the bony injury or the dressing the cause of the elevated tissue pressure?

Garfin[17] showed that in a casted extremity, 40% less volume was required to elevate intracompartmental pressures to similar levels in uncasted extremities. Therefore the threshold for intracompartmental volume increase is greatly reduced because of the volume containment of the cast. Similarly, when a constricting cast was split and spread open, this maneuver decreased compartmental pressure by 65%. Removing the cast altogether decreased the original pressures by 85%.

Tourniquets and antishock garments. In similar fashion MAST trousers[5,92] and tourniquets[21] have been implicated in the development of compartment syndrome. The use of a tourniquet can potentially produce a compartment syndrome in two ways. Tourniquets, of course, cause ischemia in the tissues distal to the level of application. The effects of prolonged ischemia and postischemic swelling have previously been discussed. However, recent studies have focused on the increased pressure effects seen by the tissue directly beneath the tourniquet.[25,87] These increased tissue pressures have led to recommendations to use a wider cuff to distribute the pressures more uniformly to the deeper tissues.[25] This recommendation also allows the use of lower inflation pressures to transmit even pressure to the deeper tissue layers.

Tourniquets will increase the local tissue pressure and there is a suggestion that elevated tissue pressure, coupled with ischemia, may act synergistically to produce significant cellular endothelial damage with redistribution of fluid from the intravascular to interstitial space.[33] This fluid transition serves to increase the intracompartmental pressure.

Maletis[47] described a 27% incidence of compartment syndrome as a complication of intravenous regional anesthesia (Bier block), using a thigh tourniquet following the reduction of tibial shaft fractures. This is compared to an incidence of between 1% and 11% compartment syndromes for those tibial fractures reduced under general anesthesia. He ascribed the high incidence of compartment syndrome to the use of the thigh tourniquet.

Compressive neuropathy at the site of a tourniquet application has been the most frequently encountered complication associated with its use.[21] However, direct pressure of sufficient magnitude applied to muscles of a compartment will have a localized ischemic effect on the compartment contents. An additive effect of the externally applied pressure to the compartment also exists with the tourniquet use.[54] The combination of internal ischemia and external compression is the mechanism for elevated compartment pressure.

The use of antishock (MAST) trousers for resuscitation of trauma victims has also been implicated in the development of compartment syndrome[1,3,5,11,88,92] and also has been known to cause a full-blown "crush syndrome" with resultant death.[20] It is suggested that antishock trousers might be contributing to the development of compartment syndrome because of a number of these were reported in normal, uninjured limbs as well as in injured extremities. The circumferential external compression is implicated. External compression of the garments decreases blood flow to the tissues by reducing the transmural pressure in the arterioles. When the transmural pressure in the arterioles cannot overcome the externally applied pressure, blood flow may stop. By exceeding the critical closing pressure of arterioles, the antishock trousers cause decreased tissue perfusion. This, in turn, leads to tissue ischemia with resultant edema and elevated compartmental pressure.[92] Authors have now recommended the use of lower inflation pressures and close observation of the extremities for patients with greater than two hours of inflation of the MAST trousers. Proper removal of the trousers should also be performed with abdominal segments deflated before lower extremity segments are removed. If the leg segments are deflated first while the abdominal portion remains inflated, venous return from the legs is prohibited. In a swollen muscle compartment, even brief venous obstruction may be sufficient to precipitate compartment syndrome.[5]

Burns and frostbite. Burns are responsible for the production of compartment syndrome in various ways. An inelastic eschar often is produced following full-thickness burns. Especially in cases where the eschar develops circumferentially, the constricting eschar decreases the compliance and volume of the involved compartments. This is the reasoning behind escharotomy.[59] It is an attempt to remove the external compressive forces that have been shown to precipitate a compartment syndrome. Burns, frostbite, and electrical injury also produce major tissue insults with resultant edema formation. It is likely that compartment syndrome develops from this combination of compression and tissue damage. It is not likely that a vascular injury plays a major role in these causes.[45] However, the progressive vascular thrombosis could potentiate the tissue ischemia and thus elevate the edema/ischemia cycle.

Congenital bands. Congenital bands, also called Streeter's dysplasia, are anomalous bands that partially or completely encircle and extremity or digit. As a digit or extremity develops shortly after birth, the constricting band will become more severe. Vascular compromise of the extremity distal to a ring constriction has been reported.[72] Impending compartment syndrome has also been noted in these cases,[99] presumably because of the inability of the compartment to adapt its volume because of the external compression of the rings. This, in effect, decreases the overall volume of the compartment with resultant increase in pressure.

Traction. Compartment syndrome has been associated with femoral fractures in children treated with Bryant's traction. The primary mechanism is thought to be a reduction in intraarterial pressure in the lower limbs being held in the overhead position. This is further aggravated by tight bandaging and hyperextension of the knee. This external compression, in essence, decreases the compliance of the compartments.[61] Similarly, an adult being placed in split

Russell's or balance suspension traction with a constricting thigh cuff could also have similar problems with external compression, thus reducing compliance of the thigh compartments. Whatever the age of the patient placed in traction, frequent neurovascular exams are warranted, and patients should be watched closely for the development of any compartmental compromise.

PATHOPHYSIOLOGY

Compartment syndromes, regardless of their causes, all have a final common pathway. This is the ischemia/edema cycle. Holden[35] suggested that a "vicious circle" begins with the injury or insult initially raising the tissue pressure. The effects of increased tissue pressure have been widely studied.

Hargens et al[25] showed that increased tissue pressure, applied to the walls of collapsible vessels, produced a corresponding increase in the pressure within those vessels. This increased tissue pressure thus increases local venous pressure only, lowering the local arteriovenous (AV) pressure gradient. No vascular occlusion occurs, and blood continues to flow down the pressure gradient from artery to vein.

$$\text{Tissue P} = \frac{1}{\text{AV pressure gradient}}$$

As seen here, tissue pressure is inversely proportional to the AV gradient. Local blood flow is determined by the local AV pressure gradient and vascular resistance.

$$\text{LBF} = \frac{\text{AV pressure gradient}}{\text{R}}$$

Changes in the local AV pressure gradient have a direct effect on local blood flow. In effect, as tissue pressure rises, the local AV pressure gradient is lowered as is the local blood flow to the tissue. It is at this point that the metabolic demands of the tissue cannot be maintained by the reduced blood flow, and ischemia results.[51] On a microcirculation level, a similar pattern is observed. Normally, capillary filtration equilibrium occurs at 13 mm Hg at the anatomic site of postcapillary venules. Net fluid filtration occurs into the tissues from the precapillary and capillary vessels, whereas net fluid absorption back into the blood occurs in the postcapillary venules where the blood pressure is less than 13 mm Hg.[24] The overall filtration force is about a −6.7 mm Hg, pulling fluid back into the capillaries at the venous end.[31]

Several changes occur with ischemia. Muscle ischemia significantly raises capillary membrane permeability to plasma proteins with the loss of colloid into the extracellular space.[12] Little of the osmotic activity of plasma proteins is available to prevent intramuscular edema. These changes result in increased filtration force and further edema formation. Because of the tight fascial enclosure, tissue pressure rises.

Without absorption of fluid back into the blood, the tissue-fluid pressure approaches intracapillary blood pressure and, as a result, the soft compressible venous end of the capillary becomes occluded.[2] This prevents the return of blood from the compartment, increasing intravascular pressure in the venous end of the capillary and further raising the tissue pressure.

When the intracompartmental pressure exceeds 30 mm Hg, lymphatic vessels probably cannot drain fluid from edematous muscle.[12] This also contributes to the vicious cycle of edema and ischemia.

Once the threshold of 30 mm Hg has been reached, small additions to intracompartmental edema or external compression will elicit large increments in intracompartmental pressure, and vulnerability to ischemic muscle necrosis rises dramatically.[64] The intracompartmental tissue pressure is usually less than the arterial blood pressure. Theoretically, the intracompartmental pressure could reach systolic blood pressure if there were disruption of a major artery. However, this is usually not the case so that the distal arterial blood flow and peripheral pulses often remain intact. Blood flow stops in the microvascular circulation when local tissue pressure exceeds the diastolic blood pressure.[2] Because the digital capillary bed drains into *extra*compartmental veins, the digital AV pressure gradient and blood flow remain intact. Thus peripheral pulses and digital circulation are poor indicators of blood flow and poor indicators of increased pressure within a compartmental space.[50]

Tissue effect

The effects of altered perfusion are time- and pressure-dependent. The effects of rising pressure are directly related to the duration and magnitude of the pressure change. Experiments[26] have shown that there is a threshold pressure of 30 mm Hg and a duration of ischemia of 8 hours. At this time significant irreversible muscle necrosis occurs with normal systemic blood pressure.[28] Higher tissue pressure requires less time to damage muscle.[51] The period of pressurization required for nerve failure is directly proportional to intracompartmental pressure. Partial conduction impairment occurs after 6 to 8 hours of pressurization at 30 mm Hg.[27] Significant irreversible damage to nervous tissue is produced at intracompartmental pressures between 30 and 40 mm Hg after 6 to 12 hours. Studies have documented that in compartment syndrome, neurologic loss is caused by an elevated tissue fluid pressure occluding the nerve/microvasculature, thus causing ischemic failure of nerve conduction.[26]

Muscle necrosis, however, is reversible even after 6 to 12 hours, providing circulation can be restored before total necrosis and fibrous replacement of the muscle occurs.[16] Therefore it is crucial to diagnose and treat the compartment syndrome as soon as possible. Circulation to ischemic muscle must be reestablished and the pressure must be released. Light microscopic evidence shows that between 4 and 6 days postfasciotomy myoblasts appear in the areas of phagocytized necrotic muscle tissue. Their origin is either from existing viable muscle cells or from satellite cells. These cells align themselves along undamaged sarcolemmal tubes. Myofilaments are then rapidly laid down on either side of these chains of nuclei. Between 6 and 8 days postfasciotomy, these chains will form myotubules containing peripheral bundles of myofibrils arranged around the central core of nuclei and cytoplasm.[79] Assuming these muscle cells can reestablish their innervation, they will continue to mature into normal muscle fibers. Muscle fibers that fail to obtain a nervous supply after injury remain at the myotubule stage and then atrophy. The nature of the repair process is usually a mixture of regeneration of muscle and fibrous tissue. However, variation in capillary perfusion between one region and another in the same muscle compartment may explain the patchy distribution of necrosis as well as muscle repair following compartment syndrome.[28]

At present, only a few studies have attempted to quantitate the cellular and biochemical limits of muscle viability as a function of different pressure relationships during ischemia. Currently, disagreement arises from the use of absolute compartment pressure measurements as a measure of tissue viability when pressure measurements are only an indirect measure of tissue viability.[26,28,51,54]

Heppenstal[33] looked at the change of delta pressure (Δp = the difference between mean arterial pressure and compartment pressure), along with the investigative technique of phosphorus nuclear magnetic resonance spectroscopy (31P−MRS). This technique monitors the metabolic state of tissue at the cellular level and is sensitive only to degrees of diminished blood flow severe enough to result in cellular metabolic derangement.[32]

The biochemical parameters that 31P−MRS measures are related to oxygen delivery. In compartment syndrome, as tissue pressure increases, the reduction in blood flow may drop so that oxygen delivery cannot be maintained below a critical level.[96] Anaerobic metabolism becomes predominant and high-energy phosphocreatinine compounds are consumed, thus decreasing the 31P−MRS spectra.

At lower Δp, less than 30 mm Hg for greater than 6 hours, there is a greater decline in the phosphocreatinine ratio and intracellular pH. Also significant is the fact that at lower Δp, the percentage recovery after fasciotomy is declined. This is the first objective criterion for defining pressure-time variables that takes into account muscle blood flow, muscle Po_2 and compartmental as well as systemic blood pressure. Data of this type are extremely important in trying to define the cellular effects of increased compartment pressure. Currently, however, the evidence will continue to indicate that significant compartmental necrosis is produced at a threshold pressure level and duration of 30 mm Hg and 8 hours. This pressure threshold is lowered under conditions of hypotension. Decompressive fasciotomy should therefore be undertaken for intracompartmental pressures of 30 mm Hg or more.

DIAGNOSIS

Prompt diagnosis is the key to management of compartment syndromes. Early decompression limits the ischemic damage and allows potential for recovery of function. The clinical findings may be so dramatic that actual pressure measurements are only confirmatory. On the other hand, in traumatized or unresponsive comatose patients, the physical examination is confusing, and one must rely on the pressure measurements to make the diagnosis. The physician must have a high clinical index of suspicion. Being aware of the potential situation in which a compartment syndrome can occur and then evaluating the patient within this context will facilitate the diagnosis.

Clinical signs and symptoms

The classic mnemonic, the "four *p*'s," is referenced here for historic purposes only. Pain, pallor, pulselessness, and paralysis, deemed as diagnostic criteria for compartment syndrome in the 1940s,[22] were based primarily on cases dealing with major vascular insufficiency. As shown earlier, pulselessness and pallor are not definitive signs of compartment syndrome. Although intracompartmental pressure may be high enough to cause ischemia of muscles and nerves by occluding microcirculation in the compartment, it only rarely is high enough to occlude the major arteries (Fig. 32-4).

Symptoms. Severe pain, resistant to analgesics, and pain that is out of proportion to what is expected from the primary problem is an excellent symptom of an impending compartment syndrome. The pain is confined to the limb involved and is nonradiating since nerve ischemia produces failure of function without loss of pain.[68] Pain is not relieved by immobilization, ice, elevation, or narcotics. Circumferential casts or dressings may actually aggravate the discomfort.

One should be aware, however, that compartment syndrome has been reported in the absence of pain.[93] This has been our experience as well. Nerve dysfunction is almost always superimposed in these cases as a peripheral sensory deficit. However, pain is usually quite clearly correlated with increasing intracompartmental pressure. Mubarak[63] showed with wick catheter measurements that pain becomes severe as pressure approaches 30 mm Hg.

Signs. A sign that most patients will exhibit is a tense, firm, swollen compartment running the length of the anatomic compartment involved. The firmness is not localized to the site of the inciting pathology, that is, a fracture or area of contusion. Conversely, if there are areas that are palpably soft, then compartment pressures are probably not elevated. Pressure will equilibrate rapidly throughout the contiguous compartment.

Pain on passive stretch of the muscles in the involved compartment is common, but it is quite subjective and unreliable.[13,63] If the injury has caused direct muscle damage, as in fractures or contusions, the stretch of this damaged

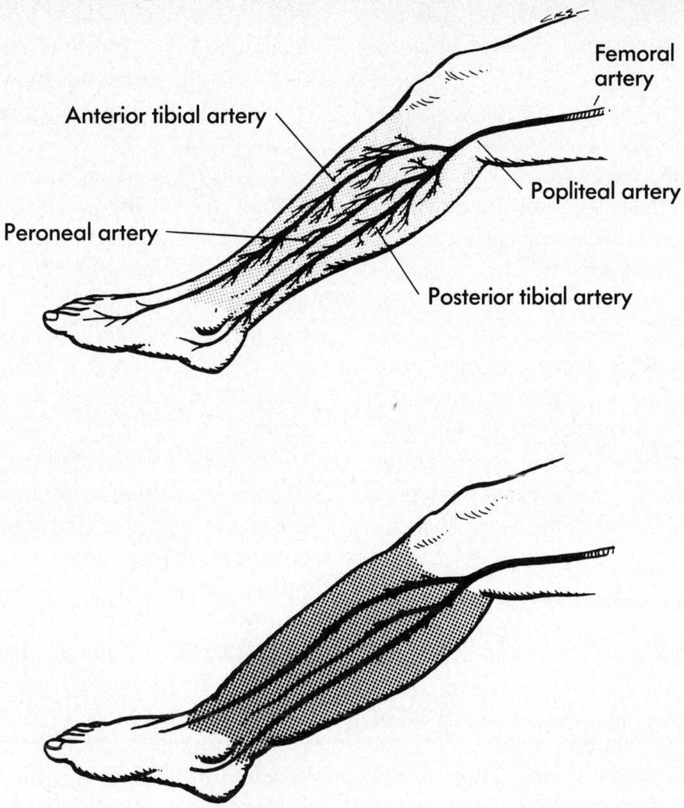

Fig. 32-4. Schematic leg compartment syndromes. Intracompartmental pressures are only rarely high enough to occlude major arteries of compartment. However, pressure is sufficient to cause ischemia of muscle and nerve by occluding microcirculation within compartment. (From Mubarak SJ and Hargens AR: Compartment syndromes and Volkmann's contracture, Philadelphia, 1981, WB Saunders Co.)

muscle will be painful, even in the absence of increased compartmental pressure. Again, sensory deficits may mask stretch pain, even with elevated compartmental pressures.[68]

A more reliable sign is a sensory deficit. Most compartments have sensory nerves that travel through the bulk of the muscular compartment. The first sign of nerve ischemia is altered sensation.[58] This is manifest by hypoesthesia and later anesthesia, with decreased sensation to light touch and pin prick. The appearance of parasthesias in the distribution of the deep peroneal nerve has been documented with pressures of greater than 30 mm Hg. It is important to check all sensory nerves since the specific nerve is indicative of which compartment is involved. However, one must be aware of the possibility of superimposed traumatic peripheral nerve deficit.

Paresis caused by compartment syndrome is a late finding and warrants emergent treatment. It is of little help in the diagnosis of early compartment syndrome.[58] Paresis may be secondary to proximal nerve injury, or muscle guarding may prevent full voluntary contraction, thus simulating paresis.

Most signs and symptoms of a compartment syndrome rely on intact sensation to the involved compartment. In patients with a coexistent nerve lesion or altered state of consciousness, we must rely on other means to make the diagnosis. The differential diagnosis of compartment syndrome includes a wide variety of conditions. Many times a compartment syndrome is superimposed on an underlying problem. Diagnosis is especially difficult when trying to differentiate compartment syndrome, arterial occlusion, and trauma-induced neuropraxia. Since signs and symptoms can overlap with these conditions, more invasive studies are often necessary to aid in the diagnosis. Arteriography, Doppler flow studies and compartment pressure measurements offer the most useful, immediate information.

Measurement of compartment pressure

The universal factor that must be present for compartment syndrome to exist is increased tissue pressure. Measurement of this pressure is the most effective means of diagnosis, especially in patients where the signs and symptoms are not clear-cut, or in patients who are comatose, unresponsive, or who act in an inappropriate fashion. Examples of patients for whom one would consider initial compartmental pressure measuring:

1. The patient who is unresponsive, whether from drug overdose or head injury

2. The unreliable, uncooperative patient whose pain response is exaggerated, such as small children or drug- or alcohol-altered adults
3. The patient with peripheral nerve injury or previous deficit where signs of nerve ischemia are unreliable[66]

Needle-injection technique. Early attempts at measuring tissue fluid pressure were made in 1889. Fine needles were inserted into the tissues and hydrostatic pressure was measured as the pressure required to inject saline. Whitesides[92] modified this method. Its primary advantage is that it is low cost and requires no special equipment other than what is found in most hospitals, offices, and emergency rooms.

The Whitesides technique is a simple system that measures the pressure necessary to overcome tissue pressure enough to inject a minute quantity of saline into the closed compartment. The technique of Whitesides is as follows:

> An 18-gauge needle is connected to a 20-ml syringe by a saline end air column. The needle is then inserted into the compartment. A second extension tube is connected to the manometer and onto a three-way stopcock. The saline extension tube with the needle is also attached to the stopcock. The stopcock is arranged so that the system is open to air at all three ports. This produces a closed system in which air is free to flow into both extension tubes as the pressure within the system increases. Increase in pressure is achieved by slowly depressing the plunger while watching the column of saline. Air pressure is raised until the saline air meniscus just moves towards the patient. This pressure is then measured on the manometer.

The most common mistake made in using the Whitesides technique is depressing the plunger of the syringe too rapidly. This will cause more saline to be injected into the compartment and makes the manometer rise rapidly, thus making the reading less accurate (Fig. 32-5). The general range of accuracy is approximately ± 3 mm Hg. However, other investigators state that there is a variability in the technique by as much as 20 to 30 mm Hg. Most authors think that the saline injection overestimates the pressures.[78] This should be reserved for instances when other equipment is not available.

Styf[86] reported increased accuracy with injection techniques when using a catheter or needle in which multiple side holes were placed. This needle facilitates use if pressure is read during fluid injection. Accuracy was also increased if, following injection of air, the air saline meniscus stopped moving, but was still concave. At this point, the plunger is just slightly withdrawn and the pressure is read when the shape of the saline meniscus changed from concave to straight.

Matsen[54,55,88] modified the needle technique to allow continuous monitoring of pressure by a slow infusion of saline. It has advantages in that it allows long-term monitoring of compartmental pressure for up to 3 days. Continuous infusion prevents the catheter tip from coagulating or plugging. The primary disadvantage is the need for an expensive precision delivery pump system, which is not necessary with other methods, namely the wick or slit catheter method. Mubarak[64] stated that another disadvantage is that it has a slower response time compared to other techniques. This makes it difficult to measure accurate changes in pressure during muscle contraction that would be a measurement needed to evaluate chronic exertional compartment syndromes.

Catheter techniques. New implanted catheter methods have been developed for the diagnosis of compartment syndrome and are very similar in methodology. The difference lies in the catheter tip itself. Both the wick catheter and slit catheter allow for long-term equilibration measurements of intracompartmental pressure, continuous monitoring during contraction and exercise, and maintenance of catheter pa-

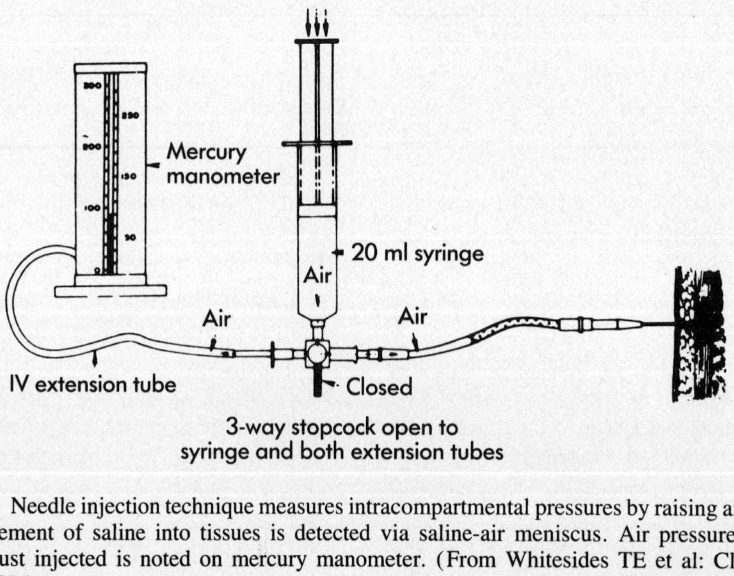

Fig. 32-5. Needle injection technique measures intracompartmental pressures by raising air pressure until movement of saline into tissues is detected via saline-air meniscus. Air pressure at which saline is just injected is noted on mercury manometer. (From Whitesides TE et al: Clin Orthop 113:43, 1975.)

tency without saline infusion.[58,62,75,78] Potential advantages of the slit catheter include more uniformity of production, which reduces the risk of leaving material behind once the catheter is removed. The slit catheter is less prone to coagulation problems as is the case with the Dexon wick catheter in which the fibers may hydrolyze and occlude the catheter orifice.[97] Dacron wick fibers are now being used and these appear to be better than the previous Dexon wick fibers[29] (Fig. 32-6).

More recently, a solid state transducer intracompartmental pressure monitor (STIC catheter) has become available, based on technology derived from the slit catheter apparatus as described by Rorabeck.[78] This is a hand-held pressure monitor with an interchangeable side port catheter attached to a syringe plunger mechanism. The technique imitates that of needle injection in which the side port catheter or needle is placed into the compartment in question. By depressing the plunger, 0.2 ml of fluid is injected and the digital readout pressure monitor is allowed to equilibrate. At the point where the digital readout stabilizes, the compartmental pressure is read. In another fashion, it can be used as a continuous pressure monitor by the use of a wick or slit catheter so that continuous pressure measurements can be made when evaluating exertional compartment syndromes or when evaluating continuous pressures in a postinjury or postsurgical situation. The advantage of this method is that the device

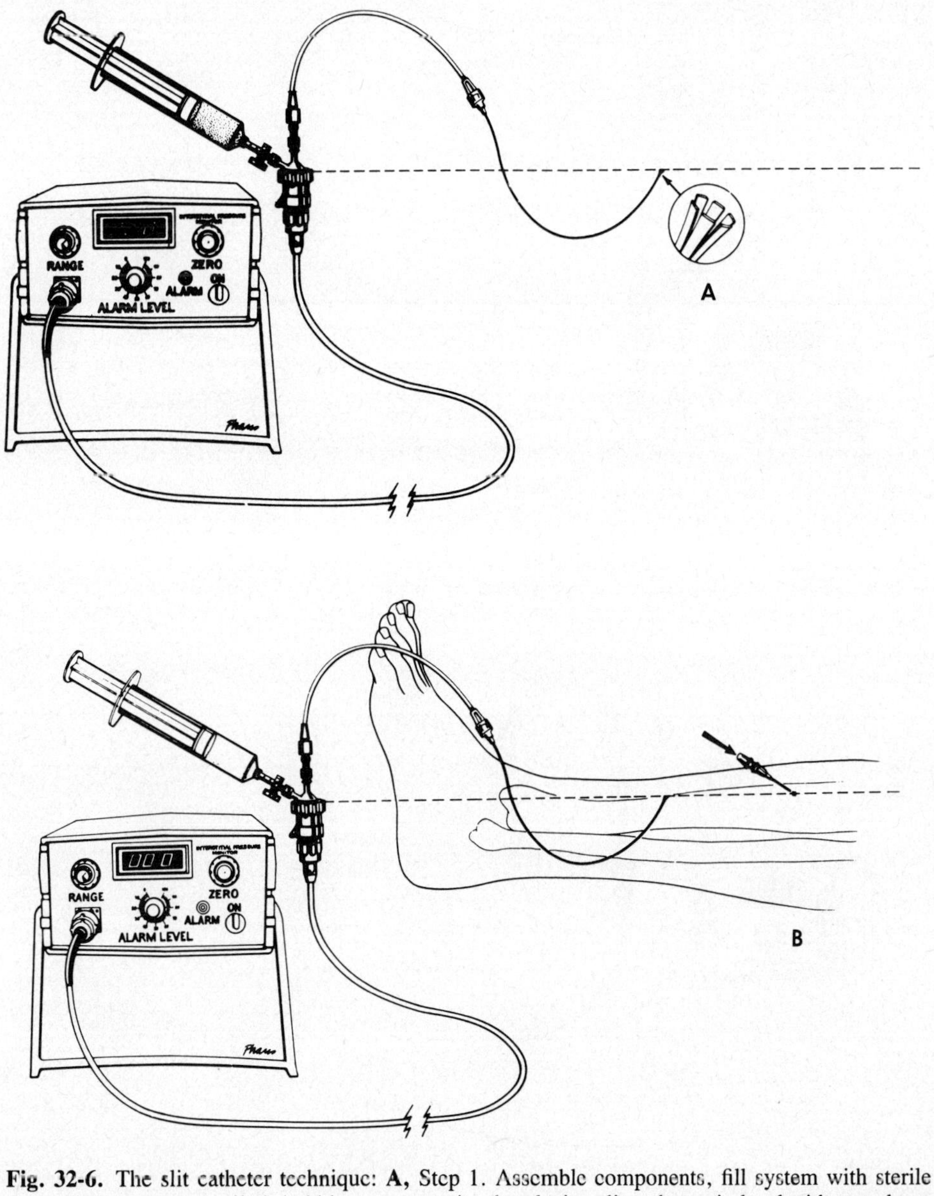

Fig. 32-6. The slit catheter technique: **A,** Step 1. Assemble components, fill system with sterile normal saline, remove all air bubbles, zero monitor by placing slit catheter tip level with transducer dome, adjust monitor "zero control" until "0.0" appears, and set alarm at desired setting. **B,** Step 2. Place transducer dome level with insertion site, prepare insertion site and insert 14-gauge catheter placement set at acute angle to long-limb axis; remove trochar. *Continued.*

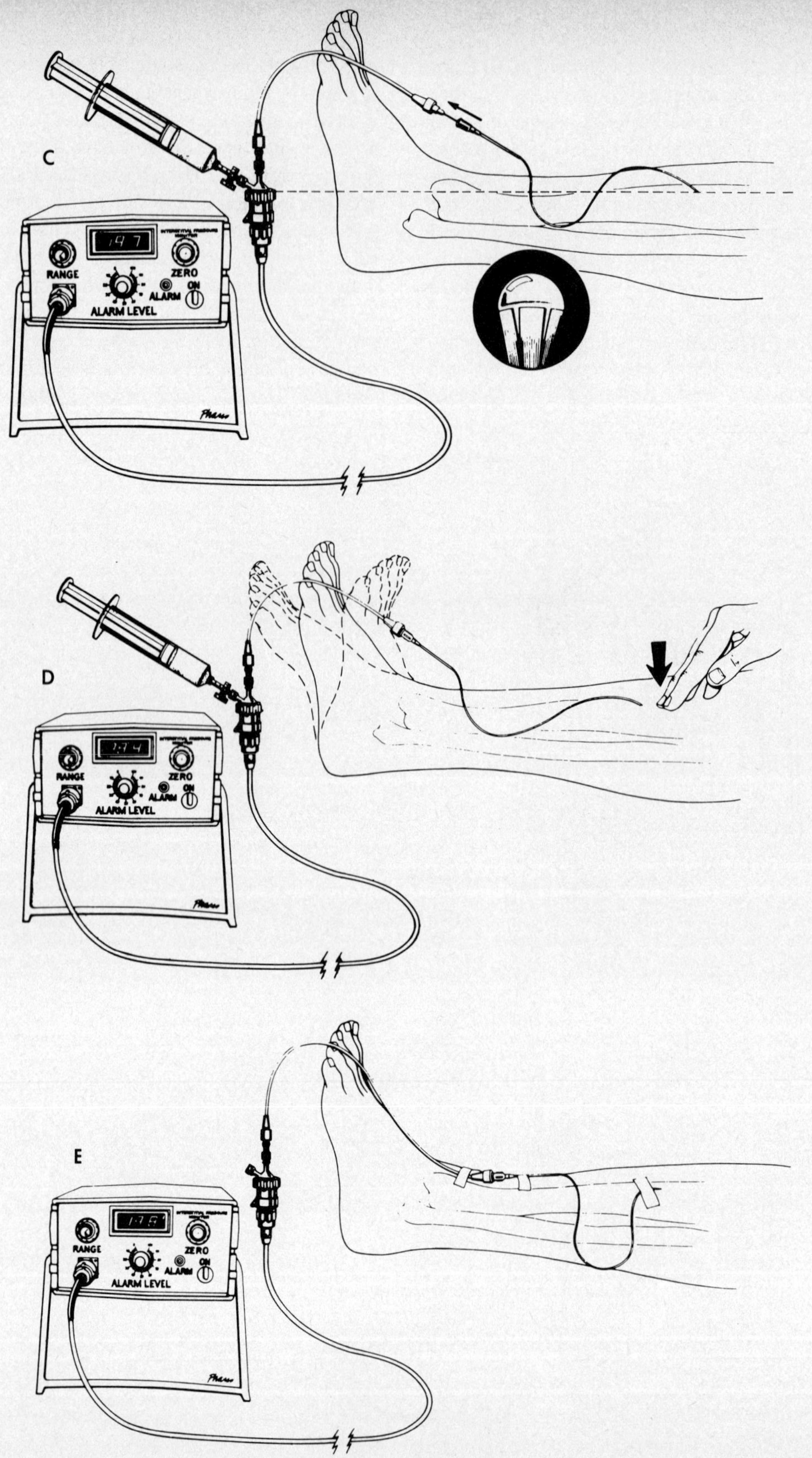

Fig. 32-6, cont'd. C, Step 3. Raise drop of saline at slit catheter tip and insert slit catheter through placement sleeve, carefully withdraw placement sleeve, and slide over slit catheter until hubs join. **D,** Step 4. Check system response by (1) plantar flexion of foot; (2) dorsiflexion of foot; and (3) digital pressure to compartment. Monitor pressure will show brisk rise in pressure readings. **E,** Step 5. Remove syringe, record intermittent or continuous pressure as required. (**A** to **E** from Mubarak SJ: Part II. A practical approach to compartment syndromes. AAOS instructional course lectures, Vol. 32, St. Louis, 1983, The CV Mosby Co.)

is totally self-contained, extremely portable, and very simple to use. Comparisons of this unit to the infusion method have shown that it is as reliable in determining compartment pressures.[40]

Difficulty in establishing a maximum tolerable compartment pressure is no doubt related to the large degree of individual variation in tolerance to elevated pressures. Other factors contributing to this dilemma are the presence of hypertension or hypotension, which may alter the compartmental pressure required to reduce blood flow, the presence of associated vasospasm and vasoconstriction, atherosclerotic disease, and arterial injury.

Progressive elevation of compartment pressure may be a more reliable sign of an evolving compartment syndrome than any absolute level of increased pressure. Serial determinations of compartment pressure, however, have the disadvantage of either requiring the presence of an indwelling catheter or multiple catheter insertions into an already potentially ischemic and compromised compartment.

Other tests

Acute compartment syndrome will raise the plasma CPK to levels of 1000 to 5000 IU. The use of this test is somewhat late since values of this magnitude indicate that massive muscle necrosis has already taken place. Other blood chemistries such as creatinine, serum potassium, SGOT, and LDH will all be elevated only if necrosis has taken place.

EMG and nerve conduction tests have been used to determine the level of nerve damage. Unfortunately, it is difficult to differentiate between a trauma-induced neuropraxia and damage from compartmental or "neural ischemia."[29] A distinct disadvantage of nerve conduction studies is that specialized equipment and personnel to perform and interpret the study are needed.

Early work has been done using Doppler venous flow (DVF) studies to evaluate evolving tibial compartment syndromes. As discussed earlier, the pathophysiology of evolving compartment syndrome emphasizes the importance of local venous hypertension, leading to a decrease in the arteriovenous pressure gradient sufficient to stop capillary flow.[2] As compartment pressure increases, the thin-walled venules collapse and thus further prevent venous flow. Loss of venous flow should occur before reduction of flow through capillary beds and subsequent tissue ischemia occurs. Loss of venous blood flow in an extremity at risk as determined by Doppler ultrasonography could be used as an early sign of an evolving compartment syndrome. In a review of 26 patients using this technique, Jones[40] showed that all patients with abnormal venous flow results had or developed neuromuscular deficits. Patients with normal DVF studies did not develop a compartment syndrome. This has a potential to become a reliable screening procedure for evolving compartment syndrome and can be done serially at the bedside in those patients whose clinical signs are equivocal. Because decreased venous flow by Doppler correlates with increasing risk of compartment syndrome, persistent decrease in DVF is an indication for direct compartmental pressure measurements and for further treatment and decompression, if indicated.

Ultrasound has also been used in conjunction with continuous compartment pressure measurements to evaluate patients who have symptoms of chronic exertional compartment syndrome. Preexercise sonography documents the anterior compartment width. Following exertion of the anterior compartment after exercise, the leg and anterior compartment are scanned again. Results have shown an average increased width of approximately 10% in active joggers with symptomatology of anterior exertional compartment syndrome.[19] This technique has advantages over CT scanning in that testing is immediate and prevents failure to detect exercise-induced volumetric changes, which may decay rapidly following exercise, before a CT scan can be obtained.[29] Diagnosis of exertional compartment syndrome of the leg is difficult to differentiate from shin splints, stress fractures, and tendinitis. When used in conjunction with compartment pressure monitoring, sonography helps differentiate between these entities and thus facilitates the decision-making process.

MANAGEMENT OF COMPARTMENT SYNDROME

As previously mentioned, the hallmark of management is having a high index of suspicion that a compartment syndrome is impending or is already established. The patients who are predisposed to this condition should be readily apparent to the physician. A thorough physical exam should document the presence or absence of peripheral pulses. If superficial pulses are absent, other causes of major arterial obstruction must be sought via Doppler instrumentation or arteriography. Conversely, the presence of distal pulses and capillary refill is no assurance that a compartment syndrome does not exist. Failure to appreciate this fact may lull one into a false sense of security and a failure to institute other diagnostic procedures and treatment. Initial management would include removing constricting splints, casts, or bandages. As noted previously, removing compression dressings or casts is an important method of reducing compartmental pressure and maintaining perfusion to the limb. The fracture reduction may be lost following removal of a cast, but limb viability takes preference.

The acute compartment syndrome is characterized by a decreased local AV pressure gradient with a resulting reduction in local tissue perfusion. The swelling in a traumatized or postoperative extremity is routinely reduced by elevating the extremity above the level of the heart to promote venous return. However, it has been shown that elevation of a limb will reduce the local AV pressure gradient significantly as compared with the AV pressure gradient at heart level. With the reduced AV pressure gradient, this increases the susceptibility of the limb to compartment syndrome by reducing the oxygen perfusion.[52,56]

The current body of evidence suggests that the decreased AV pressure gradient resulting from elevation may outweigh the beneficial effect of elevation, and that the limb should be maintained at heart level. The functional response of peripheral nerves in the upper and lower extremities has been shown to be tolerant of higher compartment pressures with the extremity kept at heart level compared with when it is elevated.[10,53] Also, this positioning promotes arterial inflow and maintains perfusion pressure within a compromised compartment.

Serial exams are of the utmost importance to monitor any progression of the neurocirculatory status. If a neurologic deficit persists without improvement for over an hour following removal of a cast and appropriate extremity positioning, then one must proceed to direct compartment pressure monitoring. If the injured compartmental pressure is greater than or equal to 30 mm Hg in a normotensive individual, then that patient now has an established compartment syndrome.

Following are indications for surgical decompression in a patient with an established compartment syndrome:[75]

1. Absolute indications
    a. Clinical signs of a compartment syndrome
    b. Elevated tissue pressure greater than 30 mm Hg in the normotensive individual
    c. Interrupted arterial circulation to an extremity for greater than 4 hours
2. Relative indications
    a. Circumferential full-thickness burns
    b. Exertional muscle overuse
    c. Limb compression syndrome

Surgical decompression

By definition, an anatomic compartment consists primarily of the muscles, arteries, veins, and nerves confined within a relatively closed osseofascial space. These boundaries may be strictly fascial or a combination of fascia and bone. The muscles in the compartment tend to act as a functional unit, whereas the nerves and arteries frequently traverse the compartment. By defining a compartment using these criteria, the human body can be divided into numerous compartments.[23] Thus any musculofascial area of the body can incur a compartment syndrome and require surgical release. Because most of the compartment syndromes occur in the forearm and the calf, the following exact surgical descriptions of technique will be concerned only with these two areas.

Forearm. Many techniques have been advocated over the years for fasciotomy of the forearm. Eaton and Green[15] were the first to describe a specific operative procedure with a longitudinal volar skin incision that crossed neither the wrist nor the elbow. The fascia is first released, followed by sectioning of the epimysium of all poorly vascularized muscle in a distal to proximal direction. Compromised muscles are decompressed, and the fascia and wounds are left open.

We recommend decompression of the volar flexor compartment performed through a standard approach of Henry.[30] It is important to realize that the volar surface contains a superficial flexor compartment as well as a deep flexor compartment and both must be decompressed. The deep compartment is most susceptible to muscle ischemia and contains the flexor pollicis longus, pronated quadratus, and the two radial profundi flexors (Fig. 32-7).

We routinely decompress the carpal canal as well as the lasertis fibrosis. An additional area for potential compression of the median nerve is the proximal edge of the pronater teres and the proximal edge of the flexor digitorum superficialis. The median nerve should be free in all areas following decompression.

Dorsal fasciotomy has been recommended in addition to the volar decompression.[18] Following volar fasciotomy, repeat pressures in the dorsal compartment should be checked. If the pressure remains greater than 30 mm Hg, fasciotomy should be carried out through a traditional dorsal Thompson approach. Skin edges are undermined and the dorsal fascia incised, being sure to decompress the mobile wad. Following decompression, pressures should be reevaluated. If obvious muscle necrosis is present, a superficial débridement should be performed. The wound is then packed open and the skin edges are placed under elastic loop tension to keep the skin margins from retracting significantly. The patient is subsequently returned to surgery in 2 to 3 days so a more substantial débridement of devitalized muscle and soft tissue can be carried out if necessary. It is possible to gradually perform a primary closure of the wound by retensioning the elastic bands over time. In this fashion, the skin edges are pulled closer and closer together until definitive approximation can be achieved (Fig. 32-8). With this approach, split-thickness skin grafts are required only occasionally. If skin grafts are to be used, further débridement may be necessary until a healthy bed of bleeding granulation tissue is present (Fig. 32-9).

Lower extremity procedures. One of the major advances in surgical technique for decompression of the lower extremity was the discovery by Seddon in 1966 that the deep posterior compartment was frequently involved and inadequately treated.[60] This further recognizes the fact that the calf consists of four compartments, and it is important to remember that rarely is only one compartment involved. Whitesides[43,92] stressed this fact of four anatomic compartments in the calf and suggested that a fibulectomy fasciotomy through a single lateral incision was an adequate means of decompressing these compartments. Pateman and Thompson[71] favored the fibulectomy approach for cases in which arterial disruption of the popliteal artery was present. The fibulectomy facilitated exposure and repair of the distal popliteal artery. They also advocated the double incision method for prophylaxis against impending compartment syndrome. Since Mubarak and Owen[65] in 1977 also recommended the double incision technique for decompression, this procedure has become fairly standard throughout most orthopedic literature (Fig. 32-10). This procedure is designed to gain access via two incisions to any or all of

A

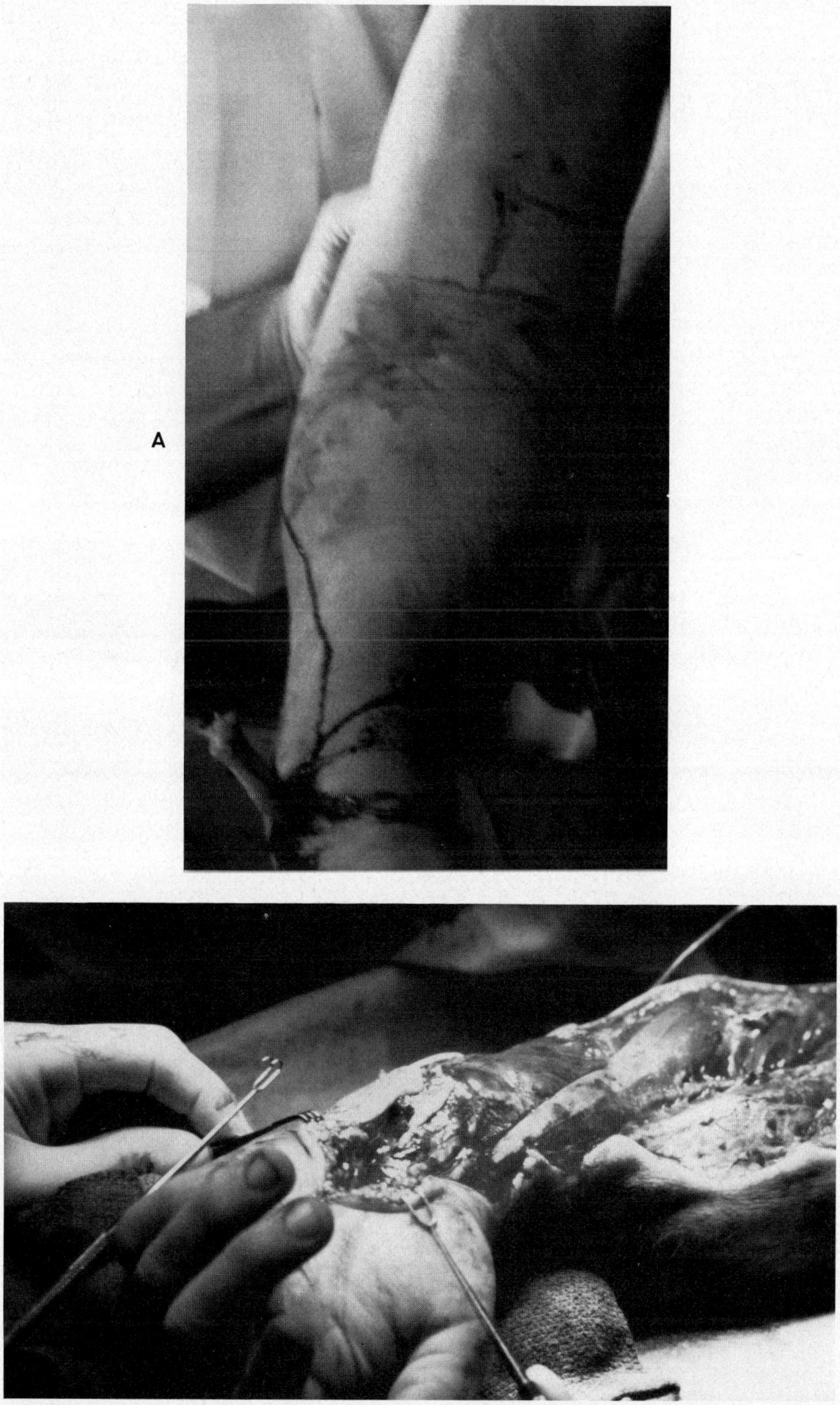

B

Fig. 32-7. A, Open forearm fracture showing grossly swollen forearm prior to fasciotomy. **B,** Volar Henry-type approach decompressing into the carpal canal as shown. Note the bulging of the muscles and severe retraction of the skin edges.

A

B

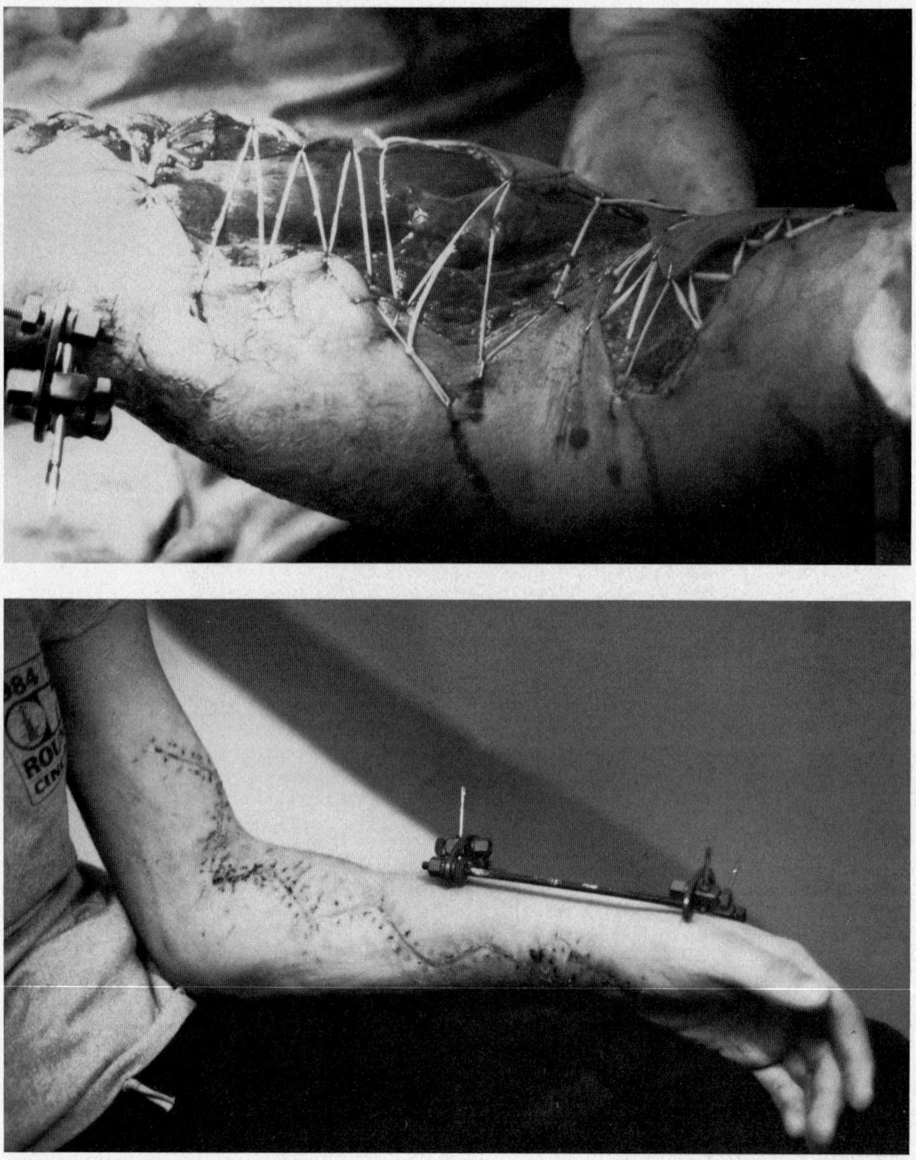

Fig. 32-8. A, To prevent severe skin retraction following fasciotomy, elastic vessel loops are stapled to the skin edges. Daily the vessel loops are tightened so as to approximate the skin edges as the swelling in the compartment subsides. **B,** Delayed primary closure was achieved without skin grafting 5 days after initial fasciotomy.

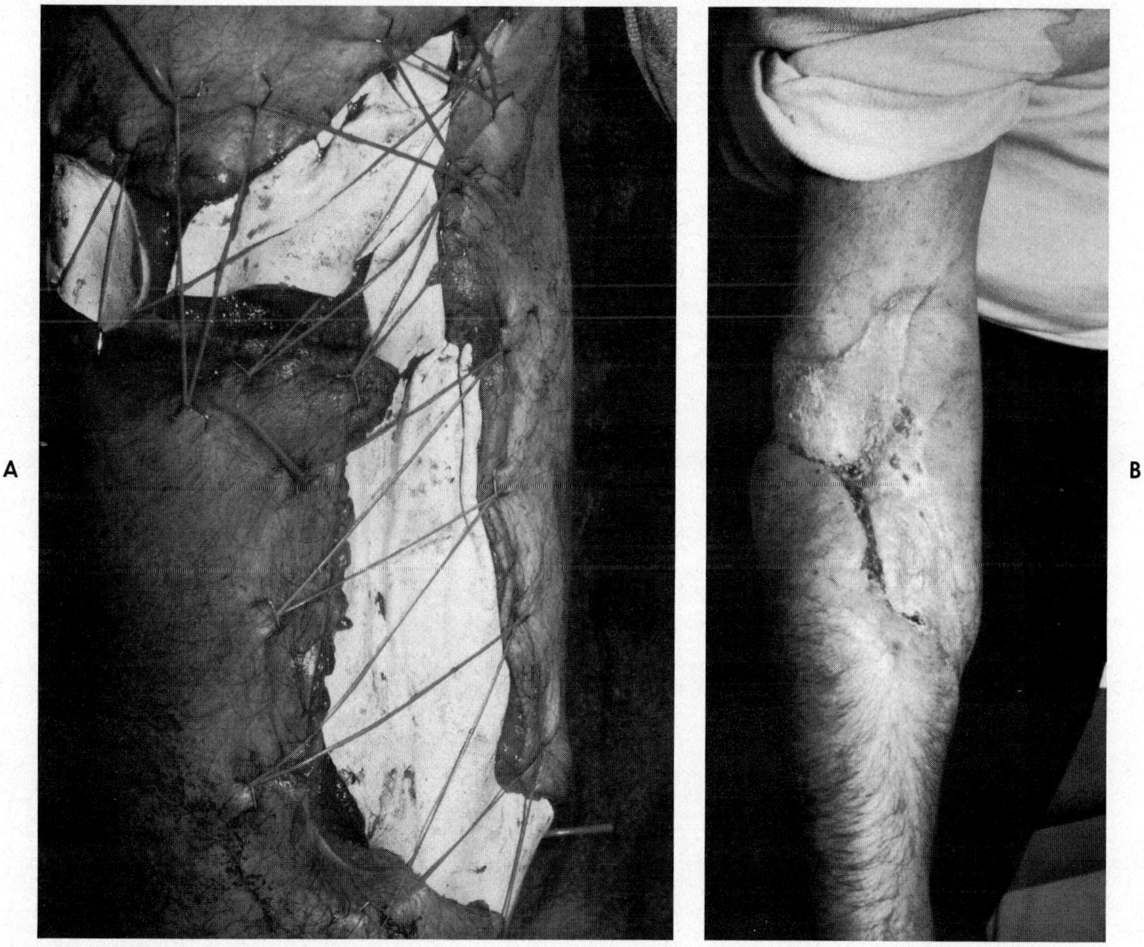

Fig. 32-9. **A,** Forearm compartment release was performed and the skin edges were apposed with vessel loops and skin staples. The wound could not be closed primarily by gradual opposition of the skin edges. **B,** Following partial apposition of the fasciotomy through the vessel loops, a skin graft was needed to achieve wound closure.

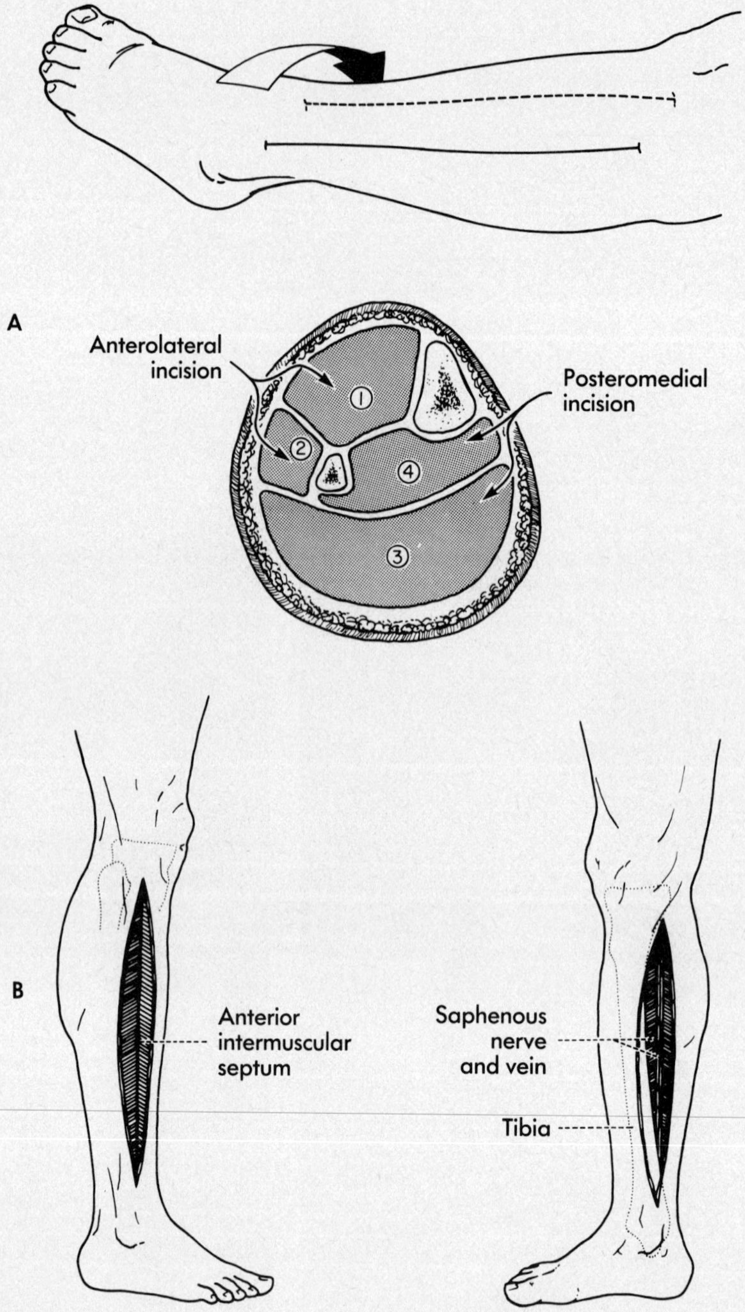

Fig. 32-10. A, Double-incision technique for performing fasciotomies of all four compartments of lower extremities. Cross-section of lower extremity showing position of anterolateral and posteromedial incisions that allow access to anterior and peroneal compartments 1 and 2 and superficial and deep posterior compartments 3 and 4, respectively. **B,** Vertical anterior incision is centered midway between tibia and fibula. Interval between anterior and lateral compartments (anterior intramuscular septum) is identified, and two fasciotomy incisions are made, one anterior and one posterior. Vertical posteromedial incision is centered 2 cm behind back of tibia. Care must be taken to avoid cutting saphenous vein and nerve. (From Rorabeck CH: Management: a practical approach to compartment syndromes. AAOS instructional course lectures, Vol. 23, St. Louis, 1983, The CV Mosby Co.)

the four compartments of the leg when these are involved with acute or chronic compartment syndromes.

The double-incision technique uses two vertical skin incisions. The first incision, along the anterolateral border of the fibula, allows access to the anterior and lateral compartments, and a second incision along the posteriomedial border of the tibia allows access to both the superficial and deep posterior compartments. The lateral incision is opened and the interval between the anterior and lateral compartments, the anterior intermuscular septum, is identified. Care should be taken to identify the superficial peroneal nerve, which lies in this interval. The fascia on either side of the septum should be incised to decompress both compartments. The vertical posteromedial incision should run the length of the compartment, and care should be taken to avoid injuring the saphenous vein and nerve. The fascia overlying the gastrocsoleus complex is divided and the muscle retracted. Deep to the gastrocsoleus lies the flexor digitorum longus and the fascia overlying it is now incised, thus completing the fasciotomy of the deep posterior compartment. There are many major advantages of the double incision technique over the fibulectomy fasciotomy technique.[75] It is simpler and requires minimal dissection. The procedure can be performed using local anesthesia if necessary. It is faster and relatively safer. The double incision method involves less risk primarily because the fascial incisions are all superficial and avoid deep neurovascular structures (Fig. 32-11). The fibula is left intact because fibulectomy in a child or adult can lead to disastrous results. This is especially true in tibia fractures where the fibula may be the only intact strut and loss of the fibula may result in serious limb reconstruction problems. Postoperatively, the wounds are managed as are the forearm fasciotomies, with sequential débridement and gradual closure.

When dealing with chronic exertional compartment syndrome, a much smaller approach to decompression can be taken. When treating a chronic anterior compartment syndrome, the length of the skin incision may be considerably shorter than for an acute syndrome.[75,77] For either anterior or lateral compartment involvement, both compartments are decompressed. The skin incision is in the midportion of the leg, halfway between the fibula and the anterior portion of the tibial crest. Muscle hernias are frequently noted in the lower third of the leg in an area overlying the anterior intermuscular septum. This is the site of emergence through the fascia of one or both sensory branches of the superficial peroneal nerve. If such a muscle hernia is present, the skin incision should be located over the hernia so that one can explore the fascial defect and easily identify the superficial peroneal nerve. Once decompression has been achieved through the use of Metzenbaum scissors pushed subcutaneously to incise the fascia, the fascial sheet is not closed since this may precipitate an acute compartment syndrome. The skin is closed in a routine fashion, and within a short time, the patient is allowed to return to full activities.

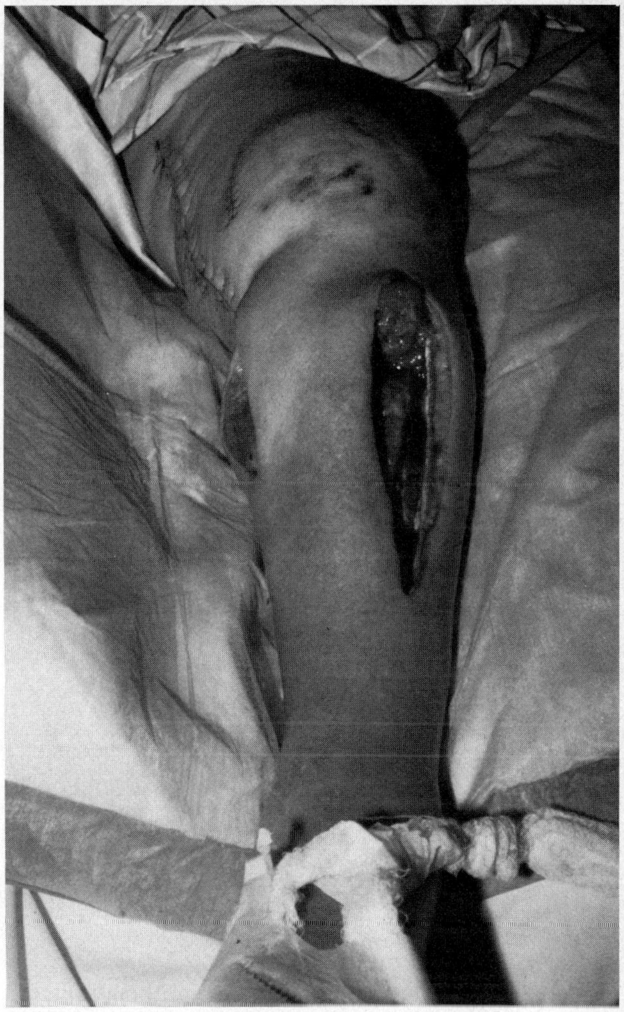

Fig. 32-11. Double-incision fasciotomy of lower extremity compartment syndrome. Both incisions were left open and skin grafting applied later. For chronic exertional compartment syndrome, the same incisions can be used opening the skin 1 to 2 cm in either direction and performing subcutaneous fasciotomies with a Metzenbaum scissor.

SUMMARY

Compartment syndrome is a condition in which high pressure, within a closed fascial space, reduces capillary blood perfusion below a level necessary for tissue viability. The local tissue ischemia produced results in further edema, thus perpetuating the edema/ischemia cycle. Intracompartmental pressure is raised through any one of a number of causes that in general terms include interstitial edema, hemorrhage, or muscle fiber swelling within the compartment. Intracompartmental edema is produced by increased capillary permeability following burn injuries, arterial drug injection, vascular reconstruction surgery, prolonged limb compression, venous obstruction, crush injuries, and perhaps venomous snake bites.[59] Muscle fiber swelling often follows long periods of ischemia with subsequent abnormal intracellular ion accumulation and water uptake. Intracompartmental pressure is also elevated by compartment volume constriction. Hemorrhage within the closed compartment space after major vessel laceration, hereditary hemorrhagic diathesis, fractures, or contusions may also produce a compartment syndrome. Finally, exercise combined with fascial inelasticity or muscle hypertrophy may cause a chronic exertional compartment syndrome.

Paramount in the diagnosis and treatment of compartment syndrome is the fact that a high index of suspicion should be maintained in the suspect patient. Clinical signs and symptoms are varied and unreliable for diagnosis of a definitive compartment syndrome. The best diagnostic study is, therefore, direct compartment pressure measuring either by needle-injection technique and wick or slit catheter measurements. For pressures greater than 30 mm Hg in a normotensive patient, immediate decompressive fasciotomy should be undertaken.[60] Ideally, with prompt diagnosis and early and effective treatment, normal function of the limb is maintained in a potentially disastrous disease process.

REFERENCES

1. Aprahamian C et al: MAST-associated compartment syndrome (MACS): a review, J Trauma 29(5):549, 1989.
2. Ashton H: The effect of increased tissue pressure on blood flow, Clin Orthop 113:15, 1975.
3. Bass RR et al: Thigh compartment syndrome without extremity trauma following application of pneumatic anti-shock trousers, Ann Emerg Med 12:382, 1983.
4. Bonutti PM and Bell GR: Compartment syndrome of the foot, J Bone Joint Surg, 68A:1449, 1986.
5. Brotman S, Browner BD, and Cox EF: MAST trousers improperly applied causing a compartment syndrome in lower extremity trauma, J Trauma 22(7):598, 1982.
6. Brower TD and Wilde AH: Femoral neuropathy in hemophilia, J Bone Joint Surg 48A:487, 1966.
7. Browne SG: The anterior tibial compartment syndrome: differential diagnosis in a Nigerian leprosarium, Br J Surg 49:429, 1962.
8. Brumback RJ: Compartment syndrome complicating avulsion of the origin of the triceps muscle: a case report, J Bone Joint Surg 69A:1445, 1987.
9. Bywaters EGL and Beall D: Crush injuries with impairment of renal function, Br Med J 1:427, 1941.
10. Chidgey LK, Szabo RM, and Kolack B: Effects of elevation on nerve function in an acute upper extremity nerve compression model, J Orthop Res 7(6):783, 1989.
11. Christensen KS: Pneumatic antishock garments (PASG): Do they precipitate lower extremity compartment syndromes? J Trauma 26:1102, 1986.
12. Courtice FC, Adams EP, and Dempsey J: The effect of ischemia on acid phosphatase β glucuronidase and lactic acid dehydrogenase in lymph from hind paw of the rabbit, Lymphology 5:67, 1972.
13. DeLee JC and Stiehl JB: Open tibia fractures with compartment syndrome, Clin Orthop 160:175, 1981.
14. Dugdale TW et al: Compartmental syndrome complicating use of the hemi-lithotomy position during femoral nailing, J Bone Joint Surg 71A:1556, 1989.
15. Eaton RG and Green WT: Epimysiotomy and fasciotomy in treatment of Volkmann's ischemia contracture, Orthop Clin North Am 3:175, 1972.
16. Eaton RG and Green WT: Volkmann's ischemia: a volar compartment syndrome of the forearm, Clin Orthop 113:58, 1975.
17. Garfin SR, Mubarak SJ, and Evans KL: Quantification of intracompartmental pressure and volume under plaster casts, J Bone Joint Surg 63A(3):449, 1981.
18. Gelbarman RH, Zakaib GS, and Mubarak SJ: Decompression of forearm compartment syndromes, Clin Orthop 134:225, 1978.
19. Gershuni DH et al: Ultrasound evaluation of the anterior musculofascial compartment of the leg following exercise, Clin Orthop 167:185, 1982.
20. Godbout B et al: Crush syndrome with death following pneumatic antishock garment application, J Trauma 24(12):1052, 1984.
21. Green TL et al: Compartment syndrome of the arm: a complication of the pneumatic tourniquet—a case report, J Bone Joint Surg 65(2):270, 1983.
22. Griffith D: Volkmann's ischemic contracture, Br J Surg 28:239, 1940.
23. Haggmark T, Jansson E, and Svane B: Cross-sectional area of the thigh muscle in man measured by computerized tomography, Scand J Clin Lab Invest 38:355, 1978.
24. Hargens AR et al: Fluid balance within the canine anterolateral compartment and its relationship to compartment syndromes, J Bone Joint Surg 60A:499, 1978.
25. Hargens AR et al: Tissue fluid pressures: from basic research tools to clinical applications, J Orthop Res 7(6):902, 1989.
26. Hargens AR and Akeson WH: Pathophysiology of the compartment syndrome. In Mubarak SJ and Hargens AR, eds: Compartment syndrome and Volkmann's contracture, Philadelphia, 1981, WB Saunders Co.
27. Hargens AR et al: Peripheral nerve conduction block by high muscle compartment pressure, J Bone Joint Surg 61:192, 1979.
28. Hargens AR et al: Quantitation of skeletal muscle necrosis in a model compartment syndrome, J Bone Joint Surg 63(4):631, 1981.
29. Hargens AR and Mubarak SJ: Laboratory diagnosis of acute compartment syndrome. In Mubarak SJ and Hargens AR, eds: Compartment syndrome and Volkmann's contracture, Philadelphia, 1981, WB Saunders Co.
30. Henry A: Extensile exposure, ed 2, Edinburgh, 1973, Churchill Livingstone, Inc.
31. Henstorf JE and Olson S: Compartment syndrome: pathophysiology, diagnosis and treatment, Surg Rounds for Orthop 1(2):33, 1987.
32. Heppenstal RB et al: Compartment syndrome: a quantitative study of high energy phosphorous compounds using p^{31} magnetic resonance spectroscopy, J Trauma 29(8):1113, 1989.
33. Heppenstal RB, Scott R, and Sapega A: A comparative study of the tolerance of skeletal muscle to ischemia, J Bone Joint Surg 63A:820, 1986.
34. Hieb LD and Alexander AH: Bilateral anterior and lateral compartment syndromes in a patient with sickle cell trait, Clin Orthop 228:190, 1988.
35. Holden CEA: Compartmental syndrome following trauma, Clin Orthop 228:190, 1988.
36. Howse AJG and Seddon H: Ischaemic contracture of muscle associated with carbon monoxide and barbiturate poisoning, Br Med J 1:192, 1966.
37. Hughes JR: Ischemic necrosis of the anterior tibial muscles due to fatigue, J Bone Joint Surg 30B:581, 1948.
38. Jepsen PN: Ischemic contracture: experimental (6) study, Ann Surg 84:785, 1926.
39. Jepsen PN: The classic ischemic contracture experimental study, Clin Orthop 113:3, 1975.
40. Jones WG, Perry MD, and Bush HL: Changes in tibial venous blood flow in the evolving compartment syndrome, Arch Surg 124:801, 1989.
41. Keim HA and Weinstein JD: Acute renal failure: a complication of spine fusion in the tuck position, J Bone Joint Surg 52A:1248, 1970.

42. Khalil IM: Bilateral compartmental syndrome after prolonged surgery in the lithotomy position, J Vasc Surg 5:879, 1987.
43. Kelly RP and Whitesides TE Jr: Transfibular route for fasciotomy of the leg, J Bone Joint Surg 49:1022, 1967.
44. Lancourt JE, Gilbert MS, and Posner MA: Management of bleeding and associated complications of hemophilia in the hand and forearm, J Bone Joint Surg 59A:451, 1977.
45. Lazarus HM and Hutto W: Electric burns and frostbite: patterns of vascular injury, J Trauma 22(7):581, 1982.
46. Madigan RR, Hanna WT, and Wallace SL: Acute compartment syndrome in hemophilia, J Bone Joint Surg 63(8):1327, 1981.
47. Maletis GF, Watson RC, and Scott S: Compartment syndrome: a complication of intravenous regional anesthesia in the reduction of lower leg shaft fractures, Orthopedics 12(6):841, 1989.
48. Mannarino F and Sexson S: The significance of interoperational pressures in the diagnosis of chronic exertional compartmental syndrome. Orthopedics 12(11):1415, 1989.
49. Matsen FA III: Compartmental syndrome: a unified concept, Clin Orthop 113:8, 1975.
50. Matsen FA III: Compartmental syndrome, New York, 1980, Grune & Stratton, Inc.
51. Matsen FA III: Practical approach to compartment syndromes. Part I. In AAOS instructional course lectures, St. Louis, 1983, The CV Mosby Co.
52. Matsen FA III, Krugmire RB Jr, and King RV: Increased tissue pressure and its effects on muscle oxygenation in level and elevated human limbs, Clin Orthop 144:311, 1979.
53. Matsen FA III et al: A model compartmental syndrome in man with particular reference to quantification of nerve function, J Bone Joint Surg 59:648, 1977.
54. Matsen FA III et al: Monitoring of intramuscular pressure, Surgery 79:702, 1976.
55. Matsen FA III, Wyss CR, and King RV: The continuous infusion technique in the assessment of clinical compartment syndromes. In Hargens AR, ed. Tissue fluid pressure and composition, Baltimore, 1981, Williams & Wilkins.
56. Matsen FA II et al: The effects of limb elevation and dependency on local arteriovenous gradients in normal human limbs with particular reference to limbs with increased tissue pressure, Clin Orthop 150:187, 1980.
57. McLaren AC and Rorabeck CH: The pressure distribution under tourniquets, J Bone Joint Surg 67(3):433, 1985.
58. Mubarak SJ: A practical approach to compartmental syndromes. Part II. In AAOS instructional course lectures, St. Louis, 1983, The CV Mosby Co.
59. Mubarak SJ: Etiologies of compartment syndrome. In Mubarak SJ and Hargens AR, eds: Compartment syndromes and Volkmann's contracture, Philadelphia, 1981, WB Saunders Co.
60. Mubarak SJ: Principles of treating compartment syndromes. In Mubarak SJ and Hargens AR, eds: Compartment syndromes and Volkmann's contracture, Philadelphia, 1981, WB Saunders Co.
61. Mubarak SJ and Hargens AR: Compartment syndromes and Volkmann's contractures, Philadelphia, 1981, WB Saunders Co.
62. Mubarak SJ et al: Muscle pressure measurement with the wick catheter. In Goldsmith HS, ed: Practice of surgery, New York, 1978, Harper & Row Publishers, Inc.
63. Mubarak SJ et al: The wick catheter technique for measurement of intramuscular pressure: a new research and clinical tool, J Bone Joint Surg 58-1:1016-1020, 1976.
64. Mubarak SJ and Owen CA: Compartment syndrome and its relation to the crush syndrome: a spectrum of the disease, Clin Orthop 113:81, 1975.
65. Mubarak SJ and Owen CA: Double-incision fasciotomy of the leg for decompression in compartment syndrome, J Bone Joint Surg 59:184, 1977.
66. Mubarak SJ et al: Acute compartment syndromes: diagnosis and treatment with the aid of the wick catheter, J Bone Joint Surg 60A:1091, 1978.
67. Murphy JB: Myositis, JAMA 63:1249, 1914.
68. Owen CA: Clinical diagnosis of acute compartment syndromes. In Mubarak SJ and Hargens AR, eds: Compartment syndromes and Volkmann's contracture, Philadelphia, 1981, WB Saunders Co.
69. Owen CA: The crush syndrome. In Mubarak SJ and Hargens AR, eds: Compartment syndromes and Volkmann's contracture, Philadelphia, 1981, WB Saunders Co.
70. Patman RD: Compartmental syndromes in peripheral vascular surgery, Clin Orthop 113:103, 1975.
71. Patman RD and Thompsen JE: Fasciotomy in peripheral vascular surgery, Arch Surg 101:663, 1970.
72. Patterson TSS: Congenital ring constrictions, Br J Plast Surg 14:1, 1961.
73. Pearson C, Adams RS, and Denny-Brown D: Traumatic necrosis of pretibial muscles, N Engl J Med 239:213, 1948.
74. Petrik ME et al: Posttraumatic gluteal compartment syndrome: a case report, Clin Orthop 231:127, 1988.
75. Rorabeck CH: Practical approach to compartment syndromes. Part III. In AAOS instructional course lectures, St. Louis, 1983, The CV Mosby Co.
76. Rorabeck CH: The pathophysiology of the anterior tibial compartment syndrome, Clin Orthop 113:52, 1975.
77. Rorabeck CH, Bourne RB, and Fowler PJ: The surgical treatment of exertional compartment syndrome in athletes, J Bone Joint Surg 67A:1245, 1983.
78. Rorabeck CH et al: Compartmental pressure measurements: an experimental investigation using the slit catheter, J Trauma 21:446, 1981.
79. Sanderson RA et al: Histologic response on skeletal muscle to ischemia, Clin Orthop 113:27, 1975.
80. Schreiber SN et al: Limb compression and renal impairment complicating narcotic overdose, J Bone Joint Surg 54A:1683, 1972.
81. Sheridan DW and Matsen FA III: An animal model of the compartmental syndrome, Clin Orthop 113:36, 1975.
82. Shires GJ et al: Alterations in cellular membrane function during hemorrhagic shock in primates, Am Surg 176:288, 1972.
83. Silbart S and Oppenheim W: Purpura fulminans: medical, surgical and rehabilitation considerations, Clin Orthop 193:206, 1985.
84. Smith B et al: Volkmann's contracture of the extraocular muscles following blowout fracture, Plast Reconstr Surg 74(2):200, 1984.
85. Stehalin A: Personal communication, March 1987.
86. Styf J: Evaluation of injection techniques in recording of intramuscular pressure, J Orthop Res 7(6):812, 1989.
87. Styf JR and Korner LM: Chronic anterior compartment syndrome of the leg, J Bone Joint Surg 68A:1338, 1986.
88. Teeny SM and Wiss DA: Compartment syndrome: a complication of the use of the MAST suit, J Orthop Trauma 1(3):236, 1987.
89. Viegas SF: Acute compartment syndrome in the thigh: a case report and review of the literature, Clin Orthop Sep(234):232, 1988.
90. Volkmann R: Die ischaemischen muskellatmungen und kontrakturen, Central f Chir, 1881, pp. 51-108 (Bick EM, trans): Clin Orthop 50:5, 1967.
91. Wallenstein RW: Results of fasciotomy in patients with medial tibial syndrome or chronic anterior compartment syndrome, J Bone Joint Surg 65A:1252, 1983.
92. Whitesides TE et al: Tissue pressure measurements as a determinant for the need of fasciotomy, Clin Orthop 113:43, 1975.
93. Whitesides TE Jr, Harada H, and Morimoto K: The response of skeletal muscle to temporary ischemia: an experimental study—Proc Am Acad Ortho Surg, J Bone Joint Surg 53A.1027, 1971.
94. Williams TM, Knopp R, and Ellyson JH: Compartment syndrome after anti-shock trouser use without lower extremity trauma, J Trauma 22(7):595, 1982.

95. Wright JG, Bogoch ER, and Hastings DE: The "occult" compartment syndrome, J Trauma 29(11):133, 1989.
96. Zatina MD et al: p^{31} nuclear magnetic resonance spectroscopy: noninvasive biochemical analysis of the ischemic extremity, J Vasc Surg 3:441, 1986.
97. Zeluff GR: Absorbable versus nonabsorbable wick material in compartment pressure monitoring, Orthop Trans 3:9, 1979.
98. Zimmerman T and Mummert K: Sickle crisis precipitated by exercise rhabdomyolysis in a patient with sickle cell trait: case report, Milit Med 139:313, 1974.
99. Zych GA and Ballard A: Congenital band causing pseudoarthrosis and impending gangrene of the leg, J Bone Joint Surg 65(3):410, 1983.

Chapter 33

VASCULAR DISEASES RELATED TO EXTREMES IN ENVIRONMENTAL TEMPERATURE

Jeffrey W. Olin
Walid Arrabi

The vast majority of cold injuries in the past have been encountered in the military population. However, with the spread of winter sports (e.g., skiing, hiking, and mountain climbing), prevalence of alcoholism, and the increasing age of the U.S. population, cold-induced injuries are more commonly encountered among the civilian population. In addition, there are various abnormal sensitivities to heat that may occur. A useful classification for vascular diseases related to extremes in environmental temperature is as follows:

1. Freezing injuries (frostbite)
2. Nonfreezing injuries (acute and chronic pernio, immersion foot, and trench foot)
3. Erythromelalgia
4. Nonspecific sensitivities to cold and heat
5. Generalized hyperthermia

This chapter will focus on the first four categories since their pathogenesis is related to alterations in peripheral circulation. Raynaud's phenomenon and disease, which are vasospastic disorders usually precipitated by cold, have been discussed in detail in Chapter 21.

Some patients are bothered by a persistent coldness in the extremities, which they attribute to circulatory problems. Often the circulation is normal and this cold sensation is caused by neural factors, vasoconstriction, or what is often called *vasomotor instability*. This is a "grab bag" term that illustrates the scientific community's lack of understanding as to why some people have cold, erythematous, or cyanotic extremities.

FROSTBITE

Frostbite is defined as a state of actual freezing of tissues resulting from exposure to cold. Frostbite is usually caused by below freezing temperatures but may occur at above freezing temperature under certain circumstances (wetness, strong wind, or high altitude).[1] While frostbite implies injury of varying degrees to superficial and deep tissues, frostnip is an injury to superficial tissues and is completely reversed with rewarming (i.e., placing hand in axilla). It has been shown experimentally that slow freezing begins in mammalian tissues when the temperature in the deeper parts reaches 10° C, and cells rarely survive when the temperature is less than 5° C.[2,3] Freezing may involve the skin, subcutaneous fat, musculoskeletal components, blood vessels, and nerves. The damage done to these tissues is directly related to the depth of the temperature and the length of exposure. The two most important environmental factors that modify the effects of frostbite are wind velocity and humidity. Wind accelerates heat loss from the victim by convection and by increasing the evaporation of sweat. The effect of wind velocity is expressed as the wind chill factor.[4,5] Moisture, as a good heat conductor, also accelerates heat loss from the skin. Wet skin cools faster than dry skin and freezes at a higher ambient temperature.[5] A number of environmental, social, and host factors have been shown to predispose tissue to cold injury either by enhancing heat loss or by decreasing body heat production. These factors include tobacco, alcohol, inappropriate clothing, underlying vascular disease, previous cold injury, fatigue, anxiety,[6] high altitude, and race (blacks may be more susceptible to cold injury than whites).[7,8]

A person's response to cold is aimed at conserving the core (internal body) temperature and the extremity viability. Assuming intact thermoregulatory mechanisms, the body reacts to cold exposure by reducing heat loss and/or augmenting heat production. Heat loss is reduced by peripheral vasoconstriction caused by sympathetic stimulation and catecholamine release. At the same time maintenance or augmentation of body heat production is accomplished by muscular activities such as shivering.[9] However, the heat production from shivering cannot be sustained for more than a few hours because of glycogen depletion, which is the source of heat energy during the shivering process. The extremities are protected by the "hunting reaction," which consists of alternating periods of vasoconstriction and vasodilation.[10,11] These cycles are irregular and last for 5 to 10 minutes. During vasodilation there is rewarming of the extremities. This recurrent rewarming is known as "cold-induced dilation" or "temperature hunting response." This serves to protect the extremities against excessive sustained vasoconstriction at minimal loss of internal body temperature.[1] However, when the body is exposed to cold of such magnitude or duration so as to threaten the internal body temperature, this mechanism fails. Since the disruption of core temperature is much more deleterious to the body than peripheral vasoconstriction, conservation of core temperatures takes precedence over rewarming of the extremities, and the hunting response is replaced by continuous and more intense vasoconstriction, thus placing the extremities at a higher risk for developing frostbite.

Pathogenesis

The exact mechanism by which freezing cold causes tissue injury is not known. Cold may directly freeze the tissues, resulting in the formation of ice crystals.[12] Ice crystals may form both intracellularly and extracellularly if freezing is rapid. The formation of intracellular crystals, as seen in rapid freezing, will disrupt cellular structures in an irreversible manner. However, in most clinical situations, freezing occurs slowly and ice crystals are formed extracellularly and, as such, cause only moderate cellular derangement.[13,14] Cellular dehydration and tissue destruction occur by a shift of water from intracellular to extracellular compartments.[15,16]

Another mechanism of tissue necrosis is related to reactive vascular changes.[1,17-19] After exposure to cold local and reflex arterial and venous constriction ensue, with resultant reduced perfusion to the affected area. Cold directly increases blood viscosity and thus causes sludging.

One of the earliest pathologic changes is endothelial cell damage with increased capillary membrane permeability (thus explaining edema formation in early frostbite). In the early thawing period vessels in the affected tissue dilate, and circulation is restored. Platelets start to aggregate and may occlude the vessels.[18] The stimulus for platelet aggregation may be prior endothelial injury. Platelet aggregation is followed by red cell aggregation, which occurs first in the venules and then in the capillaries and arterioles of the injured tissue. Because of the increased capillary permeability from endothelial injury, fluid and plasma proteins leak into the interstitial space. This resulting increase in intravascular viscosity leads to stasis and promotes further sludging. Simultaneously, rising levels of fibrinogen and lipid levels augment red cell aggregation. The net result is stasis with occlusion of the microvasculature by thrombi.

Tissues manifest variable susceptibility to frostbite. Skin, muscles, blood vessels, and nerves are highly sensitive. Connective tissue, tendons, and bones exhibit more resistance.[20]

Recent studies implicate the release of prostaglandins and thromboxane (both metabolites of arachadonic acid) in the pathogenesis of frostbite.[21] The vasoconstrictor prostaglandins (prostaglandin F_2 [PGF_2] and thromboxane B_2 [TXB_2]) have been found to be present in high levels in frostbite blister fluid. Raine et al,[22] using an experimental frostbite model, showed that antiprostaglandin agents and thromboxane inhibitors significantly improve survival of injured tissues. Further studies are needed to confirm the role of these substances in the pathogenesis and treatment of frostbite in humans.

Clinical features

Shortly after exposure to cold the patient senses pain in the affected part, which gradually progresses to numbness. Soon all sensation is lost. The frozen part looks white because of intense vasospasm. With thawing, circulation is restored to the affected parts, which then become hyperemic. Edema can develop within the first hour of thawing and may remain for days or weeks. Blisters appear within the first 24 hours and are resorbed within 1 or 2 weeks with little or no tissue loss. With mild frostbite blisters are usually large, filled with clear fluid, and extend to the tips of the digits[23] (Fig. 33-1, *A*). In severe frostbite, blisters are small, dark colored (hemorrhagic), and do not involve the tips.[9,23] The blisters may look similar to those seen in patients who have reperfusion bullae. After resorption blisters are replaced by black eschar, which can give the false impression of a deep gangrene. However, after several weeks the eschar often sloughs, and the tissues heal. An initially fragile skin covering eventually develops into a normal healthy skin. In severe and deep frostbite demarcation between viable and mummified dead tissue takes place. Amputation can be spontaneous or surgical (Fig. 33-1, *B*).

A few days after thawing a throbbing pain caused by inflammation develops and may last for weeks.[9] A persistent

A

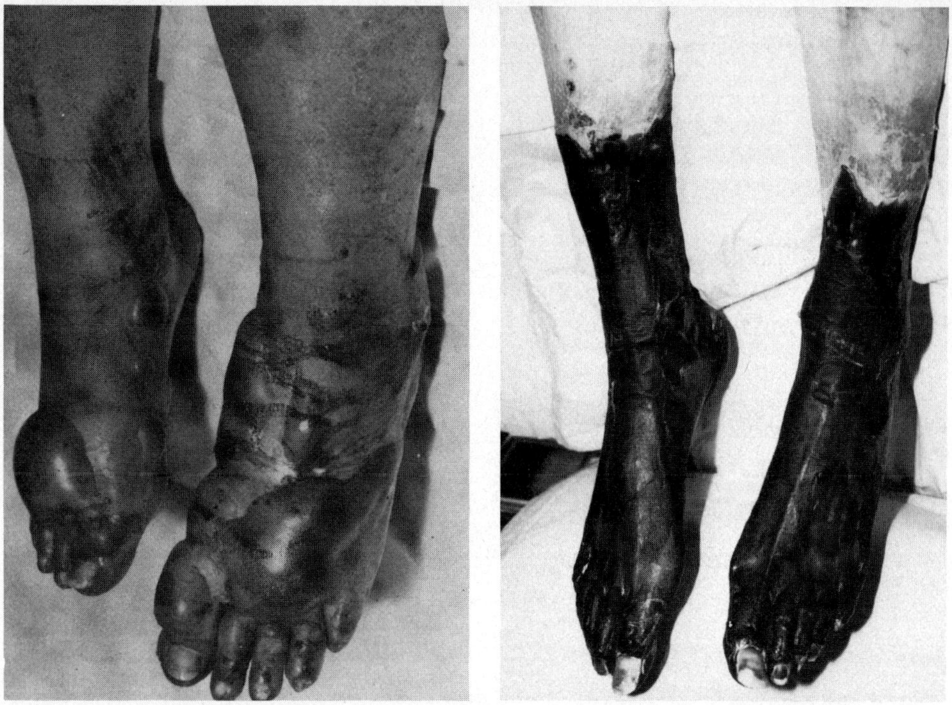

B

Fig. 33-1. A, Severe frostbite 24 hours after cold injury. Note extensive blister formation. (From Spittell JA Jr: Vascular syndromes related to environmental temperature. In Juergens JL, Spittell JA, and Fairbairn JF, eds: Peripheral vascular diseases, Philadelphia, 1980, WB Saunders Co. By permission of Mayo Foundation.) **B,** Bilateral deep frostbite resulting in bilateral gangrene. This patient required bilateral below knee amputations.

prickly pain may be present or shooting electric currentlike sensations resembling tabes dorsalis may occur, especially at night, both reflecting ischemic neuritis.[24] Hyperhidrosis and a burning sensation in the feet can occur and have been ascribed to overactivity of the sympathetic nervous system. These may respond well to sympathectomy. All patients develop some loss of touch, pain, and temperature that may later resolve or may persist indefinitely.[9]

Chronic sequelae

After frostbite up to 70% of victims develop symptoms including cold sensitivity, pain, and sensory disturbances. These symptoms may remain for years, and their presence has been reported 30 years after frostbite.[25] Color changes, hyperhidrosis, and swelling, as well as wound formation with scarring, are common. Many symptoms in postfrostbite victims resemble those seen in patients with reflex sympathetic dystrophy. Frostbite arthritis is also occasionally seen after cold injury. In children this may result in shortening and deformities of the fingers.[26] In adults clinical and radiologic features of osteoarthritis may be seen.[27,28] A rare complication of frostbite is the late development of squamous cell carcinoma at the site of injury.[29]

Diagnostic considerations

The diagnosis of frostbite is easily made, given a history of cold exposure associated with typical clinical manifestations. However, two diagnostic problems exist when evaluating a frostbite victim. These include establishing the depth of frostbite and determining tissue viability. There are two methods of classifying frostbite according to the depth of injury (Table 33-1). The first divides frostbite into four degrees and is analagous to a burn classification. The major difficulty with this classification is that it is based on the outcome of frostbitten tissue after thawing but cannot assess the depth of frostbite on appearance. The second classification may be more convenient. Superficial frostbite is differentiated from deep frostbite by palpation. In superficial frostbite deep tissues are soft while in deep frostbite, the whole part is stony hard. However, even this classification is often unreliable. Early classification has little clinical utility in terms of management decisions since all frostbite victims, except for the ones with injuries that are obviously superficial, are treated along the same lines.[5]

Early in the course of frostbite, clinical signs and symptoms do not provide a reliable way to assess tissue viability. Tissue viability is usually determined weeks or months after cold injury when the demarcation zone and sloughing of dead tissue takes place. Triple-phase bone scanning has been used in 7 patients and was found to be useful in predicting tissue viability as early as two days after cold injury.[30] More experience with this technique will be necessary to recommend its routine use in frostbite victims.

Table 33-1. Classifications of frostbite

I	II
First-degree White or yellow particles of skin with edema and hyperemia. No vesicles and no necrosis	**Superficial frostbite** Involves skin and superficial subcutaneous tissue
Second-degree Blistering and peeling	**Deep frostbite** Extends into muscle and may or may not affect bone
Third-degree Full skin necrosis with extension into the underlying subcutaneous tissue	
Fourth-degree Extension into muscle and bone with gangrene of affected parts	

Treatment

Initially, all patients with frostbite should be admitted to the hospital to evaluate the degree of injury. In mild cases the use of daily whirlpool baths with bed rest is sufficient. Treatment of deep frostbite should be considered a medical emergency since early institution of medical therapy may substantially reduce the amount of tissue loss. It is equally important to remember that thawing, which is the mainstay of therapy, should not be implemented if the patient may be reexposed to the cold. Refreezing thawed tissue promotes further tissue damage,[9] but walking on frozen limbs produces substantially less damage than walking on thawed ones.[1,20]

After transporting the victim to an adequate medical facility and removing any constricting garments, further treatment of frostbite depends on whether the tissue is still frozen or whether complete thawing has occurred. If the affected tissue is still frozen, then the most important therapeutic step is rapid rewarming of the frozen tissue. The affected part is immersed in a water bath at 38° C to 42° C (100° F to 108° F) for 15 to 30 minutes until complete thawing has occurred.[31] This is manifested by reappearance of normal color to the frozen part signifying reestablishment of blood flow. If gangrene is already present, one can hope to preserve tissue around the area of gangrene by rapid rewarming and thus limit the amount of amputation required. Rapid rewarming restores perfusion more rapidly than slow thawing at lower temperatures. Rewarming at temperatures above 42° C may increase tissue loss and is not recommended. Tissue should not be thawed by an open flame or dry heat since this may cause a burn injury. Putting ice on a frostbitten extremity will worsen the amount of injury and should never be done. When thawing is complete, the tissue should be kept dry and exposed. The thawing process is often very painful and may require the administration of narcotics for adequate pain relief. If the feet are involved, the patient should be permitted no weight bearing until healing ensues. The extremities should be elevated to minimize the amount of edema, and smoking should not be allowed under any condition.

The extremity with necrotic tissue should be cleansed for 20 minutes twice daily in a whirlpool bath with an aseptic solution at 35° C to 37° C (95° F to 99° F). Meticulous care should be taken to prevent secondary infections. Although some clinicians advocate prophylactic antibiotics in every case of frostbite, we believe that it is best to administer antibiotics only when infection occurs. To reduce the risk of infection, vesicles are left intact until they resorb spontaneously, which usually takes 1 to 2 weeks. Active exercise of the muscles, joints, and tendons is very important to prevent contractures.

Since it is difficult and sometimes impossible to assess tissue viability early in the course of treatment, and since the eventual amount of tissue loss is often much less than initially expected, an important principle in the management of frostbite injury is to avoid early débridement or amputation. Definitive débridement should be delayed until either autoamputation occurs or tissue demarcation is obvious. This may take weeks or months but is the only way now available to ensure maximum tissue preservation. It is important to appreciate that the gangrene of frostbite is often superficial.[20] Early amputation or débridement is indicated only when infected gangrene or generalized sepsis occurs.

In the literature there are conflicting reports regarding the efficacy of sympathectomy in the treatment of acute frostbite. Proponents believe it prevents ischemic tissue loss resulting from vasospasm in the area adjacent to the injured tissue. Some studies suggest that sympathectomy in the acute therapy of frostbite enhances resolution of edema and decreases tissue loss, with faster healing of the wound and fewer late sequelae.[32-35] We do not advocate early sympathectomy. Although sympathectomy is controversial in the acute phase of frostbite, there is general agreement that sympathectomy is effective for the treatment of some chronic frostbite sequela.

Low molecular weight dextran has been effective in treating animals with frostbite when they are treated early, but it has not been effective in treating humans.[36] Recently, topical applications of thromboxane inhibitors (aspirin and ibuprofen) on débrided blisters have been used with impressive results.[37,38]

Prevention of frostbite

Most cases of frostbite are preventable if appropriate measures are followed. Several thin layers of loose clothing should be worn with a first layer of water-resistant clothing (i.e., polypropylene) and an outer layer of waterproof material. Warm, loose footwear should be worn. Careful inspection and care of the feet are important, and the skin of the feet should be kept well oiled since this greatly protects the skin from low temperatures.[5] Mittens should be worn on the hands. Facial hair growth increases the likelihood of frostbite on the face because of moisture collecting on the mustache or beard.

PERNIO (CHILBLAINS)

Pernio* is a term used to denote localized inflammatory lesions of the skin as a result of an abnormal response to the cold. In the past pernio has been viewed as a skin disease, but now it is recognized as a cold-induced vascular disorder that is associated with skin manifestations.[39]

The prevalence of pernio varies considerably according to the geographic location. It is more common now in the temperate, humid climates of northwestern Europe than in the United States.[40] Winner and Cooper-Willis suggested that up to 50% of women during wartime conditions developed chilblains by the time they were 40.[41] It has been suggested that pernio is much less common than it used to be because of the availability of appropriate clothing in colder climates and because of the improvement in home and office heating. We have treated approximately 75 patients with pernio at the Cleveland Clinic from 1970 to 1986.

During exposure to cold there is increased blood viscosity resulting in a sluggish circulation in the superficial vessels accompanied by redistribution of flow to the deeper vascular network.[42] Humidity is an important predisposing factor for pernio since moisture promotes heat loss from the skin. Pernio develops only in susceptible subjects who are exposed to nonfreezing cold. Some have suggested that susceptibility seems to be related to a defective cutaneous circulation consisting of intense and prolonged vasospasm of parts of the skin during cold exposure.[5,44] This is consistent with the observation that in the same environment, subjects likely to develop pernio have cooler hands and feet than do those who are not.[5,43,44] Pernio is frequent in conditions with deficient limb circulation such as poliomyelitis, syringomyelia, and disuse phenomenon.

Pathology and pathophysiology

The vasospasm, which is induced by cold, is supplemented by structural changes in the skin that present characteristic, though not pathognomonic, histologic features. The most prominent changes are found in the dermis and subcutaneous fat and include (1) edema of the papillodermis, (2) vasculitis characterized by perivascular infiltration of the arterioles and venules of the dermis and subcutaneous fat by mononuclear and lymphocytic cells, (3) thickening and edema of the blood vessel walls, (4) fat necrosis, and (5) chronic inflammatory reaction with giant cell formation.

Not all of these changes are necessarily present, and fat necrosis and giant cell formation may be frequently absent.[45] The most consistent feature is perivascular lymphocytic or mononuclear infiltrates. In a recent study eight of nine women with pernio demonstrated histologic evidence of a lymphocytic infiltration of the blood vessel walls. While fibrinoid necrosis was not seen, some have suggested that this disease is a vasculitis.[46] The vascular changes seen on histology may also be caused by repeated episodes of vasospasm or prolonged vasospasm leading to tissue anoxia.[39]

Why one patient exposed to cold develops Raynaud's phenomenon and another pernio is not clear, but these diseases appear to be a continuum with Raynaud's phenomenon representing acute and readily reversible vasospasm and pernio representing more prolonged vasospasm with more chronic changes.

Clinical features

Pernio occurs most commonly in young women between the ages of 15 and 30 but may occur in children or adults of any age. The reason for this female predominance is not clear. It has been suggested that women have an increased responsiveness of the cutaneous circulation to cold, and the pattern of female fat distribution reduces cutaneous blood flow in some areas.[47] It has also been suggested that women who wear skirts are more exposed to the effect of cold.

Acute pernio may develop 12 to 24 hours after exposure to cold. Single and multiple erythematous, purplish edematous lesions appear accompanied by intense itching and burning. Their size varies from a few millimeters to several centimeters. The lesions tend to affect the toes and dorsa of the proximal phalanges. The fingers, nose, ears, and thighs have also been involved. Often this acute phase of pernio is bilateral and symmetrical.[5] Ulcerations may occur and are usually shallow, vary in shape and size, and may have a hemorrhagic base. The acute lesions usually disappear in 1 to 3 weeks and may not recur unless there is reexposure to cold. Acute pernio is a self-limited condition, although it may be recurrent. The legs may be slightly swollen, cool to touch, and may demonstrate varying degrees of cyanosis. Characteristically, the peripheral pulses, pulse volume recordings, and arterial pressures are normal.

Chronic pernio occurs when repeated exposure to cold results in the persistence of lesions with subsequent scarring and atrophy. Characteristically, the lesions begin in winter or fall and disappear as the warm season begins. These lesions, like those of acute pernio, often itch and burn. The natural history of pernio differs slightly depending on the age of the patient.[40] Children often have recurrences each winter for several years, and then complete recovery is the rule. In adults there is a tendency toward worsening of the pernio over the years, and this may lead to chronic occlusive vascular disease.[47] In advanced cases the seasonal variation may disappear.

Pernio has been described in association with poliomyelitis,[44] monocytic leukemia,[48,49] and with cutaneous lupus erythematosus.[50]

Erythrocyanosis[5,51] represents the nodular chronic form of pernio. Some investigators consider it a distinct though closely related condition.[40] Clinically, nodular lesions with

*Pernio is a Latin word that literally means frostbite. Its synonym, chilblain, is an Anglo-Saxon term that means cold sore.

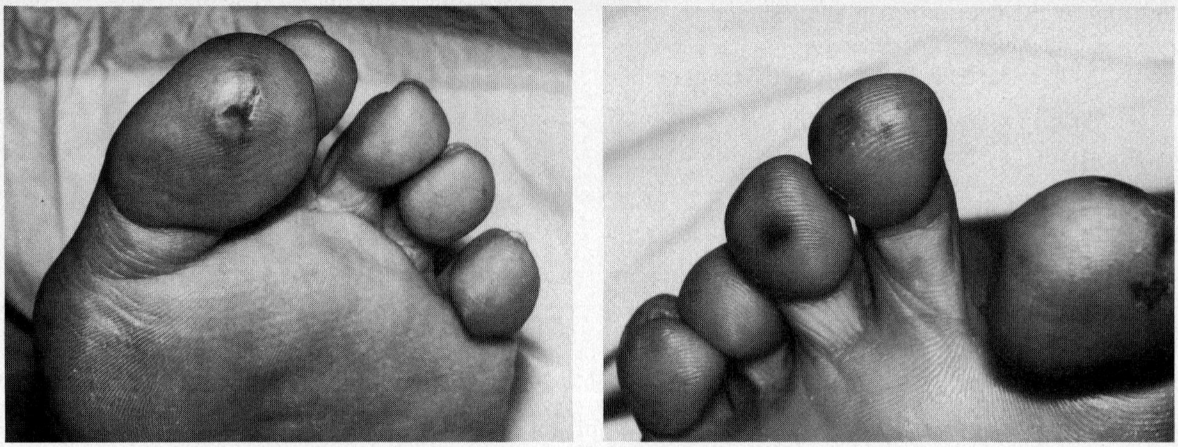

Fig. 33-2. These patients have the typical yellow-brown discoloration with shallow ulcers on the toes. This represents chronic pernio.

swelling and fibrosis appear on deeply cyanotic skin after cold exposure. These lesions occur in the lower extremities and thighs. Adolescent girls are most commonly affected.

Diagnosis

In its classic form pernio is usually not difficult to diagnose. The patient develops violet or yellow blisters, brown plaques, and shallow ulcers on the toes, which burn and itch (Fig. 33-2). These lesions first appear at the onset of winter and disappear each spring. However, in some chronic cases in which the lesions do not disappear in the warm weather or in which the lesions cause severe pigmentation and disfiguration of the lower part of the leg, the diagnosis may be more difficult.

It is beneficial to view the differential diagnosis of pernio under two main categories of diseases. The first category consists of recurrent erythematous, nodular, and ulcerative lesions that are of primary interest to the dermatologist and include four conditions: erythema induratum, nodular vasculitis, erythema nodosum, and cold panniculitis. The second category, atheromatous emboli, is of major concern to the vascular physician (see Chapter 11).

Erythema induratum (Bazin's disease) is usually, but not always, a cutaneous form of tuberculosis, which usually affects adolescent girls who develop nodular ulcerating lesions of the calves.[44,51] In biopsies from the skin caseating granulomas are present in some cases. However, mycobacterium is rarely cultured from the skin lesions. Tuberculin skin tests are usually positive. Tuberculosis is on the decline, and more cases of erythema induratum are being encountered in the absence of tuberculosis.

Nontuberculous forms of recurrent painful nodules are called nodular vasculitis.[51] No apparent cause is known. Women over the age of 30 years are usually affected. The two features that differentiate this condition from either pernio or erythema induratum are that the nodules of nodular vasculitis are extremely painful and rarely ulcerate.

Erythema nodosum may be differentiated from pernio in that it may be associated with fever, arthralgias and malaise, and a secondary underlying disease. The lesions are painful and generally do not ulcerate.

Cold panniculitis is characterized by painful nodules that appear on the skin after cold exposure. These lesions can be reproduced by the application of an ice cube. The histology of the lesion reveals fat necrosis.[52]

The palpable purpuric lesion that is sometimes present in pernio must be differentiated from other types of vasculitis, especially leukocytoclastic vasculitis. The lack of systemic manifestations and laboratory abnormalities and the relation of the lesions to cold exposure serve to separate these two conditions. Rarely, a skin biopsy may be needed to make a definitive diagnosis.

The other important entity that must be differentiated from pernio is atheromatous emboli. This presents a significant diagnostic problem in older patients because lesions produced by atheromatous emboli may appear identical to those of pernio. When a history of cold exposure is uncertain, arteriographic studies are often warranted in an attempt to demonstrate atheroma in the aorta or iliac vessels. A biopsy of these lesions establishes a definitive diagnosis in that the characteristic cholesterol clefts are present in atheromatous emboli (see Chapter 11).

Treatment

As in all cold-induced vascular disorders, prevention is the best form of treatment, and this consists of avoiding or minimizing cold exposure. When this is not feasible, adequate protection by suitable clothing forms the cornerstone of therapy. When lesions have already appeared, symptomatic therapy should be initiated. Many remedies have been used for treating pernio. They include calcium, nicotinic acid, phenoxybenzamine, and other vasodilators. The beneficial effects of these drugs are inconsistent. Ultraviolet light treatment was used 25 years ago and found to be beneficial to some patients.[53] Three doses of ultraviolet light were administered weekly at the beginning of winter.

Nifedipine was recently found to be beneficial in 10 patients with severe pernio.[54] When given at a daily dose of 60 mg, shortly after the appearance of lesions, nifedipine was shown to significantly reduce the severity of symptoms and shorten their duration in the majority of patients. Until more data are available it seems reasonable to treat patients who have chronic pernio with nifedipine or another calcium entry blocking agent. The severe itching may be treated with a local application of antipruritic agents.

In a letter to the editor[55] Ganor has reported on treating "hundreds of patients" with 0.025% fluocinolone acetonide cream under an occlusive dressing. The itch disappeared in a few days and the lesions in 1 to 2 weeks. Others have reported adverse effects with topical steroids.[56] Fitzgerald has suggested that calcium and vitamin K administered intramuscularly will cure pernio.[57] Until these dramatic results are confirmed, more conventional forms of therapy are recommended.

In severe chronic cases of pernio, sympathectomy has been used.[5,40] Although it enhances the resolution of the active lesions, it does not prevent the recurrence of new lesions, and this form of therapy is usually not necessary.

TRENCH FOOT AND IMMERSION FOOT

Trench foot is a nonfreezing cold injury resulting from exposure to cool, wet surroundings for a period of 24 hours to several days. The temperature is usually between 15° C and 0° C. Coldness alone generally will not cause trench foot. Two very important components are moisture (e.g., wet socks) and immobility. As its name indicates, this condition occurred in soldiers who were immobilized in trenches for a long period. Immersion foot is a more recent variety of nonfreezing cold injury, which was first reported during World War II in shipwreck survivors.[58] Prolonged immersion of the feet in cold or cool water is the usual initiating event. These two entities are probably different spectra of the same disease. Both conditions are primarily military injuries. However, civilian cases do occur occasionally, especially in alcoholics and in the neglected elderly.[59]

The pathophysiology of these conditions is related to cold-induced vasospasm, which results in hypoxia, endothelial injury, and capillary stasis.[60,61] Vascular occlusion and gangrene may occasionally occur.[5,60] Factors predisposing to these conditions, in addition to moisture and immobility, include dependency and fatigue.[13,58,61] Constricting footwear aggravates this condition by causing pressure necrosis on already ischemic areas.

Clinical features

There are three clinical phases in the development of these conditions.[5,58] In the initial ischemic phase (also called vasospastic or prehyperemic phase), the feet are edematous, cold to touch, and pale with patchy cyanosis. Patients note heaviness and numbness of their extremities. The pulses are often reduced or absent because of intense vasospasm. The second phase (hyperemic phase) occurs within a few hours after removal of the extremity from cold exposure and is characterized by an increase in blood flow in the extremity as a result of extreme vasodilation. This phase may persist for weeks and is characterized by the presence of red, hot extremities with marked edema. The pulses are bounding. Initially, the feet are numb, and this is replaced by an intense burning pain 8 to 10 days later. Vesicles, ulcers, and ecchymoses may develop, and in severe cases gangrene ensues. The hyperemic phase may resolve without sequelae or in severe cases may be followed by a late ischemic (posthyperemic) phase, which is characterized by cold sensitivity, numbness, and hyperhidrosis and may persist for years. Persistent pain may occur and has been attributed to either ischemic neuropathy, irritation or sensory nerve endings by scar tissue, or reflex sympathetic dystrophy.[13]

Treatment

Prophylaxis is the most important aspect in the management of immersion and trench foot because they are largely preventable conditions. Treatment of established cases consists of removing the wet, cold footwear and providing a warm environment for the victim. Affected extremities should be elevated to reduce edema.

The hyperemic stage should not be left untreated. If this phase is allowed to persist, large bullae, or blebs, rapidly occur, and massive swelling ensues. This is a reperfusion injury and can be prevented by placing the patient in a cooler environment and elevating the legs. Since the gangrene of nonfreezing cold injuries is superficial,[60] surgery should be delayed until complete demarcation and sloughing of nonviable tissues takes place. Long-term sequelae, which are related to vasospasm and sympathetic overactivity, respond well to medical and surgical sympathectomy.[5]

WARM WATER IMMERSION INJURIES

Warm water immersion injuries are primarily military injuries that are caused by protracted exposure (greater than 72 hours) to water at temperatures of 22° C to 32° C (72° F to 90° F).[62] Two distinct forms of warm water immersion injury are now recognized, warm water immersion foot and tropical immersion foot. Warm water immersion foot occurs within 3 days of contact with water and is clinically characterized by painful, white, wrinkled soles accompanied by burning sensations in the affected extremities.[62,63] Tropical immersion foot represents an extension of the injury into the ankle and dorsum of the foot and requires 3 to 7 days of continuous exposure to water to occur.[63]

Treatment consists of cessation of water exposure and elevation of the extremities when edema is present. Complete recovery from warm water immersion foot occurs in 2 to 3 days, while complete recovery from tropical immersion foot may take 7 to 10 days. Prophylaxis is of paramount importance. Silicone preparations are effective in the prevention of these conditions.[64]

ERYTHROMELALGIA (ERYTHERMALGIA)

The term *erythromelalgia* was introduced by Mitchell in 1878[65] and is a combination of three Greek words: *Erythros,* meaning red; *melos,* meaning extremity; and *algos,* meaning pain. It literally means red, painful extremities.

Ery*therm*algia is another term suggested by Smith and Allen.[66] This term was suggested because it emphasized the fact that increased temperature of the affected part is an integral part of this syndrome.

Erythromelalgia is uncommon. Brown[67] from the Mayo Clinic reported that its incidence was one in 40,000 patients seen in the 1930s. It is much less common at institutions that are not major referral centers.

A useful classification of patients with erythromelalgia is shown in the accompanying box.[5] The primary, or idiopathic, variety may occur in a simple nonfamilial form or in a familial form that has various patterns of inheritance.[68] Secondary erythromelalgia is associated with a variety of underlying conditions. Myeloproliferative disorders, primarily polycythemia vera, occur in the majority of cases.[69] In a review of 51 cases of erythromelalgia at the Mayo Clinic, 30 (59%) had a primary erythromelalgia, and in 21 (41%) the erythromelalgia was secondary to another underlying disease, mainly myeloproliferative disorders.[70] In a recent review of the world literature,[69] 61 cases of erythromelalgia were found in association with myeloproliferative disorders. Polycythemia vera accounted for 59% of these cases, essential thrombocythemia for 38%, and agnogenic myelometaplasia and chronic myelogenous leukemia in one patient each. Erythromelalgia-like eruptions have been described with the use of certain drugs, notably bromocriptine and nifedipine.[71-73]

Classification of erythromelalgia

I. ***Primary (idiopathic)***
   A. Simple nonfamilial
   B. Familial (autosomal dominant, recessive, and sex-linked)

II. ***Secondary***
   A. Associated with myeloproliferative disorders (polycythemia vera and essential thrombocythemia)
   B. Associated with other diseases
      1. Hypertension
      2. Diabetes
      3. Rheumatoid arthritis
      4. Gout
      5. Spinal cord disease
      6. Multiple sclerosis
   C. Drug induced
      1. Nifedipine
      2. Bromocriptine
      3. Pergolide

Histopathology

Because of the rarity of this condition, few histologic studies are available, and most are based on individual case reports. The histologic findings represent a spectrum that varies from completely normal histology to arteriolar occlusion with thrombus formation. This disparity may reflect a difference in histology between mild and severe cases as well as primary and secondary forms of erythromelalgia. A biopsy of two cases of primary erythromelalgia revealed normal histology with no vascular changes.[74,75] In a third case dilated and proliferating capillaries were found.[75] In patients with erythromelalgia associated with polycythemia vera and thrombocythemia, skin biopsies revealed arteriolar inflammation with sparing of the venules and capillaries.[76,77] Arteriolar occlusion by thrombi was a common finding, especially in cases associated with gangrene. These lesions were partially reversed with aspirin. In a single case report of a patient with primary erythromelalgia, there was a decreased number of nerve terminals containing acetylcholinesterase and catecholamines, compared with normal skin,[78] suggesting that a disorder of peripheral vasomotor tone exists in these patients.

Pathogenesis

The exact pathogenesis of erythromelalgia is not known. However, recently there have been advances in the understanding of this condition and several newer theories have been advocated. As with histopathology, different pathogenetic mechanisms may be operating, depending on the type of erythromelalgia present. One proposed mechanism is temperature-triggered release of vasoactive substances such as histamine, serotonin, kinins, and prostaglandins. Methysergide, a serotonin agonist, was found to be effective in treating some cases of erythromelalgia, implying that serotonin may have a role in the pathogenesis of erythromelalgia in some patients.[79]

In a study involving two patients with primary erythromelalgia, increased concentrations of prostaglandins PGE_1, PGE_2, and PGF_{12}, were demonstrated in skin profusates.[80] Prostaglandin E is a vasodilator known to cause erythema and pain in the skin. Jorgensen and Sondergaard postulate that an increased rate of synthesis of prostaglandins may be an important pathogenetic mechanism to explain some clinical features of this entity. Platelet activation with the release of various mediators including prostaglandins, especially thromboxane, may cause secondary platelet aggregation and thrombus formation in secondary forms of erythromelalgia.[77] It is noteworthy that after a single dose of aspirin, the symptoms may be relieved for 2 to 4 days, which is the duration of inhibition of the rate limiting enzyme cyclooxygenase within the platelets.

Increased limb blood flow has been demonstrated in patients with erythromelalgia. However, skin oxygenation as measured by transcutaneous oxygen diffusion was extremely reduced, indicating ischemia to the microvasculature.

Clinical features and differential diagnosis

Erythromelalgia is characterized by the clinical triad of erythema, burning pain, and increased temperature, usually of the extremities. In both the idiopathic and the secondary forms, middle-aged persons, men more than women, are affected. Rarely, the primary type may occur in children while secondary erythromelalgia usually occurs after the age of 40. The feet, especially the soles, are more commonly involved than the hands, and involvement is usually bilateral in the idiopathic variety. Asymmetric or even unilateral involvement is more common in the secondary type.[69] Recently we have treated a patient in which erythromelalgia was confined to the knee area. Gangrene is not a feature of the idiopathic variety while acryocyanosis progressing to gangrene may occur in the secondary variety.[69,77] The peripheral pulses are generally normal in the primary type and variable in secondary erythromelalgia. Usually the symptoms occur in "attacks" that last from minutes to hours and occasionally for days. The "attacks" are characteristically induced by a warm environment or exposure of an extremity to it. Exercise and dependency tend to exacerbate the symptoms. There is an individual critical skin temperature above which symptoms are induced.[81] The range of this critical temperature is 32° C to 36° C (90° F to 97° F). When the temperature is lower than the critical value, the symptoms disappear.

Erythromelalgia has been regarded as the antithesis of Raynaud's phenomenon since its symptoms are induced by warmth and relieved by exposure to the cold.[82] Patients often seek relief by exposing the affected extremity to a cooler environment (i.e., placing their extremity in cold water, walking on a cold floor barefoot or running the air conditioning at all times). Patients usually continue to suffer "attacks" with variable severity. Spontaneous remissions have been described.

The diagnosis of erythromelalgia is based on (1) erythema, (2) severe burning pain, (3) increased temperature, (4) precipitation by a warm environment, (5) relief by a cool environment, and (6) exclusion of other diseases that may mimic erythromelalgia.

Other causes of painful erythematous extremities include reflex sympathetic dystrophy, arteriosclerosis obliterans (ASO), and thromboangiitis obliterans (Buerger's disease). In ASO and Buerger's disease, although the extremities may be red and painful, they are often cool to touch, and arterial pulsations are diminished. Reflex sympathetic dystrophy (see Chapter 29) is often characterized by burning pain with swelling of the affected extremity. Usually, the affected part is cyanotic and cool but sometimes may be red and warm. There is no relationship to the temperature of the environment. Peripheral neuropathy may cause burning painful extremities, but they should not be erythematous or warm and the symptoms likewise are not temperature related. In children erythromelalgia has to be differentiated from Fabry's disease.[69]

In the majority of patients with myeloproliferative disorders, erythromelalgia preceded the clinical appearance of these disorders by several years.[69] Thus patients with erythromelalgia who are over 30 to 40 years of age should be observed by periodic blood counts.

The treatment of erythromelalgia is often difficult. In cases of secondary erythromelalgia, treatment of the underlying disease (i.e., phlebotomy of polycythemia vera and normalization of platelet count in thrombocythemia) often relieves the symptoms of erythromelalgia.[77] However, symptoms do not always correlate with the level of the hematocrit or platelet count.[69] It is important to instruct patients to avoid all potential situations that may increase peripheral vasodilation. They should try to avoid any exposure of their extremities to an increased warmth and may need to avoid exercise and alcohol because of the resultant effects on vasodilation.

Aspirin is probably the most effective modality available. Patients often demonstrate rapid and prolonged relief after a single dose of aspirin therapy. Aspirin may be effective in both the primary and secondary forms of erythromelalgia.[5] Other drugs that have been used, with variable results, include methylsergide,[79] ephedrine, propranolol,[83] phenoxybenzamine, nitroglycerin, and sodium nitroprusside.[75,84] Corticosteroids have been effective in patients with systemic lupus erythematosus and erythromelalgia.[85] Since the response to any of these drugs is unpredictable for the individual patient, trial with individual drugs for a period of 2 to 3 weeks is warranted. In some cases a combination of drugs may be successful where monotherapy has failed. Nonsteroidal antiinflammatory drugs such as indomethacin may be effective even when aspirin has not. Biofeedback was successful in one report.[86]

Surgical sympathectomy has been tried on a few patients with variable results. It cannot be recommended as a form of routine therapy in these patients.

The prognosis of a secondary erythromelalgia is that of the underlying disease. In severe refractory forms of idiopathic erythromelalgia the symptoms may be continuously debilitating, but are generally not life threatening.

COLD AND HEAT URTICARIA

Cold and heat urticaria are two forms of urticaria occurring within a larger class of urticarias induced by a variety of physical agents.

Cold urticaria (cold sensitivity)

Cold urticaria develops in response to cold exposure, such as exposure to wind, drinking cold water, or eating cold food. Patients with this disorder who swim in cold water may develop severe hypotension and could die.[40] Two forms of cold urticaria are recognized: a rare familial form transmitted as an autosomal dominant condition and a more common acquired form.

In the hereditary or familial form symptoms develop during infancy and urticaria is accompanied by fever, headache, arthralgias, and leukocytosis. The urticaria lesions are characteristically burning in nature rather than pruritic.[5] Symptoms may occur immediately after cold exposure, or there may be a delay of 9 to 18 hours between symptoms and exposure. Familial urticaria is not immunologically mediated since it cannot be passively transferred. Biopsy specimens do not show degranulation of mast cells, and histamine release often does not occur.[87]

In the acquired form of cold urticaria symptoms develop in childhood or during adult life. The vast majority of cases are idiopathic. However, cryoglobulins, cryofibrinogens, cold hemolysins, and cold agglutinins have been demonstrated especially in association with infectious mononucleosis.[88] Symptoms of pruritus and swelling appear within minutes of cold exposure and vary in severity from mild to incapacitating. In some patients symptoms resolve within weeks or months while in others they tend to remain indefinitely with exacerbations and remissions related to cold challenge. Angioedema may occasionally occur. In contrast to hereditary urticaria, acquired cold urticaria is immunologically mediated. This condition can be passively transferred by a serum factor or IgE to normal skin.[89] Degranulation of mast cells and histamine release has been demonstrated. Other released mediators included neutrophil and eosinophil chemotactic factors.[87,90,91]

The treatment for cold urticaria is uniformly disappointing. Antihistamines have been used with partial relief of symptoms in some patients. Success has been claimed in some cases with intramuscular penicillin. Oral penicillin has not been found to be helpful. Desensitization may help in some instances and consists of immersing the extremity in water at 15° C, initially for a few minutes every hour with a gradual increase in immersion periods and decrease in water temperature. Once tolerance is achieved, daily immersion is necessary to avoid relapse.

Heat urticaria (heat sensitivity)

Heat urticaria may be of two types: a generalized type also known as cholinergic urticaria and an extremely rare localized type. Cholinergic urticaria is characterized by the development of characteristic small (1 to 3 mm) pruritic urticarial lesions that persist for minutes or hours in response to an increase in core body temperature. This may be brought about by fever, exercise, exposure to hot water, or at times eating spicy food. Associated symptoms may include asthma, flushing, and syncope. Release of histamine as well as neutrophil and eosinophil chemotactic factors have been demonstrated. Patients may suffer from this disorder for months or years and then suddenly improve for no apparent reason.[92] Treatment consits of using antihistamines during or before attacks.

A localized form of heat urticaria has been described in a few patients. Itching and swelling are localized to the exposed part. Therapy consists of administration of antihistamines and/or desensitization.

REFERENCES

1. Purdue GF and Hunt JL: Cold injury: a collective review, J Burn Care Rehabil 7:331, 1986.
2. Merryman HT: Mechanics of freezing in living cells and tissue, Science 124:515, 1956.
3. Kulka JP: Histopathologic studies in frostbitten rabbits. In Ferrer MI, ed: Cold injury, New York, 1956, Josiah Macey Jr Foundation.
4. Washburn B: Frostbite: what it is and how to prevent it—emergency treatment, N Engl J Med 266:974, 1962.
5. Spittell JA Jr: Vascular syndromes related to environmental temperature, In Juergens JL, Spittell JA, and Fairbairn JF, eds: Peripheral vascular diseases, Philadelphia, 1980, WB Saunders Co.
6. Sampson JB: Anxiety as a factor in the incidence of combat cold injury: a review, Milit Med 149:89, 1984.
7. Post PW, Daniels F, and Binford RT: Cold injury and the evolution of "white" skin, Hum Biol 47:65, 1975.
8. Sumner DS, Criblez TL, and Doolittle WH: Host factors in human frostbite, Milit Med 41:454, 1965.
9. Bangs CC: Hypothermia and frostbite, Emerg Med Clin North Am 2:475, 1984.
10. Lewis T: Observations upon the reactions of the vessels of the human skin to cold, Heart 15:177, 1930.
11. Dana AS, Rex IH, and Samitz MH: The hunting reaction, Arch Dermatol 99:441, 1969.
12. Lewis RB: Local cold injury: frostbite, Milit Surg 110:25, 1952.
13. Eubanks RG: Heat and cold injuries, J Arkansas Med Soc 71:53, 1974.
14. Merryman HT: Mechanics of freezing in living cells and tissue, Science 124:515, 1956.
15. Merryman HT: Osmotic stress as a mechanism of freezing injury, Cryobiology 8:489, 1971.
16. Merryman HT: Tissue freezing and local cold injury, Physiol Rev 37:233, 1957.
17. Cummings R and Lykke AWJ: Increased vascular permeability evoked by cold injury, Patholgy 5:107, 1973.
18. Sumner DS et al: Peripheral blood flow in experimental frostbite, Ann Surg 171:116, 1970.
19. Weatherley-White RCA et al: Experimental studies in cold injury: circulatory hemodynamics, Surgery 66:208, 1969.
20. Ward M: Frostbite, Br Med J 1:67, 1974.
21. Robson MC and Heggers JP: Evaluation of hand frostbite blister fluid as a clue to pathogenesis, J Hand Surg 6:43, 1981.
22. Raine TJ et al: Antiprostaglandins and anti-thromboxanes for the treatment of frostbite, Surgical Forum 31:557, 1980.
23. Mills WJ: Frostbite: a discussion of the problem and a review of an Alaskan experience, Alaska Med 15:27, 1973.
24. Suri ML et al: Neurological manifestations of frostbite, Indian J Med Res 67:292, 1978.
25. Ervasti E: Frostbite of the extremities and their sequelae: a clinical study, Actra Chir Scand Suppl 299:1, 1962.
26. Carrera GF et al. Radiologic changes in the hands following childhood frostbite injury, Skeletal Radiol 6:33, 1981.
27. Glick R and Parhami N: Frostbite arthritis, J Rheumatol 6:456, 1979.
28. Dreyfuss JR and Glemcher MJ: Epiphyseal injury following frostbite, N Engl J Med 253:1065, 1955.
29. Eun HC, Kim JA, and Lee US: Squamous cell carcinoma in a frostbite scar. Clin Exp Dermatol 11:517, 1986.

30. Mehta RC and Wilson MA: Frostbite injury: prediction of tissue viability with triple-phase bone scanning, Radiology 170:511, 1989.
31. Fuhrman FA and Fuhrman GJ: The treatment of experimental frostbite by rapid thawing: a review and a new experimental data, Medicine 36:465, 1957.
32. Mills WJ: Frostbite: summary of treatment of the cold injured patient, Alaska Med 25:33, 1983.
33. Golding MR et al: On settling the controversy on the benefit of sympathectomy for frostbite, Surgery 56:221, 1961.
34. DeJong P et al: The role of regional sympathectomy in the early management of cold injury, Surg Gynecol Obstet 115:45, 1962.
35. Kyosola K: Clinical experience in the management of cold injuries: a study of 110 cases, J Trauma 14:32, 1974.
36. Kapur BML, Gulati SM, and Talwar JR: Low molecular weight dextran in the management of frostbite in monkeys, Indian J Med Res 56:1675, 1968.
37. Heggers JP et al: Experimental and clinical observations on frostbite, Ann Emer Med 16:1056, 1987.
38. McCauley RL et al: Frostbite injuries: a rational approach based on the pathophysiology, J Trauma 23:143, 1983.
39. McGovern T, Wright IS, and Kruger E: Pernio: a vascular disease, Am Heart J 22:583, 1941.
40. Champion RH: Cutaneous reactions to cold. In Rook DS et al, eds: Textbook of dermatology, Oxford, 1986, Blackwell Scientific Publications.
41. Winner A, and Cooper-Willis ES: Chilblains in service women, Lancet 1:663, 1946.
42. Zolar Gl and Harber LC: Reactions to physical agents. In Moschella SL and Hurley HJ, eds: Dermatology, Philadelphia, 1985, WB Saunders Co.
43. Lewis ST: Observations on some normal and injurious effects of cold upon the skin and underlying tissues: chilblains and allied conditions, Br Med J 2:837, 1941.
44. Lynn RB: Chilblains, Surg Gynecol Obstet 99:720, 1954.
45. Wall LM and Smith NP: Perniosis: a histopathological review, Clin Exp Dermatol 6:263, 1981.
46. Herman EW, Kezis JS, and Silver DN: A distinctive variant of pernio: clinical and histopathologic study in 9 cases, Arch Dermatol 117:26, 1981.
47. Jacob JR et al. Chronic pernio: a historical perspective of cold-induced vascular disease, Arch Intern Med 146:1589, 1986.
48. Mark R, Lim CC, and Borrie PF: A perniotic syndrome with monocytosis and neutropenia: a possible association with a preleukemic state, Br J Dermatol 81:327, 1969.
49. Kelly JW and Dowling JP: Pernio: a possible association with chronic myelomonocytic leukemia, Arch Dermatol 121:1048, 1985.
50. Millard LG and Rowell NR: Chilblain lupus erythematosus (Hutchinson), Br J Dermatol 98:497, 1978.
51. Montogomery H, O'Leary PA, and Barker NW: Nodular vascular diseases of the legs, JAMA 128:335, 1945.
52. Solomon LM and Beerman H: Cold panniculitus, Arch Dermatol 88:897, 1961.
53. Holti G and Ingram JT: Physiotherapy in dermatology, Lancet 1:141, 1963.
54. Dowd PM, Rustin MHA, and Lanigan S: Nifedipine in the treatment of chilblains, Br Med J 293:923, 1986.
55. Ganor S: Corticosteroid therapy for pernio, J Am Acad Dermatol 8:136, 1983.
56. Burry JN: Adverse effects of topical fluorinated corticosteroid agents on chilblains, Med J Aust, 146:451, 1987.
57. Fitzgerald KJ: Cure for chilblains, Med J Aust 1:676, 1980.
58. Francis TJR: Non-freezing cold injury: a historical review, J R Nav Med Serv 70:134, 1984.
59. Ramstead KD, Hughes RG, and Webb AJ: Recent cases of trench foot, Postgrad Med J 56:579, 1980.
60. Pruitt BA and Goodwin CW: Burns: including cold, chemical and electrical injuries. In Sabiston DC, ed: Textbook of surgery, Philadelphia, 1986, WB Saunders Co.
61. Dembert M: Medical problems from cold exposure, Am Fam Phys 25:99, 1982.
62. Allen AM and Taplin D: Tropical immersion foot, Lancet 2:1185, 1973.
63. Catterall MD: Warm water immersion injuries of the feet: a review, J R Nav Med Serv 61:22, 1975.
64. Douglas JS and Eby CS: Silicone for immersion foot prophylaxis: where and how much to use? Milit Med 137:386, 1972.
65. Mitchell SW: On a rare vasomotor neurosis of the extremities, and on the maladies with which it may be confounded, Am J Med Sci 76:17, 1878.
66. Smith LA and Allen EV: Erythermalgia (erythromelalgia) of the extremities: a syndrome characterized by redness, heat and pain, Am Heart J 16:175, 1938.
67. Brown GE: Erythromelalgia and other disturbances of the extremities accompanied by vasodilation and burning, Am J Med Sci 183:468, 1932.
68. Cohen IJK and Samorodin CS: Familial erythromelalgia, Arch Dermatol 118:953, 1982.
69. Kurzrock R and Cohen PR: Erythromelalgia and myeloproliferative disorders, Arch Intern Med 149:105, 1989.
70. Babb RR, Alarcon-Segovia D, and Fairbairn JF II: Erythromelalgia: review of 51 cases, Circulation 29:136, 1964.
71. Eisler T et al: Erythromelalgia-like eruption in Parkinsonian patients treated with bromocriptine, Neurology 31:1368, 1981.
72. Alcalay J, David M, and Sandbank M: Cutaneous reactions to nifedipine, Dermatologica 175:191, 1987.
73. Fisher JR, Padnick MB, and Olstein S: Nifedipine and erythromelalgia, Ann Intern Med 98:671, 1983.
74. Priollet P et al: Erythromelalgia without arteriolar changes, Ann Intern Med 103:639, 1985.
75. Kvernebo K and Seem E: Erythromelalgia-pathophysiological and therapeutic aspects: a preliminary report, J Oslo City Hosp 37:9, 1987.
76. Michiels JJ et al: Histopathology of erythromelalgia in thrombocythemia, Histopathology 8:669, 1984.
77. Michiels JJ et al: Erythromelalgia caused by platelet-mediated arteriolar inflammation and thrombosis in thrombocythemia, Ann Intern Med 102:466, 1985.
78. Uno H and Parker F: Autonomic innervation of the skin in primary erythromelalgia, Arch Dermatol 119:65, 1983.
79. Pepper H: Primary erythromelalgia: report of a patient treated with methylsergide maleate, JAMA 203:162, 1968.
80. Jorgensen HP and Sondergaard J: Pathogenesis of erythromelalgia, Arch Dermatol 114:112, 1978.
81. Lewis T: Clinical observations and experiments related to burning pain in the extremities and to so-called "erythromelalgia" in particular, Clin Sci 1:175, 1933.
82. Mandell F, Folkman J, and Matsumoto S: Erythromelalgia, Pediatric 59:45, 1977.
83. Bada JI: Treatment of erythromelalgia with propranolol, Lancet 2:412, 1977.
84. Ozsoylu S, Caner H, and Gokalp A: Successful treatment of erythromelalgia with sodium nitroprusside, J Pediat 94:619, 1979.
85. Alarcon-Segovia D and Diaz-Jouanen E: Erythromelalgia in systemic lupus erythematosus, Am J Med Sci 266:149, 1973.
86. Putt A: Erythromelalgia: a case for biofeedback, Nurs Clin North Am 13:625, 1978.
87. Soter NA and Wasserman SI: Cutaneous changes in disorders of altered reactivity. In Fitzpatrick TB et al eds: Dermatology in general medicine, New York, 1987, McGraw Hill Inc.
88. Lemanske RF and Bush RK: Cold urticaris in infectious mononucleosis, JAMA 247:1604, 1982.

89. Sherman WB and Seebohm PM: Passive transfer of cold urticaria, J Allergy 21:41, 1950.
90. Kaplan A et al: In vivo studies of mediator release in cold urticaria and cholinergic urticaria, J Allergy Clin Immunol 55:394, 1975.
91. Soter NA, Wasserman SI, and Austen KF: Cold urticaria: release into the circulation of histamine and eosinophil chemotactic factor of anaphylaxis during cold challenge, N Engl J Med 294:687, 1976.
92. Soter NA et al: Mast cell mediator release and alterations in lung function in individuals with cholinergic urticaria, N Engl J Med 302:604, 1980.

Chapter 34

VASCULAR TUMORS

Norman B. Ratliff
Kandice Kottke-Marchant
John R. Bartholomew

TUMORS INVOLVING MAJOR BLOOD VESSELS

Vascular neoplasia is a broad subject, too extensive to be covered in depth in a single chapter. For instance, Enzinger and Weiss in their classic text, *Soft Tissue Tumors,* devote almost all of eight chapters to this topic.[1] Therefore this chapter has been organized to concentrate on vascular neoplasms that are prone to arise in or to involve major veins or arteries, and vascular tumors that present as soft tissue masses. Most of these tumors are rare and are an unexpected finding in physical examination, arteriography, venography, computerized tomography, ultrasonography, or radiography. These tumors can lead to significant morbidity and mortality, and an understanding of their pathophysiology, clinical manifestations, diagnosis, and treatment is important to physicians caring for patients with vascular disease.

Sarcomas

Sarcomas involving the major blood vessels include the leiomyosarcomas and the intimal sarcomas. These are rare tumors, which are accompanied by diverse symptoms. The symptoms can be related to the size of the tumor and the degree of obstruction of the involved vessel, as in the case of involvement of the pulmonary artery and great veins. They may also be accompanied by nonspecific findings, including fever, weakness, and anorexia when the aorta or systemic arteries are involved.[1] Symptoms also reflect the different growth patterns of these sarcomas. Leiomyosarcomas of the vena cava and pulmonary artery grow into the lumen, obstructing the vessel, while the intimal sarcomas grow in an infiltrating pattern along the vessel wall.[1,2] In addition, in thin-walled veins leiomyosarcomas extend through the wall into adjacent structures relatively early in their course, while in arteries, with their elastic lamina, the tumor tends to remain confined to the artery much longer (Fig. 34-1).

Leiomyosarcomas. Leiomyosarcomas arising from blood vessels are rare tumors. Less than 200 cases have been reported; however, the incidence may be underestimated.[1,3] Leiomyosarcomas found in the retroperitoneum and other deep soft tissue sites may arise from blood vessels, but by the time the tumor is discovered, the vascular origin may be obscure.[1,3] The most common site of origin for leiomyosarcomas is the inferior vena cava, followed by the iliac, femoral, and saphenous veins.[1-3] When the arterial circulation is involved, the pulmonary artery is the most common site.[4]

Inferior vena cava. Leiomyosarcomas of the inferior vena cava are often large, fleshy masses that obliterate the vascular lumen and erode through the vascular wall (Fig. 34-2). Despite the slow growth of these tumors, they have usually reached considerable size by the time of diagnosis, with extensive local invasion. They can metastasize to the hepatic or renal veins, right atrium, liver, lymph nodes, kidneys, adrenal glands, ribs, and skin.[5] Of the patients with this tumor, 80% to 90% are women, with an average age of 50 years.[1] These leiomyosarcomas are difficult to diagnose because the symptoms are generally nonspecific.

Leiomyosarcomas of the inferior vena cava may be divided into superior, middle, or inferior types by their location within the inferior vena cava. This division may be helpful in classification, clinical presentation, and treatment. Leiomyosarcomas of the middle type are found in the middle third of the cava between the hepatic and renal veins, typically causing right upper quadrant pain. This pain is a nonspecific finding and can mimic cholecystitis or chole-

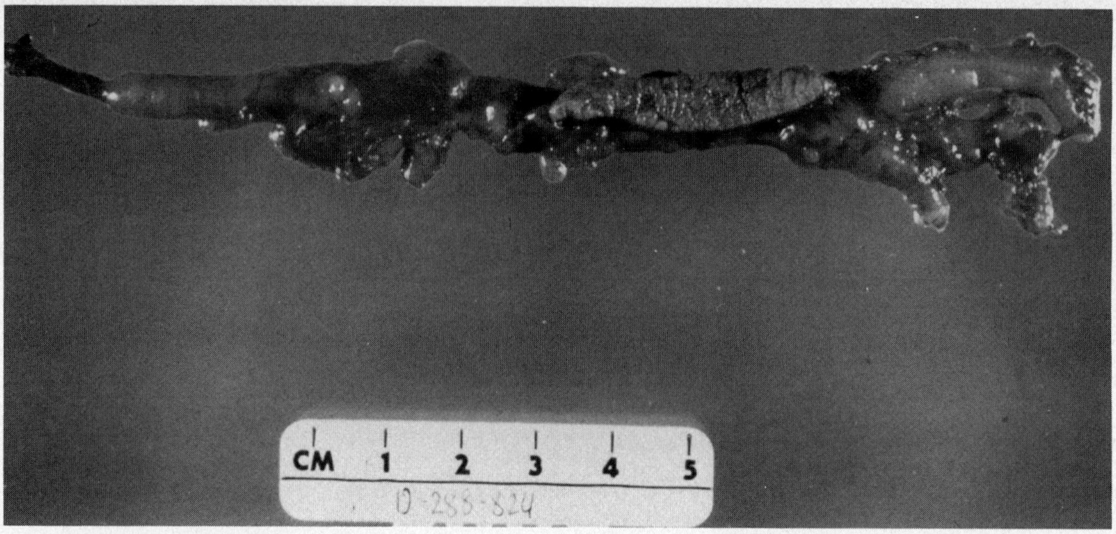

Fig. 34-1. Gross photograph of a leiomyosarcoma arising in a brachial artery. Note the apparent intravascular nature of the mass.

lithiasis. The tumor may extend into the renal veins, resulting in renal insufficiency or renal vein thrombosis. Extension into the right atrium has also been reported.[6] Tumors that arise in the superior or suprahepatic region typically develop a picture similar to Budd-Chiari syndrome because of hepatic vein obstruction or thrombosis.[7] These symptoms include jaundice, ascites, edema, and hepatomegaly. Tumors that arise in the lower third of the inferior vena cava below the renal veins often cause lower extremity edema. This may be minimal if the tumor is small or nonobstructive but can be massive if inferior vena cava obstruction is extensive or accompanied by secondary thrombosis.[7]

The diagnosis of leiomyosarcomas of the inferior vena cava is generally made at autopsy or unexpectedly during surgical exploration. An ultrasound or CT scan may be helpful, although venacavography is probably the best method to detect these rare tumors. In addition, the successful use of a transvenous biopsy to confirm the diagnosis has been reported.[6]

Treatment for leiomyosarcomas is surgical when the middle third and lower third of the inferior vena cava are involved. Tumors that arise in the superior aspect of the inferior vena cava are usually unresectable, and the effectiveness of chemotherapy or radiation therapy has not been adequately studied.[8]

Other veins. Leiomyosarcomas arise in veins other than the inferior vena cava. They also are found in the iliac, femoral, or saphenous veins and usually appear as a mass lesion. Ankle swelling and lower leg edema are the most common clinical findings. Leiomyosarcomas of the ovarian and renal veins have also been reported.[9] In contrast to leiomyosarcomas of the vena cava, the sex distribution of these tumors is almost equal. They should be treated as other leiomyosarcomas.

Pulmonary artery. Leiomyosarcomas involving the pulmonary arteries are rare.[1-3] Most of these tumors originate at the trunk of the pulmonary artery and spread in the direction of the blood flow to the left and right pulmonary arteries and to the distal pulmonary branches (Fig. 34-3). They arise during adulthood and demonstrate no sex predilection. Symptoms are related to pulmonary artery obstruction and include syncope, palpitations, dyspnea, chest pain, and overt right heart failure. In addition, intractable cough and hemoptysis have been reported.[10] Physical findings may include cyanosis, jugular venous distension, and a systolic murmur.[10] Chest x-ray films demonstrate a large cardiac silhouette or enlarged pulmonary trunk. Large filling defects near the pulmonary trunk may be seen on pulmonary angiography. Leiomyosarcomas are so unusual that the diagnosis is seldom considered until the tumor is found during surgery or autopsy.

The differential diagnosis for leiomyosarcomas involving the pulmonary artery includes pulmonary embolism, aortic stenosis, pheochromocytoma, pericardial effusion, fibrous mediastinitis, and metastatic pulmonary neoplasms.[10] The recommended treatment is surgery.

Other arteries. Leiomyosarcomas of other arteries are quite unusual. Involvement of the internal mammary artery, the inferior mesenteric artery, common iliac artery, and popliteal arteries have been reported.[9,11] Treatment for these rare tumors is surgical, although case reports have been cited in which radiation and chemotherapy have been tried in combination with surgical intervention.[9]

Intimal sarcomas. Intimal sarcomas are rare pleomorphic sarcomas that have not been further characterized. They originate in major arteries and spread in a fashion similar to that of leiomyosarcomas of the pulmonary artery.[1,2] This pleomorphic sarcoma may contain areas sugges-

A

B

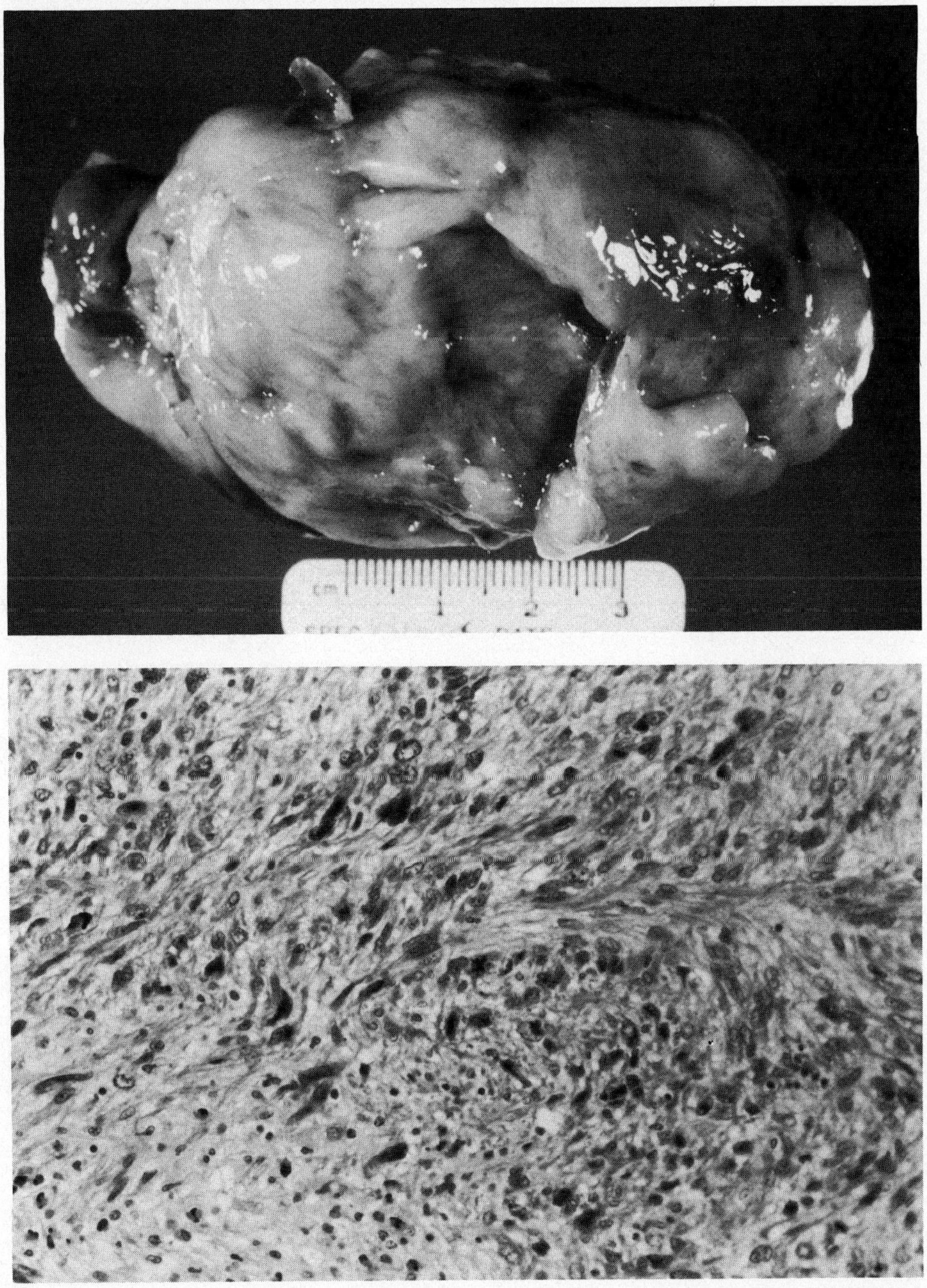

Fig. 34-2. Leiomyosarcoma of the inferior vena cava. **A,** Gross photograph demonstrating a large, lobulated tumor mass with no preservation of the vessel wall. **B,** This photomicrograph of the tumor illustrated in **A** shows typical histologic features of a leiomyosarcoma. There are fascicles and bundles of spindled neoplastic cells with prominent nuclear anaplasia. (Hematoxylin-eosin stain; ×310.)

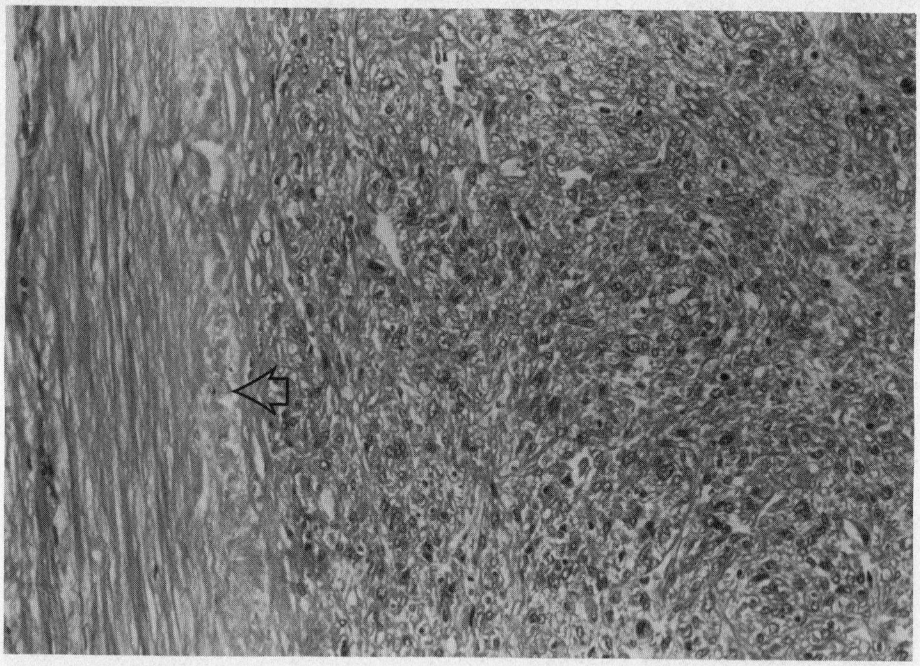

Fig. 34-3. This high-grade leiomyosarcoma of the pulmonary artery appears to arise from the vessel wall *(arrow)*. The underlying media maintains its structure. (Hematoxylin-eosin stain; ×120.)

tive of leiomyosarcoma, together with malignant fibrous histiocytoma, rhabdomyosarcoma, osteogenic sarcoma, and chondrosarcoma. The pleomorphic appearance is attested to by a plethora of synonyms, including osteogenic sarcoma, intimal sarcoma, pleomorphic chondrosarcoma, and malignant mesenchymoma. The distinctive feature of the intimal sarcomas is their growth, both within the lumen and along the surface of the blood vessel.[12] Metastases to the kidney, thyroid, pancreas, and brain have been reported.[12] The prognosis is grim.

Paragangliomas

Paragangliomas arise in association with major blood vessels and include carotid body paragangliomas, jugulotympanic paragangliomas, and mediastinal paragangliomas, also known as aortic body tumors.[1,13] Some confusion persists in the classification of these tumors. Those originating from the ear and jugular vein are commonly referred to as *glomus jugulare* or *glomus tympanicum tumors*. Paragangliomas in the mediastinum are referred to as *aortic body tumors,* while those found in the carotid body are referred to as *carotid body tumors* or *chemodectomas*. In spite of these names, which are firmly embedded in the literature, these are all paragangliomas and not true glomus tumors. A true glomus tumor originates in association with the glomus body, a specialized form of arterial venous anastomosis, important to thermal regulation.[14] True glomus tumors do not occur in association with large vessels and are characteristically found in subungual or subcutaneous sites on the extremities but may be found anywhere on the body.[15] They are usually small, only a few millimeters in size, purple, and classically very painful.

Paragangliomas arise in association with autonomic ganglia and are often classified as chromaffin or nonchromaffin tumors. The nonchromaffin tumors are concentrated in the head and neck or mediastinum, while the chromaffin tumors are generally found in the retroperitoneum. The autonomic ganglia systems, which give rise to the paragangliomas, include adrenal medulla, thoracic, intraabdominal, retroperitoneal ganglia, the vagal body, and chemoreceptors. The common histologic finding, which links the paraganglion system, is the presence of neurosecretory granules containing catecholamines.

Since any of the paragangliomas may be functional, it is advisable to assess the status of the tumor before surgery by measuring levels of urinary catecholamines and to be prepared to premedicate the patient in the same fashion as for adrenal pheochromocytoma.

Carotid body paraganglioma (chemodectoma, nonchromaffin paraganglioma, or glomus carotica). Carotid body paraganglioma arises in association with the carotid body, which is found on the posterior aspect of the bifurcation of the common carotid artery. It usually is incorporated into the adventitia of the vessel.[13,16,17] Carotid body paragangliomas are the most common of the extraadrenal paragangliomas and are frequently seen in patients living at

A

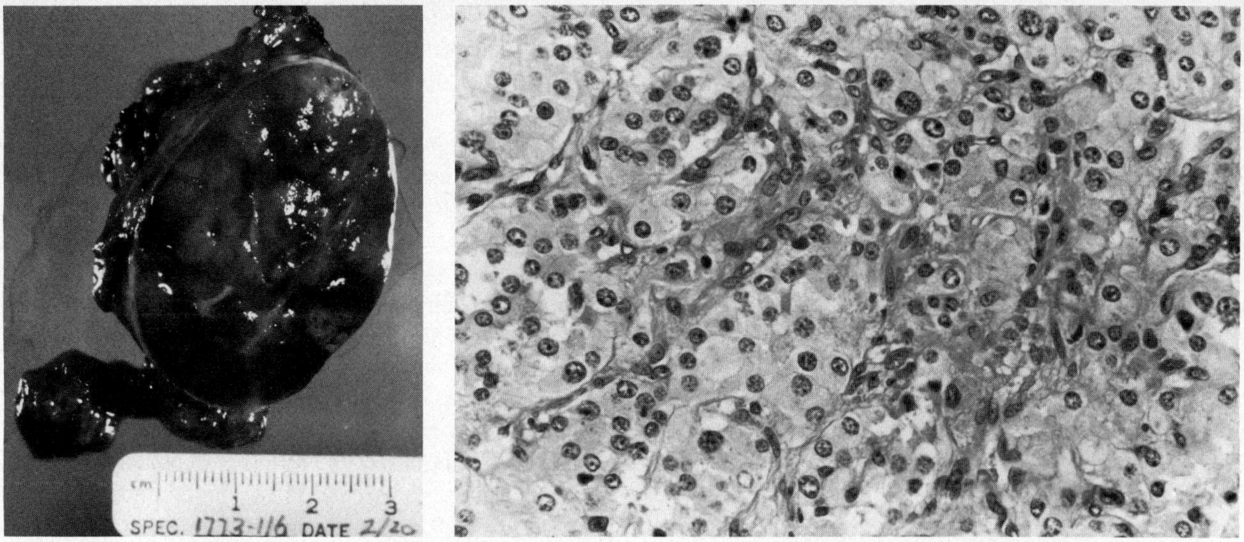

B

Fig. 34-4. Carotid body paraganglioma. **A,** This gross photograph of a large carotid body tumor demonstrates the homogeneous consistency of the tumor and its encapsulation and lack of necrosis. Despite the apparent encapsulation, these tumors may metastasize. **B,** In this photomicrograph of a paraganglioma, the tumor consists of clusters, or nests, of tumor cells with regular, round nuclei. The coarsely stippled nuclear chromatin pattern is typical of paragangliomas and other neuroendocrine tumors. (Hematoxylin-eosin stain; ×500.)

altitudes greater than 6000 feet.[17,18] In addition, they are seen in patients with cyanotic heart disease and with chronic obstructive pulmonary disease. It appears that this relationship is caused in part by continued exposure to hypoxic conditions. Males and females are about equally affected, although there are some reports indicating that females are more commonly affected at higher altitudes.[18] Carotid body tumors have been reported in children but are more frequently found in patients between 40 and 60 years of age. There may be a familial predilection, suggesting an autosomal dominant inheritance,[16,17] and when this occurs, the incidence of bilateral tumor increases dramatically.[1] Paragangliomas of all types tend to be multifocal, and a percentage of carotid body tumors are bilateral.[16]

Histologically, carotid body tumors resemble other paragangliomas regardless of their location. Clusters, or nests, of polygonal cells, referred to as "Zellballen," are surrounded by vascularized fibrous septa (Fig. 34-4). Individual cells have eosinophilic granular cytoplasm, with uniform round to oval nuclei, but occasional anaplasia and bizarre nuclei can be observed.

Although carotid body tumors may have some worrisome histologic features, they rarely demonstrate unequivocal microscopic features of malignancy. As with all neuroendocrine tumors, it is difficult to predict the biologic behavior from the microscopic appearance, and carotid body paragangliomas with no obvious malignant features may still metastasize. However, multicentric paragangliomas must be considered before concluding that a given tumor has metastasized.

Carotid body tumors usually appear as a slowly enlarging mass in the neck and are found by the patient or discovered during routine physical examination. They may be pulsatile, and a carotid bruit may be heard. These tumors are associated with symptoms resulting from their involvement of local nerves, from pressure on the hypopharynx, or invasion of the skull. These symptoms include neck or ear pain, dysphagia, tongue weakness, hoarseness, tinnitus, headache, and syncope. Vocal cord paralysis and Horner's syndrome have also been described, and hypertensive crises can occur. Carotid body tumors may be functional, and elevated levels of urinary catecholamines can be demonstrated.[19,20] Therefore preoperative evaluation with levels for the metanephrines and vanillylmandelic acids is appropriate.

The diagnosis is confirmed with selective arteriography, which classically reveals a tumor sitting in the crotch of the carotid bifurcation. Arteriography may also demonstrate a characteristic tumor blush, caused by its rich vasculature. Bilateral angiographic studies should be performed to evaluate collateral flow, to look for other paragangliomas or carotid body tumors, and to assess the extent of atherosclerosis. Ultrasonography or computed tomography may help differentiate other disease processes involving the neck. The differential diagnosis of carotid body tumors includes tuberculous lymphadenitis, branchial cleft cyst, carotid artery aneurysm, schwannoma, metastatic carcinoma, and lymphoma.

The majority of carotid body tumors are clinically benign, slow growing, and are cured by total surgical excision. A very small number behave in a malignant manner and spread to the lungs and lymph nodes, or they invade locally.[21,22] The difficulty of surgical resection is related to the degree of involvement of the carotid artery.[23] Shamblin et al classified carotid body tumors as I, II, or III, depending on their attachment to the carotid artery.[24] Group I carotid body tumors have only minimal carotid artery involvement and are easily removed surgically. Group II and III demonstrate more involvement of the carotid artery and are more difficult to remove. In addition to the degree of carotid involvement, surgery is also affected by the patient's age and underlying medical condition.[25] Complications of surgery include hemorrhage, stroke, and cranial and sympathetic nerve dysfunctions. Larger tumors are more apt to lead to cranial nerve complications, which may involve nerves VII, IX, X, and XII. The recurrent laryngeal nerve may also be affected.

Another approach to treatment involves selective intravascular embolization of the external carotid artery. This technique, using gelatin sponge emboli or particles of polyvinyl alcohol, reduces the size of the tumor by decreasing its blood supply and makes the tumor more accessible to surgery.[26,27] It may also be used in the poor surgical candidate, although it is not without some risks, including stroke. Radiation therapy has also been used in those patients who are not acceptable surgical candidates.

Recurrences, although uncommon, are more apt to happen when there is a family history of carotid body tumors or in patients with multiple paragangliomas.[23] The prognosis is excellent following surgery.

Aortic body tumors (mediastinal paragangliomas). Paragangliomas that arise from the mediastinum are associated with the pulmonary artery, aortic arch, or the sympathetic chain.[28,29] Those that originate in the pulmonary artery and aortic arch are termed aortic body tumors and are located in the anterior mediastinum. These aortic body tumors can be found wherever aortic body chemoreceptors are present,[1] and sites include the following: adjacent to the main pulmonary artery on its upper right border, in the angle between the ligamentum arteriosum and the descending thoracic aorta, and lateral to the innominate artery.

Aortic body tumors usually develop as an asymptomatic mass detected as an incidental finding on chest x-ray films. Symptoms such as pressure and hoarseness have been reported.[28,30] As with carotid body tumors, the majority of the aortic body tumors occur in people over 40, and the sex incidence is approximately equal. As with all paragangliomas, there may be an association with similar tumors at other sites.

Angiography reveals a highly vascular tumor supplied by arteries from both the aortic arch and the intercostal system with drainage into the superior vena cava.[31] Angiography should be performed in all patients who are undergoing surgical treatment. Although these tumors are histologically identical to the paragangliomas of the carotid body, aortic arch paragangliomas are more locally aggressive in their behavior.[1] Only 6% of these tumors metastasize, although up to 40% of patients may die from local invasion.[28] Complete surgical excision is the preferred treatment.

Jugulotympanic paragangliomas (glomus jugulare tumors and glomus tympanicum). Some authors refer to jugulotympanic paragangliomas as one tumor, while others separate the tumors involving the middle ear and mastoid, calling them glomus tympanicum. Tumors growing from the jugular bulb are referred to as *glomus jugulare*.[13,32,33] These tumors all arise from the paraganglia, which are associated with the auricular branch of the vagus nerve, the tympanic branch of the glossopharyngeal nerve, or the bulb of the jugular vein.

Paragangliomas are the most common neoplasms of the middle ear and the second most common nonadrenal paraganglioma.[13] The age incidence is similar to that of aortic and carotid body tumors, but in contrast to these tumors, there is a definite sex predilection for women.[32] They can be unilateral or bilateral, and a familial tendency has been reported.[34] Histologically, jugulotympanic paragangliomas are identical to carotid and aortic body paragangliomas. The incidence of metastasis is between 1% and 4%.

Patient complaints are related to the site of origin and involvement of adjacent structures. Those jugulotympanic tumors arising in the temporal bone produce symptoms related to the ear, including pulsatile tinnitus, conductive hearing loss, or vertigo. Other tumors appear as a mass in the middle ear. Jugulotympanic paragangliomas arising from the jugular bulb often produce symptoms related to involvement of the cranial nerves. The location of these tumors often makes surgical excision difficult, but they are reasonably radiosensitive.[35,36]

Leiomyomas

While 80% to 90% of the smooth muscle cell neoplasms of the great vessels are sarcomas, some are benign.[2] These leiomyomas can be distinguished from leiomyosarcomas or intimal (pleomorphic) sarcomas by the usual methods of distinguishing a benign from a malignant tumor. These include the lack of invasion of surrounding structures and the typical histology of a benign tumor. Unless one of these happens to be in a surgically inaccessible location, excision should be curative.

Papillary endothelial hyperplasia

Also known as vegetant intravascular hemangioendothelioma and intravascular angiomatosis, this peculiar lesion is one that is more likely to confuse the pathologist than the surgeon. While the cause is unknown, the evidence suggests that it is no more than an unusually prolific organizing thrombus. It is certainly not an angiosarcoma, the lesion with which it is most often confused.[37]

Papillary endothelial hyperplasia is an intravascular lesion that may develop in any vessel, including the vascular channels of a hemangioma, vascular malformations, or pyogenic granuloma.

Grossly, the lesion is typically about 2 centimeters in diameter, cystic and reddish purple, and contains clotted blood. It is surrounded by a pseudocapsule and is located inside a vessel. Occasionally, the vessel will have ruptured, allowing the lesion to extend into the surrounding tissue. It is the histology that may be confusing. Multiple small papillae lined with endothelial cells project into the lumen. The papillae may anastomose, yielding a network of small channels. While this appearance may be confused with an angiosarcoma, the lack of significant endothelial pleomorphism and mitotic activity, and the intravascular location, do not indicate angiosarcoma. The lesion is cured by simple excision, unless it is superimposed on an underlying vascular lesion.

NEOPLASMS THAT MAY PRESENT AS THROMBI

This category is composed of five neoplasms that frequently present clinically as thrombi or emboli and one variant form of thrombosis that may be misinterpreted as a neoplasm.

Low-grade endometrial stromal sarcoma

In the older literature this neoplasm is known as "endolymphatic stromal myosis." The older name reflects the delayed recognition that this is a low-grade endometrial stromal sarcoma.[38,39] This neoplasm characteristically invades lymphatic and vascular channels. It grows and permeates along those channels, thus the older name. It may present as an occlusive or stenotic lesion of pelvic veins extending into the inferior vena cava before there is any indication of a uterine neoplasm. It may be confused with a thrombus (Fig. 34-5). The clinical progression of the lesion is quite unlike a thrombus, so recognition of the entity via frozen section is not ordinarily difficult if the operating surgeon thinks of the possibility and does a biopsy.

Intravenous leiomyomatosis of the uterus

This peculiar lesion consists of the proliferation of benign uterine smooth muscle cells, analogous to the common uterine leiomyoma, but with a propensity to grow within vascular channels (Fig. 34-6). In that regard it is similar in its growth pattern to low-grade endometrial stromal sarcomas. It differs from stromal sarcomas in two important features. The cell of origin is smooth muscle, not endometrial stromal cells, and it is benign. But the growth of this strange lesion may extend, like the low-grade stromal sarcoma, via pelvic veins into the vena cava and perhaps even into the pulmonary vasculature (Fig. 34-6).[40,41]

Renal cell carcinoma

The propensity of this neoplasm to invade blood vessels is well known. As many as 30% of the renal cell carcinomas will exhibit invasion of veins in the renal pelvis at the time they are discovered. The tumor may quickly reach the renal veins and inferior vena cava and develop as an obstructive lesion, mimicking a thrombus[42] (Fig. 34-7).

Embryonal or undifferentiated sarcoma of the liver

This rare neoplasm occurs predominantly in people under 20 years of age,[43] but we have seen one case in a middle-aged individual in which the neoplasm appeared as a lesion in the right atrium and inferior vena cava with a preoperative diagnosis of cardiac myxoma and thrombus.

Cardiac myxomas

Cardiac myxomas are the most common intracardiac tumors. They occur in people of all ages, are often familial, and are found equally in both males and females. The myxomas are commonly located in the left atrium at the fossa ovalis, although they may be seen in either ventricle or in the right atrium.[44] They are usually 4 to 8 cm in diameter, globular, and may be pedunculated. Other less common primary intracardiac tumors, such as papillary fibroelastoma, angiosarcoma, and malignant fibrous histiocytoma, may also be pedunculated masses and give rise to systemic or pulmonary emboli.[45-47]

Systemic embolization to the central nervous system or kidneys is one manifestation of cardiac myxomas arising from the left side of the heart[48] (Fig. 34-8). Embolic events to the coronary arteries are also reported.[49] The usual clinical picture is similar to that of mitral valve disease with left-side heart failure and pulmonary congestion. Chest pain, arrhythmias, syncope, and noncardiac symptoms, including fever, anorexia, or weight loss, may also be seen. Pulmonary embolization or a fever of unknown origin may be other manifestations. Abnormal laboratory findings reported include an elevated hemoglobin suggesting polycythemia, elevated sedimentation rate, thrombocytopenia, or thrombocytosis.[44]

The diagnosis of myxoma must be considered in cases of systemic embolization and can be easily overlooked because of the wide variety of clinical findings and abnormal laboratory studies. A systemic illness such as a collagen vascular disease, malignancy, or endocarditis is often suspected. The M-mode or two-dimensional echocardiogram is invaluable in identifying the intracardiac mass and confirming the diagnosis. Cardiac catheterization, used more frequently in the past, is no longer essential given the reliability of the noninvasive procedures. Surgical excision is the treatment of choice.

An unusual form of myxoma, referred to as *Carney's complex* or *Carney's syndrome,* is characterized by cardiac myxomas, cutaneous myxomas, mammary myxoid fibroadenomas, spotty mucocutaneous pigmentation, primary pigmented adrenal cortical disease, large cell calcifying Sertoli cell tumors of the testes, growth hormone secreting pituitary adenomas, and psammomatous melanotic schwannomas. Systemic embolization is especially true of myxomas, which

A

B

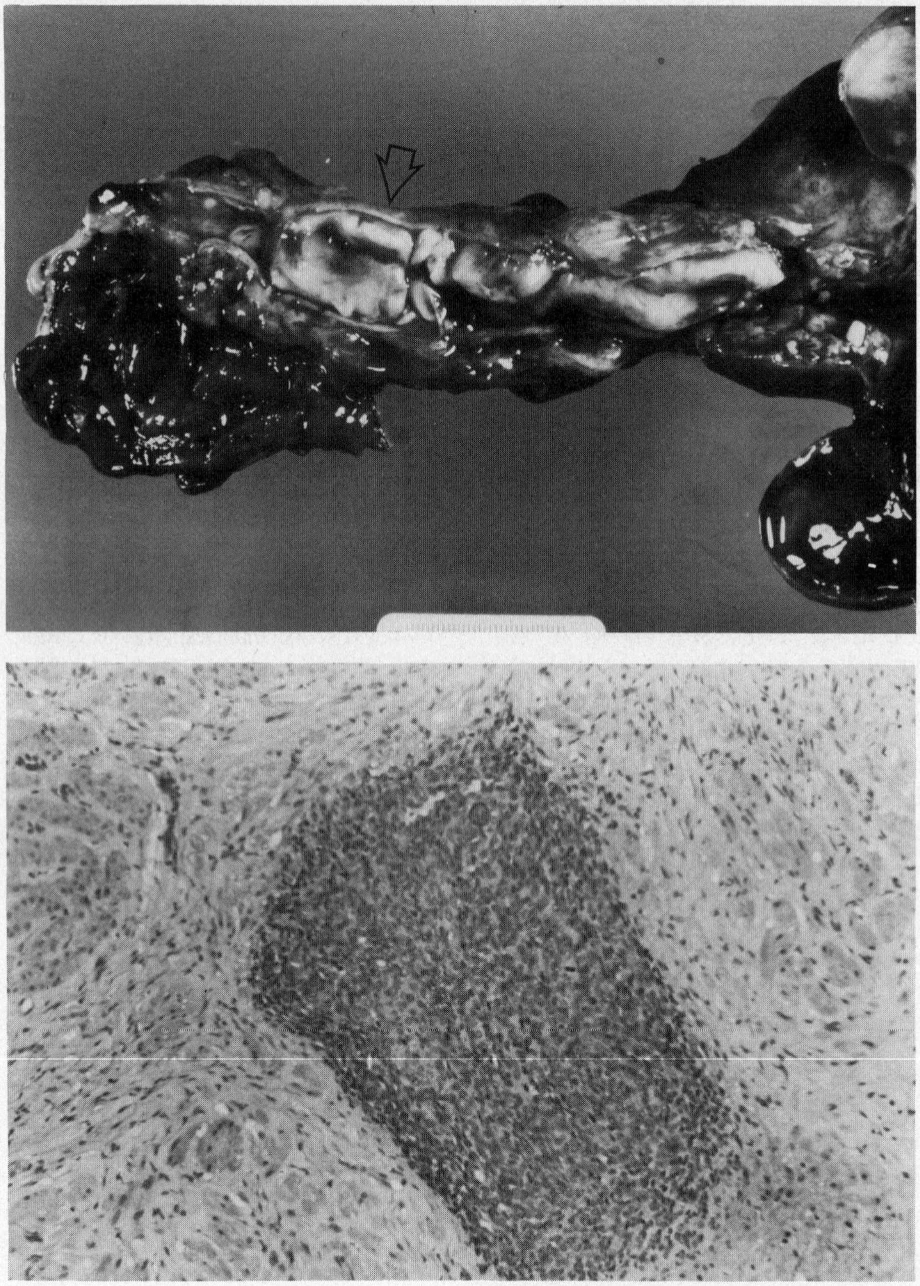

Fig. 34-5. Endometrial stromal sarcoma. **A,** This gross photograph of an endometrial stromal sarcoma shows tumor extension into an ovarian vein *(arrow)*. These tumors may often grow into and occlude pelvic veins. **B,** Histologically, endometrial stromal sarcoma consists of multiple nodules of plump, basophilic cells that invade the myometrium as well as lymphatic vessels and veins in solid cords. (Hematoxylin-eosin stain; ×200.)

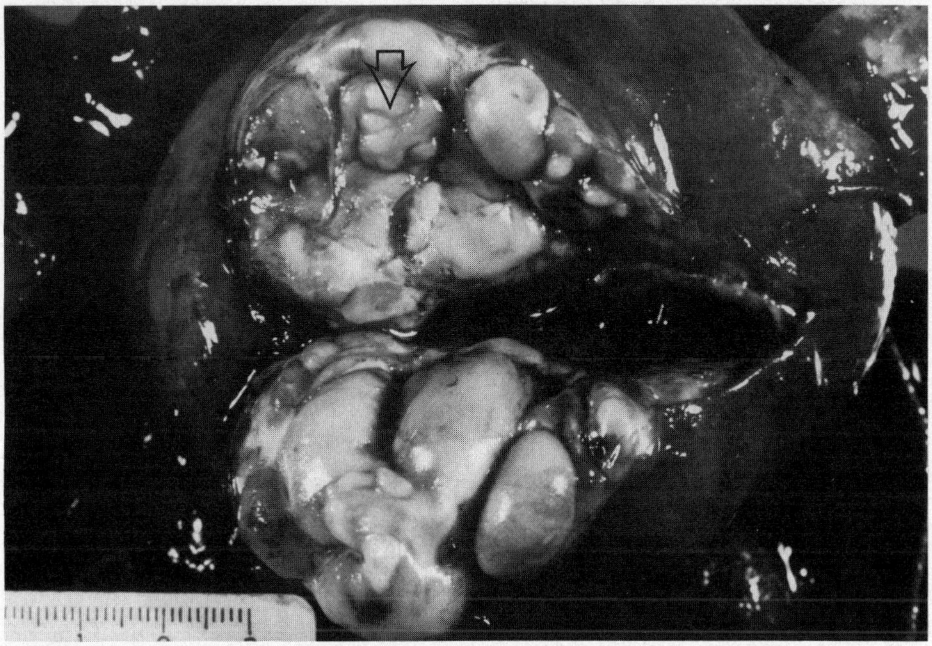

Fig. 34-6. Gross photograph of ovarian veins filled with a lobulated, bulging tumor mass *(arrow)*. This is one way in which intravenous leiomyomatosis can develop.

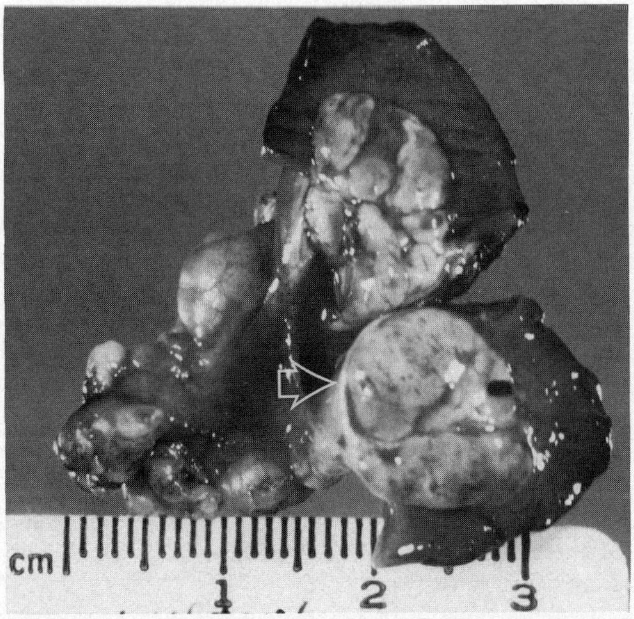

Fig. 34-7. This gross photograph dramatically demonstrates a nephrectomy specimen with renal cell carcinoma filling and distending the renal vein *(arrow)*. These tumors may grow intravascularly to fill the entire inferior vena cava and may reach the right atrium.

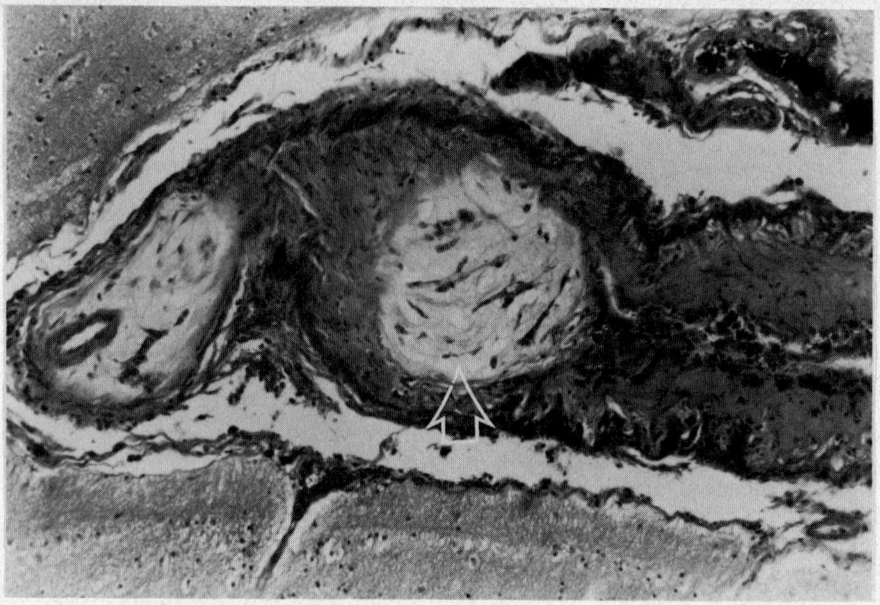

Fig. 34-8. Photomicrograph of a cerebral vessel containing an embolus *(arrow)* from a cardiac myxoma. Note the partial recanalization of the tumor embolus. (Hematoxylin-eosin stain; ×300.)

are part of this syndrome.[50,51] The complex is familial and probably autosomal dominant. It occurs primarily in young people. Individual patients usually do not manifest all of the components of the complex. In contrast to the typical cardiac myxoma, those associated with Carney's complex tend to be multicentric or multifocal and do exhibit more aggressive behavior than does the typical isolated cardiac myxoma.

VASCULAR TUMORS APPEARING AS SOFT TISSUE MASSES

Benign tumors

Cavernous hemangiomas. Cavernous hemangiomas may be deep seated. They are composed of large vascular channels that by exerting pressure on adjacent structures are locally destructive (Fig. 34-9). Thrombocytopenic purpura may complicate these hemangiomas, since it may complicate capillary hemangiomas, angiomatosis, or angiosarcomas. This syndrome is known as the Kasabach-Merritt syndrome and presents a difficult therapeutic problem because of the high risk of bleeding and infection associated with it.[1]

Arterial venous hemangiomas. These may also be in a deep location and may be associated with significant degrees of arterial venous shunting. In a deep location it is not clear whether these are truly neoplasms, as is implied by the term *hemangioma,* or whether they are really arterial venous malformations. They most commonly affect the head, neck, and lower extremities, and the larger shunts may visibly pulsate. Synonyms for this lesion include "racemose hemangioma" and "cirsoid aneurysm."[1] In addition to problems caused by the shunting, these lesions may be very painful because of pressure on adjacent nerves. The arterial venous communications are usually numerous, so ligation is not curative. Surgical excision of the lesion is often required.

Deep-seated cavernous and arteriovenous hemangiomas are the two hemangiomas that are most likely to come to the attention of the vascular physician and surgeon. The vascularity of the lesions, multiple feeding vessels, and associated bleeding problems may result in a therapeutic challenge even though they are benign.

Malignant tumors

Angiosarcoma. Angiosarcomas are rare, malignant vascular tumors of endothelial cells.[52] In contrast to other sarcomas, they have a predilection to involve skin and superficial subcutaneous tissue rather than deep soft tissue.[53] They vary from tumors resembling benign hemangiomas to very anaplastic, highly undifferentiated neoplasms, which are difficult to distinguish from carcinoma or melanoma. Angiosarcomas that arise in the setting of chronic lymphedema have been called *lymphangiosarcomas*[54] but are histologically indistinguishable from other angiosarcomas. However, since these tumors have a distinct clinical presentation, they are considered here as a separate entity.

Angiosarcomas can arise at any age, but are most often seen in the sixth and seventh decades.[52] The most common sites are the skin, especially the scalp, and subcutaneous tissue,[53,55] but they have also been described in the breast, bone, and liver.[56,57] Angiosarcomas of the liver have been

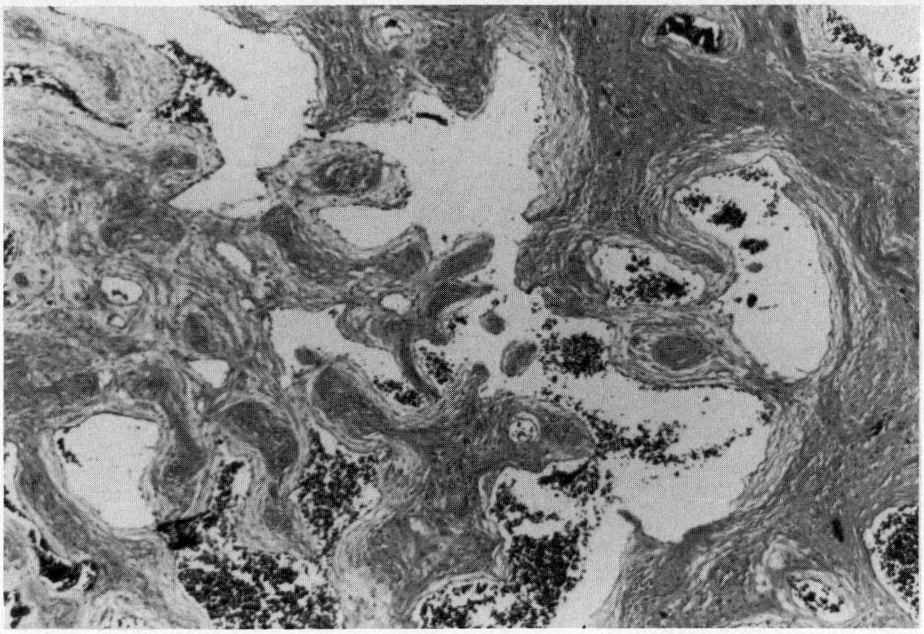

Fig. 34-9. Cavernous hemangiomas are composed of dilated, endothelial-lined vascular channels, as shown in this photomicrograph. These tumors are often located in the liver and may be either locally destructive or clinically silent. They are often incidental findings at autopsy, as in this case. (Hematoxylin-eosin stain; ×80.)

found to be associated with vinyl chloride and Thorotrast exposure.[57,58] Radiation-induced angiosarcomas have also been reported.[55]

Even though angiosarcomas are tumors of endothelial cells, tumors arising in the heart and major blood vessels are rare, comprising only 3% of all angiosarcomas.[3,59,60] Those that do arise in the major blood vessels have most often been associated with the aorta[59] but may rarely involve veins such as the superior vena cava or axillary vein.[61,62] These rare tumors can cause vascular obstruction or develop as a pulsatile mass lesion.

Manifestation of cutaneous angiosarcomas usually involves a bruiselike, firm, or ulcerated lesion on the scalp of an elderly person.[63] Angiosarcomas of the breast usually occur in reproductive-age women as rapidly growing masses that cause diffuse breast enlargement with a blue or purple discoloration of the overlying skin.[56] Symptoms of hepatic angiosarcomas are more nonspecific, including fatigue, weight loss, and abdominal pain.[57]

Grossly, angiosarcomas, regardless of location, are ill-defined hemorrhagic masses with areas of spongelike cystic spaces.[53,56] In angiosarcomas involving the skin, the overlying skin surface may be ulcerated.[53,63] Histologically, these tumors range from deceptively benign-looking neoplasms with large dilated vessels resembling hemangiomas to very high-grade tumors composed of sheets of anaplastic cells.[56] The characteristic pattern consists of an interanastomosing network of vessel-like structures lined by large cells with malignant features (Fig. 34-10). Positive identification of the cell type as endothelial is not always possible, since many angiosarcomas fail to react with immunohistochemical stains for endothelial cells, such as factor VIII related antigen.[52,64]

The prognosis in most types of angiosarcoma, whether located in the skin, breast, or liver, is relatively poor.[56,63] In a series of 72 patients with angiosarcoma of the face and scalp, Holden, Spittle, and Jones[63] found only a 12% 5-year survival rate. Angiosarcomas of the breast are among the most malignant of breast tumors, with 90% of patients dead of disease within 2 years.[56] Metastasis is usually early and is primarily hematogenous, with most of the spread occurring to the lungs, skin, and bone. However, lymph node metastasis has also been described, especially in angiosarcomas of the head and neck.[53] In cutaneous angiosarcoma, some prognostic implications can be made with tumor size when it appears. Tumors less than 5 cm have a better prognosis than larger lesions.[55] The prognosis also is better if the primary tumor can be completely excised.[55] The value of adjunct radiation or chemotherapy is minimal, since little seems to halt the progression of this highly malignant neoplasm.

Lymphangiosarcoma. Lymphangiosarcomas are highly aggressive tumors that generally arise in the setting of chronic lymphedema. Most cases are reported following the development of postmastectomy lymphedema for breast cancer and are referred to as *Stewart-Treves syndrome*[65] (Fig. 34-11). These rare tumors are found in less than 1% of all patients with breast cancer.[66]

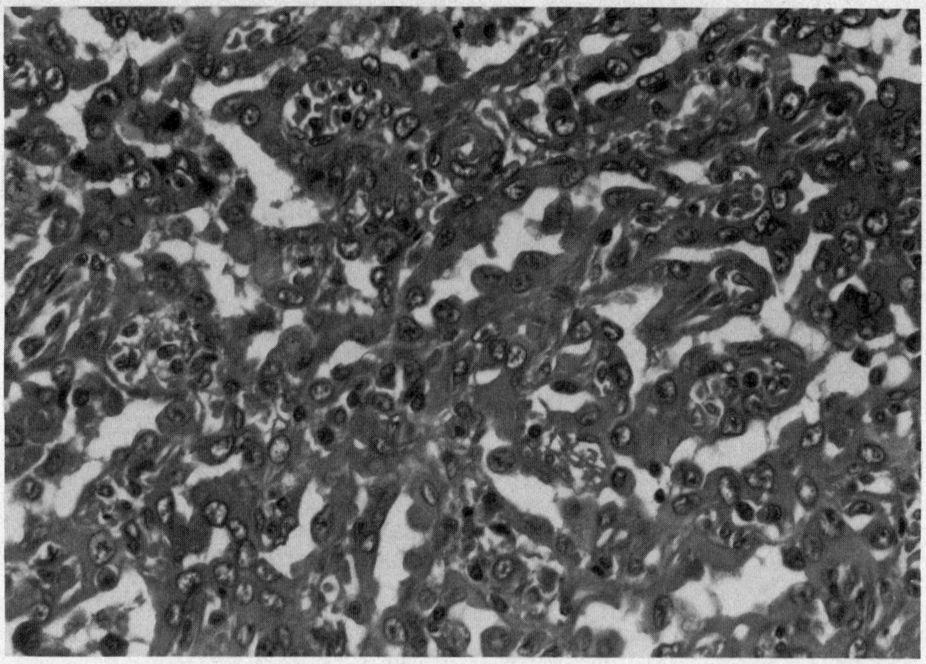

Fig. 34-10. Photomicrograph of an angiosarcoma, demonstrating the vascular-like channels lined by large, anaplastic cells. (Hematoxylin-eosin stain; ×350.)

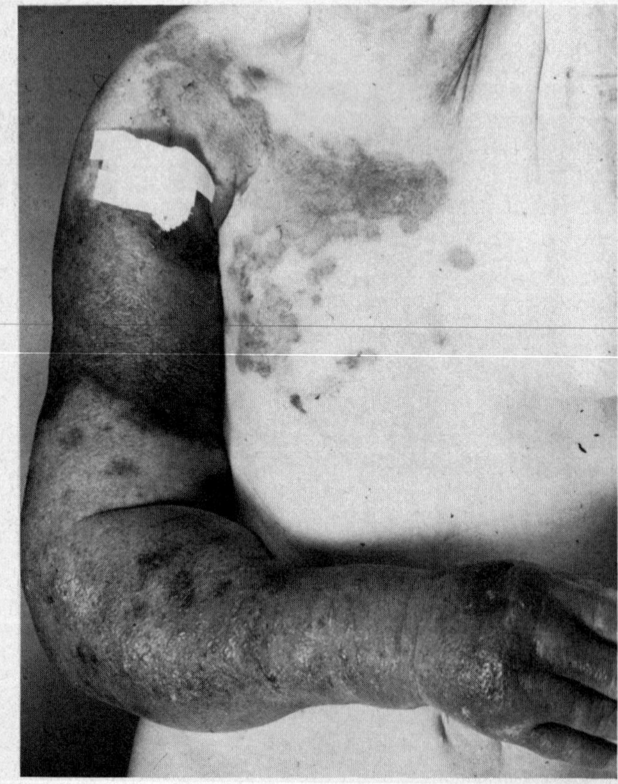

Fig. 34-11. Gross photograph of a lymphangiosarcoma arising in the right arm following mastectomy for breast carcinoma. Note the presence of lymphedema in the affected limb.

Although generally found in the upper extremity, lymphangiosarcomas are also found in the lower extremity; in areas without lymphedema; and in congenital, idiopathic, or traumatic lymphedema.[67-73]

Lymphangiosarcomas are actually angiosarcomas that arise from vascular endothelial cells and are histologically identical to angiosarcomas arising without lymphedema. They usually occur in the fifth to seventh decade of life, approximately 10 years after the original mastectomy. In the congenital, traumatic, or idiopathic setting, they may occur at a much younger age but at later intervals from the onset of lymphedema.[70]

The etiology of lymphangiosarcomas may be multifactorial and includes persistent lymphedema following radical mastectomy, radiation therapy, and local defects in cellular immunity.[67,74] Greater than 90% of all cases reported in one series were associated with a chronic lymphedematous extremity after mastectomy.[67]

Although radiation treatment is often associated with the development of lymphangiosarcomas, it is probably less important than lymphedema itself and perhaps serves only to aggravate this condition.[71,72]

Clinically, lymphangiosarcomas appear either as solitary or multiple lesions, purplish-red to bluish-red, and as macular lesions or palpable purpura and nodules. They may progress to ulcerations or become necrotic. Lymphangiosarcomas may be initially confused with an ecchymosis or cellulitis, often delaying their correct diagnosis. They frequently recur locally, following wide local excision or amputation. They spread proximally and distally and eventually metastasize to the lungs, pleura, chest wall, shoulder, liver, or bone.[1]

Current treatment methods include surgery, chemotherapy, or irradiation. Overall, all three have a poor prognosis, although amputation, including shoulder disarticulation and hindquarter or forequarter amputation, offers the best option.[67,74,75] Wide local excision is not as effective. Radiotherapy and chemotherapy have not been proven as effective, although some success has been reported by Yap et al with the use of multiple chemotherapeutic agents.[75]

Despite aggressive surgical intervention including amputation, median survival time is only 19 months in those patients who develop lymphangiosarcoma following mastectomy and 34 months following the development of these tumors in the nonmastectomy patient.[67]

Early recognition and prompt biopsy followed by aggressive surgical intervention afford the best treatment.[76] Several authors have speculated that the current trend toward the use of less radical surgical procedures involving breast cancer and the prompt treatment of cellulitis may help decrease the incidence of this condition.[73]

Kaposi's sarcoma. Kaposi's sarcoma was first described by Moritz Kaposi in 1872 and initially termed *idiopathic multiple pigmented hemorrhagic sarcoma*.[77] This tumor has been largely found in the central equatorial regions of Africa where it is endemic and represents as many as 9% of all reported malignancies.[78] Kaposi's sarcoma was considered an uncommon tumor in the United States and Europe, found mainly in the lower extremities of older men, until the recent epidemic emergence in association with the acquired immunodeficiency syndrome (AIDS).

There are four epidemiologic classifications of Kaposi's sarcoma, which include classic, or sporadic; endemic; epidemic; and that associated with immunosuppressive therapy.[79] Classic, or sporadic, Kaposi's sarcoma is a disease of elderly men found between the fifth and seventh decade of life, with a predilection for Ashkenazi Jews and southern Europeans. It is usually located on the lower extremities and generally has a relatively benign course. Endemic Kaposi's sarcoma is found in central Africa, often in younger patients. It may affect the lower extremities but can also be found in the gastrointestinal tract, lymph nodes, or bones. Four subtypes have been described, including florid, infiltrative, nodular, and lymphadenopathic.[79,80] The florid and infiltrative forms are more aggressive, rapidly growing, and deeply invasive, involving the dermis and bone, while the nodular form is generally more benign. The lymphadenopathic subtype is seen mainly in children who develop large, symmetrical tumors in their lymph nodes. Epidemic Kaposi's sarcoma is associated with AIDS and is seen most often in homosexual and bisexual men. The incidence is lower in the other AIDS risk groups—heterosexual drug addicts, blood transfusion recipients, and hemophiliacs.[81-83] This is an aggressive disease involving visceral dissemination and multiple skin lesions. The immunosuppressive form of Kaposi's sarcoma is found in renal transplant recipients or in patients who have received immunosuppressive agents for other diseases.[84]

The etiology of Kaposi's sarcoma is multifactorial. Genetic, geographic, and viral factors all play a role as well as the immunocompetence of the host.[1] Its association with AIDS is highly suggestive of a viral cause, given the high transmission rate of hepatitis B and cytomegalovirus (CMV) in this group. The immunocompetence of the host is suggested by the presence of Kaposi's sarcoma in patients receiving immunosuppressive agents and in AIDS. Genetic and geographic roles are suggested because of the striking incidence in the indigenous black population of Africa and the increase in certain other population groups including the Ashkenazi Jews and southern Europeans.

Kaposi's sarcoma is a vascular tumor of endothelial origin. Grossly, it appears on the skin or viscera as a multicentric, red-blue, purple, or reddish-brown nodule or plaque. Histologically, there are two important features, the spindle cell and the presence of vascular proliferation. Initially, an inflammatory pattern is seen with large numbers of lymphocytes, plasma cells, and large mononuclear cells. This may resemble granulation tissue. As the lesions evolve, proliferating vascular channels or capillaries are seen, and the inflammatory response diminishes. Hemosiderin deposits are noted in the dermis and give the nodules and plaques their purple or brown appearance. Later, the spindle cell, the first neoplastic element, becomes recognizable. These cells often form interlacing bundles and consist of round or oval nuclei with elongated cytoplasms. Spindle cells in Kaposi's sarcoma may resemble well-differentiated fibrosarcomas and are diagnostic for this disease.[1]

Clinically, Kaposi's sarcoma may appear as a solitary nodule or papule localized to the feet or ankles. These lesions may vary in size and may coalesce into plaques, nodules, ulcerations, or even polypoid growths (Fig. 34-12).[1] In the epidemic form lesions may be multiple and are seen on the trunk, arms, head, and neck. These lesions are occasionally symmetrical and follow the path of a superficial vein. They may be tender, painful, pruritic, and associated with edema. Over 90% of all cases involve men. An increased association with second malignancies including lymphomas, leukemia, Hodgkin's disease, melanoma, and multiple myeloma is reported.[85-87]

Visceral involvement is unusual in the classic form, but dissemination to the gastrointestinal tract, lungs, bone, liver, lymph nodes, and virtually every organ system is possible in the other types. Hemorrhages into the pulmonary or gastrointestinal tract may occur and can cause difficult management problems. Pulmonary involvement may lead to diffusion capacity abnormalities. Central nervous system involvement is rare. Classic Kaposi's sarcoma usually behaves in an indolent fashion, and a conservative approach

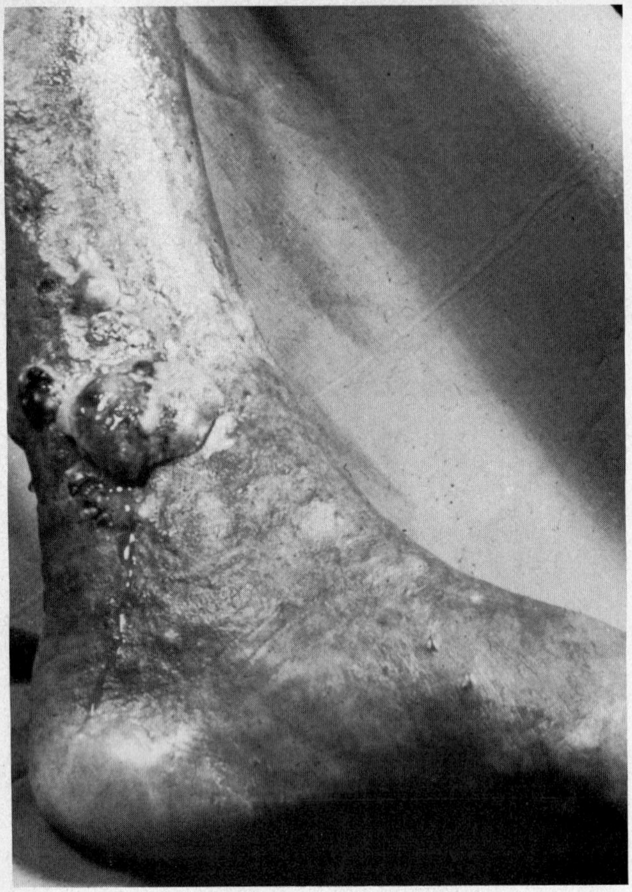

Fig. 34-12. Gross photograph of Kaposi's sarcoma involving the medial aspect of the right leg.

to treatment may be warranted. A support hose to minimize edema and localized radiation therapy may be sufficient, although surgery is used occasionally for the solitary lesions. In the classic form the prognosis is usually good, although chemotherapy or extended field radiation is needed when the tumor is more aggressive.

In the other forms of Kaposi's sarcoma a wide range of chemotherapeutic agents have been tried. These include both single agents and combined therapy using bleomycin, adriamycin, dactinomycin, vincristine, and vinblastine.[88] In the immunosuppressive form, discontinuing the drugs is necessary. In Kaposi's sarcoma associated with AIDS the use of interferon therapy is also advocated.[89] The prognosis is much worse in this group. Patients die less frequently from the tumor, however, than from the wasting, cachexia, and opportunistic infections.[88]

Hemangiopericytoma. Hemangiopericytoma is an uncommon tumor comprising only 1% of all blood vessel–related neoplasms, with a spectrum of clinical manifestations from benign to overtly malignant.[90] Hemangiopericytomas are thought to arise from pericytes, mesenchymal cells that underlie the basement membrane of capillaries.[91,92] At one time, hemangiopericytomas were thought to be related to glomus tumors, but subsequent studies have revealed the two to be separate entities.[93]

Hemangiopericytomas may occur at any age, but are most common in the fifth and sixth decades.[94,95] Rare cases have been described in infants and children,[96] although these generally behave in a benign fashion. Hemangiopericytomas are most often located in the lower extremities or retroperitoneum[90,92,94] and involve deep soft tissues or muscle. Symptoms usually are related to a painless mass, which has been enlarging slowly. Apart from the lower extremities, hemangiopericytomas can be found intracranially, where distinction from angioblastic meningiomas may be problematic.[97] Sinonasal,[98] pulmonary,[99] and pelvic or uterine hemangiopericytomas[100] have also been reported. However, Enzinger and Weiss consider uterine hemangiopericytomas to be highly vascular stromal tumors.[1] Hemangiopericytomas rarely have been described to involve large vessels such as the aorta.[101,102] Paraneoplastic syndromes, including hypoglycemia and gynecomastia, occasionally have been associated with hemangiopericytoma.[103] There is one report of a familial hemangiopericytoma occurring in three members of one family.[104]

X-ray and CT studies of hemangiopericytomas show a radiopaque soft tissue mass that often displaces adjacent structures and may rarely be calcified.[95] Pelvic tumors often have associated hydronephrosis and hydroureter.[95,100] Because of the richly vascular nature of the hemangiopericytoma, contrast-enhanced CT and angiography will show a dense, well-circumscribed stain resulting from contrast accumulation in the tumor vascular bed.[95,105] These radiologic findings are not specific for hemangiopericytoma and must be differentiated from the more common soft tissue sarcomas, such as malignant fibrous histiocytoma (MFH), liposarcoma, and synovial sarcoma. MFH can also be hypervascular like hemangiopericytomas, but liposarcomas are often hypovascular, and synovial sarcomas often contain calcified foci.[95,105]

Grossly, hemangiopericytomas are usually solitary, well-circumscribed masses with dilated vascular spaces and areas of cystic degeneration.[92,94] Histologically, hemangiopericytomas have a rich network of dilated vascular spaces, characteristically assuming a branching, or "staghorn," morphology. These vascular spaces are lined by a layer of attenuated endothelial cells (Fig. 34-13). If reticulin stains are used, each vessel-like structure is seen to be surrounded by a reticulin network, with the reticulin further outlining the individual neoplastic pericytes.[90] This pattern differs from that of angiosarcomas, where most of the cell proliferation is within reticulin-lined spaces. Features predictive of malignant behavior are not well defined, but the presence of increased mitotic rate (greater than 4 mitoses/10 high power fields) and the presence of hemorrhage and necrosis have been suggested as helpful.[92,94] The presence of metastases is the only absolute criterion for malignancy, however.

Benign hemangiopericytomas are more frequent than

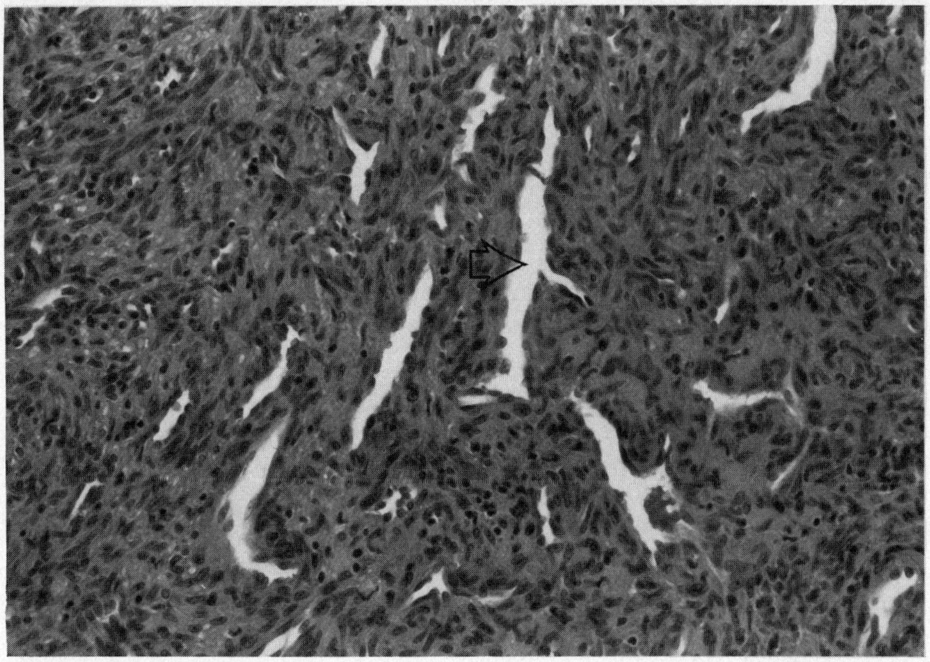

Fig. 34-13. Photomicrograph of a hemangiopericytoma showing the distinctive histologic features of this tumor. The combination of branched, or "staghorn," vessels *(arrow)* lined by low lying endothelial cells and surrounded by a highly cellular stroma. (Hematoxylin-eosin stain; ×150.)

those with malignant behavior.[92] In the literature the rate of metastases varies from 11.7%[106] to 56.5%,[107] with most being blood-borne to bone or lung. The infantile and sinonasal hemangiopericytomas, in contrast to their soft tissue counterparts, rarely recur or metastasize, regardless of histologic appearance.[96,98]

Treatment for well-differentiated hemangiopericytomas is usually complete excision, but more radical surgery may be required for tumors that display malignant features. Preoperative embolization has been employed to reduce tumor blood flow and facilitate resection.[106] Adjuvant radiation therapy and chemotherapy both have been tried, with relatively poor results.[94,106,108,109]

Hemangioendothelioma. While hemangiomas are benign vascular tumors, and angiosarcomas behave in a malignant fashion, there is a group of uncommon vascular tumors of intermediate malignancy, namely the hemangioendotheliomas. Three subtypes of hemangioendothelioma have been described, including epithelioid hemangioendothelioma (EH), spindle cell hemangioendothelioma, and malignant endovascular papillary angioendothelioma, or Dabska tumor.[110-112] These three subtypes are histologically distinct, yet all have a similar, relatively benign clinical course.

The EH is perhaps the best characterized and most frequent of the hemangioendotheliomas. It is a tumor composed of plump, epithelioid cells and is often vasocentric, most often involving a vein.[113] Originally described as a tumor of superficial and deep soft tissue,[110] it has become clear that EH may involve parenchymal sites, namely lung and liver.[114,115] Thus the intravascular bronchioloalveolar tumor (IVBAT) of the lung is now recognized to be an EH on the basis of ultrastructural and immunohistochemical studies. Likewise, EH has also been described in conjunction with large vessels,[116,117] as an osseous primary[118] and as a pleural neoplasm, grossly mimicking a mesothelioma.[119]

Epithelioid hemangioendotheliomas can arise at any age, but do not often occur in children.[113] The soft tissue type of EH may begin as a solitary, painful subcutaneous mass, while those EH associated with larger vessels may appear with obstructive vascular symptoms such as claudication or peripheral edema.[110,116,117] EH of the lung characteristically arise in young women, with chest x-ray films typically showing bilateral noncalcified parenchymal nodules.[114,119] In EH of the liver the initial symptoms are often abdominal pain and jaundice[115,120] but may also include venoocclusive symptoms.

Grossly, EH may resemble organizing thrombi, except for their tenacious attachment to the surrounding tissue[110] or may be gray or white and fibrous.[110] In the lung and liver EH often consists of multiple bulging tumor masses with central necrosis.[114,115]

Histologically, EH are composed of solid nests or sheets of plump cells with abundant eosinophilic cytoplasm resembling epithelioid cells seen in carcinoma.[110,113] Large vascular lumina are rarely, if ever, present to divulge the endothelial nature of these tumors. Rather, small intracytoplasmic lumina, sometimes containing erythrocytes, are present.[113] Frequently, these tumors can be mistaken for a carcinoma or melanoma on a histologic basis, but immunohistochemical stains with factor VIII related antigen or Ulex europaeus lectin will usually identify the endothelial nature of these tumors.[113]

The overall prognosis of soft tissue EH is quite favorable, with recurrences developing in 13% of patients and lymph node metastases in 31% of patients in one series.[113] Of those patients who developed metastases, less than one half died of disease. Because of the low-grade nature of these tumors, recommended treatment includes complete excision without adjuvant chemotherapy or radiotherapy.[113] Epithelioid hemangioendotheliomas of the lung and liver behave in a more aggressive manner than similar tumors confined to soft tissue, with a mortality of up to 65% from disease.[114,120] Liver transplantation has been successfully used as a treatment for hepatic EH, even in the presence of extrahepatic metastases.[120]

Brief mention will be made of the two other hemangioendotheliomas. A spindle cell hemangioendothelioma has recently been described by Weiss and Enzinger,[111] which appears as a slow-growing, painless nodule of the extremities or chest wall in patients of different ages. To differentiate it from EH, spindle cell hemangioendotheliomas are composed of two distinct histologic patterns: cavernous spaces resembling a hemangioma alternating with cellular areas of spindled cells with slitlike vascular spaces, resembling Kaposi's sarcoma.[111] Clinically over 50% of patients with spindle cell hemangioendothelioma experience local recurrence, but lymph node metastases and death from the disease is rare.

The malignant papillary angioendothelioma, or Dabska tumor, is a rare, low-grade angiosarcoma that appears as solitary, subcutaneous nodules in children.[112] Histologically, the Dabska tumor is distinctive, having cavernous spaces filled with tiny papillae lined by endothelial cells, some of which may display intracytoplasmic vacuolization.[121] Similar to other hemangioendotheliomas, the prognosis of the Dabska tumor appears to be good, despite the frequent presence of lymph node metastases.

REFERENCES

1. Enzinger FM and Weiss SW: Soft tissue tumors, ed 2, St Louis, 1988, The CV Mosby Co.
2. Fenoglio JJ Jr and Virmani R: Primary malignant tumors of the great vessels. In Waller BF, ed: Pathology of the heart and great vessels, vol 12, Contemporary issues in surgical pathology, New York, 1988, Churchill Livingstone, Inc.
3. McAllister HA Jr and Fenoglio JJ Jr: Tumors of the cardiovascular system, Atlas of tumor pathology, Armed Forces Institute of Pathology, 1978, Fascical 15, 2nd series.
4. Kevorkian J and Cento DP: Leiomyosarcoma of large arteries and veins, Surgery 73:390, 1973.
5. Wray RC and Dawkins H: Primary smooth muscle tumors of the inferior vena cava, Ann Surg 174:1009, 1971.
6. Pollanen M, Butany J, and Chiasson D: Leiomyosarcoma of the inferior vena cava, Arch Pathol Lab Med 111:1085, 1987.
7. Brewster DC, Athanasoulis A, and Darling RC: Leiomyosarcoma of the inferior vena cava, Arch Surg 111:1081, 1976.
8. Bailey RV et al: Leiomyosarcomas of the inferior vena cava, Ann Surg 184:169, 1976.
9. Stringer BD: Leiomyosarcoma of artery and vein, Am J Surg 134:90, 1977.
10. Shmookler BM, Marsh HB, and Roberts WC: Primary sarcoma of the pulmonary trunk and/or right or left main pulmonary artery: a rare cause of obstruction to right ventricular outflow, Am J Med 63:263, 1977.
11. Birkenstock WE and Lipper S: Leiomyosarcoma of the right common iliac artery: a case report, Br J Surg 63:81, 1976.
12. Altman NH and Shelley WM: Primary intimal sarcoma of the pulmonary artery, Johns Hopkins Med J 133:214, 1973.
13. Davis GL: Tumor and inflammatory conditions of the ear. In Gnepp DR, ed: Pathology of the head and neck, vol 10, Contemporary issues in surgical pathology, New York, 1988, Churchill Livingstone, Inc.
14. Tsuneyoshi M and Enjoji M: Glomus tumor: a clinicopathologic and electron microscopic study, Cancer 50:1601, 1982.
15. Shugart RR, Soule EH, and Johnson EW Jr: Glomus tumors, Surg Gynecol Obstet 117:334, 1963.
16. Chase WH: Familial and bilateral tumors of the carotid body, J Pathol and Bacteriol 36:1, 1933.
17. Lack EE, Cubilla AL, and Woodruff JM: Paragangliomas of the head and neck region: a pathologic study of tumors from 71 patients, Hum Pathol 10:191, 1979.
18. Saldana MJ, Salem LE, and Travezan R: High altitude hypoxia and chemodectomas, Hum Pathol 4:251, 1973.
19. Duke WW et al: A norepinephrine-secreting glomus jugulare tumor presenting as a pheochromocytoma, Ann Intern Med 60:1040, 1964.
20. Matsuguchi H et al: Noradrenaline-secreting glomus jugulare tumor with cyclic change of blood pressure, Arch Intern Med 135:1110, 1975.
21. Merino MJ and Livolsi VA: Malignant carotid body tumors: report of two cases and review of the literature, Cancer 47:1403, 1981.
22. Robertson DI and Cooney TP: Malignant carotid body paraganglioma: light and electron microscopic study of the tumor and its metastases, Cancer 46:2623, 1980.
23. Nora JD et al: Surgical resection of carotid body tumors: long-term survival, recurrence, and metastasis, Mayo Clin Proc 63:348, 1988.
24. Shamblin WR et al: Carotid body tumor (chemodectoma): clinicopathologic analysis of ninety cases, Am J Surg 122:732, 1971.
25. Meyer FB, Sundt TM Jr, and Pearson BW: Carotid body tumors: a subject review and suggested surgical approach, J Neurosurg 64:377, 1986.
26. Borges LF, Heros RC, and DeBrun G: Carotid body tumors managed with preoperative embolization, J Neurosurg 59:867, 1983.
27. Brismar J and Cronqvist S: Therapeutic embolization in the external carotid artery region, Acta Radiol Diagnosis 19:715, 1978.
28. Olson JL and Salyer WR: Mediastinal paragangliomas (aortic body tumor): a report of 4 cases and a review of the literature, Cancer 41:2405, 1978.
29. Pachter MR: Mediastinal nonchromaffin paraganglioma: a clinicopathologic study based on 8 cases, J Thorac Cardiovasc Surg 45:152, 1963.
30. Surakiatchanukul S, Goodsitt E, and Storer J: Chemodectoma of the aortic body, Chest 60:464, 1971.
31. D'Altorio RA, Rishi US, and Bhagwanani DG: Arteriographic findings in mediastinal chemodectoma, J Thorac Cardiovasc Surg 67:963, 1974.
32. Reddy EK, Mansfield CM, and Hartman GV: Chemodectoma of glomus jugulare, Cancer 52:337, 1983.
33. Alford BR and Guilford FR: A comprehensive study of tumors of the glomus jugulare, Laryngoscope 72:765, 1962.

34. van Baars F et al: Familial non-chromaffinic paragangliomas (glomus tumors): clinical aspects, Laryngoscope 91:988, 1981.
35. Brown JS: Glomus jugulare tumors revisited: a 10-year statistical follow-up of 231 cases, Laryngoscope 95:284, 1985.
36. Cole JM: Glomus jugulare tumors of the temporal bone: radiation of the glomus tumors of the temporal bone, Laryngoscope 89:1623, 1979.
37. Hashimoto H, Daimaru Y, and Enjoji M: Intravascular papillary endothelial hyperplasia: a clinicopathologic study of 91 cases, Am J Dermatopathol 5:539, 1983.
38. Hart WR and Yoonessi M: Endometrial stromatosis of the uterus, Obstet Gynecol 49:393, 1977.
39. Yoonessi M and Hart WR: Endometrial stromal sarcomas, Cancer 40:898, 1977.
40. Norris HJ and Parmley T: Mesenchymal tumors of the uterus v. intravenous leiomyomatosis: a clinical and pathologic study of 14 cases, Cancer 36:2164, 1975.
41. Harper RS and Scully RE: Intravenous leiomyomatosis of the uterus: a report of 4 cases, Obstet Gynecol 18:519, 1961.
42. Bennington JL: Tumors of the kidney. In Javadpor N and Barsky SH, eds: Surgical pathology of urologic disease, Baltimore, 1987, Williams & Wilkins.
43. Stocker JT and Ishak KG: Undifferentiated (embryonal) sarcoma of the liver: report of 31 cases, Cancer 42:336, 1978.
44. Symbas PN, Hatcher CR, and Gravanis MB: Myxoma of the heart: clinical and experimental observations, Ann Surg 183:470, 1976.
45. Shah AA et al: Malignant fibrous histiocytoma of the heart presenting as an atrial myxoma, Cancer 42:2466, 1978.
46. Harris LS and Adelson L: Fatal coronary embolism from a myxo matous polyp of the aortic valve: an unusual cause of death, Am J Clin Pathol 43:61, 1965.
47. Anderson KR, Fiddler GI, and Lie JT: Congenital papillary tumor of the tricuspid valve: an unusual cause of right ventricular outflow obstruction in a neonate with trisomy E, Mayo Clin Proc 52:665, 1977.
48. Budzilovich G, Aleksic S, and Greco A: Malignant cardiac myxoma with cerebral metastases, Surg Neurol 11:462, 1979.
49. Floriano de Morais C et al: Myocardial infarct due to a unique atrial myxoma with epithelial-like cells and systemic metastases, Arch Pathol Lab Med 112:185, 1988.
50. Carney JA: Differences between nonfamilial and familial cardiac myxoma, Am J Surg Pathol 9:53, 1985.
51. Carney JA et al: The complex of myxomas, spotty pigmentation and endocrine overactivity, Medicine 64:270, 1985.
52. Alles JU and Bosslet K: Immunocytochemistry of angiosarcomas: a study of 19 cases with special emphasis on the applicability of endothelial cell specific markers to routinely prepared tissues, Am J Clin Pathol 89:463, 1988.
53. Bardioil JM et al: Angiosarcomas of the head and neck region, Am J Surg 116:548, 1968.
54. Fisher JH: Postmastectomy lymphangiosarcoma in the lymphedematous arm: a review of 4 cases, Can J Surg 8:350, 1965.
55. Maddox JC and Evans HL: Angiosarcoma of skin and soft tissue: a study of 44 cases, Cancer 48:1907, 1981.
56. Donnell RM et al: Angiosarcoma and other vascular tumors of the breast: pathologic analysis as a guide to prognosis, Am J Surg Pathol 5:629, 1981.
57. Mark L et al: Clinical and morphologic features of hepatic angiosarcoma in vinyl chloride workers, Cancer 37:149, 1976.
58. Popper H et al: Development of hepatic angiosarcoma in man induced by vinyl chloride: Thorotrast and arsenic, Am J Pathol 92:349, 1978.
59. Kanno J, Takemura T, and Kasaga T. Malignant endothelioma of the aorta, Virchows Arch[A] 412:183, 1987.
60. Adachi K et al: Right atrial angiosarcoma diagnosed by cardiac biopsy, Am Heart J 115:482, 1988.
61. Abratt RP et al: Angiosarcoma of the superior vena cava, Cancer 52:740, 1983.
62. Alosco T et al: Angiosarcoma of the axillary vein, Cancer 64:1301, 1989.
63. Holden CA, Spittle MF, and Jones EW: Angiosarcoma of the face and scalp, prognosis and treatment, Cancer 59:1046, 1987.
64. Borgdorf WHC, Mukai K, and Rosai J: Immunohistochemical identification of factor VIII-related antigen in endothelial cells of cutaneous lesions of alleged vascular nature, Am J Clin Pathol 75:167, 1981.
65. Stewart F and Treves N: Lymphangiosarcoma in post mastectomy lymphedema, Cancer 1:64, 1948.
66. McConnell EM and Haslam P: Angiosarcoma in post-mastectomy lymphoedema: a report of five cases and a review of the literature, Br J Surg 46:322, 1959.
67. Woodward AH, Ivins JC, and Soule EH: Lymphangiosarcoma arising in chronic lymphedematous extremities, Cancer 30:562, 1972.
68. Eby CS, Brennan MJ, and Fine G: Lymphangiosarcoma: a lethal complication of chronic lymphedema—report of two cases and review of the literature, Arch Surg 94:223, 1967.
69. Merrick TA, Erlandson RA, and Hajdu SI: Lymphangiosarcoma of a congenitally lymphedematous arm, Arch Pathol 91:365, 1971.
70. MacKenzie DH: Lymphangiosarcoma arising in chronic congenital and idiopathic lymphoedema, J Clin Pathol 24:524, 1971.
71. Sordillo PP et al: Lymphangiosarcoma, Cancer 48:1674, 1981.
72. Gajarj H et al: Lymphangiosarcoma complicating chronic primary lymphoedema, Br J Surg 74:1180, 1987.
73. Schreiber H et al: Stewart-Treves syndrome: a lethal complication of post mastectomy lymphedema and regional immune deficiency, Arch Surg 114:82, 1979.
74. Tomita K et al: Lymphangiosarcoma in post-mastectomy lymphedema (Stewart-Treves syndrome): ultrastructural and immunohistologic characteristics, J Surg Oncol 38:275, 1988.
75. Yap BS et al: Chemotherapy for post-mastectomy lymphangiosarcoma, Cancer 47:853, 1981.
76. Borel Rinkes IHM and de Jongste AB: Lymphangiosarcoma in chronic lymphedema, Acta Chir Scand 152:227, 1986.
77. Kaposi M: Idiopathisches multiples pigment-sarkom der haut, Arch Derm Syph 4:265, 1872.
78. Niemi M and Mustakallio KK: The fine structure of the spindle cell in Kaposi's sarcoma, Acta Pathol Microbiol Scand 63:567, 1965.
79. Armes J: A review of Kaposi's sarcoma, Adv Cancer Res 53:73, 1989.
80. Taylor JF et al: Kaposi's sarcoma in Uganda: a clinicopathological study, Int J Cancer 8:122, 1971.
81. DeJarlais DC et al: Kaposi's sarcoma among four different AIDS risk groups, N Engl J Med 310:1119, 1984.
82. Cohn DL and Judson FN: Absence of Kaposi's sarcoma in hemophiliacs with the acquired immune deficiency syndrome, Ann Intern Med 101:401, 1984.
83. Padilla S, Rivera-Perlman Z, and Solomon L: Kaposi's sarcoma in transfusion-associated acquired immunodeficiency syndrome, Arch Pathol Lab Med 114:40, 1990.
84. Harwood AR et al: Kaposi's sarcoma in recipients of renal transplants, Am J Med 67:759, 1979.
85. Safai B et al: Association of Kaposi's sarcoma with second primary malignancies: possible etiopathogenic implications, Cancer 45:1472, 1980.
86. Law IP: Kaposi's sarcoma and plasma cell dyscrasia, JAMA 229(10):1329, 1974.
87. Gilbert TT, Evjy JT, and Edelstein L: Hodgkin's disease associated with Kaposi's sarcoma and malignant melanoma, Cancer 28:293, 1971.
88. Fauci AS et al: Acquired immunodeficiency syndrome: epidemiologic, clinical, immunologic, and therapeutic considerations, Ann Intern Med 100:92, 1984.
89. Groopman JE and Scadden DT: Interferon therapy for Kaposi sarcoma associated with the acquired immunodeficiency syndrome (AIDS), Ann Intern Med 110:335, 1989.

90. Stout AP and Murray MR: Hemangiopericytoma: a vascular tumor featuring Zimmerman's pericytes, Ann Surg 116:26, 1942.
91. Battifora H: Hemangiopericytoma: ultrastructural study of five cases, Cancer 31:1418, 1973.
92. Enzinger FM and Smith BH: Hemangiopericytoma: an analysis of 106 cases, Hum Pathol 7:61, 1976.
93. Stout AP: Tumors featuring pericytes: glomus tumor and hemangiopericytoma, Lab Invest 5:217, 1956.
94. McMaster MJ, Soule EH, and Ivins JC: Hemangiopericytoma: clinicopathologic study and long-term follow-up of 60 patients, Cancer 36:2232, 1975.
95. Lorigan JG et al: The clinical and radiologic manifestations of hemangiopericytoma, AJR 153:345, 1989.
96. Atkinson JB et al: Hemangiopericytoma in infants and children: a report of six patients, Am J Surg 148:372, 1984.
97. D'Amore ESG, Manivel JC, and Sung JH: Soft-tissue and meningeal hemangiopericytomas: an immunohistochemical and ultrastructural study, Hum Pathol 21:414, 1990.
98. Abdel-Fattah HM, Adams GL, and Wick MR: Hemangiopericytoma of the maxillary sinus and skull base, Head Neck Surg 12:77, 1990.
99. Rusch VW et al: Massive pulmonary hemangiopericytoma: an innovative approach to evaluation and treatment, Cancer 64:1928, 1989.
100. Munoz AK et al: Pelvic hemangiopericytomas: a report of five cases and literature review, Gynecol Oncol 36:380, 1990.
101. Bowles LT, Ring EM, and Hill WT: Hemangiopericytoma in a resected thoracic aortic aneurysm, Ann Thorac Surg 1:746, 1965.
102. Blenkinsopp WK and Hobs JT: Pedunculated hemangiopericytoma attached to the thoracic aorta, Thorax 21:193, 1966.
103. Howard JW and Davis PL: Retroperitoneal hemangiopericytoma associated with hypoglycemia and masculinization, Del Med J 31:29, 1959.
104. Plukker JT et al: Malignant hemangiopericytomas in three kindred members of one family, Cancer 61:841, 1988.
105. Goldman SM, Davidson AJ, and Neal J: Retroperitoneal and pelvic hemangiopericytomas: clinical, radiologic and pathologic correlation, Radiology 168:13, 1988.
106. Smullens SN et al: Preoperative embolization of retroperitoneal hemangiopericytomas as an aid in their removal, Cancer 50:1870, 1982.
107. O'Brien P and Brasfield RO: Hemangiopericytoma, Cancer 18:249, 1965.
108. Bredt AB and Serpick AH: Metastatic hemangiopericytoma treated with vincristine and actinomycin D, Cancer 24:266, 1969.
109. Mira JG, Chu FC, and Forner JG: The role of radiotherapy in the management of malignant hemangiopericytoma: report of 11 new cases and review of the literature, Cancer 39:1254, 1977.
110. Weiss SW and Enzinger FM: Epithelioid hemangioendothelioma: a vascular tumor often mistaken for a carcinoma, Cancer 50:970, 1982.
111. Weiss SW and Enzinger FM: Spindle cell hemangioendothelioma: a low grade angiosarcoma resembling a cavernous hemangioma and Kaposi's sarcoma, Am J Surg Pathol 10:521, 1986.
112. Dabska M: Malignant endovascular papillary angioendothelioma of the skin in childhood, Cancer 24:503, 1969.
113. Weiss SW et al: Epithelioid hemangioendothelioma and related lesions, Semin Diagn Pathol 3:259, 1986.
114. Dial D et al: Intravascular bronchiolar and alveolar tumor of the lung (IVBAT): an analysis of twenty cases of a peculiar sclerosing endothelial tumor, Cancer 51:451, 1983.
115. Ishak KG et al: Epithelioid hemangioendothelioma of the liver: a clinicopathologic and follow-up study of 32 cases, Hum Pathol 15:839, 1984.
116. Toursarkissian B, O'Connor WN, and Dillon ML: Mediastinal epithelioid hemangioendothelioma, Ann Thorac Surg 49:680, 1990.
117. Harris EJ Jr, Taylor LM Jr, and Porter JM: Epithelioid hemangioendothelioma of the external iliac vein: a primary vascular tumor presenting as traumatic venous obstruction, J Vasc Surg 10:693, 1989.
118. Dorfman HD, Tsuneyoshi M, and Bauer T: Epithelioid hemangioendothelioma of bone, Lab Invest 54:17, 1986.
119. Yousem SA and Hochholzer L: Unusual thoracic manifestations of epithelioid hemangioendothelioma, Arch Pathol Lab Med 111:459, 1987.
120. Marino IR et al: Treatment of hepatic epithelioid hemangioendothelioma with liver transplantation, Cancer 62:2079, 1988.
121. Manivel JC et al: Endovascular papillary endothelioma of childhood: a vascular lesion possibly characterized by high endothelial differentiation, Hum Pathol 17:1240, 1986.

Chapter 35

LEG ULCERS

Henry H. Roenigk, Jr.
Jess R. Young

Ulcerations of the lower extremity are fairly common and can present both a diagnostic and therapeutic problem to the physician. Leg ulcers are seen by both the general practitioner and the specialist. Because of the many problems involved in arriving at a proper diagnosis and course of treatment for leg ulcers, a comprehensive classification, diagnostic evaluation, and treatment program are needed for the patient who complains to the physician, "Doctor, what can you do about this ulcer I have on my lower leg?"

DIAGNOSIS OF LEG ULCERS

History

Since many leg ulcers have certain characteristic historic features, a comprehensive history of the ulcer, obtained through the following questions, is often necessary to establish a proper diagnosis:

1. What did the ulcer look like at first?
   Leg ulcers often change their appearance after secondary infection or after the application of many types of local medication, which may have been used in an attempt to heal the ulcer.
2. What started the ulcer?
   Local injury, strong medication, infection, thrombophlebitis, cold and factitial (self-induced) injury may be factors in precipitating the ulceration. Sometimes this is difficult to elicit.
3. What is the family history?
   This is particularly helpful in certain hematologic disorders (e.g., sickle cell anemia or thalassemia) and certain connective tissue disorders (e.g., systemic lupus erythematosus or rheumatoid arthritis).
4. How quickly did the ulcer develop?
   Rapidly developing ulcers suggest venous insufficiency; slowly developing ulcers suggest arterial insufficiency or malignancy.
5. How painful is the ulcer?
   Stasis ulcerations are often painless, whereas arterial ulcers are very painful. The patient with ischemic ulceration caused by arterial insufficiency often will sit in a chair all night and not elevate his legs because the dependent position gives him the best possible blood supply to his painful ulcers. Venous ulceration, on the other hand, often improves with elevation because this position relieves the edema of the surrounding tissues. Hypertensive ischemic ulcers and atrophie blanche vasculitis ulcers are very painful.
6. What drugs has the patient taken?
   It is important to obtain a complete list of all medications taken by the patient. Specific questions concerning nonprescription medications such as sedatives, sleeping pills, analgesic, and antacid medications should be included since these drugs can cause leg ulcers or lead to vasculitis with secondary ulceration.
7. Is there a history of other systemic disorders?
   A current or past history of anemia, rheumatoid arthritis, and collagen diseases often gives a clue to the cause of an unusual leg ulcer.

Physical examination

1. Where is the ulcer?
   Ulcers resulting from venous stasis are often located over the medial malleolus because this area is drained by the saphenous venous system and the perforating veins. These ulcers will usually be located over the inner aspect of the ankle but can be posterior, anterior, or lateral on occasion. Ischemic ulcers occur on areas farthest from the occluded vessel. The common location of ischemic ulcers caused by arteriosclerosis is the toes or dorsum of the foot. Hypertensive ischemic ulcers tend to occur on the lateral malleolus.
2. What is the condition of the surrounding skin?

The surrounding skin should be closely examined for stasis pigmentation, edema, varicose veins, evidence of scleroderma, petechia, or hemorrhage. The color of the skin is important. A pale color indicates poor arterial blood supply, as in ischemic ulcers.

3. Are there signs of other systemic diseases?
These will be discussed in detail later in this chapter, but a heart murmur of cardiovascular syphilis, arthritis caused by systemic lupus erythematosus, or other signs of diabetes mellitus (e.g., eyeground changes) are helpful in determining the cause of the leg ulcer.

Laboratory tests

The tests in the accompanying box are divided into three groups. Group I should be done for any leg ulcer. Groups II and III are specifically for the more unusual types of leg ulcers.

Laboratory tests

I. *Routine laboratory studies*
- A. CBC
- B. Urinalysis
- C. SMA-20
- D. Chest x-ray
- E. Bacterial culture
- F. Serologic test for syphilis (VDRL, FTA abs)

II. *Special laboratory test*
- A. Antinuclear factor/anti-DNA
- B. Serum complement
- C. Special antibody studies (ENA, SSM, SSA)
- D. Latex fixation for rheumatoid arthritis
- E. Sickle cell preparation
- F. Special hematologic tests
- G. X-rays: CT scans for malignancy, colon (ulcerative colitis), and others as indicated
- H. Fungus cultures
- I. Skin tests: PPD
- J. Urinary porphyrins
- K. Skin biopsy and special stains: H & E, I-F, acid-fast
- L. Muscle biopsy

III. *Vascular*
- A. Arterial noninvasive
  1. Doppler waveforms
  2. Segmental pressures
  3. Pulse volume recordings
- B. Venous noninvasive
  1. Doppler
  2. Duplex ultrasound
  3. Plethysmography
- C. Invasive
  1. Angiography

CLASSIFICATION OF LEG ULCERS

There are many classifications of leg ulcers.[1] Some are purely clinical and are mainly concerned with subdivision of the two major causes, arterial and venous. Some are purely histopathologic with various subdivisions of the histology of vasculitis or inflammatory skin lesions. The classifications in the box on p. 607 are a combination of clinical and histologic findings with emphasis on the clinical.

VASCULAR LEG ULCERS

Arterial leg ulcers

Leg ulcers secondary to arteriosclerosis obliterans. Arteriosclerosis obliterans (ASO), which is discussed in detail in Chapter 9, is a progressive disease that is becoming a more frequent cause of ischemic ulcers of the leg and foot. Ulceration in ASO usually appears in the terminal portions of the digits, often around the nails or in a nailbed following infection (Fig. 35-1). The ulcers are also common over bony prominences such as the first and fifth metatarsal heads, the heel, and the malleoli (Fig. 35-2). They may result from the normal pressures of shoes or may develop in corns or bunions as the result of infection or too vigorous treatment. If the ulcer is on the leg, it is usually the result of mechanical or thermal trauma.

Ischemic ulcers are usually small and shallow initially, gradually increasing in size. The base of the ulcer is often gray, yellow, or black (see Fig. 35-2) and may be covered by necrotic debris and crusted exudates. Granulation tissue is minimal or absent. The rim of the ulcer is indolent, showing no tendency for proliferation or epithelialization. There may be secondary infection, especially in diabetics. This infection usually inhibits healing and produces a chronic purulent drainage. Osteomyelitis or suppurative arthritis may complicate deep ulcerations. Common associated findings in patients with ulcerations secondary to ASO are the lack or decrease of leg pulses, atrophy of leg muscles with loss of muscle tone, deformities of the toenails, absence of hair growth on the dorsum of the foot and toes, and atrophy of the skin. Edema of the foot and leg may occur if the patient has been sitting up nightly in an attempt to relieve the pain of the ulcer.

Diagnosis. To determine the presence and severity of arterial insufficiency, no unusual or elaborate equipment is necessary although noninvasive Doppler and plethysmographic techniques are common today. An adequate evaluation may be accomplished in any physician's office. The most important finding from a physical examination is an absence or a decrease in amplitude of arterial pulsations. A good index for the severity of ischemia is a change in color of the feet with alterations in positions of the limb. After elevating the limb for about one minute, an abnormal pallor in the foot and leg will appear when there is significant ischemia. On subsequent dependence there is delay in filling of the veins beyond the normal 10-to-15-second period.

Classifications of leg ulcers

I. *Vascular*

- A. Arterial
  1. Arteriosclerosis obliterans
  2. Thromboangiitis obliterans
  3. Livedo reticularis
  4. Hypertension
  5. Chronic pernio (chronic chilblains)
- B. Venous: chronic venous insufficiency (stasis)
- C. Lymphatic: elephantiasis nostras (lymphedema)

II. *Vasculitis*

- A. Atrophie blanche
- B. Allergic vasculitis
- C. Lupus erythematosus
- D. Necrotizing angiitis
- E. Periarteritis nodosa
- F. Rheumatoid arthritis
- G. Malignant atrophic papulosis (Degos' disease)
- H. Scleroderma

III. *Hematologic*

- A. Sickle cell anemia
- B. Spherocytic anemia
- C. Thalassemia
- D. Polycythemia vera
- E. Leukemia
- F. Dysproteinemia: macroglobulinemia, cryoglobulinemia

IV. *Infectious*

- A. Fungus
  1. Blastomycosis
  2. Coccidiomycosis
  3. Histoplasmosis
  4. Sporotrichosis
  5. Maduromycosis
- B. Syphilis: secondary and tertiary
- C. Bacterial infections: primary, secondary
- D. Tuberculosis
  1. Erythema induratum
  2. Lupus vulgaris
  3. Papulonecrotic tuberculid
- E. Leprosy
- F. Atypical mycobacterial

V. *Metabolic disorders*

- A. Diabetic neurotrophic ulcer
- B. Necrobiosis lipoidica diabeticorum
- C. Pyoderma gangrenosum
- D. Gaucher's disease
- E. Gout
- F. Porphyria cutanea tarda

VI. *Tumors*

- A. Basal cell carcinoma
- B. Squamous cell carcinoma
- C. Kaposi's hemorrhagic sarcoma (classic type)
- D. Lymphoma
  1. Lymphosarcoma
  2. Mycosis fungoides
- E. Melanoma

VII. *Miscellaneous*

- A. Drugs
  1. Halogens
  2. Ergotism
  3. Methotrexate
  4. Illicit drug use
- B. Chemical burns
- C. Trophic ulcers (neuropathic)
- D. Thermal
- E. Lichen planus
- F. Weber-Christian disease (panniculitis)
- G. Acrodermatitis chronica atrophicans
- H. Insect bite
- I. Radiation
- J. Frostbite
- K. Factitial (self-induced)

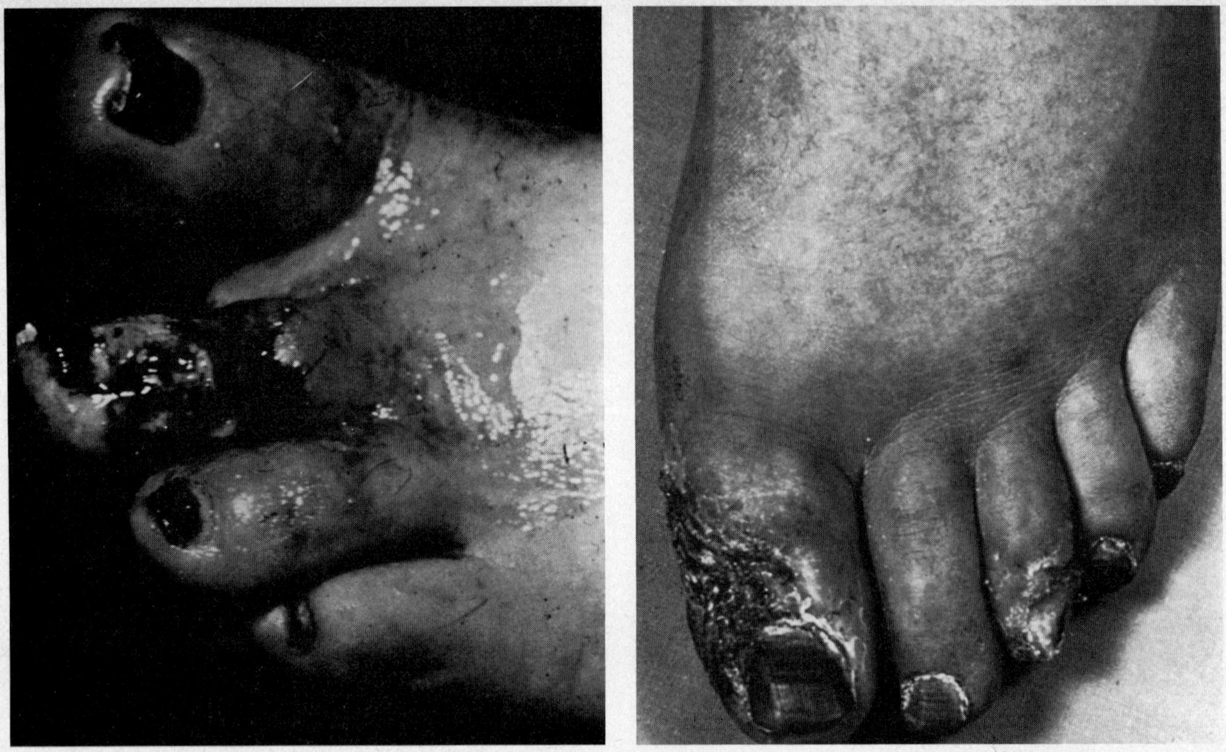

Fig. 35-1. Arteriosclerosis obliterans (ASO) ulcers of the terminal portions of the digits with necrosis of the skin.

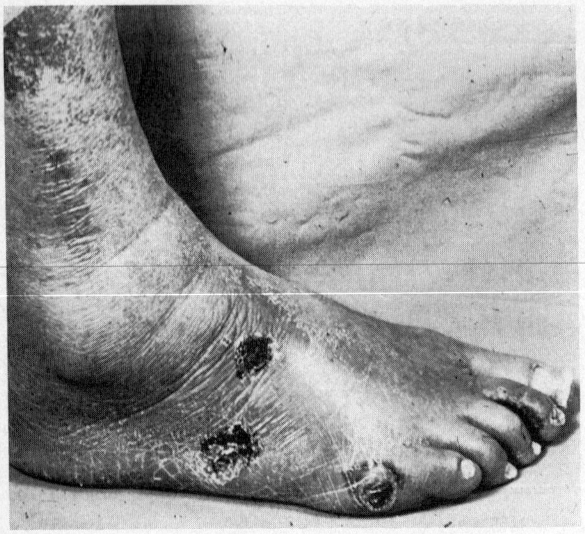

Fig. 35-2. ASO ulcers, gray or black, with poor granulation tissue in the base.

When the color does return, it may be bright red, the rubor of dependency.

Doppler measurement of ankle blood pressure will provide additional data on the severity of arterial disease. A useful ratio is a comparison of the ankle pressure, to the brachial arm pressure, or ankle-brachial index. A normal ratio is 1.0 or greater.

Arteriograms are not necessary unless arterial surgical repair of major peripheral vessels is contemplated. They then give valuable information as to the site, extent, and operability of the occlusive arterial lesions. For a more complete discussion regarding the diagnosis of ASO, see Chapter 9.

Differential diagnosis. In chronic venous insufficiency the ulcers are rarely as painful as ischemic ulcers. Dependency usually relieves the pain of ischemic ulcers while it increases the discomfort of stasis ulcers. The typical locations of the stasis ulcers in the region of the ankle, particularly just behind the medial malleolus, would be unusual sites for ischemic ulcers. The area around the stasis ulcer shows typical changes of pigmentation and induration. The base of the stasis ulcer is usually weeping and has extensive granulation tissue, while ischemic ulcers are dry with little or no granulations. Pulses are usually present in patients with stasis ulcers, but even if they are absent, the other features mentioned above should be sufficient to make the diagnosis.

Hypertensive ischemic ulcers are most commonly seen on the lateral or posterior aspect of the legs, and are usually surrounded by a bluish-red ischemic rim of tissue. The patient is hypertensive and has normal pulses.

Treatment. Patients in bed with severe ischemia should be watched carefully and protected from pressure on heels or other bony prominences by the use of padded boots, sheepskin, or a flotation mattress. Pressure from bed clothes should be prevented by the use of a foot cradle. The head of the bed should be elevated 4 to 6 inches to increase the blood flow to the feet. A warm environmental temperature helps produce reflex vasodilation.

All patients should be asked to refrain from smoking. Repeated use of analgesics may be necessary for temporary relief of ischemic pain. A tranquilizer may be helpful in alleviating the anxiety often associated with severe pain, and may potentiate the effect of the analgesics. Narcotics should be used with caution because the chronicity of the pain may lead to addiction. Systemic antibiotics are usually not necessary unless the ulcer is associated with obvious cellulitis or lymphangitis or unless there is evidence of a systemic infection with chills or fever.

The precipitating cause of many severely ischemic ulcers is trauma from mechanical, chemical, or thermal sources. Patients should therefore be given detailed instructions concerning the care of their extremities and the avoidance of further trauma. They should be carefully advised regarding care of nails, avoidance of extremes of hot and cold temperatures, and proper treatment of athlete's foot. Ingrown toenails, corns, and calluses should be treated by a physician or a podiatrist who is aware of the fact that the patient has ischemic extremities.

The value of oral vasodilator drugs is a controversial subject. Most authorities have not found them to be effective. Pentoxifylline, a hemorrheologic agent, may be helpful to some patients.

Strong chemical solutions should be avoided as applications to ischemic ulcers. Lukewarm wet dressings, or intermittent soaks using 0.9% sodium chloride, 5% boric acid solution, or Burow's compresses may promote drainage and loosen sloughs and crusts. The temperature of the solutions applied to ischemic lesions should never exceed 35° C. Maceration of viable tissue should be avoided. Culture and sensitivity studies should be made for all ulcerations, although healing is usually not promoted by antibiotic ointments unless the ulcer is grossly infected. To remove adherent necrotic crusts or eschars from ischemic ulcers, enzymatic débridement has limited value. Surgical débridement, done carefully, may help. Hydrocolloid dressings (see *Leg ulcers secondary to chronic venous insufficiency*) may also help.

Ointments containing anesthetic agents often increase tissue necrosis even though they help relieve pain, and their use should be discouraged. At no time should adhesive tape for dressings be applied directly to ischemic skin.

Skin grafting for indolent ulcers is occasionally of value, but the ulcer should be as clean as possible and should have some granulation tissue in its base before grafting is attempted.

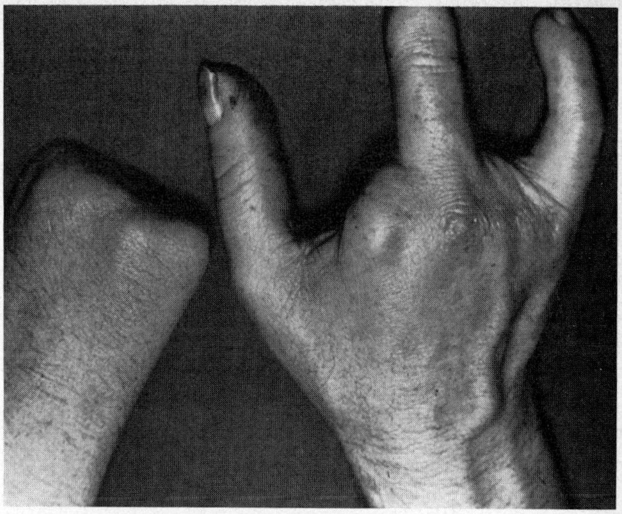

Fig. 35-3. Gangrene of the fingers resulted in multiple amputations in this man with thromboangiitis obliterans.

Surgical and nonsurgical approaches to improve arterial circulation are discussed in Chapter 9.

Leg ulcers secondary to thromboangiitis obliterans. Thromboangiitis obliterans (TAO) is a disease of the arteries and veins of the extremities and rarely of the viscera, which develops predominantly in young men and women who smoke. It is discussed in detail in Chapter 19.

Clinical features. The typical patient with TAO is a young person less than 40 years of age, who smokes, who has occlusive arterial disease distal to the popliteal artery or in the hand, and who has a history of, or presence of, a superficial thrombophlebitis.

Severe ischemic changes of ulceration and gangrene are frequent manifestations of TAO and may develop early in the disease. The toes are most commonly affected, especially around the margins of the nails. Ischemic symptoms in the upper extremities occur in about 40% of patients, especially ulcerations around the fingertips and gangrene of the fingers (Fig. 35-3). Superficial phlebitis also occurs at some stage in the disease in about 40% of patients with TAO.

Treatment. All patients with TAO should abstain from using tobacco in all forms. This abstinence should be complete and permanent, and there can be no compromise. The patient should be warned that even an occasional cigarette may be enough to cause a relapse in the disease.

Ischemic ulcers should be treated in the same manner as the ischemic ulcer of ASO. Many patients will improve markedly after the cessation of smoking, and no further measures will be needed. If significant improvement is not noted within 2 to 3 months after the patient has stopped smoking, regional sympathetic ganglionectomy should be considered. However, this sympathectomy will not be successful if the patient continues to smoke or resumes smoking.

Leg ulcers secondary to livedo reticularis. Livedo reticularis is one of a relatively uncommon group of arteriospastic disorders that may cause ischemic ulcers of the extremity because of prolonged spasm and subsequent occlusion of the arteries and arterioles. These arteriospastic disorders also include acrocyanosis and Raynaud's phenomenon. Since acrocyanosis causes no significant ischemia and no ulcerations, and since the ulcerations in Raynaud's phenomenon are usually limited to distal fingers, these two conditions will not be included in this discussion.

Pathology and pathogenesis. The changes that accompany livedo reticularis are brought about by narrowing of the arterioles that pierce the cutis from below. The narrowing can be either spastic or organic with secondary dilation of the capillaries and venules. This results in a marked slowing of blood flow. Pathologic studies may reveal no changes in the arterioles or may show proliferation of the intima and occasionally complete occlusion of some arteries.

Livedo reticularis is usually idiopathic but occasionally is associated with such diseases as atheromatous embolization, periarteritis nodosa, disseminated lupus erythematosus, and cryoglobulinemia.

Clinical features. Patients with livedo reticularis notice a persistent, bluish-red "fishnet" pattern of cyanotic mottling of the skin of the extremities. The majority are women whose symptoms are first noted between 20 and 40 years of age. The mottling may extend to the thighs and involve the arms to a lesser degree than the legs. Occasionally, it may involve the trunk, especially over the buttocks and lower abdomen. The mottling is more intense in cooler weather but never disappears entirely even in warm weather.

Many patients with livedo reticularis have no symptoms at all, while others complain of coldness, numbness, aching, or paresthesias of the feet and legs. In a few patients ulcerations of the lower legs and feet occur and continue to recur. The ulcers begin as bluish-red infarcted areas, which then break down to form irregular ulcerations from 1 to 2 cm in diameter. The ulcers are painful and resist healing.

Treatment. Since most patients with livedo reticularis are completely asymptomatic, no treatment is necessary other than reassurance. Patients with mild symptoms or patients who object to the unattractive appearance of the skin need only protect the involved areas from cold as much as possible. Vasodilating drugs such as phenoxybenzamine hydrochloride (Dibenzyline) in doses of 10 mg three or four times daily may be tried. Calcium channel blockers such as nifedipine may also be helpful. Pentoxifylline can help some patients. If ulcerations are present, they should be treated in the same manner as the ischemic ulcers of ASO. Sympathetic ganglionectomy may help resistant ulcers. Treatment of an underlying disease (i.e., systemic lupus erythematosus) can result in improvement of ulcerations.

Hypertensive leg ulcers

Pathology and pathogenesis. In severe hypertension generalized arteriolar disease occurs. There is an increase in thickness in the arteriolar wall and decrease in the diameter of the lumen. Occasionally the lumen is obstructed with thrombosis. These changes in the arterioles can result in an area of decreased blood supply to the skin. If the decrease is severe enough, or if mild trauma occurs, an area of skin infarction results, which breaks down and forms an ischemic ulcer.

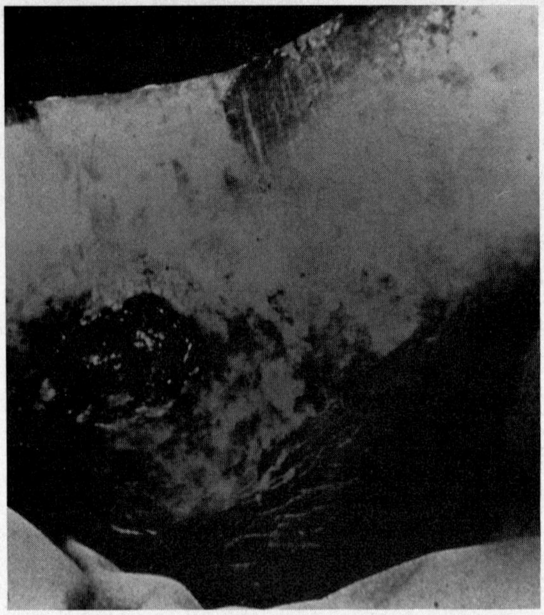

Fig. 35-4. Hypertensive ulcer over the lateral malleolus with a purplish hue around the ulcer.

Clinical features. Patients with hypertensive ulcers most often have had essential hypertension for a long time and have vascular changes in the fundi. Women in their fifth and sixth decades are most affected, although ulcers occur in men also.

Hypertensive ulcers usually originate on the lateral surface of the ankle, but may occur posteriorly or higher on the lateral calf (Fig. 35-4). An ulcer usually starts as a painful, reddish-blue plaque or as a small purpuric lesion. A hemorrhagic bleb then develops, which breaks down into a superficial ulcer. The ulcer frequently is surrounded by a cyanotic or purpuric halo, representing ischemic tissue that has not yet broken down. The ulcer may extend gradually in a serpiginous manner into this ischemic area and reach the size of 5 to 10 cm. It usually has the typical appearance of an ischemic ulcer with little granulation tissue and minimal drainage. The pain is severe, out of proportion to the size of the ulcer, and is usually the reason for seeking medical attention. There may be involvement of both legs, either simultaneously or sequentially. All lesions heal slowly, requiring weeks or months of treatment.

Treatment. It is most important that the patient's blood pressure be adequately controlled to try to retard or arrest the underlying disease process. Healing of hypertensive ulcers is slow at best, but may be impossible without adequate treatment of the blood pressure.

Since the hypertensive ulcer is secondary to ischemia, the same plan of treatment outlined for the treatment of the arteriosclerotic ulcer applies. Treatment should be directed at increasing the blood supply, relieving pain, clearing up any local infection, and protecting the leg from any further injury. The patient should not smoke.

Leg ulcers secondary to chronic pernio (chronic chilblains). When a person susceptible to chronic pernio is exposed repeatedly to cold, severe arteriospasm can result in ulcerative cutaneous lesions on the toes and lower legs. These ulcers tend to heal during the warm season and to recur during the cool months.

Pathology and pathogenesis. The vascular changes in chronic pernio are most likely caused by the repeated episodes of arteriospasm that occur on cold exposure. Intimal proliferation, thickening of arterial walls, and periarterial and perivenous infiltrations of lymphocytes, monocytes, and neutrophilic leukocytes may be seen. The arterial spasm also produces ischemic changes in the tissues with varying degrees of chronic inflammatory reactions.

Clinical features. The typical patient with chronic pernio is a young man or woman with recurring, painful ulcerations of the toes, feet, or legs. Early in the disease the ulcers appear at the onset of cold weather and disappear in the summer, but later these seasonal effects may not be so prominent. Following cold exposure, small, (5 to 15 mm) red, elevated lesions can be seen on the toes and occasionally on the dorsum of the feet and toes. Blisters then form on these lesions within a few days, and the color changes to a blue or violet hue. The blisters then form a superficial, painful ulcer with a hemorrhagic base. Often 15 to 20 ulcers are present at a time. After 3 to 5 weeks, these lesions heal spontaneously, leaving permanent pigmented and scarred areas. Successive crops of lesions may appear.

Treatment. The most important feature of treatment in chronic pernio is the avoidance of exposure to cold. If cold cannot be avoided, adequate protection should be sought by dressing warmly and by not exposing the affected areas to the cold. Oral vasodilators may be tried, but usually are not effective. Calcium channel blockers such as nifedipine are the treatment of choice. The use of ultraviolet-B (UVB) phototherapy before cold exposure may prevent the development of chronic pernio lesions. Sympathectomy should be done for lesions that do not respond to conservative measures, but it will not give permanent protection from recurrence of the lesions.

Leg ulcers secondary to chronic venous insufficiency. Stasis dermatitis and ulceration are the most frequent complications of chronic venous insufficiency. The stasis ulcer is the most common type of leg ulcer. Chronic venous insufficiency accounts for approximately 10% of admissions to large general hospitals; much time has been lost from work and large sums of money have been spent every year for treatment, and many of these persons become totally disabled from their diseases.

Pathology and pathogenesis. An understanding of the pathogenesis of the stasis ulcer will help in planning more effective treatment for the patient.[2,3]

The veins of the leg can be grouped into the deep, the superficial, and the communicating (perforating) veins. The deep veins consist of the tibial, peroneal, and sural veins of the calf, and the popliteal and femoral veins of the thigh. They lie in the muscular compartment of the leg, well supported by the deep fascial layer. The superficial veins, the greater and lesser saphenous veins, lie in the subcutaneous compartment beneath the skin and have little external support. The communicating veins perforate the deep fascial layer and join the superficial to the deep veins. Each perforating vein has a valve that allows blood to pass only from the superficial system to the deep system.

The venous pressure in the leg is normally low during walking or exercise because compression of the calf muscles forces the blood upward while the vein valves prevent retrograde flow. When extensive thrombophlebitis of the deep veins occurs, however, many valves are destroyed during the healing process and the venous walls are weakened. This results in incompetence in the deep and perforating veins, producing an ambulatory venous hypertension. This abnormally high venous pressure upsets the normal capillary fluid exchange. There is excessive loss of fluid from the bloodstream to the extracellular spaces, and congestion and edema eventually develop. The accumulation of protein-rich fluid and the impairment in the exchange of oxygen and metabolites lead eventually to the typical changes of chronic venous insufficiency. These stasis changes are often aggravated by scratching, overtreatment, or sensitization to the many proprietary preparations applied to the leg before the patient seeks professional help.

Stasis ulcer itself is an uncommon complication of varicose veins but is often associated with incompetent perforating veins that lead into the area of the ulcer.

Clinical features. Stasis ulcerations usually occur in the region of the ankle over the medial malleolus (Fig. 35-5). They rarely occur on the feet, upper leg, or thigh and often develop in areas of indurated cellulitis or dermatitis. There is usually brown pigmentation in the surrounding skin, and the affected leg is often edematous. The ulcers may develop spontaneously or may be secondary to minor trauma such as bumping, scratching, or kicking. The size of the ulcer varies greatly, and if neglected, the ulcer may extend until most of the circumference of the leg is involved. The base of the ulcer is usually moist with extensive granulations, and is often secondarily infected. The ulcers may or may not be painful and are never as painful as ischemic ulcers. The discomfort is often much relieved by rest and elevation, which is in contrast to the marked increase of pain of ischemic ulcerations on elevation. After an ulceration has healed, there is a tendency to recurrence in the same area.

Differential diagnosis. In any type of ulcer the presence of a history of thrombophlebitis or edema, the presence of

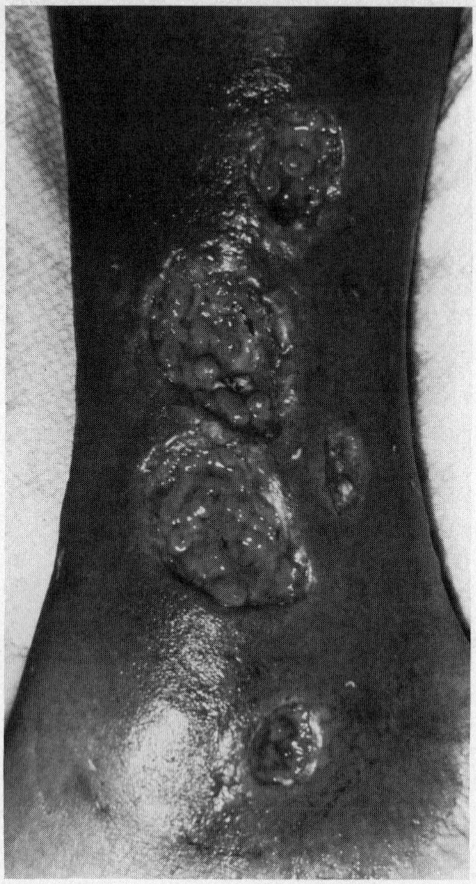

Fig. 35-5. Severe generalized chronic venous stasis with eczematous changes, edema, and ulcerations.

varicose or dilated veins, and the presence of stasis pigmentation, induration, and dermatitis will make chronic venous insufficiency the chief suspect in the search for the cause of the ulcer.

Arteriovenous fistula should be considered in all cases of chronic venous insufficiency. The history of a penetrating injury and the presence of a thrill and bruit may indicate a traumatic arteriovenous fistula. Increased length and circumference of the limb, the presence of hemangiomas and other vascular anomalies, and dilated veins in unusual places may indicate a congenital arteriovenous fistula.

It is important to differentiate between ischemic ulcers caused by ASO or TAO and stasis ulcers. Ischemic ulcers usually develop more distally on the feet and toes; they are more painful, and some relief is obtained by dependency. If ischemic ulcers do develop on the leg, they are usually the result of trauma. Pulses are absent in ischemic ulcers, and there are no signs of chronic venous insufficiency.

Hypertensive ischemic ulcers are usually found on the lateral or posterior aspect of the lower leg, are very painful, and often are surrounded by a purplish, cyanotic rim of ischemic tissue.

In lymphedema there is diffuse thickening and prominence of the skin and subcutaneous tissue that is not a feature of the edema of chronic venous insufficiency. On elevation the edema of lymphedema may not change at all, while chronic venous insufficiency edema usually subsides promptly with rest and elevation of the extremities. The typical stasis changes of dilated veins, pigmentation, dermatitis, and ulceration almost never occur as complications of lymphedema.

Treatment of acute stasis dermatitis. If weeping acute dermatitis accompanies the stasis ulcer, the leg is best treated by bed rest and wet compresses. The compresses should be changed every 2 to 3 hours. The wet dressings should not be enclosed in a plastic covering since this will result in maceration of tissues and will prevent the evaporation necessary to promote the healing process. The following solutions are suggested for compresses: (1) aluminum acetate (Burow's solution) 0.5%, (2) isotonic saline solution 0.9%, or (3) acetic acid solution 1%. Between compresses a drying antiinflammatory topical steroid or steroid/antibiotic ointment or cream will help clear the dermatitis.

Treatment of subacute stasis dermatitis. When the acute phase of the dermatitis has subsided and the patient becomes more ambulatory, recurrence of edema after prolonged standing must be prevented. If this is not done, acute dermatitis may promptly recur. The use of a modified Unna paste boot dressing is ideal in this situation.[4] These flesh-colored roll bandages are impregnated with a uniformly spread paste of zinc oxide, calamine, glycerin, and gelatin. Their use eliminates the need for bed rest or extensive hospital care.

To apply the Unna boot the leg is first cleansed with lukewarm water or mineral oil to remove any debris or previous medication (Figs. 35-6 and 35-7). Any of the following topical medications may then be applied to the leg: (1) gentian violet 1% (Fig. 35-8), (2) fluocinolone acetonide (Synalar) cream or ointment 0.025% (or any other topical corticosteroid preparation), or (3) topical antibiotics alone, such as ointments containing polymyxin B, bacitracin, and neomycin (Polysporin, Neosporin), erythromycin (Ilotycin), or gentamicin sulfate (Garamycin).

The modified Unna boot is applied from an area just proximal to the toes to just below the popliteal space (Figs. 35-9 to 35-12). The foot should be kept at a right angle to minimize chafing. A circular turn is made with the bandage around the foot, and it is then directed obliquely over the heel as would be done in applying an elastic bandage. This is repeated until the calf has been adequately covered. The first layers of the boot should be snug, and the bandage roll should be cut frequently during its application to ensure a flat surface. It should be applied in a "pressure gradient manner" with the greatest pressure applied at the ankle and lower third of the leg with progressively diminishing pressure over the upper two thirds of the leg. At no time should the bandage be given any reverse turns because the resulting ridges may cause discomfort and skin irritation as the band-

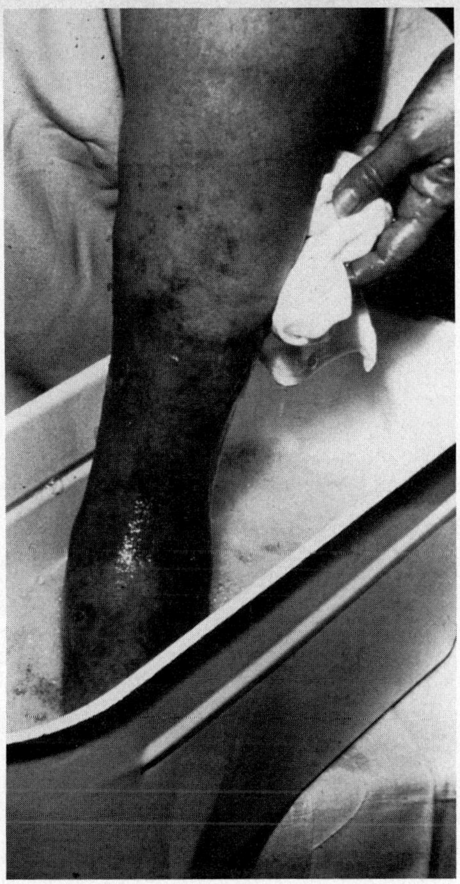

Fig. 35-6. Application of the Unna boot. The ulcer is first cleaned of previous medication.

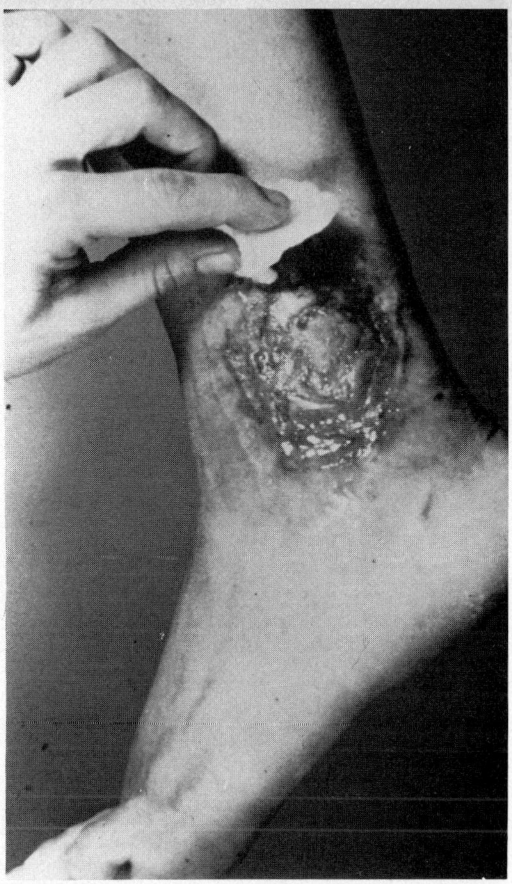

Fig. 35-7. Mineral oil cleansing of the ulcer.

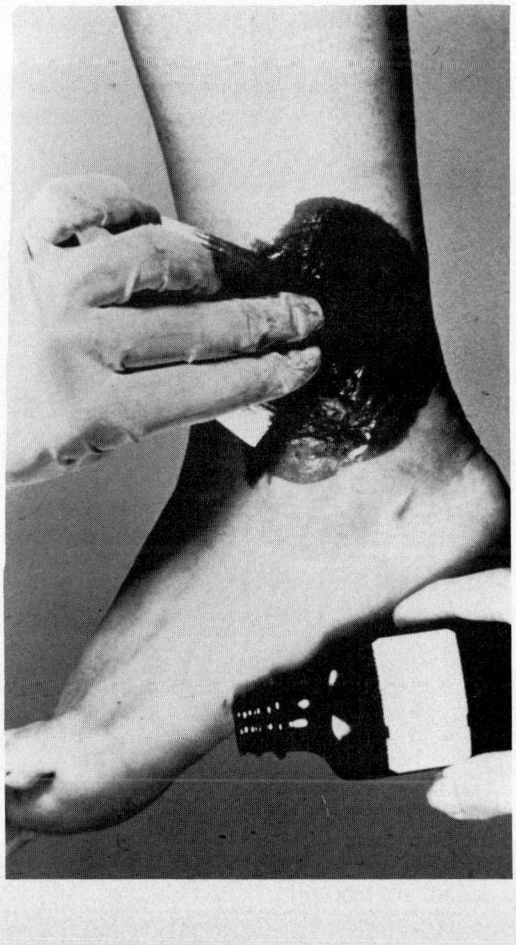

Fig. 35-8 Application of gentian violet to the ulcer and surrounding skin.

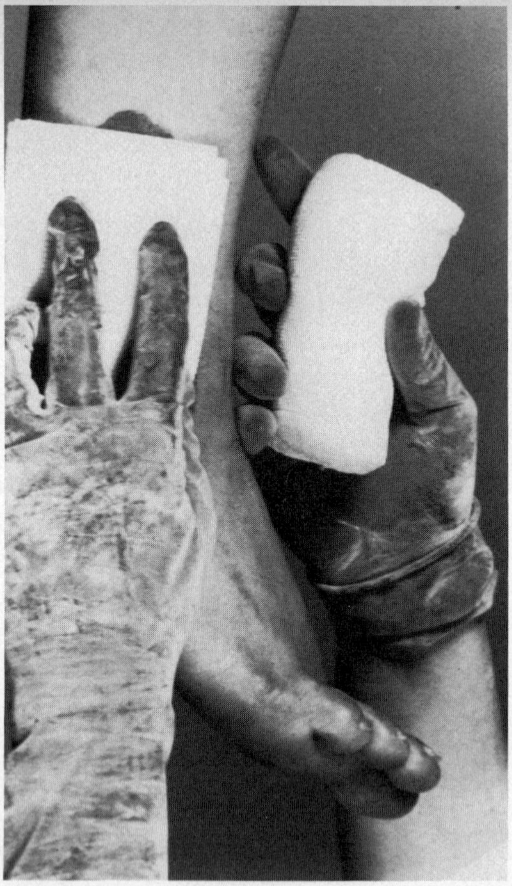

Fig. 35-9. Gauze applied to ulcer. This is followed by applications of Unna paste boot.

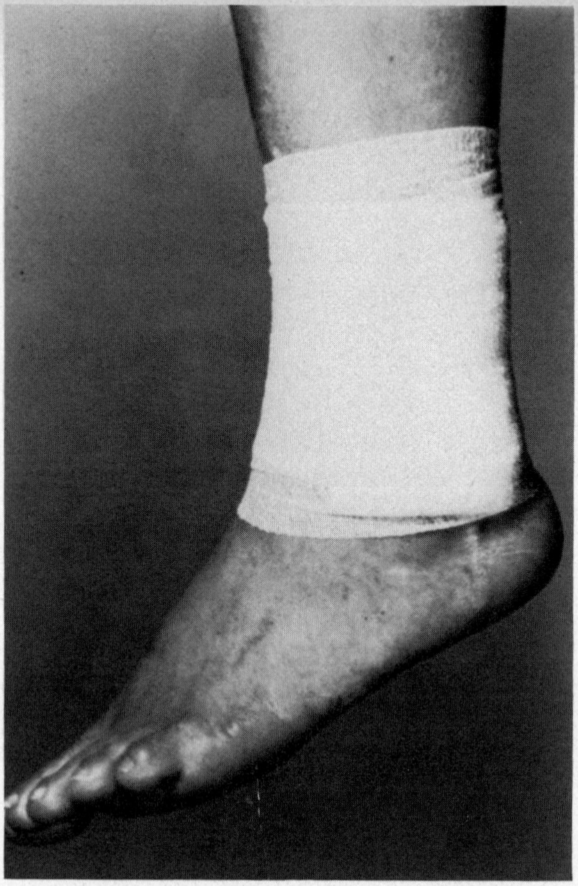

Fig. 35-10. Initial application of Unna paste boot.

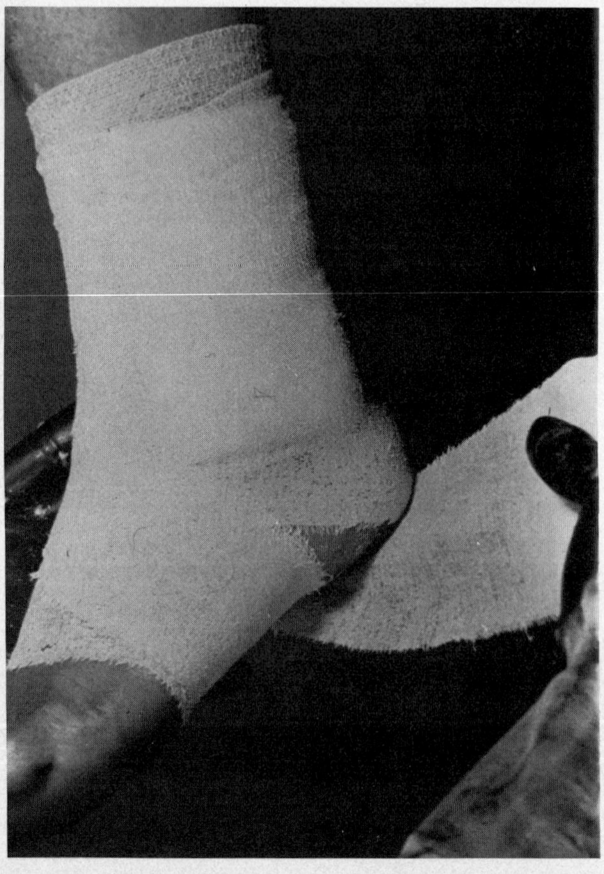

Fig. 35-11. Application of Unna paste boot with increased pressure over ankle and foot.

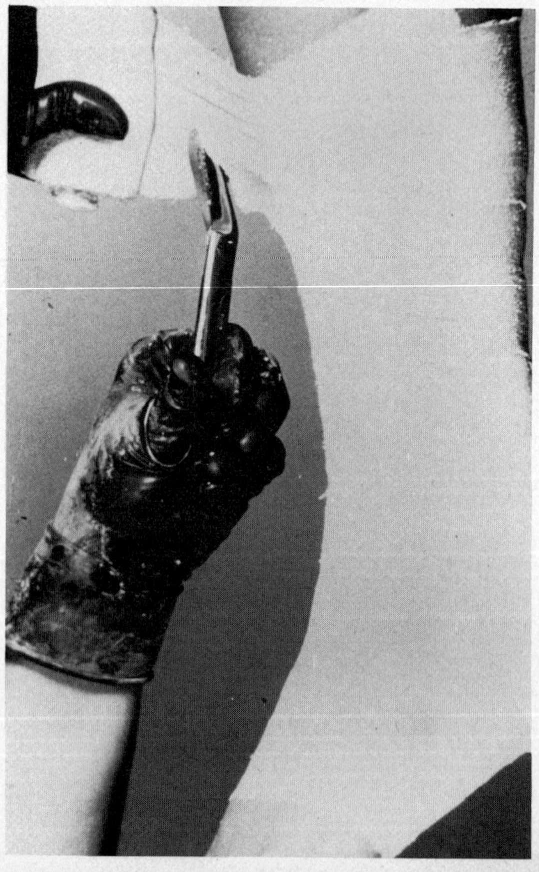

Fig. 35-12. Completion of the Unna paste boot up to the knee.

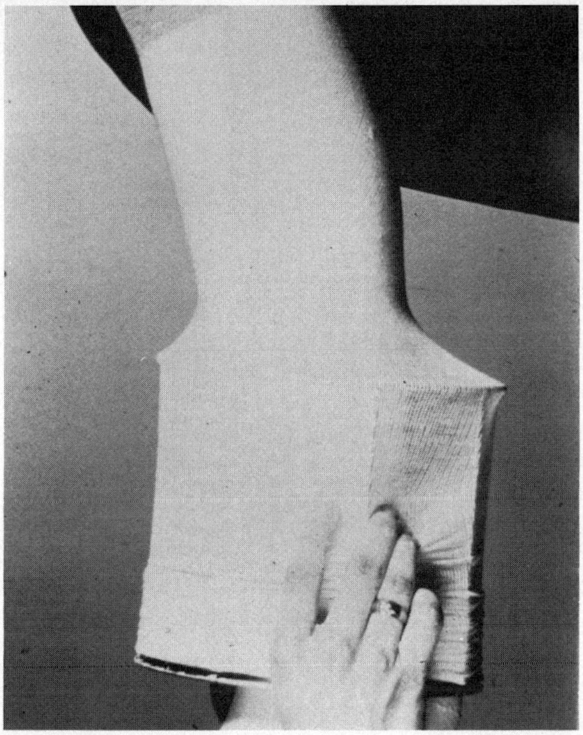

Fig. 35-13. Application of tubegauze over the Unna boot.

age hardens. Care should be taken not to apply the bandage too loosely or too tightly, and each turn should overlap the preceding turn. A double layer of Tubegauze is placed over the Unna boot and secured at the upper and lower limits with tape (Figs. 35-13 to 35-15). The tape should not be placed directly on the skin. This dressing is usually changed at weekly intervals unless excessive drainage necessitates changing every 3 to 5 days.

Even though the Unna boot is effective, there are problems associated with it including a long learning curve for correctly applying the cast, maceration of the skin when drainage is excessive, and inability to observe or bathe the leg while the cast is on. Because of these problems we have recently tried, and have been favorably impressed with, an alternative to the boot. This consists of an absorbent dressing (Allevyn, supplied by Smith and Nephew Medical, Massillon, Ohio) (Fig. 35-16), which is held in place by a light white compression liner (Fig. 35-17). During the day when the patient is active, the compression liner is covered by a heavy support stocking with a posterior zipper (Fig. 35-18). This appears to be a simple, easy-to-learn, and effective option to the Unna boot. The patients are enthusiastic about the program because the dressing is less bulky

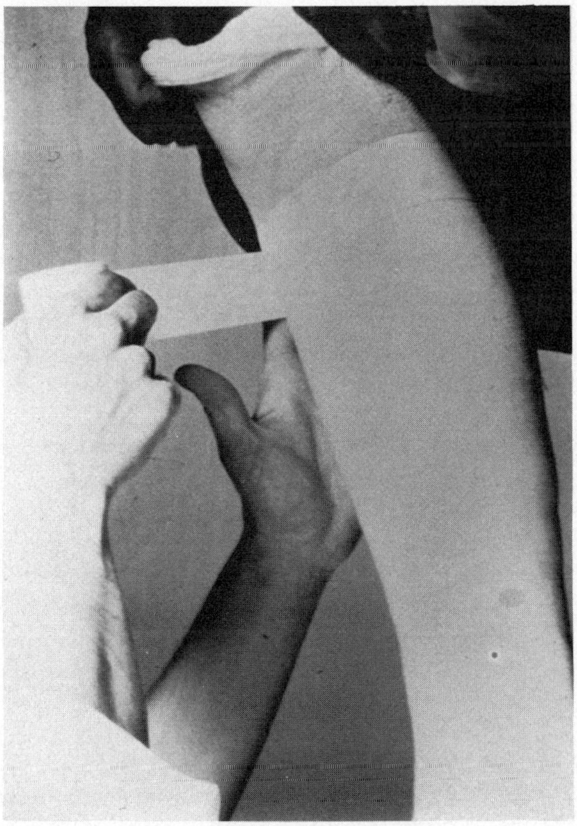

Fig. 35-14. Taping of the tubegauze dressing in place.

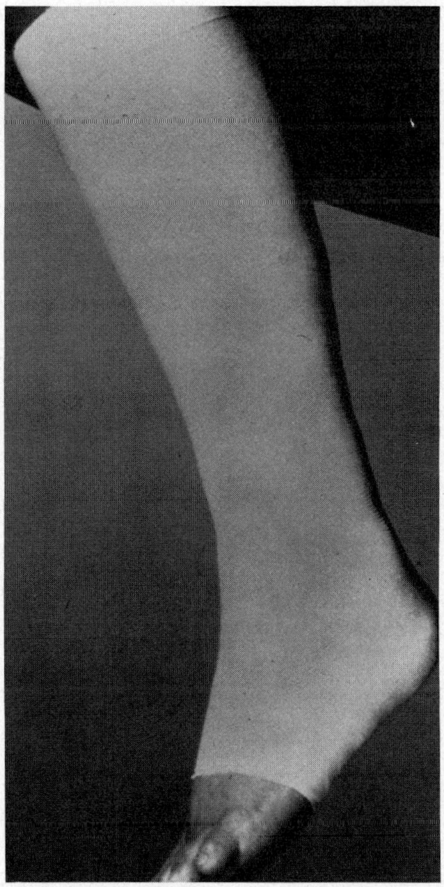

Fig. 35-15. Completed Unna boot dressing.

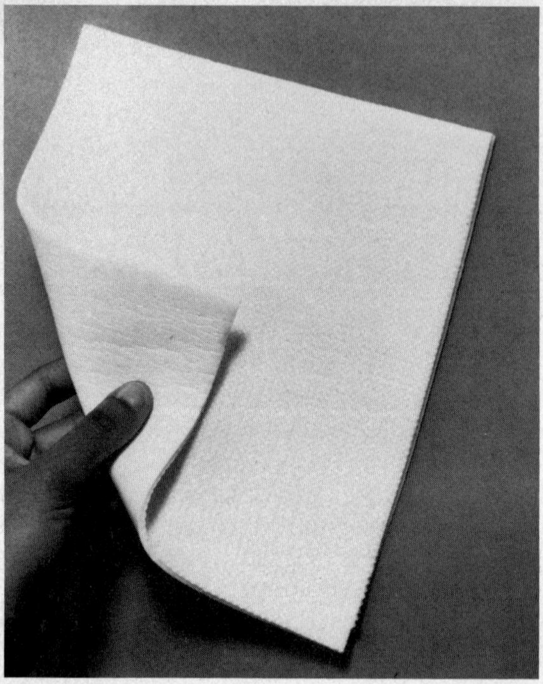

Fig. 35-16. This absorbent dressing (Allevyn) is applied to the draining stasis ulcer.

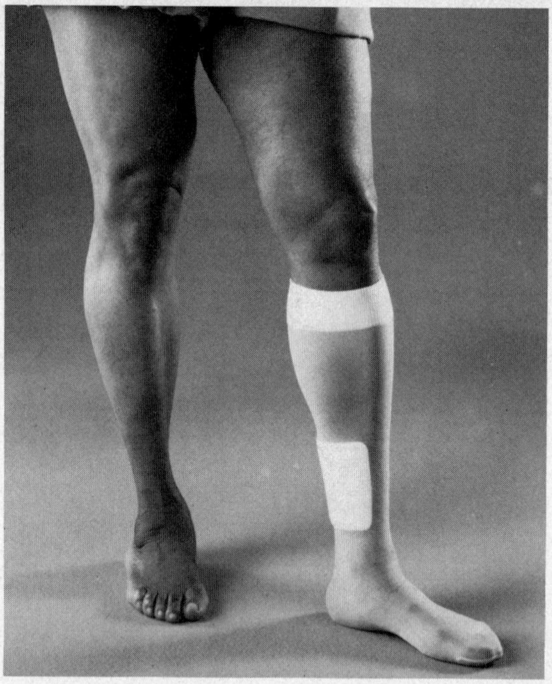

Fig. 35-17. The absorbent dressing is held in place by a light white compression liner.

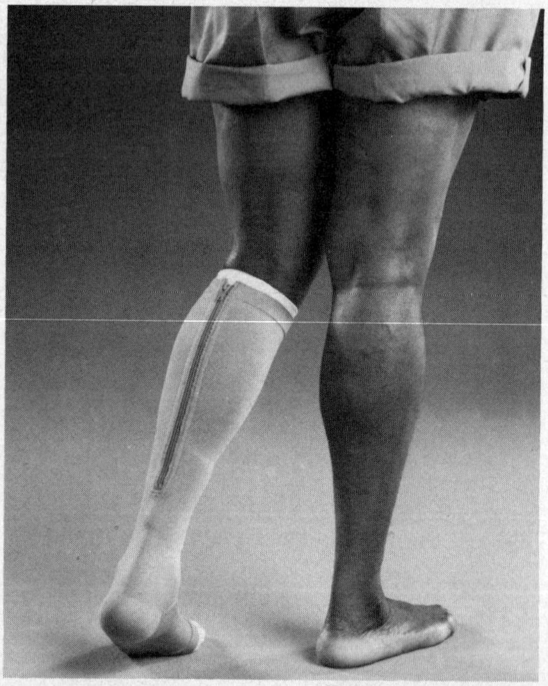

Fig. 35-18. The compression liner is covered by a heavy support stocking with a posterior zipper. (Liner and stocking supplied by Jobst Institute, Toledo, Ohio.)

and the dressing can be removed nightly to bathe the leg.

Treatment of stasis ulcers. The general principles of management of a stasis ulcer are the same as those for subacute stasis dermatitis.[5] The ulcer is cleansed and gently débrided. If there is considerable secondary infection, an occlusive dressing should not be applied. Bed rest and compresses are recommended as mentioned previously until the infection subsides. Pyogenic crusts should be removed, and any drainage should be cultured before antibiotic therapy. Topical antibiotic ointments may be used between the compresses. If cellulitis, lymphangitis, or septicemia are present, systemic antibiotic therapy is indicated. The choice of antibiotics should be dictated by the culture and sensitivity reports. The Unna boot is used in the manner outlined in the section on subacute stasis dermatitis.

Débridement of ulcers. Topical enzymes,[6] antibiotics, and other agents are often used to débride leg ulcers and develop a healthy granulation tissue. Another excellent method of local débridement is the application of topical viscous lidocaine (Xylocaine) and the use of a small, sharp curet to remove the eschar that adheres to the granulation tissue and inhibits reepithelialization of the ulcer. Occasionally, forceps and small scissors can be used to cut away thicker eschar that cannot be removed by the curet.

Use of benzoyl peroxide. Benzoyl peroxide, a potent oxidizing agent widely used in treating acne vulgaris, has been reported to give excellent results in promoting gran-

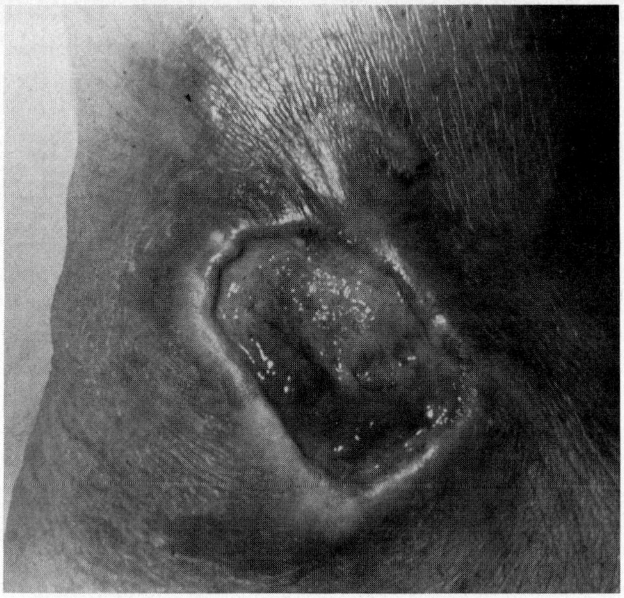

Fig. 35-19. Chronic venous stasis ulcer before benzoyl peroxide dressing is applied. Poor granulation tissue.

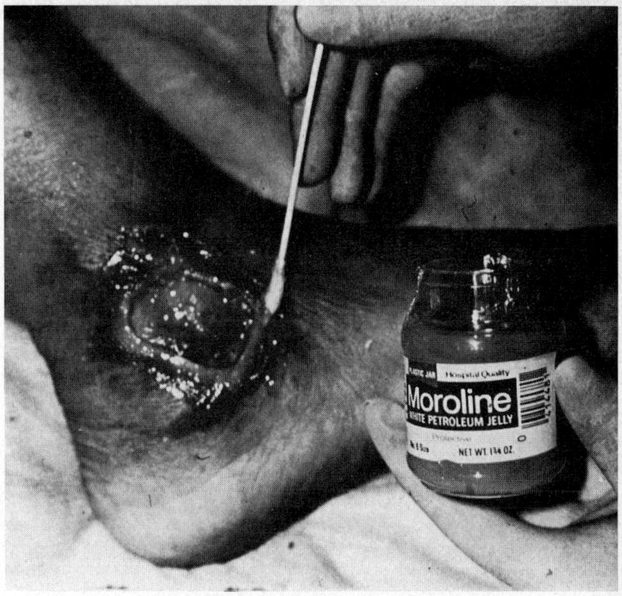

Fig. 35-20. Application of Vaseline around the edge of the ulcer.

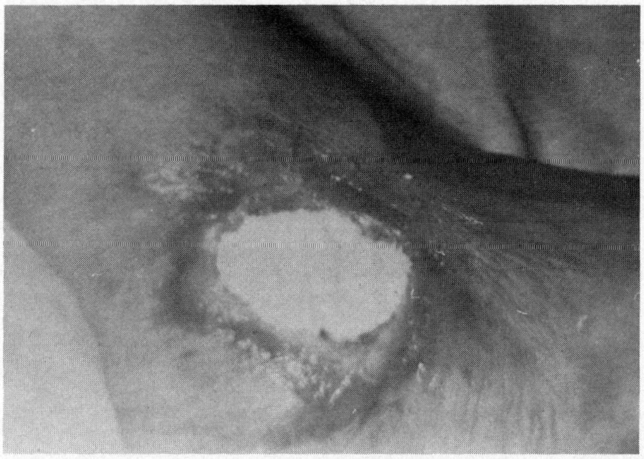

Fig. 35-21. A piece of terrycloth is soaked with 20% benzoyl peroxide.

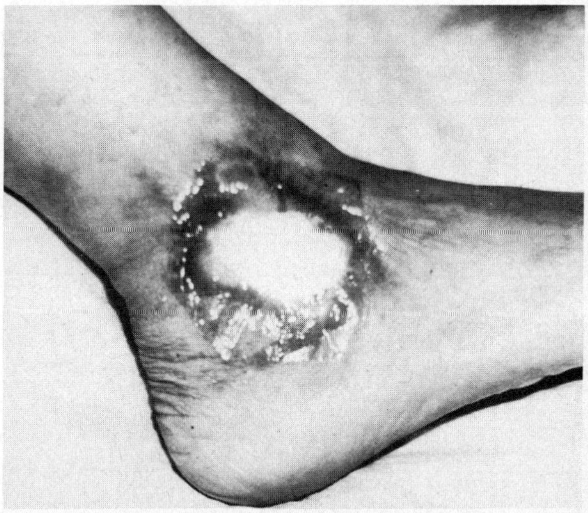

Fig. 35-22. Saran wrap placed over the benzoyl peroxide–soaked cloth on the ulcer.

ulation tissue in ulcers[7] (Fig. 35-19). Lotion with 10% benzoyl peroxide is commonly available, but a special preparation of a 20% lotion works better. The normal skin margins of the ulcer are protected with Vaseline (Fig. 35-20), because 20% benzoyl peroxide can be irritating to normal skin. A piece of terrycloth cut in the exact shape of the ulcer is moistened with normal saline solution, impregnated with 20% benzoyl peroxide lotion (Fig. 35-21), and applied to the ulcer. The ulcer with 20% benzoyl peroxide is then occluded with plastic wrap (Fig. 35-22) and wrapped with gauze. The dressings are changed every 6 to 8 hours, if possible, which can be done as outpatient treatment with a reliable patient. Initially, there is some local pain and irritation, but soon the infection starts to clear, and the rolled borders of the leg ulcer flatten and begin good reepithelialization (Fig. 35-23). Excessive granulation tissue at epithelial borders may be cauterized with 10% silver nitrate solution. The wounds may eventually completely cover with a combination of epithelium and scar (Figs. 35-24 and 35-25). Benzoyl peroxide probably acts by providing bactericidal action, stimulating granulation tissue, releasing oxygen into tissue, and débridement.

Dextran polymer beads. This treatment consists of applying a thick layer of a three-dimensional network of porous dextran polymer beads, 0.1 to 0.3 mm in diameter, to the ulcer. DuoDerm beads work in a similar fashion in absorbing

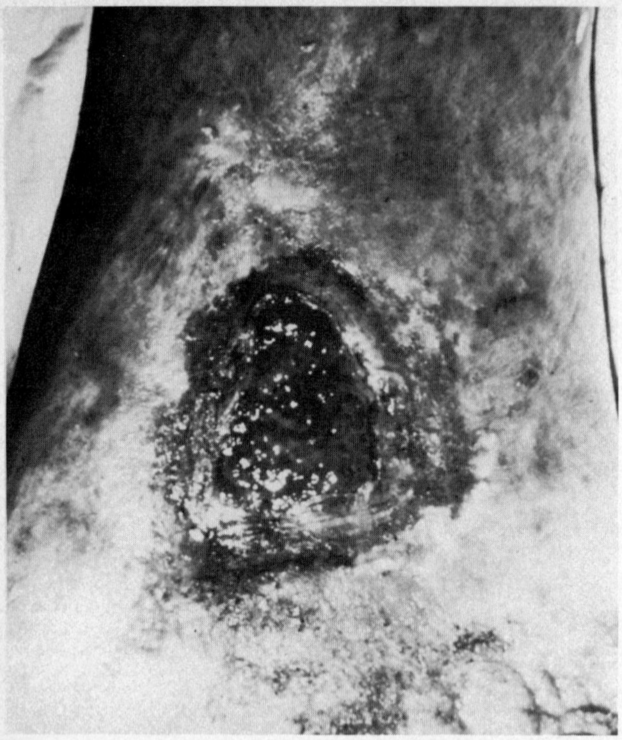

Fig. 35-23. Increased granulation tissue, flattening of borders, and beginning healing of ulcer.

wound debris. The beads are highly hydrophilic and absorb fluid until saturated, swelling in the process. When placed on a discharging ulcer surface, the beads absorb the exudate, bacteria, and tissue degradation residues from the ulcer surface.

New wound dressings. In the past few years, new dressings have been developed that do more than just cover the wound and keep it clean.[8,9] These occlusive or semiocclusive dressings vary in the degree of débridement, cleansing, and wound granulation that speed the healing process.[10-12] It is well accepted that epithelial migration occurs more readily in a moist environment such as that created by occlusive dressings. Some examples are Opsite, Tegaderm (polyrethan) Bioclusive, Vigilon (polyethylene oxdihydrogel with polyethylene film backing, thicker hydrogel films on both sides, and gel in the middle), and DuoDerm (hydrocolloid material surrounded by an inert, hydrophobic polymer that is adhesive).[13-16]

Most of these dressings, except DuoDerm and Vigilon, will transport water,[17] and all except DuoDerm will transport oxygen. They all absorb bacteria, except Vigilon, and only DuoDerm is not transparent. All except Vigilon are self-adhesive to the skin. There is excessive accumulation of fluid under some of these dressings, especially Opsite. There can be exacerbation of infection and cellulitis if these dressings are used on an infected leg ulcer. They are best used

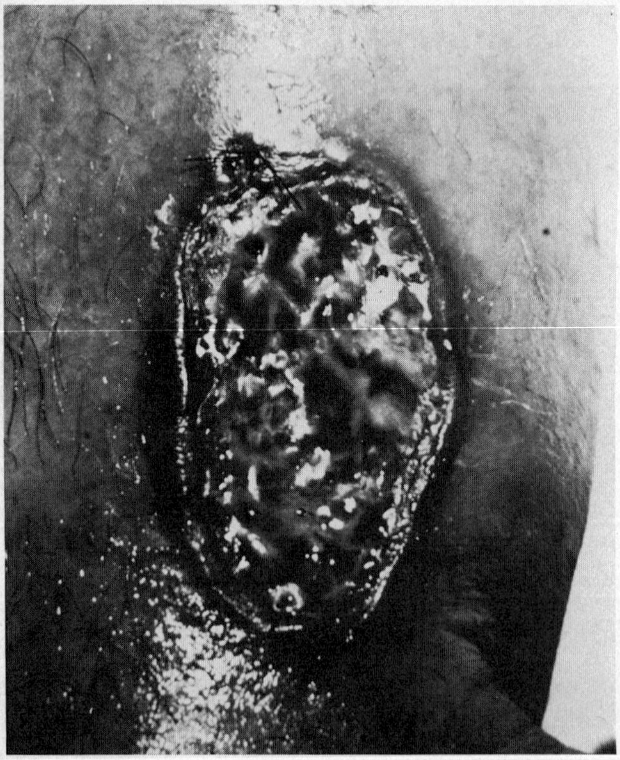

Fig. 35-24. Venous stasis ulcer before 20% benzoyl peroxide.

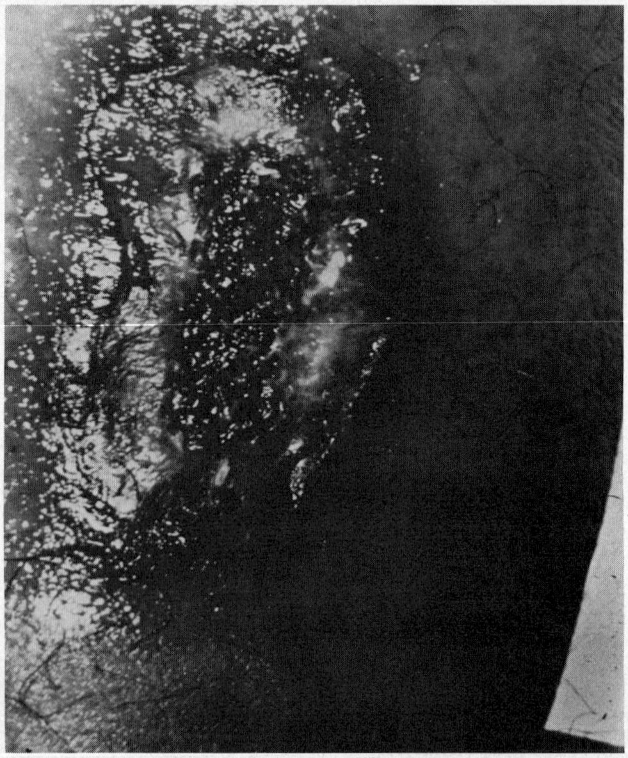

Fig. 35-25. Ulcer beginning to heal and new epithelium from edges.

when all infection is cleared, and there is good granulation tissue and reepithelialization is sought. Although these new dressings are physiologically better for wound healing, some clinical trials have indicated that ulcer healing is equally effective with the older elastic compressive dressing. These agents can be used under an Unna boot but should be changed every 2 to 3 days.

Once the edema is gone and the infection has cleared, new granulation tissue will start to appear with the above techniques. These dressings, and even benzoyl peroxide applications, can be administered at home. Continued bed rest with elevation is recommended unless an Unna boot or heavy support stocking is used over the dressing, in which case the patient can ambulate normally. Once the granulation tissue fills the ulcer, then reepithelialization will start from the edges of the ulcer and occasionally from islands of granulation tissue in the center of the ulcer. If rapid reepithelialization is occurring, continued use of wound dressings and Unna boot will result in complete healing of the ulcer with a combination of scar tissue and new epithelium.

Surgical management. The final goal in the treatment of all leg ulcers is to provide adequate skin coverage to the ulcer. With ulcers that have poor granulation tissue, with necrotic or fibrotic tissue at the border that shows no sign of epithelial ingrowth after conservative measures, more aggressive surgical approaches to growing skin over the ulcers must be considered.

When healthy granulation tissue has become established in the ulcer base and the surrounding inflammation has subsided, the patient is ready for pinch grafting if this is the planned surgical procedure. The donor area (usually on the anterior thigh) is prepared by shaving, if necessary, and washing with Betadine soap. Sterile technique is maintained when working in the donor area, but strict sterile technique is not necessary in the recipient site.

Circular areas of 5 to 10 mm are marked in parallel rows on the upper thigh with gentian violet. These areas are elevated by intradermal injections of 1% lidocaine beneath each circle. This serves two purposes: anesthesia and elevation of the skin for easy removal of small epidermal or dermal grafts. Anesthesia can also be produced by using a field block. In such a case, elevations should be produced by injection of sterile saline under each circle. A curved needle or tip of a 30-gauge needle is placed at the center of a circle and is used to further tent up the skin. A single-edged razor blade or No. 15 scalpel blade is used to cut a split-thickness graft. The depth of the pinch graft should be 1 to 2 mm or to middermis. Subcutaneous fat taken with the graft interfaces with the "take" and may produce undue scarring in the donor area. It is wise to take grafts first from the most dependent area of the donor site so that blood does not obscure the operative field.

As grafts are removed, they are placed in a Petri dish containing gauze moistened with saline. When an assistant is available, these can be transferred to him or her for placement on the ulcer. When performing the procedure without an assistant, the practitioner cuts all grafts first and then moves them to the recipient area to avoid contaminating the donor area by to and from movement with each graft. The recipient site is cleaned, and a curette is used to stimulate mild bleeding.

With a 25-gauge needle or forceps, the grafts are placed on the ulcer bed next to, but not touching, each other until the defect is covered. The placement of the pinch grafts can be facilitated by their marking with gentian violet on the epidermal side. After placement of the grafts, the practitioner must allow 1 to 2 mm at the margins of the ulcer because epithelium growing in from the edges of the ulcer may prevent the border grafts from taking.

The area is then sprayed with Skin Prep, a spray adhesive dressing or a topical antibiotic is carefully applied over the grafts. A semipermeable membrane, such as Vigilon or Op-Site, is then applied on the grafted ulcer with its edges extending approximately 3 cm beyond the margin of the ulcer.

To prevent the grafts from tenting up and losing contact with the ulcer base, gauze cut to the approximate size of the ulcer is placed over the ulcer bed. A circular thick gauze slightly larger than the ulcer is prepared to protect the grafts and provide pressure to the tissue surrounding the ulcer. An elastic dressing is wrapped around the ulcer directly over the gauze to apply minimal pressure.

The donor area should first be sponged free of blood, and then gentian violet applied to the area. This is covered with a semipermeable dressing and a bandage. Alternatively, each removed site in the donor area can be sutured with a 4-0 nylon stitch.

The patient should be kept strictly at bed rest for 72 hours with limited ambulation in a wheelchair with the leg elevated.

The ulcer is examined through the adhesive membrane at 48 hours and daily thereafter. If fluid collects beneath the membrane it may be punctured and the fluid drained. If infection develops, the membrane should be removed. However, with an adequate pressure dressing, any fluid that forms tends to drain from under the edges of the membrane. The membrane is removed from the ulcer 7 to 10 days after grafting. Should any of the grafts become dislodged, they are repositioned and the wound is redressed. Once the semipermeable membrane is removed, the wound is dressed by applying a 4×4 inch gauze pad and elastic bandage. This dressing is changed three times a day. Periods of ambulation may be started a week after grafting; however, elevation of the leg should be continued until healing is complete—usually a matter of 2 to 4 weeks.

If the donor sites are sutured, then the sutures should be removed 10 to 14 days after grafting. If the donor sites are left to heal by secondary intention, gentian violet should be placed on the area twice a day until dry crusts form. This area usually heals with minimal scarring.

Ceilley, Rink, and Zueklhe[18] treated 75 patients with a total of 130 ulcers of various causes by pinch grafting and found that most patients had better than 75% of graft "takes" by the fifth postoperative day. The most impressive results were seen in the stasis and posttraumatic groups. The least impressive results were seen in the group with ischemia; however, even in this group 50% of the ulcers were successfully grafted. Of the 75 patients, 15 had recurrences of ulceration in the grafted area in less than 12 months. Most of these recurrences were in the group with ischemia, and they usually took place within 1 month of grafting. They found no significant correlation of recurrence with age, duration of ulceration, or size of the ulcer. Gilmore and Wheeland[19] and Wheeland[20] found similar results with pinch grafts.

When there is adequate granulation tissue in the ulcer bed, an alternative to pinch grafting is the split-thickness skin graft (Fig. 35-26). The technique is similar to grafts placed in other areas of the body. The anterior thigh is usually chosen as the donor site.

The response to porcine xenografts has proved to be a reliable guide to successful autografting.[21] Lyophilized porcine skin, commercially available in sterile packages, is reconstituted in normal saline and applied to the wound. Adherence or loss of the xenograft is obvious within 24 hours. If the graft adheres, it is allowed to remain for 1 to 3 days. Autografting is undertaken within 72 hours of successful adherence. If the xenograft does not adhere, it is removed, and topical measures to improve the bed of the ulcer are reinstituted. A trial of the xenograft can be done again 2 to 3 days later.

For ulcers with exposed bone or tendon, fully vascularized full-thickness skin and subcutaneous tissue must be applied. Split-thickness skin grafts do not become revascularized when placed upon exposed bone denuded of its periosteum, or on tendon denuded of paratendon. This situation is not too common with leg ulcers, but when it does occur, it is usually over an exposed tibia. Full-thickness vascularized tissue may be provided by local flaps (Fig. 35-27), cross-leg pedicle flaps, or by the application of distant tissue in the form of a free flap transfer revascularized by microvascular technique. Such procedures require a skilled surgeon experienced in flap surgery.

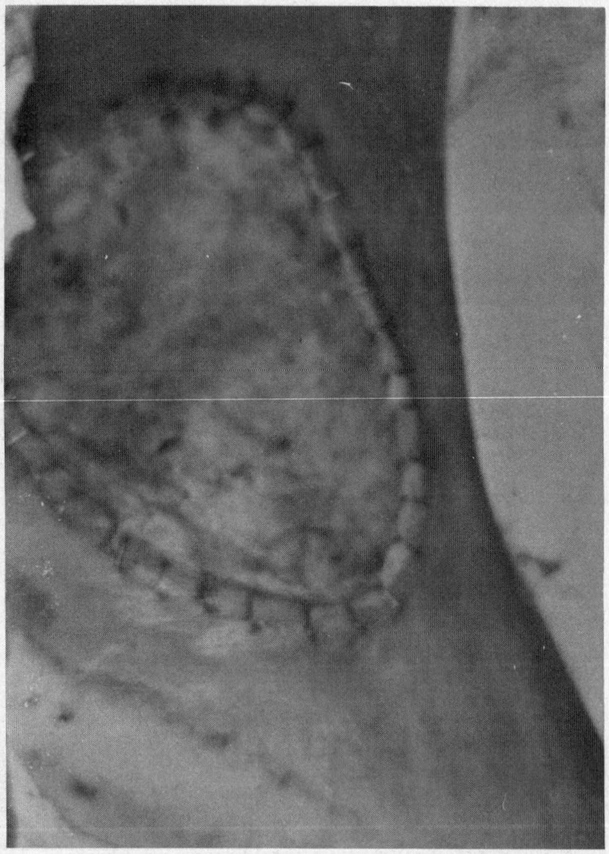

Fig. 35-26. Split-thickness skin graft to leg ulcer.

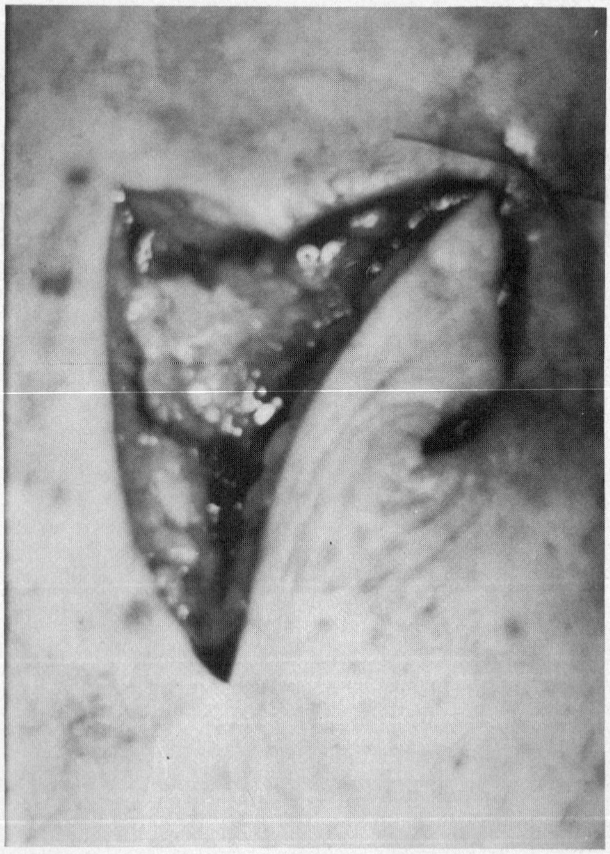

Fig. 35-27. Local rotational flap used to close an ulcer and anterior tibial surface.

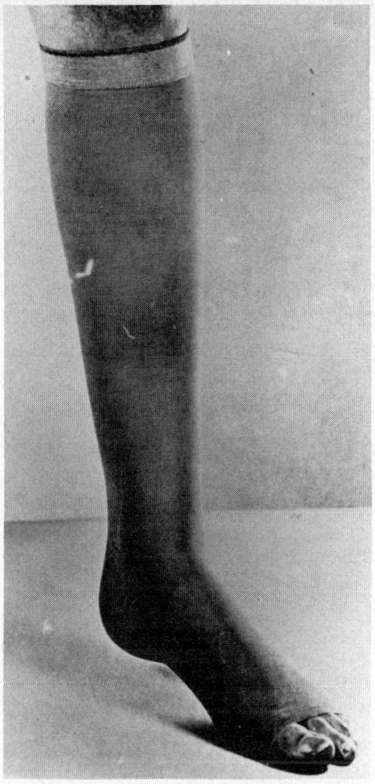

Fig. 35-28. Pressure gradient supportive stocking for chronic venous stasis problems.

Treatment of generalized eczematization. In patients with severe stasis dermatitis and ulceration, a generalized eczematous eruption may develop as a sensitization or id reaction. This can often be controlled by topical corticosteroids and antihistamines such as cyproheptadine (Periactin), 4 mg four times daily, or other antihistamines. It may be necessary in severe cases to give systemic corticosteroids orally or intramuscularly.

Treatment of neurodermatitis. Because of lichenification of "habit scratching," an associated neurodermatitis of the legs may develop. If this occurs, the application of fluocinolone acetonide (Synalar) or other potent topical corticosteroids under plastic food wrap at bedtime may be helpful. Intralesional injection of triamcinolone acetonide (Kenalog Parenteral) suspension (10 mg/ml) into localized neurodermatitis may bring more prompt relief of the pruritus.

Treatment of chronic venous insufficiency. After the acute and subacute stages of dermatitis have subsided and the cellulitis and ulcerations have healed, the treatment of chronic venous insufficiency is not finished. The patient must be impressed with the fact that he or she has a lifelong problem and that continuous supportive measures will be necessary to prevent future complications.

Elastic bandages and proprietary elastic stockings are usually not satisfactory for most of these patients. Individually measured, "pressure-gradient" supportive stockings, such as the Jobst stocking,* are preferred (Fig. 35-28). Directions for Jobst stocking measurements are furnished

*Jobst Institute, Box 653, Toledo, Ohio 43601.

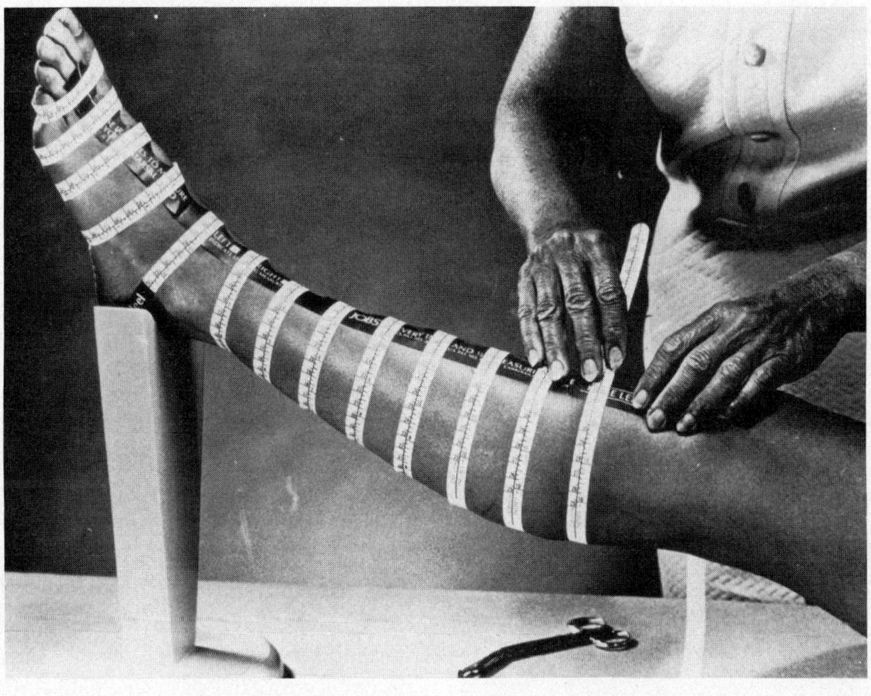

Fig. 35-29. Measurement for the Jobst stocking.

by the company (Fig. 35-29). Measurement should be made only after all edema has subsided or after the patient's legs have been mechanically pumped to make them edema free. There are other types of good supportive stockings such as Camp stockings, Sigvaris 902 series stockings, or Medi-Strumpf stockings.

The patient should put on the supportive stockings before arising and remove them just before retiring. It is usually necessary to purchase new stockings every 3 to 4 months because the stockings will stretch out.

Lymphatic leg ulcers

Lymphedema of an extremity is a swelling of the soft tissues caused by an accumulation of tissue fluid. This condition is described in detail in Chapter 27. True, uncomplicated lymphedema, regardless of its cause, is not usually associated with ulcerations. When ulcers do occur, they are usually the result of trauma (Fig. 35-30). In rare patients lymphangiosarcoma may develop in a lymphedematous limb, and this tumor may ulcerate. For this reason any unusual appearing ulcer in a patient with lymphedema should be biopsied. The treatment of ulcerations in lymphedema is similar to that described for stasis ulcers. These ulcers are usually resistant to treatment, and often must be treated by skin grafts. The treatment of lymphedema is outlined in Chapter 27.

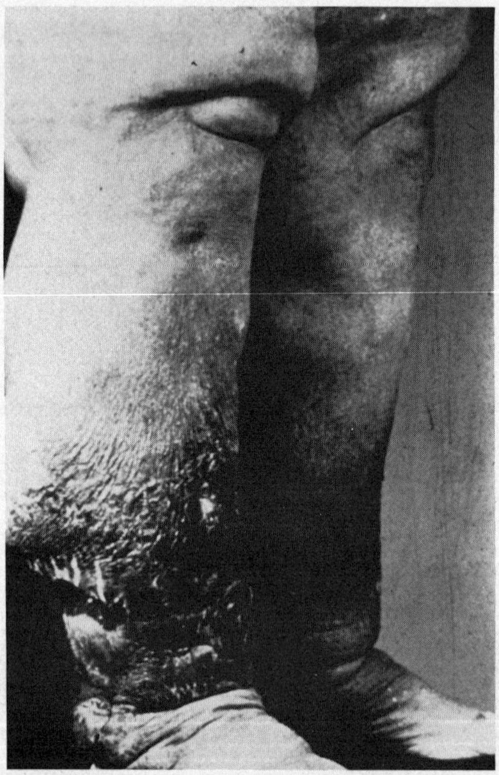

Fig. 35-30. Chronic lymphedema with ulceration.

LEG ULCERS SECONDARY TO VASCULITIS

Vasculitis is an ill-defined term and if used alone includes all inflammatory reactions around and within all blood vessels. Vasculitis as used here, or angiitis, refers to the hypersensitivity vasculitis group with the primary inflammatory processes involving small- and medium-size blood vessels. This results in necrosis, fibrinoid degeneration, hyalinization, and a granulomatous reaction. Those vascular inflammations secondary to embolus or inflammation in neighboring tissues are not included. Vasculitis of the skin is usually the cutaneous sign of a complex benign or malignant pathologic process, which may herald a systemic disorder. The vasculitis lesion that ulcerates may thus be the initial sign of a severe systemic disease.

Many different terms have been applied to the entity of vasculitis, including polyarteritis nodosa, hypersensitivity angiitis, Wegener's granulomatosis, allergic granulomatosis, and necrotizing vasculitis. The term vasculitis is often used to refer to a hypersensitivity or allergic reaction to drugs. The reaction is primarily in the small blood vessels of the skin. Leg ulcers resulting from a vasculitis may be associated with other generalized disorders such as systemic lupus erythematosus or rheumatoid arthritis.

The different types of vasculitis are based primarily on histopathologic criteria. The size of the blood vessel involved (small or large), the types of inflammatory cells (polymorphonuclear leukocytes, lymphocytes, or granulomatous lesions), and the evidence of or lack of necrosis of blood vessel walls determine the category of the lesion. Thus the skin biopsy becomes essential in the diagnosis of vasculitis. Biopsies are best taken from fresh, early (less than 24 hours old) papular purpuric lesions. It is often necessary to biopsy two or three different lesions to get the proper diagnosis. It is also important that the biopsy be deep and that the specimen have good subcutaneous fat and even muscle. Excision biopsy rather than punch biopsy is preferred. For a classification of vasculitis see Chapter 20.

Cutaneous features of vasculitis

Cutaneous lesions of vasculitis vary from erythematous macules to purpura, to hemorrhagic vesicles, and to urticarial, nodular, and eventually necrotic lesions and ulceration. The lower extremities are most often involved, but any portion of the skin may develop lesions, which may or may not be painful (Figs. 35-31 to 35-33).

Although the specific types of vasculitis have certain distinguishing clinical and histologic features, some types of cutaneous vasculitis are identified by the presence of many palpable purpuric lesions. The number of these depends on the stage of destruction and the size of blood vessels involved.

When the arterioles of the superficial dermis are affected, as in hypersensitivity angiitis, the skin manifestations begin as small urticarial or erythematous maculopapular lesions, which usually become petechial but in which brown pig-

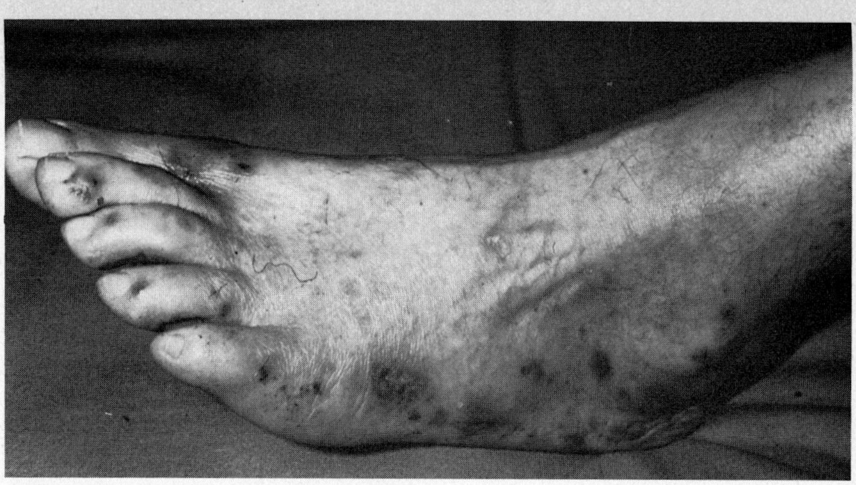

Fig. 35-31 Vasculitis with purpura and small ulcerations on the feet.

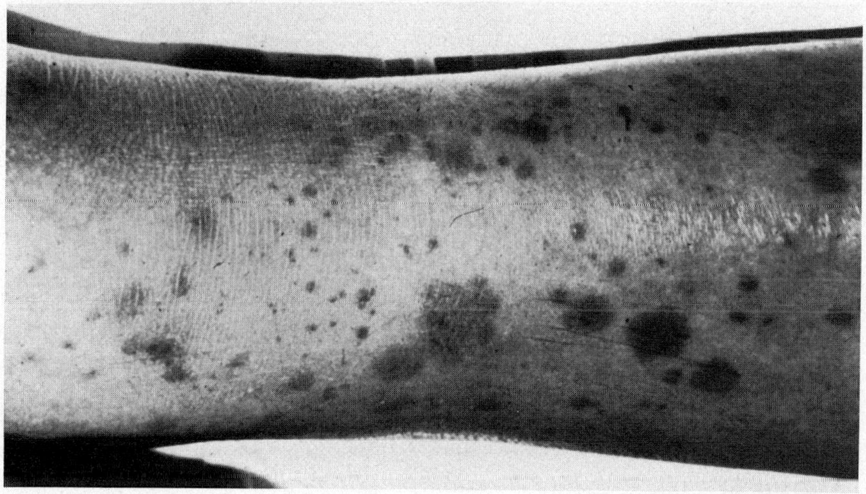

Fig. 35-32. Cutaneous vasculitis with palpable purpura on lower legs.

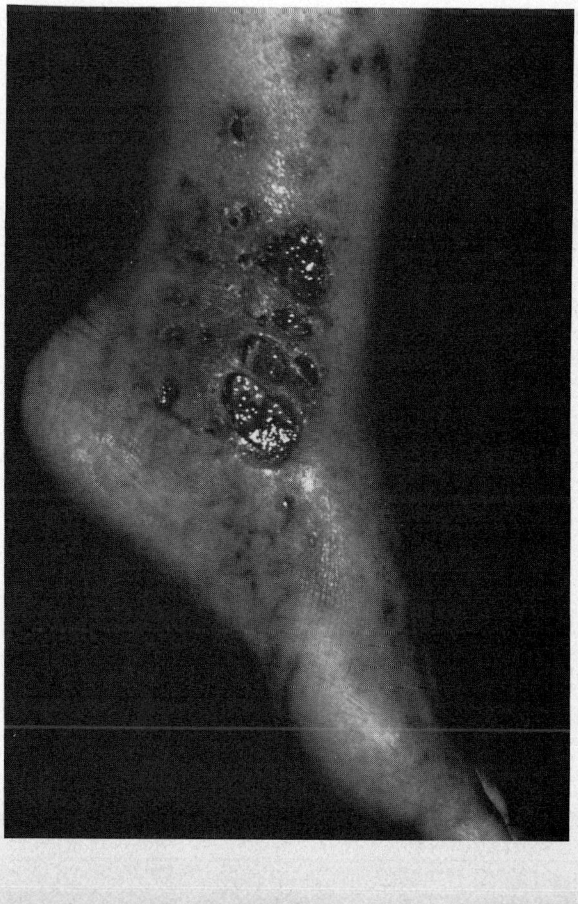

Fig. 35-33. Vasculitis with larger ulcerations, which simulate chronic venous stasis ulcers.

mentation may develop as they evolve. The petechiae are almost always palpable. The raised lesions are indicative of more exudative and inflammatory response than is produced by simple vascular or thrombocytopenic purpura. The petechiae of bacterial endocarditis are also palpable but usually show a halo of erythema. The hemorrhagic lesions vary from pinpoint size to several centimeters in diameter and may result in blood-filled bullae or extensive areas of superficial hemorrhage or gangrene. The overlying damage epidermis will usually break down and ulcerate at this point.

The site where most of these lesions occur is the lower extremities, concentrated around the ankles and dorsa of the feet (see Figs. 35-31 to 35-33). Other areas of the body are more rarely affected.

Systemic features of vasculitis

Systemic manifestations are common in vasculitis. Fever is a common but nonspecific symptom in up to 75% of patients. Musculoskeletal pain and symptoms of peripheral neuropathy occur early in the majority of patients. Renal disease occurs in most patients and is a common cause of death. The pathologic manifestations may be varied in the kidney, but a needle biopsy, including direct immunofluorescence studies, is often helpful in establishing a diagnosis of systemic vasculitis. Gastrointestinal symptoms also vary depending on the size of the vessel affected. Abdominal pain, steatorrhea, or acute cholecystitis may lead to abnormal liver function tests or a picture of hepatitis. Pancreatitis and diabetes may appear as a manifestation of pancreatic vasculitis. Myocardial infarction is one of the more common causes of death from systemic vasculitis, but individual episodes are often clinically silent. Asymptomatic pericarditis may be present. Hypertension may be severe and probably caused by renal cortical ischemia. Pulmonary infiltrations are more often found in the granulomatous forms of vasculitis and may be associated with a blood eosinophilia. Almost any manifestation of brain involvement may be found when central nervous vasculitis is present. The multifocal nature of the neurologic signs is a clue to their cause, cranial nerve and cortical hemisphere involvement predominating.

For a more detailed account of the clinical features, diagnosis, and treatment of the various vasculitides, see Chapter 20.

HEMATOLOGIC LEG ULCERS

Leg ulcers secondary to sickle cell anemia

Chronic leg ulcers are very common in sickle cell anemia (homozygous hemoglobin S disease) (Fig. 35-34). The incidence ranges between 25% and 75% and is more common in older patients. The ulcers usually have sharply defined edges and are single, but they may be multiple and bilateral. They most often occur in the lower leg around the malleoli. The ulcers are usually sharply marginated, round or oval, and may be shallow or deep. The borders may be elevated or irregular. The base usually shows granulation tissue and is occasionally covered with dried serous or seropurulent crust.

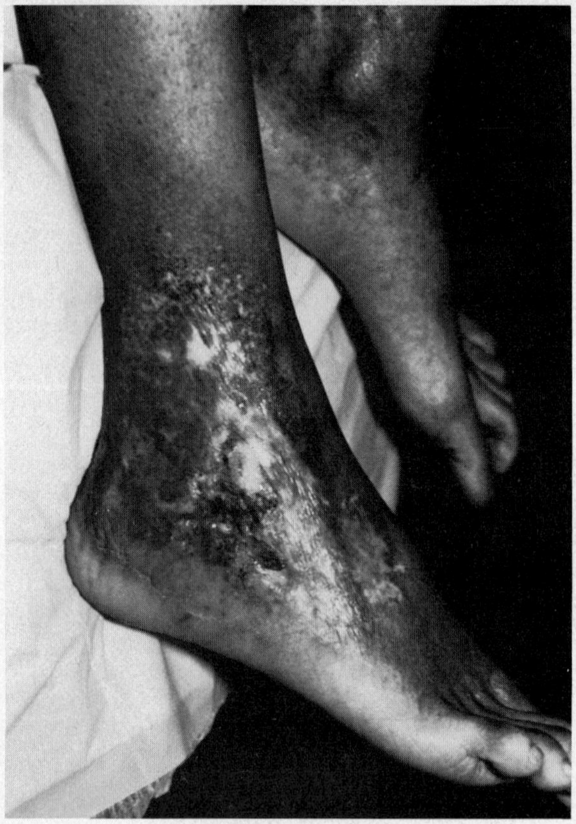

Fig. 35-34. Sickle cell anemia with scarring and ulceration around the ankle.

The mechanism leading to the development of sickle cell ulceration is the lowered oxygen tension and/or the low pH that is present in areas of stasis. This causes erythrocytes containing hemoglobin S to form intracellular hemoglobin tactoids that change the shape of the red cells to the sickle form. These sickled cells are more rigid, or less deformable, than normal cells. Increased viscosity results, and microthrombosis may occur. This in turn aggravates the stasis, setting up a vicious circle, which may result in ulceration.

The diagnosis of sickle cell anemia is readily confirmed by complete blood count, including a reticulocyte count and hemoglobin electrophoresis. There is no normal adult hemoglobin; there is an 80% to 90% hemoglobin S with the remainder fetal hemoglobin.

These ulcers are very resistant to healing. Unless the patient receives multiple transfusions of normal blood, maintaining the hemoglobin at about 10 g or above, the ulcers will not heal. Skin grafting has been successful if the hemoglobin is maintained at a near-normal level, but unfortunately the graft often breaks down when the transfusions are discontinued.

Similar types of leg ulcers are uncommon but may occur

in the older age group of patients who have a combination of abnormal hemoglobins, such as hemoglobin SC disease or hemoglobin S-thalassemia disease. As a general rule, these leg ulcers do not occur in patients who maintain a hemoglobin above 9 g.

Leg ulcers secondary to hereditary spherocytosis

In hereditary spherocytosis it is the red cell membrane and not the hemoglobin molecule that is abnormal. The exact nature of this membrane defect is obscure, but the increased tendency to sphere and the increased viscosity seen with normal red cells at a low pH are exaggerated in hereditary spherocytosis. Furthermore, the defective cells are spheroidal even at a normal pH. Trapping occurs in the spleen because of lower pH that occurs in that organ, and a similar effect can be presumed for areas of stasis such as the lower legs.

In most patients with a severe form of hereditary spherocytosis, leg ulcers are uncommon because many of the patients have had a splenectomy before reaching middle age. Leg ulcers are common in patients who have a moderately severe degree of hereditary spherocytosis that has persisted for many years.

Leg ulcers secondary to thalassemia

Thalassemia, sometimes referred to as *Mediterranean anemia,* occurs in both homozygous and heterozygous forms and with varying degrees of severity. In thalassemia major (Cooley's anemia) leg ulcers have been reported but are uncommon. In the very mildest forms of thalassemia minor, that is, in those patients who are totally asymptomatic and have no hemolytic process, leg ulcers do not occur. In the intermediate forms of thalassemia minor, however, leg ulcers may occur in a small percentage of patients (less than 5%). In these patients the hemoglobin is usually 9 g or less. The mechanism of leg ulcers is probably inadequate tissue oxygenation caused by the lower than normal concentration of hemoglobin A that characterizes this disorder.

Leg ulcers secondary to polycythemia vera, leukemia, and dysproteinemia

Other hematologic disorders such as polycythemia vera, chronic leukemia, and dysproteinemia occasionally produce leg ulcers.

In patients with polycythemia vera there is an increase in the viscosity of the blood and usually an increase in the number of platelets. Venous stasis and venous thromboses are not uncommon in these patients, and stasis ulcers may occur. Deep venous thromboses of the lower extremities may render treatment of the stasis ulcer more difficult.

Leg ulcers are uncommon in patients with either acute or chronic leukemia, and when present, are usually caused by trauma with secondary infection. The leukemic cells do not combat infection as well as normal white blood cells.

Various types of dysproteinemia may be associated with leg ulcers. Patients with cryoglobulinemia of moderate or marked severity may have stasis pigmentation, superficial skin ulceration, and necrosis. Gangrene of the digits may also be present. Serum viscosity is markedly increased and aggravated by coldness of the extremities. The most effective immediate therapy is plasmapheresis, which will reduce the viscosity. The extremities can be provided with a warm environment by using an electric blanket and a heat cradle.

Leg ulcers are uncommon in patients with Waldenström's macroglobulinemia even though the serum viscosity is high. In those patients with cryomacroglobulinemia, leg ulcers are more frequent. Patients with the usual type of multiple myeloma, such as IgG and IgA, rarely have leg ulceration. Even those with myeloma kidney and/or amyloidosis have no problems with leg ulcers.

LEG ULCERS SECONDARY TO INFECTIONS

Whatever their original cause, leg ulcers usually become infected secondarily because of exposure to pathogenic bacteria on the surface of the skin. It must be remembered, however, that infection may be the primary etiologic factor as well as a secondary invader.

Leg ulcers secondary to fungal infections

Pathogenic fungus infections are categorized as superficial or deep. The superficial infections usually invade only the stratum corneum and epidermis and produce macerations or pustules in the groin or feet. Ulcerations are not a feature of these superficial infections. The deep fungal infections may produce granulomatous ulcerative lesions on the skin, but they are also responsible for more serious internal infections involving the lungs, brain, and other vital organs.

There are two distinct types of deep fungal infections of the skin. The rarer form, the chancriform syndrome, is an example of primary cutaneous inoculation. It usually follows trauma to the skin with an introduction of pathogenic organisms into the tissues. At the site of inoculation an area of erythema and induration develops. In 1 to 2 weeks a chancre appears followed by lymphangitis and lymphedema of the involved limb. The more common form of the deep fungal infections is associated with systemic involvement. The appearance of the lesion is usually a papular pustular nodule that enlarges peripherally to form an elevated ulcerated verrucous granuloma. The greatest activity of the infection occurs at the periphery, which is clearly demarcated from normal skin. The deep fungi, which may produce a lower extremity ulceration, include blastomycosis (Fig. 35-35), coccidioidomycosis, histoplasmosis, and sporotrichosis. These can be differentiated by direct examination (smear), fungal culture characteristics, and identification of the organism on biopsy of the lesion with periodic acid-Schiff (PAS) stain. Treatment is with systemic antifungal therapy such as Amphotericin B or Ketoconazole (Nizoral).

Leg ulcers secondary to syphilis

Even today syphilis in all its stages must be considered the "great masquerader," as it was 50 years ago. Although

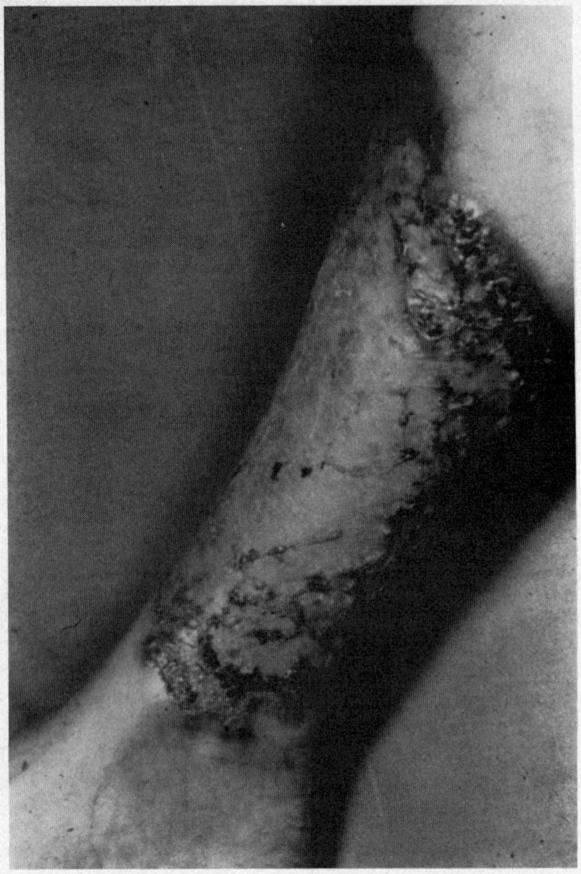

Fig. 35-35. Blastomycosis of the lower leg with an expanding ulceration with a verrucous border.

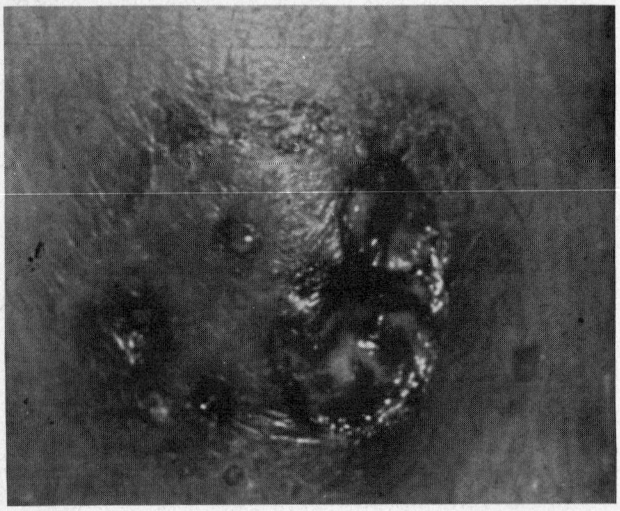

Fig. 35-36. Syphilitic gumma of the leg with ulceration.

primary and secondary lesions of syphilis do not often appear as leg ulcers, the tertiary stage has several clinical forms that may present as leg ulcers. With the advent of AIDS, syphilis is increasing again.

Syphilitic gumma (Fig. 35-36), a late form of syphilis, develops as a deep subcutaneous fixed nodule or plaque that may be singular or multiple. The lesions often ulcerate and extrude a thick sanguinous secretion. The ulcers are clearly demarcated, deep, and have a purulent base. They heal from the base and leave a contracted scar.

The causative organism, *Treponema pallidum,* is not identified on direct examination of the tissue. Serologic tests for syphilis usually show high titers. The fluorescent treponemal antibody (FTA) absorption test is positive. A tissue biopsy of the nodule or ulcer shows a granulomatous process that extends from the dermis into the subcutaneous tissue. Epithelial cells and giant cells are numerous. Massive caseation necrosis appears, typically in the center of the granulomatous lesion. The U.S. Public Health Service recommends treatment of this disorder with 6.0 to 9.0 million units of benzathine penicillin.

Leg ulcers secondary to bacterial infections

Bacterial infections of the lower extremities are not often the primary cause of leg ulcers (Fig. 35-37) but often are secondary contaminants. The recognition of these organisms is important, because eradication is at times necessary before other medical or surgical management of the leg ulcer can be accomplished.

Ulcers of the leg often become secondarily infected and produce an increased inflammation of the ulcer and surrounding tissue. The clinical signs are erythema, edema, and either a purulent exudate or a heavy eschar with pronounced peripheral inflammation. The bacterial flora of the vascular ulcers can be polymicrobial. The most common significant bacteria are *Staphylococcus aureus* and *Escherichia coli*. Appropriate cultures and antibiotic sensitivity testing are indicated.

Treatment of secondary bacterial infection usually consists of local measures. Wet compresses with one of the following agents are helpful: (1) Burow's solution, (2) potassium permanganate solution 1:10,000 in saline, (3) 3% silver nitrate, (4) 1% acetic acid solution, and (5) 3% boric acid solution.

Local débridement of the ulcer with curette is helpful in removing the thick eschar and infection. This is often very painful and may have to be done with the patient under general anesthesia. Prior application of viscous Xylocaine may make the procedure more tolerable to the patient.

Systemic antibiotics (IV) are indicated after appropriate cultures have been taken if cellulitis or evidence of systemic infection is present.

Leg ulcers secondary to tuberculosis

Primary lesions of tuberculosis are quite rare today but can be a cause of leg ulcers. Secondary forms of tuberculosis, or so-called tuberculids, are a more common cause of leg ulcers.

Primary tuberculosis. Lupus vulgaris of the lower extremity is rare. It appears as a well-demarcated reddish-brown patch or patches containing small papules (Fig.

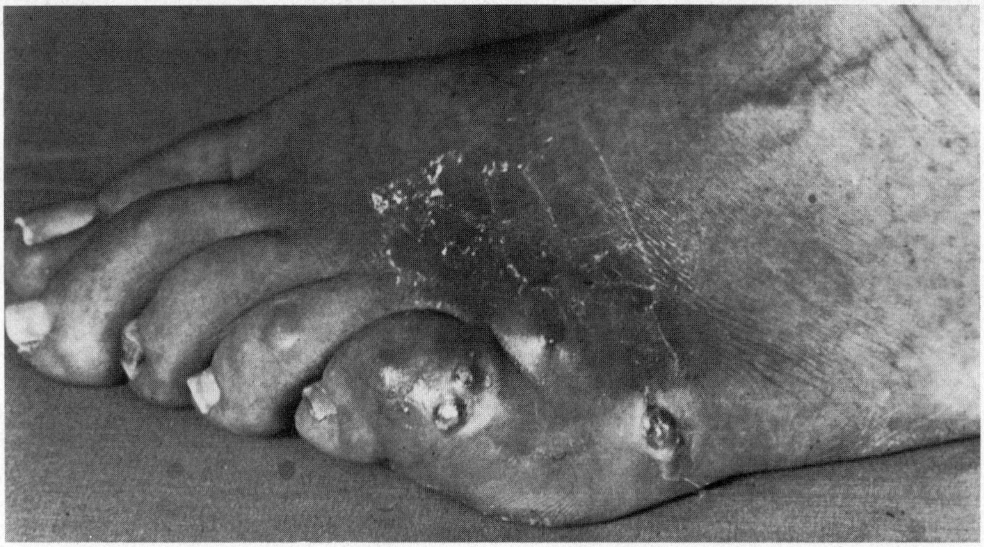

Fig. 35-37. Bacterial infection of the foot with cellulitis and ulceration caused by intraarticular infection of cortisone.

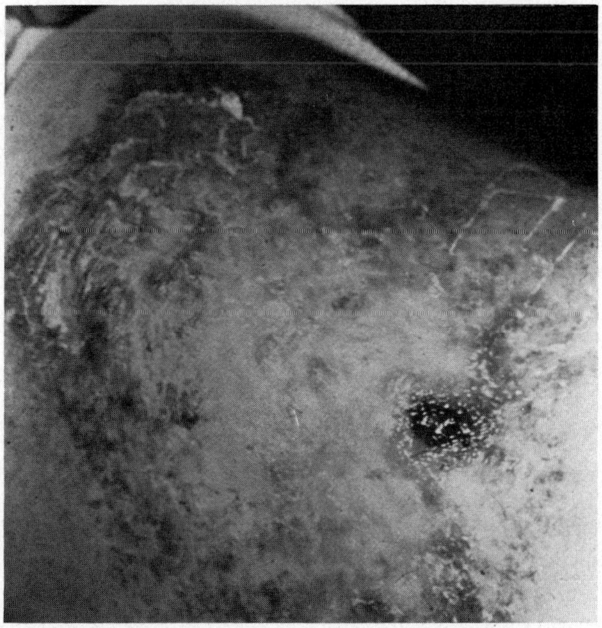

Fig. 35-38. Lupus vulgaris of the thigh with ulceration.

35-38). The papules show positive dioscopy (a yellow-brown color when a glass slide is pressed against them). These yellow lesions gradually become atrophic and show multiple areas of ulceration. Occasionally the borders develop a verrucal growth. A biopsy shows a typical tubercle with moderate caseation in the upper dermis. Acid-fast stains reveal the presence of small numbers of tubercle bacilli. Squamous cell carcinomas may occur in these chronic lesions.

The initial signs of tuberculosis verrucosa cutis usually are a single verrucous plaque with an inflammatory border and superficial pustules. The histologic pattern shows inflammatory reaction with caseation necrosis. Acid-fast stains reveal more tuberculosis bacilli than are seen in lesions of lupus vulgaris. The treatment of these two disorders is generally with the systemic antituberculosis drugs.

Secondary forms of tuberculosis (tuberculids). In the past tuberculids were thought to represent hematogenous dissemination of tubercle bacilli from a visceral focus into the skin. Over the years four disorders have been classified as tuberculids: erythema induratum (Fig. 35-39), papulonecrotic tuberculid (Fig. 35-40), lichen scrofulosorum, and lupus miliaris disseminatus faciei. These disorders are now thought to represent different diseases and are not necessarily secondary to tuberculosis, although they have histologic features similar to tuberculosis.

LEG ULCERS SECONDARY TO METABOLIC DISEASES

Leg ulcers secondary to pretibial myxedema

Pretibial myxedema typically occurs in about 3% of patients with toxic diffuse goiters. The characteristic lesions are firm, nonpitting, and irregular swellings, nodules, or plaques that are flesh colored and waxy and have a "pigskin" appearance. They may appear during the hyperthyroid stage, but often first appear following iodine-131 or surgical treatment of thyrotoxicosis.

The soft tissue lesions of pretibial myxedema do ulcerate, but infrequently. Treatment with Cordran tape or intralesional triamcinolone suspension often produces resolution of the lesions.

Leg ulcers secondary to lichen amyloidosis

Amyloid may be deposited in the skin in patients with more serious underlying conditions. Lichen amyloidosis,

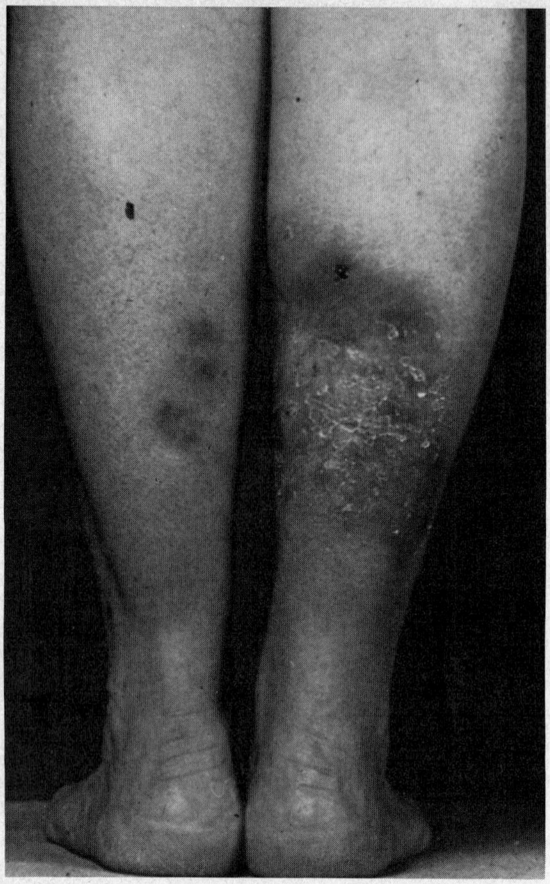

Fig. 35-39. Erythema induratum of posterior calf area.

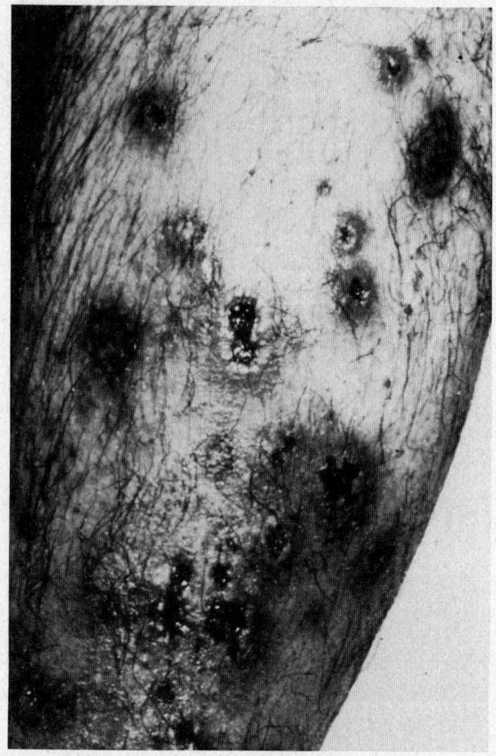

Fig. 35-40. Papulonecrotic tuberculid of the lower legs.

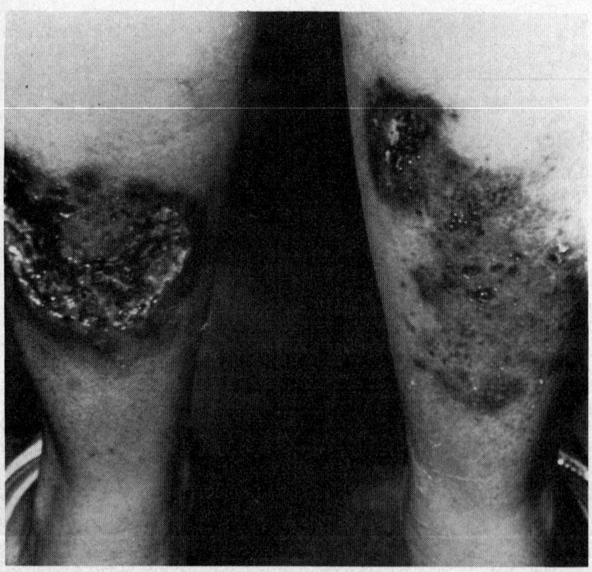

Fig. 35-41. Pyoderma gangrenosum. Note ulcerations with rolled granulomatous borders on lower legs.

however, is a benign localized deposition of amyloid, usually in the lower extremity, which rarely ulcerates. The eruption consists of discrete, firm papules that vary in color from red to reddish brown, and which may coalesce to form plaques.

Differential diagnosis includes lichen planus and lichen simplex chronicus. Skin biopsy confirms the diagnosis by using special stains (crystal violet, methyl violet, Thioflavin-T) that demonstrate the fibrous glycoprotein of amyloid in the upper dermis. Treatment of the lesions can be with intralesional steroids or dermabrasion destruction of the papules. The lesions are difficult to treat.

Leg ulcers secondary to pyoderma gangrenosum

Acute necrotizing ulcerations of the lower extremity with a rolled vegetating border are suggestive of pyoderma gangrenosum (Fig. 35-41), and investigation for possible gastrointestinal disease often discloses chronic ulcerative colitis.

The skin lesions usually begin as erythematous papulonodules that enlarge rapidly into plaques up to 12 cm or more in diameter. The active border is deeply violaceous red and the central portion is necrotic and ulcerated. A halo of erythema surrounds the lesion. Lesions of pyoderma gangrenosum are often extremely painful, and although they usually occur on the lower part of the leg, they may occur anywhere on the body.

Bacteriologic cultures of the ulceration often are sterile or grow contaminant organisms. Skin biopsy from the edge of the ulcer shows considerable proliferation of the epidermis (pseudocarcinomatous hyperplasia) and necrosis with chronic inflammatory cells in the dermis. The biopsy is not diagnostic of pyoderma gangrenosum, but helps to exclude other causes. Special stains (e.g., PAS, Giemsa) should be done to rule out deep fungus or other infectious source.

Although pyoderma gangrenosum was considered at one time pathognomonic of an underlying chronic ulcerative colitis, today other conditions such as regional enteritis, gastric ulcer, empyema, diabetes mellitus, and chronic debilitating infections may be associated with it.[22] Therapy is directed primarily at the underlying systemic disorder.

Leg ulcers secondary to porphyria cutanea tarda

Porphyria cutanea tarda (PCT) is an abnormality of porphyrin metabolism that results in cutaneous lesions and increased urinary excretion of uroporphyrins and coproporphyrins. The majority of patients have abnormal liver functions because of an excessive use of alcohol, toxins, or drugs.

The clinical features include fragility of the skin and bulla formation of the sun-exposed areas, especially the hands. Healing of bullae results in scar formation and milia. Hyperpigmentation, hypertrichosis, and morphea-like plaques are other features.

Ulcerations of the hands are common but ulcers of the lower extremity are not a common feature of PCT.

Leg ulcers secondary to Gaucher's disease

Skin changes in the chronic form of Gaucher's disease are usually a brownish or brownish-yellow pigmentation on the face, body, or legs. The lesions usually do not ulcerate but resemble Schamberg's pigmented purpura.

Leg ulcers secondary to gout

Gout is a form of recurrent arthritis associated with hyperuricemia that results in deposits of crystals of monosodium urate in joints and subcutaneous tissue. These will occasionally develop on the leg, especially around the malleolus, and may ulcerate and simulate a stasis ulcer or a rheumatoid nodule that can ulcerate. The more common locations of tophaceous deposits are the helix of the ear, hands, and elbows.

Skin biopsy may be necessary to identify the crystals of monosodium urate. Formalin fixation will dissolve away most urate crystals; therefore, fixation of skin biopsies in absolute ethanol is required for the preservation of crystals in histologic material.

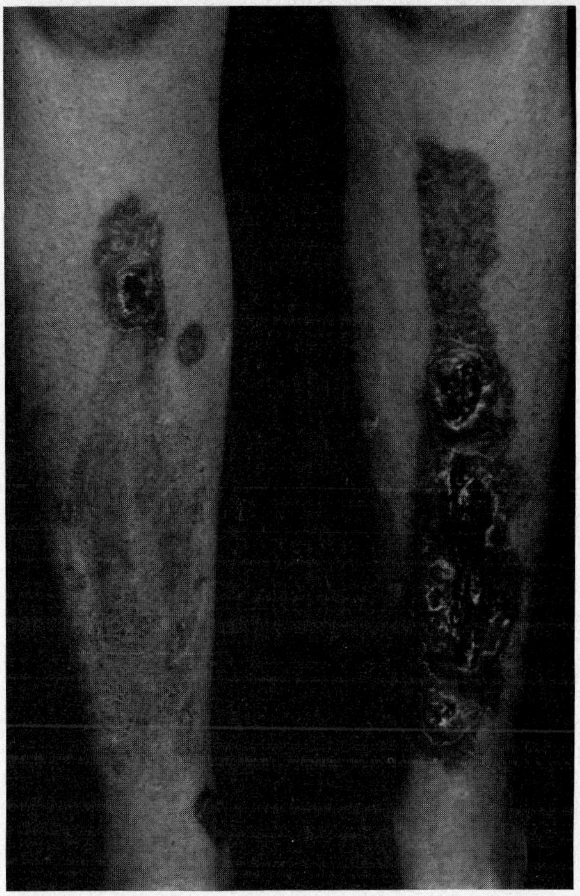

Fig. 35-42. Necrobiosis lipoidica diabeticorum of the anterior tibial areas with ulcerations in a diabetic.

Leg ulcers secondary to diabetes mellitus

Cutaneous disorders often found in diabetics include pruritus, bacterial and fungal infections, pigmentation, xanthomatous lesions, and dermal changes secondary to vascular disease and neurotrophic disorders. These skin clues are important because they may help detect unsuspected diabetes mellitus in its early stages. Many of these lesions are impossible to treat effectively unless the underlying diabetes is detected and treated.

Leg ulcers secondary to necrobiosis lipoidica diabeticorum. Necrobiosis lipoidica diabeticorum (NLD) is a rare but almost certain diagnostic sign of underlying diabetes mellitus. NLD occurs in approximately 0.3% of all diabetics. It is somewhat more frequent in females under the age of forty. If the glucose tolerance test is normal, a cortisone glucose tolerance test may detect latent diabetes mellitus.

The clinical lesions are usually located on the anterior surface of the legs (Fig. 35-42), but they may be located on any portion of the skin, including the scalp. They are atrophic yellow or orange depressed areas with telangiectatic blood vessels coursing through them. They vary in number

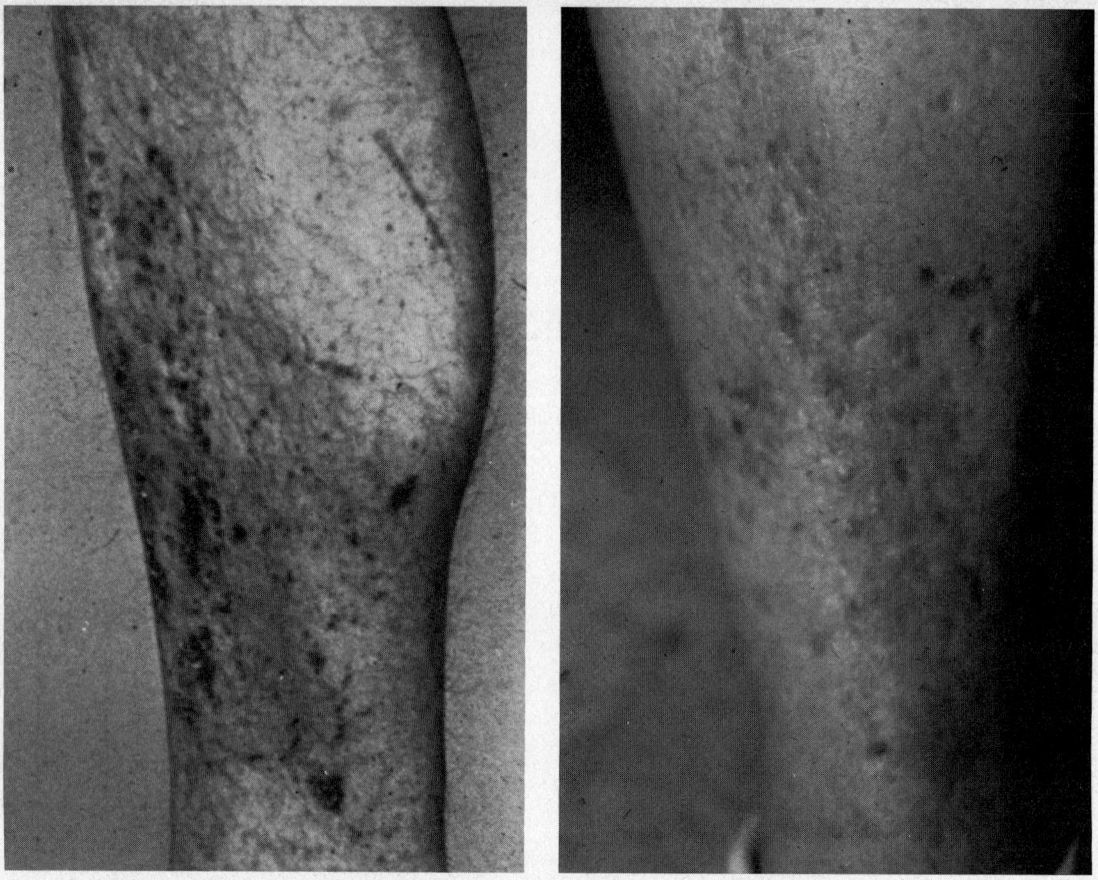

Fig. 35-43. Diabetic dermopathy on the anterior tibial surfaces with indentation and ulcerations.

from one to several and are usually asymptomatic and present only a cosmetic problem. Occasionally trauma or therapy that is too vigorous causes ulceration of the NLD lesion. Degeneration of the dermal connective tissue is probably caused by proliferative angiitis and obliterative changes in the arterioles.

Treatment of NLD is difficult and often not necessary. The lesions are only of cosmetic concern. Control of diabetes mellitus does not prevent the extension of lesions of NLD. Topical corticosteroids with occlusion or Cordran tape may produce some improvement. Intralesional corticosteroids may also prevent extension of the lesion. Caution must be taken with the use of vasoconstrictive corticosteroids in a lesion with impaired circulation. Often the NLD lesions may ulcerate after intralesional steroids. Ulcerated NLD lesions, if they are small, will heal with 3% topical gentian violet and Unna boots. Large ulcerations usually require excision of the entire lesion and split-thickness skin grafting. Lesions may persist for years and result in fibrosis and involution.

Leg ulcers secondary to diabetic dermopathy. Multiple, discrete, atrophic, pigmented macular lesions can occur on the anterior tibial surface of the lower extremities of a diabetic patient (Fig. 35-43). The lesions are usually asymptomatic but have been known to ulcerate and resemble areas of trauma.

The histopathologic features include proliferation and thickening of small blood vessels in the upper dermis and may be analogous to those vessel changes in neuropathy, nephropathy, and retinopathy. There is no specific treatment except local measures such as compresses, topical antibiotics, and gentian violet to heal the ulcerated lesions.

Leg ulcers secondary to bullae diabeticorum. Blisters and bullae that appear mainly on the legs have been described in diabetics.[23] The bullae are predominantly subepidermal and histologically contain proteinaceous fluid, fibrin threads, and scanty polymorphonuclear cells. The lesions are probably multifactorial in origin, but diabetic microangiopathy seems to be the most potent factor. Local care will heal the lesion.

LEG ULCERS SECONDARY TO TUMORS

Almost any type of tumor, whether primary in the skin or metastatic, may occur on the lower extremities. The tumors may ulcerate and have the appearance of a stasis ulcer that fails to respond to the usual modes of treatment. The importance of the history, especially a history of previous radiation therapy to the leg, is important.

Biopsy is always indicated when a tumor is suspected. If the lesion is ulcerated, the advancing border may be more revealing than the atrophic and possibly infected center of the scar. A deep wedge biopsy is preferred over a punch biopsy.

Leg ulcers secondary to basal cell carcinoma

Basal cell carcinoma of the lower extremity is a relatively rare and frequently misdiagnosed skin lesion. Because the most common sites for basal cell carcinoma are the exposed areas of the head and neck, the clinical index of suspicion is low when it occurs on the legs.

The lesions may vary in size from a 1 to 2 mm skin-colored papule with slight telangiectasia to a large, eroded, and ulcerating lesion several centimeters in diameter.

The treatment of choice for small basal cell carcinomas (less than 1 cm in diameter) is surgical electrocautery and curettement. Because lesions on the legs may be larger and healing may be a problem, primary excision or excision and grafting may be the treatment of choice.

Leg ulcers secondary to keratoacanthoma

Keratoacanthoma is a benign skin tumor that clinically and histologically resembles a squamous cell carcinoma. There are two types of keratoacanthomas—localized and generalized (rare).

The lesion consists of a firm, hemispheric nodule, 1 to 2 cm in diameter, which in its center has a horn-filled crater. The sites of predilection are exposed areas such as the face and the dorsa of the hands, but the lesions may occur on the legs as ulcerative tumor lesions.

A true keratoacanthoma, if left untreated, will usually undergo spontaneous involution within several months and leave an atrophic scar. Because there is often a problem in clinical differentiation from squamous cell carcinoma, the treatment of choice is usually complete primary excision of the lesion. This gives the best cosmetic results and leaves a good specimen for the pathologist to evaluate. Intralesional 5-fluorouracil will also cause regression of lesions that are not suitable for surgery.

Leg ulcers secondary to squamous cell carcinoma

Squamous cell carcinoma may occur anywhere on the skin as well as on mucous membranes. It may begin to develop as a senile keratosis or leukoplakia and is most common on the face, neck, and hands.

Most commonly, the lesion consists of a shallow ulcer surrounded by a wide, elevated, and indurated border. Occasionally, raised, fungoid, verrucous lesions without ulceration occur. The lesions are more common on exposed areas such as the face, hands, and arms, and are related to the total amount of solar exposure to the skin. Radiation therapy to the face for acne often predisposes the patient to squamous cell carcinoma. It is also a common complication of excessive radiation on the leg or foot, which may have been given years earlier for a neurodermatitis or a plantar wart. Squamous cell carcinoma can also occur in old injuries such as scars, burn wounds, or chronic ulcers.

Verrucous carcinoma frequently occurs on the foot or leg and appears as a persistent wart. Deep histologic sections show this malignant tumor. Mohs' chemosurgery is the treatment of choice. Complete excision of the primary lesion is necessary. Occasionally, amputation of a portion of the leg is necessary. Lymph node dissection of local and distal nodes is sometimes indicated. Recurrent lesions are treated with chemotherapy and sometimes with deep x-ray therapy.

Leg ulcers secondary to Kaposi's hemorrhagic sarcoma

The cutaneous lesions of classic type Kaposi's sarcoma (not AIDS related) most frequently begin on the lower extremity, especially the feet (Fig. 35-44). Later lesions may spread to involve any area of the body. The earliest lesion may be a reddish-brown nodule or groups of nodules that resemble a dermatofibroma. The lesions may be unilateral, but usually they are bilateral and symmetrical. There is an associated brawny edema of the legs. The process tends to extend along veins and lymphatic vessels. Purpura and eventual ulceration of lesions often result. Chronic lymphedema is frequently present.

Treatment includes superficial x-ray therapy, injections of cytotoxic agents, and local treatment with laser or electrodesiccation and cautery.

Leg ulcers secondary to lymphoma

The term *lymphoma* designates a group of malignant disorders that arise from the lymphoreticular system and

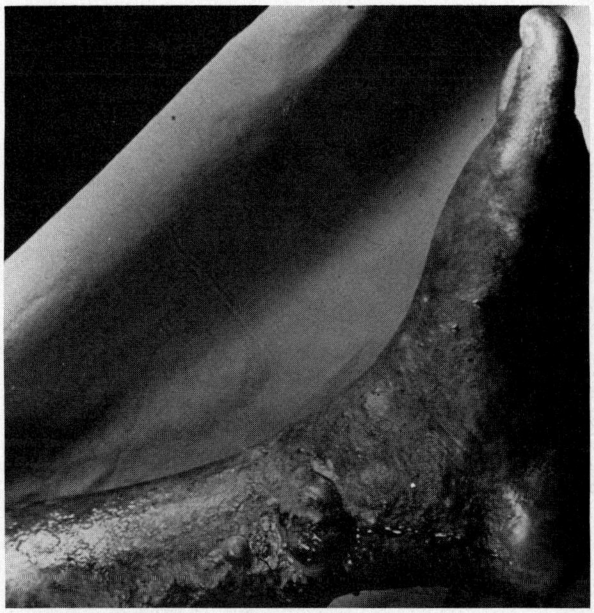

Fig. 35-44. Kaposi's hemorrhagic sarcoma of the lower extremity with fungating and ulcerating tumors.

appear with both cutaneous and visceral infiltration of these abnormal cells. Lymphomas may start from a solitary lesion, but usually the lesions are multiple from the beginning. The lesions may first develop as ulcerations of the lower extremities.

The proper diagnosis is established by an adequate skin or lymph node biopsy, hemogram, bone marrow biopsy, chest x-ray, and CT scans.

The histologic classification varies depending on the predominant cell patterns (T or B cell) and immaturity of cell types. Hodgkin's disease rarely produces skin lesions, but there are skin manifestations of other types of lymphoma. The most common type affecting the skin is mycosis fungoides (cutaneous T-cell lymphoma). Mycosis fungoides primarily involves the skin, but in the late stages it may invade lymph nodes and other internal organs.

Mycosis fungoides is usually divided into three stages: the eczematous or premycotic stage, the infiltrative stage, and the tumor stage. The erythroderma or exfoliative type may be associated with abnormal cells in the peripheral blood called Sézary cells.

The eczematous stage of mycosis fungoides is very similar to eczema, neurodermatitis, psoriasis, parapsoriasis variegata, or parapsoriasis en plaques and may go undiagnosed for 10 to 20 years. There may be scaling patches with variable colors from red to purple. The plaque, or infiltrative stage, shows irregularly shaped, well-demarcated, slightly indurated plaques. There may be some central clearing, and lesions may resemble tinea corporis. The tumor stage consists of tumors of various sizes and round or lobulated brownish-red tumors. These tumors often undergo ulceration (Fig. 35-45).

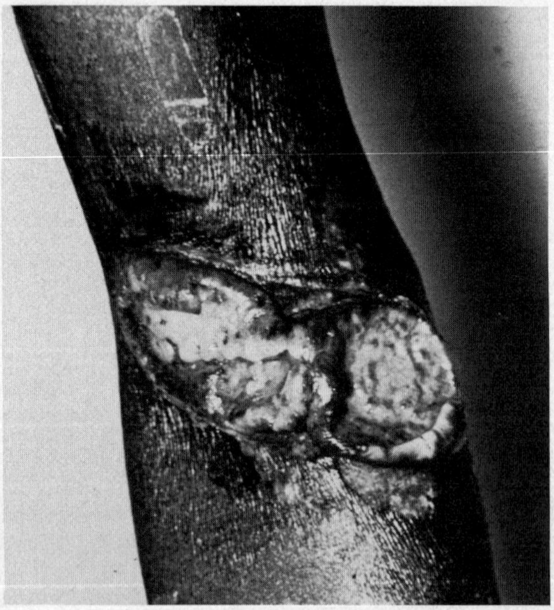

Fig. 35-45. Ulcerative tumor lesion of mycosis fungoides lymphoma.

In the rare form of mycosis fungoides d'emblée, the tumors of the skin develop without previous presence of erythematous or plaque lesions.

Treatment of mycosis fungoides depends on the stage of the disease. Early eczematous lesions respond to topical corticosteroids and UVB (ultraviolet B) phototherapy. The plaque stage responds well to photochemotherapy such as PUVA (psoralen and ultraviolet A) or to topical nitrogen mustard. Combination therapy with PUVA and interferon also works well. Total body electron beam therapy has a high cure rate but also results in considerable morbidity. Late stages are treated with various combinations of chemotherapeutic agents.

Hemangiolymphangioma leg ulcers

This form of tumor is composed largely of dilated and cystic lymphatic vessels combined with dilated blood vessels. The lesions are superficial or deep. The superficial lesions are called *lymphangioma circumscriptum* and are characterized by the presence of groups of small, thick-walled vesicles resembling frog's spawn. The vesicles may have a dark blue color because of red cells mixed in with lymph. The deep type of lesion is called *lymphangioma cavernosum,* and the lesions are more nodular and tumor-like. They also are a deeper reddish-blue. The lesions may ulcerate and drain lymph fluid to the skin.

Treatment is primary excision if the lesions are small or CO_2 laser to larger lesions. They need not be removed.

Malignant melanoma leg ulcers

Malignant melanoma is a vicious tumor that often arises from the skin, occasionally having its origin in a junctional or compound nevus. It often develops in a nevus that the patient has had for many years. There is a sudden increase in size of the lesion, elevation, change in pigmentation, bleeding, or ulceration (Fig. 35-46). The majority of malignant melanomas begin on the lower extremities. The tumor may also appear in the skin as a metastatic melanoma and no primary lesion may ever be discovered.

Melanomas are divided into three clinicopathologic categories, which correlate fairly well with prognosis. The flat, spreading lesions have been designated as superficial spreading melanoma, the nodular lesions as nodular melanoma, and those arising in the melanotic freckles of Hutchinson (lentigo maligna) as lentigo maligna melanoma. Nodular melanoma appears to have the poorest prognosis, whereas lentigo maligna melanoma has the best. All deeply pigmented lesions that could possibly be malignant melanoma must have a biopsy. If the suspicion of melanoma is strong, a wide excision should be done as the initial diagnostic biopsy. If the diagnosis of melanoma is doubtful, a 4 mm punch biopsy is adequate.

The histologic depth of the melanoma (Levels I-V) also correlates well with the prognosis and dictates the extent of treatment needed. Initial treatment is wide excision with

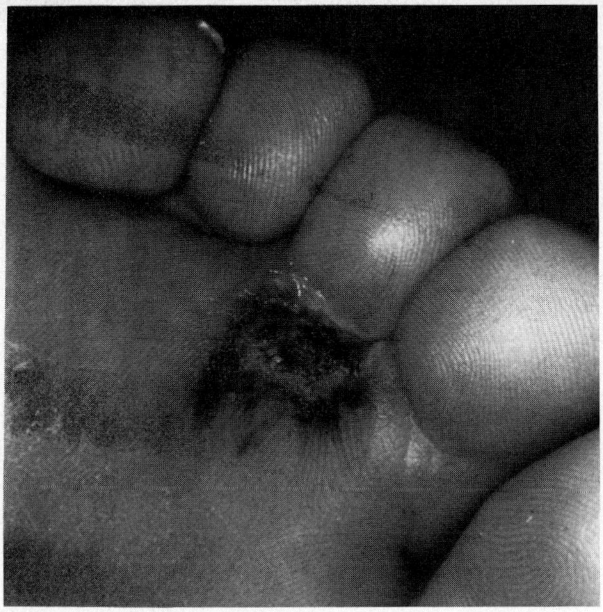

Fig. 35-46. Malignant melanoma of the sole of the foot with early ulceration.

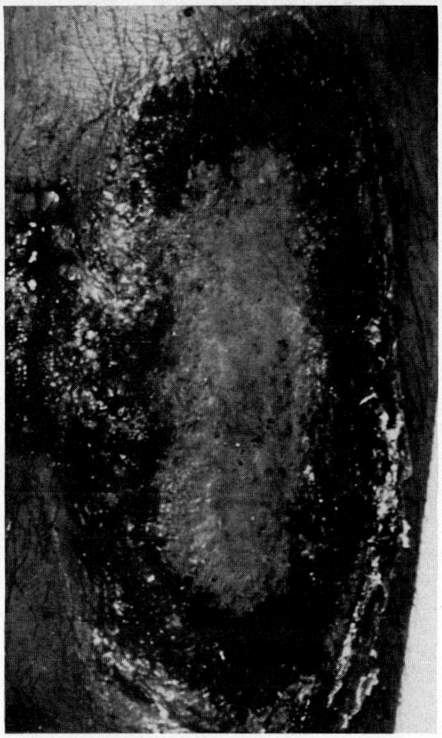

Fig. 35-47. Bromoderma with ulceration of the leg that simulates a deep fungal infection.

primary closure with a skin graft. Lymph node removal is done in Level IV and V melanomas. Immunotherapy, chemotherapy, x-ray, and other experimental forms of therapy are used for late-stage melanoma, but prognosis is poor. Early recognition, public education about early signs, and avoidance of sunlight has improved the prognosis in recent years.

LEG ULCERS SECONDARY TO MISCELLANEOUS CAUSES

Leg ulcers secondary to drugs

Many sedatives and analgesic medications contain bromide compounds. These were used much more commonly 30 years ago, but are still available in some nonprescription medications. Both bromide and iodide compounds can produce similar types of leg ulcers, although iodides tend to produce an acneform or follicular, pustular, bullous, and later fungating hemorrhagic ulcer (Fig. 35-47). The bromide and iodide lesions may also resemble erythema nodosum or the lesions of tertiary syphilis. One characteristic of these lesions, which are often found on the anterior tibial surface, is extreme local pain. Serum bromide or iodide levels in the blood are increased. Treatment consists of discontinuing the bromide or iodide and substituting another halogen such as sodium chloride. Granulomatous bromodermas are usually very slow to heal.

Ergot occasionally, particularly in America, may cause eruptions that result from ergoted grain. The lesions are bullous and pustular and may become gangrenous ulcers. Similar conditions may be produced by ergotamine tartrate.

Methotrexate has become an accepted drug in the treatment of various neoplastic disorders and for many years has been used to manage severe treatment-resistant psoriasis vulgaris. Many different routes (intravenous, oral, intramuscular) and dosage schedules (weekly or daily) have been advocated. Well-recognized adverse effects occur in the rapidly dividing organ systems of the body (bone marrow, gastrointestinal tract). In patients who take an overdose of methotrexate, severe painful oral mucosal ulcerations and spontaneous, painful ulcerations of plaques or psoriasis often develop on their skin (Fig. 35-48). Laboratory studies may show a leukopenia, thrombocytopenia, and anemia. Leukovoran factor may be effective if given within a few hours after an overdose of methotrexate. Ulcerations of the psoriatic plaques will heal slowly with conservative topical therapy.

Leg ulcers secondary to burns

Chemical. Levophed and other vasopressor drugs are used for restoring blood pressure in controlling certain acute hypotensive states. These drugs are powerful peripheral vasoconstrictors, and it is usually recommended that they be administered in a large antecubital vein. When there is extravasation of the solution into the tissue, which might happen if given into a smaller vein in the legs, local necrosis of tissue can result in ulceration (Fig. 35-49). These ulcers usually require grafting to heal.

Several other drugs such as radiopaque dyes used for

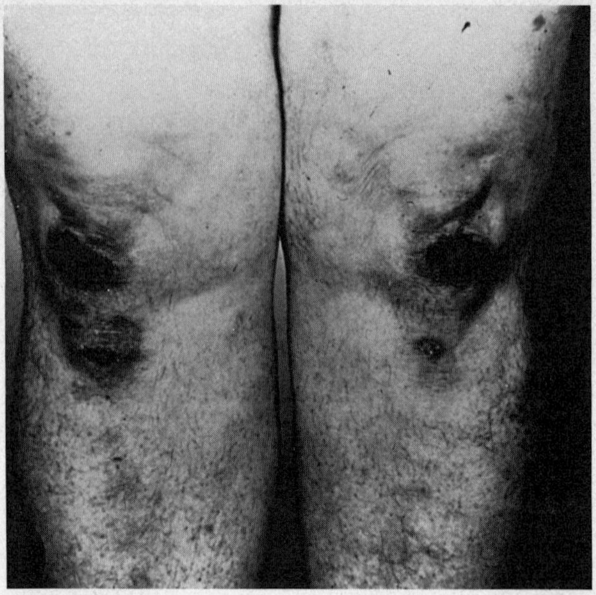

Fig. 35-48 Ulceration of psoriatic plaques on both knees caused by an overdose of methotrexate.

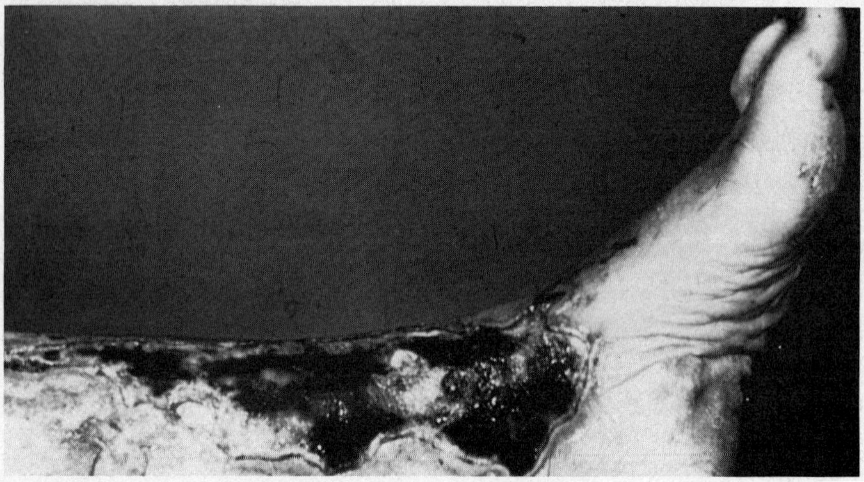

Fig. 35-49. Large necrotic ulcer of leg caused by an infiltration of Levophed into subcutaneous tissue.

arteriograms and nitrogen mustard can produce similar local tissue necrosis and ulceration.

Thermal. Thermal burns, which are third degree, extending to full skin thickness, should be treated by skin grafting. Small ulcerations may heal with conservative management.

Leg ulcers secondary to radiation

Ionizing radiation has been used for years to treat both benign and malignant lesions of the skin. In previous years many benign disorders such as acne, warts, and hypertrichosis in young individuals were treated with large doses of ionizing radiation. These patients begin to show the cumulative effects of the radiation 20 years later. Some of the ulcerations may turn into basal cell or squamous cell carcinomas.

After a single exposure of the skin to a dose of 1000 R or above an acute dermatitis with erythema followed by blistering, pain, edema, necrosis, and ulceration may develop. The roentgen ulcer may take 6 to 8 weeks to develop after the acute phase subsides. The ulcer is characterized by a punched-out appearance, dirty granulating base, undermining of the borders, and extreme pain. The ulcers may enlarge for a time, then heal partially, break down inter-

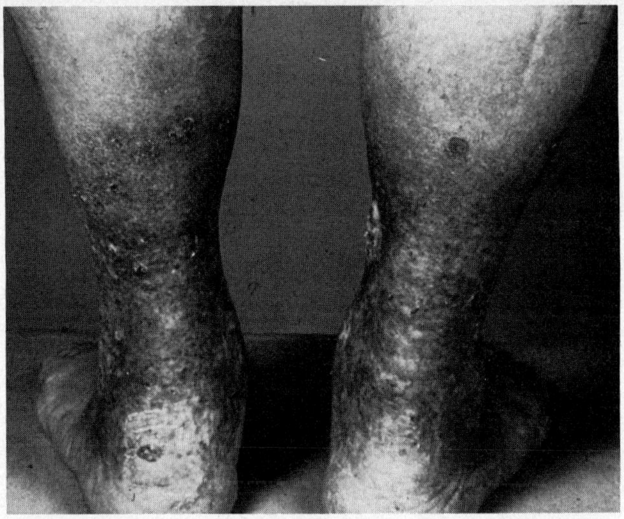

Fig. 35-50. Chronic radiation dermatitis of the legs with ulceration.

mittently, and finally heal with deforming scarring.

Chronic radiation dermatitis shows progressive hypopigmentation, loss of appendages, and atrophy of the epidermis and dermis. Later hyperpigmentation and hypopigmentation and superficial telangiectasia develop. The skin is very susceptible to minor trauma, and ulceration of chronic radiation dermatitis is quite common (Fig. 35-50).

Radiation carcinoma of the skin can occur many years after ionizing radiation. These cancers may first appear as hyperkeratotic plaques or as a chronic nonhealing ulcer. Skin biopsy to make the proper diagnosis and then aggressive destruction or excision and grafting of the tumor is the best treatment.

Decubitus leg ulcers

Decubitus ulcers or pressure sores are most frequently seen in debilitated patients in the older age group and especially in patients with neurologic problems. The ulcers usually result from prolonged application of pressure concentrated in a relatively small area of the body and is sufficient enough to compress the capillary circulation, causing tissue damage and necrosis[24] (Fig. 35-51).

The major emphasis in any decubitus ulcer care program must be ulcer prevention. The skin of all patients, particularly those with high risk for decubitus ulcer development, must be watched constantly. Once any area of skin becomes reddened, pressure on this area must be minimized 100% of the time. The patient should be turned at least every 2 hours while he or she is awake, and the time of turning should be recorded on a "turning sheet." If this regimen is followed, decubitus ulcers will not develop.

Other measures can be used to aid in the program:

1. A foam rubber mattress template with a silicone gel flotation pad insert works very well, providing the foam rubber mattress is placed on a regular mattress and is covered by one sheet. The flotation pad is inserted in this foam rubber mattress, encased in a stocking net. The pad should never be covered with a pillow case, nor should Chuxs be used.
2. An air mattress may help if the apparatus is not defective, if the patient does not weigh too much, and if only one sheet is applied over the mattress. If Chuxs are needed, the air mattress does not work well.
3. A sheepskin will offer protection if the patient does not sweat excessively. It is especially good for protecting the heels and elbows. If Chuxs are needed under the buttocks, the sheepskin is not effective.
4. Protective boots help protect the feet and heels.
5. If the patient is elderly or has dry skin, a skin lotion with a lanolin base should be used instead of soap for his or her daily bath (soap tends to dry out the skin).
6. The skin can be sprayed with tincture of benzoin to protect it. The sprayed area should be covered with powder afterward.
7. Castellani's paint or gentian violet is effective if there is weeping from the reddened areas.

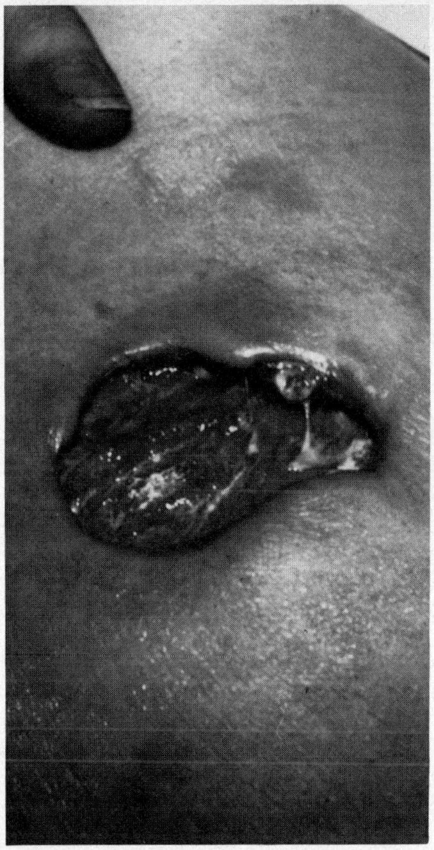

Fig. 35-51. Chronic decubitus ulcers of the leg in an older person confined to bed.

8. A waterbed may be effective in minimizing pressure, but some patients suffer fear and insecurity while in the bed. An inexpensive waterbed can be devised by removing the air valve from an ordinary camping air mattress, filling the mattress with water, clamping it tight, and using an electric blanket beneath the mattress to keep the water at body temperature.

All of the measures used in the treatment of reddened areas are also effective in the treatment of open ulcerations. However, when the ulcer is present, minimizing pressure on the area 100% of the time becomes absolutely mandatory. Any or all of the following measures may be tried, but their effectiveness is variable.

1. A heat lamp may be set up about 12 inches from the area and used for 15 minutes, four times daily.
2. The edges of the open areas may be painted with tincture of benzoin.
3. After cleansing, Burow's solution or potassium permanganate (1:10,000) soaks may be used several times daily.
4. After cleansing, a mixture of equal amounts of milk of magnesia and granulated sugar is applied to the area. The ulcer is cleansed and the mixture is applied daily.
5. Elase ointment can be used if débridement is a problem. The ulcer in the surrounding area must be watched carefully when this is used because of the danger of sensitization.
6. Ichthyol 10% in Lassar's paste may be spread thickly on a gauze sponge large enough to cover the ulcer and its borders. This sponge should be pressed firmly against the skin. The area should be covered with a large, soft dressing such as an ABD pad, which should be changed every day. When changing the dressing, any adherent paste can be removed easily with a gauze sponge saturated with mineral oil.
7. Oxygen therapy can be tried for very deep and draining areas. The areas are irrigated with hydrogen peroxide and then washed. A hole is punched in the bottom of a large wax paper cup or container, and then an oxygen catheter with 100% oxygen running is placed in the bottom of this container. The open mouth of the container is placed against the ulcer for a 15- to 20-minute period daily.
8. Hydrocolloid dressing such as DuoDerm may be placed over the ulcer and changed every 3 to 4 days. This will clean up the area and stimulate granulation tissue (see the section on stasis ulcers).
9. Surgical treatment is often necessary if these measures fail to promote healing of the ulcer. Split-thickness or full-thickness skin grafts may fill the ulcer after it has been surgically débrided. Full-thickness skin flaps are often preferred if good skin is available locally.

Leg ulcers secondary to lichen planus

Lichen planus is a papulosquamous dermatitis of unknown cause that usually appears as a generalized eruption. The diagnostic lesion is a small, flat-topped, polygonal, violaceous papule that later becomes brownish and may leave hyperpigmentation. Histopathology of a typical skin lesion confirms the diagnosis.

Hypertrophic lichen planus most commonly affects the shins and ankles. The lesions are thickened, warty hypertrophic plaques covered with fine adherent scales. Lichen planus may appear with bullae and ulceration confined to the feet and toes, permanent loss of toenails, and a cicatricial alopecia of the scalp. The chronic, painful ulceration of the feet is often a diagnostic problem and may have a surrounding area of atrophic depigmented skin. Treatment consists of either systemic or intralesional corticosteroids.

Leg ulcers secondary to erythema nodosum

Erythema nodosum is a common cause of nodules on the lower leg and often is mistaken for superficial thrombophlebitis. It usually does not ulcerate, but if the lesions do ulcerate, a diagnosis of erythema induratum should be considered. The cause of erythema nodosum is variable, with streptococcal infections and drug sensitivity (iodides, sulfonamides, and penicillin) being the most common causes. Other diseases that may underlie the eruption are tuberculosis, sarcoidosis, deep fungal infections, ulcerative colitis, rheumatic fever, lymphogranuloma venereum, leprosy, and syphilis. Very often no underlying cause of the nodosum lesions is found, and symptomatic therapy with aspirin, antihistamines, or corticosteroids may be indicated.

Leg ulcers secondary to panniculitis (Weber-Christian disease)

Relapsing febrile nodular nonsuppurative panniculitis consists of crops of painful subcutaneous nodules, usually occurring on the thighs and buttocks. Fever and generalized malaise may accompany the attacks, and occasionally severe leukopenia may also be present. The lesions usually do not ulcerate, but there have been cases of ulceration on thighs from the fat necrosis. Skin biopsy shows a nonspecific fat necrosis, depending on the stage of the disease when the biopsy is taken. There are numerous lymphocytes throughout the fat and also a secondary vascular inflammatory reaction. There are many other forms of panniculitis, which are subdivided mainly on histologic changes. They all produce nodules and ulcer-like lesions on the lower legs.

Scleroderma leg ulcers

Scleroderma (progressive systemic sclerosis) is a chronic disease that often begins in the skin or small blood vessels. It progresses to form diffuse, hard, ivory-colored areas, in addition to a hidebound appearance of the hands and face. Internal organs (esophagus, heart, kidneys) may also become involved, and death may ensue.

Skin biopsy is often diagnostic of scleroderma with edema, homogenization, fibrosis, and sclerosis of the collagen. The glandular structures (sweat glands) in the dermis become atrophic and are bound down by the sclerosis of the collagen.

Digital ischemia is a prominent feature of scleroderma, especially of the fingertips, but painful ulcerations may also occur on the lower extremity over the medial and lateral malleolus.

Leg ulceration in rheumatoid arthritis

Necrotizing vasculitis may occur in rheumatoid arthritis as it does in other autoimmune diseases; ischemic ulcerations may occur, primarily on the lower legs. Rheumatoid ulcers tend to be associated with subcutaneous rheumatoid nodules, which also may undergo necrosis and ulcerate. Avoidance of high-dose corticosteroids or rapid withdrawal of corticosteroid is important in these patients. Surgical excision of the rheumatoid nodule that has ulcerated is indicated. Control of the rheumatoid arthritis with corticosteroids and immunosuppressants, such as methotrexate,[25] may help the ulceration heal. Skin grafting is often needed, but failure of a skin graft to take is not uncommon.

Factitial leg ulceration

Ulceration of the lower extremity that is caused by the patient may be one of the most difficult types of leg ulcer to diagnose correctly. The ulcerations may develop many bizarre patterns, mainly because of the multiple methods of producing the ulcerations. Many patients produce the ulcers by picking or probing with their fingers, but more commonly some device is used, including a syringe and needle (containing medicine or sputum), probes, scissors, sticks, acids, chemicals, or cigarettes (Fig. 35-52). Once the diagnosis is suspected the acceptance of the diagnosis by the patient and/or the family is at times even more difficult than is proving the diagnosis.

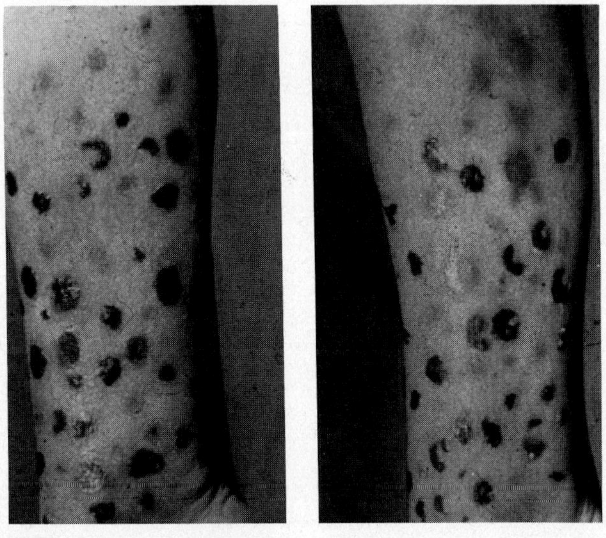

Fig. 35-52. Facticial ulcers of the legs caused by repeated burns by the patient with a cigarette.

One method of proving a factitial cause is to have the ulcerations completely occluded with a nonremovable type of dressing (Unna boot) for several weeks. The factitial ulcer will usually heal, only to reoccur once the patient can get at the skin. A laissez-faire attitude toward the disease on the part of the patient and any peculiar affects that have been noticed will reinforce the suspected diagnosis.

These patients tend to go to many doctors and may be difficult patients to handle. Psychiatric consultation is only partially helpful.

REFERENCES

1. Roenigk HH Jr and Young JR: Leg ulcers: medical and surgical management, Hagerstown, Md, 1975, Harper & Row.
2. Krull EA: Chronic cutaneous ulcerations and impaired healing in human skin, J Am Acad Dermatol 12:394, 1985.
3. Lottie T et al: The pathogenesis of venous ulcers, J Am Acad Dermatol 16:877, 1987.
4. Hendricks WM and Swallow RT: Management of stasis leg ulcers with Unna boots versus elastic support stockings, J Am Acad Dermatol 12:90, 1985.
5. Witkowski JA and Parish LC: Cutaneous ulcer therapy, Int J Dermatol 25:420, 1986.
6. Westerhof W et al: Controlled double-blind trial of fibrinolysin-desoxyribonuclease (Elase) solution in patients with chronic leg ulcers who are treated before autologous skin grafting, J Am Acad Dermatol 17:32, 1987.
7. Coleman GJ and Roenigk HH Jr: Topical therapy of leg ulcers with 20% benzoyl peroxide lotion, Cutis 21:491, 1978.
8. Falanga V: Occlusive wound dressings, Arch Dermatol 124:872, 1988.
9. Falanga V, Zitelli JA, and Eaglstein WH: Wound healing, J Am Acad Dermatol 19:559, 1988.
10. Freidman S and Su D: Hydrocolloid occlusive dressing management of leg ulcers, Arch Dermatol 120:1329, 1984.
11. Varghese MC et al: Local environment of chronic wounds under synthetic dressings, Arch Dermatol 122:52, 1986.
12. Katz S et al: Semipermeable occlusive dressings, Arch Dermatol 122:58, 1986.
13. Alper JC et al: Moist wound healing under a vapor-permeable membrane, J Am Acad Dermatol 8:347, 1983.
14. Alper JC et al: Use of the vapor permeable membrane for cutaneous ulcers: details of application and side effects, J Am Acad Dermatol 11:858, 1984.
15. Eaglstein WH: Experiences with biosynthetic dressings, J Am Acad Dermatol 12:434, 1985.
16. Eaglstein WH et al: Optimal use of an occlusive dressing to enhance healing, Arch Dermatol 124:392, 1988.
17. Angermeier MC, Alper JC, and Urbaniak HS Jr: Vapor-permeable membrane therapy for ulcers or osteomyelitis, J Dermatol Surg Oncol 10:384, 1984.
18. Ceilley RI, Rink MA, and Zueklhe RL: Pinch grafting for chronic ulcers of liver extremities, J Dermatol Surg Oncol 3:303, 1977.
19. Gilmore WA and Wheeland RG: Treatment of ulcers on legs by pinch grafts and a supportive dressing of polyurethane, J Dermatol Surg Oncol 8:177, 1982.

20. Wheeland RG: The technique and current status of pinch grafting. J Dermatol Surg Oncol 13:873, 1986.
21. Dinner MI and Peters CR: Surgical management of ulcers on the lower limbs. J Dermatol Surg Oncol 4:696, 1978.
22. Perry HO and Brunsting LA: Pyoderma gangrenosum, Arch Dermatol 75:380, 1957.
23. Cantwell AR and Marty W: Idiopathic bullae in diabetics, Arch Dermatol 96:42, 1967.
24. Witkowski JA and Parish LC: Histopathology of the decubitus ulcer, J Am Acad Dermatol 6:1014, 1982.
25. Espinoza LR et al: Oral methotrexate therapy for chronic rheumatoid arthritic ulcerations, J Am Acad Dermatol 15:508, 1986.

Chapter 36

THE SWOLLEN LIMB

William F. Ruschhaupt III

The patient with a swollen limb is a common problem for the practicing physician.[1] Swelling, like fever, should not be considered a disease in itself, but rather a sign of an underlying disorder. Although the disorder is often minor, at times edema may indicate a serious disease process. It is important to recognize, though, that all swelling is not edema. The finding of swelling or edema should alert the physician to seek the cause.

PHYSIOLOGIC PRINCIPLES

The process that leads to finding the correct cause of a swollen limb must be built on an understanding of the factors affecting edema formation.[2] Edema represents an increase in the interstitial (extravascular) component of the extracellular fluid volume. There are many systemic influences, such as renal salt and water balance, and physiologic concepts, such as effective blood volume or adequacy of arterial vascular filling, which will not be discussed here, but do affect edema formation systemically. However, there is a need to review six factors affecting edema formation in an extremity. Four are major physiologic principles: capillary blood pressure, plasma colloid oncotic pressure, tissue colloid oncotic pressure, and tissue pressure itself. The other two factors are changes in capillary permeability and obstruction of lymphatic flow, either of which can occur uniquely in the affected limb. None of these factors is routinely measured or quantified for the clinician.

Interstitial fluid contains all the components found in blood plasma except the amount of protein. The principal physiologic processes that account for the dynamics of interstitial fluid within any extremity are filtration and reabsorption. Filtration is the process that occurs on the arterial end of the capillary system, while reabsorption is thought to occur on the venous side of the capillary system. Changes in any of the six physiologic factors affecting the extracellular fluid volume can result in edema formation in the affected limb.

Capillary blood pressure

Arterial blood pressure is the driving force for filtration in the arterial portion of the capillary system. As blood passes through the normal arterial bed and begins to enter the venous side, the effects of arterial blood pressure are diminished. Working in conjunction with the one-way valve system of the deep veins of an extremity, the muscles of that extremity are the pump for the venous side of the circulation. Normal capillary venous pressure is therefore physiologically lower than normal capillary arterial pressure, facilitating reabsorption of interstitial fluid, if all other factors are static. However, a static state is never achieved in the dynamics of human physiology. At any given time, either filtration or reabsorption is occurring predominantly. If local venous pressure increases, as with a deep vein occlusion, then the localized central venous pressure in that extremity would be increased and transmitted in a retrograde fashion. An increase in capillary venous blood pressure would occur. In this setting reabsorption would then be decreased, and an increase in the interstitial fluid (edema) would follow.

Colloid oncotic pressure

Oncotic pressure in the extracellular fluid compartments is created by the concentration of electrolytes, glucose, urea, and proteins within the extracellular fluid. The relatively large protein molecules of the plasma exert their osmotic influence within the capillary system because of their inability to pass through the capillary walls. Plasma has a relatively high concentration of the osmotically active proteins, whereas interstital fluid has a relatively low concentration. In the normal state, low concentrations of osmotically active proteins in the interstital fluid rarely favor an increase in the interstital fluid volume at either side of the capillary bed. Therefore in the normal state, if there is no change in the number of protein molecules within the interstitial fluid, the concentration of proteins in the plasma would be highest on the venous side of the capillary bed. Reabsorption of the interstitial fluid on the venous side would again be favored.

Interstitial tissue pressure

The area available within the tissues of an extremity for interstital fluid volume is limited. When the volume increases above its normal level, the pressure within the space increases. Obviously, this increasing pressure must be overcome by the forces favoring filtration if any further accumulation of interstitial fluid is to continue. However, in the normal state, tissue pressure is not high in any of the extremities and can be easily exceeded by the dynamics of capillary arterial pressure.

Capillary permeability

The permeability of the capillary walls to plasma proteins has already been mentioned. The capillary membrane is semipermeable, but any change in this condition would allow for a variation in flow of fluid from the normal pathways. Increasing capillary permeability to proteins would allow plasma proteins to exit the intravascular space for the extravascular space, thus critically changing colloid oncotic pressures in the plasma and interstitial fluid. Plasma colloid oncotic pressure is the major driving force for reabsorption of interstitial fluid. This change would critically favor edema formation.

Lymphatic flow

The lymphatic system is a direct outflow system for the interstitial fluid. However, lymphatic fluid contains large amounts of protein. The walls of the lymphatic system are permeable to protein, but the capillary walls are not. When the flow of lymph from an extremity is obstructed or inadequate, there are several factors that favor edema. Not only is edema caused by the direct obstruction of the lymphatic flow, but also the protein content of the interstitial fluid increases. This gives rise to an increase in interstitial colloid oncotic pressure, thus decreasing the pressure gradient favoring reabsorption on the venous side of the capillary bed.

CLINICAL APPROACH

The history and physical examination remain the cornerstones for the diagnosis of the swollen limb. The findings are important in determining what additional tests are necessary to confirm the diagnosis.

History

The acuity of onset of swelling in an extremity is a strong clue to its cause. Sudden onset of swelling over several hours or days suggests an acute process such as deep vein thrombophlebitis, cellulitis, compartment syndrome, or gastrocnemius muscle rupture. A gradual, progressive onset over several weeks to months suggests lymphedema, chronic venous insufficiency, some systemic process, or exposure to particular medications. Edema that occurs intermittently and then resolves, but continues to recur is typical for the limb swelling seen with recurrent episodes of lymphangitis and cellulitis.

Edema is usually worse at the end of the day and improved by morning. Redistribution occurs as a result of the recumbent position during sleep. If the patient is unable to sleep or rest horizontally, this diurnal variation may be lost. As the duration of the edema continues and the cause persists, daily variation will tend to diminish over time.

The presence or absence of pain can be helpful in arriving at the correct diagnosis. Painful swelling of a limb suggests thrombophlebitis, cellulitis, compartment syndrome, muscle rupture, or reflex sympathetic dystrophy. The swelling caused by lymphedema and the swelling from systemic causes should be painless.

Systemic symptoms are important. A history of swelling associated with a high fever and shaking chills directs the clinician to an infectious source such as recurrent cellulitis, lymphangitis, or septic phlebitis. Nonseptic deep vein thrombophlebitis may be associated with a low-grade fever, but it does not produce a high fever or chills.

The patient should be questioned regarding predisposing conditions that may have contributed to the development of the swollen leg such as prolonged plane flights, automobile trips, any period of prolonged immobility, trauma, accidents, operations, or childbirth.

Physical examination

One of the most obvious findings on physical examination is whether swelling involves one limb or both. The division of the causes of limb swelling into causes for unilateral and bilateral swelling forms the basis for the discussion of specific causes in subsequent portions of this chapter.

The appearance of the skin of the involved limb gives many clues to the underlying causes. Frequently, comparison with the opposite extremity is helpful in determining the change from normal appearance. A reddened area, perhaps with red tender streaks leading away from the area, is highly suggestive of cellulitis with lymphangitis. A more elongated raised area of redness with a palpable cord is suggestive of a superficial thrombophlebitis. A reddish-blue hue to the extremity suggests the presence of a proximal deep vein thrombophlebitis. Ecchymoses would indicate trauma or a ruptured muscle.

The location of the swelling is of particular importance. Swelling in the calf or thigh in the absence of ankle or foot edema indicates a local process within those muscle groups or regions and not a true edematous process. A ruptured medial head of the gastrocnemius, traumatic hematoma, or an osteogenic sarcoma can develop in this way. Involvement of the foot, resulting in a typical dorsal hump, and involvement of the toes is a sign of lymphedema. An enlarged limb that spares the foot and toes suggests lipedema.

Edema of the upper extremity vs edema of the lower extremity helps to create some interesting contrasts. Acute deep vein thrombophlebitis of the upper extremity is usually secondary to thoracic outlet syndrome or to iatrogenic causes from the use of intravenous catheters. Swelling is usually the first manifestation of the problem. By contrast acute deep vein thrombophlebitis in the lower extremity is variable in terms of its frequency of producing edema, not only at the time of onset but also through its course. The lower extremity is frequently the site of chronic venous insufficiency as a result of prior deep vein thrombophlebitis, yet venous insufficiency and stasis symptoms are unusual sequelae in the upper extremity. Lymphedema in the lower extremity is about equally distributed between primary and secondary causes, whereas in the upper extremity, lymphedema is almost always secondary in nature.

Diagnostic tests

Following a thorough history and physical examination, the noninvasive vascular laboratory can play a critical role in the differential diagnosis of various causes of the swollen extremity. Negative as well as positive studies can be significant to the clinician. The diagnosis of proximal deep vein thrombophlebitis can be firmly established in a good noninvasive vascular laboratory with the use of duplex ultrasonography. In the lower extremities, this noninvasive study can accurately identify the presence or absence of deep vein thrombophlebitis in the popliteal, superficial femoral, common femoral, and iliac veins. The technique can also detect the presence of a Baker's cyst or popliteal artery aneurysm. While this technique is not as accurate for consistent demonstration of a calf vein thrombophlebitis, if the patient has a swollen leg from at least the knee distally, then a negative study implies that proximal deep vein thrombophlebitis is not the cause of that swelling.

If the noninvasive laboratory does not have duplex ultrasonography, then various plethysmographic techniques can be accurate in the diagnosis of proximal deep vein thrombophlebitis. It is important, however, that an ongoing quality control program exists in those laboratories, since these techniques are technician dependent for accuracy.

If the noninvasive vascular laboratory is unavailable, then standard radiographic contrast venography should be used to establish the presence or absence of acute deep vein thrombophlebitis.

Other studies are also used for assessing the swollen limb. Computerized tomography (CT) scanning and magnetic resonance imaging (MRI) are particularly useful in evaluating localized masses or unusual causes. When looking for systemic causes, electrocardiogram, chest x-ray, urinalysis, complete blood cell count, electrolytes, renal function tests, and hepatic function tests are necessary.

CAUSES OF UNILATERAL SWOLLEN LIMB

(see the accompanying box)

Acute deep vein thrombophlebitis (Chapter 24)

Of the three most common vascular causes of the swollen limb (deep vein thrombophlebitis, chronic venous insufficiency, and lymphedema), acute deep vein thrombophlebitis can have the most dramatic onset. Swelling, bluish-red discoloration, and prominent veins may be associated with acute deep vein thrombophlebitis and may or may not be accompanied by or preceded by pain.

Chronic venous insufficiency (Chapter 26)

One of the results of an acute deep vein thrombophlebitis can be the development of chronic venous insufficiency. Damage to the valves in the venous system can cause a stasis syndrome to develop with pigmentation, dermatitis, edema, cellulitis, and ulceration. It is important to note that stasis cellulitis is a nonbacterial inflammatory process.

Lymphedema (Chapter 27)

The third most common vascular cause of limb swelling is lymphedema. Lymphedema has a slow, insidious onset, unless it is related to an acute surgical or traumatic disruption of the lymphatic system. Lymphedema should be categorized into either primary or secondary types. Depending on the age of the patient at the onset of the lymphedema and its duration, an aggressive search for the underlying cause may be necessary. It is important to recognize that lymphedema always begins in the most distal portion of the ex

Causes of unilateral swollen limb

Acute deep vein thrombophlebitis
Chronic venous insufficiency
Lymphedema
Cellulitis
Abscess
Osteomyelitis
Charcot's joint
Popliteal cyst
Popliteal artery aneurysm
Trauma
Compartment syndrome
Vascular anomalies
Thermal injury
Tumors
Dependency
Disuse
Gastrocnemius rupture
Revascularization
Retroperitoneal fibrosis
Factitial

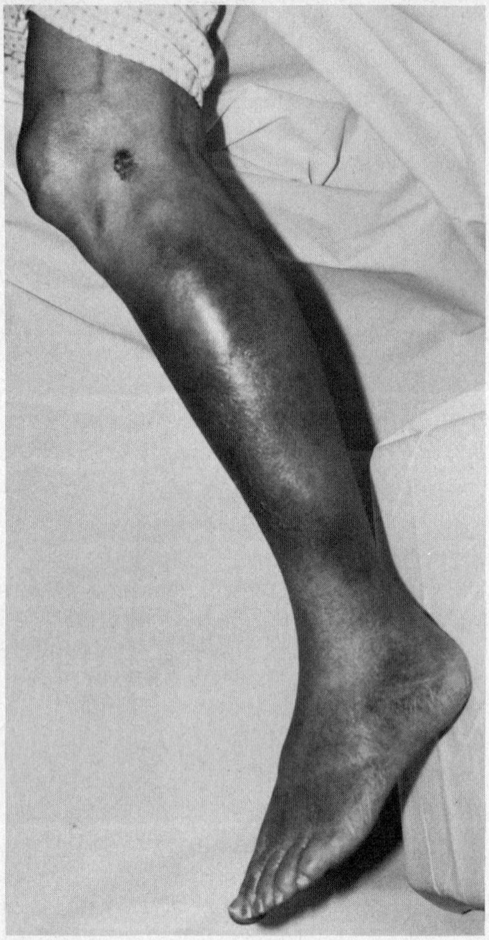

Fig. 36-1. Cellulitis. Notice the skip areas of involvement in the foot and leg.

tremity; therefore careful observation of the hand or foot is important in discovering this entity early.

Cellulitis

Cellulitis is the most common infectious cause of limb swelling (Fig. 36-1). Cellulitis can occur as a single isolated event or a series of recurrent events and is regularly misdiagnosed (usually as recurrent thrombophlebitis or worsening chronic venous insufficiency). Cellulitis occurs when there is a portal through the normal skin barriers for bacteria to enter and to release their toxins in the subcutaneous tissues. The acute onset with swelling, localized redness, and pain is also frequently associated with systemic signs of high fever, shaking chills, and sweats. The redness does not have to be uniform and often does have skip areas. Regional lymph nodes can also be tender and enlarged.

Cellulitis generally responds well to antibiotic therapy, and improvement can be quite rapid, especially with intravenous therapy. The key to preventing recurrent attacks of cellulitis lies in adequate antibiotic therapy for the initial event, as well as in the recognition and appropriate management of the portal of entry through the skin.

Of all the portals of entry, the most commonly overlooked are the skin cracks and fissures that occur in the skin between the toes as a result of tinea pedis. Without recognition and treatment of this fungal infection of the skin, recurrent episodes of cellulitis will occur. Recurrent episodes of cellulitis and accompanying lymphangitis can produce severe secondary lymphedema as a result of the destruction and scarring of the lymphatic vessels in the involved extremity. Other portals of entry for recurrent cellulitis include the sites of drug abuse, contusions, abrasions, ulcerations, ingrown toenails, and hangnails.

Unfortunately, many episodes of cellulitis go unrecognized because a diagnosis of deep vein thrombophlebitis is erroneously made. Because many physicians in the past have treated deep vein thrombophlebitis not only with anticoagulants but also with antibiotics, the "phlebitis" responds to this therapy, and the cellulitis is not recognized. The problem with this approach is that episodes recur because the portal of entry has not been eliminated.

Abscess

Abscesses rarely develop from a cellulitic process, but instead they follow a deep-seated infection, which can occur as a result of some sort of puncture wound. Swelling of the involved limb is most frequently localized with early abscess formation but can be significant enough to give the appearance of a generalized edematous process. The principles of management of this entity are recognition of the problem, obtaining adequate cultures, adequate incision and drainage of the abscess, and appropriate antibiotic therapy.

Osteomyelitis

Osteomyelitis is the third infectious process that can produce limb swelling. Again the swelling occurs usually in the distal portion of an extremity. The diabetic patient with diabetic neuropathy and neurotrophic ulcers represents an ideal setting for this infection to occur, but any patient with a severe peripheral neuropathy is susceptible. Patients with sickle cell anemia are also prone to develop osteomyelitis, particularly from *Salmonella* organisms. With hematogenous osteomylitis, any of the long bones of the extremity are common targets.

Charcot's joints (Chapter 38)

In Charcot's neuropathic arthropathy, the joints are not only swollen, but they are also usually deformed. The swelling can be easily noticed and is initially accompanied by localized warmth. The swelling and warmth can extend proximally from the involved joint and can produce localized tenderness on examination in an otherwise neuropathic distal portion of an extremity. Such a picture is not only frequently clinically confusing but also radiographically confusing. On plain films it is often difficult, if not impossible, to separate the early Charcot's joint from osteomyelitis since the neuropathic extremity is a prime setting for either process. Further radiographic investigations may be necessary, including various nuclear medicine scanning techniques, which may or may not shed further light on the matter. MRI also holds some promise for resolving these diagnostic conflicts before proceeding with exploratory surgical intervention.

Popliteal cysts

Popliteal cysts (Baker's cysts) may produce localized swelling in an extremity behind the knee or swelling distally with the signs and symptoms of deep vein thrombosis.[4] The latter occurs when there is compression of the popliteal vein. Dissection of a Baker's cyst, without rupture, into the muscles of the lower extremities can also produce swelling. If a popliteal cyst ruptures, the signs and symptoms are difficult to distinguish from a deep vein thrombosis. Indeed, an acute deep vein thrombophlebitis can result from compression by a large popliteal cyst. Physical examination should suggest the presence of a popliteal cyst in either the swollen leg or the nonswollen leg, particularly in a patient with either rheumatoid arthritis or long-standing degenerative joint disease involving the knee. A popliteal cyst can be accurately diagnosed by ultrasound examination in the vascular laboratory, but occasionally arthrography may be needed to solidify the diagnosis. This is especially true if the cyst has ruptured.

Popliteal artery aneurysm (Chapter 17)

Just as large popliteal cysts can cause venous compression, so can large popliteal artery aneurysms produce increased venous hypertension by this same mechanism. Persistent restriction of outflow of the venous system in an extremity will create the factors that favor distal edema formation and in some cases be the initial manifestation of this significant arterial problem.

Trauma

Severe trauma leading to fractures and even disruption of skin integrity is an obvious cause of a swollen limb. In such a setting the clinician is faced with the task of determining whether or not thrombophlebitis or cellulitis might be associated with the trauma. Incidental or unnoticed trauma can also produce limb swelling (Fig. 36-2). In most instances this is more localized and may or may not be accompanied by ecchymoses.

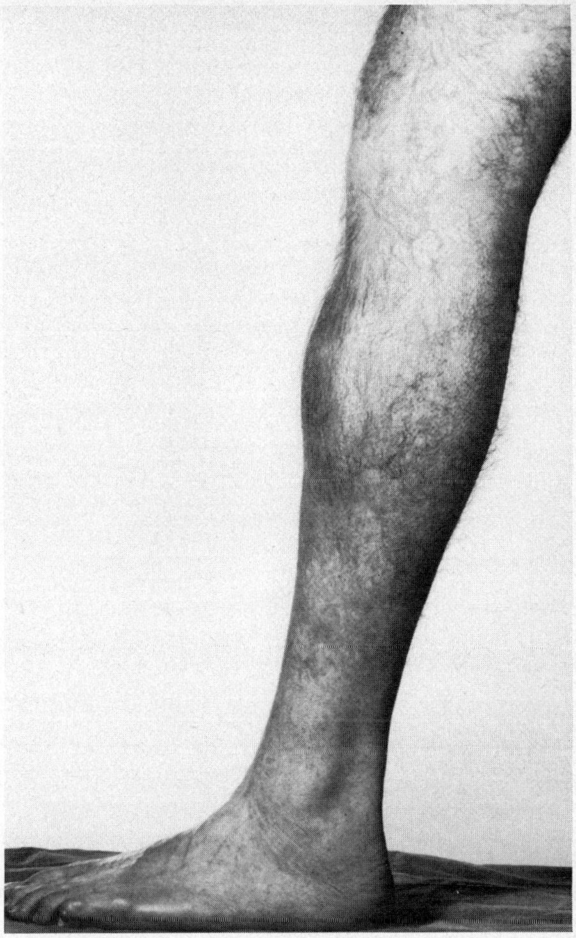

Fig. 36-2. Traumatic hematoma on anterior tibial surface, which did not produce compartment syndrome, but which did require drainage.

Compartment syndrome (Chapter 32)

Sudden occlusion of an artery by thrombosis or embolism can lead to severe pain, induration, and edema. Compartment syndromes can occur because of the local tissue response to severe hypoxemia or to restoration of blood flow to an ischemic extremity. In a relatively fixed, enclosed area, the compartment's ability to accommodate a sudden increase in volume is limited. This is particularly true if there are other mechanical factors such as trauma or encasement in bandages or dressings. These syndromes are most commonly seen in the lower extremity but can occur in the arms as well. Fasciotomy, either prophylactic or therapeutic, is occasionally necessary in the management of the compartment syndrome.

Vascular anomalies (Chapter 30)

The principle that not all swelling is edema is clearly demonstrated in patients with vascular anomalies. Hyperthophied extremities or muscle groups caused by either congenital or acquired arteriovenous fistulas are typical examples (Fig. 36-3). Physical findings of a thrill or bruit in the area can suggest the presence of an arteriovenous fistula. Increased temperature locally may also occur, and occasionally congestive heart failure and cardiac enlargement may be found.

Klippel-Trenaunay syndrome is a distinct clinical triad of varicose veins, port-wine stain (nevus flammeus), and

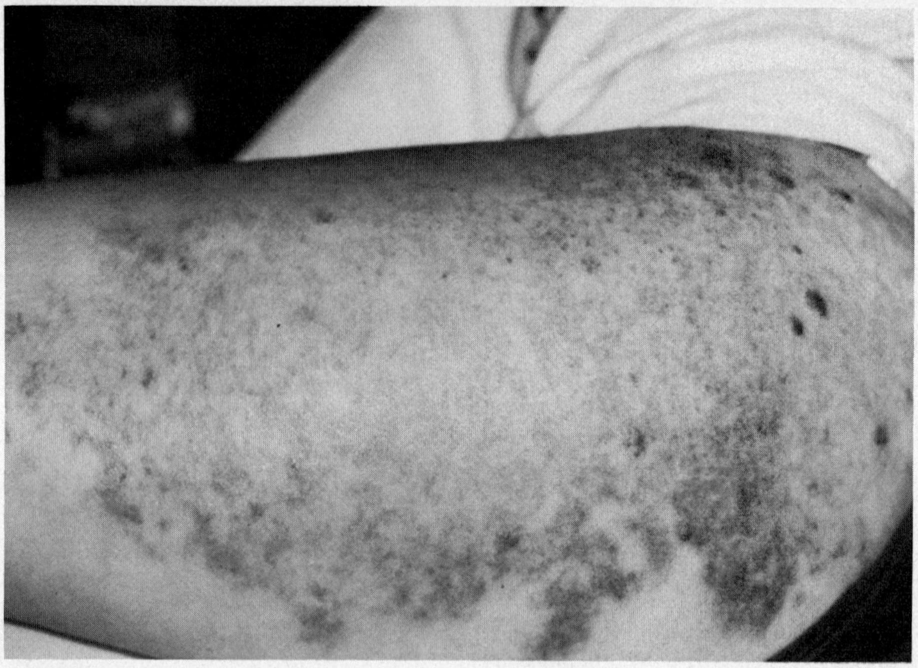

Fig. 36-3. Capillary venous hemangioma involving lateral proximal thigh and hip region.

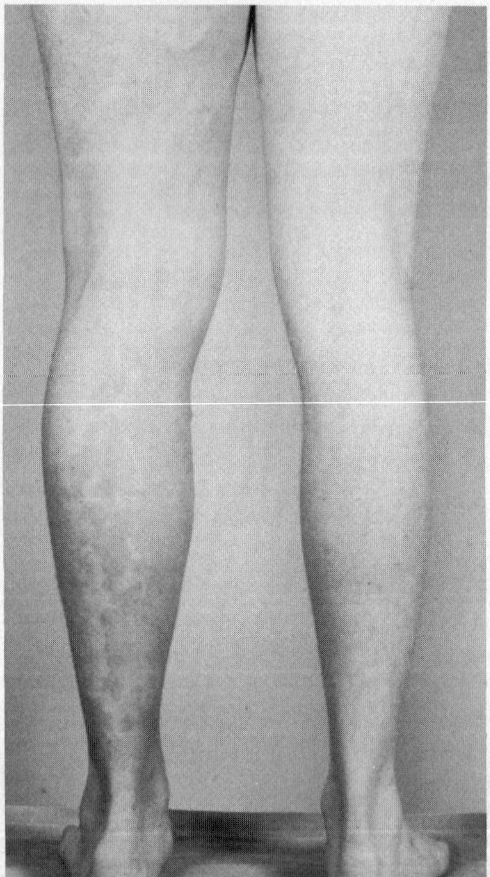

Fig. 36-4. Klippel-Trenaunay syndrome. Varicose veins, cutaneous hemangioma (port-wine stain), and muscular hypertrophy.

muscular hypertrophy (Fig. 36-4). This syndrome has been associated with the occurrence of arteriovenous fistulas, as well as the agenesis of the deep venous system.[5] It is important to recognize the latter since surgical ligation and stripping of varicose veins in these patients can result in severe chronic venous insufficiency.

Thermal injury

Exposure to severe heat, as well as cold, can produce a swollen limb. There is a common mechanism for edema formation in heat or cold injury. The major change occurs as a result of damage to the capillary membrane. Thermal injury increases capillary permeability, resulting in greater flow of plasma proteins from the intravascular space into the interstitial fluid. With severe cold exposure, edema does not occur until rewarming takes place.

Tumors

Limb swelling can be produced by a variety of tumors, both benign and malignant. Cavernous hemangiomas and others vascular tumors are discussed in Chapter 34. Any tumor of bone, muscle, tendon, cartilage, nerve, blood, or lymphatic vessel can produce a swollen extremity.[3]

Dependency

Both unilateral and bilateral limb swelling can be caused by dependency. Unilateral leg swelling secondary to dependency is frequently seen with severe arterial insufficiency. The patient will have rest pain and/or ischemic ulcerations and will be unable to sleep lying flat. The patient will dangle one foot over the side of the bed throughout the

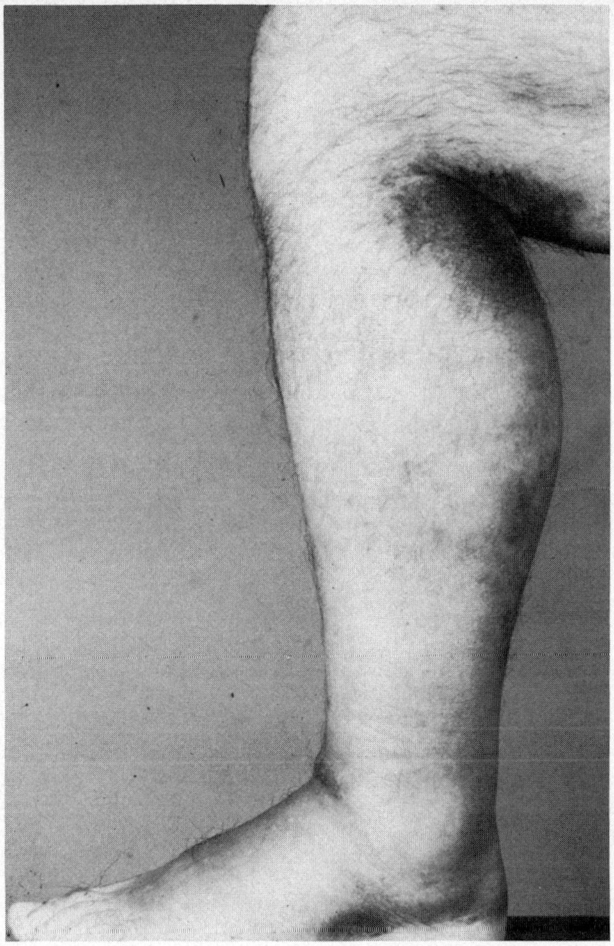

Fig. 36-5. Ruptured medial head of gastrocnemius. Ecchymoses in popliteal fossa and malleoli (below).

night, resulting in prolonged dependency and edema. Similarly, prolonged use of crutches with one leg dependent or a prolonged disuse of an extremity will result in limb swelling.

Gastrocnemius rupture

The weekend athlete who has a history of sudden onset of pain in the calf and subsequent leg swelling is a classic example of a patient with a rupture of the medial head of the gastrocnemius muscle. However, this injury can occur by falling off a curb or down a step. There is usually a history of a specific event. Some patients describe hearing a "snap" or "pop" with a sudden onset of severe pain in the calf and an inability to bear weight on the involved leg. The tear in the medial head of the gastrocnemius causes swelling to develop promptly, and within several days ecchymosis can occur around both the medial and lateral side of the ankle and foot (Fig. 36-5). The ecchymosis is the result of gravitational dissection of blood from the torn muscle through the muscle tissue planes and can take a characteristic crescent shape beneath the malleoli.

It is important to recognize the clinical picture and to treat appropriately. This syndrome in the past has been confused with acute deep vein thrombophlebitis and treated with anticoagulants. This leads to further hemorrhage into the calf. Treatment with casting for this problem promotes the development of acute deep venous thrombophlebitis. The appropriate treatment consists of the application of ice packs to the calf during the first 24 to 48 hours and elevation. This should be followed with avoidance of all weight bearing on the leg for a few days and later progressive ambulation. Gradual stretching exercises in a physical therapy program may be helpful. As the patient returns to weight bearing, a lift in the heel of the shoe of the involved leg avoids severe stretching of the gastrocnemius. The patient is advised to avoid physical activity with quick stop-and-go actions for the duration of the recovery process. Following recovery, an ongoing stretching program before and after any exercise is critical.

Revascularization

There are several mechanisms for limb swelling following revascularization of an extremity. Besides the trauma of surgical incisions, revascularization creates a pathophysi-

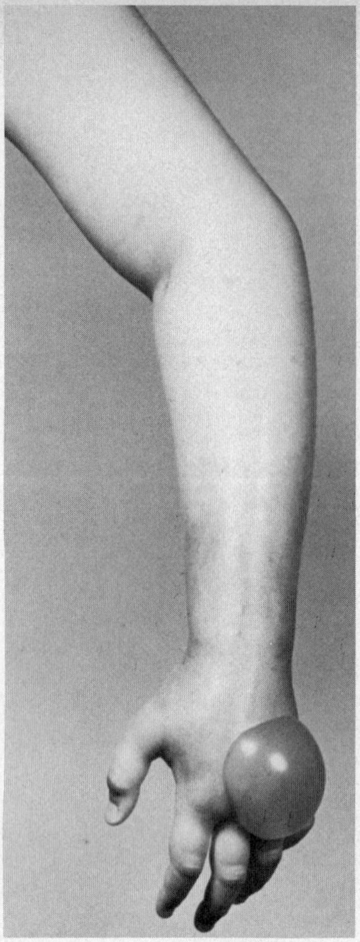

Fig. 36-6. Revascularization bullae following arterial revascularization.

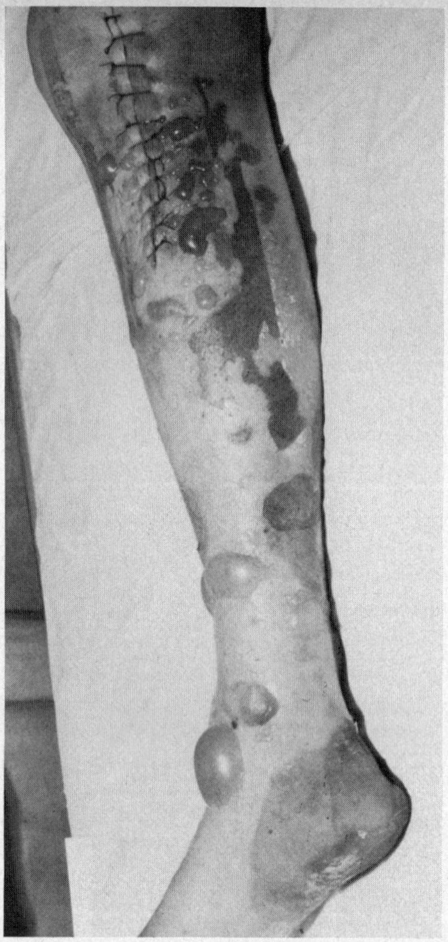

Fig. 36-7. Revascularization bullae following successful femoral-popliteal bypass.

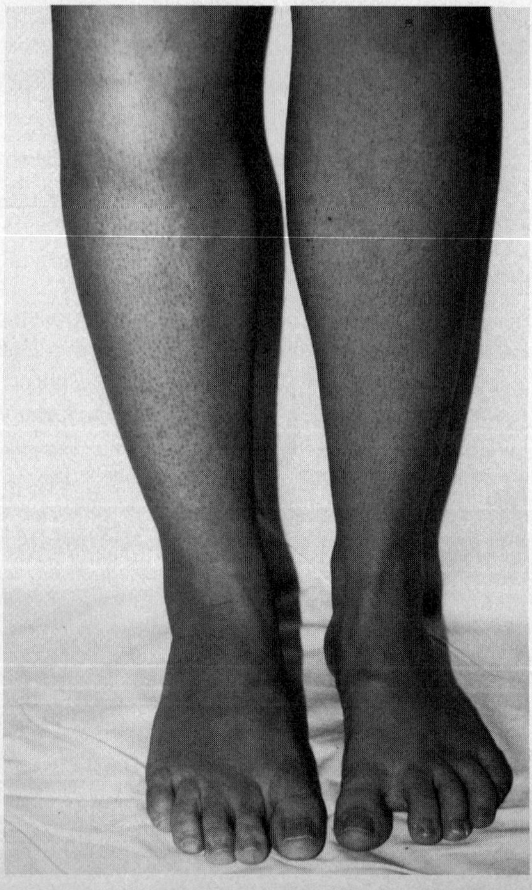

Fig. 36-8. Factitial edema. Note distinct circumferential mark from tourniquet constriction on proximal right calf.

ology similar to that discussed in the section on thermal injury. In the presence of severe, usually chronic, ischemia in an extremity the capillary membrane is damaged and permeability to plasma proteins is altered. Once revascularization occurs, not only is there increased intravascular pressure affecting a damaged capillary membrane, but also the increased permeability allows greater egress of the plasma proteins from the intravascular space. Occasionally, the factors favoring edema formation are so strong that in addition to generalized leg swelling, actual bullous formation occurs (Figs. 36-6 and 36-7).[2] These bullae can resolve quietly and require only clean dressings following spontaneous rupture.

Retroperitoneal fibrosis

In retroperitoneal fibrosis, involvement of the venous and lymphatic vessels in the retroperitoneal space can produce lower extremity swelling. Lower extremity swelling can be either unilateral or bilateral. Retroperitoneal fibrosis can be idiopathic or can occur secondary to the use of methysergide (Sansert) for the treatment of migraine headache. Occasionally a positive response can be obtained with the use of steroids for retroperitoneal fibrosis.

Factitial limb swelling

Factitial limb swelling can be very difficult to diagnose and treat. Factitial edema is self-induced by a constrictive garment, strap, or device. The history is confusing because the edema has a fluctuating pattern in terms of its occurrence and its relationship to activity or time of day. The problem can continue for many months or years before being suspected. The most helpful clue on physical examination is a distinct, sharp demarcation at the edge of the edema and evidence of skin marks correlating with the type and location of constricting device used to produce the swelling (Fig. 36-8).[2] Treatment of this entity requires the involvement of multiple clinical disciplines including psychiatry and the building of support networks for the patient.

CAUSES OF BILATERAL SWOLLEN LIMB

(see the accompanying box)

Causes of bilateral swollen limb

- Congestive heart failure
- Cirrhosis
- Protein deficient states
- Acute glomerulonephritis
- Cushing's syndrome
- Pregnancy
- Obesity
- Lipedema
- Dependency
- Pretibial myxedema
- Drug-induced
- Idiopathic cyclic edema

Congestive heart failure

Limb edema can be associated with congestive heart failure, may be very subtle, and may not be associated with the typical findings of dyspnea on exertion, orthopnea, or paroxysmal nocturnal dyspnea. In older people limb edema frequently occurs concurrently with chronic obstructive pulmonary disease and congestive heart failure. In this setting, edema can be an early manifestation.

Cirrhosis

Because of many dilated venous tributaries and multiple small arterial venous fistulas, hepatic cirrhosis is commonly associated with an increased total blood volume with decreased effective blood volume. When combined with alterations in serum albumin levels there is further activation of the salt and water retaining mechanisms of the body. Peripheral edema is usually seen in this condition only when both mechanisms are present and hypoalbuminemia is readily detected.[6]

Protein deficiency states

In protein deficiency states such as severe malnutrition or protein-losing gastroenteropathy, the marked decrease of plasma proteins results in a decrease in the plasma colloid oncotic pressure. These changes in plasma colloid oncotic pressure significantly enhance the increase in interstitial fluid accumulation. Nephrotic syndrome results in edema through the same changes in plasma proteins. However, the cause of the hypoproteinemic state is the markedly increased renal loss of protein in the urine, not secondary to decreased synthesis or intake.

Acute glomerulonephritis

In the presence of abnormal renal function, not only are there hemodynamic factors causing edematous states but also intrinsic changes in the kidney that favor edema formation. Acute glomerulonephritis appears to create a primary renal avidity for sodium and water, in addition to changes in capillary permeability and their secondary hemodynamic changes.[6] Hematuria, proteinuria, and hypertension are usually also present with the edema.

Cushing's syndrome

Cushing's syndrome is the result of increased production of cortisol (hydrocortisone) by the adrenal gland. The syndrome can also be produced by ingestion of hydrocortisone-containing or producing drugs. Although cortisol normally increases solute free water clearance, at high concentrations cortisol favors tubular sodium reabsorption. It is this mineralocorticoid activity of high levels of cortisol that leads to edema formation.

Idiopathic cyclic edema

Idiopathic cyclic edema is poorly understood and not well recognized. The diagnosis is made after other causes of edema have been excluded. It affects almost exclusively women who are usually 20 to 40 years of age. They may be mildly obese and may have associated psychosomatic complaints or disorders. The typical location for the edema is in both the upper and lower extremities as well as the face. The edema appears to be directly related to the upright position, and a 2- to 4-pound weight gain throughout the day can occur. This syndrome is not to be confused with the fluid retention associated with the menstrual cycle. There are no definitive pathophysiologic mechanisms to explain idiopathic edema. Several mechanisms have been proposed including secondary hyperaldosteronism, excessive secretion of antidiuretic hormone, orthostatic change in capillary membrane permeability, estrogen/progesterone hormone imbalance, abnormal albumin metabolism, and even defects in the vasomoter tone of the capillary venous system. The number of treatments suggested is greater than the number of explanations for this syndrome. Suggested treatments have included restrictive salt and water intake, bed rest, weight loss, the use of elastic support stockings, and modified psychotherapy. Numerous medications have been reported to be effective, including progesterone, spironolactone, thiazide, other diuretics, propranolol, captopril, and dextroamphetamine. With such a wide array of suggested pathophysiology and treatments, it is fortunate that idiopathic cyclic edema tends to subside in a self-limiting course from a few months to several years.[7]

Pregnancy

In contrast to disease processes that create swollen extremities, pregnancy causes peripheral vasodilation, which creates a decrease in the effective blood volume. This, in turn, leads to sodium and fluid retention. There appears to be some compensatory mechanism that does not allow the sodium retention to progress to the same degree as seen in individuals with abnormal disease states and similar pathophysiology.[8] In addition, during pregnancy the gravid uterus can compress the lower venous collecting system, thus increasing distal venous pressure.

Obesity

Obesity appears to be associated with sodium and fluid retention. Multiple mechanisms have been suggested for this including increased peripheral vasodilation with increased surface area of the interstitial spaces. Obesity also creates bilateral "swelling," with the deposition of fat in the subcutaneous tissues, giving the appearance of enlargement to the extremity.

Lipedema

Lipedema is a bilateral and symmetric deposition of fat in the lower extremities in a very characteristic pattern (Fig. 36-9). The excess fat deposits are noted in the buttocks and legs, but they stop at the ankles; the feet are spared. The enlargement of the extremities is nonpitting unless there is

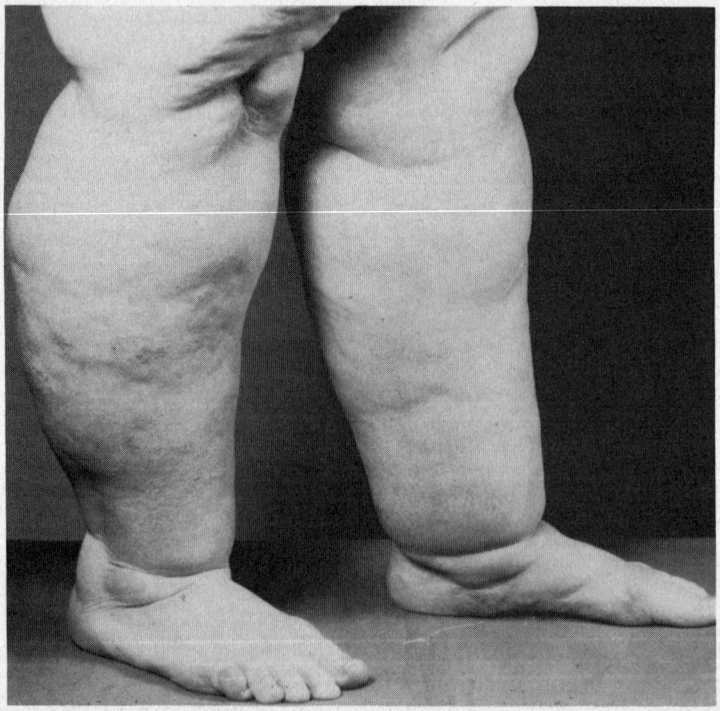

Fig. 36-9. Lipedema. Bilateral, symmetrical deposition of fat with no involvement of the feet.

an associated fluid retention syndrome. This was first described by Allen and Hines in 1940, with little additional description or information written about this distinct entity since that time.[9] Lipedema occurs almost exclusively in women, and there may be a familial tendency. Patients complain of swelling, pain, and tenderness in the involved areas, especially if they have mistakenly been told to wear heavy elastic support stockings.

Dependency

Dependency warrants mentioning again as a mechanism for bilateral edema formation. Prolonged sitting or standing will result in some degree of edema in almost everyone. Patients with severe rheumatoid or osteoarthritis and patients confined to a wheelchair or chair because of a stroke, amputation, or paraplegia are especially prone to develop dependent edema. Dependency because of ischemic pain can cause marked swelling. These tendencies are aggravated by excessive salt intake or warm weather and can occur before or during menstruation or during pregnancy.

The recognition of dependent edema is important not only to avoid unnecessary testing or invasive procedures but also to focus on the treatment of the underlying cause of the dependency.

Pretibial myxedema

Hyperthyroidism may be associated with the development of pretibial myxedema. Skin changes occur on the pretibial regions or on the dorsa of the feet (Fig. 36-10). The tissue appears to be raised, thickened, or infiltrated but without true pitting. Evidence of pretibial myxedema can occur during active hyperthyroidism or even after treatment. The process appears self-limited, and spontaneous resolution can occur.

Drug-induced edema

Drugs can cause bilateral soft, pitting edema in the dependent portions of the extremities.[4] The edema resolves after the drug is withdrawn. Many hormonal drugs including corticosteroids, estrogens, progesterones, and testosterone can cause edema. The nonsteroidal antiinflammatory drugs have also been implicated. Examples include phenylbutazone (Butazolidin), ibuprofen (i.e., Advil or Motrin), sulindac (Clinoril), as well as most of the other nonsteroidal antiinflammatory drugs. Antihypertensive drugs can also cause this syndrome, including methyldopa (Aldomet), hydralazine (Apresoline), diazoxide (Hyperstat), clonidine (Catapres), and reserpine (Serpasil). The antibiotics with a

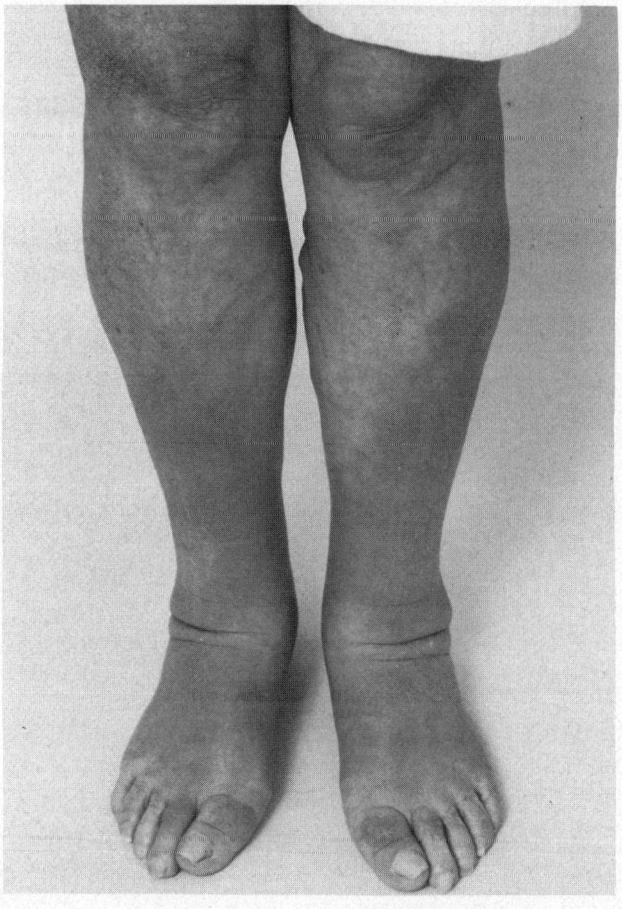

Fig. 36-10. Pretibial myxedema with slightly hyperpigmented, thickened skin over distal portion of lower legs and feet.

high-sodium content have also been reported to produce edema, especially carbenicillin. Edema can also result from taking antidepressants, especially the monoamine oxidase inhibitors.

CONCLUSION

Although the seemingly simple segregation of causes by bilateral vs unilateral involvement might be the most obvious of divisions, clinicians, particularly those who see patients with vascular diseases regularly, are presented with challenging situations that overlap any arbitrary categorization. Patients who have undergone an amputation can only develop unilateral lower extremity swelling, although the cause is one that ordinarily would cause bilateral swelling.

Patients who develop bilateral swelling may have simultaneous or concurrent processes of two normally unilateral causes. An example of simultaneous processes would be the patient who develops bilateral leg swelling caused by a deep vein thrombosis involving the inferior vena cava or the deep veins of both legs. This is not an uncommon occurrence in patients who have underlying cancers. Another example of concurrent activity of related processes is the presence of chronic venous insufficiency in one extremity and the new onset of acute deep vein thrombophlebitis in the other.

Separate causes for limb swelling can occur both simultaneously as well as concurrently. An example of this is the patient with a pelvic cancer that results in secondary lymphedema in one leg and a deep vein thrombophlebitis in the other. These types of unfortunate events do occur and challenge the clinician, not only in terms of diagnosis, but also in terms of management.

The patient with a swollen limb is not only a common problem for the practicing clinician but is also a diagnostic challenge. To accept the challenge and to properly care for the patient, the clinician must have an understanding of the many causes of leg swelling. With this foundation, a thorough history and complete physical examination along with certain tests will allow the clinician to arrive at the correct diagnosis.

REFERENCES

1. Dale WA: The swollen leg. In Ravitch MM, ed: Current problems in surgery, Chicago, 1973, Yearbook Publishers, Inc.
2. Ruschhaupt WF: Differential diagnosis of edema of the lower extremities. In Spittell JA: Clinical vascular disease, Philadelphia, 1983, FA Davis Co.
3. Taylor JS and Young JR: The swollen limb: cutaneous clues to diagnosis and treatment, Cutis 21:553, 1978.
4. Lofgren KA: Varicose veins. In Juergens JL, Spittell JA, and Fairbairn JF, eds: Peripheral vascular disease, ed 5, Philadelphia, 1980, WB Saunders Co.
5. Fairbairn JF: Clinical manifestations of peripheral vascular disease. In Juergens JL, Spittell JA, and Fairbairn JF, eds: Peripheral vascular disease, ed 5, Philadelphia, 1980, WB Saunders Co.
6. Braunwald E: Edema. In Braunwald E et al, eds: Harrison's principles of internal medicine, ed 11, New York, 1987, McGraw-Hill, Inc.
7. Feldman HA, Jayakumar S, and Puschett JB: Idiopathic edema: a review of etiologic concepts and management, Cardiovasc Med 3:475, 1978.
8. Schrier RW: Body fluid volume regulation in health and disease: a unifying hypothesis, Ann Intern Med 113:155, 1990.
9. Allen EV and Hines EA Jr: Lipedema of the legs: a syndrome characterized by fat legs and orthostatic edema, Proc Staff Meet Mayo Clinic 15:184, 1940.

Chapter 37

VASCULAR DISEASES OF THE UPPER LIMB

Thom W. Rooke
Anthony W. Stanson

A wide variety of pathologic conditions can affect the arteries, veins, and lymphatic vessels of the upper limb. Although the overall incidence of vascular disease is less in the upper limb than that in the lower limb (largely because of the lower incidence of atherosclerosis and venous thrombosis), the frequency of certain conditions (i.e., cold-induced vasospasm or occupational occlusive disease) is substantially higher for the upper limb. The clinical spectrum of upper limb vascular disease is extremely diverse. Some conditions cause symptoms that are minimal and a little more than a nuisance, while others may result in limb loss or severe disability.

ARTERIOSCLEROSIS AND ARTERIAL OBSTRUCTIVE DISEASES

Atherosclerosis

Atherosclerosis affects the arteries of the upper limb, although it affects them less frequently than it does those of the lower limbs. Exact figures for the incidence of upper extremity atherosclerosis are difficult to obtain. One report from Cincinnati described a 20-year experience with 6149 limbs affected by arterial occlusive disease. Of these only 288 (4.7%) were upper limbs.[1] In most of these cases the occlusive process was thought to be atherosclerosis, although documentation of this was usually unavailable. A similar low incidence of clinically significant upper extremity atherosclerosis was also observed during a 20-year series from the Mayo Clinic.[2] Based upon these studies and others it is reasonable to estimate that serious atherosclerosis is at least 20 times less frequent in the upper extremity than in the lower extremity. The reasons for the lower incidence in the upper limbs is unknown.

The mechanisms underlying atherosclerosis formation are complex and have been discussed in Chapter 7. Risk factors for upper extremity atherosclerosis are probably the same as those for atherosclerosis elsewhere—namely family history of atherosclerosis, male gender, smoking, hypertension, diabetes, and increased lipids. Some forms of trauma may also predispose to the formation of atherosclerosis-like lesions. The relative contribution made by each of these factors remains uncertain.

Atherosclerosis in the upper limb occurs more frequently (and severely) in proximal than in distal vessels. The subclavian (or innominate) and axillary arteries are most commonly affected (Fig. 37-1) whereas disease development distally is unusual.[3] Atherosclerosis of the aortic arch may also limit blood flow to the upper extremities, particularly if it (1) involves the orifice of the vessels coming off the arch or (2) results in aortic aneurysm formation or dissection (the latter may cause subsequent obstruction of the brachiocephalic vessels). Other complications of atherosclerosis include *atheroemboli* (which typically originate from fragmenting plaques and ulcers) and thrombosis (which may occur spontaneously at sites where plaques rupture or cause vessel stenosis).

Symptoms. The symptoms of upper extremity atherosclerosis are similar to those produced by atherosclerosis in the leg and are influenced not only by the level and severity of the arterial occlusion but also by the extent of arterial collateralization. *Claudication** occurs when arm exercise increases the muscular demand for blood beyond that which can be supplied via the diseased arteries and collaterals. The limb is asymptomatic at rest, but muscle fatigue, pain, or

*This is actually a misnomer, since the Latin root from which it is derived refers to a limping gait.

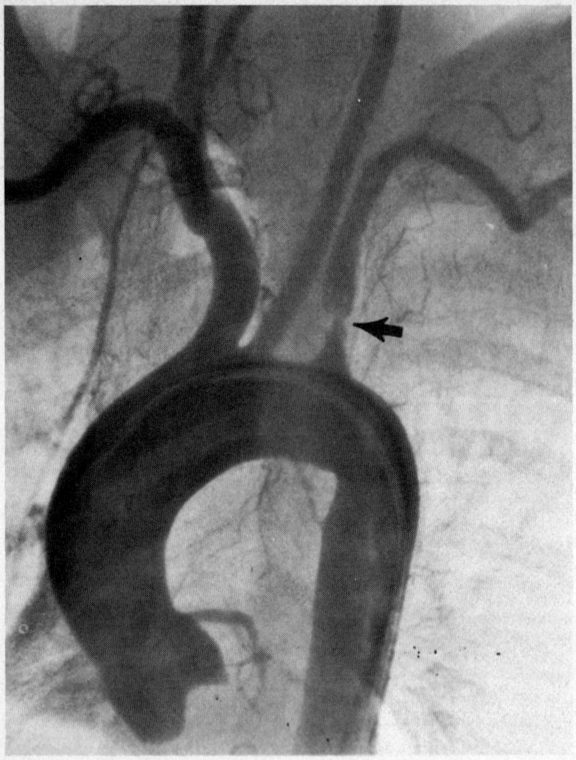

Fig. 37-1. Arch aortogram. Stenotic lesion of the proximal left subclavian artery *(arrow)* is atheromatous disease.

cramping develop during exercise. *Rest pain* occurs when the blood supply is insufficient to meet the resting metabolic demands of the limb (i.e., *ischemia*). If untreated, rest pain may lead to subsequent tissue breakdown, ulceration, and gangrene. *Atheroemboli* may cause small areas of infarction, particularly in the distal portion of the fingers. The *subclavian steal syndrome* occurs when subclavian obstruction develops proximal to the origin of the carotid or vertebral artery, thus creating a situation in which the arm may be perfused by retrograde carotid or vertebral flow. Physical activity involving the affected limb increases the demand for limb blood flow and in doing so augments the "steal" from the neural circulation, which may lead to the development of central nervous system symptoms.

Evaluation. When upper extremity atherosclerosis is suspected, the history and physical examination should include an assessment of (1) the presence of atherosclerosis in other vessels, especially the coronary and renal arteries and the arteries of the lower extremity, (2) cardiovascular risk factors that can be potentially modified such as smoking, hypertension, hyperlipidemia, and poor control of diabetes, and (3) the degree of disability or discomfort produced by the occlusive disease. Each of these factors (along with other aspects of the patient's overall health status) will influence therapeutic decisions.

Functional testing plays an important role in the assessment of obstructive lesions (see Chapter 3). Segmental pressures (obtained from inflatable cuffs placed at various levels along the arm) can be measured and compared with the pressure in the contralateral arm or in the legs; this provides information about the location and severity of the disease. In situations where the degree of obstruction is insufficient to affect resting blood pressure, a drop in pressure may be observed following exercise of the limb. Other standard noninvasive vascular laboratory studies (e.g., pulse volume recordings, Doppler waveform analysis, transcutaneous oxygen tension measurements, and skin temperature recordings) can provide variable degrees of potentially useful information and may be performed if available.

Arteriography remains the gold standard for imaging the arteries of the upper extremity and should be used to evaluate atherosclerosis when indicated. Angiographic studies must include an arch aortogram with additional selective injections and filming. Two-dimensional real-time ultrasound and Doppler technology and magnetic resonance imaging are becoming increasingly attractive as alternatives in certain situations, especially for screening purposes.

Therapy. Significant atherosclerotic disease has traditionally been treated surgically. *Bypass operations,* using conduits such as saphenous veins, hypogastric artery, or synthetic grafts, can be performed.[4,5] Local endarterectomy may be useful in situations where focal disease is present.[6,7] *Stellate ganglion sympathectomy* is occasionally a useful adjunct to revascularization, especially when ischemia is severe and the small, more distal vessels of the hands or arms are also obstructed.[8] Balloon *angioplasty,* mechanical *atherectomy,* and recanalization using laser, hot-tipped catheters, or other means may be employed in some situations, although the potential for embolization into the cerebral arteries makes work with these devices dangerous when used on lesions proximal to the carotid or vertebral arteries.[9] Conservative therapy involving risk factor reduction and regular upper extremity exercise is an option in most cases and should be employed whenever possible. Except for the long-term benefits derived from the use of drugs that help to reduce such risk factors as hyperlipidemia, hypertension, and elevated blood sugar, there has been little success using medical pharmacology (such as vasodilators) in the treatment of upper extremity atherosclerosis.

Emboli

Clinically significant emboli to the upper extremity occur 5 to 10 times less frequently than emboli to the lower extremity.[10] Thrombotic material originating within the heart accounts for most (up to 90%) of these emboli[11]; conditions predisposing to embolization include atrial fibrillation, myocardial infarction, cardiomyopathy, congestive heart failure, rheumatic valvular disease, cardioversion, prosthetic valves, cardiac surgery or catheterization, and others.[12] Vegetations associated with endocarditis and atrial myxoma are other potential causes of cardiac-derived emboli, and may give rise to mycotic aneurysms (Fig. 37-2).

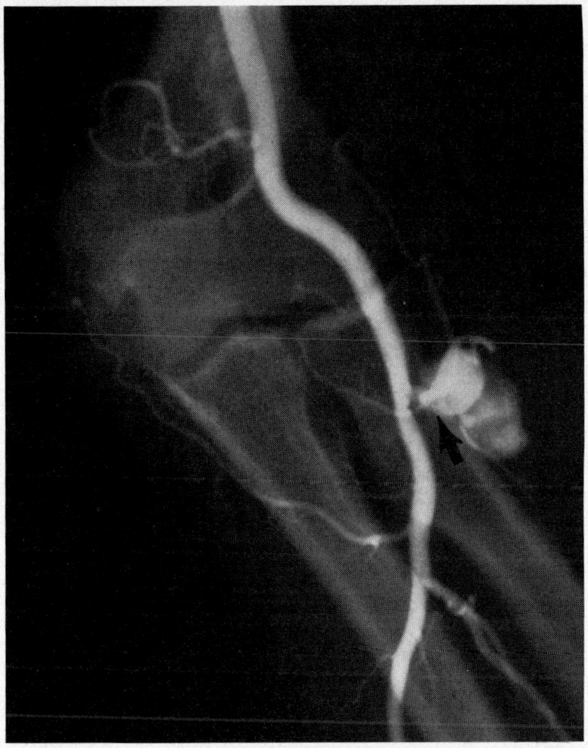

Fig. 37-2. Arm arteriogram. Mycotic aneurysm at the proximal radial artery *(arrow)* in a patient with bacterial endocarditis.

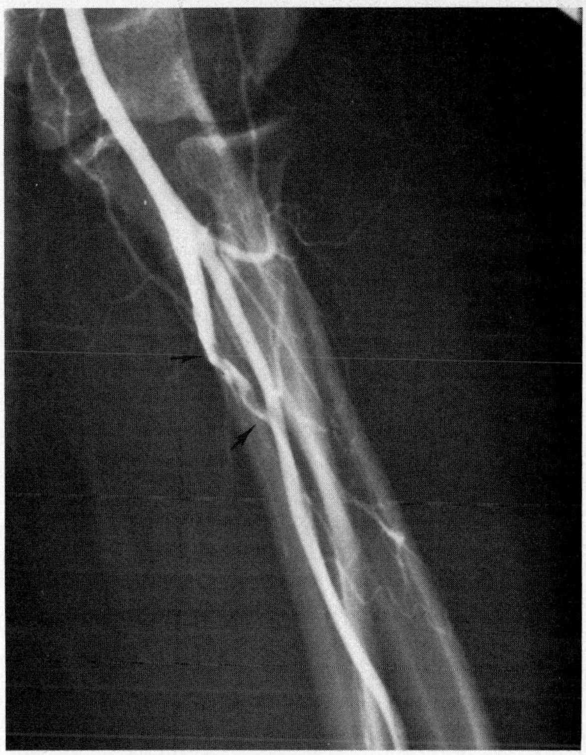

Fig. 37-3. Arm arteriogram. Embolus in proximal ulnar artery *(arrows)*. This was a complication from a proximal subclavian atheromatous stenosis.

Noncardiac sources of emboli include aneurysms of the aorta (or major branch vessels) and complicated arterial plaques (Fig. 37-3). These lesions frequently give rise to microemboli composed largely of platelets and plaque components such as cholesterol. Rarely, paradoxical emboli may pass from the venous circulation across a patent foramen ovale and lodge in the upper extremity.[13]

Emboli to large- or medium-size vessels usually appear as acute arterial occlusion. Typically, there is a discrete point beyond which pulsations are diminished or lost. The extremity becomes cool, painful, pale, mottled, or discolored. Over time both sensation and motor function may become impaired. When ischemia is severe, acute arterial occlusion constitutes a true medical emergency, which can lead to limb loss. However, if collateral vessels around the obstructed site are present, acute arterial occlusion may be relatively asymptomatic. Microemboli tend to shower the distal extremity and cause skin discoloration, pain, and small areas of cutaneous infarction. Repeated episodes of microembolization to the same area are common. Although often serious, microemboli are less likely than large emboli to cause limb loss.

Evaluation. The diagnosis of acute arterial embolic occlusion can usually be made on clinical grounds alone, especially when there is sudden onset of ischemia in a patient known (or found on subsequent examination) to have a cardiac problem predisposing to emboli. It is essential to assess the severity of limb ischemia since this dictates the course and speed of therapy. Noninvasive vascular laboratory studies are rarely necessary. Angiography may be indicated, especially when a structural problem with the artery (such as aneurysm or stenosis) is suspected at or above the level of the occlusion. A thorough cardiac examination is required when emboli may have originated in the heart. Two-dimensional real-time echocardiography (either transthoracic or transesophageal) appears to be the best technique for identifying potential cardiac sources in these patients.[14,15]

Therapy. The patient with acute arterial occlusion should be heparinized immediately if no contraindications are present. Steps to diagnose and localize the embolus should be performed promptly because of the potential seriousness of the situation. If ischemia is severe, and the embolus appears to be relatively proximal in location, balloon catheter embolectomy should be attempted as soon as possible (flow must be restored within 6 to 12 hours to prevent or minimize permanent damage). In cases of suspected embolism, this can be done without preceding angiography.[16] If embolectomy fails or if the artery has underlying structural problems, arteriography and revascularization surgery can be performed. Lysis of the emboli, using lytic agents such as streptokinase, urokinase, or tissue plasminogen activator (administered systemically or via a catheter placed in the artery), is also an option in certain patients.[17] The restoration of flow following a period of ischemia may be accompanied by muscle swelling and the development of compartment syndrome in up to 10% of patients.[12,18] When embolization is not limb threatening, conservative measures may be employed initially. These include anticoagulation, positioning of the limb into a slightly dependent position, protection of the limb from trauma, and prevention of heat loss. Spontaneous lysis, recanalization, or the development of collateral vessels may occur from hours to weeks and result in significant clinical improvement.

Microemboli are usually best treated by immediate anticoagulation and conservative measures. The cardiac or vascular source of emboli must be identified and treated appropriately to prevent recurrences. Depending on their etiology and the response to treatment, long-term therapy with warfarin or antiplatelet agents may be indicated.

Despite the institution of therapeutic measures, upper extremity embolization often necessitates a minor (46% incidence in one series) or major (16%) amputation.[19] Even when the limb has been successfully treated, there is a high (approximately 25%) mortality rate in these patients resulting from emboli affecting other organs.[19]

Inflammatory disorders

The vasculitides (conditions in which blood vessel inflammation is the primary process) comprise a large group of systemic disorders that encompass an extremely broad spectrum of causes, pathologies, and clinical manifestations. Involvement of the upper extremity with arteritis, either as an isolated finding or as part of the systemic disorder, is a relatively infrequent occurrence. Unfortunately, the vasculitides of the upper extremity are a difficult group of diseases to classify or discuss for several reasons: (1) Most types of vasculitides are rare, and it is unusual for those investigating them to obtain a large series. Many conclusions about specific forms of vasculitides are therefore based upon findings from small series or even case reports. (2) For virtually all types of vasculitides, the underlying cause is unknown. (3) Diseases with different clinical pictures may have nearly identical pathologic findings. (4) The criteria used to diagnose many forms of vasculitides are often poorly defined and unclear. (5) Vasculitis terminology is nonuniform and confusing. In other words a multitude of different names are used by various authorities to describe the same diseases.

The histopathologic findings in vasculitis are highly variable. Inflammation is (by definition) present at some time in all types and includes such nonspecific findings as edema, deposition of fibrin and complement, and infiltration by various inflammatory cells.[20] Inflammation (which can be diffuse or focal) may involve the entire thickness of the vessel wall uniformly, or it may predominate in certain layers. Intraluminal thrombosis may occur. In some types granulomas form. When the integrity and structure of the vessel are destroyed by inflammation, the vasculitis is said to be *necrotizing*.

It is perhaps easiest to classify the vasculitides of the upper extremity according to the size of the involved vessel.

Small vessels. Many systemic disorders may have as part of their presentation a small vessel vasculitis involving the upper extremity. This type of vasculitis is frequently associated with rheumatic diseases such as systemic lupus erythematosus, rheumatoid arthritis, dermatomyositis, mixed connective tissue diseases, and scleroderma.[21] Other types such as erythema nodosum and hypersensitivity angiitis may be associated with various systemic disorders or can occur de novo. Circulating factors (such as cryoglobulins, hepatitis A antigen, myeloma proteins, macroglobulins, and others) and various drugs or medicines may also be associated with vasculitis.[22-24] Autoimmunity is thought to play an etiologic role in many, if not most, situations.[25] The tissues most frequently involved are the skin and joints, although damage to other structures can occur. Fingers and hands (Fig. 37-4) are usually affected but the entire upper limb may be involved. Clinical (primarily dermal) manifestations of disease include urticaria, rashes, livedo, purpura, Raynaud's phenomenon, hemorrhage, infarction, ulceration, and gangrene.

Medium-size vessels. Periarteritis nodosa is the classic example of a vasculitis that affects medium-size vessels, although small vessels are frequently involved as well. The disease is idiopathic but resembles serum sickness in many ways, which suggests a possible autoimmune origin. A role for infective agents has also been postulated. Similar diseases that rarely affect medium and small vessels of the upper extremity (and which may be variants of periarteritis nodosa) include such entities as Wegener's granulomatosis, lymphomatoid granulomatosis, Kawasaki disease,[26] and Churg-Strauss syndrome. These diseases typically involve the skin (necrosis or gangrene) and may produce neuropathy.

Large vessels. Large vessel vasculitides that affect the upper limb include Takayasu's arteritis (Fig. 37-5), temporal arteritis (Fig. 37-6), Behçet's syndrome, Cogan's syndrome, and the arteritis associated with relapsing polychondritis and various seronegative spondyloarthropathies. Takayasu's[27] and temporal arteritis are probably the most common and important of these. Both can affect the aorta and large branch vessels and appear pathologically similar, with granulomatous and nongranulomatous inflammation tending to involve the entire thickness of the arterial wall. However, Takayasu's arteritis tends to affect patients who are younger (under 40 years of age) and frequently female (female-to-male ratio is 5:1), while temporal arteritis affects those who are older (over 55 years of age) and less often female (female-to-male ratio of 2:1). Takayasu's arteritis appears to affect the upper extremity more frequently than temporal arteritis does. The symptoms of these diseases are typically those of upper extremity arterial occlusive disease, namely arm claudication, rest pain, or tissue breakdown. Aneurysm formation involving the brachiocephalic vessels (and the associated complications of acute arterial occlusion or distal embolization) may also occur.

A

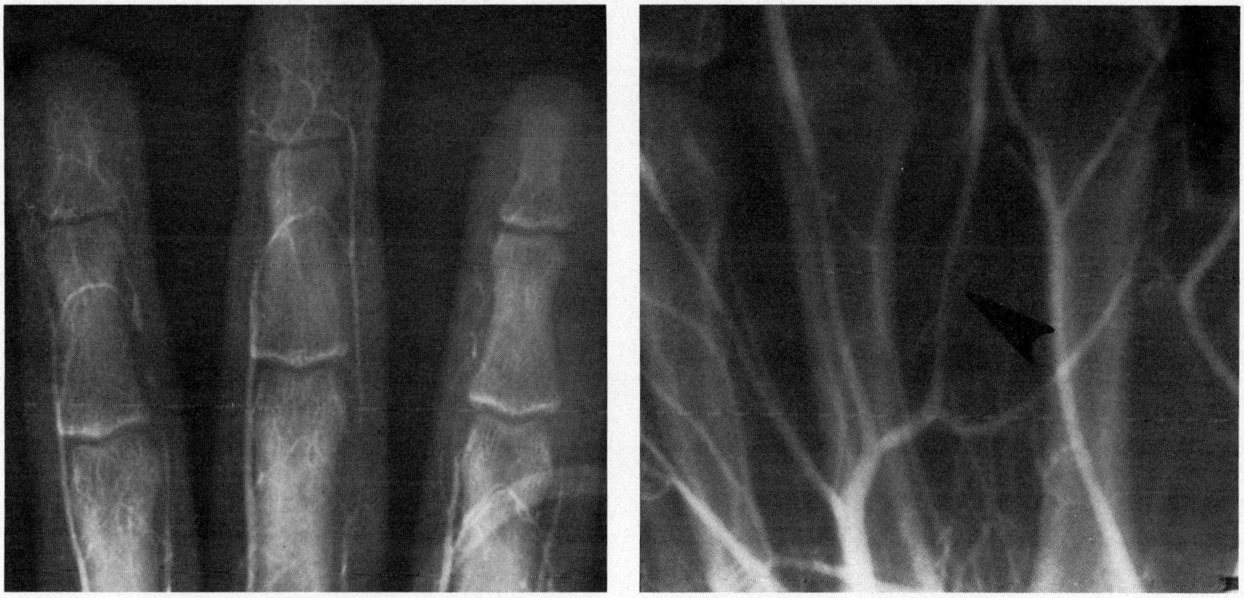

B

Fig. 37-4. Hand arteriogram. Vasculitis of an indeterminate type in a young female. **A,** Digital artery occlusions and segments of stenoses. **B,** Metacarpal artery with smooth-walled narrowing *(arrowhead)*. A similar finding is present in two adjacent arteries.

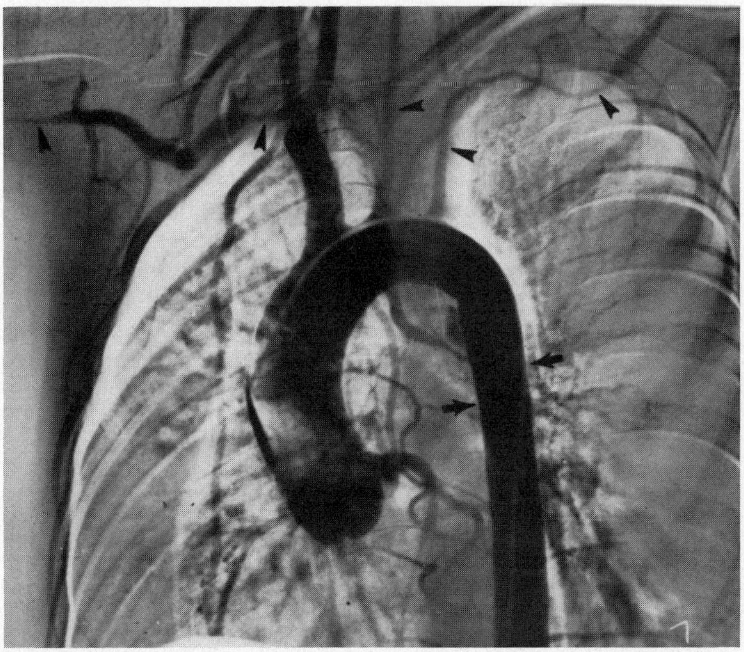

Fig. 37-5. Arch aortogram of patient with Takayasu's disease. The segments of stenoses *(arrowheads)* of the brachiocephalic arteries are typical for a giant cell type of arteritis. Because the left common carotid artery (and proximal left subclavian artery) is involved, the angiographic findings are specific for Takayasu's arteritis. Note also the irregularity of the aortic wall *(arrows)*.

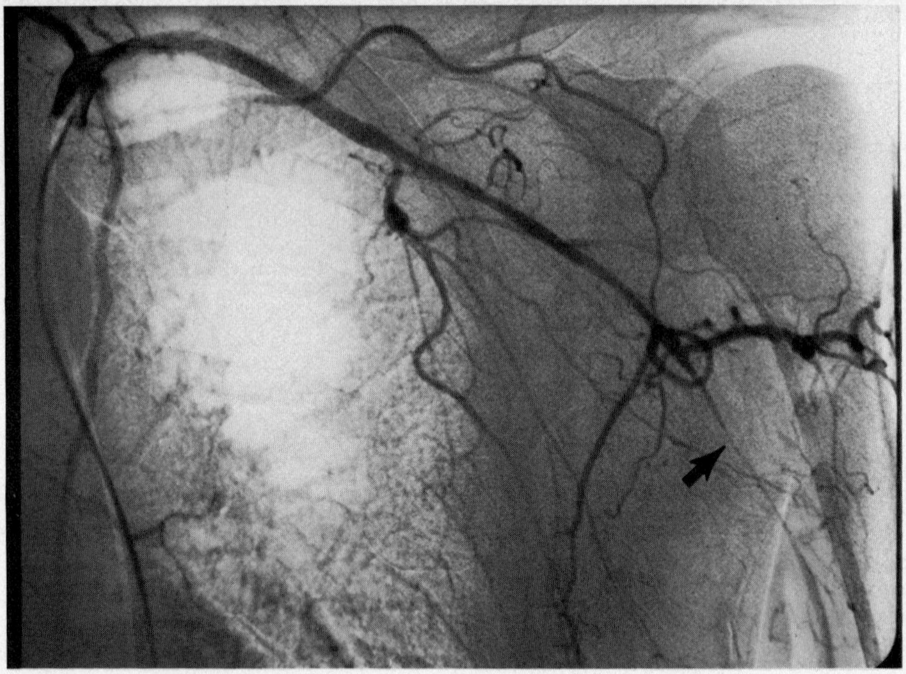

Fig. 37-6. Left subclavian arteriogram of patient with temporal arteritis. Axillary and proximal brachial *(arrow)* arteries have segments of smooth-wall narrowing and tapered stenosis.

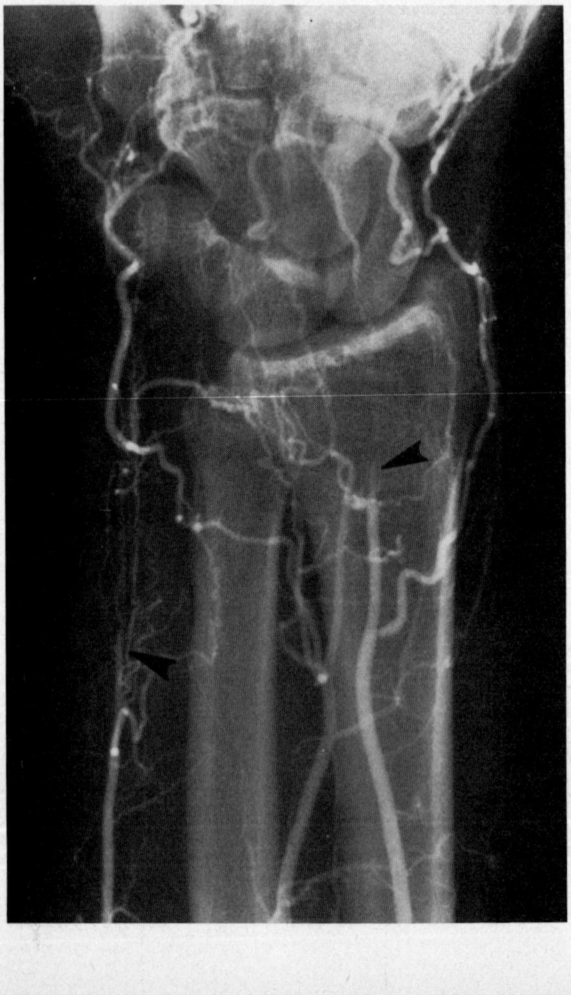

Fig. 37-7. Arm arteriogram at the wrist. Buerger's disease in a young male smoker. The tapered occlusions of the ulnar and radial arteries *(arrowheads)* in conjunction with distal arterial occlusions and skip areas of normal arterial segments are typical angiographic findings.

Buerger's disease. Buerger's disease (thromboangiitis obliterans) is an unusual entity that is probably best classified as a vasculitis, although not all authorities agree.[9,28] Patients are usually male (80% to 90%) and young (under 50 years of age), suggesting that youth and male gender are important risk factors; other factors such as heredity, race, and geography may also be involved. The cause of Buerger's disease is unknown, but tobacco abuse appears to play a critical role.

The disease affects the small- and medium-size arteries of the limbs early in its course and may progress to involve the large arteries (Fig. 37-7) as well as veins.[29-31] Pathologically, the disease is *panvasculitis* in which the lumen typically contains thrombus with organizing fibroblasts and other cellular elements (including giant cells), while the intima, media, and adventitia demonstrate various degrees of thickening and infiltration by inflammatory cells. Unlike other types of vasculitis Buerger's disease rarely has systemic manifestations or involvement of blood vessels outside of the extremities. The clinical signs and symptoms are similar to those of occlusive disease from other causes, although often more severe. Gangrene with subsequent amputation (autoamputation or surgical) of fingers, hands, or arms is not unusual.

Evaluation. The history and physical examination are helpful in assessing patients with vasculitis. Antecedent illness, smoking habits, a history of drug or medication use, and associated medical conditions (such as the presence of a rheumatic disease) should be sought. Vasculitis occurring elsewhere in the body must be identified and evaluated as necessary. The distribution and appearance of cutaneous findings may provide helpful clues. When large vessels are involved, pulses may be reduced and bruits heard. Laboratory tests, especially the erythrocyte sedimentation rate, can be very helpful. Abnormalities in hepatic or renal function may provide clues to the presence of vasculitis in these organs. In many cases, especially with small-vessel processes involving the skin, biopsy is the only way to confirm the diagnosis. Biopsy should be obtained from a clinically involved area when possible. When it is not possible, blind biopsy of the testicle, muscle, or nerve may be attempted. Arteriography is indicated in many cases of large- and medium-size vessel disease, not only to make the diagnosis but also to plan surgery.

Therapy. Treatment depends on the type of vasculitis present. In many situations the condition will resolve spontaneously and conservative measures are therefore all that is necessary. Discontinuation of tobacco use typically leads to marked improvement, especially in Buerger's disease. Prednisone and various immunosuppressive agents are useful in a variety of disease types. The dosage and duration of therapy is largely determined by the clinical response, although changes in the erythrocyte sedimentation rate may also be used to guide treatment. The occlusive symptoms of Takayasu's and temporal arteritis have been shown to stabilize and resolve following adequate steroid therapy. Some types of vasculitis are life-threatening because of their systemic effects, and balancing the therapeutic benefits of steroids or immunosuppressive agents against their toxicity can be difficult. Trimethoprim-sulfamethoxazole has been reported to be efficacious in patients with Wegener's granulomatosis,[32] but the role of antibiotics in other conditions is questionable. When aneurysms or fixed stenotic lesions have developed, surgical repair or revascularization is an option, especially after the inflammatory process is resolved or controlled.[33]

Traumatic and occupational disease

A significant amount of upper extremity vascular disease occurs as a result of trauma, which can be acute or chronic.

Acute trauma. Of the 66,000 surgical procedures performed annually in the United States for the repair of damaged blood vessels, an appreciable number involve the upper extremity. *Penetrating wounds* caused by bullets, knives, and punctures predominate and may affect the blood vessels of the limb at any level. Vascular disruption usually causes obvious problems, but damage from penetrating wounds may be occult in up to 25% to 35% of injuries.[34] Secondary thrombosis or aneurysm (either true or false) formation[35] can complicate matters. *Blunt trauma* resulting from high-impact deceleration, crush injuries, or blows to the arm also occur frequently. Thrombosis is probably the most common sequela, but hemorrhage, spasm, stenosis, or aneurysm formation,[36,37] is possible. *Iatrogenic injuries* are seen with increasing frequency as medicine becomes more procedure oriented. Catheterization procedures involving the arm[38] (especially those performed via a brachial or axillary vascular access site) and nonvascular surgical procedures on the upper extremity are the usual causes, but occasionally arterial punctures for blood gas determinations, direct pressure measurements, or even phlebotomy can produce significant vascular injury.[39] Vascular injuries related to intravascular drug use are also increasing in frequency.[40] *Miscellaneous* pathologic conditions caused by acute trauma include *fat embolization* (which follows injury to bones and adjacent blood vessels) and *compression syndromes* (which occur when edema or swelling cause extrinsic compression of blood vessels sufficient enough to impair flow). Fasciotomy may be required to relieve a compression syndrome and restore circulation.

Chronic trauma. Repeated episodes of trauma may also injure arteries. Arterial occlusive complications related to intermittent periods of arterial compression caused by the thoracic outlet syndrome are common. Exposure to *chronic vibration* (which occurs in workers using chain saws, jack hammers, and drills) provides another example of ischemia caused by recurrent low-level trauma.[41-45] Histopathologic changes in the small arteries of affected individuals include hypertrophy of smooth muscle cells, periarterial fibrosis, demyelination and loss of periarterial nerve fibers, increases in collagen-containing connective tissues, and loss of elastic fibers. These changes (and others) result in arterial narrowing, luminal obstruction, vasospasm, and thrombosis (Fig. 37-8). For reasons that are not well understood, patients with vibratory-induced disease may also have increased blood viscosity. The use of antifibrin agents to reduce the viscosity has been investigated.[46] Generalized abnormalities in sympathetic nerve function also occur. The *hypothenar hammer syndrome,* in which the hands develop ulnar arterial irregularities (Fig. 37-9) or occlusion (Fig. 37-10) as a result of excessive use in activities such as squeezing or pounding, represents another syndrome produced by chronic trauma.[47,48] Similar types of small vessel arterial occlusive, thrombotic, and vasospastic problems have also been observed in typists, piano players, baseball and hockey players, and in virtually every occupation or hobby wherein strenuous use of the hands occurs.[49]

The evaluation of patients with vascular trauma involving the upper extremity should include both functional and im-

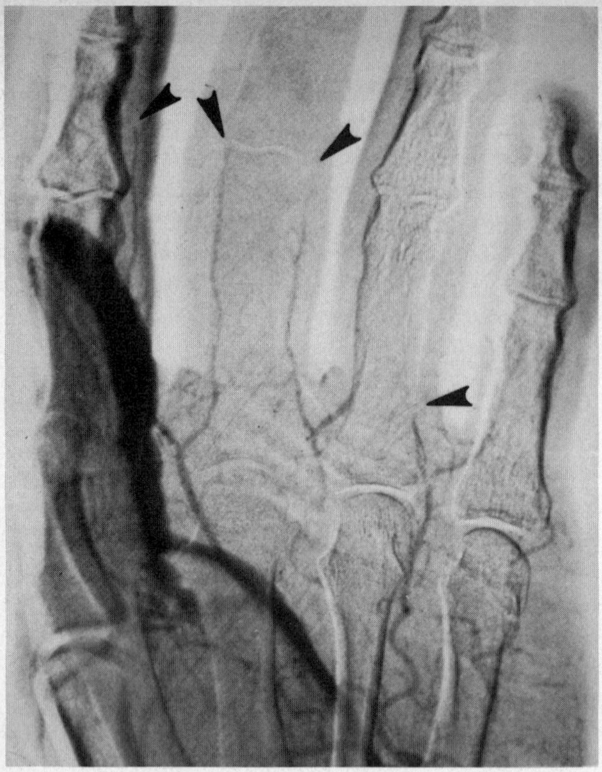

Fig. 37-8. Hand arteriogram of patient with chronic vibration injury. Multiple digital artery occlusions *(arrowheads)* and preceding irregular, stenotic segments indicate a long exposure to vibration tools.

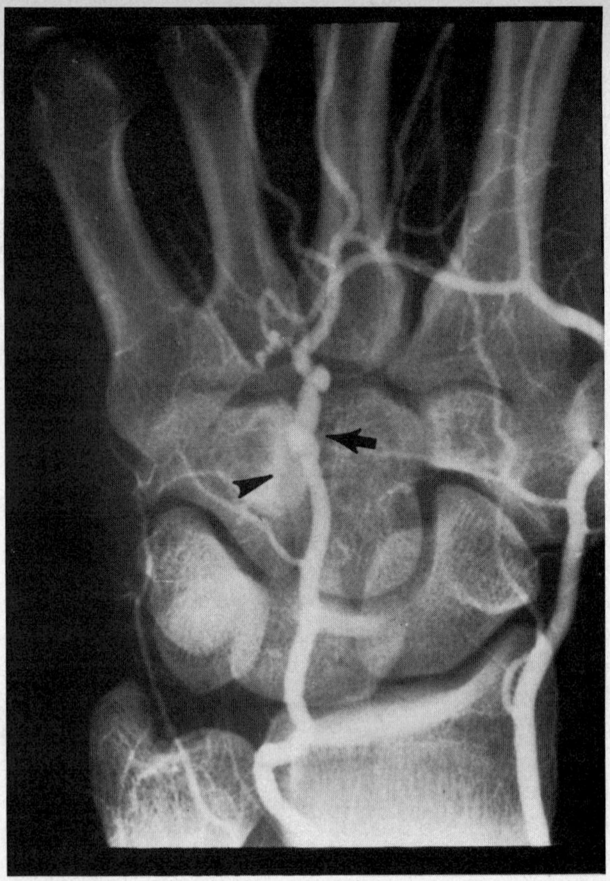

Fig. 37-9. Hand arteriogram. Ulnar artery injury from using the hand as a "hammer." The irregularities *(arrow)* of the short arterial zone over the hook of the hamate bone *(arrowhead)* are the result of repeated trauma.

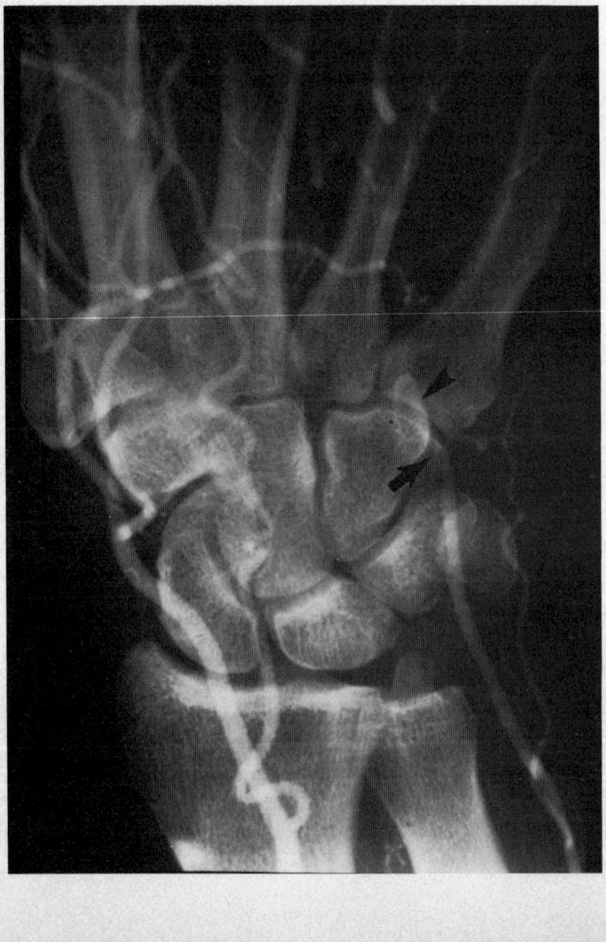

Fig. 37-10. Hand arteriogram. Ulnar artery occlusion *(arrow)* from trauma (hammer-hand) occurs over the hamate bone hook *(arrowhead)*.

aging studies when necessary. Noninvasive functional testing, described earlier in this chapter, is especially important in those patients for whom disability is an issue.[50-52] The liberal use of arteriography has been recommended for ruling out or evaluating vascular injury.[34,53] The roles of duplex scanning,[54] computerized tomography, and magnetic resonance imaging in the diagnosis and evaluation of vascular trauma are expanding and may soon replace arteriography in many situations.

The treatment of traumatic and occupational diseases involves several steps. The most important is to eliminate the source of vibration or trauma. Structural repair or bypass of the affected arteries using microsurgical techniques may be indicated.[55] The use of vasodilators to combat spasm may offer some therapeutic benefit in selected patients (see the upcoming section on vasospasm).

Miscellaneous conditions. A variety of miscellaneous pathologic processes can obstruct the arteries of the upper limb. For example, various *degenerative arteriopathies* (as occur with diseases such as the Marfan syndrome, so-called "cystic medial necrosis," and a multitude of congenital or acquired conditions involving abnormalities in collagen or elastic tissue composition) may result in aneurysm formation or dissection involving the upper extremity. Arteries such as the brachial artery may rarely be subject to *entrapment*.[56] *Fibromuscular dysplasia* occasionally occurs in the arteries of the upper limb, especially the axillary artery.[57] *Medial calcification,* although seldom a clinical problem, is sometimes incidentally noted on x-ray films of the arm.[58] *Coagulopathies* (including thrombocytosis and the various platelet disorders) may complicate certain systemic illnesses or can appear as isolated entities. Either way they may contribute to thrombosis and subsequent occlusion of large or small arteries. *Malignancy* can cause thrombosis through unexplained mechanisms.[59-61]

Venous disease

In comparison to the lower limbs, the upper limbs are rarely affected by venous disease. The most common venous problem is *thrombosis,* which may be superficial or deep. Usual causes of *superficial venous thrombosis* include systemic illnesses such as malignancy or inflammatory bowel disease, intravenous infusion or injection of irritating drugs, and direct (usually blunt) trauma. *Deep venous thrombosis* may also be caused by any of the factors that produce superficial venous thrombosis. In addition, venous compression (as occurs with any form of thoracic outlet obstruction), indwelling catheters,[62] pacemaker leads,[63] or vigorous use of the upper extremity[64,65] can contribute to thrombosis. Clotting abnormalities may play a role in the cause of either superficial or deep venous thrombosis.

Significant upper extremity deep venous clotting occurs most commonly in the axillary and subclavian veins, although thrombosis of the superior vena cava may also produce symptoms in the upper limb. The clinical manifestations of venous thrombosis include pain and/or swelling at (and distal to) the site of venous occlusion; tender, palpable veins; and cyanotic discoloration of the skin. The severity of symptoms depends on how acute and extensive the thrombosis is. When it is massive, there may be extreme swelling, skin breakdown, and gangrene. Pulmonary embolism from upper extremity deep venous thrombosis may occur in up to 12% of patients.[38]

The diagnosis of upper extremity deep venous thrombosis has traditionally required venography, but recent advances in ultrasonic imaging combined with Doppler (i.e., duplex scanning) have made this the preferred test in many situations.[66,67] Treatment of venous thrombosis depends on the severity and location of the clot. As with cases of superficial venous thrombosis that occur elsewhere in the body, superficial venous thrombosis of the upper limb usually responds well to topical heat and antiinflammatory drugs. On the other hand, acute deep venous thrombosis is usually treated with anticoagulants (heparin initially and then warfarin for 6 to 12 weeks). Thrombolysis using any of the currently available lytic agents is also an option.[63,68] For chronic occlusion surgical venous bypass is a potential option.

Occasionally *extrinsic compression* of the brachial veins will mimic venous thrombosis. Tumors, aneurysms of the brachiocephalic arteries, and structural abnormalities of the thoracic outlet do this most commonly. Eliminating the cause of compression is usually sufficient to treat this condition.

NEUROVASCULAR COMPRESSION

The so-called "thoracic outlet syndrome" actually refers to a group of clinical conditions that result from compression of the neurovascular bundle supplying the upper extremity. Symptoms may vary, depending on whether the artery, vein, or nerve is the major affected structure. In many subjects two or even all three components are involved to some degree, thereby complicating the clinical picture. It is estimated by some that 97% of all symptoms in patients with thoracic outlet syndrome are related to compression of the nerves within the brachial plexus, while 2% are caused by venous compression and 1% by arterial compression.[69] Others[70] argue that mild vascular compression may mimic the symptoms of nerve compression. They cite a low incidence of positive electromyographic findings as evidence against significant primary neurologic involvement in most cases (Roos[71] offers opposing arguments as to why nerve involvement might not produce electromyographic changes). Matters are further confused by the fact that 50% to 60% of asymptomatic normal subjects (especially those who are young or athletic) have evidence of intermittent, positional arterial compression.[72] Thus while neurovascular compression appears well established as the cause of thoracic outlet syndrome, the exact pathophysiologic mechanisms by which signs and symptoms are produced remain unclear.

The neurovascular bundle is especially susceptible to

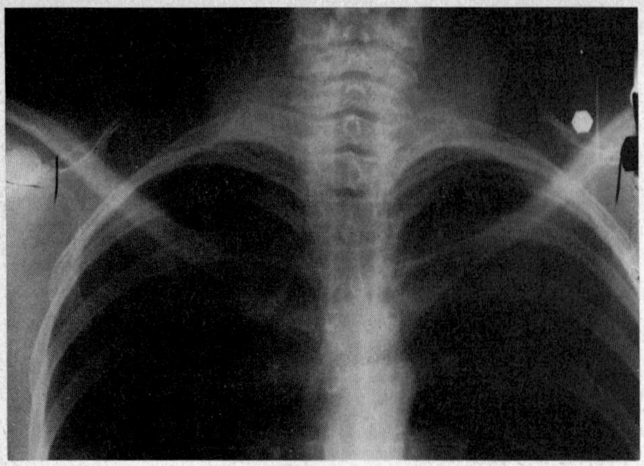

Fig. 37-11. Cervical rib on the right compromises the thoracic outlet.

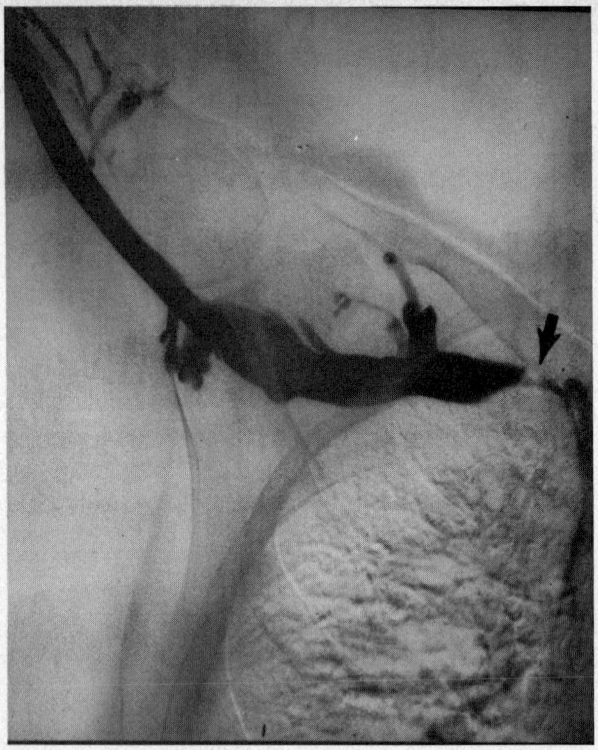

Fig. 37-12. Right arm venogram in abduction. Stenosis *(arrow)* at the junction of the axillary and subclavian segments. A cervical rib had been resected several months earlier. Venous obstruction resulted from postoperative fibrosis.

compression at three sites along its exit path from the thorax.[70] These sites (costoscalene, costoclavicular, and retropectal) usually provide minimal room for the neurovascular bundle even in normal individuals. Minor anatomic variations can subsequently reduce these openings further and cause neurovascular impingement. Most authorities agree that the costoclavicular position is the most frequent site of compression.[70] Cervical ribs (Fig. 37-11) are common in patients with thoracic outlet syndrome. They occur in up to 1% of the population but cause symptoms in only 5% to 10% of subjects having them.[73] In 50% of cases cervical ribs occur unilaterally.[70] The ribs may be complete (i.e., they have a bony articulation with the first rib), but in most cases they are incomplete and connect to the first rib via a dense fibromuscular band; however, the ability to cause compression may be similar in both situations.

Other forms of congenital fibrous bands can also occur and cause compression, with nine separate types described.[71] Other factors responsible for compression include hypertrophic muscles (especially the scalenus anterior); congenital variations in the origin and insertion of various muscles; clavicle or first rib bony abnormalities; trauma, including fractures and "whiplash"-type cervical injuries; poor posture[74,75]; scoliosis; tumors; changes after surgery; muscular dystrophy; and a host of others.[72] Minimal trauma or strain involving the head, neck, or shoulder precipitates the initial appearance of thoracic outlet syndrome in up to 60% of patients.[69]

Symptoms

Because neurovascular compression may affect arteries, veins, or nerves, it is not surprising that the clinical manifestations of thoracic outlet syndrome are extremely diverse. Symptoms of *nerve compression* include numbness, pain, and paresthesias that usually affect the hands and fingers but may involve the entire arm. Weakness is seen less frequently and may be difficult to separate from pain. Symptoms of *arterial compression and obstruction* include cold hands or fingers, arm claudication, aching pain, pallor or cyanosis, Raynaud's phenomenon (in up to 15% of patients), distal embolization, and skin breakdown or ulceration.[70] Symptoms of *venous compression and obstruction* (Fig. 37-12) include swelling edema, pain, and cyanosis. The fact that certain symptoms (e.g., pain, swelling, or Raynaud's syndrome) can be caused by compression of either nerves or blood vessels makes it difficult to identify the involved structure on the basis of symptoms alone. Some symptoms may be intermittent, positional, and mild (reflecting compression that occurs in certain positions only) while others may be constant and debilitating (suggesting either chronic compression or failure to recover fully between episodes of intermittent compression).

Several complications appear to be directly related to neurovascular compression (Fig. 37-13).[76] The arterial wall can become inflamed, thickened, and adherent to surrounding structures at the site of compression.[72] Atherosclerosis development is possible. The vessel may also dilate and become ectatic or aneurysmal. These aneurysms are typically fusiform in shape and may be lined by mural thrombus. Complications of these aneurysms include embolization of thrombotic materials, thrombosis causing acute arterial occlusion, or rarely spontaneous rupture. The major venous complication caused by thoracic outlet compression is thrombosis with subsequent limb swelling. As previously

A

B

C

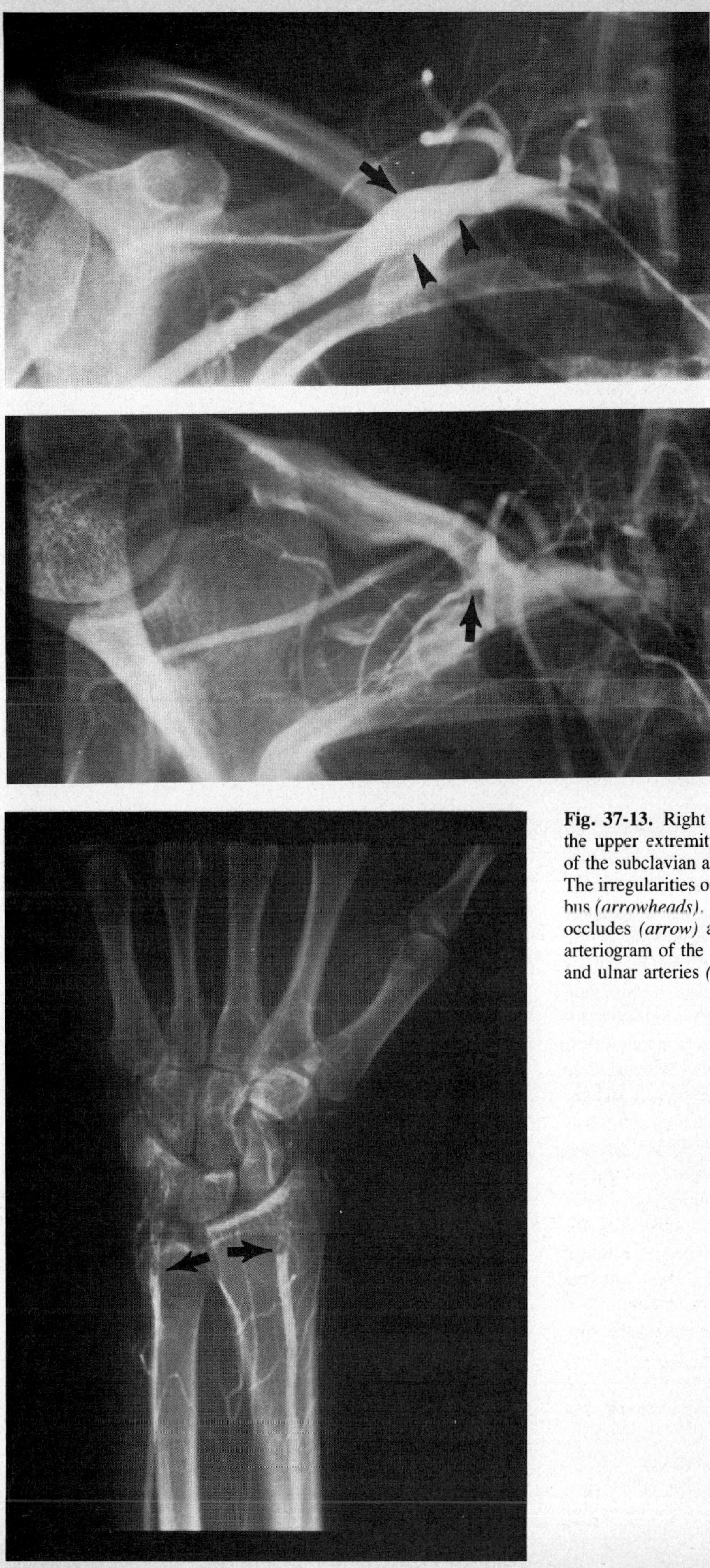

Fig. 37-13. Right subclavian arteriogram. **A,** Neutral position of the upper extremity. Fusiform aneurysm *(arrow)* at the junction of the subclavian and axillary artery segments over a cervical rib. The irregularities on the inferior border of the aneurysm are thrombus *(arrowheads)*. **B,** Abduction of the arm. The subclavian artery occludes *(arrow)* at its crossing with the cervical rib. **C,** Hand arteriogram of the same patient. Embolic occlusions of the radial and ulnar arteries *(arrows)*.

noted, nerve dysfunction (documented by electromyography) is an unusual complication of chronic or intermittent compression.

Evaluation

There is universal agreement about the importance of a good history and physical examination in the workup of the patient with suspected thoracic outlet syndrome. The history should include a careful review of (1) the symptoms involved and the circumstances under which they occur (such as which limb position causes symptoms), (2) how long the symptoms have been present and what factor(s) such as strain or trauma precipitated the initial appearance, (3) the degree of disability or discomfort caused by the problem, and (4) other medical conditions that could be factors. The physical examination should include a search for cervical ribs, hypertrophied muscles, subclavian artery aneurysm, distal emboli, and hand or digital ischemia. A good neurologic examination is essential to search for problems such as cervical disk disease or carpal tunnel syndrome. The role of maneuvers designed to demonstrate the positional loss or attenuation of pulses (such as hyperabduction or Adson's maneuver) is controversial. Some authorities feel that many of these are totally unreliable, being falsely negative or positive in too many patients to be of clinical value.[71] Others assign high importance to their use.[70] The key fact on interpreting these tests is the association between a limb position and the development of the patient's usual symptoms. When present, this association is generally significant. Because of the difficulty in proving its presence, thoracic outlet syndrome is frequently a diagnosis of exclusion. One first demonstrates that the disease is consistent with thoracic outlet syndrome and then rules out other potential causes.

The role of many laboratory and imaging tests in the evaluation of thoracic outlet syndrome is often minimal. A chest or cervical x-ray film may be useful for identifying cervical ribs. Most authorities suggest arteriograms only for selected patients, such as those with bony abnormalities, neurologic involvement, arterial insufficiency (with possible atherosclerosis), subclavian aneurysm, or evidence of emboli. Arteriography should not be used to make the diagnosis of thoracic outlet syndrome but rather to identify a fixed vascular abnormality or emboli. Noninvasive laboratory tests are also of limited value, although duplex (ultrasound/Doppler) scanning may have some utility, especially for documenting or assessing stenosis, poststenotic dilation, aneurysm formation, and mural thrombus. The roles of electromyography[77] and somatosensory evoked potentials[78] in diagnosing brachial plexus involvement remain unclear.

Therapy

Conservative measures such as stretching exercises (or other forms of physical therapy), analgesics, and avoidance of positions that cause neurovascular compression may be all that is necessary in mild cases of thoracic outlet syndrome. When this fails or the symptoms are severe, surgery is usually indicated. A variety of operations designed to relieve the compression or to repair damaged blood vessels can be performed, depending on the exact problems present. The surgical details are beyond the scope of this work (see Chapter 28). Resection of ribs (first or cervical) or fibrous bands is usually performed.[70] If subclavian aneurysm formation has occurred, the aneurysm should be resected and replaced by a graft.[72] Nonaneurysmal poststenotic dilation may resolve following the repair of the stenosis or rib resection. However, at what point a reversible poststenotic dilation becomes an irreversible aneurysm is uncertain. Sympathectomy is sometimes performed along with rib resection or other corrective procedure.[79] Venous obstruction can be treated with thrombectomy[80] or thrombolysis.[81] This may be done as an isolated procedure or in conjunction with thoracic outlet decompression.

VASOSPASM

Cutaneous vasoconstriction occurring in response to ambient temperature changes is a normal physiologic mechanism necessary for thermal regulation. When it occurs inappropriately or is excessively intense, it may become pathologic, causing a condition referred to as *Raynaud's syndrome* or *phenomenon*.* Raynaud's syndrome most often affects the upper limb. It may be caused by or associated with a systemic disorder (secondary Raynaud's syndrome), or it can occur as an isolated entity (primary Raynaud's syndrome).

In both the primary and secondary forms of Raynaud's syndrome, females are affected more often than males. Attacks are usually triggered by exposure to the cold or emotional stress.[82] Episodes are most often bilateral, but in some situations (usually with secondary disease) they may be unilateral or even confined to a single digit. During an attack the affected skin typically turns white and may become numb or painful. As the episode progresses the discolored areas may become cyanotic and develop rubor before returning to normal. Digital ulcerations are rare in the primary form but occur frequently and can be severe in the secondary disease. The clinical manifestations and consequences of the disease are often determined by the associated conditions. In primary Raynaud's syndrome the symptoms are usually stable and may be little more than a nuisance, while in some forms of secondary Raynaud's syndrome (e.g., scleroderma) severe and debilitating sequelae may evolve.

*Various authorities have attempted to differentiate between the terms *Raynaud's syndrome, Raynaud's phenomenon,* and *Raynaud's disease,* using Raynaud's disease to describe the primary condition and Raynaud's syndrome or phenomenon to describe secondary conditions. We prefer to use Raynaud's syndrome or phenomenon for any episodic, inappropriate, or severe episode of cutaneous vasoconstriction. Whenever possible, secondary Raynaud's syndrome should be described in terms of the causative or associated condition such as "posttraumatic Raynaud's syndrome," or "Raynaud's syndrome secondary to scleroderma."

The pathophysiology of Raynaud's syndrome is poorly understood (see Chapter 21). Many patients appear to have abnormalities in adrenergic function that cause increased vasomotor tone and sensitivity to cold,[83] but the nature of these abnormalities remains obscure. Blood viscosity may also be elevated in some subjects.[84,85] Patients with primary Raynaud's syndrome usually have patent large and small arteries, although those with long-standing disease often demonstrate some evidence of intimal thickening and occasionally show fixed digital artery obstruction.[86] In contrast, patients with secondary disease may have considerable vascular obstruction in the involved extremities. This reflects the fact that vascular occlusive processes related to atherosclerosis, arteritis, thoracic outlet syndrome, embolic occlusions, or rheumatic or occupational diseases are often associated with Raynaud's syndrome. Certain drugs, especially β-blockers, nicotine,[87] and ergotamine-containing compounds[88] may also predispose to vasospasm.

Diagnosis

The diagnosis of Raynaud's syndrome is made largely on clinical grounds. Laboratory study of these patients has traditionally been unsatisfying. Tests to screen for the possibility of large vessel occlusive disease should be performed on all patients. Provocative testing to document and assess abnormal vasoconstriction is often of limited value because of the difficulty in reliably reproducing symptoms in a laboratory setting. In our noninvasive vascular laboratory we immerse the patient's hands in ice water for 30 seconds and document the time required for digital temperature to recover. Normal individuals usually do this in 10 minutes or less, while more prolonged rewarming periods are typically required for patients with clinical evidence of Raynaud's syndrome. Other investigators have used different forms of cold challenge including total-body cooling[89] and have also explored alternative methods for studying the changes in blood flow such as venous occlusion plethysmography,[90] laser-Doppler velocimetry,[91,92] pulse volume recordings, xenon-131 washout,[93] photoplethysmography,[94] and thermography.[95,96] No laboratory method of assessment has emerged as clearly superior at this time.

Therapy

The treatment of Raynaud's syndrome remains a difficult problem. In cases of secondary Raynaud's syndrome, treatment of the underlying condition should be attempted whenever possible. Simple conservative measures such as dressing warmly, avoiding unnecessary exposure to the cold, and intermittently warming the hands[97] may improve matters substantially. Occasionally, moving to a warmer climate may be necessary. Biofeedback is effective in a number of cases.[98] Avoiding drugs with a potential for causing vasoconstriction (e.g., β-blockers, nicotine, and ergotamine) is important. Certain vasodilators may help, especially nifedipine,[99-101] prazosin,[102,103] and possibly ketanserin.[104,105] Interruption of sympathetic nerves to the upper extremity, either through ganglionic injection or surgical sympathectomy, is an option for patients with severe and debilitating symptoms.[106]

ARTERIOVENOUS FISTULAS, MALFORMATIONS, AND VASCULAR TUMORS

Upper extremity arteriovenous fistulas may be *acquired* or *congenital* (see Chapter 30). Acquired arteriovenous fistulas usually result when trauma to the arm disrupts an artery and adjacent vein, allowing blood to flow between the two. These abnormal communications are often occult at first but tend to enlarge from weeks to months and may eventually carry a significant amount of blood. Symptoms of arteriovenous fistulas depend on the blood flow. They may be totally asymptomatic, or they can produce pain, swelling, discoloration, abnormal pulsations of the affected arms, increased limb growth, ischemia distal to the fistula, and elevated skin temperatures. Common types of injury that lead to fistula formation include gunshot and knife wounds, bone fractures, catheterization procedures involving the arm, and surgery.[107] One of the most common forms of upper extremity arteriovenous fistula are those created intentionally for use in hemodialysis.[108]

Congenital arteriovenous malformations (Fig. 37-14) encompass a wide spectrum of lesions in which abnormal arteriovenous shunting may be present. These include *arteriovenous fistulas,* certain tumorlike growths such as *hemangiomas* (which may be arterial, venous, capillary, or mixed, depending on which type of vessel the lesion developed from*), and various forms of *angiodysplasias*. Other benign and malignant tumors (such as hemangiosarcomas, lymphosarcomas, or any large vascular tumor) may be associated with abnormal arteriovenous shunting of blood. Numerous schemes have been developed for naming and categorizing these anomalies, none of which are totally satisfactory. The term *arteriovenous malformation* can therefore be used generically to include all significant congenital vascular lesions, with additional modifying terms affixed as needed.

The diagnosis of arteriovenous fistula or malformation is usually suspected on the basis of the above-mentioned physical findings. Arteriography may be necessary to define the extent of the fistula, especially if surgery is contemplated. In arteriovenous malformations involving small vessels (especially those that grow rapidly) biopsy may be necessary to ensure that the malformation is not caused by a malignancy. Treatment is by surgical ligation or removal of the fistula (or tumor) when possible.[109] Traumatic arteriovenous fistulas can usually be repaired surgically without undue difficulty. However, in many cases of congenital malformation the lesion is too extensive to remove. Various

*Some authors prefer to group all large vessel hemangiomas under the term "cavernous hemangioma."

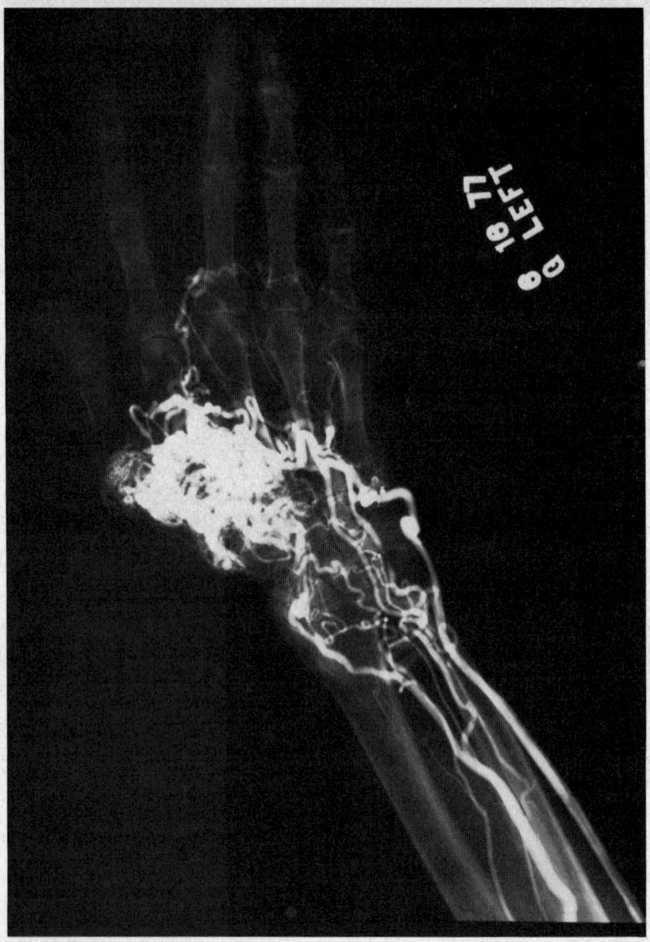

Fig. 37-14. Hand arteriogram. Arteriovenous malformation diffusely involving the wrist and radial aspect of the hand. The lesion involves bones and soft tissues. There is also venous shunting.

embolization techniques have been tried. Unfortunately, while these procedures may temporarily reduce fistula flow, the lesions tend to recur or enlarge, making them difficult to eliminate completely.

LYMPHATIC DISEASE

Upper extremity lymphatic disorders include *lymphangitis* and *lymphatic obstruction*. Lymphangitis (i.e., lymphatic inflammation) usually results from bacterial or fungal entry into the lymphatic vessels via sites of localized infection in the hands or fingers, but it may also be triggered by the direct injection of irritants (such as contrast material for radiologic studies) into the lymphatic vessels. Lymphangitis manifests itself clinically with fever, localized pain and tenderness, and signs of lymphatic inflammation such as red streaks extending up the skin of the arm. In cases of infective lymphangitis, streptococcus is the usual cause and the use of penicillin or other antibiotics with an appropriate spectrum of activity is therefore indicated.[110] Repeated episodes of lymphangitis may lead to loss or blockage of the lymphatic vessels.

Lymphatic obstruction in the upper extremity may occur secondary to a wide variety of disorders. In the United States the leading cause has been surgical disruption of lymphatic vessels or radiation-induced lymphatic fibrosis occurring as a result of surgical mastectomy and adjuvant radiation therapy for breast cancer.[111] Other common causes of lymphatic obstruction include congenital abnormalities or deficiencies of lymph vessels, recurrent episodes of lymphangitis, and blockage by various types of tumors (local or metastatic). In many tropical countries lymphatic infiltration with various parasites is the leading cause of lymphatic obstruction.[112] The swelling that develops throughout the arm as the result of lymphatic obstruction is referred to as *lymphedema*. The diagnosis of lymphedema is made by (1) ruling out other causes of upper limb swelling and (2) radionuclide lymphatic scanning *(lymphoscintigraphy)* to confirm the lack of vessel patency.[113,114] *Lymphangiography* is probably best avoided because of the potential for causing lymphangitis with additional loss of lymphatic vessels. The treatment of lymphatic obstruction in lymphedema can be difficult. Conservative measures include periodic limb elevation, protection of the involved arm from injury, use of prophylactic antibiotics to prevent infection, and the wearing of an elastic compression garment (sleeve) to reduce and control swelling.[115] Externally applied intermittent compression devices ("lymphatic pumps") are of value in certain situations.[116] For patients with proximal obstruction of large lymphatic vessels, bypass operations are a possibility.

REFERENCES

1. Welling RE et al: Obliterative arterial disease of the upper extremity, Arch Surg 116:1593, 1981.
2. Laroche GP et al: Chronic arterial insufficiency of the upper extremity, Mayo Clin Proc 51:180, 1976.
3. Crawford ES et al: Thrombo-obliterative disease of the great vessels arising from the aortic arch, J Thorac Cardiovasc Surg 43:38, 1962.
4. Grant KC: Experience with distal in-situ vein grafts, Can J Surg 30:163, 1987.
5. Hallett JW: Trends in revascularization of the lower extremity, Mayo Clin Proc 61:369, 1986.
6. Carlson RE et al: Innominate endarterectomy: a 16-year experience, Arch Surg 112:1389, 1977.
7. Ekestrom S, Liljequist L, and Nordhus O: Surgical management of obliterative disease of the brachiocephalic trunk, Scand J Thorac Cardiovasc Surg 17:305, 1983.
8. Williams SJ: Chronic upper extremity ischemia: current concepts in management, Surg Clin North Am 66:355, 1986.
9. Gomes AS: Arteriography in the diagnosis and management of vascular disorders of the upper extremity. In Machleder HI, ed: Vascular disorders of the upper extremity, New York, 1983, Futura Publishing Co, Inc.
10. Fogarty TJ: Arterial embolism. In Dale A, ed: Management of arterial occlusive disease, Chicago, 1971, Year Book Medical Publishers, Inc.
11. Shoor PM and Fogarty TJ: Acute arterial insufficiency. In Miller DC and Roon AS, eds: Diagnosis and management of peripheral vascular disease, Menlo Park, Calif, 1982, Addison-Wesley Publishing Co, Inc.
12. Green RM, DeWeese JA, and Rob CG: Arterial embolectomy before and after the Fogarty catheter, Surgery 77:24, 1970.
13. Meister SG et al: Paradoxical embolism: diagnosis during life, Am J Med 53:292, 1972.
14. Seward JB et al: Transesophageal echocardiography: technique, anatomic correlations, implementation, and clinical applications, Mayo Clin Proc 63:649, 1988.
15. Shub C: The role of echocardiography in clinical practice. In Spittell JA, ed: Clinical medicine, Philadelphia, 1982, Harper & Row, Publishers, Inc.
16. Fairbairn JF, Joyce JW, and Pairolero PC: Acute arterial occlusion of the extremities. In Juergens JL, Spittell JA, and Fairbairn JF, eds: Peripheral vascular diseases, Philadelphia, 1980, WB Saunders Co.
17. Sullivan KL, Sminken SL, and White RI: Treatment of a case of thromboembolism resulting from thoracic outlet syndrome with intraarterial urokinase infusion, J Vasc Surg 7:568, 1988.
18. Savelyev VS, Zatevakhin II, and Stephanov NV: Artery embolism of the upper limbs, J Surg 81:367, 1977.
19. Machleder HI: Etiology and management of major arterial and venous occlusive processes involving the upper extremity. In Machleder HI, ed: Vascular disorders of the upper extremity, New York, 1983, Futura Publishing Co, Inc.
20. Sheps SG and McDuffie FC: Vasculitis. In Juergens JL, Spittell JA, Fairbairn JF, eds: Peripheral vascular diseases, Philadelphia, 1980, WB Saunders Co.
21. Machleder HI: Vaso-occlusive disorders of the upper extremity, Curr Probl Surg 25:1, 1988.
22. Levo Y et al: Association between hepatitis B virus and essential mixed cryoglobulinemia, N Engl J Med 296:1501, 1977.
23. Brouet JC et al: Biologic and clinical significance of cryoglobulins: a report of 86 cases, Am J Med 57:775, 1974.
24. McDuffie FC et al: Hypocomplementemia with cutaneous vasculitis and arthritis: possible immune complex syndrome, Mayo Clin Proc 48:340, 1973.
25. Mills JL et al: Upper extremity ischemia caused by small artery disease, Ann Surg 206:521, 1987.
26. Ames EL et al: Bilateral hand necrosis in Kawasaki syndrome, J Hand Surg 10A:391, 1985.
27. Hall S et al: Takayasu arteritis, Medicine 64:89, 1985.
28. Juergens JL: Thromboangiitis obliterans. In Juergens JL, Spittell JA, and Fairbairn JF, eds: Peripheral vascular diseases, Philadelphia, 1980, WB Saunders Co.
29. McKusick VA et al: Buerger's disease: a distinct clinical and pathological entity, JAMA 181:5, 1962.
30. Lambeth J and Yong NK: Arteriographic findings in thromboangiitis obliterans, AJR 109:553, 1970.
31. Rivera R: Roentgenographic diagnosis of Buerger's disease, J Cardiovasc Surg 14:40, 1973.
32. DeRemee RA, McDonald TJ, and Weiland LH: Wegener's granulomatosis: observations on treatment with antimicrobial agents, Mayo Clin Proc 60:27, 1985.
33. Leitner DW, Ross JS, and Neary JR: Granulomatous radial arteritis with bilateral, nontraumatic, true arterial aneurysms within the anatomic snuffbox, J Hand Surg 10A:131, 1985.
34. Trunkey DD and Lim RC: Vascular trauma. In Miller DC and Roon AJ, eds: Diagnosis and management of peripheral vascular disease, Menlo Park, Calif, 1982, Addison-Wesley Publishing Company, Inc.
35. Kutsal A and Kivanc O: A case of ulnar aneurysm: clinical and surgical considerations, J Cardiovasc Surg 29:326, 1988.
36. Ho PK et al: Aneurysms of the upper extremity, J Hand Surg 12A:39, 1987.
37. Ho PK, Dellon AL, and Wilgis EF: True aneurysms of the hand resulting from athletic injury: report of two cases, Am J Sports Med 13:136, 1985.
38. Horattas MC et al: Changing concepts of deep venous thrombosis of the upper extremity: report of a series and review of the literature, Surgery 104:561, 1988.
39. Rooke TW: Vascular complications of interventional procedures. In Holmes DR Jr and Vlietstra RE, eds: Interventional cardiology, Philadelphia, 1989, FA Davis Co.
40. Benitez PR and Newell MA: Vascular trauma in drug abuse: patterns of injury, Ann Vasc Surg 1:175, 1986.
41. Nasu Y and Ishida K: Follow-up study of patients with vibration syndrome in Japan, Scand J Work Environ Health 12:313, 1986.
42. Pyykko I et al: Vibration syndrome among Finnish forest workers: a follow-up from 1972 to 1983, Scand J Work Environ Health 12(4):307, 1986.
43. Brubaker RL, Mackenzie CJ, and Hutton SG: Vibration-induced white finger among selected underground rock drillers in British Columbia, Scand J Work Environ Health 12:296, 1986.
44. Engstrom K and Dandanell R: Exposure conditions and Raynaud's phenomenon among riveters in the aircraft industry, Scand J Work Environ Health 12:293, 1986.
45. Yu ZS et al: Epidemiologic survey of vibration syndrome among riveters, chippers and grinders in the railroad system of the People's Republic of China, Scand J Work Environ Health 12:289, 1986.
46. Nasu Y: Defibrinogating therapy for peripheral circulatory disturbance in patients with vibration syndrome, Scand J Work Environ Health 12:272, 1986.
47. Pineda CJ et al: Hypothenar hammer syndrome: form of reversible Raynaud's phenomenon, Am J Med 79:561, 1985.
48. Savader SJ, Savader BL, and Drewry GR: Hypothenar hammer syndrome with embolic occlusion of digital arteries, Clin Radiol 39:324, 1988.

49. McCarthy WJ et al: Upper extremity arterial injury in athletes, J Vasc Surg 9:317, 1989.
50. Bovenzi M: Finger thermometry in the assessment of subjects with vibration-induced white finger, Scand J Work Environ Health 13:348, 1987.
51. Ekenvall L: Clinical assessment of suspected damage from hand-held vibrating tools, Scand J Work Environ Health 13:271, 1987.
52. Paterson C: Canadian compensation law and vibration-induced white finger. A revised description, Scand J Work Environ Health 12:402, 1986.
53. McCready RA, Procter CD, and Hyde GL: Subclavian-axillary vascular trauma, J Vasc Surg 3:24, 1986.
54. Gooding GA: Sonography of the radial artery at the wrist, AJR 150:629, 1988.
55. Slavin SA: Microvascular reconstruction of the hand, Clin Plast Surg 10:139, 1983.
56. Talha H et al: Brachial artery entrapment: compression by the supracondylar process, Ann Vasc Surg 1:479, 1986.
57. Garrett HE, Hodosh S, and DeBakey ME: Fibromuscular hyperplasia of the left axillary artery, Arch Surg 94:737, 1967.
58. Lie JT and Juergens JL: Degenerative arterial diseases other than atherosclerosis. In Juergens JL, Spittell JA, and Fairbairn JF, eds: Peripheral vascular diseases, Philadelphia, 1980, WB Saunders Co.
59. Albin G et al: Paraneoplastic digital thrombosis: a case report, Angiology 37:203, 1986.
60. Petri M and Fye KH: Digital necrosis: a paraneoplastic syndrome, J Rheumatol 12:800, 1985.
61. Taylor LM Jr et al: Digital ischemia as a manifestation of malignancy, Ann Surg 206:62, 1987.
62. Curelaru I et al: Dynamics of thrombophlebitis in central venous catheterization via basilic and cephalic veins, Acta Chir Scand 150:285, 1984.
63. Bradof J, Sands MJ Jr, and Lakin PC: Symptomatic venous thrombosis of the upper extremity complicating permanent transvenous pacing: reversal with streptokinase infusion, Am Heart J 104:190, 1982.
64. Stevenson IM and Parry EWA: Radiological study of the aetiological factors in venous obstruction of the upper limb, J Cardiovasc Surg (Torino) 16:580, 1975.
65. Campbell CB et al: Axillary, subclavian, and brachiocephalic vein obstruction, J Surg 82:816, 1977.
66. Falk RL and Smith DF: Thrombosis of the upper extremity thoracic inlet veins: diagnosis with duplex Doppler sonography, AJR 149:677, 1987.
67. Sullivan ED, Peter DJ, and Cranley JJ: Real-time B-mode venous ultrasound, J Vasc Surg 1:465, 1984.
68. Drury EM et al: Lytic therapy in the treatment of axillary and subclavian vein thrombosis, J Vasc Surg 2:821, 1985.
69. Roos DB: Thoracic outlet syndromes. In Machleder HI, ed: Vascular disorders of the upper extremity, New York, 1983, Futura Publishing Co, Inc.
70. Fairbairn JF, Campbell JK, and Payne WS: Neurovascular compression syndromes of the thoracic outlet. In Juergens JL, Spittell JA, and Fairbairn JF, eds: Peripheral vascular diseases, Philadelphia, 1980, WB Saunders Co.
71. Roos DB: Thoracic outlet and carpal tunnel syndromes. In Management of neurovascular diseases involving the upper extremity, Philadelphia, 1984, WB Saunders Co.
72. Kieffer E: Arterial complications of thoracic outlet syndrome. In Bergen Y, ed: Evaluation and treatment of upper and lower extremity circulatory disorders, Orlando, Fla, 1984, Grune & Stratton, Inc.
73. Roos DB: Congenital anomalies associated with thoracic outlet syndrome, Am J Surg 132:771, 1976.
74. Priest JD: The shoulder of the tennis player, Clin Sports Med 7:387, 1988.
75. Bouhoutsos J, Morris T, and Martin P: Unilateral Raynaud's phenomenon in the hand and its significance, Surgery 82:547, 1977.
76. Scher LA et al: Vascular complications of thoracic outlet syndrome, J Vasc Surg 3:565, 1986.
77. Daube JR: Nerve conduction studies in the thoracic outlet syndrome, Neurology 25:347, 1962.
78. Machleder HI et al: Somatosensory evoked potentials in the assessment of thoracic outlet compression syndrome, J Vasc Surg 6:177, 1987.
79. Dunant JH: Thoracic outlet syndrome: treatment of vascular complications, Vasa 14:51, 1985.
80. DeWeese JA, Adams JT, and Gaiser DL: Subclavian venous thrombectomy, Circulation XLI, XLII (II): 158, 1970.
81. Steed DL et al: Streptokinase in the treatment of subclavian vein thrombosis, J Vasc Surg 4:28, 1986.
82. Freedman RR and Ianni P: Role of cold and emotional stress in Raynaud's disease and scleroderma, Br Med J 287:1499, 1983.
83. Freedman RR et al: Increased alpha-adrenergic responsiveness in idiopathic Raynaud's disease, Arthritis Rheum 32:61, 1989.
84. Okada A et al: Usefulness of blood parameters, especially viscosity, for the diagnosis and elucidation of pathogenic mechanisms of the hand-arm vibration syndrome, Scand J Work Environ Health 13:358, 1987.
85. Sandhagen B and Wegener T: Blood viscosity and finger systolic pressure in primary and traumatic vasospastic disease, Ups J Med Sci 90:55, 1985.
86. Lewis T: The pathological changes in the arteries supplying the fingers in warm-handed people and in cases of so-called Raynaud's disease, Clin Sci 3:287, 1938.
87. Bovenzi M: Finger systolic pressure during local cooling in normal subjects aged 20 to 60 years: reference values for the assessment of digital vasospasm in Raynaud's phenomenon of occupational origin. Int Arch Occup Environ Health 61:179, 1988.
88. Siefert KB et al: Bilateral upper extremity ischemia after administration of dihydroergotamine-heparin for prophylaxis of deep venous thrombosis, J Vasc Surg 8:410, 1988.
89. Engelhart M, Nielsen HV, and Kristensen JK: The blood supply to fingers during Raynaud's attack: a comparison of laser-Doppler flowmetry with other techniques, Clin Physiol 5:447, 1985.
90. Halperin JL, Cohen RA, and Coffman JD: Digital vasodilatation during mental stress in patients with Raynaud's disease, Cardiovasc Res 17:671, 1983.
91. Goodfield MJ, Hume A, and Rowell NR: The effect of simple warming procedures on finger blood flow in systemic sclerosis, Br J Dermatol 118:661, 1988.
92. Wollersheim H, Reyenga J, and Thien T: Laser Doppler velocimetry of fingertips during heat provocation in normals and in patients with Raynaud's phenomenon, Scand J Clin Lab Invest 48:91, 1988.
93. Olsen N and Petring OU: Vibration elicited vasoconstrictor reflex in Raynaud's phenomena, Br J Ind Med 45:415, 1988.
94. Cooke ED, Bowcock SA, and Smith AT: Photoplethysmography of the distal pulp in the assessment of vasospastic hand, Angiology 36:33, 1985.
95. Dupuis H: Thermographic assessment of skin temperature during a cold provocation test, Scand J Work Environ Health 13:352, 1987.
96. Belcaro G et al: Infrared and ELC thermography in the assessment of the digital rewarming curve after a finger-cooling test: a preliminary report, Panminerva Med 27:33, 1985.
97. Goodfield MJ and Rowell NR: Hand warming as a treatment for Raynaud's phenomenon in systemic sclerosis, Br J Dermatol 119:643, 1988.
98. Freedman RR: Long-term effectiveness of behavioral treatments for Raynaud's disease, Behav Res Ther 18:387, 1987.
99. Nilsson H et al: The effect of the calcium-entry blocker nifedipine

on cold-induced digital vasospasm: a double-blind crossover study versus placebo, Acta Med Scand 221:53, 1982.
100. Rodeheffer RJ et al: Controlled double-blind trial of nifedipine in the treatment of Raynaud's phenomenon, N Engl J Med 308:880, 1983.
101. Pin PG, Sicard GA, and Weeks PM: Digital ischemia of the upper extremity: a systematic approach for evaluation and treatment, Plast Reconstr Surg 82:653, 1988.
102. Lewis P et al: Nifedipine in patients with Raynaud's syndrome: effects on radial artery blood flow, Eur Heart J 8:83, 1987.
103. Waldo R: Prazosin relieves Raynaud's vasospasm, JAMA 241:1037, 1979.
104. Arneklo-Nobin B, Elmer O, and Akesson A: Effect of long-term ketanserin treatment on 5-HT levels, platelet aggregation and peripheral circulation in patients with Raynaud's phenomenon: a double-blind, placebo-controlled cross-over study, Int Angiol 7:19, 1988.
105. Lagerkvist BE and Linderholm H: Cold hands after exposure to arsenic or vibrating tools: effects of ketanserin on finger blood pressure and skin temperature, Acta Pharmacol Toxicol (Copenh) 58:327, 1986.
106. van de Wal HJ et al: Thoracic sympathectomy as a therapy for upper extremity ischemia: a long-term follow-up study, Thorac Cardiovasc Surg 33:181, 1985.
107. Miller DR and Malki A: Large saccular aneurysm and A-V fistula of the brachial vessels, J Cardiovasc Surg (Torino) 26:605, 1985.
108. Kherlakian GM et al: Comparison of autogenous fistula versus expanded polytetrafluoroethylene graft fistula for angioaccess in hemodialysis, Am J Surg 152:238, 1986.
109. Wilgis EFS: Tumors. In Vascular injuries and diseases of the upper limb, Boston, 1983, Little, Brown & Co, Inc.
110. Schirger A: Lymphedema, Cardiovasc Clin 13:293, 1983.
111. Kobayashi MR and Miller TA: Lymphedema, Clin Plast Surg 14:303, 1987.
112. Lymphatic filariasis—tropical medicine's origin will not go away, Lancet 1:1409, June 20, 1987.
113. Samuels LD: Lymphoscintigraphy, Lymphology 20:4, 1987.
114. Ohtake E and Matsui K: Lymphoscintigraphy in patients with lymphedema: a new approach using intradermal injections of technetium-99m human serum albumin, Clin Nucl Med 11:474, 1986.
115. Stillwell GK: Management of arm edema. In Stoll BA, ed: Breast cancer management: early and late, Chicago, 1977, Heinemann Medical and Year Book Medical.
116. Zanolla R et al: Evaluation of the results of three different methods of postmastectomy lymphedema treatment, J Surg Oncol 26:210, 1984.

Chapter 38

DIABETIC FOOT LESIONS

Marvin E. Levin

The human foot is a mechanical marvel. It consists of 26 bones, 29 joints, 42 muscles, and innumerable tendons and ligaments. In a lifetime this phenomenal machine, with its multiple moving parts, walks over 100,000 miles—four times around the world. It is exposed to significant pressures. The forefoot and hallux bear the stepping off, or dynamic pressure. In normal individuals the average dynamic pressure, the stepping off pressure, is 3.59 kg/cm^2 over the first metatarsophalangeal joint, 6.21 kg/cm^2 over the second metatarsophalangeal joint, and 5.84 kg/cm^2 over the hallux.[1] The threshold for static, standing pressure, abnormality is 1.75 kg/cm^2.[2] The threshold level for dynamic forefoot pressure abnormality is 10 kg/cm^2.[3] Pressures above these values would be considered abnormal. The diabetic tends to have increased foot pressures, and this can be demonstrated even in diabetics with early sensory neuropathy.[4] In diabetics with ulceration there are significantly higher pressures.[5] Most of the diabetic ulcerations occur at the areas of maximum pressure, the metatarsal heads. Foot problems are common in the population at large; however, the diabetic is especially vulnerable because of increased pressures and the complications of arteriosclerosis obliterans (ASO) and peripheral neuropathy. The combination of these factors compounded by infection can lead to gangrene and amputation.

Diabetes is one of the oldest diseases known. The *Papyrus Ebers* of 1500 BC mentions its symptoms and suggests treatment. However, the history of gangrene of the feet goes back to biblical times, where, in II Chronicles 16:12-14, the first case of gangrene, possibly caused by diabetes, is described: "In the 39th year of his reign King Asa became affected with gangrene of his feet; he did not seek guidance from the Lord but resorted to physicians. He rested with his forefathers in the 41st year of his reign."

Whether or not King Asa did indeed have diabetic gangrene is a moot point. Certainly in biblical times there was not much one could do for a foot lesion except to pray. Even in the late 1800s the famous surgeon, Ambroise Paré said, "I dressed [the wound] and God healed it." Today, however, the skills of multiple medical disciplines are significantly reducing amputation rates. With increasing awareness of diabetic foot problems and improved treatment, amputation rates will continue to decrease.

This chapter is devoted to describing the pathogenesis of diabetic foot lesions and providing information on management so that the goal of decreasing amputation can be realized.

EPIDEMIOLOGY

Today there are approximately 14 million diabetics in the United States. We can expect to see this number increase since the diabetic population is increasing by 6% per year and doubling every 15 years.[6] By the turn of the century there will be 20 million diabetics in this country. This increasing diabetic population is caused by a decrease in fetal mortality and a prolonged life span, which has been increased by the discovery of insulin, antibiotics, and antihypertensives. Of these, antibiotics are probably the most significant. McDermott and Rogers stated that curing all cancers would add 2 years to the life expectancy for Americans, but the introduction of antibiotics has added 10 years.[7] However, these added years have not always been quality years for the diabetic since they have resulted in a multitude of complications, not the least of which are foot problems. The diabetic who is most likely to develop a foot lesion is over age 40. Today 90% of the diabetics in this country are over age 40.[8] Of all diabetics, 15% will develop a foot ulcer during their lifetime.[9] Most of these are the result of peripheral neuropathy and the insensate foot. Peripheral neuropathy is extremely common in the diabetic type I patients with the incidence gradually increasing with age and duration. After 20 years of diabetes 42% of diabetics have evidence of peripheral neuropathy.[10]

Of diabetics, 8% have ASO at the time of diagnosis, 15% after 10 years, and 45% after 20 years.[11] Kreines et al reviewed the natural history of ASO in type II diabetics.[12] Of diabetics, 20% will enter the hospital because of foot problems.[13] Of these patients, 30% have symptomatic ASO, and 7% will require vascular surgery or amputation.[13]

Race

Race may play a significant role in the number of amputations required by the diabetic population. A 2.3 times greater incidence of amputation in blacks, compared with whites, was found in South Carolina[14] and a 1.4 times greater incidence in nonwhites, compared with whites, in New Jersey.[15] One study suggested that the increased prevalence of hypertension and smoking in blacks may be a contributory factor.[16] The Pima Indians in the Southwest have shown an exceptionally high rate, a 3.7 times greater incidence than whites.[17]

Age

In comparing age groups researchers have found the amputation rate in the 45- to 64-year-old group is two to three times higher, compared with nondiabetics. In those over 65 it is seven times higher.[14] Of all lower extremity amputations, 96% occur in those over age 45 and 64% in those 65 years of age or older.[18] Younger diabetics may also undergo amputation. I have seen an above-knee amputation needed because of atherosclerosis in a 27-year-old type I diabetic.

Sex

Diabetes has been a great equalizer between the sexes when looking at ASO alone. The ratio of ASO in nondiabetic men as compared with that in women is 30:1. However, in the diabetic the ratio of men to women is approximately 2 :1. The risk for lower extremity amputation has been found to be from 1.4 to 2.6 times greater for men than for women with diabetes.[14,15,17] In a series of 20 consecutive diabetic amputations performed in 1988 at our university hospital, there were an equal number of men and women. Sex per se may not be a factor. Men are more likely to traumatize their feet. They do more physical work than women, are on their feet more, thereby subjecting them to a greater degree of trauma.

Type of diabetes

The overall number of amputations performed is greater in type II patients than in type I. This is largely because type II patients are older and greater in number. After adjusting for age there may be a slightly increased incidence of amputations in type I patients.[8,18]

AMPUTATION

More than 50,000 major diabetic amputations were reported in 1985 in the United States.[18] The cost of an amputation can be very expensive. Mackey et al, at the University of Minnesota, reported an average cost of $40,000 per amputation.[19] In the 1988 review of 20 diabetics undergoing amputation at our university hospital, there was an average hospital stay of 22.85 days, with a range of 10 to 45, and an average in-hospital cost of $24,430, with a range of $7,000 to $44,800. The age of the patients undergoing amputation ranged from 40 to 82 years, with an average age of 63.7 years. Based on 50,000 plus amputations at an average cost of approximately $25,000 each, $1.2 billion is spent annually on amputations. This figure does not include the surgeon's fee, cost of rehabilitation, possible loss of job, disability and welfare payments, and Medicare payments for patients who go on Medicare before age 65 as a result of amputation. As the population ages and medical costs rise, these numbers will increase. However, the increasing numbers of educational programs in foot care and the use of therapeutic shoes have demonstrated a reduction in the number of amputations being performed annually. Several recent studies have shown a reduction of 50% in the amputation rate when special foot care programs are initiated. Davidson et al[20] and Edmonds et al[21] have decreased their amputation rate by 50% and Assal et al have decreased their center's amputation rate by 83%.[22]

The long-term and short-term outlook for the diabetic undergoing amputation has always been poor. In the preantibiotic era the principal cause of in-hospital mortality in patients with diabetic gangrene was toxemia and infection.[23] With the availability of antibiotics and newer management techniques, a mortality rate of 50% in 1935[24] had fallen to 3% in the 1980s.[25] Bodily and Burgess reported that their in-hospital mortality had decreased to 1.5%.[26] They felt that this improvement was the result of better cardiovascular support and early rehabilitation.[26] The amputation site is also a critical factor in predicting mortality. Rosenberg and Shah found that midthigh amputations were twice as lethal as below-knee amputations.[27] Age was a factor after age 60, and obesity led to a somewhat increased mortality.[27] The high frequency of in-hospital mortality and the relative short-term survival rate in all these reports was the result of the high incidence of cardiac and renal disease. For example, in the series of Rosenberg and Shah 90% of those who died had associated heart disease.[27]

Fearon et al found local complication rates of 18% and systemic complication rates of 36%. Complications included such problems as gastrointestinal bleeding, myocardial infarction, congestive heart failure, and cerebral vascular accidents.[25] The surgeon and surgical house officers who must spend most of their hospital day in the operating room do not have the time, and frequently do not have the expertise, to manage the systemic and metabolic problems of the diabetic after surgery. In the diabetic patient the major postoperative problem is not the operative site but the control of blood glucose and the management of medical problems such as cardiac and renal difficulties, which require the constant attention of trained medical personnel. It is therefore my strong opinion that any diabetic patient undergoing surgery should be returned to the medical division for postoperative care.

The long-term outlook for the diabetic amputee has not improved significantly since Silbert's report of 1952, when he found in a follow-up study of 294 cases a 65% survival rate for 3 years but only a 41% survival rate at the end of 5 years.[28] Ecker and Jacobs found data similar to those of Silbert 18 years later. In their series of 103 patients they found only a 61% survival rate 3 years after the first amputation.[29]

Because of the high mortality in this group of diabetics, many of them do not live long enough to undergo a second amputation. For those who do, the long-term outlook for the second leg is poor. This poor prognosis for the second leg is not new. Marchal de Calvi in 1864 stated that "often the opposite leg is affected, gangrene sets in and soon the patient succumbs to horrible suffering. Having relieved him only of his local affliction (by amputation), I have done nothing but mutilate him."[30] This problem still exists. On the average, 42% of these patients will have amputation of the remaining leg in 1 to 3 years and 56% in 3 to 5 years.[28,29,31-33] The dismal outlook for the contralateral leg reported in the 1960s has not improved over the past two decades. In the 1980 report of Ebskov and Josephsen,[34] the high risk of a contralateral amputation was still present with an incidence of 11.9% within 1 year, 17.8% after 2 years, 27.2% after 3 years, and 44.3% at 4 years. A contributing factor is the increased load pattern on the remaining foot. Larsen, Christiansen, and Ebskov[35] concluded that regulation of pedal load pattern on the remaining foot had a considerable curative and preventive effect in preventing and healing ulcerations. This redistribution of pressures is accomplished with shoes fitted with special insoles designed to redistribute pressure.

Infection is one of the major reasons for amputation in the contralateral leg. Kucan and Robson, in a 3-year follow-up study of 45 patients, found that 49% of the patients developed a severe infection involving the contralateral foot within 28 months.[36]

PATHOGENESIS

The foot of the diabetic is especially prone to atherosclerosis and neuropathy. The signs and symptoms of either

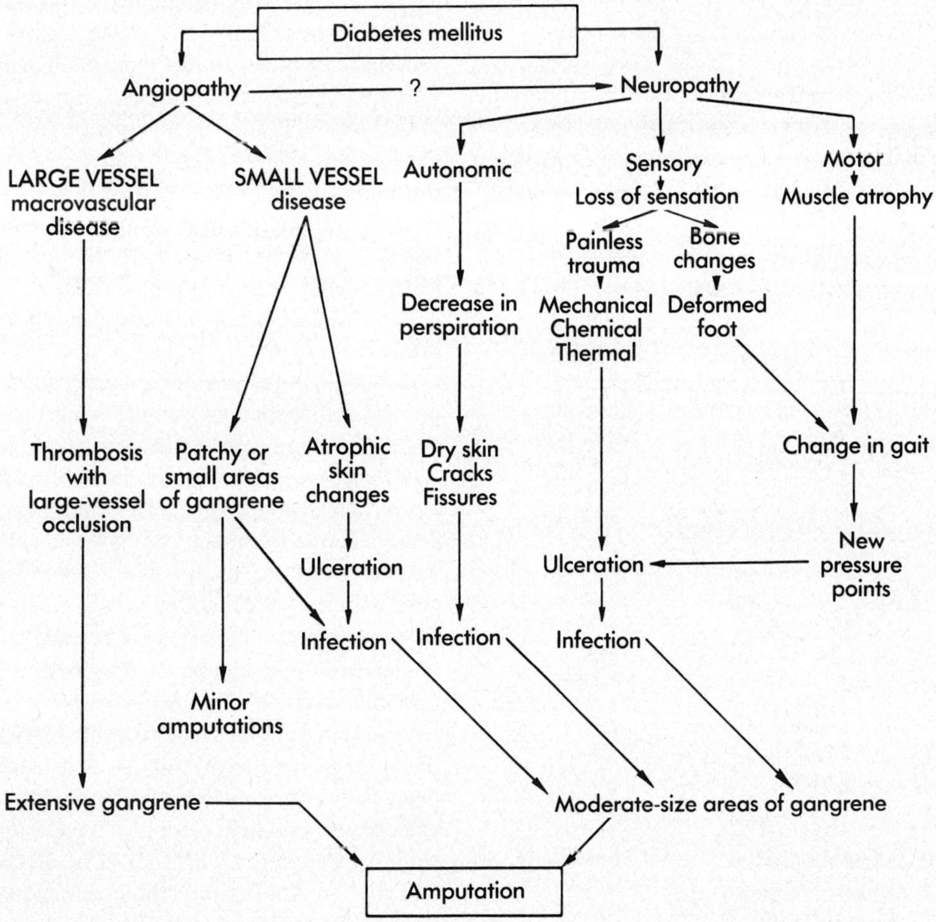

Fig. 38-1. Pathogenesis of diabetic foot lesions. (From Levin ME and O'Neal LW: The diabetic foot, ed 4, St Louis, 1988, The CV Mosby Co.)

ischemia or neuropathy may predominate; however, neither is ever present to the total exclusion of the other. The clinical picture is therefore the result of complications stemming from one or more of these factors (Fig. 38-1). Peripheral neuropathy is the leading cause of most diabetic foot lesions. Impaired blood flow to the injured or lacerated areas prevents healing and, in the presence of infection, limits the delivery of antibiotics. The most important effect of peripheral neuropathy on the diabetic foot is the loss of sensation, making the foot vulnerable even to trivial trauma. A break in the skin, though inconspicuous and miniscule, can become a portal of entry for bacteria. Once infection develops in the diabetic foot the final cataclysmic events of gangrene and the need for amputation result. Fig. 38-1 outlines the pathogenesis of diabetic foot lesions.

Peripheral vascular disease

ASO involves both large and small vessels. The pathogenesis of atherosclerosis in diabetes mellitus has recently been reviewed by Colwell et al[37] and is discussed in Chapter 7. The deposits of lipids, cholesterol, calcium, and smooth muscle cells and platelets in the plaques, are qualitatively the same in the diabetic and nondiabetic, although quantitatively much greater in the diabetic. There are, however, important differences. These are listed in Table 38-1. In the diabetic the vessels involved are primarily those below the knee, the tibial and peroneal arteries. In the series of Janka, Standl, and Mehnert the overall prevalence of isolated proximal vascular disease involving femoral and iliac vessels was 5.8% in the diabetic, the same percentage as in the general population. They concluded that proximal vascular disease in the diabetic may represent the atherosclerotic process with coexisting diabetes but did not necessarily represent diabetogenic macroangiopathy.[38] While this may be true, it is my clinical impression that there is acceleration of this atherosclerotic process, even in these larger vessels. Atherosclerotic involvement of the larger proximal vessels, iliac, and femoral vessels is definitely accelerated by smoking. For example, we recently saw a type I 27-year-old patient, diabetic since age 5, who had been a heavy smoker since age 13. At age 27 he developed intermittent claudication in his right leg. Vascular laboratory studies demonstrated a right superficial femoral artery obstruction (Fig. 38-2). It was felt that his prolonged heavy smoking had contributed significantly to his proximal artery atherosclerotic process.

Table 38-1. Differences in diabetic and nondiabetic arteriosclerosis obliterans

Arteriosclerosis	Diabetic	Nondiabetic
Clinical	More common Younger patient More rapid	Less common Older patient Less rapid
Male:female	2:1	30:1
Occlusion	Multisegmental	Single segment
Vessels adjacent to occlusion	Involved	Not involved
Collateral vessels	Involved	Usually normal
Lower extremities	Both	Unilateral
Vessels involved	Tibial Peroneal Small Arteriole	Aortic Iliac Femoral
Gangrene	Patchy areas of foot and toes	Extensive
In hospital mortality with amputation	1.5%-3%	Significantly less

Modified from Levin ME: The diabetic foot: pathophysiology, evaluation and treatment. In Levin ME and O'Neal LW, eds, The diabetic foot, ed 4, St. Louis, 1988, The CV Mosby Co.

Further evidence of which vessels are involved is demonstrated by the type of vascular surgery that is performed in these patients. While vascular surgery of all types is more common in the diabetic than in the nondiabetic, the procedure most frequently performed in the diabetic is tibioperoneal bypass surgery, involving the vessels below the knee. Vascular surgery performed on the diabetic lower extremity is approximately 10% aortofemoral bypass, 40% femoropopliteal bypass, and 70% tibioperoneal bypass.[39] The experience with percutaneous angioplasty is limited. It tends to be less applicable in the diabetic because the atherosclerotic process occurs most often in the smaller vessels. Large and small vessel disease do not necessarily progress at the same rate. It is not uncommon, for example, for small vessels in the toes to have evidence of ischemia, while the dorsalis pedis or posterior tibial pulses may be present and of adequate quality. Approximately one third of the diabetic population may have small areas of gangrene with palpable dorsalis pedis or posterior tibial pulses. Fig. 38-3 illustrates a significant decrease in toe pressure with a normal ankle pressure.

Microangiopathy is not a significant factor in the pathogenesis of diabetic foot lesions. While there may be capillary basement membrane thickening, there is no evidence that this contributes to the foot lesions. This has been noted by LoGerfo and Coffman.[40] They stressed that in many instances there are enough patent vessels at the ankle to allow vascular surgery. This is usually a tibioperoneal bypass surgery with the bypass to the tibial vessels at the ankle. Vascular surgery techniques are discussed in Chapter 9.

Ischemia or gangrene of the toes can result from four possible causes: (1) atherosclerosis with thrombosis, (2) microthrombi formation resulting from infection (Fig. 38-4), (3) cholesterol emboli, and (4) drugs, which can decrease blood flow. Microthrombi secondary to infection can convert the small vessels in the toes to end-arteries with resulting gangrene of the toes (Fig. 38-5). Cholesterol emboli that break off from atheromatous plaques in the proximal larger vessels can also cause cyanosis and gangrene of the toes. This results in the blue or purple toe syndrome. The toe takes on a deep purplish discoloration, and gangrene

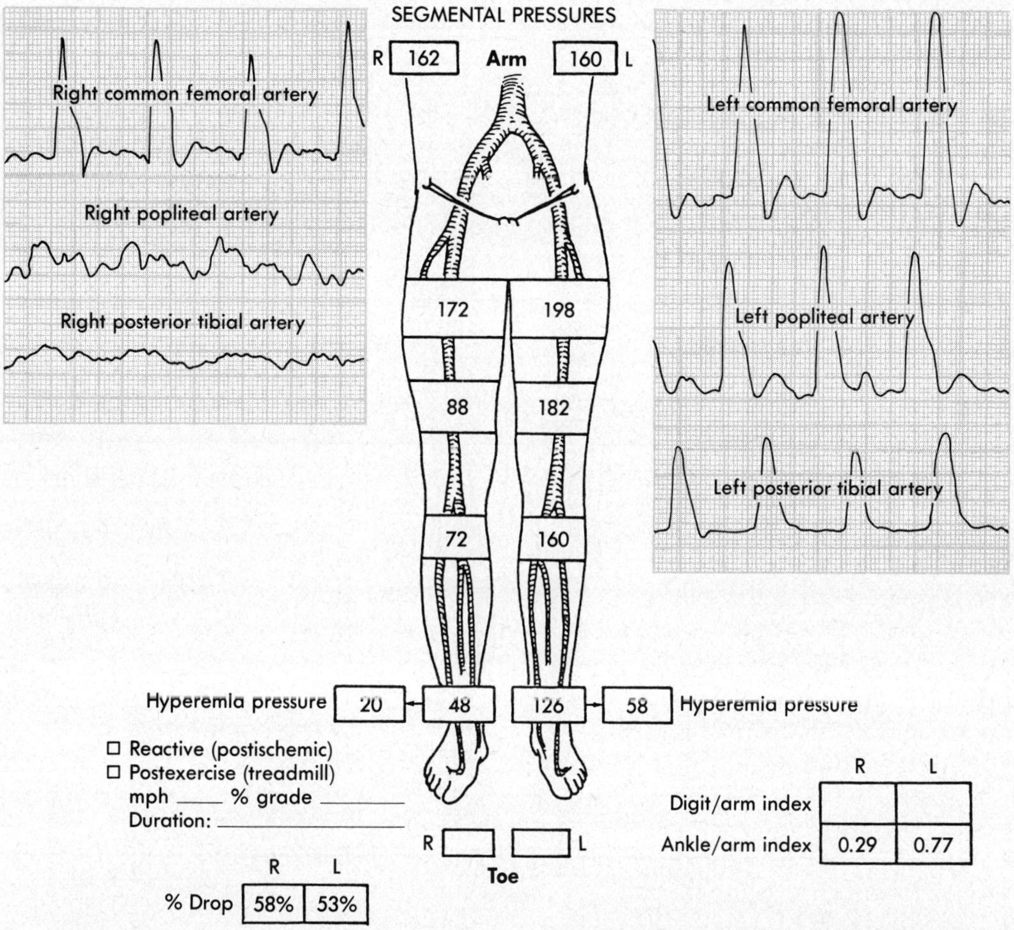

Fig. 38-2. Severe peripheral vascular disease in 27-year-old man. Doppler pressures reveal evidence of right superficial femoral artery obstruction. Note blunted waveforms in right popliteal and right posterior tibial arteries, with ankle/arm index of only 0.29. Patient had been diabetic since age 5 and was heavy smoker since early teens. He required right femoral-popliteal Goretex bypass graft. (From Levin ME and O'Neal LW: The diabetic foot, ed 4, St Louis, 1988, The CV Mosby Co; courtesy Dr. Charles B. Anderson, Department of Surgery, Washington University School of Medicine, St Louis.)

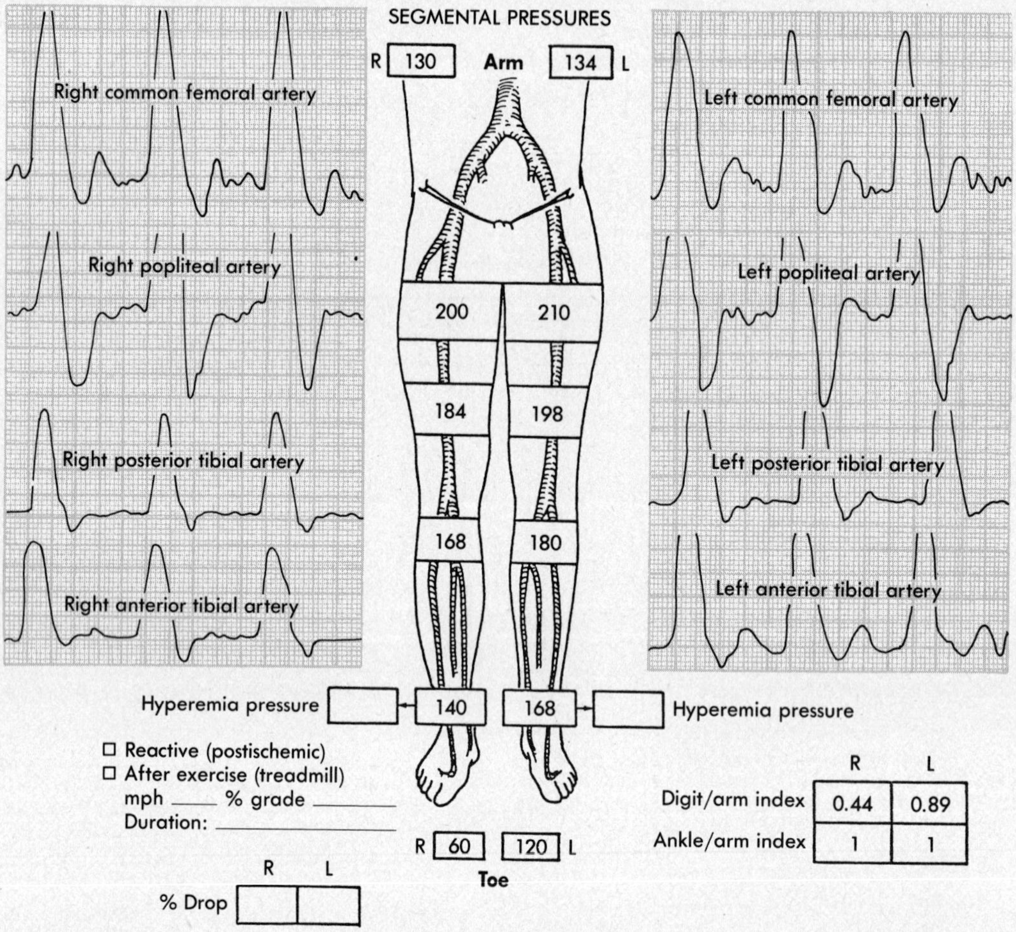

Fig. 38-3. Doppler waveforms in lower extremity of 62-year-old woman with type II diabetes, who had ischemic changes in right great toe. Note normal ankle/arm indexes but low pressure in right great toe. Low toe pressure and normal ankle pressure confirm small-vessel disease of great toe. (From Levin ME and O'Neal LW: The diabetic foot, ed 4, St Louis, 1988, The CV Mosby Co.)

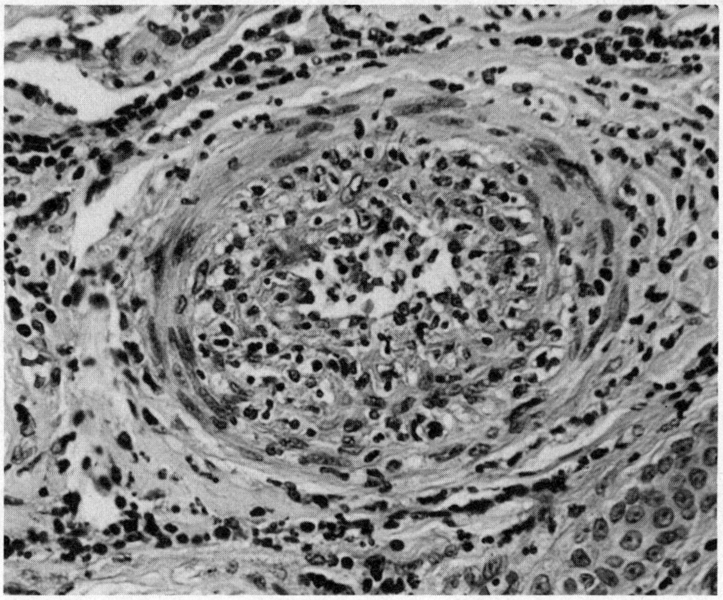

Fig. 38-4. Obliteration of lumen of small dermal arteriole by intimal hyperplasia and septic thrombus. Note cellular evidences of inflammation in areolar tissues near arteriole. This arteriole was about 1 mm from margin of area of dry gangrene. (From Levin ME and O'Neal LW: The diabetic foot, ed 4, St Louis, 1988, The CV Mosby Co.)

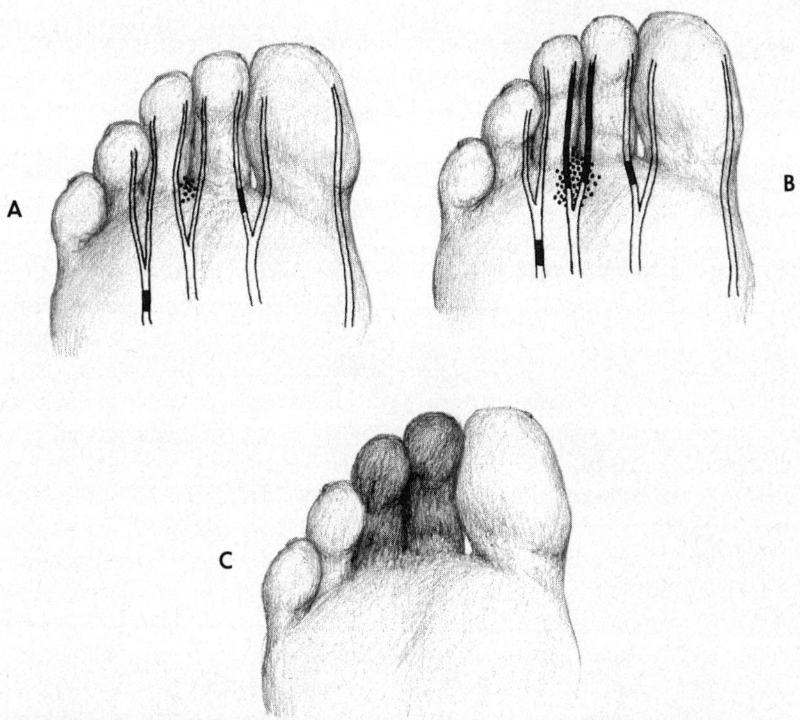

Fig. 38-5. Schematic drawings of mechanism whereby advancing infection causes obliteration of small arteries that have been converted into end-arteries by arteriosclerotic disease process, with resultant gangrene. **A,** Early web-space infection in foot with patchy segmental arteriosclerotic occlusion of digital and metatarsal vessels. **B,** Thrombosis of arteries adjacent to web-space infection. **C,** Gangrene of second and third toes. (From Levin ME and O'Neal LW: The diabetic foot, ed 4, St Louis, 1988, The CV Mosby Co.)

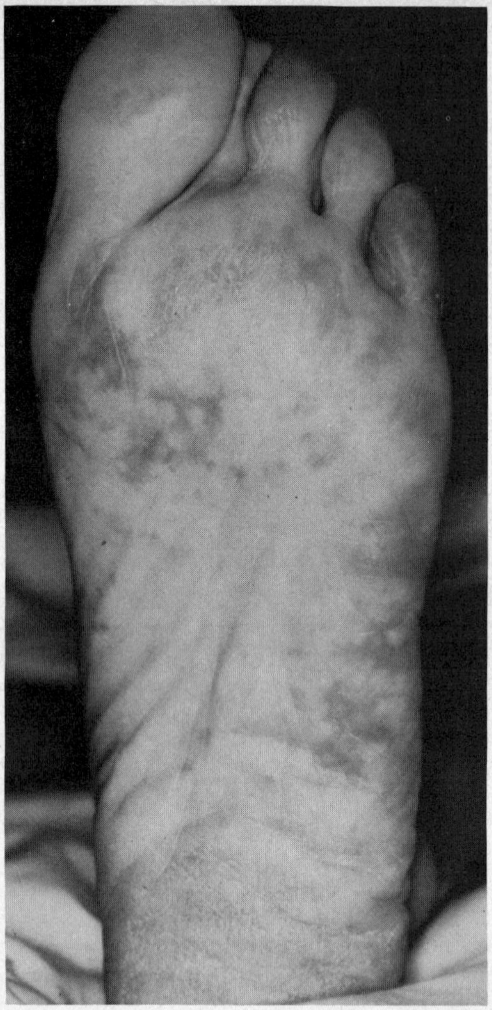

Fig. 38-6. Cyanotic changes in the fifth toe and livedo reticularis pattern of the foot secondary to cholesterol emboli from atheroscleromatous plaque shown in Fig. 38-7. (Courtesy Dr. Gregorio Sicard, Department of Surgery, Washington University School of Medicine, St Louis.)

can develop. On occasion these toes can be revascularized. Cholesterol emboli to the foot also result in painful petechia and a livedo reticularis pattern (Fig. 38-6). The atheromatous plaques may be present in the aorta, iliac, or more distant vessels. The syndrome is characterized by the sudden onset of pain in the toe. Leg and thigh myalgias may be present if muscular arteries are involved. When digital artery blood flow becomes sluggish, the toe may become bluish-purple. A sharp demarcation frequently occurs between normally perfused skin and ischemic areas. Many of these patients have received anticoagulation therapy with warfarin.[41] It is therefore extremely important to periodically check the toes and feet of patients receiving anticoagulants. However, all patients with this syndrome are not receiving anticoagulant therapy. Repeated attacks of acute ischemic changes occurring bilaterally, the development of painful cyanotic toes, petechiae, and a livedo reticularis pattern strongly suggest microemboli.

A 60-year-old man developed a painful, cyanotic fifth toe on his right foot and painful petechial lesions on both feet. These did not blanch on compression. He also complained of myalgias of the lower extremities. An angiogram (Fig. 38-7) showed a large atheromatous plaque in the left lateral wall of the infrarenal portion of the aorta with ulceration. Fig. 38-6 shows a purplish discoloration of his right fifth toe and a livedo reticularis pattern on the sole of the foot. The patient underwent successful removal of this ulcerated plaque. The treatment in such cases is vascular surgery with removal of the plaques, thereby preventing further embolization. In the study of Fisher et al[42] patients with multilevel atherosclerotic occlusive disease had their peripheral lesions treated first. In this small series the authors had no morbidity or mortality. Recurrent embolization did not occur during the follow-up period of 8 to 24 months.

Finally, certain drugs can affect ASO and cause gangrenous changes in the toes. Vasopressors such as dopamine (Intropin) frequently are used to treat shock. Because of the norepinephrine-like and vasoconstrictive effects of these agents, ischemic gangrene can develop in the toes and feet, particularly in diabetics who already have peripheral arterial insufficiency. Dopamine exerts positive inotropic effects by direct action on the adrenergic receptors. When sufficiently large doses of these inotropic drugs are administered, the predominant effect is vasoconstriction in all vascular beds.[43] Dopamine should be used with caution and in as low a dose as possible. If a patient is in shock, the risk/benefit ratio would dictate the use of inotropic drugs despite the peripheral vascular risks; however, the feet of these patients must be observed daily. Peripheral circulation can also be impaired by the use of β-blockers, which are commonly used for treatment of angina and hypertension. Zacharias et al[44] found peripheral vascular complications to be a side effect in 22 of 305 patients treated with a β-blocker. This mechanism appears to result from unopposed α-vasoconstriction subsequent to β-blockade.

Diabetes is a hypercoagulable state resulting in increased blood viscosity[45] and impaired blood flow in the microvascular vessels. The increase in hypercoagulability or blood viscosity is caused by several factors. Increased platelet hyperactivity has been well documented.[37] Elevated levels of fibrinogen have been reported, and a decrease in fibrinolysis has been documented in diabetes mellitus and may play a role in the increased fibrinogen levels.[46] Small et al have shown that there is an increase in fibrinolysis in poorly controlled NIDD patients who are treated with insulin.[47] Von Willebrand's factor is elevated.[48] Increase in red cell rigidity has also been demonstrated.[49] An increased tendency toward hypercoagulability has been demonstrated in smokers, compared with control subjects.[50] All of these factors can lead to an increase in blood viscosity and a decrease in blood flow.

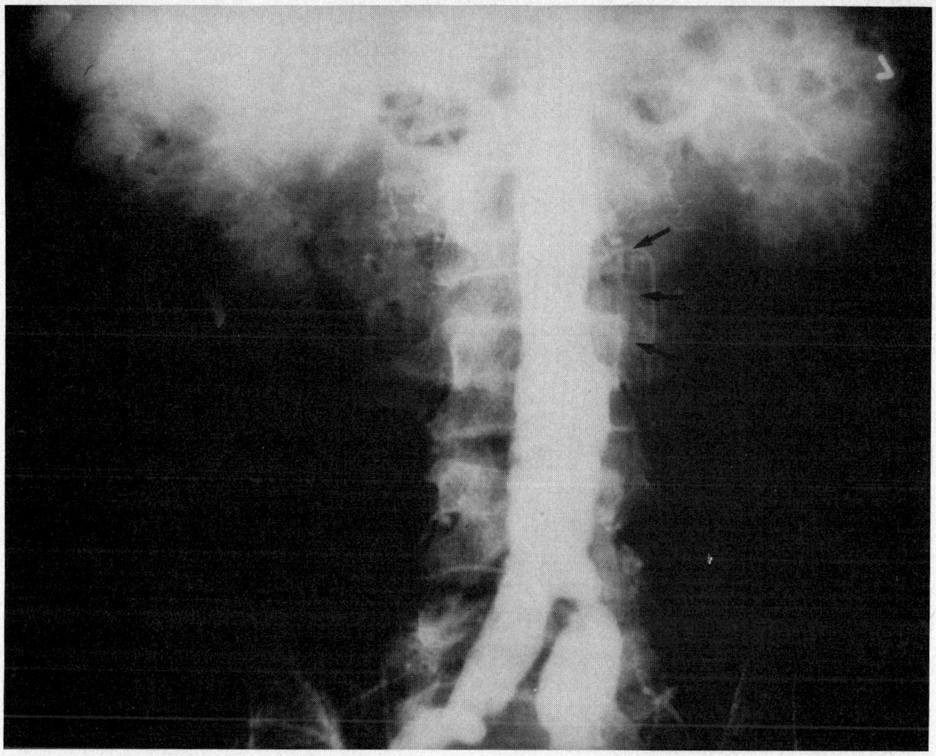

Fig. 38-7. Arteriogram showing large filling defect caused by an atheroscleromatous plaque of the aorta just inferior to the renal artery in a patient showing evidence of cholesterol emboli to the foot. (Courtesy Dr. Gregorio Sicard, Department of Surgery, Washington University School of Medicine, St Louis.)

Risk factors. Listed in the accompanying box are the risk factors in the development of diabetic arterial disease. Age, duration, and genetic factors may well be the most important factors, but unfortunately, they cannot be corrected. However, certain risk factors can be altered. Of the correctable risk factors, smoking tops the list.[51] The physiologic effects of smoking on blood flow were shown many years ago by the study of Allison and Roth.[52] An excellent review of the consequences of smoking has been written by Couch.[53] Pollin[54] has estimated that cigarette smoking causes an estimated 325,000 to 355,000 deaths annually in the United States. This is more than all other drug and alcohol abuse deaths combined; seven times more than all automobile fatalities per year; more than eleven times all reported deaths caused by acquired immunodeficiency syndrome; and more than all American military fatalities in World War I, World War II, and Vietnam combined.[54] A clinical series from New Zealand found that cigarette smoking was 2.5 times as frequent in persons who were diabetic and had ischemia and gangrene as in a control series of persons without diabetes.[55] In an analysis of smoking habits in a large series of men with ASO, only 2.5% were nonsmokers.[56] Recently, Kannel,[57] in a 26-year follow-up study of the Framingham study of 5209 subjects, found that cigarette smoking together with impaired glucose tolerance and

Risk factors for diabetic macrovascular arteriosclerosis

1. Genetic predisposition
2. Age
3. Duration of diabetes
4. Smoking
5. Hypertension
   a. Systolic blood pressure
   b. Diastolic blood pressure
6. Hypercholesterolemia
7. Hypertriglyceridemia
8. Hyperglycemia
9. Miscellaneous risk factors
   a. Hyperinsulinemia
   b. Inotropic drugs
   c. β-blockers

Modified from Levin ME: The diabetic foot: pathophysiology, evaluation and treatment. In Levin ME and O'Neal LW, eds, The diabetic foot, ed 4, St. Louis, 1988, The CV Mosby Co.

hypertension were powerful predisposing factors in ASO. Cigarette smoking approximately doubled the risk in both sexes. The impact was discernible into advanced age and was dose related. Mortality was increased twofold to fourfold in men and women, respectively, predominantly because of coexisting cardiovascular disease.

Experience strongly confirms that patients who smoke and have chronic occlusive arterial disease affecting the extremities do not do well. A single cigarette can cause narrowing of the arteries and reduction of blood flow, which may last as long as one hour or more.[58]

The mechanisms by which smoking is atherogenic is unknown but may be related to intimal injury from increased levels of carboxyhemoglobin.[59] Smoking has been demonstrated to affect platelet function and increase the tendency toward thrombus formation.[60] The series of Beach and Strandness[61] on ASO and associated risk factors in diabetics showed a high correlation between smoking and atherosclerosis. They found this to be one of the most important risk factors and presented evidence to show that the cessation of smoking was associated with a decrease in the progression of atherosclerosis. Another effect of smoking is its possible influence on prostacyclin (PGI_2), an important prostaglandin that prevents platelet aggregation and promotes vasodilation. Nadler, Velasco, and Horton[62] have shown that cigarette smoking inhibits prostacyclin formation. In their study smoking tobacco with nicotine abolished the PGI_2 response to norepinephrine. Their observations suggest that inhalation of nicotine-containing tobacco smoke reduces vascular PGI_2 production and that this may be a factor in developing accelerated cardiovascular disease.

Although the nicotine and carbon monoxide content of cigarette smoke has been felt to be the major risk, a recent paper by Kaufman et al has shown that patients who smoked cigarettes with a reduced amount of nicotine and carbon monoxide did not have any lower risk factor for myocardial infarction than did those who smoked the cigarettes containing a larger amount of those substances.[63] This was recently confirmed by Palmer, Rosenberg, and Shapiro who found that smoking "low yield" cigarettes did not lower the risk of a first nonfatal myocardial infarction.[64]

Cigarette smoking may also contribute to the pathogenesis of atherosclerosis through its effect on lipid metabolism. The study of Brischetto et al showed the plasma lipid and lipoprotein profiles of cigarette smokers from randomly selected families to be abnormal.[65] The study demonstrated that those who smoked had higher plasma cholesterol, triglycerides and VLDL levels, and a lower HDL cholesterol concentration.[65]

An increased hypercoagulability has been found in chronic smokers, compared with nonsmokers.[50] It became pronounced immediately after smoking three cigarettes.[50] The group who smoked had higher plasma fibrinogen, lower plasminogen and plasminogen activator, and higher plasma viscosity.[50] After smoking three cigarettes there was an increase in platelet aggregation, von Willebrand's factor, and a decrease in red blood cell deformability.[50]

A possible miscellaneous effect of smoking is altered insulin absorption. Evidence suggests that the absorption of insulin in smokers may be impaired from subcutaneous sites because of the peripheral vasoconstriction caused by nicotine.[66]

Hypertension is also a risk factor that can be controlled. Control of both systolic and diastolic pressure is important. There is no question that a strong correlation exists between hypercholesterolemia and cardiovascular disease. However, not all authorities have found a correlation between peripheral ASO and hypercholesterolemia.[17,38] Nevertheless, any patient with elevated cholesterol values should be treated.

The role of hyperglycemia in the pathogenesis of atherosclerosis is also debatable. Nelson et al[17] have found a correlation between hyperglycemia and ASO. Others, however, have not found a strong correlation.[38,61,67] Vaccaro et al found no increase of ASO with impaired glucose tolerance.[68] Experimentally, Lorenzi, Cagliero, and Toledo have shown glucose toxicity for human endothelial cells in culture.[69] On the other hand, Weimann, Lorch, and Baumgartner have not demonstrated that high glucose concentrations influenced replication of prostacyclin release of human endothelial cells.[70] The question of glucose toxicity on the endothelium still remains in limbo. Nevertheless, every effort should be made to control the blood sugars because uncontrolled diabetes may result in increased triglycerides, which may adversely affect the endothelium.

Hyperglycemia leads to increased glycosylation cross-linkage of collagen and stiffness in the arterial wall.[71] Binding of advanced glycosylation end products to macrophages results in increased synthesis and release of interleukin-1, which can also stimulate the arterial wall smooth muscle proliferation.[71]

Hyperinsulinemia can also be a risk factor in the pathogenesis of atherosclerosis. Hyperinsulinemia is common in type II patients who have insulin resistance. It is also common in type I patients because the insulin is administered subcutaneously and does not initially pass through the liver for removal. Of insulin secreted by the pancreas 50% is removed by one pass through the liver. Insulin is a growth hormonelike factor and has been found by several investigators to stimulate the duplication of smooth muscles and their migration into the lumen.[72,73] This process plays a major role in the formation of the atherosclerotic plaque. Evidence of atherosclerosis caused by hyperinsulinemia has been reported to occur in the presence of normal glucose tolerance. Zavaroni et al[74] found that a group of "healthy persons" with hyperinsulinemia and normal glucose tolerance had an increase in vascular risk factors and triglycerides and lower HDL concentrations. In the experimental diabetic BB rat, Larson and Haudenschild found a genetic predilection, sensitivity of the vascular smooth muscle cells to insulin, and a dissociation of this effect from hyperglycemia.[75]

Adiposity, and especially the fat distribution, is a vascular risk factor. Distribution of body fat has been found to be an independent predictor of metabolic aberrations, including cardiovascular morbidity and mortality.[76] Abdominal or truncal obesity has been associated with hyperinsulinemia, hypertriglyceridemia, decreased HDLs, and hypertension.[77,78] Peiris et al measured intraabdominal fat, using computerized tomography.[79] They found that intraabdominal fat deposition constitutes greater cardiovascular risk than obesity alone. They also reached the conclusion that hyperinsulinemia may constitute an important component of increased vascular risk associated with abdominal obesity.[79]

In summary, the development of ASO in the diabetic obviously stems from a wide combination of risk factors.

Signs and symptoms of arteriosclerosis obliterans (ASO). The subjective (symptoms) and objective (signs) findings of ASO are listed in the accompanying box. Intermittent claudication is a common symptom associated with diabetic ASO. In the Framingham study diabetes was associated with twofold to threefold excess risk of intermittent claudication for both sexes.[80] An excess risk for intermittent claudication was observed in men receiving oral hypoglycemic therapy and in women receiving insulin or oral agents. Diabetics with intermittent claudication were at an especially high risk of cardiovascular events.[80] The word *claudication* comes from the Latin, meaning "to limp." The patient with claudication may limp; however, more characteristically he or she stops to rest. The pain or discomfort is usually localized in the calf, is characterized by pain associated with walking, and is relieved by cessation of walking without the need to sit down. The discomfort associated with intermittent claudication must be distinguished from pain in the leg with walking, which can result from degenerative arthritic changes; disk disease; tumors of the spinal cord, particularly the cauda equina; thrombophlebitis; anemia; and even myxedema.

Signs and symptoms of ASO in the lower extremity

1. Intermittent claudication
2. Cold feet
3. Nocturnal pain
4. Rest pain
5. Nocturnal and rest pain relieved with dependency
6. Absent pulses
7. Blanching on elevation
8. Delayed venous filling after elevation
9. Dependent rubor
10. Atrophy of subcutaneous fatty tissues
11. Shiny appearance of skin
12. Loss of hair on foot and toes
13. Thickened nails, often with fungal infection
14. Gangrene
15. Miscellaneous
    a. Blue-toe syndrome
    b. Acute vascular occlusion

Modified from Levin ME: The diabetic foot: pathophysiology, evaluation and treatment. In Levin ME and O'Neal LW, eds, The diabetic foot, ed 4, St. Louis, 1988, The CV Mosby Co.

Pain with walking resulting from these causes is referred to as *pseudoclaudication*. Differentiation from ischemic claudication and pseudoclaudication can be made by history alone. Patients with claudication caused by ischemia simply need to stop walking and rest for a minute or two and then proceed. Patients with pseudoclaudication usually require 15 to 20 minutes of rest and frequently give a history of having to sit down, change position, flex or extend their back to get relief. The symptom of intermittent claudication depends on ischemia in the muscle. Because of the small-muscle mass in the foot some investigators believe that claudication is infrequent in the foot.

Some diabetics, despite significant ASO, may not have symptoms of intermittent claudication because of the loss of pain sensation. This stresses the need for routine examination of the diabetic's lower extremity for signs of ASO, even though the patient is not complaining of symptoms. Improvement in intermittent claudication can be achieved with cessation of smoking and supervised training and exercise programs.[81]

Cold feet are a common complaint in patients with ASO. It is cold feet that prompt the diabetic to resort to using hot water bottles and heating pads. This can result in severe burns to a foot that has become insensitive to heat because of peripheral neuropathy. For example, normal skin at a moderate ambient temperature of 70° F, or 21.1° C, needs less than 1 ml/100g/min of blood flow to function normally.[82] This need can be met in the presence of even advanced ASO. However, if the skin is heated to 104° F, or 40° C, which can easily be achieved with a hot water bottle or heating pad, a blood flow ten times greater than normal is required.[82] In the face of severe vascular disease this need cannot be met, and skin breakdown, blistering, ulceration, or gangrene can result.

Rest pain usually indicates at least two hemodynamically significant arterial blocks in a series. Rest pain is caused by nerve ischemia and is persistent with peaks of intensity. It is worse at night and may require the use of narcotics for relief. Rest pain is decreased by dependency of the legs. Therefore the patient often sleeps in a chair, and edema of the leg, secondary to constant dependency, is common.

Nocturnal ischemic pain is a form of neuritis that usually precedes rest pain. It occurs at night or during sleep because the circulation is essentially of the core variety, with very little perfusion of the lower extremity. Ischemic neuritis thus produced becomes intense and disrupts sleep. The patient invariably gains relief by standing up or dangling his or her feet over the edge of the bed and on occasion by walking a few steps. This activity increases the cardiac output, leading to improved perfusion of the lower extremities and relief of the ischemic neuritis. If vascular lesions that produce rest

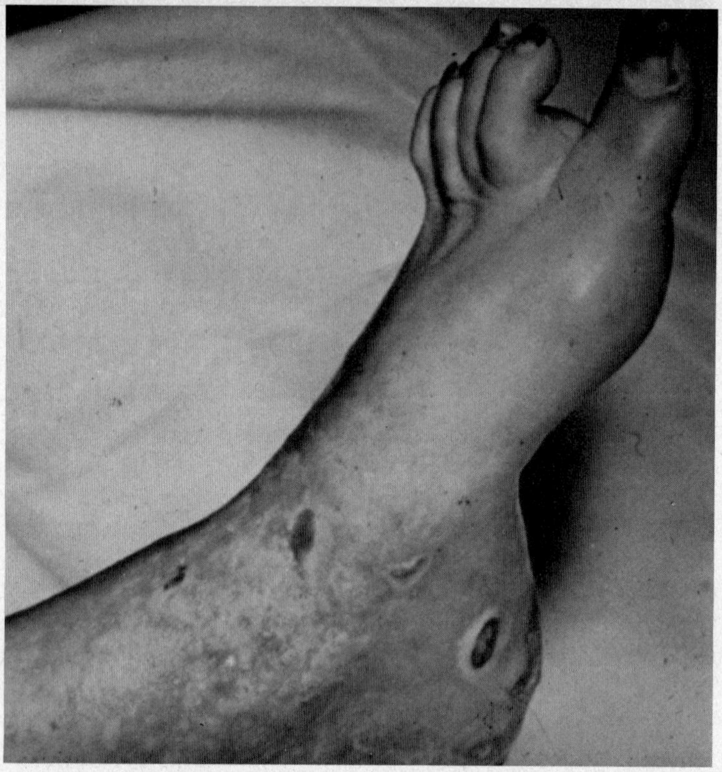

Fig. 38-8. Classic diabetic foot with ischemic skin changes: atrophy of subcutaneous tissues, hair loss on dorsum of foot, thickening of nails, atrophy of interosseus muscles resulting in cocked up toes, and commonly seen superficial ulcerations. (From Levin ME and O'Neal LW: The diabetic foot, ed 4, St Louis, 1988, The CV Mosby Co; courtesy John F. Fairbairn II, M.D., Mayo Clinic, Rochester, Minn., and The Upjohn Company, Kalamazoo, Mich.)

and nocturnal pain are not corrected by vascular surgery, gangrene almost always develops, necessitating amputation. Rest pain and nocturnal pain are therefore indications for angiography and, when possible, vascular surgery. Diabetics with severe ASO and ischemia may not experience rest pain or night pain because of peripheral neuropathy, again stressing the need for examining the lower extremity on a routine basis. Nocturnal leg pain may also be caused by peripheral neuropathy. The nocturnal pain of neuropathy can be differentiated from that of ischemia simply by history. The patient with nocturnal neuropathic pain will get up and walk to alleviate his or her discomfort, while the patient with ischemic pain sits up all night with the legs dependent. Absent pulses are significant evidence of ASO. Examination of the patient with intermittent claudication involving the calf muscle may reveal both a femoral and pedal pulse but no popliteal pulse. The pedal pulses are present because of the collateral vessels in these patients. After a brisk walk the foot will pale and become pulseless.

Further ischemic changes are characterized by shiny, atrophic cool skin. As vascular insufficiency progresses there is loss of hair on the dorsum of the foot. Thickening of the nails is also influenced by the arterial insufficiency. These nails frequently have fungal infections. In addition, the nails tend to grow more slowly when the blood supply is decreased. Ischemia leads to atrophy of the subcutaneous tissue. The skin appears to be tightly drawn over the foot, and ulceration can occur from minor trauma to this atrophic skin. Fig. 38-8 illustrates the typical diabetic foot afflicted with ASO and neuropathy.

In the diabetic most of the changes of ischemia occur slowly, although the possibility of sudden occlusion from emboli or complete thrombosis must always be considered. The signs and symptoms of a sudden arterial occlusion are usually called the *five p's* (see the box on p. 681). The extent of ischemia and the final outcome depend on the collateral circulation and the time elapsing from the onset of acute occlusion to treatment. Most sudden occlusions are the result of emboli, but they can occur from thrombosis at the site of an atherosclerotic plaque. These occlusions must be treated as soon as possible since peripheral nerves and skeletal muscle have less resistance to ischemia than skin and bone. Malan and Tattoni have indicated that irreversible changes of skeletal muscle and peripheral nerves occur after 4 to 6 hours of severe ischemia.[83] Pain from embolism is usually more severe and sudden in onset than pain from

The five *p*'s of acute arterial occlusion in the lower extremity

1. Pain: sudden onset
2. Pallor: waxy
3. Paresthesias: numbness
4. Pulselessness: no pulse below block
5. Paralysis: sudden weakness

thrombosis. Pallor is also more severe with embolism than with thrombosis. With embolism the affected extremity is waxlike and lemon yellow. With thrombosis the extremity appears less cadaverous and tends to be somewhat cyanotic. The paresthesia is caused by peripheral nerve ischemia. The management of acute arterial occlusion is discussed in Chapter 12.

Peripheral neuropathy

The first description of the manifestations of diabetic neuropathy was made by Marchal de Calvi in 1864.[30] Now over 100 years later, despite much research and many publications, the exact cause of diabetic neuropathy remains unexplained. The pathogenesis is undoubtedly multifactorial. A decreased blood flow in the vasonervorum caused by vascular narrowing of the vessel or increased blood viscosity is a factor. Another possible factor under investigation is the trapping of immunoglobulins on peripheral nerve myelin.[84] This does not occur in the brain and may account for the fact that there are rarely central nervous system neuropathies.[84]

Metabolic change is probably the most significant factor.[85,86] Glucose enters the nerve without the need for insulin. It is then converted by the enzyme aldose reductase to the polyols, sorbitol, and fructose. It has been postulated that when high levels of polyols or glucose are present, there is a decrease of *myo*-inositol in the nerves. *Myo*-inositol appears to be important for nerve membrane function and nerve conduction.[85] The use of aldose reductase inhibitors to prevent the conversion of glucose to sorbitol and fructose has been shown to improve motor nerve conduction. Sural nerve biopsy specimens from patients with diabetic neuropathy treated the aldose reductase inhibitor, sorbinil, showed regeneration and repair of myelinated fibers.[87] Recently Dyck et al biopsied the sural nerve of diabetic patients treated with sorbinil. Despite improved motor nerve conduction they did not find any significant change in levels of *myo*-inositol, casting doubt on its importance.[88]

Increased levels of polyols diffuse very poorly out of the nerve, resulting in a hyperosmotic effect, which causes edema of the nerve. Edema of sural nerves has been confirmed by Griffey et al.[89] This group, using magnetic resonance spectroscopy, found that the sural nerves of patients with peripheral neuropathy were edematous and treatment with sorbinil decreased this edema.[89] This was probably accomplished by a decrease in the levels of sorbitol and fructose, thus decreasing hyperosmolality and decreasing the influx of water.

There are a number of syndromes associated with diabetic neuropathy.[90] The most common of those involving the foot are distal symmetric sensorimotor polyneuropathies, resulting in pain; paresthesias; muscle atrophy; the loss of sensation; autonomic neuropathy with dry, scaly feet; radiculopathy; and entrapment syndromes. An important entrapment syndrome affecting the foot is the tarsal tunnel syndrome. This results from compression of the posterior tibial nerve at the tarsal tunnel or of the plantar nerves. This causes sensory impairment in the sole of the foot and weakness of the intrinsic pedal musculature. It usually occurs unilaterally. This differentiates it from the metabolic bilateral symmetric polyneuropathy. Its symptoms are burning pain and paresthesias at the ankle and plantar surface of the foot.[91]

Diabetic patients with peripheral neuropathy do not always have neuropathy because of diabetes. These patients, like any nondiabetic individual, may have neuropathy resulting from a number of other causes (see the accompanying box). Neoplastic effects may result from humoral causes or direct nerve compression. Recently we saw a lady with diabetes and peripheral neuropathy. Her neuropathy, being unilateral, was atypical. Further evaluation revealed a meningioma of the spinal cord. Treatment for diabetic peripheral neuropathy in this patient would have resulted in a misdiagnosis.

As noted in Fig. 38-1, neuropathy can ultimately result in amputation, through various pathways. These include the loss of autonomic, sensory, or motor nerve function. Autonomic involvement results in decreased perspiration. This leads to dryness, cracking, and fissuring of the skin, which

Causes of peripheral neuropathy

1. Diabetes mellitus
2. Alcoholism
3. Herniated nucleus pulposus
4. Heavy metals
5. Vitamin deficiencies
6. Collagen disease
7. Pernicious anemia
8. Malignancy
9. Pressure neuropathy
10. Uremia
11. Porphyria
12. Hansen's disease (leprosy)
13. Drugs

Modified from Levin ME: The diabetic foot: pathophysiology, evaluation and treatment. In Levin ME and O'Neal LW, eds, The diabetic foot, ed 4, St. Louis, 1988, The CV Mosby Co.

can be portals of entry for bacteria. Autonomic dysfunction can also lead to the loss of the flare reaction.[92] Any noxious stimuli to the skin results in an increased blood flow. In the diabetic with significant foot lesions, this autonomic effect is blunted, thereby impeding wound healing. Orthostatic hypotension, a complication of autonomic involvement, may lead to a decrease in pressure and arterial perfusion with standing.

The most important neuropathic factor is the loss of pain and temperature sensation. The patient with nerve impairment develops an insensate foot that endures painless trauma from mechanical, chemical, or thermal sources, frequently resulting in ulceration and infection (see Fig. 38-1).

Painless mechanical trauma can occur from a variety of causes. The most common is walking. The repetitive stress of walking results in callus buildup and hot spots. Because there is no pain, the patient continues to walk. The callus builds up, and pressure necrosis and ulceration result. Abnormally high pressures, especially under the forefoot, have been found in such feet.[5]

Trauma from painless puncture wounds is not rare. Fig. 38-9 shows a carpenter's nail deep in the tissues of the foot of a 45-year-old who required insulin for 10 years. He had a small, painless draining area on his foot for approximately 1 month and sought medical attention only because the area had failed to heal. The dorsalis pedis and posterior tibial pulses were of good quality. However, vibratory sense and pain and touch sensation were markedly diminished. Radiographs of the foot revealed the carpenter's nail, which must have been present for at least a month without any discomfort to the patient. The area involved had caused severe osteomyelitis and was ultimately amputated.

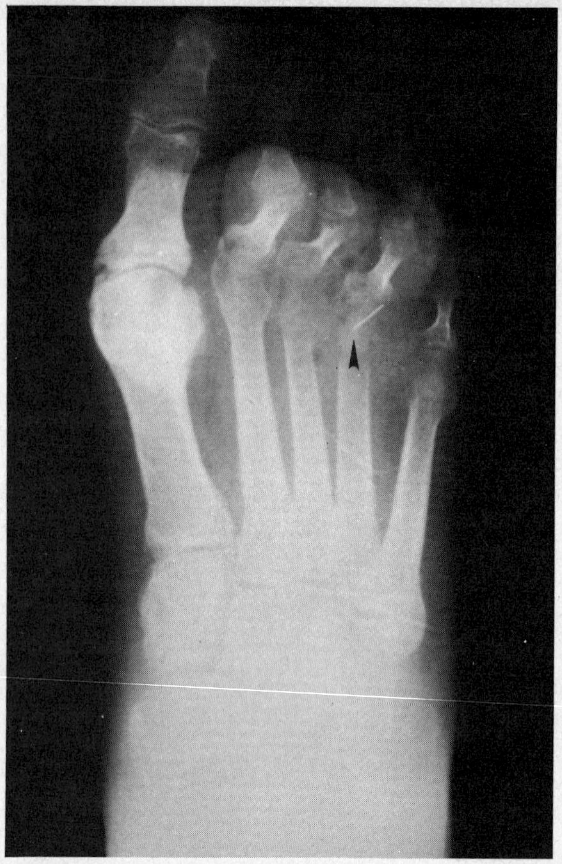

Fig. 38-9. Carpenter's nail present for approximately 1 month in tissues of foot of an insulin-requiring diabetic patient. He had no knowledge of having stepped on this nail, nor did he have any pain or discomfort. (From Levin ME and O'Neal LW: The diabetic foot, ed 4, St Louis, 1988, The CV Mosby Co; courtesy Dr. J. Joseph Marr, Sr. Vice President, Discovery Research Searle, Skokie, Ill.)

I would agree with Dr. Paul Brand, who stated that "the diabetic who claims his shoes are killing him may well be right." Painless ulceration from ill-fitting shoes may become infected; gangrene may follow, and amputation may be necessary. Ulcers most often occur on the side of the foot (Fig. 38-10). The number of foreign objects found in patients' shoes that they have walked on without pain or awareness is legion. To mention only a few, there are pebbles, coins, and unbelievably large objects such as doll chairs and shoehorns (Figs. 38-11 and 38-12).

Another extreme example of painless trauma is noted in Fig. 38-13, *A*. This shows ulceration over the Achilles tendon of a patient who kept the back of his heel against a chair while on jury duty. Blisters developed, ulcerated, and penetrated to the Achilles tendon. The patient's physician advised using a Band-Aid and returning to work. Fortunately the patient sought a second opinion, and a skin-graft flap procedure was done, and the ulceration healed (Fig. 38-13, *B* and *C*).

Another common cause of painless injury results from "home surgery." Because persons with diabetic neuropathy feel no pain, they frequently cut their calluses too deep and their nails too close, resulting in ulceration and infection. Fig. 38-14 shows an infected and gangrenous great toe that resulted from a patient practicing "home surgery." Even though she was partially blind, she attempted to cut the nail and in doing so, cut into the tissue. This resulted in infection, gangrene, and partial amputation.

Chemical trauma results from the use of callus and corn removers. It has also occurred from soaking the feet in chemical solutions and strong antiseptics.

Thermal injuries are quite common in the insensitive diabetic foot. Fig. 38-15 shows gangrene of the toes of a diabetic who had soaked his cold foot in a bucket of hot water. Fortunately the patient had good dorsalis pedis and posterior tibial pulses and had a successful midtarsal amputation. The fact that only the toes became gangrenous is good evidence for the existence of small vessel disease. Severe burns have occurred in patients with insensitive feet who have walked on hot sandy beaches, or other hot surfaces. We have seen a number of these patients ultimately require amputation. Diabetic patients going to the beach or

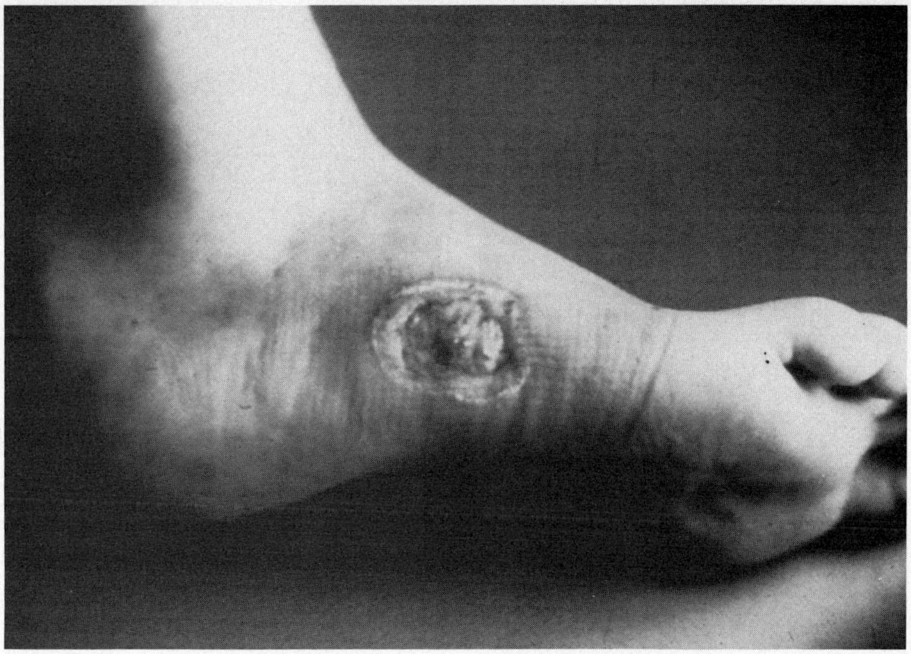

Fig. 38-10. Ulceration on the side of the foot, suggestive of an ill-fitting shoe.

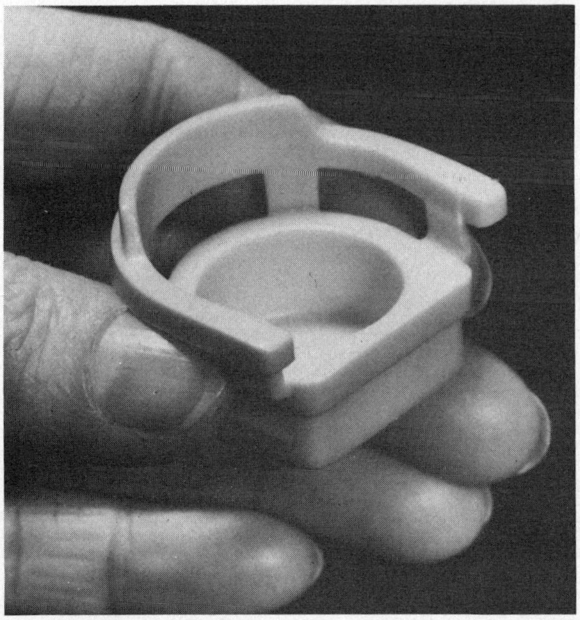

Fig. 38-11. Doll's chair measuring 2.5 by 3.8 cm found in patient's shoe. He had worn the shoe all day without being aware of chair's presence because of almost total absence of sensory perception produced by severe diabetic neuropathy. (From Levin ME and O'Neal LW: The diabetic foot, ed 4, St Louis, 1988, The CV Mosby Co.)

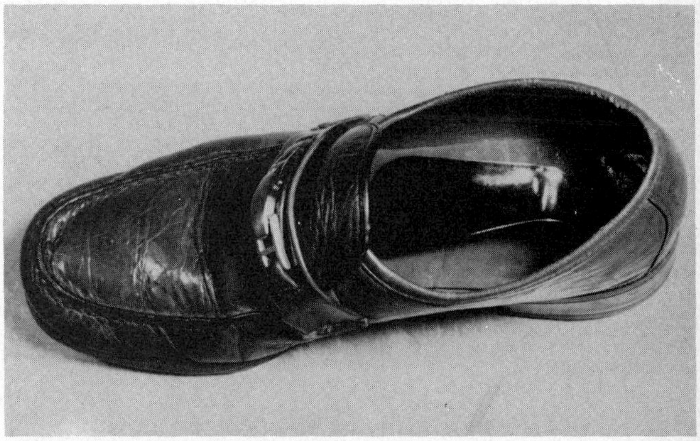

Fig. 38-12. Shoehorn in shoe worn by patient who, because of insensitive foot resulting from diabetic neuropathy, was unaware of its presence until removing shoe at end of day. (From Levin ME and O'Neal LW: The diabetic foot, ed 4, St Louis, 1988, The CV Mosby Co.)

A

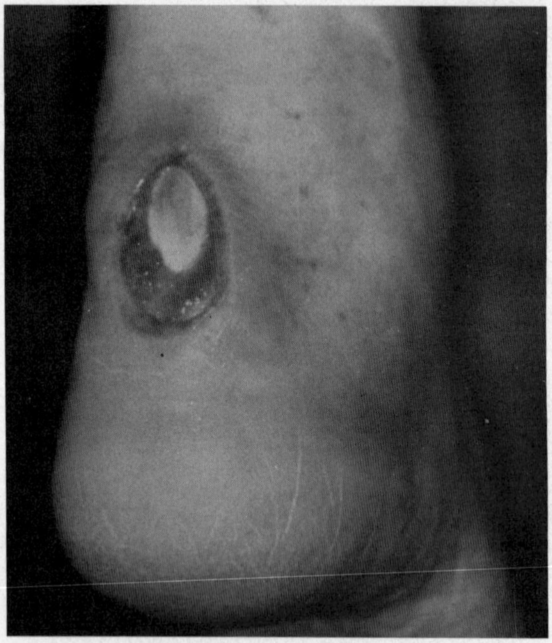

Fig. 38-13. A, Ulceration resulting from breakdown of painless blister that penetrated to Achilles tendon. **B,** Outline of skin flap for treatment of ulceration **(A)**. **C,** Healed skin-flap graft for treatment of ulceration **(A)**. (From Levin ME and O'Neal LW: The diabetic foot, ed 4, St Louis, 1988, The CV Mosby Co; courtesy Dr. Leroy Young, Department of Plastic Surgery, Washington University School of Medicine, St Louis.)

B

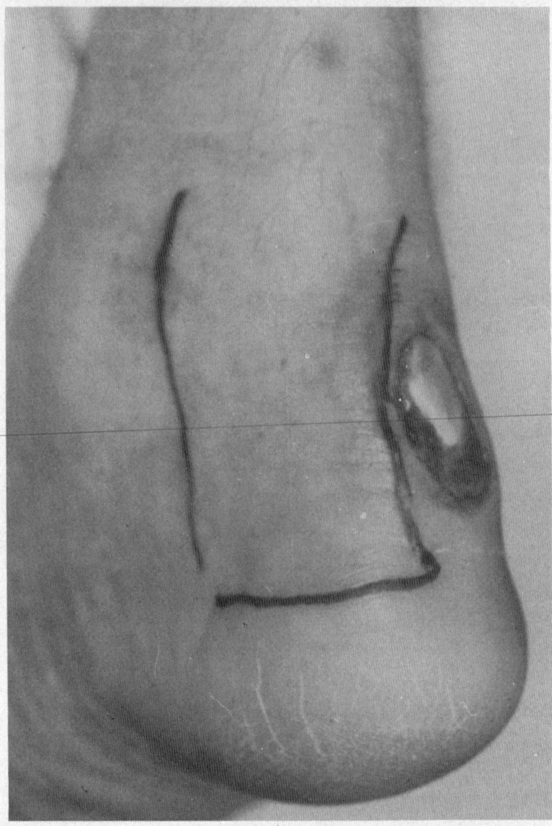

C

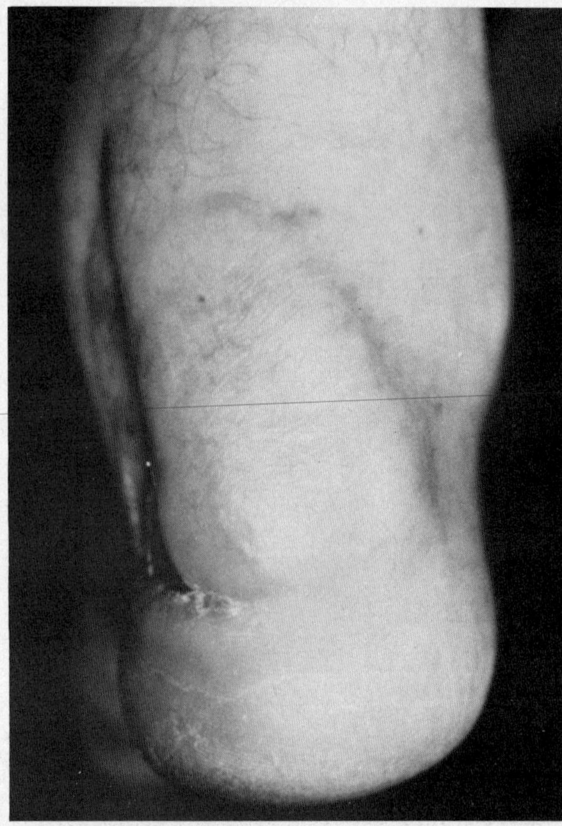

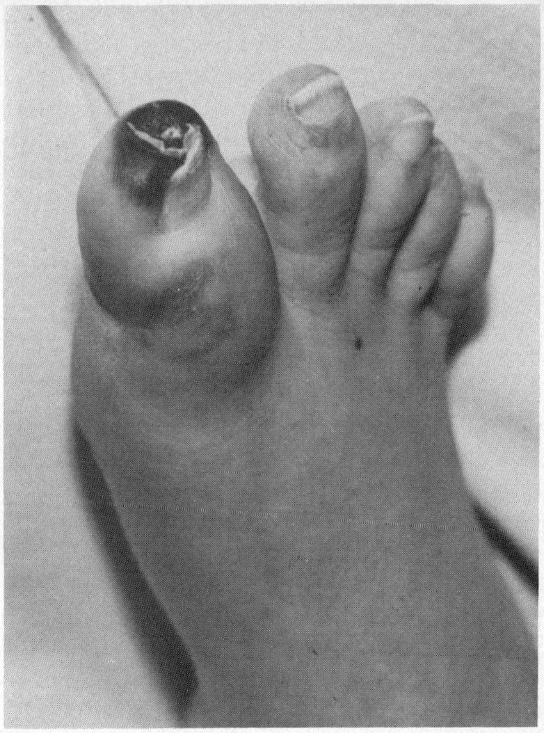

Fig. 38-14. Gangrenous toes resulting from patient's attempt at home surgery. Toenail was cut too deep, became infected, and gangrene developed. (From Levin ME and O'Neal LW: The diabetic foot, ed 4, St Louis, 1988, The CV Mosby Co.)

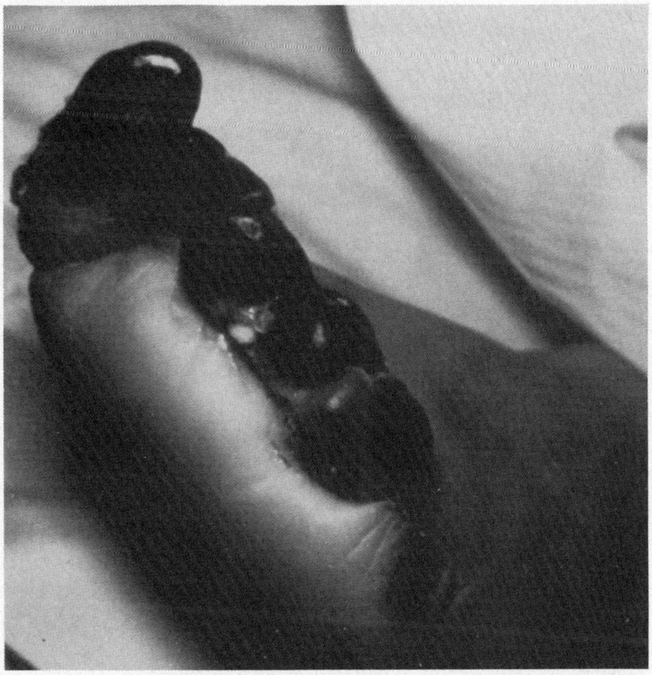

Fig. 38-15. Gangrene in toes of patient who had soaked his cold foot in hot water. (From Levin ME and O'Neal LW: The diabetic foot, ed 4, St Louis, 1988, The CV Mosby Co.)

to swimming pools should wear protective footwear. Patients who have placed their feet in front of the fireplace to warm them have sustained severe burns, not an uncommon occurrence. Perhaps the most dramatic case of painless thermal injury that I have encountered was in a diabetic patient who had a previous below-knee amputation. He had purchased a riding lawn mower, and in positioning the "good leg," he inadvertently placed it on the manifold, which became extremely hot. Only when he smelled "something burning" did he look down to discover that his shoe and foot were on fire. Unfortunately, subsequent amputation of his remaining foot was necessary.

Signs and symptoms of diabetic neuropathy. The signs and symptoms of diabetic peripheral neuropathy are listed in the accompanying box. Diabetic neuropathy in the lower extremity is bilateral and tends to be symmetric. The sensory involvement is characterized by two major system complexes. One consists of pain and paresthesias. The other, paradoxically, consists of a decreased or absent sensation of touch, pain, and temperature. The paresthesias may be manifested as tingling or burning. Many patients exhibit marked hyperesthesias of the feet and legs, which may be so great that they cannot stand even the lightest touch such as sheets or pajamas. Treatment for this extreme sensitivity, which may involve the entire trunk, other than control of the blood sugar and the use of pharmacologic agents, consists of wearing firmly fitting hose or even a body stocking. Putting these on is very uncomfortable but once they are applied, there is no longer any contact with movable clothing, and the patient is much more comfortable. The pain of peripheral neuropathies may be severe, knifelike, or shooting. It can be almost constant and frequently is more severe at night. The pain may be severe enough to require narcotics for relief. A great deal of caution must be observed in prescribing narcotics for these patients, since the treatment may be long, and drug habituation or addiction can develop. The decrease in sensory perception is not only manifested by loss of pain and temperature sensation, but can also be manifested by a "dead feeling" in the feet, giving the sensation of walking on an unusual surface such as cushions.

Signs and symptoms of neuropathy in the diabetic foot and leg

1. Paresthesia
2. Hyperesthesia
3. Hypoesthesia
4. Radicular pain
5. Loss of deep tendon reflexes
6. Loss of vibratory and position sense
7. Anhidrosis
8. Heavy callus formation over pressure points
9. Trophic ulcers
10. Infection complicating trophic ulcers
11. Foot drop
12. Changes in shape of foot produced by:
    a. Muscle atrophy
    b. Changes in bone and joints
13. Radiographic signs:
    a. Demineralization
    b. Osteolysis
    c. Charcot's joint

Modified from Levin ME: The diabetic foot: pathophysiology, evaluation and treatment. In Levin ME and O'Neal LW, eds, The diabetic foot, ed 4, St. Louis, 1988, The CV Mosby Co.

Radicular pain, or mononeuropathy, in the lower extremity is not uncommon. One example is the relatively frequent occurrence of diabetic femoral neuropathy, or L-3 radiculopathy, which is characterized by low back pain that may be of sudden onset. The pain extends into the anterior part of the thigh and is associated with paresthesias and sensory loss in that area. There may be weakness of flexion at the hip, extension of the knee (quadriceps weakness), and adduction of the thigh. The knee jerk may be significantly decreased or absent. Radicular pain must always be differentiated from root pain produced by other causes, such as a ruptured disk, arthritis, or tumor. Although peripheral symmetric polyneuropathy is metabolic in origin, the mononeuropathies are most likely the result of thrombi in a vessel of the vasonervorum. Over a period of weeks or months this will recanalize, nerve function will return, and the pain will disappear.

In evaluating sensation in the foot, it is important not only to do the physical examination but also to take a careful history. For example, changes in shoe size can be a tip-off to the development of neuropathy. Dr. Paul Brand has pointed out that with loss of sensation a patient tends to purchase a smaller shoe size. The smaller size is no longer uncomfortable because the patient has lost sensation. In fact, the correct size feels too large to the patient. The patient should be asked, as part of the history, whether he or she has had a change in shoe size.

Foot deformities. Muscle atrophy caused by involvement of the motor nerves leads to an imbalance of the interosseous muscles in the foot. This frequently leads to cocked up toes. Ulceration may occur on the tips and tops of the toes, and because of thinning of the fat pad underneath the first metatarsal-phalangeal joint, ulceration may occur in this area (Fig. 38-16). Prevention of ulceration in these areas requires straightening out of these cocked up, or claw, toes at a time when circulation is good. However, if this cannot be done, then it is important to make sure the toe box of the shoe is large enough to accommodate the top of these deformed toes. Cushioned insoles should be worn to protect the tips of these toes.

The most extreme example of diabetic foot deformity is the Charcot's foot or neuroarthropathy. The incidence of Charcot's foot is most common in the fifth and sixth decades and increases with the duration of diabetes. It is essentially

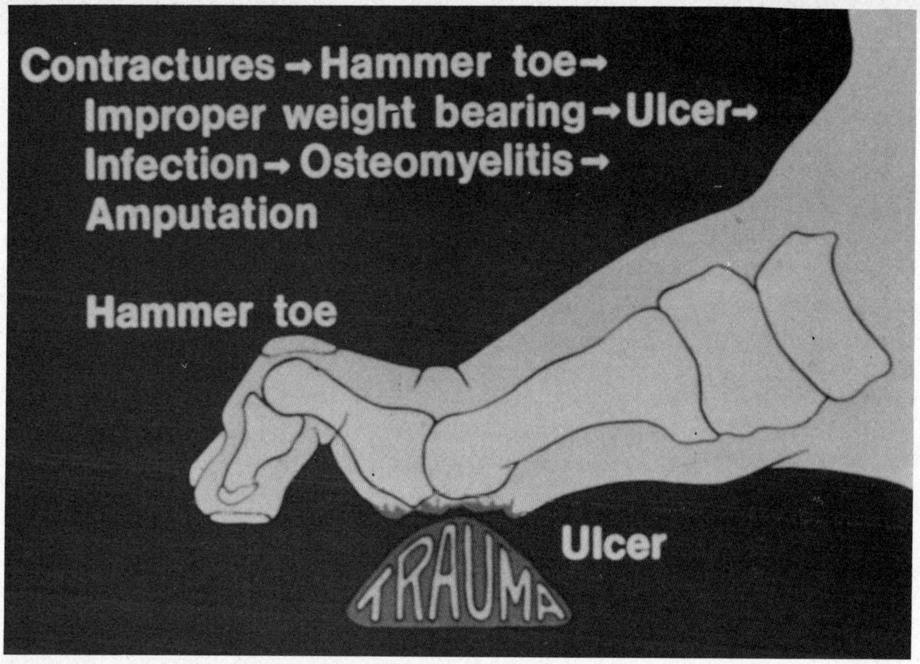

Fig. 38-16. Progression of contractures leading to hammer toes, ulceration, and infection. (From Levin ME and O'Neal LW: The diabetic foot, ed 4, St Louis, 1988, The CV Mosby Co; courtesy the Michigan Diabetes Research and Training Center, Ann Arbor, Mich., 1983, The University of Michigan.)

the same in both sexes and is bilateral in approximately one third of all cases. The average duration of diabetes before the development of this lesion is 12 years. In Boehm's series the duration of the disease ranged between 2 and 20 years.[93] However, it may occur in the younger diabetic patient and in the patient with diabetes of recent onset. It has even been reported as the initial clinical manifestation of diabetes. There appears to be no significant relationship between the development of Charcot's foot and the degree of blood glucose control. Radiographically, the sites most often affected in diabetic patients are the smaller joints of the foot, particularly the tarsometatarsal joints and, to a lesser extent, the joints of the metatarsophalangeal area, and the ankle.[94]

Classically, Charcot's foot develops as an acutely hot, erythematous, and swollen foot with bounding pulses and prominent veins. Despite what is written in some textbooks, patients with Charcot's foot frequently have moderate pain and discomfort. It may be difficult to differentiate the warm, red Charcot's foot from cellulitis. However, the patient with Charcot's foot is afebrile, and the white blood cell count is normal. The sedimentation rate may be slightly elevated. The neuropathic component to the development of Charcot's foot probably stems from involvement of the autonomic nervous system. The result is the equivalent of sympathectomy to the arteries in the foot. The arteries dilate and A-V shunts have been demonstrated in these feet.[95] X-ray examination in the acute stage usually reveals no bony abnormality (Fig. 38-17, *A*). If the patient continues to walk, there can be gradual dissolution and fragmentation of the distal ends of the metatarsals (Fig. 38-17, *B*) and the ankle bones. The distal ends of the metatarsals become pointed, the "peppermint stick sign," as if the ends of the bone were licked away.[96] The x-ray films also show the absence of calcification in the interosseous arteries, further evidence that there is no significant vascular insufficiency. It is felt that the increased circulation causes reabsorption of the bone. Evidence that increase in circulation contributes to the Charcot's foot has been suggested by the report of Edelman et al.[97] These authors reported three cases of Charcot's foot that developed following successful peripheral vascular surgery. These cases demonstrate the important role of increased blood flow in the absorption of calcium from the bones in the foot, their collapse, and the development of Charcot's foot. Because there is relative insensitivity in these feet, patients continue to walk, subsequently developing the so-called stress fractures and further bone destruction. Treatment for these patients in the acute stage is nonweight bearing, frequently with the aid of a contact cast. If the process is allowed to progress, the arch collapses and the foot becomes everted and shortened and takes on a clubfoot shape. The arch is lost and takes on a rocker bottom configuration (Fig. 38-18). It is the plantar area of the arch that breaks down and becomes ulcerated (Fig. 38-19). Ul-

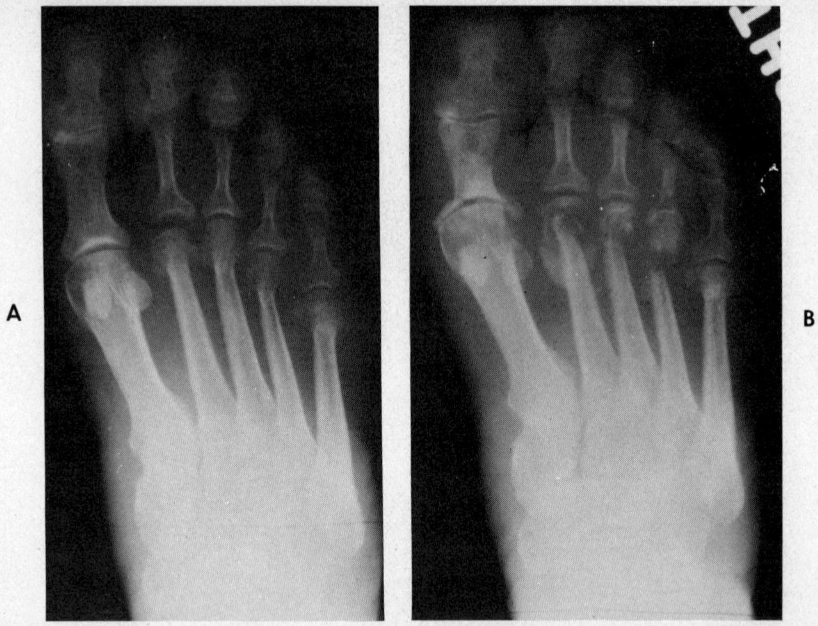

Fig. 38-17. **A,** Foot of 60-year-old man with known diabetes of 4 years' duration. **B,** Same foot, 3 months later, showing classic osteolytic bone changes of diabetic neuropathy involving distal segment of the metatarsals. (From Levin ME and O'Neal LW: The diabetic foot, ed 4, St Louis, 1988, The CV Mosby Co; courtesy Dr. Robert Karsh, Washington University School of Medicine, St Louis.)

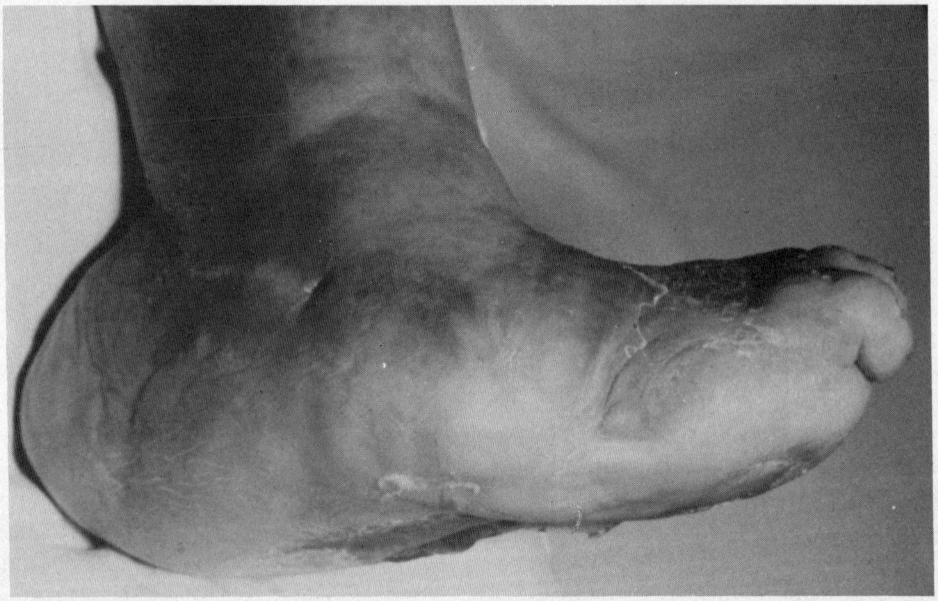

Fig. 38-18. Clubfoot appearance of Charcot's foot, with collapse of the tarso-metatarsal joints. (From Levin ME and O'Neal LW: The diabetic foot, ed 4, St Louis, 1988, The CV Mosby Co.)

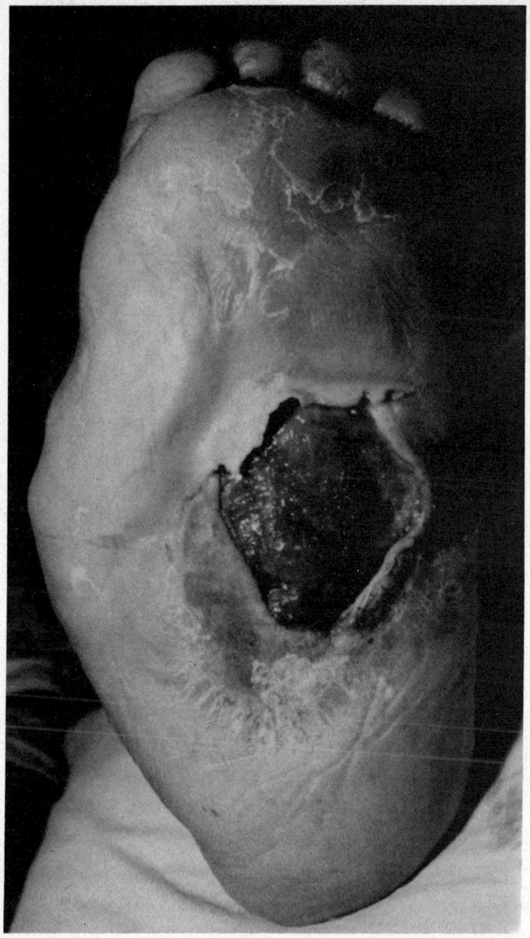

Fig. 38-19. Massive ulcer on plantar surface of arch in patient with Charcot's foot (Fig. 38-18). (From Levin ME: Pathophysiology of diabetic foot lesions. Reprinted by permission from Clinical diabetes mellitus: a problem-oriented approach, J. Davidson, 1986, © 1986 by Thieme Medical Publishers, Inc., New York.)

ceration on the plantar surface in the area of the arch is a classic sign of Charcot's foot.

Because of bone destruction in Charcot's foot, it is sometimes difficult to distinguish between osteoarthropathy and osteomyelitis. If there is no portal of entry or ulceration overlying the area of bone destruction and there are other findings compatible with Charcot's foot, the most likely diagnosis is neuroarthropathy. However, osteomyelitis must always be ruled out. Routine imaging techniques have not always been conclusive. Recently, the combined use of leukocyte and bone imaging has helped to make this distinction. Using this technique, Splittgerber et al[98] found that bone imaging frequently demonstrated increased activity in both osteoarthropathy and osteomyelitis. However, leukocyte imaging showed increased activity in only the cases of osteomyelitis. There was minimal or no activity in the cases with osteoarthropathy.[98] In a larger series of 35 cases Schauwecker et al also found the use of leukocyte scanning useful for evaluating osteomyelitis in the presence of osteoarthropathy.[99]

Infection

Infection is the third major factor in the pathogenesis of diabetic foot lesions and when associated with ischemia, frequently leads to amputation.[100] Breaks in the skin, which may be almost imperceptible, such as cracks, fissures in calluses, and major wounds, such as neurotrophic foot ulcers, act as portals of entry for bacteria. A variety of factors contribute to the diabetic's difficulty in handling infection. In the nondiabetic, infection leads to increased blood flow. In the diabetic, however, infection frequently leads to microthrombi formation in the small arterioles, which further impairs circulation (see Fig. 38-4).[101] When this occurs in the small arteries of the toes, it can convert the vessels into end-arteries, resulting in gangrene of the toes (see Fig. 38-5). Vascular disease impairs the delivery of antibiotics and oxygen to the affected areas. Impaired autonomic neurogenic vascular responses has already been mentioned. Leukocyte function is frequently impaired with defective adherence, diapedesis, chemotaxis, phagocytosis, and microbicidal activity of leukocytes in diabetic patients, particularly in those with uncontrolled diabetes and ketosis.

Most diabetic foot infections are polymicrobial.[102] It is not unusual to culture four to five organisms from these wounds. These may be gram-negative or gram-positive organisms, aerobes and anaerobes. The most common gram-positive aerobes are *Staphylococcus aureus,* group B streptococcus, and enterococcus. The most common gram-negative aerobes are *Escherichia coli, Proteus, Klebsiella, Enterobacter, Pseudomonas,* and other enteric bacilli. The most common gram-positive anaerobes are *Peptostreptococcus* and *Clostridium*. The most common gram-negative anaerobe is *Bacteroides fragilis*. Among the anaerobes, *B fragilis* is extremely common. Finegold has found 95% of diabetic foot ulcers to be infected with it.[103] Many of the polymicrobial flora occurring in the diabetic foot are gas formers. Extensive gas formation frequently can be demonstrated by soft tissue x-rays. When gas is present it indicates virulent infection frequently caused by E. coli, *Proteus,* or *Bacteroides*. Gas formation does not necessarily indicate that a clostridial infection is present. However, if it is, the prognosis is extremely poor.

The culturing technique is extremely important.[104] Culturing for anaerobes is particularly difficult. Special bedside kits for the collection of specimens likely to contain anaerobes should be used, such as anaerobic transport vials.* Infected ulcers or open sinuses may appear to be only superficial, and simple swabbing of these areas may not reflect the nature of deeper tissue infection. Curettage or needle aspiration are the most reliable methods. If grossly necrotic tissue is present or there is eschar overlying the ulceration,

*Gibco Laboratories, Lawrence, Massachusetts.

the overlying tissue should be removed during débridement and the underlying necrotic tissue cultured both for anaerobes and aerobes. It is critically important in the treatment of infection that the necrotic material be vigorously removed, and débridement carried deep enough to identify all areas of infection. Superficial débridement will result only in delay and inaccurate evaluation of the extent of the infection, its degree, and the types of organisms involved.

Osteomyelitis is common in the diabetic foot. It is sometimes difficult to establish a diagnosis of osteomyelitis. The use of ultrasonography, CT scanning, or assessment by nuclear-type procedures is helpful, using indium-labeled white blood cell scans. When indicated, bone biopsy and culture may be helpful.

Treatment. The use of a variety of oral antibiotics can be satisfactory in treating superficial infections. Recently the effectiveness of ciprofloxacin in these infections has been demonstrated.[105] However, when a significant or deep infection is suspected, hospitalization and parenteral antibiotics are the treatments of choice. Because impaired circulation, which is so frequently present in these patients, limits the delivery of antibiotics, they should be given parenterally. In addition, the antibiotic of choice may be available only in a parenteral form.

Treatment should begin with broad-spectrum antibiotics, while waiting for the culture results. The definitive antibiotics of choice will depend on the nature of the infection and the organisms that are identified. Because of the difficulty in obtaining totally accurate cultures, clinical judgment may become important in the choice of antibiotics. In the face of severe infection, the use of a second- or third-generation cephalosporin is indicated. The presence of *Pseudomonas* may require an aminoglycoside. However, aminoglycosides can be associated with nephrotoxicity, and this becomes extremely important in the diabetic who frequently has impaired renal function. Daily peak and trough levels are critically important as are frequent measures of BUN and creatinine values. Ototoxicity may also occur. One of the best treatments for *Bacteroides* is metronidazole (Flagyl). Because the treatment of infection can be difficult and the numerous antibiotics available confusing, consultation with an expert in infectious disease should be considered.

SPECIAL DIABETIC FOOT PROBLEMS

The heel

The heel of the diabetic is particularly vulnerable to trauma. The heel is exposed to a great deal of pressure, resulting in callus buildup. As the callus becomes thicker it tends to crack and becomes a source of infection. When the heel is infected, the infection tends to penetrate deeply. The skin of the heel is tightly bound by numerous vertical septa extending through the subcutaneous tissue to the surface of the calcaneus. These septa result in formation of small cylinders that are packed with fatty tissue. These small fat-containing tubes act like shock absorbers on heel impact. With ischemic changes there is atrophy of the subcutaneous fatty tissue, thus decreasing the shock absorber-like effect. When the skin covering the heel is destroyed, much of the subcutaneous fat colliquates, and the septa are disrupted. If healing does occur, a tight scar will result, which makes the heel susceptible to further trauma.

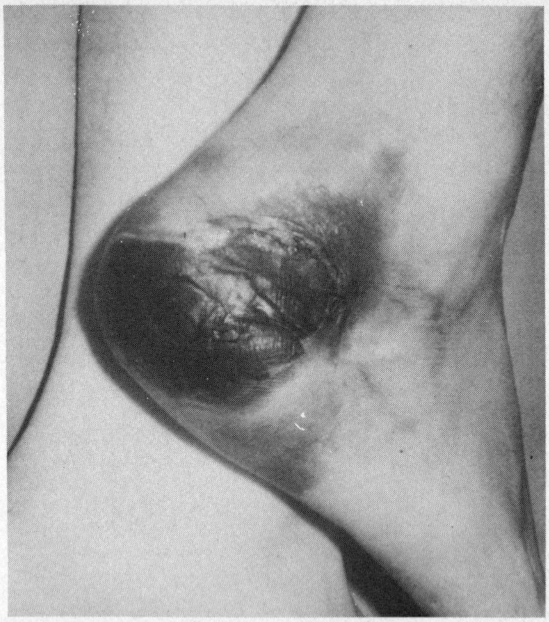

Fig. 38-20. Gangrene of heel of bedridden diabetic patient caused by weight of immobile neuropathic foot on mattress. (From Levin ME and O'Neal LW: The diabetic foot, ed 4, St Louis, 1988, The CV Mosby Co.)

When the diabetic is required to have bed rest for any length of time, such as when hospitalized, particular attention must be paid to the heel. Because of loss of sensation, the patient tends to keep the heels in the same position. This results in pressure necrosis, skin breakdown, infection, and gangrene (Fig. 38-20). Needless to say, prevention is the solution to this problem. The use of heel protectors or foam rubber or egg crate-type sponge rubber mattresses is essential. The available heel protectors may not always stay in place, therefore daily checks of the protector and the heel are necessary.

Painful neuropathy

One of the most difficult therapeutic problems confronting the physician is the diabetic with painful neuropathy. Despite a long list of treatments (see the box on p. 691) none have proved totally successful. Some are totally ineffective, and those that have shown some benefit can have significant side effects. Fortunately in most patients with painful neuropathy, the pain and paresthesias disappear with time, months to years. The loss of sensation is permanent. The apparent success of some treatments in uncontrolled studies can be attributed to the coincidental disappearance

Treatments for painful diabetic neuropathy

1. Megavitamins
2. B_{12} injections
3. Neuroleptics
   a. Phenytoin (Dilantin)
   b. Carbamazepine (Tegretol)
4. Tricyclics
5. Blood sugar control
6. Aldose reductase inhibitors
7. Nonsteroidal drugs
8. Pentoxifylline (Trental)
9. Mexiletine (Mexitil)
10. Capsaicin
11. Transcutaneous electrical nerve stimulation (TENS)

of pain while taking the treatment. Injections of B_{12} and megavitamins do not work. Phenytoin (Dilantin) is one of the oldest recommended treatments for painful neuropathy and has been reported to be more effective in women than in men.[106] However, controlled studies have not found phenytoin to be effective.[107] Furthermore, phenytoin can have significant side effects, not the least of which is severe exfoliative dermatitis. Carbamazepine (Tegretol) has been reported to help in some patients with painful peripheral neuropathy. However, this drug must be used with caution because of its many side effects. In the study of Rull et al[108] side effects occurred in 28 of 30 patients. Tricyclics, especially amitriptyline, alone or in combination with fluphenazine hydrochloride (Prolixin), have been the current treatment of choice.[109] Success with tricyclics or in combination with fluphenazine hydrochloride can occur within several days. However, it may require several weeks to achieve the result. Because tricyclics may have some cardiac side effects, these drugs should be used cautiously and should be closely monitored in patients who have cardiac disease. Recent investigations have shown no adverse cardiac effects from the use of tricyclic drugs in moderate doses in patients with cardiac disease. In fact this class of drugs has been found to have an antiarrhythmic effect. Veith et al[110] have shown that the tricyclic antidepressants had no effect on left ventricular ejection fraction at rest or during maximum exercise. Premature ventricular contractions were reduced by imipramine (Tofranil) but were not consistently changed by doxepin.[110] In the study of Giardina et al[111] imipramine hydrochloride was evaluated for its cardiovascular effects in 44 depressed patients. Imipramine prolonged the PR, QRS, and QT intervals; increased the heart rate; and lowered T wave amplitude. However, no patient developed high-grade arterioventricular block or severe intraventricular conduction abnormalities. Tricyclic drugs may also have an anticholinergic effect and should be used with caution in patients in whom anticholinergic drugs could be contraindicated, for example, patients with prostatism. Fluphenazine hydrochloride (Prolixin) may also cause signs and symptoms of parkinsonism, and its use should be carefully monitored.

Control of blood sugar remains one of the most important treatments for diabetic neuropathy, and motor nerve conduction velocities have been shown to improve with improved glucose levels.[112] However, development of peripheral neuropathy has been found at the time of control of the blood sugar.

The use of aldose reductase inhibitors to relieve pain is still experimental, and at present the Food and Drug Administration has not released them for clinical use. Feeding *myo*-inositol to a streptozotocin diabetic mouse improved motor nerve conduction.[113] However, there are no human studies using *myo*-inositol. Because *myo*-inositol has not been clearly evaluated in humans, I would not recommend its use at this time.

Several new drugs have been added to the list of treatments for painful diabetic peripheral neuropathy. Cohen and Harris reported subjective improvement in six of seven patients who had painful neuropathy and were treated with pentoxifylline (Trental).[114] Kalmanshon et al reported a single case of intractable painful diabetic neuropathy that had a dramatic response to pentoxifylline therapy.[115] Theoretically the improvement in these cases would be the result of a decreased viscosity and an improved blood flow in vasonervorum. Newrick et al have suggested impaired blood flow through the vasonervorum by demonstrating an abnormal nerve vein oxygen gradient in patients with diabetic neuropathy.[116]

Nonsteroidal antiinflammatory drugs have also been demonstrated to be helpful in the treatment of painful neuropathy. In a small series of 18 males Cohen and Harris found that eight of the patients were improved with ibuprofen or sulindac vs a placebo.[117]

Mexiletine is an antiarrhythmic drug that has been found to decrease the pain of diabetic neuropathy.[118] This group conducted a randomized double-blind crossover study to evaluate the effectiveness of this drug in relieving painful diabetic neuropathy. Nineteen patients were evaluated every 2 weeks for symptoms of pain, dysesthesia, parethesias, nightly exacerbation of symptoms, and sleep disturbances. The patients also recorded the extent of their pain on a graphic visual analogue rating scale. During treatment subjective symptoms improved in all patients except one. Mexiletine did not improve any of the objective signs of nerve function, deep tendon reflexes or vibration threshold variation, or hemoglobin A_1C. The exact mechanism is unknown. However, Dejgard, Petersen, and Kastrup point out that mexiletine has a sodium channel blocking effect that is important to its function and is the electrophysiologic basis of the drug's antiarrhythmic action.[118] Thus the effect of the drug may be the result of inhibition of the spontaneous activity in regenerating nerve fibers. It is contraindicated in preexisting second- or third-degree AV block unless the patient has a pacemaker. Larger carefully controlled clinical trials with this agent are indicated.

The use of topically applied capsaicin (Axsain) is the most recent addition to the long list of drug treatments for painful peripheral neuropathy. Capsaicin is the pungent ingredient of hot peppers of the genus *Capsicum*.[119] While capsaicin is a new treatment for painful neuropathy, it has been in use for over a decade in neural science research to probe the function of unmyelinated and thinly myelinated afferent neurons. Capsaicin appears to be selective for type C nociceptive neurons and depletes them of the neural transmitter, substance P, thus preventing the transmission of pain impulses. A multicenter, double-blind, randomized, vehicle-controlled trial evaluating the safety and efficacy of topical capsaicin (0.075%) in patients with confirmed painful diabetic neuropathy has been carried out by Chad et al.[120] Seventy-one percent of the capsaicin-treated patients and 42% of the vehicle-alone patients showed an overall improvement in their pain. This drug is applied topically four times a day to the painful area. Skin irritations have been noted with the use of capsaicin.

Transcutaneous electrical nerve stimulation (TENS) has been postulated to relieve pain by stimulation of large myelinated afferent A fibers that, when properly stimulated, inhibit transmission of nociceptive impulses by the A-delta and C nerve fibers. Inhibition of the C fibers, which carry the pain impulses, could help relieve pain. This theory was first suggested by the classic paper of Melzack and Wall.[121]

Toenails

Abnormalities of the toenails are common in the diabetic.[101] The nails are frequently thickened (Fig. 38-21). The markedly thickened nail, onychogryphosis, frequently occurring with fungal infection, is a potential hazard. This nail can get hooked in bedding or stockings, causing avulsion of the nail. Furthermore, the nail can cause severe pressure necrosis, subungual hemorrhage, ulceration, and infection of the nailbed. The patient may have nails that are markedly curved. These are particularly hazardous to the diabetic (Fig. 38-22). Older patients frequently neglect to trim their toenails or have them trimmed. Nails that curve in may cut into an adjacent toe with resulting ulceration (Fig. 38-23). Ingrown toenails are a potential source of infection, either by growing into the skin or because patients may attempt to do "home surgery" to remove the ingrown nail (see Fig. 38-14). The resulting infection of the foot can make amputation necessary.

EXAMINATION OF THE DIABETIC FOOT

One of the most important aspects of the office or clinic visit is the examination of the diabetic's foot and leg. Despite the problems associated with the diabetic foot, it is frequently the most neglected part of the examination. The low rate of foot inspection in a clinic setting has been documented by Cohen, who found that only 15% to 19% of patients who entered the examining room had their feet inspected.[122] In the review of Bailey, Yu, and Rayfield only 12.3% of the diabetic patients' feet were examined.[123] The foot and lower extremity of the diabetic should be examined at every routine office visit at least three or four times a year and more often when indicated. This examination should include not only the removal of shoes and stockings but also the trousers or pantyhose as well. It is only in this setting that the lower extremity can be properly examined. Patients are reluctant to remove their shoes and stockings

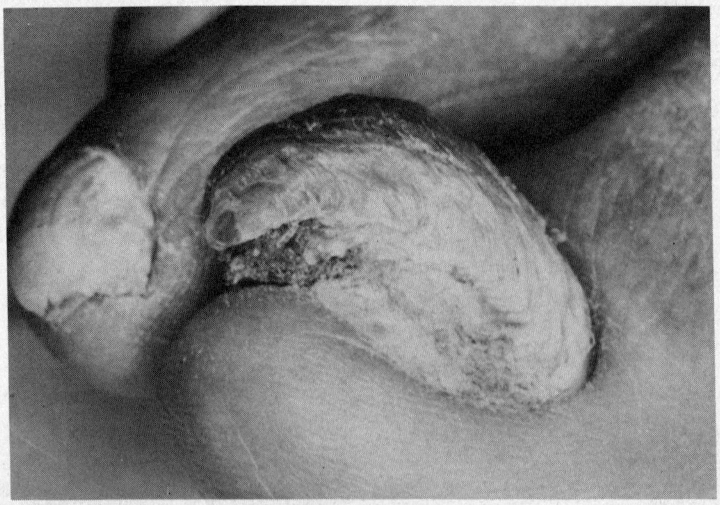

Fig. 38-21. Onychogryphosis. In diabetic patient infection may begin in debris covering nailbed. This type of nail easily hooks bedding, socks, or furniture, causing avulsion of nail and trauma to proximal nail fold. (From Levin ME and O'Neal LW: The diabetic foot, ed 4, St Louis, 1988, The CV Mosby Co.)

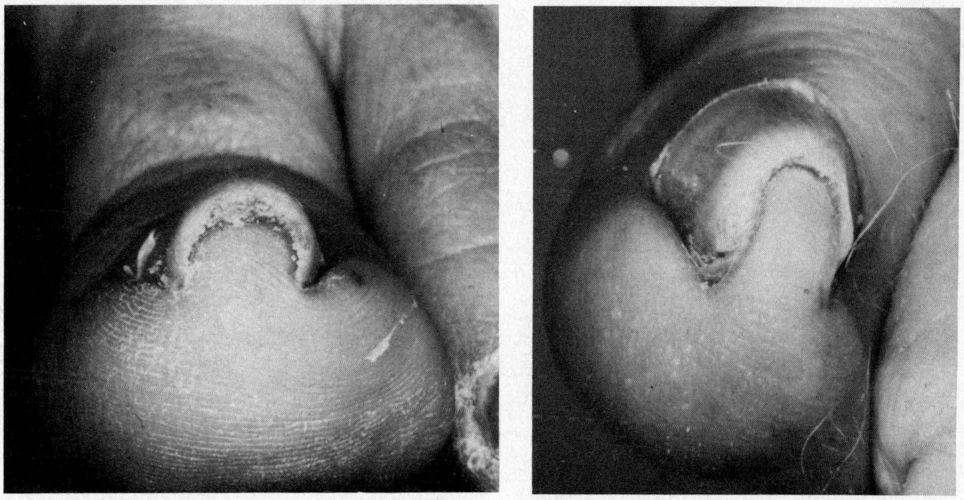

A B

Fig. 38-22. Type of nail **(A)** that is particularly hazardous in diabetic patient. It starts from wide base at nail root and incurves distally, pinching nailbed **(B)**. These two nails form arcs of greater than 200 degrees at distal toe. If neglected, medial and lateral nail margins may meet beyond distal toe, forming full circle and brittle claw. (From Levin ME and O'Neal LW: The diabetic foot, ed 4, St Louis, 1988, The CV Mosby Co.)

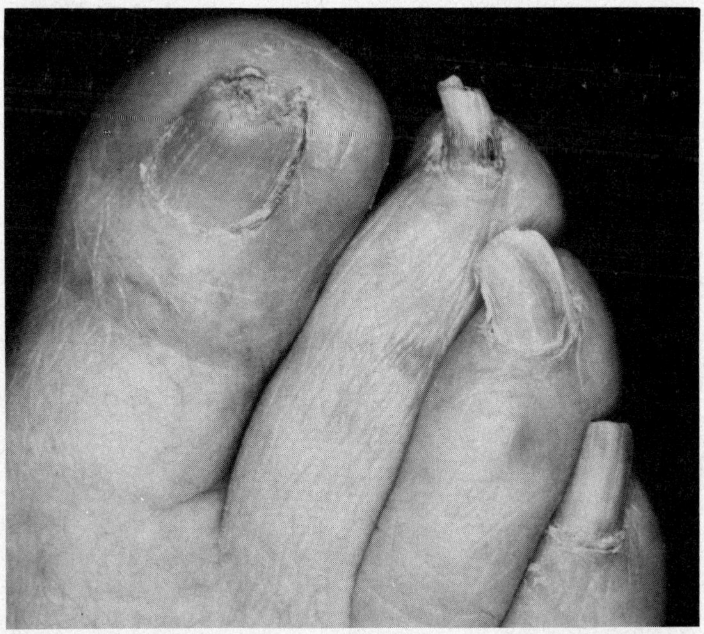

Fig. 38-23. Toes of obese diabetic patient with onychomycosis of nail of hallux and incurving distal growth of all nails. Nails have grown long because of neglect. Note that nail of third toe gouges skin of second toe. (From Levin ME and O'Neal LW: The diabetic foot, ed 4, St Louis, 1988, The CV Mosby Co.)

because they seldom feel pain or discomfort and therefore assume that all is well. Secondly, it is embarrassing to many of these patients to remove their shoes and stockings. However, if this is not done on a routine basis, lesions will be missed, treatment delayed, and amputation may be the result. Examination of the foot and lower extremity includes inspection, palpation, and a neurologic and vascular examination.

Inspection

Simply inspecting the legs and feet will give many clues to the vascular status. Evidence of significant ischemia in the foot includes the loss of hair on the dorsum of the foot and toes, skin that is shiny and atrophic and appears to be drawn tightly around the foot because of loss of the subcutaneous fat layers, and dependent rubor. All of these findings are indicative of severe peripheral arterial disease. One of the simplest evaluations for vascular insufficiency is to measure delayed capillary filling time. This is done by having the patient lie on his or her back, raising the legs to a 45-degree angle, and keeping them in this position until the feet blanch. Then have the patient sit upright, and dangle the legs. By measuring the time required for capillary filling one can estimate the degree of vascular insufficiency. Normal capillary filling time is 10 to 15 seconds. A filling time over 40 seconds indicates very severe ischemia. The extremity with severe ASO will develop dependent rubor. Patients with varicose veins may also have dependent rubor. Shiny atrophic skin, pallor on elevation, delayed filling time, and dependent rubor are the hallmarks of significant lower extremity vascular insufficiency. Details of the vascular examination can be found in Chapter 2.

Inspection between the toes is of the utmost importance. Soft corns and heloma molle, with ulceration occurring between the toes, usually the fourth and fifth, are caused by friction of the adjacent head of the proximal phalanx of the fifth toe (Fig. 38-24).

Fig. 38-25 shows an example of a painless interdigital ulcer in an elderly woman. When this patient came into the office and was asked to remove her shoes and socks, she refused, saying that her feet felt fine and that she had no problems with them. After much insistence she removed her shoes and stockings, and the ulcer was identified. When asked how long she had the ulcer the patient looked down and with great surprise stated that she did not know that she had an ulcer because she had felt no pain. Foot inspection frequently will reveal interosseous muscle atrophy with resulting contractions, hammer and cocked up toes. Because ulcerations can occur at the tip and top of the toes (see Fig. 38-16), I refer to this as the "tip-top toe ulcer syndrome." These patients need a special shoe with an insole to protect the tips of the toes and a toe box big enough to accommodate these cocked up toes.

Painless blisters may occur because of friction. However, other bullous lesions are peculiar to the diabetic. These are referred to as *bullosis diabeticorum,* which consists of two types, the acute superficial blister, which heals rapidly (Fig. 38-26) and a deeper hemorrhagic type, which tends to go

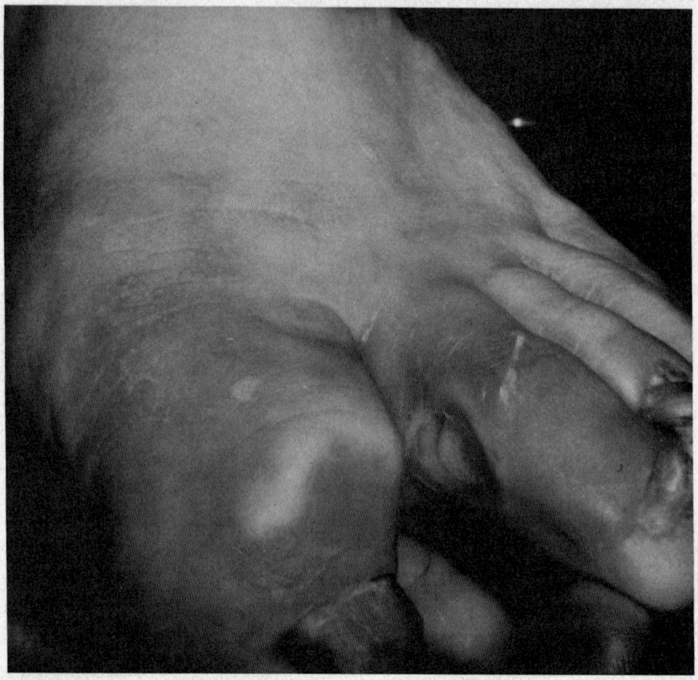

Fig. 38-24. Heloma molle of base of second toe from pressure of deformed adjacent interphalangeal joint of hallux. (From Levin ME and O'Neal LW: The diabetic foot, ed 4, St Louis, 1988, The CV Mosby Co.)

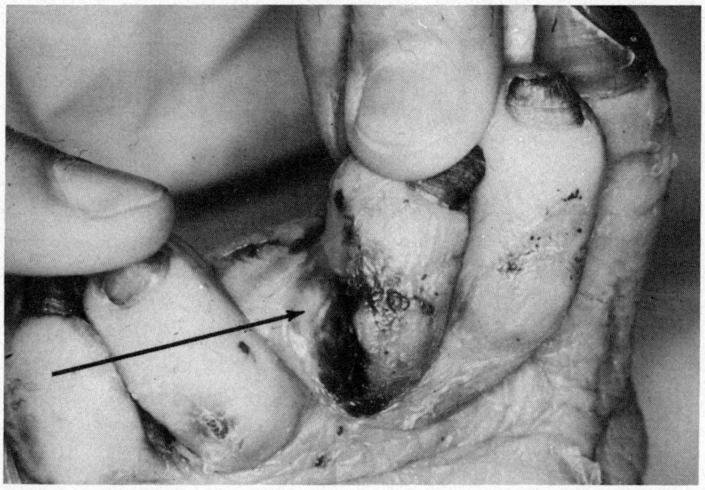

Fig. 38-25. Painless interdigital ulcer in elderly diabetic woman. Arrow points to exposed tendon, indicating depth of ulceration. This painless ulcer was found on routine foot examination. (From Levin ME and O'Neal LW: The diabetic foot, ed 4, St Louis, 1988, The CV Mosby Co.)

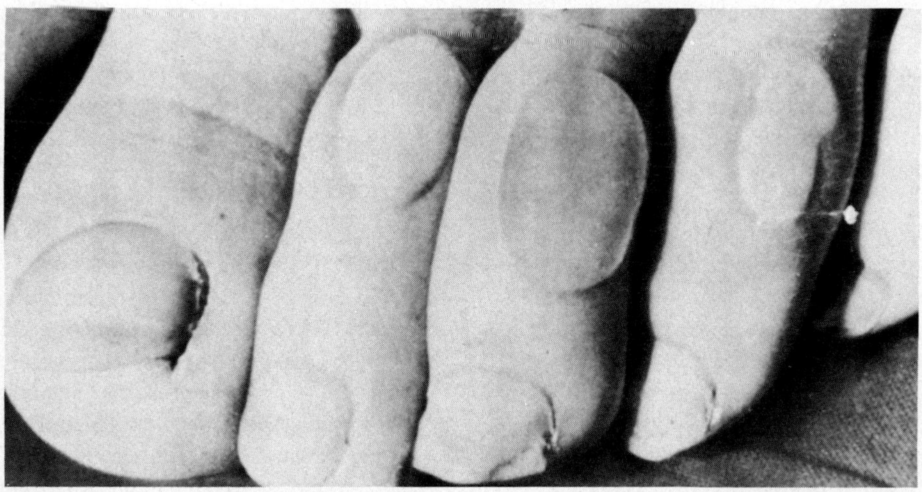

Fig. 38-26. Characteristic bullosis diabeticorum seen on toes of diabetic individual. (From Allen GE and Hadden DR: Br J Dermatol 82:216, 1970.)

on to superficial necrosis of the skin. The mechanism for the development of these lesions is unkown. Allen and Hadden[124] stress that the condition should be recognized because the treatment course and prognosis differ from those of ischemic and neuropathic lesions. Jelinek has authored an excellent text on diabetic skin lesions.[125]

Palpation

Touching the skin is a simple and important part of the examination. The experienced hand and eye (see inspection) are extremely important in the evaluation of ASO. Palpation consists of evaluating the pulses—the femorals, popliteals, dorsalis pedis, and posterior tibial. Auscultation for bruits will help identify the presence of atheromatous plaques and narrowing of the arterial lumen. One of the most important aspects of palpation is detecting whether the skin is warm or cool. Sophisticated instruments are available for quantitative measurements of skin temperature, for example, the Mikron digital infrared thermometer.* The approximate cost is $1800. This is a useful instrument for doing research but it is not necessary for routine examination of the foot. Palpation with the palm or back of the hand is sufficient. When indicated, a hand-held Doppler, relatively inexpensive and easy to use, should be employed in evaluating the peripheral vascular status. The use of Doppler and other laboratory techniques for evaluating ASO can be found in Chapter 3.

Sensory examination

While a variety of sophisticated techniques are available for measurement of vibratory sense (large nerve fibers), such as the biothesiometer,† a simple tuning fork with a 128 cycle is sufficient. This examination should include vibratory sense, not only at the ankle and tibia but also at the tips of the toes. Once the patient can no longer feel the vibration, the examiner can apply the tuning fork to the same area of his or her own foot to see whether further vibrations can be detected.

The examination to assess the ability to perceive temperature, a small nerve fiber modality, can also be carried out. Guy et al found the lateral aspect of the foot to be the most sensitive location for the measurement of thermal sensation.[126] These authors noted loss of thermal sensation in all feet with neuropathic ulcerations and in feet with Charcot's joint. When thermal sensitivity was compared with vibratory perception threshold, it was found that thermal sensitivity was sometimes selectively affected, especially in those patients with painful neuropathy, suggesting that the small fibers are more vulnerable in the diabetic.[126] Quantitative measurements of thermal sensation can be made with sophisticated instruments such as the Marstock stimulator.‡ This consists of a metal plate through which a current of 3 amperes is delivered. The patient presses a switch as soon as the plate feels warm. The current is then reversed to change the temperature to cool. The device gives an objective and quantitative measure of temperature sensation.[127] However, using test tubs of cold and warm water is a simple, qualitative, and reasonable means of detecting thermal sensation.

Sensory evaluation to perceive protective sensation is frequently carried out by using a pin. This is an inadequate way to evaluate sensation since it will vary with each investigator, depending on how forcefully one uses the pin. Today's state-of-the-art evaluation for the ability to perceive touch is done using the Semmes Weinstein monofilaments.* These filaments come in three different thicknesses, 4.17, 5.07, and 6.10. The monofilament is simply placed against the skin and pressure applied until the filament buckles (Fig. 38-27). The monofilament is usually applied to the bottom of the foot and to different areas. The patient should be able to identify the area being touched. The patient should also be able to detect the presence of the monofilament at the time it buckles. A thickness of 5.07 is equal to 10 g of linear pressure and is the limit used to determine protective sensations.

While there is variability from patient to patient, the natural history of loss of peripheral nerve function is as follows: Vibratory sense is usually the first to be lost, followed by loss of reflexes (the Achilles reflex is usually the first to go), and finally, loss of sensations of pain and touch.

MANAGEMENT OF THE DIABETIC FOOT

Improvement of circulation

Improvement and maintenance of the blood flow will depend on a variety of approaches. It begins with controlling the vascular risk factors, which has been previously discussed. Vasodilators do not work.[128] Sympathectomy rarely has any value in the treatment of these patients. The vascular insufficiency, as previously noted, is caused primarily by atherosclerotic narrowing of the vessels and not vasospastic disease. In addition, because of the frequent involvement of the autonomic nervous system in these patients, many have already had autosympathectomy.

Hemorrheologic agents can decrease viscosity and improve blood flow in the microcirculation. Pentoxifylline (Trental) increases the flexibility of red and white blood cells. A red cell measures 7.4 microns; a white cell is slightly larger. A capillary lumen is only 3 to 5 microns. Therefore the red and white cells must change their shape to move through the smaller capillaries. Roeren, LeVeen, and Nugent,[129] using photoplethysmography found increased blood flow to the toes in diabetics treated with pentoxifylline. After 3 months of treatment, the diabetic patients reported a decrease in symptoms of paresthesias. The ankle-brachial indexes showed no significant effect, thus indicating that the effect of pentoxifylline was on the microcirculation. However, Schwartz et al found pentoxifylline to increase Doppler

*Mikron Instrument Company, Box 211, Ridgeway, NJ 07451.
†Biomedical Instruments, Newburg, Ohio.
‡Somedic, Stockholm, Sweden.

*These may be obtained from the Gillis W. Long Hansens Disease Center, Nylon Filament Project, Carville, Louisiana 70721.

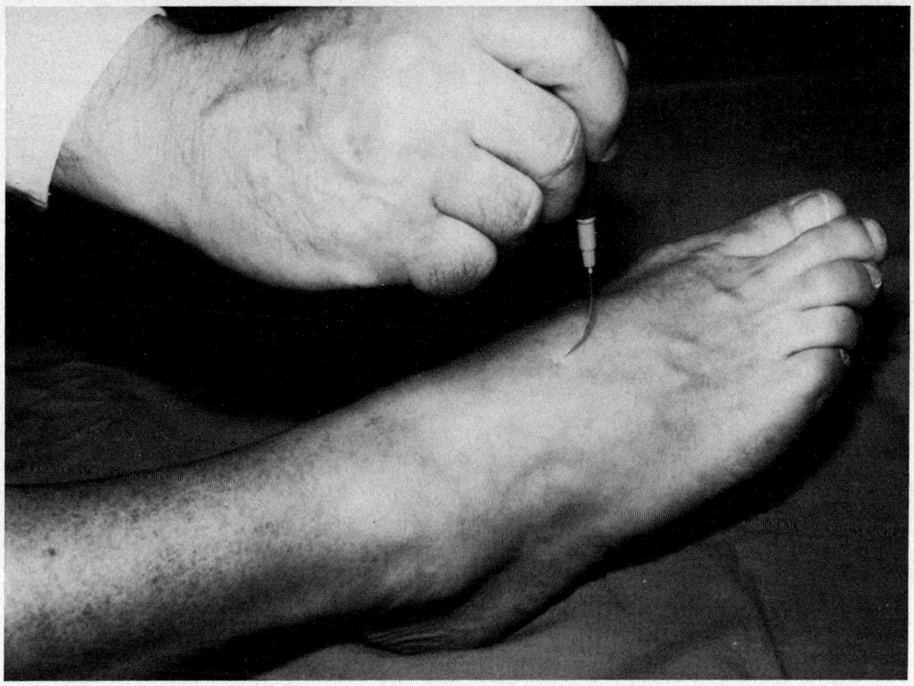

Fig. 38-27. Semmes-Weinstein monofilament being used to evaluate sensory perception. Patient should be able to detect sensation at the time the monofilament buckles. The 5.07 filament equals 10 grams of linear strength to buckle and represents the threshold for loss of touch sensation. (From Levin ME: State of the art: on the evaluation, prevention, and treatment of diabetic foot lesions, J Diabetic Complications 3:211, 1989.)

waveforms.[130] Because it increases the flexibility of the red and white cells[131,132] and decreases fibrinogen levels,[133] this drug may be helpful in decreasing blood viscosity thereby increasing blood flow. Currently the use of pentoxifylline in the United States has been approved only for the treatment of intermittent claudication. In Canada it has also been approved for treatment of ischemic trophic foot ulcers. It may prove to be beneficial in the treatment of the chronic ischemic foot in patients who are not candidates for vascular surgery. Anecdotally, reports have found pentoxifylline to be beneficial in the healing of superficial ulcerations around the ankle and tip of the toes caused by vascular insufficiency. Because pentoxifylline takes 2 to 3 months to achieve its effect, it is not the treatment for major plantar ulcers.

The ultimate improvement in circulation is achieved through vascular surgery. This is discussed in Chapter 9. Angiography is required preoperatively to establish the location of the block and the feasibility of vascular surgery. The diabetic with peripheral arterial disease frequently has renal disease with an elevated blood urea nitrogen (BUN) level and creatinine. These patients can suffer renal shutdown following the administration of contrast media. To avoid this complication these patients should be kept well hydrated before the procedure, and the use of temporally close contrast studies should be avoided. The use of the newer "low osmolality" nonionic contrast agents may help decrease the side effects of these agents. However, they do not appear to have decreased the incidence of renal shutdown. Recent evidence has shown that renal failure was the same whether the contrast material had high or low osmolarity.[134] This was confirmed in the study of Schwab et al.[135] Parfrey et al found the risk for diabetics with preexisting renal insufficiency was approximately 9% lower than had been previously reported.[136] However, in this series the lower incidence of renal failure could be attributed to the fact that there were few patients with severe renal failure, defined as serum creatinines over 5 mg/dl, and the patients were not randomly selected so there could be physician bias. The risk of renal shutdown can be minimized by patient selection, hydration, and decreasing the dose of contrast material. Cigarroa et al decreased their incidence of contrast nephropathy by using a formula to calculate a contrast material "limit" in patients with renal disease.[137] Furthermore, if one extremity is being evaluated, it is not necessary to use enough contrast material to visualize both extremities.

Because most vascular occlusions in the diabetic occur below the knee, transcutaneous angioplasty in these vessels is limited. However, an 85% primary success rate has been reported in a small series.[138]

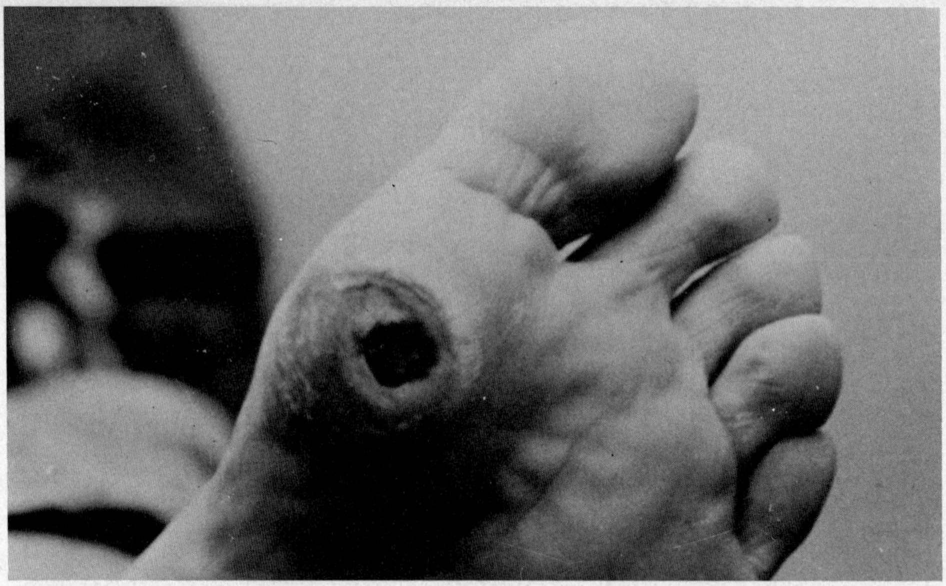

Fig. 38-28. Classic neuropathic diabetic foot ulcer. Note ulceration in callus is well circumscribed. Lesion is painless. (From Levin ME and O'Neal LW: The diabetic foot, ed 4, St Louis, 1988, The CV Mosby Co; courtesy the Michigan Diabetes Research and Training Center, Ann Arbor, Mich, 1983, The University of Michigan.)

Treatment of diabetic neurotrophic foot ulcers

Ulcers occur in the diabetic because of repetitive stress on insensitive feet. In addition, patients who develop ulcers have increased foot pressures.[5] When repetitive stress continues, the foot develops hot spots, pressure necrosis, and ultimately ulceration. This occurs most often at the sites of the most pressure and excessive callus buildup. Fig. 38-28 is the classic diabetic neurotrophic foot ulcer, sometimes referred to as *malperforans ulcer*. When a patient develops an ulceration on the dorsum of the foot, it is caused by trauma. When the ulcer is on the side of the foot (see Fig. 38-10), it is almost always caused by an ill-fitting shoe.

Listed in the accompanying box are the approaches to the aggressive treatment of diabetic neurotrophic foot ulcers. The treatment of these ulcers requires establishment of depth and degree of ulceration. What may appear to be a superficial ulceration may only be the tip of the iceberg. There may be penetration deep into the tissues. Fig. 38-29, *A*, shows what appears to be a relatively small ulcer on the plantar surface of this 60-year-old woman's foot. She had been diabetic for 20 years and had severe peripheral neuropathy with an insensate foot. She had stepped on a nail and developed a painless ulceration, which she treated with a variety of "home remedies." When the wound failed to heal after several weeks she sought medical attention. The wound appeared to be a small superficial ulcer. However, extensive débridement revealed infection penetrating deep into the interfacial spaces (Fig. 38-29, *B*). Fortunately, the patient's circulation was good. She responded to parenteral antibiotic therapy, and a skin graft was successful. A number of lessons can be learned from this case. First, patients should not go barefoot; second, one should not assume that the ulceration is superficial and treat it with topical agents; and third, vigorous débridement must be done to establish the degree of penetration, and then the ulcer must be treated accordingly. After adequate débridement the final ulcer will be larger than the original ulcer. All the necrotic material should be removed. Surgical débridement is preferred over whirlpool. X-rays are necessary in every case of foot ul-

Primary treatment of foot ulcers

1. Evaluation
   a. Clinical appearance
   b. Depth of penetration
   c. Radiologic appearance
2. Metabolic control
3. Débridement
4. Bacterial cultures (aerobic and anaerobic)
5. Antibiotics
6. Avoidance of soaking the feet
7. Nonweight bearing
   a. Bed rest
   b. Contact casting
8. Improvement in circulation (vascular surgery)
9. Posthealing treatment

Modified from Levin ME: The diabetic foot: pathophysiology, evaluation and treatment. In Levin ME and O'Neal LW, eds, The diabetic foot, ed 4, St. Louis, 1988, The CV Mosby Co.

A

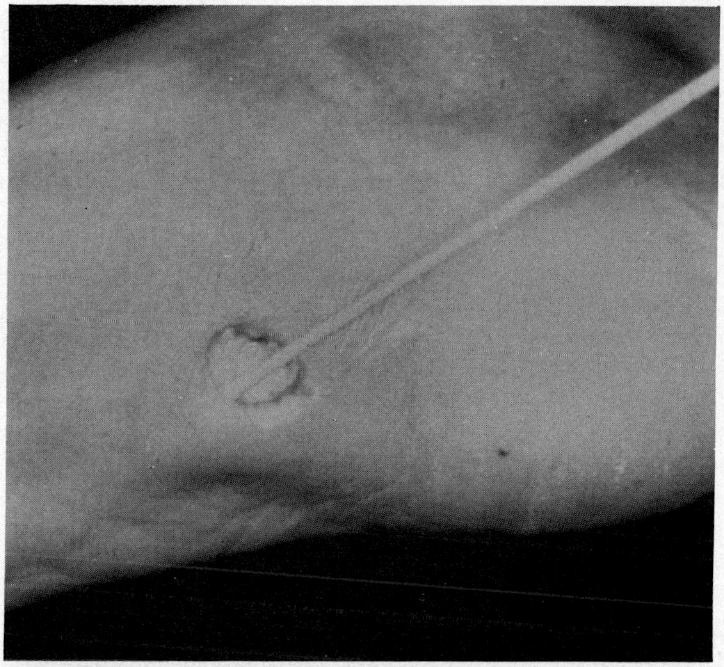

B

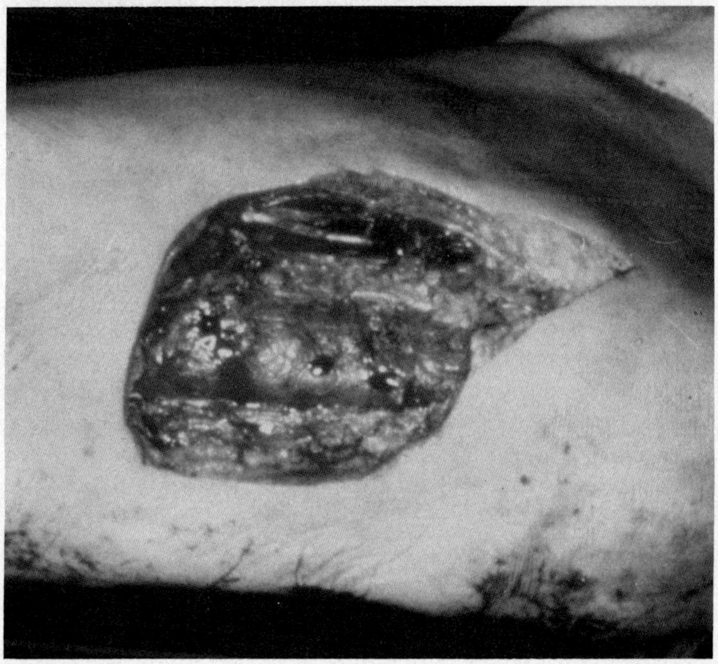

Fig. 38-29. A, Ulcer appears to be small and superficial on plantar surface of foot. **B,** Exploration of ulcer reveals infection to penetrated tissues and interfascial plane. (From Levin ME and O'Neal LW: The diabetic foot, ed 4, St Louis, 1988, The CV Mosby Co.)

ceration to rule out osteomyelitis and the presence of foreign objects (see Fig. 38-9). Metabolic control is essential because white cells do not function well in the face of hyperglycemia or ketosis.

Adequate surgical débridement is necessary in every case for establishing the depth of the ulcer and for proper cultures. Débridement needs to be done vigorously. The surgeon must be sure to explore deep into the tissues for infection. Taylor and Porter have demonstrated that aggressive foot débridement, and when indicated, revascularization, resulted in long-term salvage of 73% of threatened limbs even in high-risk patients.[139] Cultures should be taken both aerobically and anaerobically. The choice of parenteral or oral antibiotics will depend on medical judgment, however, it should be kept in mind that the treatment of a significant infection requires a high concentration of antibiotics. In the face of significant peripheral vascular disease this cannot be achieved with oral antibiotics. Furthermore, the antibiotic of choice frequently can only be given parenterally. If an oral antibiotic is chosen, patients must be cautioned to look for evidence of increasing infection, such as pain, redness, or lymphangitis. Patients should be instructed to call their physician at once should any of these signs or symptoms develop. Patients receiving oral antibiotics should be seen every 48 to 72 hours, since there can be a very rapid spread of the infection in the diabetic foot.

Soaking the feet has no benefit although it has been a traditional approach.[140] Soaking may lead to maceration and further infection. Because the foot is insensitive, soaking may occur in water that is too hot, resulting in severe burns. Chemical soaks can also result in burns.[140] Nonweight bearing is essential. These patients have insensitive feet and, since the ulcers do not hurt, the patient continues to walk, resulting in an increase in pressure necrosis, preventing healing. The use of crutches and wheelchairs is seldom successful in achieving total and consistent nonweight bearing. The best method for nonweight bearing in appropriately selected patients is the use of the contact cast.[141-144] The contact cast allows the patient to be ambulatory, but still essentially nonweight bearing, by redistributing the weight, thereby decreasing the pressure on the ulcer area. Mueller et al conducted the first prospective control trial and conclusively demonstrated the value of total contact casting (TCC) vs traditional dressing treatment (TDT).[143] In comparable groups they demonstrated that in the TCC group there was 90% healing requiring 42 ± 29 days, compared to the TDT group of which there was only a 32% healing with a 65 ± 29 days range of healing. The patients in the TDT group were instructed in nonweight bearing, use of wet-to-dry saline dressings, wearing special shoes with insoles, and healing sandals. However, these patients were all found to be noncompliant.

Contraindications for total-contact casting have been reviewed by Sinacore.[144] These include active or acute infection, osteomyelitis, ulcer depth greater than ulcer width, excessive edema, blindness or obesity, patients with Doppler indexes less than 0.45, and noncompliance.

When an ulcer does not heal despite good metabolic control, nonweight bearing, débridement, and parenteral antibiotics, one should consider vascular surgery for improving inadequate circulation. Fig. 38-30, *A*, shows an ulceration on the plantar surface of the heel. The patient had an insensitive foot and a shoe that had a rough area in the heel. He was hospitalized and the usual aggressive approaches described earlier were carried out. Débridement was continued to the periosteum of the calcaneus, yet healing did not occur. As a last resort vascular surgery was undertaken. Since the patient had received a kidney transplant because of renal failure, a nephrologist was called in for consultation before an angiogram was obtained. An angiogram (Fig. 38-30, *B*) showed the transplanted kidney in the left iliac fossa, a good aorta and iliac vessels, moderate atherosclerosis in both superficial femoral arteries, and occlusion of both left and right tibial and peroneal vessels at their origins (Fig. 38-30, *C*). The patient underwent a left popliteal-posterior tibial bypass (Fig. 38-30, *D*). His left ankle Doppler index, which measured 0.66 preoperatively, probably an erroneously high reading because of incompressible vessels, had now risen to 0.95. Within 3 weeks, the plantar ulcer had completely healed (Fig. 38-30, *E*). Techniques for vascular surgery are discussed in Chapter 9.

The importance of treating neurotrophic foot ulcers by improving circulation is shown in the study of Sage and Doyle.[145] They believe, and I agree, that the degree of ischemia and not necessarily the extent of the ulcer is one of the most significant factors in evaluating the potential outcome of treatment. Their success rate in the ischemic group was 25%. The success rate of the nonischemic group was 83%. Classifications were based on Doppler studies and physical examination.

The efficacy of hyperbaric oxygen in treating diabetic foot ulcers continues to be investigated. The use of topical hyperbaric oxygen has been reported, in some studies, to be a successful form of therapy.[146,147] However, Leslie et al have noted that these studies either were retrospective, uncontrolled, or that the assignment of subjects to oxygen therapy vs control therapy was apparently arbitrary. They conducted a prospective and randomized study of 28 diabetic patients treated with topical hyperbaric oxygen. These patients were observed for a 14-day period. At 7 days and 14 days there were no differences in the type of microorganisms isolated by curettage. Changes in ulcer size did not differ between the control and the topical hyperbaric oxygen group. It was their conclusion that the healing of diabetic neurotrophic ulcers was not accelerated by topical hyperbaric oxygen.[148] Baroni et al treated 18 hospitalized adult diabetic patients who developed gangrenous lesions of the foot. In a hyperbaric chamber these were compared with a group of 10 diabetic patients with comparable foot lesions

A

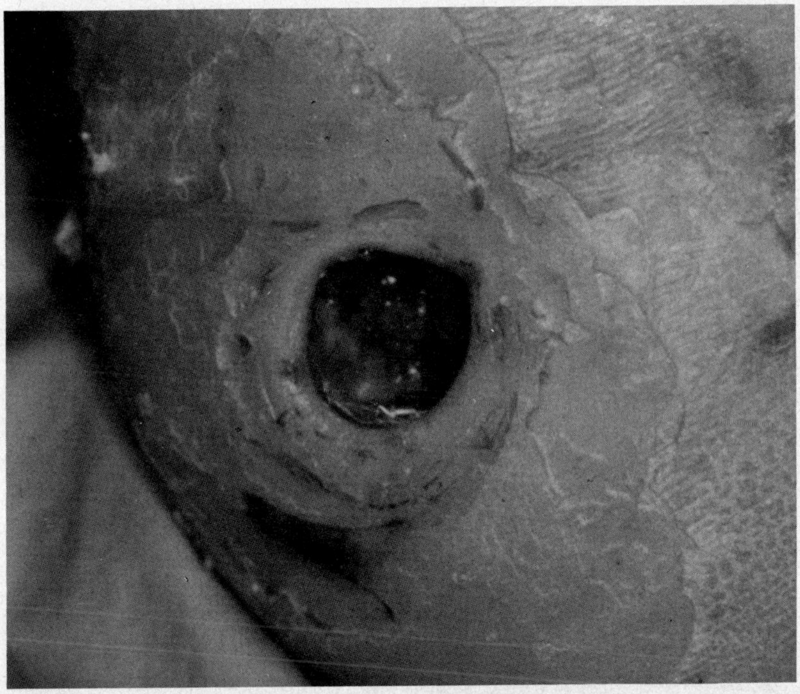

B

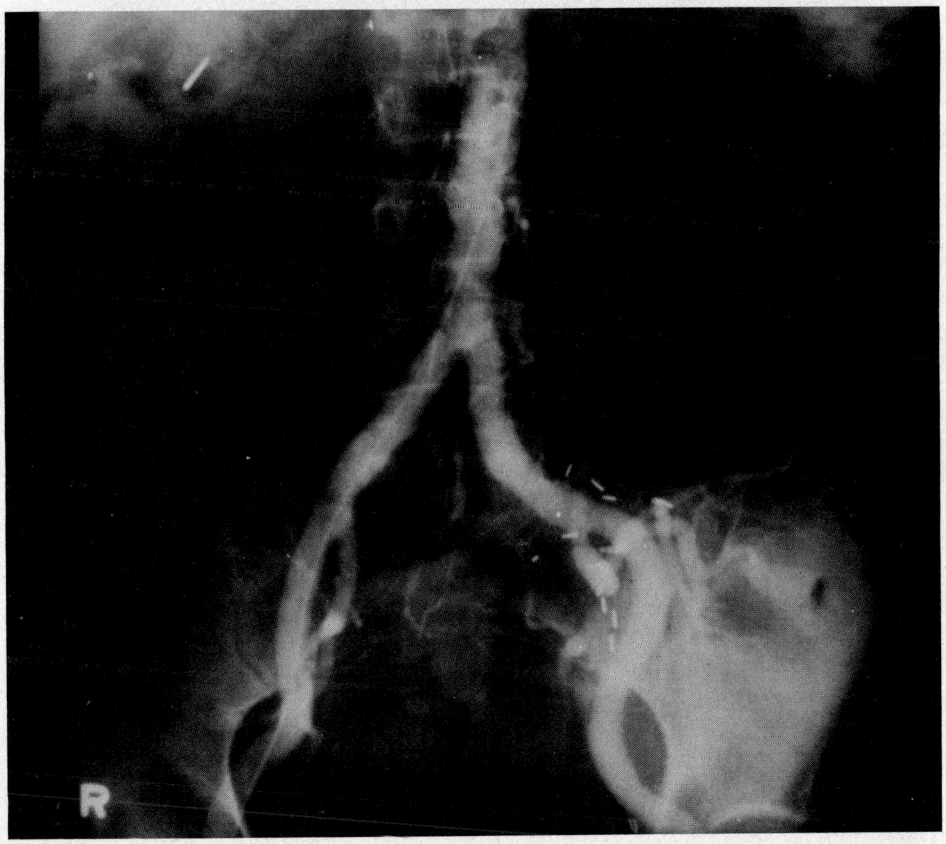

Fig. 38-30. A, Ulceration of plantar surface of heel, which was débrided to periosteum of calcaneus. **B,** Arteriogram of patient with ulcer (**A**). Arteriogram revealed normal aorta and iliac arteries. Previously transplanted kidney is noted on left side of pelvis

Continued.

C

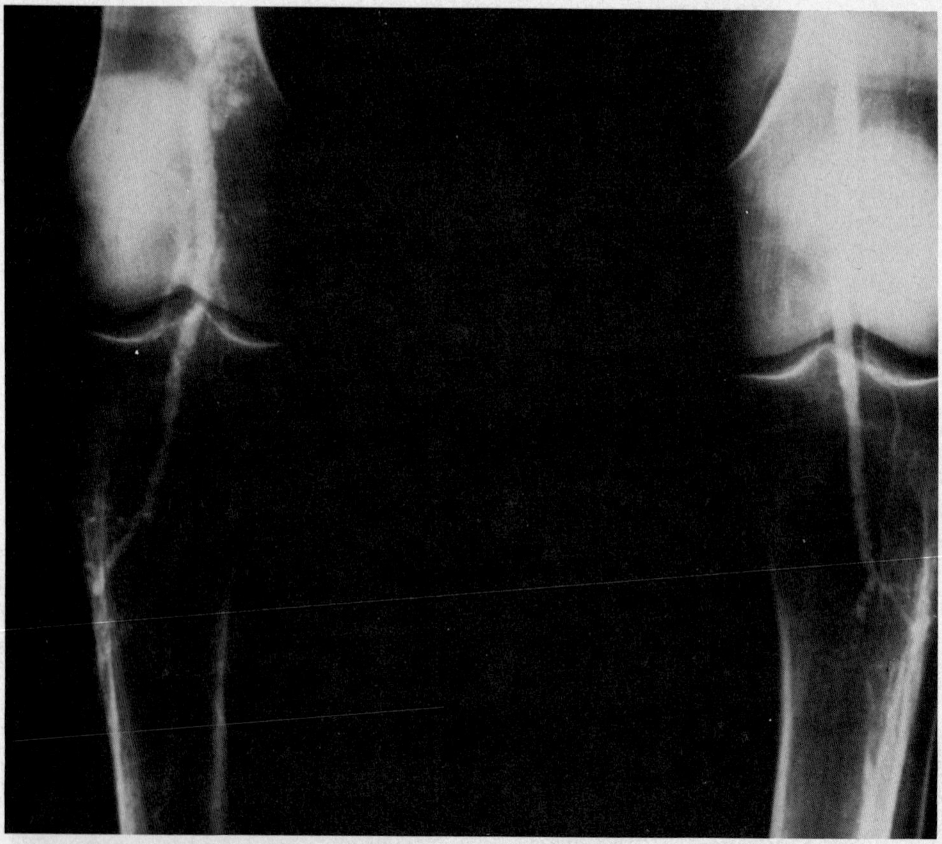

D

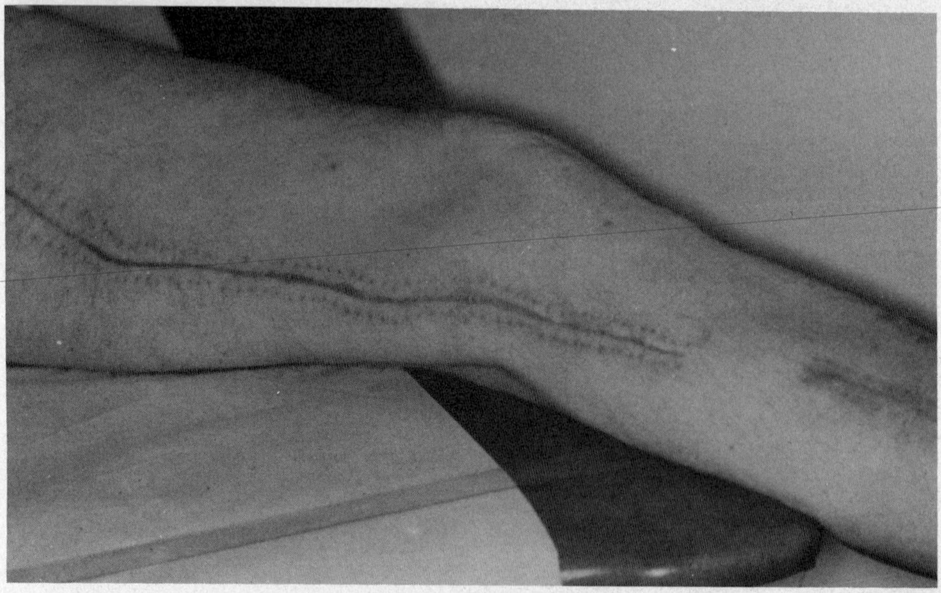

Fig. 38-30, cont'd. C, Arteriogram shows occlusion of both left and right tibial and peroneal vessels at their origin. **D,** Extent of surgery for popliteal posterior tibial bypass. **E,** Healed ulcer 3 weeks after vascular surgery. (From Levin ME and O'Neal LW: The diabetic foot, ed 4, St Louis, 1988, The CV Mosby Co; courtesy Dr. Gregorio Sicard, Department of Surgery, Washington University School of Medicine, St Louis.)

E

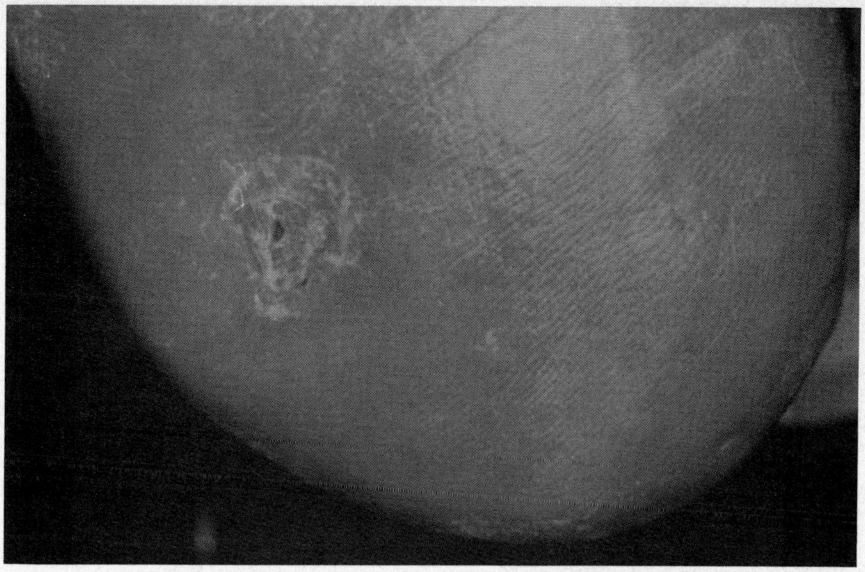

Fig. 38-30, cont'd. E, For legend see opposite page.

not treated in the chamber.[149] They found that hyperbaric oxygen treatment drastically reduced leg amputations. While it was stated that the patients had macroangiopathy and Doppler studies, none were reported. Furthermore, in this study the patients were apparently not randomized. Confirmation of the use of the hyperbaric chamber for the treatment of diabetic neurotrophic foot ulcers will require larger and better controlled study.

Topical treatment of foot ulcers

While a variety of topical agents, proteolytic enzymes, and topical antibacterials have been used to treat diabetic foot ulcers, I believe that this represents only adjunct therapy. The initial use of these preparations and allowing the patient to walk delays more aggressive therapy and can result in the loss of a foot.

A topical treatment that is currently under investigation is platelet derived growth factor (PDGF) or wound healing factor.[150] Daily application of PDGF will stimulate angiogenesis, scar tissue formation, and epithelialization. Preliminary trials have suggested beneficial effects from this form of therapy. It must be kept in mind that this type of therapy is used in conjunction with the aggressive types of treatment previously noted. There are many impediments to wound healing (see the accompanying box) and when applicable, each of these must be addressed.

Impediments to wound healing

Vascular

Atherosclerosis
Increased viscosity

Neurologic

Insensate foot
Deformed foot
Decreased flare reaction

Infection

Poor blood supply
Microthrombi
Hyperglycemia
Decreased PMN function
Polymicrobial infection

Mechanical

Weight bearing on ulcer
Improperly fitted shoes

Treatment after diabetic neurotrophic foot ulcers are healed

Even though a neurotrophic foot ulcer has healed, the job has not been completed. The underlying causes of the ulceration, such as foot deformities, calluses, and increased pressure, are still present. Therefore special measures are necessary to protect the vulnerable sites of previous breakdown. This requires reeducation of the patient in walking, teaching him or her to take shorter steps, and frequently a change in jobs is necessary. Special shoes are very important.

Special shoes

Special shoes for patients who have cocked up toes has been discussed. The patient with a markedly deformed foot,

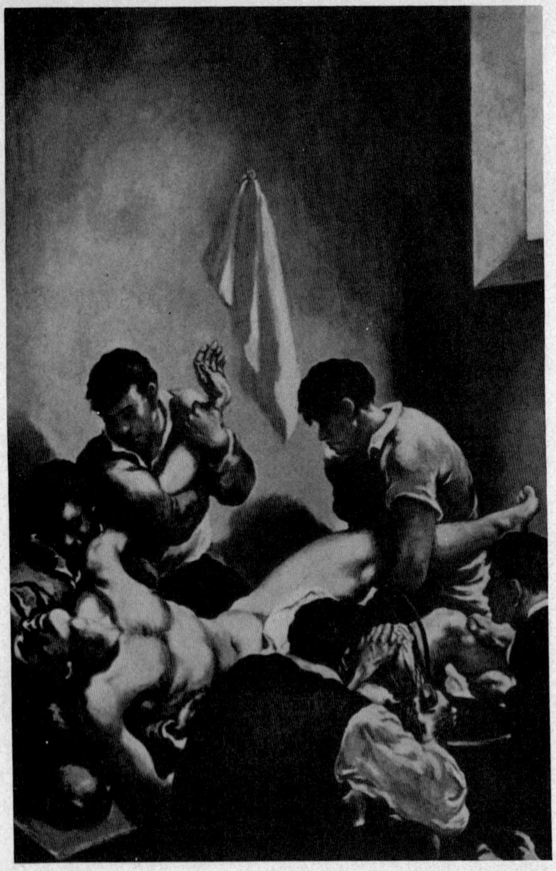

Fig. 38-31. Painting depicts agonies of patient undergoing amputation in ancient time. Formerly amputations were performed only with alcohol as an anesthetic. Many people died during this guillotine operation, some even died of shock and terror before the operation began! (Painting by Italian Count Gregorio Calvi de Bergolo in 1953. From the International Museum of Surgical Sciences and Hall of Fame. International College of Surgeons, Chicago.)

such as Charcot's foot, needs a specially molded shoe. The use of special therapeutic shoes is critically important in preventing ulcerations or recurrence of ulcers. This frequently requires an extra-depth shoe with a plasticlike material, frequently a plastazote insert, to redistribute the weight and to prevent recurrence of ulceration. This was clearly demonstrated at a study at King's College in London, which showed an 83% recurrence of ulcers when patients returned to wearing their regular shoes. However, with the use of special shoes there was only a 17% recurrence.[21] The importance of therapeutic shoes is being recognized with increasing frequency. Footwear management has been reviewed by Coleman.[151]

Teamwork

Teamwork in the management of the diabetic foot is not that depicted in Fig. 38-31. The goal of teamwork is to save the diabetic foot and leg, not to remove it. It is obvious that treatment of diabetic foot problems can be quite complex, requiring many medical disciplines (see the accompanying box).

Team members involved in the care of the diabetic foot

1. Primary physician
2. Endocrinologist
3. Diabetologist
4. Nurse educator
5. Podiatrist
6. Infectious disease specialist
7. Radiologist
8. Neurologist
9. Vascular surgeon
10. Orthopedist
11. Pedorthist
12. Orthotist
13. Social worker
14. Home care nurse

Modified from Levin ME: The diabetic foot: pathophysiology, evaluation and treatment. In Levin ME and O'Neal LW, eds, The diabetic foot, ed 4, St. Louis, 1988, The CV Mosby Co.

The primary physician's most important task is examining the foot at every visit and educating the patient in foot care. Unfortunately, this is done infrequently. Foot inspection can save many feet and prevent multiple hospitalizations. Because diabetic neuropathy or ASO cannot be totally prevented, the best approach toward saving the diabetic foot is patient education. The primary physician who does not do this loses the advantage of the adage, "an ounce of prevention is worth a pound of cure."

The nurse educator and trained assistant are important members of the team. They not only educate the patient about the various aspects of diabetes, but they also examine the feet and teach foot care. Many times the podiatrist is the first to detect a neurotrophic foot lesion and occasionally the first to diagnose the patient's diabetes. The podiatrist may be able to correct the presenting foot lesion, such as cocked up toes or chronic recurrent ingrown toenails. The podiatrist's role in patient education in foot care is paramount. The frequency of neuropathic syndromes and their differential diagnoses may require a neurologist. The vascular surgeon's role in revascularizing feet and legs has saved many a patient from amputation. The orthopedist frequently sees the patient because of foot deformities. The expertise of the orthopedist in prophylactic or other corrective surgery is of the utmost importance. Other important members of the team treating diabetic foot deformities consist of the certified pedorthist and orthotist. These specialists in fitting prophylactic shoes are extremely important. The physical therapist may have two roles. In medical centers where contact casting is practiced, it is frequently the physical therapist who is trained to apply these special casts. When amputations occur, the physical therapist's skills, together with those of the specialist in physical medicine, are required for rehabilitation. Treatment of diabetic neuropathic lesions can be prolonged, and since hospital stays must be shortened, many patients require home nursing care services. The home care nurse may be needed to carry out prolonged parenteral antibiotic therapy, change dressings, and observe the clinical course of the patient at home, thus shortening the hospital stay.

Financial problems resulting from loss of a job can be monumental. The social worker becomes an important team member in these cases.

Patient education

Of all the approaches to saving the diabetic foot, the most important is patient education. Despite our current knowledge and good diabetic control, physicians cannot totally prevent atherosclerosis and peripheral neuropathy. However, the patient can be educated in proper foot care, learning how to prevent injury to insensitive feet and detect foot lesions as early as possible.

At the time of the office visit, and while the shoes and socks are off, the nurse and physician should review the *do's* and *dont's* of foot care with the patient. This cannot be done by simply handing the patient a sheet of instructions. The instructions must be explained and questions encouraged and answered. If this is done, the patient will have a better understanding of the importance of foot care. The list of instructions that I use for patient education is given in the accompanying box. Patients should be instructed to look not only at their feet but also to inspect between the toes. Patients with impaired vision, extreme obesity, or arthritis cannot inspect their feet adequately. These inspections can be carried out by a family member. For patients who cannot see their feet because of obesity or arthritis, a mirror can be placed on the floor, allowing them to inspect the bottom of the foot. The feet should be kept clean and the patient should be cautioned to dry carefully between the toes. Moisture left in these areas can lead to maceration and infection.

Because autonomic neuropathy leads to the inability of the foot to perspire, the skin becomes dry, flaky, and cracked. The application of a very thin coat of lubricating material to the foot after bathing helps to seal in the moisture. It is moisture rather than the oil itself that keeps the skin pliable and decreases the dryness. Any type of cream can be used. Each practitioner has his or her favorite. Even such exotic oils as mink oil have been suggested.[152] It is very important that lubricants not be placed between the toes where extra moisture can accumulate and lead to maceration.

Extremes of temperature should be avoided. Many pa-

Patient instructions for the care of the diabetic foot

1. Do not smoke.
2. Inspect the feet daily for blisters, cuts, and scratches. The use of a mirror can aid in seeing the bottom of the feet. Always check between the toes.
3. Wash feet daily and dry carefully, especially between the toes.
4. Avoid extremes of temperature. Test water with hand or elbow before bathing.
5. If feet feel cold at night, wear socks. Do not apply hot water bottles or heating pads. Do not soak feet in hot water.
6. Do not walk on hot surfaces such as sandy beaches or on the cement around swimming pools.
7. Do not walk barefoot.
8. Do not use chemical agents for the removal of corns and calluses. Do not use corn plasters. Do not use strong antiseptic solutions on the feet.
9. Do not use adhesive tape on the feet.
10. Inspect the inside of shoes daily for foreign objects, nail points, torn linings, and rough areas.
11. If your vision is impaired, have a family member inspect feet daily, trim nails, and buff down calluses.
12. Do not soak feet.
13. For dry feet use a very thin coat of a lubricating oil or cream. Apply this after bathing and drying the feet. Do not put the oil or cream between the toes. Consult your physician for detailed instructions.
14. Wear properly fitting stockings. Do not wear mended stockings. Avoid stockings with seams. Change stockings daily.
15. Do not wear garters.
16. Shoes should be comfortable at time of purchase. Do not depend on them to stretch out. Shoes should be made of leather. Running or special walking shoes may be worn after checking with your physician.
17. Do not wear shoes without stockings.
18. Do not wear sandals with thongs between the toes.
19. In wintertime take special precautions. Wear wool socks and protective foot gear, such as fleece-lined boots.
20. Cut nails straight across.
21. Do not cut corns and calluses. Follow instructions from your physician or podiatrist.
22. Avoid crossing your legs since this can cause pressure on the nerves.
23. See your physician regularly and be sure that your feet are examined at each visit.
24. Notify your physician or podiatrist at once should you develop a blister or sore on your feet.
25. Be sure to inform your podiatrist that you are a diabetic.

Modified from Levin ME: The diabetic foot: pathophysiology, evaluation and treatment. In Levin ME and O'Neal LW, eds, The diabetic foot, ed 4, St. Louis, 1988, The CV Mosby Co.

tients with cold insensitive feet caused by ASO have incurred severe burns by soaking them in water that is too hot (see Fig. 38-15) and using heating pads or hot water bottles. The water temperature should be tested before bathing. This should be done with the elbow, not with the hand, which may also have developed insensitivity because of peripheral neuropathy. Cement around swimming pools and hot, sandy beaches are other areas frequently not suspected of being extremely hot and potentially disastrous for the diabetic. Many diabetic patients with insensitive feet have suffered severe burns secondary to walking on these surfaces. Patients should be advised to wear protective footwear at the beach and pool.

Chemical burns can occur from chemical agents used to remove corns and calluses. The use of these substances should be avoided. The diabetic should inspect the inside of the shoes daily for foreign objects, nail points that have protruded through, and torn linings. Some of the unusual items found in shoes resulting in foot trauma are listed in this chapter.

A critically important part of the diabetic's educational program is instruction in proper footwear. The shoes should be comfortable at the time of purchase and the patient should not depend on them to "stretch out." However, shoes that feel comfortable at the time of purchase may actually be too small since the patient with an insensitive foot cannot detect discomfort. New shoes should be worn only a few hours a day. The shoes should be made of leather and not synthetic materials. However, running or walking shoes may reduce the rate of callus buildup.[153] Patients with foot deformities should wear special therapeutic or molded shoes. The patient should be instructed not to wear thongs. Fig. 38-32 shows an ulceration between the first and second toes of a patient who had worn thonged sandals.

The patient should be taught the proper method of cutting nails straight across or following the curve of the nails but never to cut deep into the corners. Improper trimming can result in an ingrown toenail. Recurring ingrown toenails may be treated conservatively, but they are always a potential source of infection and, when indicated, should receive definitive therapy, usually surgical intervention by either the patient's surgeon or podiatrist. Patients must be instructed repeatedly not to do home surgery. Serious complications can result when the patient cuts on insensitive feet (see Fig. 38-14).

Calluses should not be cut by the patient. Pumice stones, emery boards, and callus files can be used, but if the calluses are particularly thick, they should be trimmed by a physician, surgeon, or podiatrist.

Patients should be reminded to inform any physician working with their feet that they are diabetic so that the physician can take the necessary precautions.

The effectiveness of total foot care programs has been previously noted.[20-22] Lippmann has reduced the amputation rate of 8 to 15 cases a year to zero with a special foot care program implemented in nursing homes.[154]

PATIENT ADHERENCE

Despite the most detailed and repeated instructions, many patients will not adhere to a good foot care program. For instance, it is very difficult to convince some women to forego wearing fashionable high-heeled shoes despite their lament that "these shoes are killing me," which in fact may be more truth than cliche. And, as previously noted, despite warnings, many patients succumb to that irresistible urge to do "home surgery." For many patients going barefoot "feels too good to give up," or they are simply not motivated enough to put on their shoes for their own protection. Ces-

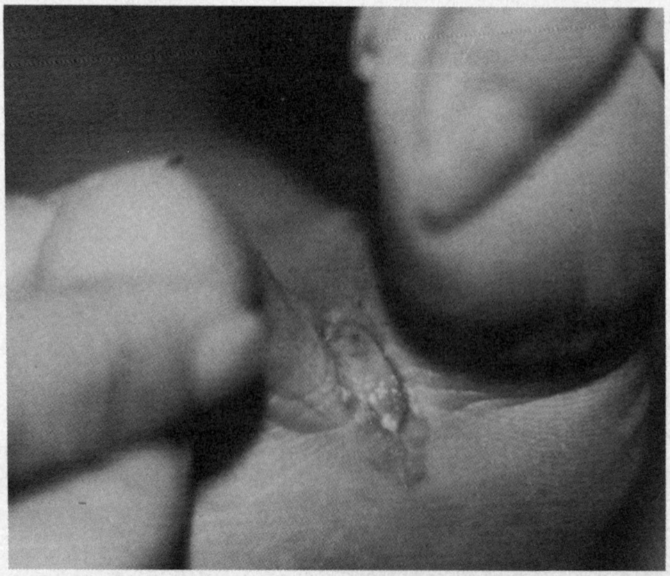

Fig. 38-32. Ulceration between toes from wearing thongs. (From Levin ME and O'Neal LW: The diabetic foot, ed 4, St Louis, 1988, The CV Mosby Co.)

sation of smoking is almost impossible for many patients. It is not unusual for a physician to visit a patient after amputation and find him or her lying in bed, smoking. When the danger and risk to the remaining limb is explained for the "hundredth time," the response is usually "You're right, Doc. I know smoking can cause the loss of the other leg. I am going to quit smoking—some day."

For all the reasons listed, and despite the constant efforts of health care professionals, patient adherence is difficult to accomplish. The problem is compounded even further by patients who do not keep their clinic appointments. Miller found that an intensified foot care program resulted in approximately two-thirds fewer hospital admissions of those patients with diabetic foot problems who faithfully participated in the program, compared with patients who did not attend the clinic on a regular basis.[155] Without patient cooperation adherence to good foot care cannot be achieved; but with the continued efforts of the physician and assistants, patient adherence can be greatly improved.

Rehabilitation following lower limb amputation in the diabetic

Unfortunately all amputations cannot be prevented. Therefore rehabilitation becomes an important facet in the overall management of the diabetic amputee. If we achieve our goal of reducing the amputation rate by 50%, we will still have 25,000 plus diabetic amputations per year. A significant number of these patients can benefit from a prosthetic rehabilitation program.

Following amputation, the goal is to furnish and train a diabetic amputee with a prosthesis, and most importantly, to return the patient to his or her previous life-style. However, not all amputees are candidates for a prosthesis. General contraindications for prosthetic fitting are: (1) chronic and progressive mental deterioration; (2) advancing neurologic disorders such as parkinsonism or stroke; (3) chronic pulmonary obstructive disease; (4) a patient who has not walked for long periods before amputation; (5) when the other extremity is affected by impending gangrene, ulceration, and infection; (6) when there is irreducible pronounced knee flexion contractures in below-knee amputees and hip flexion contractures in above-knee amputees; and (7) when cardiac disease with congestive heart failure or angina is present.[156]

It must be kept in mind that diabetic patients with ASO also have a high incidence of coronary artery disease. The use of a prosthesis increases energy requirements and work load. For example, a normal patient, when walking, requires 0.16 ml of oxygen per meter per kilogram. The individual with a below-knee amputation requires 0.26 ml of oxygen, and an above-knee amputee requires 0.35. A bilateral above-knee amputee requires 0.72.[156] Many diabetics cannot handle this increased work load and some only with extreme difficulty, even taking into account the fact that patients with amputations tend to walk at a much slower rate. A nonamputee will walk at 82 meters per minute, approximately 3 miles per hour, a below-knee amputee at 45 meters per hour, an above-knee amputee at 36 meters per hour, and a bilateral above-knee amputee at 22 meters per hour.[156] Careful evaluation of the cardiac status therefore becomes critically important.

Advanced age is not necessarily a contraindication to prosthetic fitting nor is a history of myocardial infarction from which the patient has recovered. However, special consideration must be given to these patients.

In general if the patient has walked before amputation and has learned to walk with a walker after the operation, he or she should be able to manage a below-knee prosthesis. The use of an above-knee prosthesis presents a more difficult problem since the energy cost is higher and control of the prosthetic knee requires neuromuscular coordination, which is often beyond the ability of the elderly amputee. The decision as to whether the amputee can be fitted with a prosthesis or not can often be made early in the postoperative period.

While there may be some variability in techniques for fitting prostheses, they are basically the same in all institutions. To prepare the stump for a prosthesis, a balloon pressure device is applied to decrease edema and promote healing for early fitting. The techniques of prosthetic fitting are not covered in this chapter since they are basically the same in most physical therapy departments. However, there are different types of prostheses, and the choice of a prosthesis depends on the patient's life-style. Amputees can resume many of their previous physical activities, such as bicycle riding and playing golf; even competitive golf can be accomplished.*

An important part of the rehabilitation program is the patient's understanding of the prosthesis, its capabilities and limitations. Use of the prosthesis depends to a significant degree on the patient's motivation. However, motivation alone is not enough. Many patients feel that an artificial limb will restore normal gait. They must understand that a prosthesis will feel heavy, walking will require more energy, and there will be some physical discomfort. They must learn the skill of prosthetic walking before a gait becomes automatic. Dispelling the unrealistic expectations and proper psychologic preparation are vital to prevent disappointment and rejection.

It is obvious that the total rehabilitation of the diabetic amputee requires a coordinated team (see the box on p. 708). The team required for successful rehabilitation consists initially of physicians; surgeons; diabetologists; and internists, or primary physicians, whose role must be to prepare the patient physically and emotionally for the amputation. Thus rehabilitation must begin before the amputation. Time may be a limiting factor in this preparation. Because of the emotional state associated with an impending

*Information on the proper prosthesis for the golfer can be obtained from the National Amputee Golf Association (NAGA), P.O. Box 1228, Amherst, NH 03031.

Rehabilitation team

Primary physician
Surgeon
Physical medicine expert
Physiatrist
Physical therapist
Prosthetist
Psychologist
Sex therapist
Occupational therapist
Social worker

amputation, the disturbed patient and family may be limited in their ability to understand the initial information. The surgeon must also prepare the patient and family for the amputation. The surgeon must be knowledgeable regarding future prosthetic fitting so that the bone and skin flaps will be appropriate. A psychologist, when necessary, should see these patients during the rehabilitation period to help with their emotional state and to provide reassurance and training. A physiatrist, physical therapist, and prosthetist are essential members of the team. An often neglected part of the patient's rehabilitation is instruction in how to manage sex following an amputation. A sex therapist can be a very important member of the team since emotional, esthetic, and functional difficulties related to the amputation can result. Finally, a social worker may be necessary since an amputation has a major socioeconomic impact on the patient's life-style.

SUMMARY

The pathogenesis of diabetic foot lesions is multifactorial. Physicians involved in the management of the diabetic foot must understand the pathogenesis and risk factors involved so that whenever possible the development of foot problems can be prevented or delayed. Management is complicated and consultation can help save the foot. The physician who does not seek help is not being fair to himself or herself or to the patient. Aggressive treatment of foot ulcers, the use of special shoes, and patient education have been stressed. Taking all of these factors into consideration, the goal of all physicians and clinics managing the diabetic foot should be to reduce their amputation rate by at least 50%. This goal is a realistic one and can be achieved.

REFERENCES

1. Sanders LJ: Personal communication, June 3, 1989.
2. Betts RP et al: Static and dynamic foot pressure measurements in clinical orthopaedics, Med Biol Eng Comput 18(5):674, 1980.
3. Betts RP, Franks CI, and Duckworth T: Analysis of pressures and loads under the foot. I. Quantitation of the dynamic distribution, Clin Phys Physiol Meas 1:101-12, 113-24, 1980.
4. Boulton AJM et al: Abnormalities of foot pressure in early diabetic neuropathy, Diabetic Med 4(3):225, 1987.
5. Boulton AJM et al: Dynamic foot pressure and other studies as diagnostic and management aids in diabetic neuropathy, Diabetes Care 6:26, 1983.
6. Crofford OB: Report of the National Commission on Diabetes to the Congress of the United States, U.S. Department of Health, Educational Welfare Publication NIH pub. no. 67-1018, Washington, D.C., 1975, U.S. Government Printing Office.
7. McDermott W and Rogers DE: Social ramifications of control of microbial disease, Johns Hopkins Med J 151:302, 1982.
8. Drury TF, Danchik KM, and Harris MI: Chapter VII. Sociodemographic characteristics of adult diabetes. In Harris MI and Hammer RF, eds, Diabetes in America, Bethesda, Maryland, 1985, NIH pub. no. 85-1468, p. 1.
9. Palumbo PJ and Melton LJ III: Chapter XV. Peripheral vascular disease and diabetes. In Diabetes in America: Diabetes data compiled in 1984, Washington, D.C., U.S. Government Printing Office, 1985, NIH pub. no. 85-1468, p. 1.
10. O'Brien IAD and Corrall RJM: Epidemiology of diabetes and its complications, N Engl J Med 318:1619, 1988.
11. Melton LJ III et al: Incidence and prevalence of clinical peripheral vascular disease in a population-based cohort of diabetic patients, Diabetes Care 3:650, 1980.
12. Kreines K et al: The course of peripheral vascular disease in non-insulin dependent diabetes, Diabetes Care 8(3):235, 1985.
13. Block P: The diabetic foot ulcer: a complex problem with a simple treatment approach, Milit Med 146(9):644, 1981.
14. Most RS and Sinnock P: The epidemiology of lower extremity amputations in diabetic individuals, Diabetes Care 6:87, 1983.
15. Miller AD et al: Diabetes related lower extremity amputations in New Jersey: 1979-1981, J Med Soc of New Jersey 82:723, 1985.
16. Ogbuawa B, Williams JT, and Henry WL: Diabetic gangrene in black patients, South Med J 75:285, 1982.
17. Nelson RG et al: Lower-extremity amputation in NIDDM: 12 year follow-up study in Pima Indians, Diabetes Care 11:8, 1988.
18. Bild DE et al: Lower-extremity amputation in people with diabetes: Epidemiology and prevention, Diabetes Care 12:(1)24:31, 1989.
19. Mackey WC et al: The costs of surgery for limb-threatening ischemia, Surgery 99(1):26, 1986.
20. Davidson JK et al: Assessment of program effectiveness at Grady Memorial Hospital-Atlanta. In Steiner G and Lawrence PA, eds, Educating diabetic patients, New York, 1981, Springer-Verlag.
21. Edmonds ME et al: Improved survival of the diabetic foot: The role of a specialized foot clinic, Q J Med 60(232):763, 1986.
22. Assal JP et al: Patient education as the basis for diabetes care in clinical practices, Diabetologia 28:602, 1985.
23. Mandelberg A and Sheinfeld W: Diabetic amputations: amputation of lower extremity in diabetes—analysis of one hundred twenty-eight cases, Am J Surg 71:70, 1944.
24. Levin CM and Dealy FN: The surgical diabetic: a five year survey, Ann Surg 102:1029, 1935.
25. Fearon J et al: Improved results with diabetic below-knee amputations, Arch Surg 120:777, 1985.
26. Bodily KC and Burgess EM: Contralateral limb and patient survival after leg amputation, Am J Surg 146:280, 1983.
27. Rosenberg MW and Shah DM: Bilateral blue toe syndrome: a case report, JAMA 243:365, 1980.
28. Silbert S: Amputation of the lower extremity in diabetes mellitus: a follow-up study of 294 cases, Diabetes 1:297, 1952.
29. Ecker LM and Jacobs BS: Lower extremity amputation in diabetic patients, Diabetes 19:189, 1970.
30. Marchal de Calvi CJ: Recherches sur les accidents diabeques, Paris, 1864, P. Asselin.
31. Cameron HC, Lennard-Jones JE, and Robinson MD: Amputations in the diabetic: outcome and survival, Lancet 2:605, 1964.
32. Goldner MG: The fate of the second leg in the diabetic amputee, Diabetes 9:100, 1960.

33. Hoar CF and Torres J: Evaluation of below the knee amputation and the treatment of diabetic gangrene, N Engl J Med 266:440, 1962.
34. Ebskov B and Josephsen P: Incidence of reamputation and death after gangrene of the lower extremity, Prosthet Orthot Int 4:77, 1980.
35. Larsen K, Christiansen JS, and Ebskov B: Prevention and treatment of ulcerations of the foot in unilaterally amputated diabetic patients, Acta Orthop Scand 53:481, 1982.
36. Kucan JO and Robson MC: Diabetic foot infections: fate of the contralateral foot, Plast Reconstr Surg 77:439, 1986.
37. Colwell JA et al: New concepts about the pathogenesis of atherosclerosis in diabetes mellitus. In Levin ME and O'Neal, LW, eds, The diabetic foot, ed 4, St Louis, 1988, The CV Mosby Co.
38. Janka HU, Standl E, and Mehnert H: Peripheral vascular disease in diabetes mellitus and its relation to cardiovascular risk factors: screening with Doppler ultrasonic technique, Diabetes Care 3:207, 1980.
39. Levin ME and Sicard GA: Evaluating and treating diabetic peripheral vascular disease. Part I: Clin Diab 5(3):62, 1987.
40. LoGerfo FW and Coffman JD: Vascular and microvascular disease of the foot in diabetes, N Engl J Med 311:1615, 1984.
41. Moldveen-Geromimus M and Merriam JC Jr: Cholesterol embolization: from pathologic curiosity to clinical entity, Circulation 35:946, 1967.
42. Fisher DF et al: Dilemmas in dealing with the blue toe syndrome: aortic versus peripheral source, Am J Surg 148:863, 1984.
43. Golbranson FL et al: Multiple extremity amputations in hypotensive patients treated with dopamine, JAMA 243:1145, 1980.
44. Zacharias FJ et al: Propranolol in hypertension: a study of long-term therapy, 1964-1970, Am Heart J 83:755, 1972.
45. Prentice CRM and Lowe GDO: Blood viscosity and the complications of diabetes, Adv Exp Med Biol 164:99, 1984.
46. Geiger M and Binder BR: Plasminogen activation in diabetes mellitus, J Biol Chem 259:2976, 1984.
47. Small M et al: Enhancement of fibrinolysis after insulin administration in NIDDM, Diabetes Care 9(2):216, 1989.
48. Borkenstein MH and Muntean WE: Elevated factor VIII activity and factor VIII-related antigen in diabetic children without vascular disease, Diabetes 31:1006, 1982.
49. Sargent WQ: Hemorheology. In Levin ME and O'Neal LW, eds, The diabetic foot, ed 4, St. Louis, 1988, The CV Mosby Co.
50. Belch JJF et al: The effects of acute smoking on platelet behavior, fibrinolysis and haemorheology in habitual smokers, Thromb Haemost 51(1):6, 1984.
51. Gordon T and Kannel WB: The Framingham Study: predisposition to atherosclerosis in the head, heart and legs, JAMA 221:661, 1972.
52. Allison RD and Roth GM: Central and peripheral vascular effects during cigarette smoking, Arch Environ Health 14:189, 1970.
53. Couch NP: On the arterial consequences of smoking, J Vasc Surg 3:807, 1986.
54. Pollin W: The role of the addictive process as a key step in causation of all tobacco-related disease, JAMA 252:2874, 1984.
55. Delbridge L, Appleburg M, and Reeve TS: Factors associated with the development of foot lesions in the diabetic, Surgery 93:78, 1983.
56. Juergens JL and Bernatz PE: Atherosclerosis of the extremities. In Juergens JL et al, eds, Peripheral vascular disease, Philadelphia, 1980, WB Saunders Co.
57. Kannel WB: Cigarette smoking and peripheral arterial disease, Prim Cardiol 12(3):13, 1986.
58. Fairbairn JH II and Juergens JL: The principles of medical treatment. In Juergens JL et al, eds: Peripheral vascular disease, Philadelphia, 1980, WB Saunders Co.
59. Wald N et al: Association between atherosclerotic disease and carboxy-hemoglobin levels in tobacco smokers, Br Med J 1:761, 1973.
60. Levine PH: An acute effect of cigarette smoking on platelet function: a possible link between smoking and arterial thrombosis, Circulation 48:619, 1973.
61. Beach KW and Strandness DE Jr: Arteriosclerosis obliterans and associated risk factors in insulin dependent diabetics, Diabetes 29:882, 1980.
62. Nadler JL, Velasco JS, and Horton R: Cigarette smoking inhibits prostacyclin formation, Lancet 1:1248, 1983.
63. Kaufman DW et al: Nicotine and carbon monoxide content of cigarette smoke and the risk of myocardial infarction in young men, N Engl J Med 308:409, 1983.
64. Palmer JR, Rosenberg L, and Shapiro MB: "Low yield" cigarettes and the risk of nonfatal myocardial infarction in women, N Engl J Med 320:1569, 1989.
65. Brischetto CS et al: Plasma lipid and lipoprotein profiles of cigarette smokers from randomly selected families: enhancement of hyperlipidemia and depression of high-density lipoprotein, Am J Cardiol 52:675, 1983.
66. Klemp P and Stagbert B: Smoking reduces insulin absorption from subcutaneous tissue, Br Med J 284:237, 1982.
67. Pirart J: Diabetes mellitus and its degenerative complications: a prospective study of 4,400 patients observed between 1947 and 1973. II, Diabetes Care 1:252, 1978.
68. Vaccaro O et al: Peripheral arterial circulation in individuals with impaired glucose tolerance, Diabetes Care 8(6):594, 1985.
69. Lorenzi M, Cagliero E, and Toledo S: Glucose toxicity for human endothelial cells in culture: delayed replication, disturbed cell cycle, and accelerated death, Diabetes 34:621, 1985.
70. Weimann BJ, Lorch E, and Baumgartner HR: High glucose concentrations do not influence replication and prostacyclin release of human endothelial cells, Diabetologia 27:62, 1984.
71. Brownlee M, Cerami A, and Vlassara H: Advanced glycosylation end products in tissue and the biochemical basis of diabetic complications, N Engl J Med 318(20):1315, 1988.
72. Capron L et al: Growth-promoting effects of diabetes and insulin on arteries: an in-vivo study of rat aorta, Diabetes 35:973, 1986.
73. Sato Y et al: Experimental atherosclerosis-like lesions induced by hyperinsulinism in Wistar rats, Diabetes 38:91, 1989.
74. Zavaroni I et al: Risk factors for coronary artery disease in healthy persons with hyperinsulinemia and normal glucose tolerance, N Engl J Med 320(11):702, 1989.
75. Larson DM and Haudenschild CC: Activation of smooth muscle cell outgrowth from BB/Wor rat aortas, Diabetes 37:1380, 1988.
76. Lapidus L et al: Distribution of adipose tissue and risk of cardiovascular disease and death: a 12 year follow-up of participants in the population study of women in Gothenburg, Sweden, Br Med J (Clin Res) 289:1257, 1984.
77. Haffner SM et al: Hyperinsulinemia, upper body adiposity and cardiovascular risk factors in non-diabetics, Metabolism 37:333, 1988.
78. Anderson AJ et al: Body fat distribution, plasma lipids, and lipoproteins, Arteriosclerosis 8:88, 1988.
79. Peiris AN et al: Adiposity, fat distribution, and cardiovascular risk, Ann Intern Med 110:867, 1989.
80. Brand FN, Abbott RD, and Kannel WB: Diabetes, intermittent claudication, and risk of cardiovascular events: the Framingham Study, Diabetes 38:504, 1989.
81. Jonason T et al: Effect of physical training on different categories of patients with intermittent claudication, Acta Med Scand 206:253, 1979.
82. Lippmann HI: The foot of the diabetic. In Brodoff BM and Bleicher SJ, eds: Diabetes mellitus and obesity, Baltimore, 1982, Williams & Wilkins.
83. Malan E and Tattoni G: Physio-anatomopathology of acute ischemia of the extremities, J Cardiovasc Surg 4:212, 1963.
84. Brownlee M, Vlassara H, and Cerami A: Trapped immunoglobulins on peripheral nerve myelin from patients with diabetes mellitus, Diabetes 35:999, 1986.
85. Greene DA, Lattimer SA, and Sima AAF: Sorbitol, phosphoinositides, and sodium-potassium-ATPase in the pathogenesis of diabetic complications, N Engl J Med 316(10):599, 1987.

86. Harati Y: Diabetic peripheral neuropathies, Ann Intern Med 107:546, 1987.
87. Sima AAF et al: Regeneration and repair of myelinated fibers in sural-nerve biopsy specimens from patients with diabetic neuropathy treated with sorbinil, N Engl J Med 319(9):548, 1988.
88. Dyck PJ et al: Nerve glucose, fructose, sorbitol, myo-inositol, and fiber degeneration and regeneration in diabetic neuropathy, N Engl J Med 319(9):542, 1988.
89. Griffey RH et al: Diabetic neuropathy: structural analysis of nerve hydration by magnetic resonance spectroscopy, JAMA 260(19):2872, 1988.
90. Greene DA: Neuropathy in the diabetic foot: new concepts in etiology and treatemnt. In Levin ME and O'Neal LW, eds: The diabetic foot, ed 4, St. Louis, 1988, The CV Mosby Co.
91. Aguayo AJ: Neuropathy due to compression and entrapment. In Dyck PJ, Thomas PK, and Lambert EH, eds: Peripheral neuropathy, Philadelphia, 1975, WB Saunders Co.
92. Parkhouse N and LeQuesne PM: Impaired neurogenic vascular response in patients with diabetes and neurogenic foot lesions, N Engl J Med 318:1306, 1988.
93. Boehm JJ: Diabetic charcot's joint, N Engl J Med 267:185, 1962.
94. Sinha SK, Frykberg RG, and Kozak GP: Neuroarthropathy in the diabetic foot. In Kozak GP, ed: Clinical diabetes mellitus, Philadelphia, 1982, WB Saunders Co.
95. Boulton AJM, Scarpello JHB, and Ward JD: Venous oxygenation in the diabetic neuropathic foot: evidence of arterial venous shunting, Diabetologia 22:6, 1981.
96. Robillard R, Gagnon P, and Alaries R: Diabetic neuroarthropathy: a report of four cases, Can Med Assoc J 91:795, 1964.
97. Edelman SV et al: Neuroosteoarthropathy (Charcot's joint) in diabetes mellitus following revascularization surgery: three case reports and a review of the literature, Arch Intern Med 147:1504, 1987.
98. Splittgerber GF, et al: Combined leukocyte and bone imaging used to evaluate diabetic osteoarthropathy and osteomyelitis, Clin Nucl Med 14:156, 1989.
99. Schauwecker DS et al: Combined bone scintigraphy and Indium-III leukocyte scans in neuropathic foot disease, J Nucl Med 29:1651, 1988.
100. Klamer TW et al: The influence of sepsis and ischemia on the natural history of the diabetic foot, Am Surg 53:490, 1987.
101. O'Neal LW: Debridement and amputation. In Levin ME and O'Neal LW, eds, The diabetic foot, ed 4, St. Louis, 1988, The CV Mosby Co.
102. Sapico FL et al: The infected foot of the diabetic patient: quantitative microbiology and analysis of clinical features, Rev Infect Dis 6(suppl 1):S171, March-April, 1984.
103. Finegold SM: Anaerobic bacteria: their role in infection and their management, Postgrad Med 81(8):141, 1987.
104. Little JR and Kobayashi GS: Infection of the diabetic foot. In Levin ME and O'Neal LW, eds: The diabetic foot, ed 4, St. Louis, 1988, The CV Mosby Co.
105. Peterson LR et al: Therapy of lower extremity infections with ciprofloxacin in patients with diabetes mellitus, peripheral vascular disease, or both, Am J Med 86:801, 1989.
106. Ellenberg M: Treatment of diabetic neuropathy with diphenylhydantoin, New York State J Med 68:2653, 1968.
107. Saudek CD, Werns S, and Reidenberg MM: Phenytoin in the treatment of diabetic symmetrical polyneuropathy, Clin Pharmacol Ther 22(2):196, 1977.
108. Rull JA et al: Symptomatic treatment of peripheral diabetic neuropathy with carbamazepine (Tegretol): double blind crossover trial, Diabetologia 5:215, 1969.
109. Davis JL et al: Peripheral diabetic neuropathy treated with amitriptyline and fluphenazine, JAMA 238:2291, 1977.
110. Veith RC et al: Cardiovascular effects of tricyclic antidepressants in depressed patients with chronic heart disease, N Engl J Med 306:954, 1982.
111. Girardina EV et al: The electrocardiographic and antiarrhythmic effects of imipramine hydrochloride at therapeutic plasma concentrations, Circulation 60:1045, 1979.
112. Ward JDN: Improvement in motor nerve conduction following treatment in newly diagnosed diabetics. In Camerini-Davalos RA and Cole HS, eds: Vascular and neurologic changes in early diabetes, New York, 1973, Academic Press, Inc.
113. Winegard AI and Greene DA: Diabetic polyneuropathy: the importance of insulin deficiency, hyperglycemia and alterations in myoinositol metabolism in its pathogenesis. N Engl J Med 295:1416, 1976.
114. Cohen KL and Harris S: Pentoxifylline and diabetic neuropathy: Letter to the editor, Ann Intern Med 107(4):600, 1987.
115. Kalmansohn RB et al: Treatment of diabetic neuropathy with pentoxifylline: case report, Angiology 39(4):371, 1988.
116. Newrick PG et al: Clinicopathological correlates of human diabetic neuropathy (abstract), Diabetes 36(suppl 1):86A, 1987.
117. Cohen KL and Harris S: Efficacy and safety of nonsteroidal anti-inflammatory drugs in the therapy of diabetic neuropathy, Arch Intern Med 147:1442, Aug 1987.
118. Dejgard A, Petersen P, and Kastrup J: Mexiletine for treatment of chronic painful diabetic neuropathy, Lancet 2:9, 1988.
119. Holzer P: Peppers, capsaicin and the gastric mucosa: Letter to the editor, JAMA 261(22):3244, 1989.
120. Chad DA et al: Treatment of painful diabetic neuropathy with topical capsaicin: a double-blind multicenter investigation, Diab. Program of the 49th Annual Meeting of The American Diabetes Association 38(suppl 2):26A, June 1989 (abstract 104).
121. Melzack R and Wall PD: Pain mechanisms: a new theory, Science 150:971, 1965.
122. Cohen SJ: Potential barriers to diabetes care, Diabetes Care 6:499, 1983.
123. Bailey TS, Yu HM, and Rayfield EJ: Patterns of foot examination in a diabetes clinic, Am J Med 78:371, 1985.
124. Allen GE and Hadden DR: Bullous lesions of the skin in diabetes (bullous diabeticorum), Br J Dermatol 82:216, 1970.
125. Jelinek JE, ed: Diabetes and the skin, Philadelphia, 1985, Lea & Febiger.
126. Guy RJC et al: Evaluation of thermal and vibration sensation in diabetic neuropathy, Diabetologia 28:131, 1985.
127. Fruhstorfer H, Lindblom U, and Schmidt WG: Method for quantitative estimation of thermal thresholds in patients, J Neurol Neurosurg Psychiatry 39:1071, 1976.
128. Coffman JD: Vasodilator drugs in peripheral vascular disease, N Engl J Med 300:713, 1979.
129. Roeren T, LeVeen RF, and Nugent L: Photoplethysmographic documentation of improved microcirculation after Pentoxifylline therapy, Angiology 39(11):929, 1988.
130. Schwartz RW et al: Pentoxifylline increases extremity blood flow in diabetic atherosclerotic patients, Arch Surg 124(4):434, 1989.
131. Franzini E, Martin FM, and Chan MT: Leukocyte filterability: its measurement in the laboratory and effects of pentoxifylline, Clin Hemorheology 8:477, 1988.
132. Matrai A and Ernst E: Pentoxifylline improves white cell rheology in claudicants, Clin Hemorheology 5:483, 1985.
133. Ferrari E et al: Effects of long-term treatment (4 years) with pentoxifylline on heamorhoeological changes and vascular complications in diabetic patients, Pharmatherapeutica 5(1):26, 1987.
134. Davidson CJ et al: Cardiovascular and renal toxicity of a nonionic radiographic contrast agent after cardiac catheterization: a prospective trial, Ann Intern Med 110:119, 1989.
135. Schwab SJ et al: Contrast nephrotoxicity: a randomized controlled trial of a nonionic and an ionic radiographic contrast agent, N Engl J Med 320:149, 1989.
136. Parfrey PS et al: Contrast material-induced renal failure insufficiency, or both: a prospective controlled study, N Engl J Med 320:143, 1989.

137. Cigarroa RG et al: Dosing of contrast material to prevent contrast nephropathy in patients with renal disease 86:649, 1989.
138. Schwarten DE and Cutcliff WB: Arterial occlusive disease below the knee: treatment with percutaneous transluminal angioplasty performed with low profile catheters and steerable guide wires, Radiology 169:71, 1988.
139. Taylor LM Jr and Porter JM: The clinical course of diabetics who require emergent foot surgery because of infection or ischemia, J Vasc Surg 6:454, 1987.
140. Levin ME and Spratt IL: To soak or not to soak, Clin Diabetes 4:44, 1986.
141. Boulton AJM et al: Use of plaster casts in the management of diabetic neuropathic foot ulcers, Diabetes Care 9:149, 1986.
142. Helm PA, Walker SC, and Pullium G: Total contact casting in diabetic patients with neuropathic foot ulcers, Arch Phys Med Rehabil 65:691, 1984.
143. Mueller MJ et al: Total contact casting in treatment of diabetic plantar ulcers: controlled clinical trial, Diabetes Care 12(6):384, 1989.
144. Sinacore DR: Total contact casting in the treatment of diabetic neuropathic ulcers. In Levin ME and O'Neal LW, eds, The diabetic foot, ed 4, St. Louis, 1988, The CV Mosby Co.
145. Sage R and Doyle D: Surgical treatment of diabetic foot ulcers: a review of forty-eight cases, J Foot Surg 23:102, 1984.
146. Diamond E et al: The effect of hyperbaric oxygen on lower extremity ulcerations, J Am Podiatr Med Assoc 72:180, 1982.
147. Heng MCY, Pilgrim JP, and Beck FW: A simplified hyperbaric oxygen technique for leg ulcers, Arch Dermatol 120:640, 1984.
148. Leslie CA, et al: Randomized controlled trial of topical hyperbaric oxygen for treatment of diabetic foot ulcers, Diabetes Care 11(2):111, 1988.
149. Baroni G et al: Hyperbaric oxygen in diabetic gangrene treatment, Diabetes Care 10:(1)81, 1987.
150. Knighton DR et al: Classification and treatment of chronic nonhealing wounds: successful treatment with autologous platelet-derived wound healing factors (PDWHF), Ann Surg 204:322, 1986.
151. Coleman WC: Footwear in a management program of injury prevention. In Levin ME and O'Neal LW, eds, The diabetic foot, ed 4, St. Louis, 1988, The CV Mosby Co.
152. Bernstein RK: Two tips for care of the diabetic foot, Diabetes Care 8:525, 1985.
153. Soulier SM: The use of running shoes in the prevention of plantar diabetic ulcers, J Am Podiatr Med Assoc 76:395, 1986.
154. Lippmann HI: Must loss of limb be a consequence of diabetes mellitus, Diabetes Care 2:432, Sept-Oct 1979.
155. Miller LV: Evaluation of patient education: Los Angeles County Hospital experience, report of National Commission on diabetes to the Congress of the United States, U.S. Department of Health, Education and Welfare, NIH pub. no. 76-1021, Vol 3, Part V, Washington, D.C., 1975.
156. Steinberg FU: Rehabilitation of the diabetic amputee and neuropathic disabilities. In Levin ME and O'Neal LW, eds, The diabetic foot, ed 4, St. Louis, 1988, The CV Mosby Co.

Chapter 39

THE MANAGEMENT OF SYNTHETIC GRAFT INFECTION FOLLOWING ABDOMINAL AORTIC AND LOWER EXTREMITY ARTERIAL RECONSTRUCTION

Patrick J. O'Hara

Arterial reconstruction for the treatment of aneurysmal or occlusive disease of the aortoiliac and femoral distal systems has allowed longer and more productive lives for countless patients since the introduction of vascular surgery more than 35 years ago. Initially, arterial reconstruction was limited to procedures utilizing autogenous tissue alone. However, these methods, which include endarterectomy as well as bypass and patch angioplasty using arterial or venous graft material, have significant limitations. While still the ideal graft material for use in many situations such as femorodistal bypass operations, autogenous arterial substitutes may not be uniformly available or adequate. The long-term durability of endarterectomy, especially in infrainguinal arterial reconstructions, has often been disappointing. Furthermore, autogenous reconstruction is rarely an option in the treatment of patients with aortoiliac aneurysmal disease. Consequently, the introduction of high-quality synthetic arterial graft material has enormously increased the versatility and durability of many vascular reconstructions.

A serious liability associated with synthetic graft material, however, is its susceptibility to infection. Although its incidence is low, arterial prosthetic graft infection is one of the most feared complications in vascular surgery because its management is usually difficult and involves significant risks of mortality and morbidity.[1]

It is likely that the number of synthetic vascular reconstructions required will probably continue to increase because of the aging population with its reservoir of arterial disease and increasing reliance on interventional techniques. Furthermore, as the useful life expectancy of patients with treated vascular disease increases, the population with implanted synthetic grafts requiring reoperation for revision or disease progression will also grow. As a result, although the incidence of arterial prosthetic graft infection is low, the physician caring for patients with vascular disease should anticipate the need for guidelines in the management of synthetic graft infections.

Because of the substantial morbidity associated with the current standard treatment of arterial prosthetic graft infection, considerable controversy exists regarding the optimal management of such patients. Much of this controversy appears to center upon the definition and extent of synthetic graft sepsis. Szilagyi et al[2] characterized arterial prosthetic graft sepsis on the basis of the depth of clinical wound infections. Grade I patients were those in whom only the dermis was affected. Grade II patients had wound infections extending into the subcutaneous tissue without directly involving the arterial implant. Among Grade III patients the synthetic arterial graft was grossly involved in the infection. All Grade I and II patients healed without difficulty and probably did not have actual arterial prosthetic graft sepsis. All of the significant morbidity in the Szilagyi et al series was observed among the Grade III patients. Other factors that are likely to influence the clinical course of patients with synthetic arterial infection include the virulence of the microorganism involved, the size of the inoculum, the extent of synthetic graft and native tissue involvement, the quality of the host response, and the adequacy of antimicrobial and surgical therapy. For the purposes of this analysis, arterial prosthetic graft infection is defined as the contamination of synthetic graft material with a sufficient inoculum of microorganisms to allow its colonization.

ANATOMIC CLASSIFICATION AND INCIDENCE

The reported rate of occurrence of prosthetic graft infection depends upon the anatomic location of the implanted synthetic. The incidence of graft infection involving the abdominal aorta is documented in several series to range from 0.27% to 2.34%. When arterial reconstruction is confined to the aortoiliac system, requiring only an abdominal or flank incision, the reported incidence ranges from 0% to 1.2%. However, if aortofemoral reconstruction, which requires one or more additional groin incisions, is performed, the reported incidence is greater, ranging from 0.47% to 3.0% (Table 39-1).[2-9] In the Cleveland Clinic experience, from 1961 through February 1985, the overall incidence of aortic prosthetic graft infection irrespective of groin incision requirement was 0.77%.[7,8] This figure should be regarded as a minimum value since it is possible that some patients who acquired graft infection at the Cleveland Clinic may have subsequently sought treatment elsewhere. If the synthetic vascular reconstruction was confined to the aortoiliac region, requiring only an abdominal or flank incision, the incidence of graft infection was 0.43%. However, if extension to the femoral region was required, the incidence of graft sepsis rose significantly ($P < 0.01$) to 1.34%. In general, extension of an aortic synthetic reconstruction to the femoral region appears to increase the risk of graft sepsis by a factor of 2 to 3 (Table 39-1).

Patients with associated graft enteric communications form an important subgroup of those with aortic graft infection.[10,11] Among this group with graft enteric fistulae, exposure of the prosthetic material to the lumen of the gastrointestinal tract has taken place. While graft enteric communication can occur in any portion of the gastrointestinal tract, the most common site involves the proximal aortic anastomotic region and the fourth portion of the duodenum. The minimal institutional incidence of graft enteric fistula formation in the Cleveland Clinic series was 0.36% (13/3652) of aortic reconstructions.[7,8]

In the femoroperipheral position, including femorofem-

Table 39-1. Incidence of prosthetic graft infection in the aortoiliofemoroperipheral positions in seven published reports

Author	Year	No. of patients	Graft location	No. of infections	Incidence (%)
Hoffert, Gensler, and Haimovici[3]	1965	128	AI and AF	2	1.56
		69	FP	9	13.0
Fry and Lindenauer[4]	1967	890	AI and AF	12	1.34
Szilagyi et al[2]	1972	1662	AI and AF	23	1.38
		418	AI	3	0.7
		1244	AF	20	1.6
		380	FP	9	2.4
Goldstone and Moore[5]	1974	423	AI and AF	9	2.13
		163	AI	2	1.2
		260	AF	7	3.0
		54	FP	2	3.7
Lorentzen et al[6]	1985	1922	AI and AF	45	2.34
		425	AI	0	0
		1497	AF	45	3.0
		489	FP	17	3.5
O'Hara et al[7,8]	1986	3652	AI and AF	28	0.77
		2306	AI	10	0.43
		1346	AF	18	1.34
Edwards et al[9]	1987	1829	AI and AF	5	0.27
		769	AI	0	0
		1060	AF	5	0.47
		583	FP	17	2.9

AI, Aortoiliac.
AF, Aortofemoral.
FP, Femoroperipheral.

oral transpubic reconstructions when the data are reported, the published incidence of prosthetic graft infection ranges from 2.4% to 13% (Table 39-1).[2,3,5,6,9] The observed increase in the rate of graft sepsis involving infrainguinal reconstructions probably reflects the larger proportion of operations requiring a groin incision. Other factors probably include the closer proximity of the synthetic graft to the body surface as well as to infected ischemic lesions involving the lower extremity.

NATURAL HISTORY

It has been a longstanding surgical observation that, once entrenched, sepsis tends to persist in the region of a foreign body until the infected foreign material is removed. Correspondingly, when synthetic graft sepsis is established, microorganisms are able to thrive in the avascular interstices of the graft material where blood-borne antibiotics and host defenses are unable to penetrate in sufficient concentration to completely eradicate them.

For a variable time, the synthetic graft material colonized by the microorganisms in the host tissues may coexist in symbiotic balance. However, if the original inoculum is large or if the population of infecting microorganisms overwhelms host defenses, the sepsis may progress along the synthetic graft. The rate of progression probably depends on at least three factors: (1) the size of the infecting inoculum, (2) the virulence of the infecting organism, and (3) the quality of the local environment. The graft environmental quality is related to its incorporation, local vascularity, local antibiotic concentration, and host resistance. A large inoculum of a virulent organism in the presence of a compromised host and fresh nonincorporated graft will likely lead to rapid progression. In contrast, a small inoculum of an indolent organism involving a well-incorporated graft in a noncompromised host may be tolerated for an extended period.

The consequences of established synthetic graft infection that has progressed sufficiently to be clinically apparent include both local and systemic effects. When local sepsis has progressed to the anastomosis of the synthetic graft to involve the native artery, proteolytic enzymes weaken the host vessel at the suture line, leading to separation, leak, and pseudoaneurysm formation. Further progression of this process can lead to complete anastomotic disruption with massive hemorrhage. Other late systemic effects of sepsis include bacteremia and septic emboli from continuous seeding of the intravascular space from the infected arterial prosthesis. Eventually, metastatic abscess formation may be observed. As the septic process overwhelms the host, multisystem failure may eventuate in death.

To interrupt this downward spiral, the septic focus must be identified and eliminated early while the host organism, with adequate support, can still respond. Consequently, if prosthetic graft sepsis is clearly established, removal of the infected synthetic material and adequate débridement and drainage is usually required. In a clinical setting, however, accurate determination of the extent of graft sepsis is often difficult.

ETIOLOGY AND PATHOGENESIS

Etiology, defined as the cause of disease, may be contrasted with pathogenesis, defined as the mode of origin or development of a morbid process. The etiologic agent of clinical graft infections is usually single or multiple bacteria, although fungal graft infections are being reported with increasing frequency.[12-14] Ultimately, the mechanism of prosthetic graft infection involves the contamination of the synthetic material with a sufficient inoculum of microorganisms to allow its colonization. The prosthetic contamination may be primary, occurring at the time of implantation, or secondary, occurring at a later time after a period of sterile function. While occasionally obvious, it may be nearly impossible to differentiate primary contamination with an indolent organism from secondary contamination.

Primary contamination of a prosthetic arterial graft may occur directly because of a break in sterile technique at the time of surgical implantation. The graft itself may be contaminated if the package integrity is violated or the graft sterilization is outdated. Other potential sources of synthetic graft contamination at the time of implantation include contact with the skin, bacteria in lymphatic channels, especially in the inguinal region in the presence of lower extremity lesions, and hematogenous seeding from bacteremia.

A previously noninfected graft may become secondarily infected as a result of direct contamination in either the early or late postoperative period. In the early postoperative period, synthetic graft exposure to the environment may occur as a result of wound complications, such as superficial wound infection or fat necrosis, especially in the femoral region in obese individuals. Chronic serous drainage from groin incisions, or lymph fistulae, may lead to secondary infection of underlying synthetic graft material. Mechanical erosion of the overlying skin, especially if the graft is tunneled too superficially in thin individuals, may also lead to skin slough and graft exposure. In the late postoperative period, the synthetic graft may be directly contaminated by extension of an adjacent abscess to the synthetic material, such as in the presence of acute appendicitis or diverticulitis. Alternatively, exposure of the body or shaft of the graft to the lumen of the gastrointestinal tract, or graft-enteric erosion, may cause late direct secondary graft infection. Indirect contamination of a prosthetic arterial graft may occur by hematogenous seeding from bacteremia. Some evidence suggests that large arterial prostheses may not become entirely endothelialized in humans even after several months.[15] Other experimental evidence from a study using a canine model suggests that synthetic graft material has continued susceptibility to colonization from bacteremic origin probably because of incomplete healing.[16] Graft colonization

Table 39-2. Culture results among patients with infected arterial prosthetic grafts in the aortoiliofemoral region in seven published reports

Author	Year	No. of patients	Graft location	Staphylococcal species (%)	Nonstaphylococcal species (%)	Unknown/no growth (%)
Fry and Lindenauer[4]	1967	12	AI and AF	67	25	8
Conn et al[18]	1970	11	AI and AF	27	73	0
		7	FP	43	57	0
Szilagyi et al[2]	1972	29	AI and AF	45	48	7
		10	FP	50	30	20
Goldstone and Moore[5]	1974	27	AI, AF, and FP	67	26	7
Bandyk et al[19]	1984	30	AF	50	40	10
Lorentzen et al[6]	1985	62	AF and FP	74	21	5
O'Hara et al[7,8]	1986	84	AI and AF	35	46	19

AI, Aortoiliac.
AF, Aortofemoral.
FP, Femoroperipheral.

from bacteremia appears to be especially likely in the first few weeks after implantation into the canine model.[17]

BACTERIOLOGY

The culture results among patients with infected arterial prosthetic grafts in the aortoiliofemoral region in seven published reports spanning the years 1967 through 1986 are summarized in Table 39-2.[2,4-8,18,19] Staphylococcal species, either alone or in combination with other organisms, were isolated in 27% to 74% of the patients reported. Nonstaphylococcal species accounted for 21% to 73% of the positive cultures. With the exception of one series, in which identifiable microorganisms were isolated from all patients with clinical graft infection, the remaining series had incidences from 5% to 20% of unknown or no-growth culture results despite clinical evidence of graft infection. This observed disparity in culture results emphasizes the difficulty inherent in comparing culture data obtained from patients with synthetic graft infection over widely varying times. The culture results may be influenced by the culture method used, the antibiotic therapy employed, the anatomic location of the graft, and the mechanism of graft inoculation, among other factors.

The role of bacterial culture results in the diagnosis and treatment of prosthetic graft infection is complicated by the fact that microorganisms can be isolated from arterial tissue and explanted arterial synthetic grafts in the absence of clinical signs of graft sepsis. Ernst et al reported a 15% incidence of positive cultures of aneurysm contents and an 11% incidence of positive intestinal bag content cultures among patients undergoing abdominal aortic aneurysm repair. Gram-positive organisms comprised 81% of the isolates, with *Staphylococcus epidermidis* being most common. However, the incidence of clinical graft sepsis in that series was only 2.5%.[20] Ilgenfritz and Jordan reported 19.6% of 56 patients undergoing abdominal aortic aneurysm repair yielded positive aneurysm wall and content cultures, but no patient developed clinical graft sepsis over a mean 24.5-month follow-up period. Again, *S. epidermidis* was the most common microorganism isolated in 6 of 11 patients.[21] Similarly, McAuley, Steed, and Webster reported a 14% incidence of positive cultures among 64 patients operated on for abdominal aortic aneurysm, with no graft infections observed over a 25-month follow-up period. Of the microorganisms, 73% were gram-positive, and most were sensitive to the prophylactic antibiotic given.[22] In an interesting study, MacBeth et al cultured the arterial walls of 88 patients undergoing clean elective arterial reconstructive procedures yielding positive cultures in 43%. The most common organism isolated was *S. epidermidis* in 71% of the positive cultures.[23]

Brook, in a 10-year review of specimens of aortofemoral graft infection, documented the presence of anaerobic bacteria in 13 of 16 specimens (81%).[24] Specialized culture techniques are required to isolate these fastidious organisms. Whether these organisms represent the cause of the graft sepsis or secondary contamination from a gastrointestinal or genitourinary source remains speculative.

More recent studies have emphasized the importance of *S. epidermidis* in the pathophysiology of late prosthetic graft infection. Prosthetic material may be colonized by slime-producing, low-virulence microorganisms, such as *S. epidermidis*, as a bacteria-laden biofilm at the time of implantation. This biofilm, consisting of a polysaccharide matrix referred to as *glycocalyx*, permits adhesion to the biomaterial surface and protects the microorganism from host defenses.[25] The relatively low number of microorganism colonies localized in the adherent biofilm may lie dormant for long periods, living in a symbiotic relationship with the host organism without inciting an inflammatory response. Routine microbiologic culture techniques will often fail to grow bacteria, perhaps accounting for some of the unknown or no-growth culture results listed in Table 39-2. Specialized microbiologic culture techniques designed to disrupt the biofilm are necessary to recover organisms from the involved prosthetic material.[26] *S. epidermidis* has been shown to be

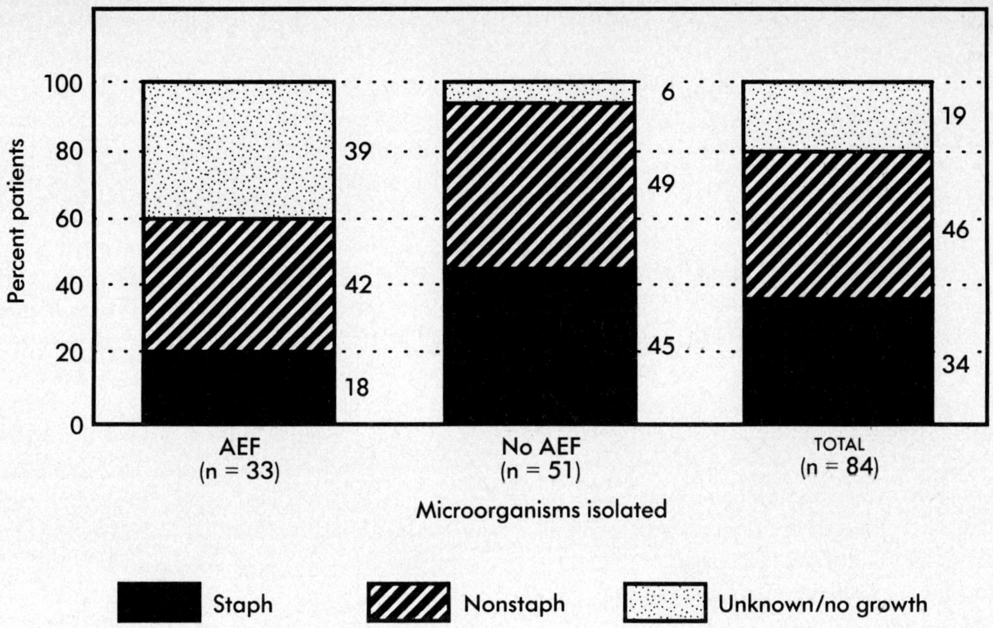

Fig. 39-1. Microorganisms isolated from patients with abdominal aortic graft sepsis treated at the Cleveland Clinic, 1961-1985. (*AEF*, Aortoenteric fistula; *Staph*, staphylococcal species.) (Data from O'Hara PJ et al, J Vasc Surg 3:725, 1986.)

capable of producing acute graft infections with perigraft inflammation and anastomotic disruption.[27] Kaebnick et al[25] studied synthetic graft material from aortofemoral and femoropopliteal reconstructions that showed no clinical evidence of graft infection but did require revision for pseudoaneurysm formation or graft thrombosis. A sensitive culture method using tryptic soy broth and ultrasonic oscillation to disrupt the adherent graft surface biofilm was used. Microorganisms were isolated from 79% of the graft samples, and *S. epidermidis* was the prevalent isolate. Microorganisms were isolated from 90% of the pseudoaneurysm grafts and 69% of thrombosed grafts, leading the authors to conclude that low-virulence organisms can colonize vascular prostheses and not provoke signs of graft infection. They proposed that anastomotic pseudoaneurysm may be the sequela of a bacteria-laden biofilm infection.[25] Bergamini, using a canine model, tested the feasibility of excision of an *S. epidermidis*-infected vascular prosthesis followed by immediate in situ replacement with another synthetic prosthesis. He concluded that prosthetic replacement of Dacron prosthesis infected by *S. epidermidis* as a bacteria-laden biofilm can result in early graft healing, but persistent colonization of one third of replacement grafts signifies that recurrent clinical infection remains a risk.[28]

Another factor that may influence the disparity of reported culture results is the mechanism of graft infection. Series including a high proportion of patients whose graft infections are secondary to aortoenteric fistulae or contamination from a genitourinary source are likely to report a high incidence of gram-negative bacterial isolates.

Microorganisms isolated by standard culture techniques in a series of 84 patients with infected abdominal aortic grafts managed at the Cleveland Clinic from 1961 through February 1985 are summarized in Fig. 39-1.[7,8] In the entire series, the predominant organism was *Staphylococcus*, which either alone or in combination with other organisms was isolated from 34% of the patients. Nonstaphylococcal organisms, isolated from 46% of the patients, consisted of *Serratia*, *Proteus*, *Escherichia coli*, *Pseudomonas*, *Klebsiella*, *Enterobacter*, *Bacteroides*, α-hemolytic *Streptococcus*, *Citrobacter*, Enterococcus, *Salmonella*, and *Candida*. Nineteen percent had either unknown organisms or no growth and probably included some missed biofilm-laden graft infections. When the subset of patients with aortoenteric fistulae is contrasted to the group without this complication, the nonstaphylococcal isolate percentage remains about the same. However, the aortoenteric fistulae group has a lower incidence of staphylococcal microorganism isolation (18% vs 45%) and a higher incidence (39% vs 6%) of unknown organisms or no growth. The entire significance of this finding is not fully explained but probably reflects differing mechanisms of graft contamination. Aortoenteric fistulae probably occur because of erosion of the synthetic graft into the lumen of the adjacent bowel, whereas aortic graft infection in the absence of aortoenteric fistula formation likely represents contamination from a nonenteric source.

Geary et al, in a canine study comparing the effects of graft infection involving autogenous vein and polytetrafluoroethylene when infected with *S. epidermidis* or *Pseudomonas aeruginosa*, emphasized the relative importance of the infecting organism in the outcome of graft sepsis. The authors concluded that *S. epidermidis* is a less virulent organism that may persist in graft walls, despite negative cultures, whereas *P. aeruginosa* is a highly virulent organism that can disrupt native artery and vein grafts and anastomoses.[29]

PREDISPOSING FACTORS

Factors that predispose to synthetic graft infection may be viewed as patient-related or procedure-related features. Patient factors refer to characteristics of the individual patient with vascular disease and are independent of the surgical procedure itself. Technical factors relate to the characteristics of the surgical procedure and its sequelae.

The major patient factors are obesity, associated systemic illness, poor nutritional status, and a bacteremic source. Obesity has long been recognized to contribute to an increased incidence of perioperative complications. Wound complications are common because increased retraction is required, and procedures require more time than usual. Furthermore, thick subcutaneous tissue is relatively avascular and provides a favorable environment for bacterial growth. Thick intertriginous folds, especially in the groin area, interfere with optimal surgical skin preparation and later with wound hygiene. Wound complications in the groin region can lead to involvement of the underlying synthetic material. Associated systemic illness, such as diabetes mellitus or chronic renal failure, may be associated with poor wound healing characteristics and impaired host defenses. Poor nutritional status is often observed among patients with vascular disease, who are often elderly and debilitated. This can lead to hypoproteinemia and anergy, predisposing to poor wound healing and diminished resistance to infection. Kwaan, Dahl, and Connolly[30] reported on deficiencies in the immune status (as estimated by serum albumin levels, total lymphocyte counts, immunoglobin assays, and cutaneous sensitivity tests) of 12 patients with clinical prosthetic graft sepsis. Adjunctive parenteral nutritional support produced enhancement of immune responses and accelerated recovery. Finally, patients with peripheral vascular disease commonly exhibit sources of bacteremia, such as ischemic septic foci in the lower extremity. Local sepsis should be controlled by drainage and débridement, in addition to appropriate antibiotic coverage, before synthetic arterial reconstruction to minimize systemic bacteremia.

Technical factors that, in theory, predispose to the development of synthetic graft sepsis include breaks in sterile technique, emergency operation, the need for reoperation, prolonged operative time, the requirement for a groin incision, and technical misadventures. Adequate sterile technique requires attention to detail to avoid contamination. Emergency operations are frequently associated with both hemorrhage and hypoperfusion and may require rapid prepping and draping. Extra vigilance is required in the emergency setting. The relationship of the need for reoperation to prosthetic graft sepsis is not as clear. In the Cleveland Clinic series of abdominal aortic graft infections, patients who had aortoenteric fistulae had 1.3 reoperations before the onset of sepsis, whereas patients who had nonaortoenteric fistulae had 2.3 reoperations.[7,8] This observation suggests that contamination at the time of reoperation may play a role in the pathogenesis of aortic graft infections not associated with aortoenteric fistula. Durham, Malone, and Bernhard[31] reported that positive arterial cultures obtained at the initial vascular reconstruction had no predictive value regarding the development of subsequent graft infection. In contrast, positive arterial cultures obtained at a subsequent vascular operation were associated with a significant increase in the incidence of graft infection in that group. Long-term antibiotic therapy was suggested for the latter group. Prolonged operative time exposes the wound and synthetic graft to ambient bacteria for a long period, increasing the inoculum of microorganisms. The requirement for a groin incision, as described earlier, increases the incidence of graft infection by a factor of approximately two. Technical misadventures, leading to injury of the gastrointestinal or genitourinary tracts, can expose the prosthetic graft material to contamination from these sources. A history of previous abdominal surgery may increase the risk of enterotomy and may indicate consideration of alternative methods of exposure, such as the retroperitoneal approach to the abdominal aorta in selected patients.

CLINICAL MANIFESTATIONS

The clinical manifestations and course of prosthetic graft infection may be quite variable. Patients may develop systemic or local symptoms occurring early or late in the course of the graft infection. Furthermore, the clinical course may be rapid and fulminant or long and indolent. In addition, some patients who initially exhibit a less aggressive clinical picture may progress rapidly to a major complication such as rupture of an anastomotic pseudoaneurysm or massive gastrointestinal hemorrhage. These variations probably depend on the interaction of several variables such as the size of the inoculum and virulence of the infecting microorganism, host resistance, mechanism of graft infection, and the anastomotic location of the involved prosthetic graft.

The initial symptoms and physical findings observed among a series of 84 patients with abdominal aortic prosthetic graft infection managed at the Cleveland Clinic from 1961 through February 1985 are presented in Fig. 39-2.[7,8] Fever was the most common symptom demonstrated by 42% of the entire series. Gastrointestinal bleeding occurred in 37% of the entire series but was especially predominant among patients with aortoenteric fistula, occurring in 79% of that subgroup. Only 10% of patients with aortic graft infection in the absence of aortoenteric fistula developed gastrointestinal bleeding. Patients with intraabdominal synthetic arterial prostheses who have fever, or other evidence of occult sepsis, and gastrointestinal bleeding should be considered to have an aortoenteric fistula until proven otherwise by endoscopy or surgical exploration. Such patients may initially have a relatively small "herald" gastrointestinal

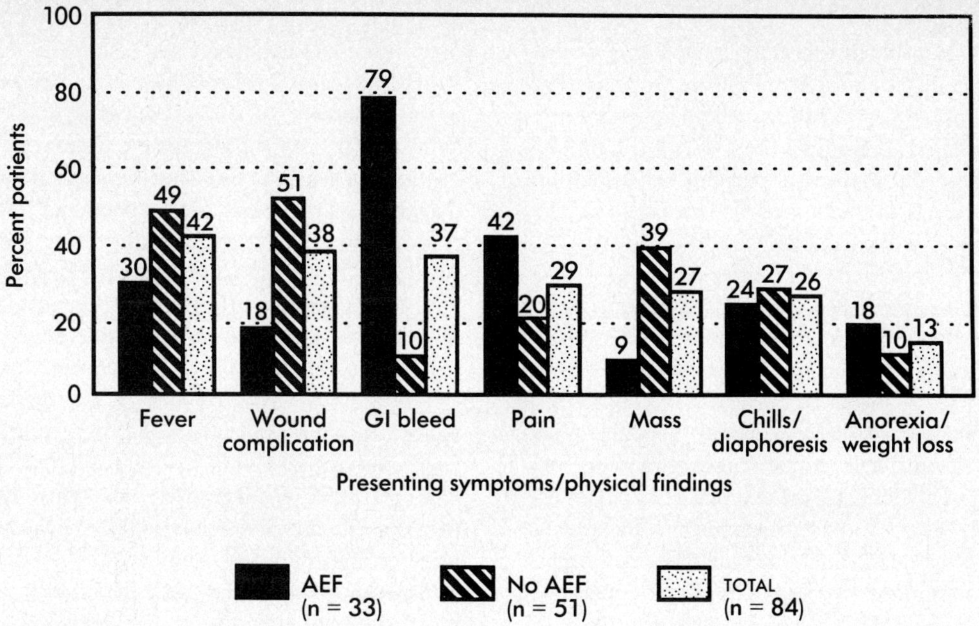

Fig. 39-2. Presenting symptoms and physical findings among patients with abdominal aortic graft sepsis treated at the Cleveland Clinic, 1961-1985. (*GI*, Gastrointestinal; *AEF*, aortoenteric fistula.) (Data from O'Hara PJ et al, J Vasc Surg 3:725, 1986.)

hemorrhage, which stops temporarily. As the septic process progresses at an unpredictable rate, however, rupture of the aortic anastomosis into the gastrointestinal tract may result, manifested as sudden, massive, exsanguinating gastrointestinal bleeding. Other symptoms of systemic sepsis, such as chills and diaphoresis or anorexia and weight loss, were more evenly distributed between the two subgroups. The mean interval from the time of graft implantation to the onset of symptoms of graft sepsis was 41 months, with a range of 0 to 224 months.

In the Cleveland Clinic series, the physical findings noted most commonly among patients with abdominal aortic graft sepsis were the presence of wound hematoma or draining sinus tract, which occurred in 38% of the entire series.[7,8] Fifty-one percent of patients with abdominal aortic graft infection in the absence of aortoenteric fistula had wound complications, whereas only 18% of the aortoenteric fistula subgroup had these findings. Abdominal pain or the discovery of a mass, suggesting pseudoaneurysm or abscess formation, occurred in 27% of the entire series. In contrast, these findings were present among 39% of the patients without aortoenteric fistula but appeared in only 9% of the patients with aortoenteric fistula. These distinctions are likely to reflect the difference in the pathogenesis of graft infection between the two subgroups.[7,8]

In the infrainguinal position the usual signs of prosthetic graft sepsis are wound complications, pain or mass from abscess or pseudoaneurysm formation, or graft thrombosis. Less commonly, late systemic symptoms such as fever, chills, or anorexia may be observed. Very late manifestations of prosthetic graft sepsis, regardless of location, are those associated with overwhelming sepsis, such as metastatic abscess formation and multisystem failure. At this stage the prognosis for patient salvage, even with aggressive intervention, is poor.

DIAGNOSIS

The diagnosis of prosthetic graft sepsis may be obvious, as in the case of a patient with purulent drainage around an exposed synthetic prosthesis. However, some patients with a history of previous prosthetic graft placement may develop more generalized systemic symptoms suggestive of sepsis. In this setting it may be difficult to differentiate primary or secondary graft infection from sepsis as a consequence of other possible causes.

The objectives of the diagnostic workup of a patient being evaluated for prosthetic graft sepsis are the establishment of an accurate diagnosis of graft infection and the determination of the extent of the prosthetic graft involvement. Diagnostic studies helpful in achieving these objectives can be grouped into preliminary and subsequent studies.

The preliminary studies begin with a carefully conducted history and physical examination, which, coupled with a high index of suspicion, can often establish the diagnosis. Baseline lower extremity noninvasive arterial examinations, consisting of plethysmographic and Doppler pressure studies, are usually obtained to document the extent of associated occlusive vascular disease. The results of these objective studies are especially helpful later if autogenous or extra-anatomic bypass procedures are required. Routine laboratory examination, in addition to standard blood chemistry determinations, should include initial blood, urine, sputum, and wound cultures for both aerobic and anaerobic microorganisms. Early nutritional assessment, including evaluation of serum protein and transferrin levels as well as anergy testing, is advisable, especially if the patient appears chronically ill or debilitated. If facilities are available, early consultation with an infectious disease specialist can be helpful, especially with regard to monitoring the antibiotic therapy and the developing culture data.

If the diagnosis is still uncertain after preliminary diagnostic studies are accomplished, gastrointestinal endoscopy should be performed to rule out an associated graft enteric fistula. This procedure is mandatory in the evaluation of a patient who has previously undergone aortic graft placement and who has evidence of gastrointestinal bleeding. Visualization of the prosthetic graft material on endoscopic examination is pathognomonic for the diagnosis of graft enteric fistula. The procedure should be extended to include the fourth portion of the duodenum, since this area is the most common location for the development of aortoenteric or graft enteric fistulae.

Other subsequent diagnostic studies include angiography, which only rarely is able to demonstrate a graft enteric fistula. It is more commonly required to plan alternative revascularization, which may be necessary if infected synthetic graft material requires removal. Ultrasonography can yield information regarding the specific nature of a palpable mass, which may be an abscess, hematoma, or pseudoaneurysm. While gastrointestinal contrast studies are rarely helpful, magnetic resonance imaging (MRI) or computed tomography (CT) scanning of the abdomen and pelvis is often very helpful.[32] These newer imaging techniques are able to accurately demonstrate a perigraft fluid or gas collection as well as pseudoaneurysm formation. In the late postoperative period following abdominal aortic graft placement, the demonstration of periprosthetic gas has been reliably associated with prosthetic graft infection, presumably caused by gas-forming microorganisms.[33,34] CT scan-guided fine-needle aspiration of perigraft fluid collections can yield fluid, which may be sent for appropriate microbiologic culture studies.[35] Care must be taken during this procedure, however, to ensure that microorganisms are not introduced into the perigraft area leading to secondary contamination of a previously sterile prosthesis. In the early postoperative period, however, loculated periprosthetic air is a common and innocuous finding on CT scans of the aortic graft bed, especially following repair of abdominal aortic aneurysms larger than 6 cm in diameter. In a study by O'Hara et al, 65% (17/26) of patients undergoing elective abdominal aortic aneurysm repair had periprosthetic air demonstrated on initial CT scan on the third postoperative day. By the seventh postoperative day only 38% (9/24) of patients available for follow-up scanning had residual perigraft air and complete resolution was noted in all patients in the study group on late CT scans 52 days following aortic graft placement.[36]

Radionuclide scanning has been proposed as a useful method of diagnosing synthetic graft infection. The results of gallium scanning have been disappointing, however, particularly because of difficulties in interpretation, especially in the abdomen.[37] Radiolabeled leukocyte scanning, using ^{111}In- or ^{99}Tc- labeled autologous leukocytes, had been suggested as a sensitive and specific method applicable for the diagnosis of prosthetic graft infection.[38,39] In a subsequent report Sedwitz et al concluded that in the absence of clinical suspicion, the indium-111 leukocyte scan does not reliably predict prosthetic graft infection because of the low specificity of the test in the early postoperative period.[40] A new scanning techique using ^{111}In- labeled, human polyclonal IgG appears to show promise as a reliable method to diagnose vascular graft infections. In a preliminary report by LaMuraglia et al, 10 of 10 patients with positive scan results had confirmed localized graft infections, whereas 14 of 15 patients with negative scans had no vascular infections identified during follow-up study.[37]

Sinography may play a limited role in the diagnosis of prosthetic graft infection among patients with a wound sinus tract. A carefully performed sinogram may demonstrate tracking to the synthetic biomaterial and may delineate the proximal extent of a perigraft sinus. This information may be useful in planning treatment, especially if it demonstrates extension to involve the body of an aortofemoral graft.

Ultimately, the diagnosis of graft infection may be suspected on clinical grounds yet remain unconfirmed despite a thorough diagnostic evaluation. In these situations surgical exploration under sterile conditions in the operating room may be required to establish the diagnosis and ascertain the extent of the prosthetic involvement. In the clinical setting of an open wound with underlying but not exposed synthetic graft material, great care should be taken to avoid contamination of the graft. However, if the synthetic graft is exposed to the enviroment, unincorporated, or surrounded by cloudy fluid, prosthetic graft sepsis must be strongly suspected. Patients who have undergone placement of an intraabdominal aortic prosthetic graft and who subsequently develop gastrointestinal bleeding present a particular diagnostic dilemma. If the patient is actively bleeding and unstable, urgent laparotomy is required for diagnosis as well as treatment. However, if the patient is stable, aggressive nonoperative evaluation to rule out aortoenteric fistula is required. If the usual evaluation, including upper gastrointestinal endoscopy, is negative, diagnostic laparotomy to rule out aortoenteric fistula may be required. A recent study by Pabst et al, however, documents the low yield of such procedures. The authors conclude that laparotomy to exclude aortoenteric fistula appears to be unwarranted when appropriate diagnostic efforts to demonstrate the lesion do not reveal any abnormality, and there is no evidence of occult sepsis.[41]

OBJECTIVES IN TREATMENT

The principal objectives in the treatment of prosthetic graft sepsis are the control of hemorrhage, if present; the control of local and systemic sepsis; the provision of adequate perfusion; and the provision of adequate support both in the early and late phases of therapy.[8] The first priority of treatment is the preservation of the patient's life. The second priority is the preservation of functional limbs. Optimal treatment accomplishes both goals.

Patients with prosthetic graft infection, acute hemorrhage, and hemodynamic instability require urgent surgical exploration in conjunction with aggressive volume resuscitation. In the early postoperative period hemorrhage manifested by profuse bleeding from an infected wound indicates disruption of the underlying graft-to-artery anastomosis. This is more common among patients infected with virulent organisms such as *Pseudomonas*. Commonly, in this situation the patient's host artery or autogenous graft material is autolyzed and friable. Acute infection-induced hemorrhage occurring later, when overlying tissue is healed, is more likely to appear as an expanding pseudoaneurysm manifested as a painful enlarging mass in the abdomen, groin, or popliteal space, depending on the location of the involved anastomosis. In either case, isolation of the inflow and outflow vessels should be performed expeditiously. This may be difficult in patients who have undergone several previous operations. Temporary arterial control may be facilitated by use of intravascular occluding balloon catheters.

Once acute hemorrhage is controlled, or if it is not a factor, the next major objective is the control of systemic and local sepsis. Systemic sepsis is treated by the intravenous infusion of microorganism-specific antibiotics. The optimum dosage is best monitored by antibiotic blood level determinations. Ideally, adequate tissue levels should be attained by the time of surgical exploration. Local sepsis is optimally controlled by application of the general surgical principle of adequate débridement and drainage with obliteration of dead space.

Perhaps the most difficult and fundamental problem in the treatment of prosthetic graft sepsis is the accurate determination of the depth and extent of the local sepsis and consequently the adequacy of excisional therapy. This observation may explain the disparity in reported results of treatment of graft sepsis with excisional and nonexcisional methods. In general, however, in the presence of well-established prosthetic graft sepsis, especially with involvement of the surrounding host tissues, local control usually demands removal of all the infected synthetic material.[7,8,42,43] When doubt exists regarding the involvement of prosthetic material, it seems best to remove it completely, especially if the infected area is relatively inaccessible or difficult to closely monitor, such as in the retroperitoneum or pelvis. Failure to adequately control the local sepsis usually leads to persisting infection and eventual disruption of the arterial closure.

Ideally, local débridement should remove all necrotic and infected material with the goal of eliminating, or at least minimizing, residual microorganism inoculum to allow antibiotic and host defenses an opportunity to eradicate the remaining pathogens. Infected arterial wall must be removed and closure carried out in grossly healthy tissue with monofilament suture material. Dead space may be managed by placement of an omental pedicle in the aortic bed or by rotation of local muscle flaps, such as the sartorius, used in the treatment of infections in the groin region. Drainage of the retroperitoneum is usually best managed by sump drains brought out through the flank or through a groin incision, whereas drainage of groin or extremity incisions can usually be accomplished through conventional methods. The skin is usually left open to heal by secondary intention.

Once the infected synthetic material is removed, the extremities should be inspected for viability. If they are viable, no further reconstruction should be carried out in the acute phase. Ideally, when the sepsis is eradicated and all the wounds are healed, vascular reconstruction may be reconsidered if necessary.[43] If, conversely, the extremities are nonviable after removal of the infected graft, or if it is apparent on preoperative clinical assessment that the limbs are dependent on the infected graft for survival, alternative revascularization will be required. When feasible, autogenous reconstruction, consisting of endarterectomy, autogenous arterial or venous grafting, autogenous arterial or venous patch angioplasty, or combinations of these techniques, all employing monofilament suture material, are preferred. Considerable innovation is often required. When autogenous reconstruction is not feasible, extraanatomic bypass in noninfected tissue planes may be required. The most commonly employed extraanatomic synthetic bypass procedures employed for lower extremity revascularization are the axillofemoral or axillobifemoral graft and the femorofemoral graft. In some instances innovative combinations of autogenous reconstruction and synthetic extraanatomic bypass procedures may be employed to solve a particular revascularization need.[42,44]

The fourth major objective in the management of prosthetic graft sepsis is the provision of adequate early and late support. In practice, support is provided concurrently with diagnostic and therapeutic measures. Early basic physiologic assistance consisting of respiratory and hemodynamic support is frequently required, especially if the patient has severe systemic sepsis. Renal failure is a common complicating factor, and provisions for dialysis may be required. An important consideration is early attention to the issue of nutritional support. Many of these patients will have prolonged impairment of gastrointestinal function and coexisting high metabolic requirements, thus requiring total parenteral nutrition. Nutritional assessment early in the course of the illness with evaluation of circulating protein levels and immunocompetence is essential. In the later phases of therapy, as with any prolonged and debilitating illness, continued physical therapy and psychologic support is necessary, especially if amputation has been required.

Because of the risk of persisting sepsis and exsanguinating hemorrhage associated with established but inadequately treated prosthetic graft infection, especially when the aortoiliac system is involved, definitive therapy is preferred if it is technically possible and the patient represents an acceptable risk for intervention. Traditionally, definitive treatment has involved the complete removal of all infected synthetic material, débridement of all involved host tissues, and autogenous or extraanatomic synthetic revascularization in the clean tissue planes when reperfusion is necessary for limb viability. This approach, if carried out early enough in the course of the illness, appears to most reliably yield optimal results.[7,8,42,43,45] However, if the excisional approach is not feasible, a therapeutic compromise may be required.

When graft infection involves an entire aortobiliac graft, excision of the contaminated prosthesis and axillobifemoral grafting is the treatment of choice. Closure of the aortic stump is carried out with at least two layers of monofilament permanent suture. Autogenous pledgets of saphenous vein or fascia lata may sometimes be required to prevent the sutures from cutting through friable aortic tissue and to ensure a hemostatic closure.[46] The use of a seromuscular jejunal patch has also been proposed to provide healthy, well-vascularized tissue to the aortic stump closure in an attempt to control persisting sepsis and reduce the incidence of aortic stump disruption.[11,47] If the infection involves an entire aortobifemoral graft, bilateral axillofemoral or axillopopliteal bypass grafts are required for lower extremity revascularization. If only the femoral anastomosis of an aortobifemoral graft is infected, it may be possible to remove only the infected portion.[43,48,49] This is accomplished by first exploring the limb through a clean flank incision. If no involvement is noted at that level, the limb is divided, and healthy, noninfected tissue is interposed between the divided ends. After the flank wound is closed and isolated with occlusive dressings, the infected femoral portion of the graft is removed. Lower extremity revascularization, if required, may be accomplished either by means of an obturator foramen bypass or more commonly by axillofemoral or axillopopliteal bypass in noninfected tissue planes. Synthetic graft infections involving femorofemoral or femoropopliteal grafts are also managed by removal of the infected portion of the prosthetic and autogenous or extraanatomic synthetic revascularization if necessary. The lateral approach to the popliteal artery, as described by Veith et al, may be particularly helpful in this situation.[50]

Autogenous reconstruction methods have been emphasized as particularly useful in the management of patients with arterial prosthetic graft infection.[51,52] These consist of endarterectomy and the use of autogenous arterial and venous grafts. Sources of autogenous arterial graft material include hypogastric artery and also endarterectomized occluded superficial femoral artery. The greater and lesser saphenous and the cephalic venous systems provide a ready source of autogenous vein graft material. Frequently, a combination of techniques may be tailored to a particular clinical situation.

Although complete excision of all infected synthetic material appears to be the most reliable method to manage infected arterial prosthetic grafts, it is, nevertheless, associated with considerable mortality and morbidity, especially when the infected grafts are in the aortic position.[1,7,8,42,53-55] Furthermore, complete prosthetic excision is not always possible, as in the case of graft infection following thoracoabdominal aortic aneurysm repair. Additionally, some patients are too debilitated or refuse to accept excisional treatment. As a result there has been interest in nonexcisional

Table 39-3. Results of selected reports of local or nonexcisional treatment of infected synthetic arterial grafts

Author	Year	No. of patients	Locations	Treatment	Follow-up period	Recurrence/death
Kwaan and Connolly[56]	1981	10	A, E, and I	M and L	1-4 yr	0/0
Thomas and Baird[57]	1986	6	A	R and D	1.5-5 yr	2/0
Vollmar and Kogel[58]	1987	7	A	R	1-3 yr	—/1
Walker et al[59]	1987	23	A	R	Mean 5.2 yr	—/7
Samson et al[60]	1988	34	I and E	L	Mean 4 yr	9/—
Tobin[61]	1988	1	A	L	7 mo	0/0
Ammar and Turrentine[62]	1989	3	A and I	M	Mean 45.3 mo	0/0
Atnip[63]	1989	1	A	R	2.5 yr	0/0
Dagher and Stueber[64]	1989	3	I and U	M	Mean 11 mo	0/0
Mixter et al[65]	1989	31	A, I, E, and T	M	Mean 36 mo	1/0

A, Aortic.
E, Extraanatomic.
I, Infrainguinal.
U, Upper extremity.
T, Thoracic.
M, Muscle flap.
L, Local irrigation; dressings; drainage; closure.
R, Regraft in situ.
D, Direct suture without excision.

forms of therapy in which the infected prosthesis is left in place. The reported methods, summarized in Table 39-3, include treatment with antibiotics alone, local irrigation with antibiotic solution, coverage with rotational flaps or other forms of soft tissue graft coverage, direct suture repair of aortoenteric fistulae, and graft excision with in situ synthetic replacement.[56-65] While many of the results are impressive, the series are relatively small and poorly controlled and the follow-up care is relatively limited. In clinical practice, recurrence or persistence of sepsis in the synthetic material is commonly observed when nonexcisional therapy is employed, often with catastrophic consequences.* The Cleveland Clinic experience with nonexcisional treatment of infected abdominal aortic prostheses, although small, has been disappointing. From 1961 through February 1985, nine patients with aortoenteric fistulae underwent operations in which all the involved prosthetic material was not removed. Three had contaminated grafts replaced with new prosthetic grafts in the same location. Three others had correction of infected false aneurysms by placement of another prosthetic graft. An additional three patients each underwent aortoenteric fistula repair without removal of the aortic graft. One of these nine patients was lost during follow-up care subsequent to hospital discharge 114 days after operation. The remaining eight patients all died within 1 month following surgical treatment.[7,8] Vetsch et al has reported that, in the dog, in situ replacement of vascular prostheses infected by *Staphylococcus epidermidis* can result in graft healing with normal anastomotic bonding.[66]

In theory, if the graft infection is confined to an adherent biofilm and is completely excised with the original graft, some patients may be adequately treated by in situ graft replacement and long-term antibiotic suppression. Unfortunately, it is difficult, in the clinical setting, to reliably identify those patients who may be safely treated by nonexcisional methods. It seems clear that more late follow-up data are needed to evaluate the effectiveness of nonexcisional methods, and if such an approach is chosen, very close long-term follow-up care is mandatory.

The Cleveland Clinic experience in the surgical management of 84 patients with infected synthetic grafts in the aortic position from 1961 through February 1985 is summarized in Fig. 39-3.[7,8] Fifty-four patients (64%) were managed by total graft removal and extraanatomic bypass, while 13 (15%) patients underwent graft removal alone. Eight patients (10%) were treated by partial graft removal with extraanatomic bypass. One patient in this last group had a contaminated groin segment of an aortofemoral graft removed with anastomosis of the noninfected proximal iliac limb to the host iliac artery. Nine other patients (11%), just described, underwent miscellaneous nonexcisional treatment.

The influence of the treatment sequence used among patients treated for abdominal aortic graft infection at the Cleveland Clinic from 1961 through February 1985 is depicted in Fig. 39-4.[7,8] Thirty-two patients without aortoenteric fistulae were managed by total excision of the infected abdominal aortic grafts and extraanatomic bypass. Of these patients, 17 had combined operations in which infected grafts were first removed and then extraanatomic revascularization performed at the same operation. The other 15 patients underwent preliminary, staged extraanatomic by-

*References 1, 7, 8, 42, 43, 45.

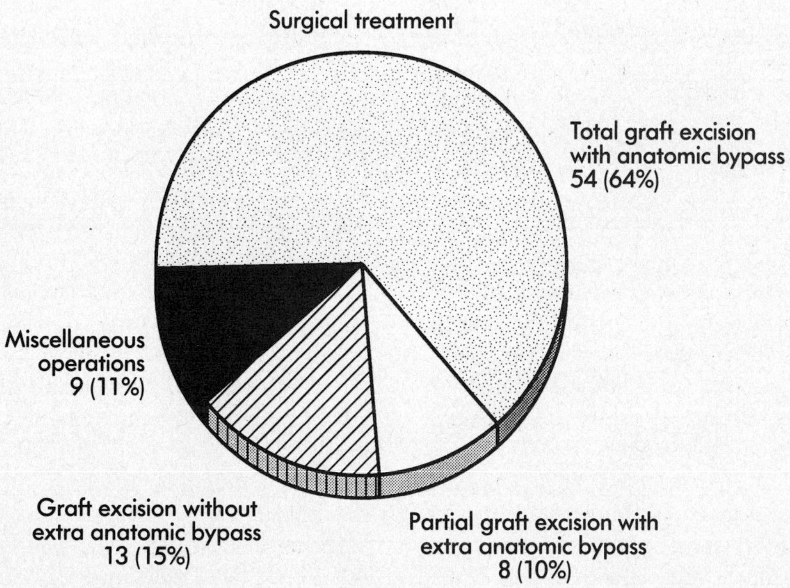

Fig. 39-3. Surgical treatment of patients with abdominal aortic graft sepsis at the Cleveland Clinic, 1961-1985. (There were no survivors in the *Miscellaneous operations* group.) (Data from O'Hara PJ et al, J Vasc Surg 3:725, 1986.)

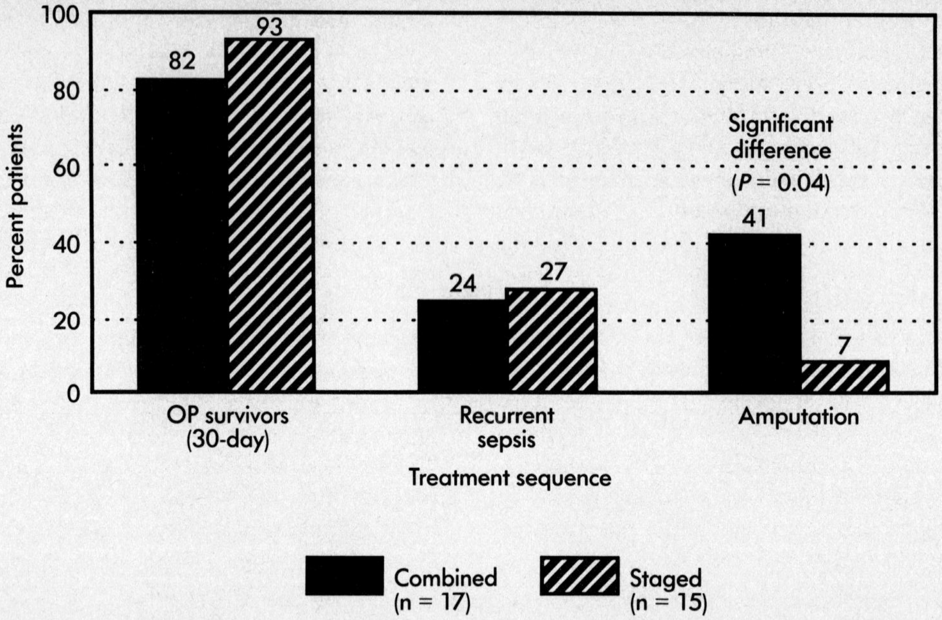

Fig. 39-4. Comparison of survival, recurrent graft sepsis, and associated amputation between staged and combined extraanatomic bypass and graft excision groups at the Cleveland Clinic, 1961-1985. (*OP*, Operative.) (Data from O'Hara PJ et al, J Vasc Surg 3:725, 1986.)

pass with subsequent infected graft removal as a second procedure. No difference in the incidence of recurrent sepsis, operative mortality, or 1-year survival was demonstrated between the combined and staged groups. Moreover, amputations were necessary in fully 41% of the patients in the combined group but in only 7% of those in the staged group. This difference was statistically significant ($P = 0.04$).[7,8] Consequently, when the clinical situation permits, preliminary extraanatomic bypass should precede the removal of an infected arterial prosthesis when the need for alternative revascularization is apparent, a recommendation supported by other investigators.[49,67-69] Hemorrhage or hemodynamic instability, often associated with aortoenteric fistulae, mandates urgent exploration and precludes the staged approach, however.

RESULTS

It is difficult to evaluate with accuracy the results of treatment of arterial prosthetic graft infection for several reasons. Primarily, since the incidence is low, most published reports are based on either anecdotal information or on small series of patients. Because graft sepsis is unusual, reports containing a relatively large number of patients may encompass a long span of time during which other advances may obscure the effect of a particular form of therapy on the eventual outcome. Furthermore, accurate diagnosis and staging is difficult to establish, especially early on, while the clinical course and outcome may be influenced by a variety of uncontrolled variables. These include the location and extent of graft sepsis, the mechanism of graft infection, and the host response capability, which is, in turn, influenced by the presence of concurrent associated disease and the nutritional state of the patient. In the ideal situation the influence of these and other variables may be controlled by the use of prospective, randomized clinical trials. However, such studies would be anticipated to require a prohibitive amount of time to complete, even by busy clinical centers, and will likely remain logistically impractical for the foreseeable future.

Such inadequacies notwithstanding, a review of the data suggests that no current treatment is completely satisfactory.[1,10] Mortality among patients who develop synthetic graft sepsis remains high, especially when it involves the aortoiliac region. Aortoenteric fistula formation carries an especially ominous prognosis.[7,8,10,42] Among survivors, morbidity, usually in the form of amputation, is considerable. For these reasons, controversy over the methods of optimal management continues.

The data in Table 39-4 summarize the results of eight published reports on series of patients managed with infection in synthetic arterial prostheses in the aortoiliac, aortofemoral, or femoroperipheral (including femorofemoral) locations from 1965 through 1987.[2-4,6-9,18,70] Although graft sepsis is less common in the aortoiliofemoral region than in the femoroperipheral region, the mortality is usually approximately twice as high among the aortic patients. Mortality ranges from 20% to 75% in the aortoiliofemoral group and from 0% to 29% in the femoroperipheral group. The number of amputations is difficult to express as a percent because of the inability to determine the number of limbs at risk in all of the published reports. In addition, it was not always possible to determine from the published series

Table 39-4. Eight published reports on patients with prosthetic graft infection in the aortoiliac, aortofemoral, or femoroperipheral position who died or required amputation

Author	Year	No. of patients	Graft location	No. of deaths (%)	No. of amputations
Hoffert, Gensler, and Haimovici[3]	1965	2	AI and AF	1 (50)	2
		9	FP	2 (22)	6
Fry and Lindenauer[4]	1967	12	AI and AF	9 (75)	1
Conn et al[18]	1970	11	AI and AF	6 (55)	2
		7	FP	2 (29)	4
Szilagyi et al[2]	1972	29	AI and AF	14 (48)	4
		10	FP	0 (0)	5
Lorentzen et al[6]	1985	45	AI and AF	13 (29)	10
		17	FP	3 (18)	9
O'Hara et al[7,8]	1986	84	AI and AF	58 (69)	23
Edwards et al[9]	1987	5	AF	1 (20)	2
		17	FP	3 (18)	2
Kikta et al[70]	1987	32	FP	7 (22)	26

AI, Aortoiliac.
AF, Aortofemoral.
FP, Femoroperipheral.

whether the number of amputations were tabulated for all patients in a series or for merely the operative survivors. Furthermore, some patients, especially in the aortoiliofemoral group, required unilateral amputations, while others required bilateral procedures or did not survive long enough to undergo amputation. In the Cleveland Clinic series of aortic graft infections, a total of 23 patients (27%) required major amputations, 9 of which were bilateral. This figure probably represents a minimal incidence because several of the 61 remaining patients who did not undergo amputation failed to survive long enough after treatment of the infected prosthetic graft to permit definitive treatment of their ischemic limbs.[7,8] In the femoroperipheral group, however, the amputations were likely to be unilateral. Among this group, the amputation rate, determined by dividing the number of amputations by the number of patients in the series or the number of limbs at risk, if known, ranged from 12% (2/17) to 79% (26/33). The wide discrepancy in amputation rates in the femoroperipheral graft infection group in part reflects the underlying indication for the original graft. If done for limb salvage, subsequent revascularization options after graft removal are severely limited.

The primary causes of death in the Cleveland Clinic series of patients with abdominal aortic synthetic graft infection are illustrated in Fig. 39-5. Systemic sepsis with multisystem failure was the most frequent cause of death, responsible in 31 patients (53%), whereas cardiac complications, renal failure, and miscellaneous causes accounted for the remaining deaths. Eight (32%) of the 25 deaths of patients with aortoenteric fistulae were caused by ruptured aortic closures, which occurred at a mean interval of 94 days after graft removal and probably reflect persisting sepsis in the aortic stump suture lines. This complication led to 22% (13/58) of the deaths in the entire series.[7,8]

In the Cleveland Clinic report of patients with synthetic graft infections involving the aortoiliofemoral locations, the early and late mortality rates were calculated by the life table method producing cumulative survival cures (Figs. 39-6 to 39-8).[7,8] For the entire series cumulative survival at 30 days, 1 year, and 5 years was 72%, 42%, and 18%, respectively (see Fig. 39-6). The 30-day operative survival rate among patients with aortoenteric fistulae was 49%, which was significantly less ($P = 0.003$) than that (86%) of those patients without this complication (see Fig. 39-7), a disparity documented by other observers.[42] This difference represented operative mortality, since beyond the perioperative period no statistical difference in late mortality between the two groups could be demonstrated. One-year survival of patients treated since 1980 (54%) was significantly improved ($P = 0.035$) when compared with that of patients treated before 1980 (31%), although there was no demonstrable difference in survival between the groups at sample times later than 1 year (see Fig. 39-8).[7,8]

PREVENTION

Prevention of prosthetic graft sepsis assumes paramount importance because, despite optimal early and aggressive therapy, synthetic graft infection is associated with substantial mortality and morbidity. Problem areas in the prevention of synthetic graft infection can be addressed in the preoperative, intraoperative, and postoperative phases of care.

Of primary concern in the preoperative period is control of local sepsis. Patients with arterial occlusive disease who have undrained infections involving the lower extremity, often in the plantar space, must undergo early, adequate drainage and débridement. The dual objectives are the prevention of local spread leading to extensive tissue necrosis,

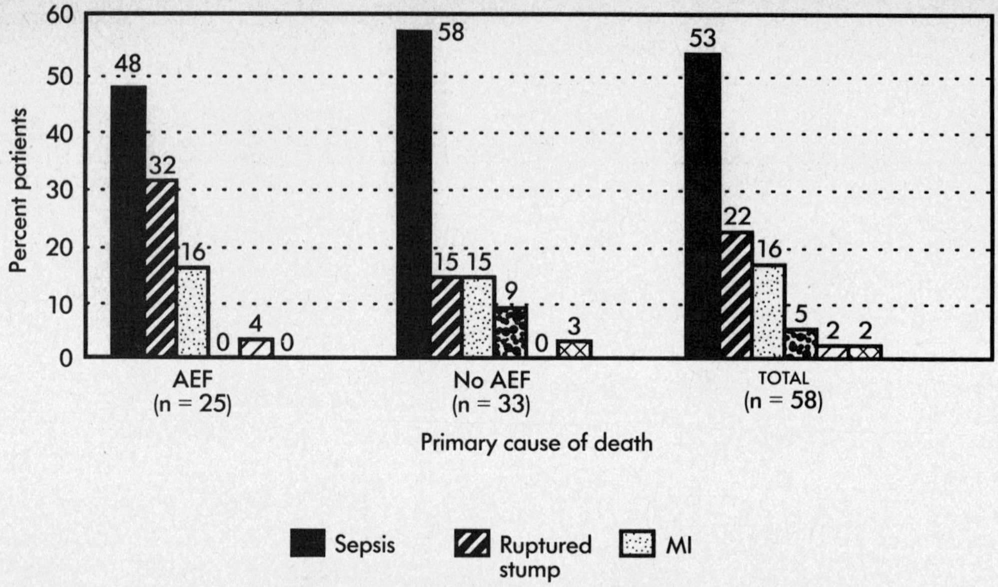

Fig. 39-5. Primary cause of death among patients with abdominal aortic graft sepsis treated at the Cleveland Clinic, 1961-1985. (*AEF*, Aortoenteric fistula; *CHF*, congestive heart failure, *ARF*, acute renal failure; *MI*, myocardial infarction; *Ca*, carcinoma; *TAA*, thoracoabdominal aortic aneurysm.) (Data from O'Hara PJ et al, J Vasc Surg 3:725, 1986.)

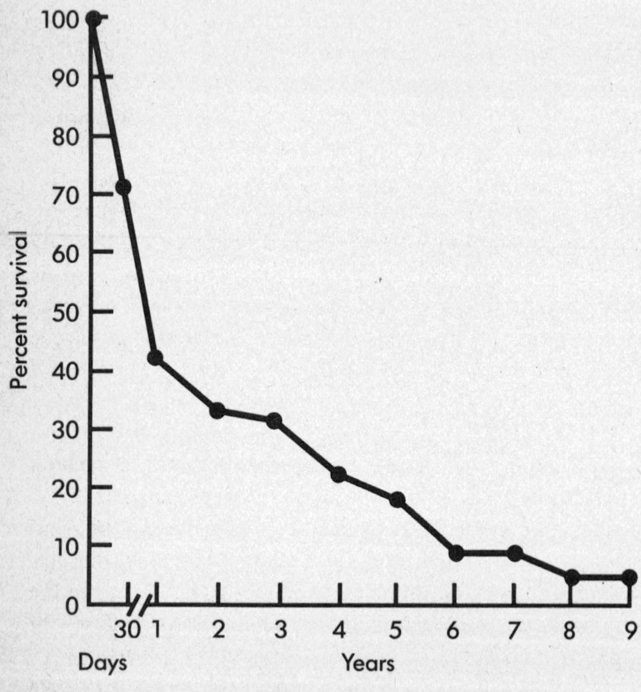

Fig. 39-6. Life table analysis of cumulative survival for 84 patients with infected abdominal aortic grafts. (From O'Hara PJ et al, J Vasc Surg 3:725, 1986.)

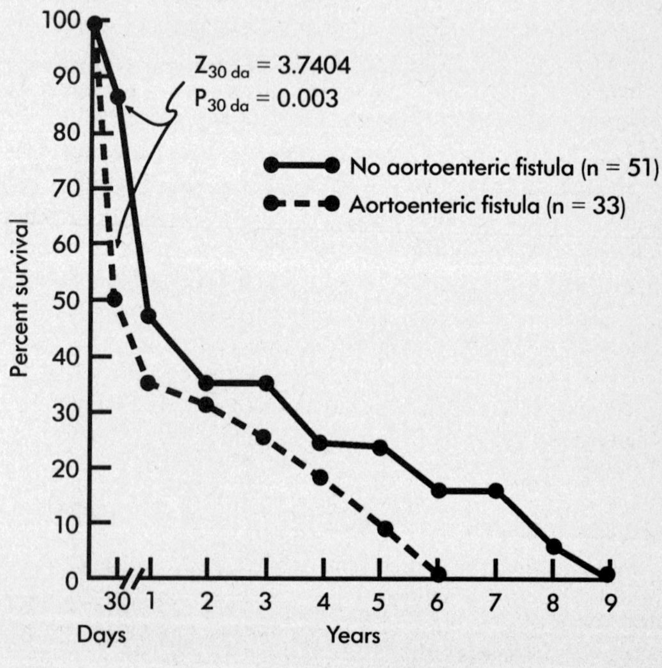

Fig. 39-7. Life table analysis of cumulative survival for patient subsets with and without aortoenteric fistulae. (From O'Hara PJ et al, J Vasc Surg 3:725, 1986.)

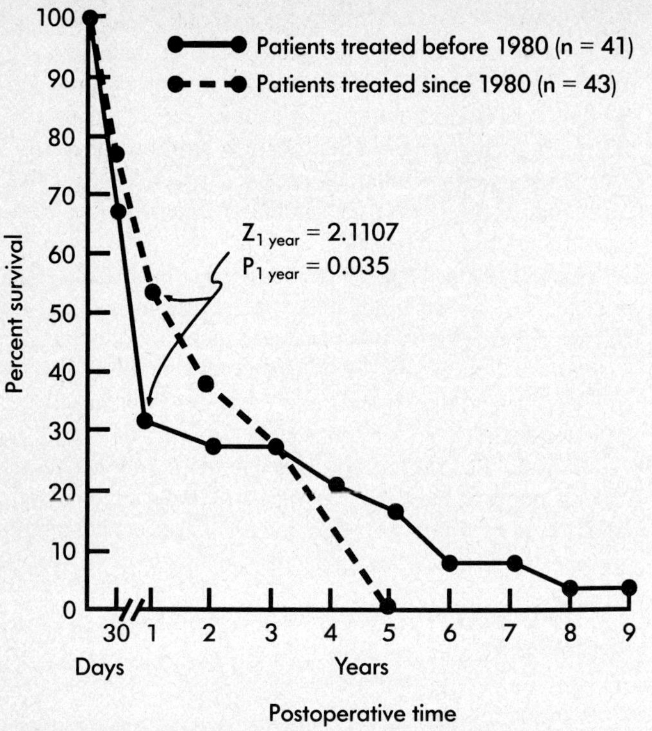

Fig. 39-8. Comparison of cumulative survival (by life table) for patient subsets treated before and after 1980. (From O'Hara PJ et al, J Vasc Surg 3:725, 1986.)

which may preclude limb salvage despite successful revascularization, and the prevention of bacteremia leading to potential seeding of implanted prosthetic material. Simultaneous intravenous, culture-specific antibiotic therapy is also required. Other potential sources of bacteremia, such as poor oral hygiene, should be corrected if the clinical situation permits. Control of associated diseases, such as diabetes mellitus and cardiac or renal failure, should be obtained. As time permits, the patient's nutritional status should be optimized, especially if anergy is documented.

Intraoperative measures include the use of prophylactic antibiotic coverage. The spectrum should be broad enough to cover staphylococcal species as well as those organisms likely to cause bacteremia in the particular clinical setting encountered. Antibiotic therapy is begun preoperatively and supplemented periodically during the procedure to maintain adequate blood and tissue levels. Strict adherence to the principles of surgical asepsis is mandatory, and particular vigilance is required when the operation is lengthy. Meticulous surgical technique and efficient organization are required to avoid complications and to minimize operative time. The groin incision should be used with care after precautions to ensure optimal skin preparation have been taken. As in all clinical medicine, good judgment is required to ensure an optimal outcome. Except in unusual circumstances, it is probably unwise to combine gastrointestinal or genitourinary procedures with vascular operations in which synthetic graft material is utilized because of the potential for contamination.

In the postoperative phase, antibiotic coverage should be continued until all central intravenous lines and indwelling urinary catheters are removed and the risk of bacteremia is no longer a factor. Antibiotic coverage is usually continued until open wounds are closed, especially if they are in close proximity to the synthetic graft material. Personnel caring for the patient should avoid unnecessary wound manipulation. Prompt management of complications, such as colon ischemia or wound infection, should be undertaken before the sepsis has extended to involve and colonize the adjacent synthetic graft. Wound seromas in the vicinity of synthetic graft material will usually resolve spontaneously in weeks to months. Repeated aspiration should be avoided because the procedure runs the risk of introducing sepsis, and the seroma usually will reaccumulate. If a lymph fistula occurs, treatment with local antiseptic ointment and systemic antibiotics until the fistula resolves usually is sufficient. However, if the drainage persists longer than approximately one week, or if a seroma is large, uncomfortable, or poses a risk of spontaneous rupture, surgical exploration with ligation or excision and sclerosis is indicated to prevent retrograde contamination of and colonization of the underlying graft material. On occasion, graft replacement has been advocated.[71]

CONTROVERSIES AND FUTURE DEVELOPMENTS

The mortality and morbidity associated with prosthetic graft infection is high despite aggressive traditional therapy. For this reason, controversy exists regarding optimal treatment. Some areas of investigation have been discussed in preceding sections of this chapter; other areas of continuing debate remain to be settled by further study. Because the problem of prosthetic graft infection is multifaceted, it is likely that no single approach to management will be adequate for all clinical situations.

The relative indications for graft excision and extraanatomic bypass, as opposed to in situ synthetic graft replacement or local, nonexcisional treatment of synthetic graft infection, remain to be precisely defined. Accurate and reliable guidelines to determine which patients will require delayed or immediate revascularization after synthetic graft removal are required. This information could be used to facilitate the clinical decision to proceed with staged extraanatomic bypass before the removal of an infected aortic graft. The question of the optimal route and duration of antibiotic therapy required to completely eradicate residual infection remains incompletely answered. A related question concerning the safe interval required before placing a new synthetic graft in the bed of a previously excised, infected prosthetic was addressed by Reilly, Ehrenfeld, and Stoney. In a report on seven patients who underwent late reinsertion of a prosthetic graft in the aortic position at a mean interval of 14.5 months following a previous removal of an infected aortic prosthesis, six were well at a mean follow-up interval of 57 months postoperatively. One patient died 1 month following regrafting. The authors concluded that a reimplantation interval of 6 to 12 months may be safe.[72]

The current recommended approach at the Cleveland Clinic for the treatment of infected arterial grafts, when the diagnosis is certain, consists of complete removal of all the infected synthetic graft material. This does not necessarily mean removal of the entire graft if infection can reliably be excised by partial graft removal. If revascularization is necessary, it is accomplished using autogenous tissue if feasible. If autogenous tissue is not available or adequate, extraanatomic bypass with synthetic material may be required. If the requirement for revascularization is certain or nearly so, and the patient's clinical status permits, the revascularization is carried out before the graft excision to minimize ischemic time. Appropriate antibiotic coverage to achieve adequate tissue levels is used until all wounds are closed and there is no further evidence of residual sepsis. When the clinical situation does not permit this approach, or if the diagnosis of graft infection is in doubt, conservative, nonexcisional approaches may be attempted. However, the patient must be carefully observed and followed-up on for an indefinite period because of the risk of late recurrence or emergence of graft sepsis.

Future developments, which may offer promise in the prevention and treatment of arterial prosthetic graft infections, involve various forms of synthetic graft modification. These methods include endothelial seeding techniques, antibiotic bonding or impregnation procedures, and the development of prosthetic materials that inhibit bacterial adhesion to the synthetic graft.

The development of techniques for endothelial seeding of synthetic vascular grafts by several investigators may lead to the evolution of infection-resistant arterial substitutes.[73-75] Birinyi et al concluded that endothelial cell seeding improved resistance of a polytetrafluoroethylene vascular graft to late bacterial challenge in a dog model.[76] Jarrell et al reported that Dacron grafts coated with basement membrane human collagen and seeded with cultured human endothelial cells could establish a complete monolayer of endothelial cells 30 minutes after seeding.[77] These studies suggest the potential for clinical application of endothelial seeding techniques in the future. However, based upon studies in the New Zealand white rabbit, Buckels, Nordestgaard, and Wilson have suggested that the resistance to bacteremic graft infection may be unrelated to neointimal formation and may be caused by filling of the graft interstices with protein coagulum.[78]

Antibiotic bonding to synthetic grafts may be facilitated by pretreating the grafts with a surfactant, such as tridodecylmethylammonium chloride or benzalkonium chloride.[79-83] Other methods include an antibiotic bonding collagen release system[84] or the addition of antibiotics directly to the blood used for preclotting the graft.[85,86] Such methods may offer promise in the treatment of established graft infections or in the prevention of contamination of noninfected grafts. Problems remain, however, in controlling the rate of effluence as well as the blood and local tissue levels of the antibiotic. Furthermore, the antibiotic cannot be changed after the graft is implanted.

Various synthetic graft materials may have differing propensities for bacterial adherence. Silicone coating of Dacron material significantly reduced the rate of adherence to *Staphylococcus epidermidis* strains, in a study by Harris and Martin, and may have a role in the development of an infection-resistant arterial prosthesis.[87]

It appears that more study is needed to permit adequate understanding of the pathogenesis of synthetic arterial graft infection to facilitate its prevention and to allow the development of more effective therapeutic alternatives.

REFERENCES

1. Bunt TJ: Synthetic vascular graft infections. I. Graft infection, Surgery 93:733, 1983.
2. Szilagyi DE et al: Infection in arterial reconstruction with synthetic grafts, Ann Surg 176:321, 1972.
3. Hoffert PW, Gensler S, and Haimovici H: Infection complicating arterial grafts, Arch Surg 90:427, 1965.
4. Fry WJ and Lindenauer SM: Infection complicating the use of plastic arterial implants, Arch Surg 94:600, 1967.
5. Goldstone J and Moore WS: Infection in vascular prostheses: clinical manifestations and surgical management, Am J Surg 128:225, 1974.
6. Lorentzen JE et al: Vascular graft infection: an analysis of sixty-two graft infections in 2411 consecutively implanted synthetic vascular grafts, Surgery 98:81, 1985.
7. O'Hara PJ et al: Surgical management of infected abdominal aortic grafts: review of 25-year experience, J Vasc Surg 3:725, 1986.
8. O'Hara PJ: Surgical management of infected abdominal aortic grafts. In Cowgill LD, ed: Cardiac surgery: state of the art reviews, Philadelphia, 1987, Hanley & Belfus, Inc.
9. Edwards WH et al: Primary graft infections: J Vasc Surg 6:235, 1987.
10. Bunt TJ: Synthetic vascular graft infections. II. Graft-enteric erosions and graft-enteric fistulas, Surgery 94:1, 1983.
11. Buchbinder D et al: Pathologic interactions between prosthetic aortic grafts and the gastrointestinal tract: clinical problems and a new experimental approach, Am J Surg 140:192, 1980.
12. Pasternak BM, Samson R, and Karp MP: Fungal infection of a vascular prosthesis, Surgery 85:586, 1979.
13. Dosher W, Krishnasastry KV, and Deckoff SL: Fungal graft infections: report and review of the literature, J Vasc Surg 6:398, 1987.
14. Anderson J and Kron IL: Treatment of *Aspergillus* infection of the proximal aortic prosthetic graft with associated vertebral osteomyelitis, J Vasc Surg 1:579, 1984.
15. Berger K, Sauvage LR, and Wood SJ: Healing of arterial prostheses in man: its incompleteness, Ann Surg 175:118, 1972.
16. Goeau-Brissonniere O et al: Experimental colonization of an expanded polytetrafluoroethylene vascular graft with *Staphylococcus aureus*: a quantitative and morphologic study, J Vasc Surg 5:743, 1987.
17. Leport C et al: Experimental colonization of a polyester vascular graft with *Staphylococcus aureus*: a quantitative and morphologic study, J Vasc Surg 8:1, 1988.
18. Conn JH et al: Infected arterial grafts: experience in 22 cases with emphasis on unusual bacteria and technics, Ann Surg 171:704, 1970.

19. Bandyk DF et al: Aortofemoral graft infection due to *Staphylococcus epidermidis*, Arch Surg 119:102, 1984.
20. Ernst CB et al: Incidence and significance of intra-operative bacterial cultures during abdominal aortic aneurysmectomy, Ann Surg 185:626, 1977.
21. Ilgenfritz FM and Jordan FT: Microbiological monitoring of aortic aneurysm wall and contents during aneurysmectomy, Arch Surg 123:506, 1988.
22. McAuley CE, Steed DL, and Webster MW: Bacterial presence in aortic thrombus at elective aneurysm resection: is it clinically significant? Am J Surg 147:322, 1984.
23. MacBeth GA et al: The relevance of arterial wall microbiology to the treatment of prosthetic graft infections: graft infection vs. arterial infection, J Vasc Surg 1:750, 1984.
24. Brook I: Role of anaerobic bacteria in aortofemoral graft infection, Surgery 104:843, 1988.
25. Kaebnick HW et al: The microbiology of explanted vascular prostheses, Surgery 102:756, 1987.
26. Bergamini TM et al: Identification of *Staphylococcus epidermidis* vascular graft infections: a comparison of culture techniques, J Vasc Surg 9:665, 1989.
27. Martin LF et al: Vascular prosthetic infection with *Staphylococcus epidermidis*: experimental study of pathogenesis and therapy, J Vasc Surg 9:464, 1989.
28. Bergamini TM et al: Infection of vascular prostheses by bacterial biofilms, J Vasc Surg 7:21, 1988.
29. Geary KJ et al: Differential effects of a gram-negative and a gram-positive infection on autogenous and prosthetic grafts, J Vasc Surg 11:339, 1990.
30. Kwaan JHM, Dahl RK, and Connolly J: Immunocompetence in patients with prosthetic graft infection, J Vasc Surg 1:45, 1984.
31. Durham JR, Malone JM, and Bernhard VM: The impact of multiple operations on the importance of arterial wall cultures, J Vasc Surg 5:160, 1987.
32. Olofsson PA et al: Diagnosis of prosthetic aortic graft infection by magnetic resonance imaging, J Vasc Surg 8:99, 1988.
33. Haaga JR et al: CT detection of infected synthetic grafts: preliminary report of a new sign, AJR 121:317, 1978.
34. Pliskin M and Rogers WH: Diagnosis of aortic graft infection, Radiology 133:798, 1979.
35. Katz BH, Black RA, and Colley DP: CT-guided fine needle aspiration of a periaortic collection, J Vasc Surg 5:762, 1987.
36. O'Hara PJ et al: Natural history of periprosthetic air on computerized axial tomographic examination of the abdomen following abdominal aortic aneurysms repair, J Vasc Surg 1:429, 1984.
37. LaMuraglia GM et al: Utility of the indium 111-labeled human immunoglobulin G scan for the detection of focal vascular graft infection, J Vasc Surg 10:20, 1989.
38. Serota AJ et al: Uptake of radiolabeled leukocytes in prosthetic graft infection, Surgery 90:35, 1981.
39. Brunner MC et al: Prosthetic graft infection: limitations of indium white blood cell scanning, J Vasc Surg 3:42, 1986.
40. Sedwitz MM et al: Indium 111-labeled white blood cell scans after vascular prosthetic reconstruction, J Vasc Surg 6:476, 1987.
41. Pabst TS et al: Gastrointestinal bleeding after aortic surgery: the role of laparotomy to rule out aortoenteric fistula, J Vasc Surg 8:280, 1988.
42. Reilly LM et al: Late results following surgical management of vascular graft infection, J Vasc Surg 1:36, 1984.
43. Turnipseed WD et al: Arterial graft infections: delayed immediate vascular reconstruction, Arch Surg 118:410, 1983.
44. Baird RJ et al: Ascending aorta to bifemoral bypass: a ventral aorta, J Vasc Surg 3:405, 1986.
45. Edwards MJ, Richardson JD, and Klamer TW: Management of aortic prosthetic infections, Am J Surg 155:327, 1988.
46. Cogbill TH: Secure aortic stump closure with autogenous vein pledgets, Surgery 96:940, 1984.
47. Shah DM et al: Clinical use of the seromuscular jejunal patch for protection of the infected aortic stump, Am J Surg 146:198, 1983.
48. Bennion RS et al: Surgical management of unilateral groin infection after aortofemoral bypass, Surg Gynecol Obstet 156:724, 1983.
49. Casali RE et al: Infected prosthetic grafts, Arch Surg 115:577, 1980.
50. Veith FJ et al: Lateral approach to the popliteal artery, J Vasc Surg 6:119, 1987.
51. Ehrenfeld WK et al: Autogenous tissue reconstruction in the management of infected prosthetic grafts, Surgery 85:82, 1979.
52. Seeger JM et al: Autogenous graft replacement of infected prosthetic grafts in the femoral position, Surgery 93:39, 1983.
53. Martin-Paredero V et al: Fate of aortic graft removal, Am J Surg 146:194, 1983.
54. Yeager RA et al: Aortic and peripheral prosthetic graft infection: differential management and causes of mortality, Am J Surg 150:16, 1985.
55. Dougherty SH and Simmons RL: Infections in bionic man: the pathobiology of infections in prosthetic devices. II, Curr Probl Surg 19:265, 1982.
56. Kwaan JHM and Connolly JE: Successful management of prosthetic graft infection with continuous povidone-iodine irrigation, Arch Surg 116:716, 1981.
57. Thomas WEG and Baird RN: Secondary aorto-enteric fistulae: towards a more conservative approach, Br J Surg 73:875, 1986.
58. Vollmar JF and Kogel H: Aorto-enteric fistulas as postoperative complication, J Cardiovasc Surg 28:479, 1987.
59. Walker WE, et al. The management of aortoduodenal fistula by in situ replacement of the infected abdominal aortic graft. Ann Surg 205.727, 1987.
60. Samson RH et al: A modified classification and approach to the management of infections involving peripheral arterial prosthetic grafts, J Vasc Surg 8:147, 1988.
61. Tobin KD: Aortobifemoral perigraft abscess: treatment by percutaneous catheter drainage, J Vasc Surg 8:339, 1988.
62. Ammar AD and Turrentine MW: Exposed synthetic vascular grafts of the groin: graft preservation by means of tensor fasciae latae flap, J Vasc Surg 10:202, 1989.
63. Atnip RG: Mycotic aneurysms of the suprarenal abdominal aorta: prolonged survival after in situ aortic and visceral reconstruction, J Vasc Surg 10:635, 1989.
64. Dagher FJ and Stueber K: Use of muscle flaps to salvage prosthetic vascular grafts, Contemp Surg 35:31, 1989.
65. Mixter RC et al: Rotational muscle flaps: a new technique for covering infected vascular grafts, J Vasc Surg 9:472, 1989.
66. Vetsch R et al: Anastomotic tensile strength following in situ replacement of an infected abdominal aortic graft, Arch Surg 124:425, 1989.
67. Trout HH, Kozloff L, and Giordano JM: Priority of revascularization in patients with graft enteric fistulas, infected arteries, or infected arterial prostheses, Ann Surg 199:669, 1984.
68. Reilly LM et al: Improved management of aortic graft infection: the influence of operation sequence and staging, J Vasc Surg 5:421, 1987.
69. Spanos PK et al: The management of infected abdominal aortic grafts and graft-enteric fistulas, Ann Surg 183:397, 1976.
70. Kikta MJ et al: Mortality and limb loss with infected infrainguinal bypass grafts, J Vasc Surg 5:566, 1987.
71. Blumenberg RM, Gelfand ML, and Dale WA: Perigraft seromas complicating arterial grafts, Surgery 97:194, 1985.
72. Reilly LM, Ehrenfeld WK, and Stoney RJ: Delayed aortic prosthetic reconstruction after removal of an infected graft, Am J Surg 148:234, 1984.
73. Graham LM et al: Expanded polytetrafluoroethylene vascular prostheses seeded with enzymatically derived and cultured canine endothelial cells, Surgery 91:550, 1982.
74. Herring M, Gardner A, and Glover J: A single staged technique for seeding vascular grafts with autogenous endothelium, Surgery 84:498, 1978.

75. Stanley JC et al: Enhanced patency of small diameter, externally supported Dacron iliofemoral grafts seeded with endothelial cells, Surgery 92:994, 1982.
76. Birinyi LK et al: Increased resistance to bacteremic graft infection after endothelial seeding, J Vasc Surg 5:193, 1987.
77. Jarrell BE et al: Use of an endothelial monolayer on a vascular graft prior to implantation: temporal dynamics and compatibility with the operating room, Ann Surg 203:671, 1986.
78. Buckels JAC, Nordestgaard AG, and Wilson SE: Microporous vascular grafts do not require neointima for resistance to bacteremic infection, J Vasc Surg 5:198, 1987.
79. Shue WB et al: Prevention of vascular prosthetic infection with an antibiotic-bonded Dacron graft, J Vasc Surg 8:600, 1988.
80. Greco RS et al: Prevention of vascular prosthetic infection by benzalkonium-oxacillin bonded polytetrafluoroethylene graft, Surg Gynecol Obstet 155:28, 1982.
81. Greco RS and Harvey RA: The role of antibiotic bonding in the prevention of vascular prosthetic infections, Ann Surg 195:168, 1982.
82. Harvey RA and Greco RS: The noncovalent bonding of antibiotics to a polytetrafluoroethylene-benzalkonium graft, Ann Surg 194, 1981.
83. Greco RS et al: The application of antibiotic bonding to the treatment of established vascular prosthetic infection, Arch Surg 120:71, 1985.
84. Moore WS et al: Development of an infection-resistant vascular prosthesis, Arch Surg 116:1403, 1981.
85. Powell TW, Burnham SJ, and Johnson G: A passive system using rifampin to create an infection-resistant vascular prosthesis, Surgery 94:765, 1983.
86. White JV et al: Simple methods for direct antibiotic protection of synthetic vascular grafts, J Vasc Surg 1:372, 1984.
87. Harris JM and Martin LF: An in vitro study of the properties influencing *Staphylococcus epidermidis* adhesion to prosthetic vascular graft materials, Ann Surg 206:612, 1987.

INDEX

C

D

E

G

H

H

N

O

Q

R

W

X

Y

Z